The ASCRS Manual of Colon and Rectal Surgery

Preface

In continuation with the first two volumes, the third edition of the American Society of Colon and Rectal Surgeons' (ASCRS) Manual is again abstracted from and a companion to the third edition of the *ASCRS Textbook of Colon and Rectal Surgery* (Steele, Hull, Read, Saclarides, Senagore, Whitlow, eds. New York: Springer, 2016). The manual serves as a readily available, easy-to-access, and succinct resource for all providers caring with colorectal disease.

The collective goal for the third edition of the *ASCRS Textbook of Colon and Rectal Surgery* was to provide a valuable resource for surgeons and health-care providers who care for patients with colorectal disease at all stages of their careers. In line with previous editions, we aimed to build upon the collective experience and expertise from national and international experts in the field, providing a completely revamped, up-to-date tome covering the wide breadth of colorectal disease organized around the "pillars" of colorectal surgery including perioperative care (including endoscopy), anorectal disease, benign disease (including inflammatory bowel disease), malignancy, pelvic floor disorders, and a "miscellaneous" section that covers aspects both inside and beyond the operating room that are pertinent to providers at every level. In addition, each chapter contains several *key concepts* that succinctly depict the major learning objectives for individual sections and are in line with the Core Curriculum for Colon and Rectal Surgery provided by the Association of Program Directors in Colon and Rectal Surgery and the key topics used by the American Board of Colon and Rectal Surgery.

Each chapter in the manual has been abstracted, edited, and reviewed by the textbook authors and manual editors. Many diagrams, figures, and algorithms have been retained from the textbook, as they are felt to help with patient care. In an effort to continue to build and expand upon the education platform across the ASCRS, the manual serves as a bridge between the journal (*Diseases of the Colon and Rectum*), the ASCRS textbook, and other resources such as CARSEP and CREST. Further information, including more in-depth technical, scientific, and expert opinion, as well as references, are available and can always be accessed through any of our other resources and programs. It is our sincere wish that this manual will serve as a relevant and practical tool to provide information and recommendations and ultimately help improve the care and outcome for our patients.

Cleveland, OH, USA — Scott R. Steele, MD
Cleveland, OH, USA — Tracy L. Hull, MD
Chicago, IL, USA — Neil Hyman, MD
Worcester, MA, USA — Justin A. Maykel, MD
Gainesville, FL, USA — Thomas E. Read, MD
New Orleans, LA, USA — Charles B. Whitlow, MD

Contents

Contributors

Cary B. Aarons, MD Division of Colon and Rectal Surgery, Hospital of the University of Pennsylvania, Philadelphia, PA, USA

Maher A. Abbas, MD, FACS, FACRS Al Azhra Hospital Dubai, Dubai, UAE

Karim Alavi, MD, MPH Department of Surgery, University of Massachusetts Medical School, Worcester, MA, USA

Dennis K. Ames, JD La Follette, Johnson, Dehaas, Fesler & Ames, Santa Ana, CA, USA

Glenn T. Ault, MD, MSEd Division of Colorectal Surgery, Department of Surgery, University of Southern California, Los Angeles, CA, USA

Jennifer M. Ayscue, MD, FACS, FASCRS Section of Colon & Rectal Surgery, Department of Surgery, MedStar Washington Hospital Center, Washington, DC, USA

Amir L. Bastawrous, MD, MBA, FACS, FASCRS Swedish Cancer Institute, Swedish Colon and Rectal Clinic, Seattle, WA, USA

Joshua I. S. Bleier, MD, FACS, FASCRS Department of Surgery, Hospital of the University of Pennsylvania/Pennsylvania Hospital, Philadelphia, PA, USA

Liliana Bordeianou, MD, MPH Department of General Surgery, Massachusetts General Hospital, Boston, MA, USA

Raul Martin Bosio, MD, MSBS ProMedica Physicians General Surgery, Sylvania, OH, USA

W. Donald Buie, MD, MSc, FRCSC, FACS, FASCRS Department of Surgery, Foothills Medical Centre, University of Calgary, Calgary, AB, Canada

Jamie A. Cannon, MD Division of Gastrointestinal Surgery, Department of Surgery, University of Alabama at Birmingham, Birmingham, AL, USA

Evie H. Carchman, MD Department of Surgery, University of Wisconsin – School of Medicine and Public Health, Madison, WI, USA

Joseph C. Carmichael, MD Department of Surgery, University of California, Irvine, Orange, CA, USA

Peter A. Cataldo, MD, FACS, FASCRS Department of Surgery, University of Vermont Medical Center, University of Vermont College of Medicine, Burlington, VT, USA

Thomas E. Cataldo, MD, FACS, FASCRS Division of Colon and Rectal Surgery, Department of Surgery, Beth Israel Deaconess Medical Center, Harvard Medical School, Boston, MA, USA

Andrea Cercek, MD Department of Medicine, Memorial Sloan Kettering Cancer Center, New York, NY, USA

Bradley J. Champagne, MD, FACS, FASCRS Fairview Medical Center, Cleveland, OH, USA

Department of Colorectal Surgery, Cleveland Clinic, Cleveland, OH, USA

George J. Chang, MD, MS Department of Surgical Oncology, The University of MD Anderson Cancer Center, Houston, TX, USA

Dorin T. Colibaseanu, MD Department of Surgery, Mayo Clinic, Rochester, MN, USA

Kyle G. Cologne, MD Department of Surgery, Division of Colorectal, University of Southern California Keck School of Medicine, Los Angeles, CA, USA

Tara M. Connelly, MD, MB, BCh, MSc Department of Colorectal Surgery, University Hospital Limerick, Limerick, Ireland

Jennifer S. Davids, MD Department of Surgery, University of Massachusetts Memorial Medical Center, Worcester, MA, USA

Bradley R. Davis, MD, FACS, FASCRS Department of Surgery, Section of Colorectal Surgery, Atrium Health, Carolinas Medical Center, Charlotte, NC, USA

Kurt Davis, MD Department of Surgery, Lousiana State University Health School of Medicine, New Orleans, LA, USA

Conor P. Delaney, MD, PhD Department of Colorectal Surgery, Digestive Disease Institute, Cleveland Clinic, Cleveland, OH, USA

Eric J. Dozois, MD Department of Surgery, Mayo Clinic, Rochester, MN, USA

Jonathon Efron, MD Department of Surgery, Johns Hopkins Hospital, Johns Hopkins University, Baltimore, MD, USA

Peter F. Ehrlich, MD, MSc Section of Pediatric Surgery, University of Michigan C.S. Mott Children's Hospital, Ann Arbor, MI, USA

Marwan Fakih, MD Department of Medical Oncology and Therapeutic Diagnostics, City of Hope Medical Center, Duarte, CA, USA

Daniel L. Feingold, MD, FACS, FASCRS Department of Surgery, Columbia University, New York, NY, USA

Alessandro Fichera, MD, FACS, FASCRS Department of Surgery, University of North Carolina, Chapel Hill, NC, USA

Todd D. Francone, MD, MPH Department of General Surgery, Section of Colorectal Surgery, Massachusetts General Hospital, Boston, MA, USA

Charles M. Friel, MD, FACS, FASCRS Department of Surgery, University of Virginia Medical Center, Charlottesville, VA, USA

Wolfgang B. Gaertner, MSc, MD, FACS, FASCRS Department of Colon & Rectal Surgery, University of Minnesota, Minneapolis, MN, USA

Julio Garcia-Aguilar, MD, PhD Department of Surgery, Memorial Sloan Kettering Cancer Center, New York, NY, USA

Kelly A. Garrett, MD, FACS, FASCRS Department of General Surgery, Section of Colon and Rectal Surgery, Weill Cornell Medical College, New York Presbyterian Hospital, New York, NY, USA

Stephen R. Gorfine, MD Division of Colorectal Surgery, Department of Surgery, The Mount Sinai Hospital, New York, NY, USA

Brooke Gurland, MD Colorectal Surgery, Stanford University, Stanford, CA, USA

Eric M. Haas, MD, FACS, FASCRS Division of Colon and Rectal Surgery, Houston Methodist Hospital, Houston, TX, USA

The University of Texas Medical School, Houston, TX, USA

LLP LTD, Houston, TX, USA

Jason Hall, MD, MPH, FACS, FASCRS Division of Colon and Rectal Surgery, Boston University Medical Center, Boston, MA, USA

Tufts University School of Medicine, Boston, MA, USA

Karin M. Hardiman, MD, PhD Division of Colorectal Surgery, University of Michigan, Ann Arbor, MI, USA

Dana M. Hayden, MD, MPH Department of General Surgery, Loyola University Medical Center, Maywood, IL, USA

Charles P. Heise, MD, FACS, FASCRS Department of Surgery, University of Wisconsin – School of Medicine and Public Health, Madison, WI, USA

Alan J. Herline, MD Department of Surgery, Georgia Regents University, Augusta, GA, USA

Daniel O. Herzig, MD, FACS, FASCRS Division of Gastroenterology and General Surgery, Department of Surgery, Oregon Health and Science University, Portland, OR, USA

Rebecca E. Hoedema, MS, MD, FACS, FASCRS Department of Colon and Rectal Surgery, Spectrum Health/Ferguson Clinic, Grand Rapids, MI, USA

Stefan D. Holubar, MD, MS, FACS, FASCRS Department of Colorectal Surgery, Cleveland Clinic, Cleveland, OH, USA

Tracy L. Hull, MD Department of Colorectal Surgery, Cleveland Clinic, Cleveland, OH, USA

Steven R. Hunt, MD Division of General Surgery, Section of Colon and Rectal Surgery, Department of Surgery, Barnes Jewish Hospital, Washington University School of Medicine, St. Louis, MO, USA

Neil Hyman, MD, FACS, FASCRS Section of Colon and Rectal Surgery, University of Chicago Medicine, Chicago, IL, USA

Eric K. Johnson, MD, FACS, FASCRS Department of Colorectal Surgery, Cleveland Clinic, Cleveland, OH, USA

Andreas M. Kaiser, MD, FACS, FASCRS Keck Medical Center of the University of Southern California, Los Angeles, CA, USA

Matthew F. Kalady, MD, FACS, FASCRS Department of Colorectal Surgery, Digestive Disease Institute, Cleveland Clinic, Cleveland, OH, USA

Brian R. Kann, MD, FACS, FASCRS Department of Colon and Rectal Surgery, Ochsner Medical Center, New Orleans, LA, USA

Muneera R. Kapadia, MD, MME Department of Surgery, University of Iowa Hospitals and Clinics, Iowa City, IA, USA

Kevin R. Kasten, MD Department of Surgery, Section of Colorectal Surgery, Atrium Health, Carolinas Medical Center, Charlotte, NC, USA

Brody School of Medicine, East Carolina University, Greenville, NC, USA

Gregory D. Kennedy, MD, PhD Department of Surgery, University of Alabama-Birmingham, Birmingham, AL, USA

Jason D. Keune, MD, MBA Department of Surgery, St. Louis University School of Medicine, St. Louis, MO, USA

Cindy J. Kin, MD, MS Department of Surgery, Stanford University School of Medicine, Stanford, CA, USA

P. Ravi Kiran, MBBS, MS Division of Colorectal Surgery, Department of Colorectal Surgery, Columbia University Medical Center and Mailman School of Public Health, New York, NJ, USA

Center for Innovation and Outcomes Research, New York Presbyterian Hospital/Columbia University Medical Center, New York, NY, USA

Walter A. Koltun, MD, FACS, FASCRS Department of Surgery, Division of Colon and Rectal Surgery, Milton S. Hershey Medical Center, Penn State College of Medicine, Hershey, PA, USA

Mukta K. Krane, MD, FACS Department of Surgery, University of Washington Medical Center, Seattle, WA, USA

Anjali S. Kumar, MD, MPH, FACS, FASCRS Department of Medical Education and Clinical Sciences, Elson S. Floyd College of Medicine, Washington State University, Everett, Spokane, Tri-Cities, Vancouver, WA, USA

Alex Jenny Ky, MD, FACS Mount Sinai School of Medicine, New York, NY, USA

Frederick R. Lane, MD Kendrick Colon and Rectal Center, Franciscan St. Francis Health, Indianapolis, IN, USA

Erin O. Lange, MD, MSPH Department of Surgery, University of Washington Medical Center, Seattle, WA, USA

Sang W. Lee, MD, FACS, FASCRS University of Southern California, Los Angeles, CA, USA

Martin Luchtefeld, MD, FACS, FASCRS Department of Colon and Rectal Surgery, Spectrum Health/Ferguson Clinic, Grand Rapids, MI, USA

Kim C. Lu, MD, FACS, FASCRS Division of Gastrointestinal and General Surgery, Department of Surgery, Oregon Health & Science University, Portland, OR, USA

Anthony R. MacLean, MD, FRCSC, FACS Department of Surgery, Foothills Medical Centre, University of Calgary, Calgary, AB, Canada

Helen M. MacRae, MD, MA, FRCSC, FACS Department of Surgery, Mount Sinai Hospital, Toronto, ON, Canada

Najjia N. Mahmoud, MD Division of Colon and Rectal Surgery, Department of Surgery, University of Pennsylvania Health System, Philadelphia, PA, USA

Christopher R. Mantyh, MD Department of Surgery, Duke University Medical Center, Durham, NC, USA

Jorge Marcet, MD Department of Surgery, Tampa General Hospital, Tampa, FL, USA

David J. Maron, MD, MBA Department of Colorectal Surgery, Cleveland Clinic Florida, Weston, FL, USA

Dipen C. Maun, MD Kendrick Colon and Rectal Center, Franciscan St. Francis Health, Indianapolis, IN, USA

Justin A. Maykel, MD Division of Colon and Rectal Surgery, University of Massachusetts Memorial Medical Center, Worcester, MA, USA

Michael F. McGee, MD, FACS, FASCRS Section of Colon and Rectal Surgery, Division of Gastrointestinal and Oncologic Surgery, Department of Surgery, Northwestern Memorial Hospital, Chicago, IL, USA

M. Shane McNevin, MD, FACS, FASCRS Sacred Heart Hospital, Spokane, WA, USA

Genevieve B. Melton, MD, PhD Division of Colon & Rectal Surgery, Department of Surgery, University of Minnesota Medical Center, Minneapolis, MN, USA

John Migaly, MD, FACS, FASCRS Division of Advanced GI & Oncologic Surgery, Duke University Medical Center, Durham, NC, USA

Steven Mills, MD Department of Surgery, University of California, Irvine, Orange, CA, USA

Husein Moloo, MD, MSc, FRCS Department of Surgery, Ottawa Hospital Research Institute, University of Ottawa, Ottawa, ON, Canada

Roberta Muldoon, MD Department of Surgery, Vanderbilt University Hospital, Nashville, TN, USA

Matthew G. Mutch, MD, FACS, FASCRS Section of Colon and Rectal Surgery, Department of Surgery, Washington University School of Medicine, St. Louis, MO, USA

Garrett M. Nash, MD, MPH Department of Surgery, Memorial Sloan Kettering Cancer Center, New York, NY, USA

Guy R. Orangio, MD, FACS, FASCRS LSU Department of Surgery: Chief Section of Colon and Rectal Surgery, University Medical Center New Orleans, New Orleans, LA, USA

Emmanouil P. Pappou, MD, PhD Department of Colorectal Surgery, Columbia University, New York, NY, USA

Ian M. Paquette, MD Department of Surgery, Division of Colon and Rectal Surgery, University of Cincinnati Medical Center, Cincinnati, OH, USA

Marie Fidela R. Paraiso, MD Department of Obstetrics and Gynecology, Cleveland Clinic, Cleveland, OH, USA

W. Brian Perry, MD, FACS, FASCRS Audie L. Murphy VA Medical Center, San Antonio, TX, USA

Matthew M. Philp, MD, FACS, FASCRS Division of Colon and Rectal Surgery, Temple University Hospital, Philadelphia, PA, USA

Vitaliy Y. Poylin, MD, FACS, FASCRS Division of Colon and Rectal Surgery, Department of Surgery, Beth Israel Deaconess Medical Center, Harvard Medical School, Boston, MA, USA

Isabelle Raîche, MD, FRCS Department of Surgery, The Ottawa Hospital, University of Ottawa, Ottawa, ON, Canada

Jan Rakinic, MD, FACS, FASCRS Section of Colorectal Surgery, Department of Surgery, Southern Illinois University, Springfield, IL, USA

Thomas E. Read, MD, FACS, FASCRS Division of Gastrointestinal Surgery, University of Florida College of Medicine, Gainesville, FL, USA

Scott E. Regenbogen, MD, MPH Division of Colorectal Surgery, University of Michigan, Ann Arbor, MI, USA

Rocco Ricciardi, MD, MPH Massachusetts General Hosptal, Boston, MA, USA

Howard M. Ross, MD, FACS, FASCRS Department of Surgery, Division of Colon and Rectal Surgery, Temple University Hospital, Philadelphia, PA, USA

Andrew Russ, MD Department of Surgery, University Colon and Rectal Surgery, University of Tennessee Medical Center, Knoxville, TN, USA

Tushar Samdani, MD, MS, DNB(Surgery), MRCS(Edin) Department of Colorectal Surgery, Medstar Saint Mary's Hospital, Leonardo Town, MD, USA

Dana R. Sands, MD, FACS, FASCRS Department of Colorectal Surgery, Cleveland Clinic Florida, Weston, FL, USA

Giulio A. Santoro, MD, PhD Treviso Regional Hospital Italy, Treviso, Italy

Stephen M. Sentovich, MD, MBA Department of Surgical Oncology, City of Hope, Duarte, CA, USA

Matthew L. Silviera, MD Division of General Surgery, Section of Colon and Rectal Surgery, Department of Surgery, Barnes Jewish Hospital, Washington University School of Medicine, St. Louis, MO, USA

Michael J. Snyder, MD, FACS, FASCRS Department of Surgery, University of Texas Health Science, Houston, TX, USA

Mattias Soop, MD, PhD Department of Surgery, Salford Royal NHS Foundation Trust, Salford, UK

Manchester Academic Health Science Center, The University of Manchester, Manchester, UK

Constantine P. Spanos, MD, FACS, FASCRS Department of Colorectal Surgery, Keck School of Medicine, University of Southern California, Los Angeles, CA, USA

Department of Surgery, Aristotelian University of Thessaloniki, Panorama-Thessaloniki, Greece

Scott R. Steele, MD, MBA, FACS, FASCRS Department of Colorectal Surgery, Cleveland Clinic, Cleveland, OH, USA

David B. Stewart, Sr., MD, FACS, FASCRS Section Chief, Colorectal Surgery, University of Arizona - Banner University Medical Center, Tucson, AZ, USA

Scott A. Strong, MD, FACS, FASCRS Division of GI and Oncologic Surgery, Northwestern Medicine, Chicago, IL, USA

Daniel H. Teitelbaum, MD Section of Pediatric Surgery, University of Michigan C.S. Mott Children's Hospital, Ann Arbor, MI, USA

Amy J. Thorsen, MD University of Minnesota, Minneapolis, MN, USA

Konstantin Umanskiy, MD, FACS, FASCRS Department of Surgery, University of Chicago, Chicago, IL, USA

Cecile A. Unger, MD, MPH Department of Obstetrics and Gynecology, Cleveland Clinic, Cleveland, OH, USA

Michael A. Valente, DO, FACS, FASCRS Department of Colorectal Surgery, Digestive Disease Institute, Cleveland Clinic, Cleveland, OH, USA

H. David Vargas, MD, FACS, FASCRS Department of Colon and Rectal Surgery, Ochsner Medical Center, New Orleans, LA, USA

Madhulika K. Varma, MD Division of Colon and Rectal Surgery, University of California-San Francisco, San Francisco, CA, USA

Martin R. Weiser, MD Department of Surgery, Memorial Sloan Kettering Cancer Center, New York, NY, USA

Mark L. Welton, MD, MHCM Corporate Department, Fairview Health Services, Minneapolis, MN, USA

Mark H. Whiteford, MD, FACS, FASCRS Providence Portland Medical Center, Providence Cancer Center, Portland, OR, USA

The Oregon Clinic, Gastrointestinal and Minimally Invasive Surgery, Portland, OR, USA

Oregon Health & Science University, Portland, OR, USA

Charles B. Whitlow, MD Department of Colon and Rectal Surgery, Ochsner Medical Center, New Orleans, LA, USA

Elizabeth C. Wick, MD Division of General Surgery, University of California San Francisco, San Francisco, CA, USA

Kirsten Bass Wilkins, MD, FACS, FASCRS Department of Surgery, RWJ Barnabas Health, Edison, NY, USA

Y. Nancy You, MD, MHSc Department of Surgical Oncology, University of Texas MD Anderson Cancer Center, Houston, TX, USA

Massarat Zutshi, MD Department of Colorectal Surgery, Lerner College of Medicine, Cleveland Clinic, Cleveland, OH, USA

Part I

Perioperative/ Endoscopy

1 Anatomy and Embryology of the Colon, Rectum, and Anus

Joseph C. Carmichael and Steven Mills

Key Concepts

- The dentate line represents a true division between embryonic endoderm and ectoderm.
- The location of the anterior peritoneal reflection is highly variable and can be significantly altered by disease such as rectal prolapse.
- The right and left ischioanal space communicate posteriorly through the deep postanal space between the levator ani muscle and anococcygeal ligament.
- The junction between the midgut (superior mesenteric artery) and the hindgut (inferior mesenteric artery) leads to a potential watershed area in the area of the splenic flexure.
- There is a normal, three-stage process by which the intestinal tract rotates during development beginning with herniation of the midgut followed by return of the midgut to the abdominal cavity and ending with its fixation.

Anatomy of the Anal Canal and Pelvic Floor

- The "anatomic" anal canal begins at the dentate line and extends to the anal verge.
- The "surgical" anal canal extends from the anorectal ring to the anal verge.
- The surgical anal canal is formed by the internal anal sphincter (IAS), external anal sphincter (EAS), and puborectalis (Fig. 1.1).
- The surgical anal canal is longer in males than in females. It averages 4.4 cm in males and 4.0 cm in females. Its length does not change with age.
- MR imaging shows that the anterior and posterior external anal sphincter length (not including puborectalis) was significantly shorter in women.
- The anal canal forms proximally where the rectum passes through the pelvic hiatus and joins with the puborectalis muscle and be thought of as a "tube within a tube."
- The inner tube is the visceral smooth muscle of the IAS and longitudinal layer that is innervated by the autonomic nervous system.
- The outer muscular tube consists of somatic muscles including the components of the puborectalis and EAS and is responsible for voluntary control.
- The EAS extends distal to the IAS, and the anal canal terminates at the anal verge where the superficial and subcutaneous portions of the external anal sphincter join the dermis.

J. C. Carmichael (✉) · S. Mills
Department of Surgery, University of California, Irvine, Orange, CA, USA
e-mail: jcarmich@uci.edu

S. R. Steele et al. (eds.), *The ASCRS Manual of Colon and Rectal Surgery*,
https://doi.org/10.1007/978-3-030-01165-9_1

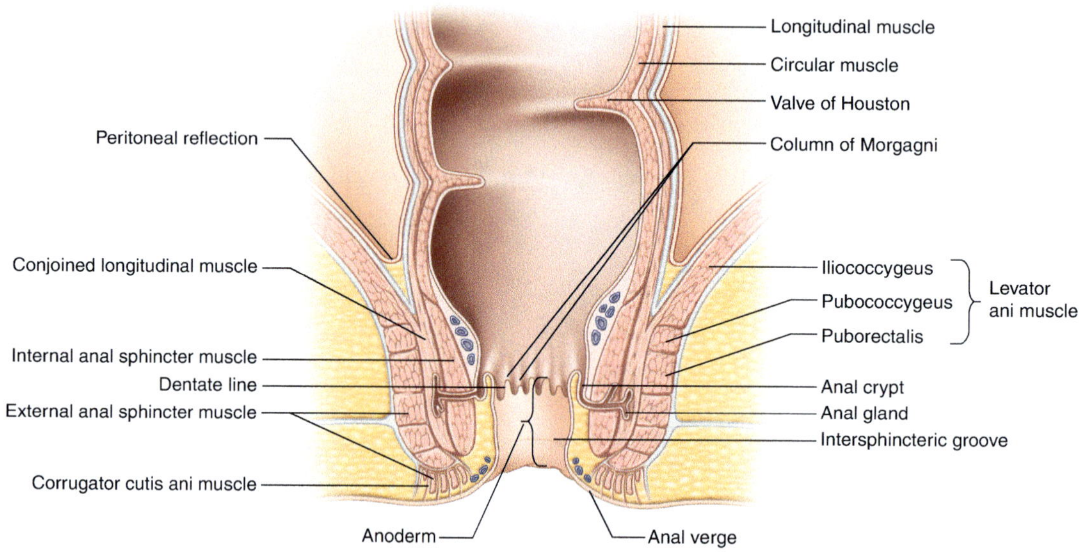

Fig. 1.1 Anal canal

Anal Canal Epithelium

- The proximal anal canal is lined by the columnar epithelium of the rectal mucosa.
- Six to twelve millimeter proximal to the dentate line, the anal transition zone (ATZ) begins, which is an area of gradual transition of columnar epithelium to squamous epithelium.
- The columns of Morgagni are redundant columns of tissue with anal crypts at their base. This forms the rippled dentate line (or pectinate line) which can be most easily identified – anal crypts are connected to underlying anal glands which are the presumed source of sepsis in the majority of anorectal abscesses and fistula. On average, there are six anal glands surrounding the anal canal (range 3–12) that are more concentrated in the posterior quadrants.
- All glands have a crypt but not all crypts have a gland. Some crypts are connected to multiple glands. The anal gland ducts proceed inferior and lateral from the anal canal and enter the submucosa where two-thirds enter the internal anal sphincter and half terminate in the intersphincteric plane.
- Distal to the dentate line, the anoderm begins and extends for approximately 1.5 cm. Anoderm has squamous histology and is devoid of hair, sebaceous glands, and sweat glands. At the anal verge, the anal canal lining becomes thickened and pigmented and contains hair follicles – this represents normal skin.
- The dentate line represents a true division between embryonic endoderm and ectoderm. Proximal to the dentate line, the innervation is via the sympathetic and parasympathetic systems, with venous, arterial, and lymphatic drainage associated with the hypogastric vessels. Distal to the dentate line, the innervation is via somatic nerves with blood supply and drainage from the inferior hemorrhoidal system.

Internal Anal Sphincter

- The internal anal sphincter is the downward continuation of the circular smooth muscle of the rectum. It terminates approximately 1 cm proximal to the distal aspect of the external anal sphincter producing a palpable intersphincteric groove on physical exam. Imaging studies show that the IAS is approximately 2 mm in thickness and 35 mm in length on average.

Conjoined Longitudinal Muscle

- The anatomy and function of the perianal connective tissue plays a significant role in normal anorectal function. The conjoined longitudinal muscle (or conjoined longitudinal coat) lies in between the internal and external anal sphincters. It begins at the anorectal ring as an extension of the longitudinal rectal muscle fibers and descends caudally joined by fibers of the puborectalis muscle.
- At its most caudal aspect, some of the conjoined longitudinal muscle fibers (referred to as *corrugator cutis ani muscle*) traverse the distal external anal sphincter and insert into the perianal skin, and some enter the fat of the ischiorectal fossa. Some fibers of the conjoined longitudinal muscle interlace in a network within the subepithelial space and have been referred to as Treitz's muscle. They have also been referred to *corrugator cutis ani*, *musculus submucosae ani*, *mucosal suspensory ligament*, and *musculus canalis ani*.
- Possible functions of the conjoined longitudinal muscle include attaching the anorectum to the pelvis and acting as a skeleton that supports and binds the internal and external sphincter complex together.

External Anal Sphincter

- The external anal sphincter (EAS) is composed of striated muscle that forms an elliptical tube around the internal anal sphincter and conjoined longitudinal muscle.
- Goligher demonstrated that the external anal sphincter was truly a continuous sheet of skeletal muscle extending up to the puborectalis and levator ani muscles. While the external anal sphincter does not have three distinct anatomic layers, it is not uncommon to see the proximal portion of the EAS referred to as deep EAS, the midportion referred to as the superficial EAS, and the most distal aspect as the subcutaneous EAS.
- The mid-EAS has posterior attachment to the coccyx via the anococcygeal ligament, and the proximal EAS becomes continuous with the puborectalis muscle. Anteriorly, the proximal EAS forms a portion of the perineal body with the transverse perineal muscle.
- There are gender differences in the morphology of the anterior external anal sphincter that have been demonstrated on imaging. The normal female external anal sphincter has a variable natural defect (in 75% of nulliparous women) occurring along its proximal anterior length below the level of the puborectalis sling. Knowledge of this is important in interpreting anal ultrasound for fecal incontinence.
- The external anal sphincter is innervated on each side by the inferior rectal branch of the pudendal nerve (S2 and S3) and by the perineal branch of S4. There is substantial overlap in the pudendal innervation of the external anal sphincter muscle on the two sides which enables reinnervation to be partially accomplished from the contralateral side following nerve injury.

Perineal Body

- The perineal body represents the intersection of the external anal sphincter, superficial transverse perinei, deep transverse perinei, and bulbospongiosus (also referred to as bulbocavernosus) muscles (Fig. 1.2). Recent research suggests that the transverse perinei (TP) and bulbospongiosus (BS) muscles contribute significantly to anal incontinence. It has been proposed that the EAS, TP, and BS muscles be collectively referred to as the "EAS complex muscles."

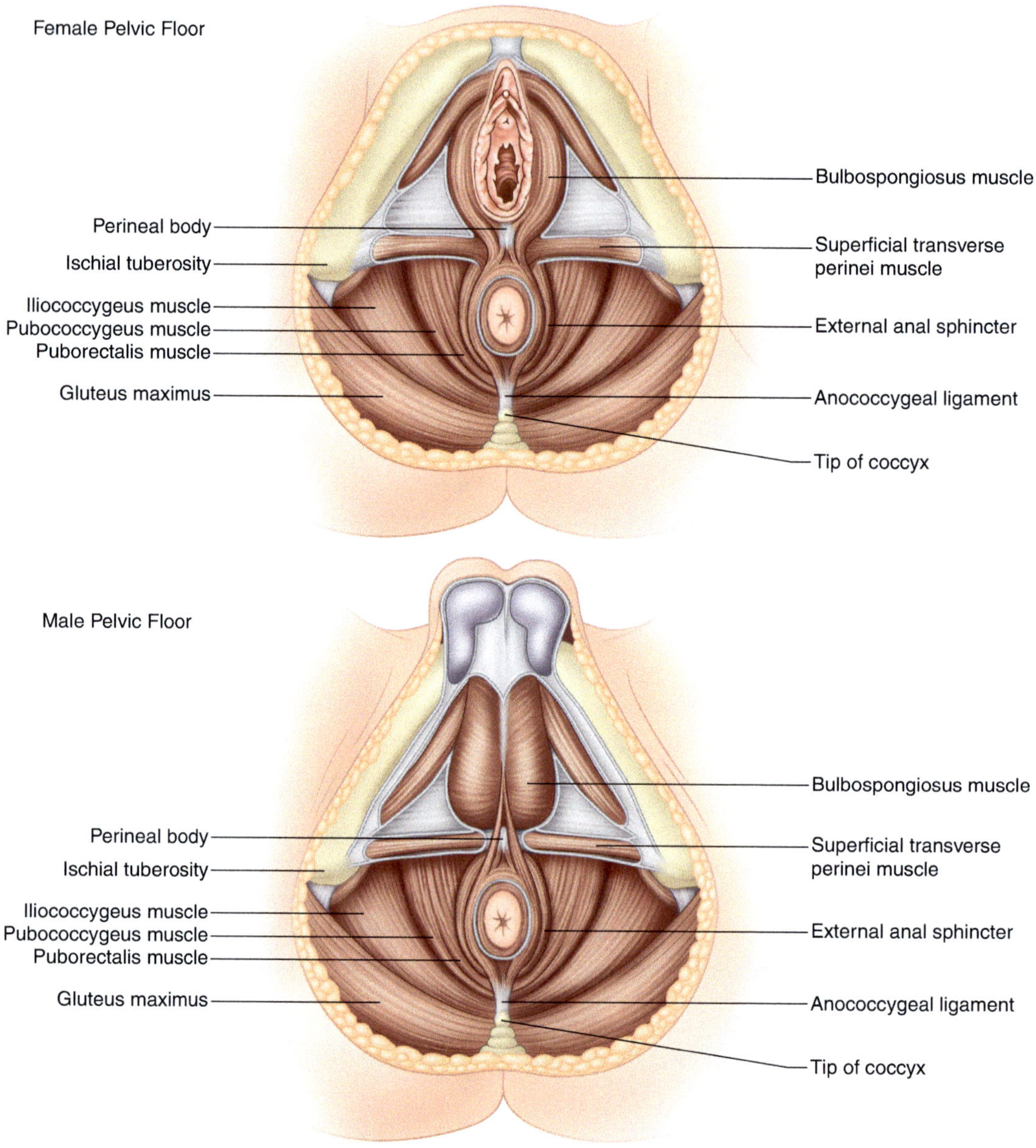

Fig. 1.2 Pelvic floor muscles

Pelvic Floor Muscles

- In addition to the anal sphincter and perineal body, the levator ani (LA) muscles contribute to pelvic organ support.
- The LA has three subdivisions including the pubococcygeus (aka pubovisceral), puborectalis, and iliococcygeus.
- In vivo MRI measurements in women have shown distinct, visible muscle fascicle directions for each of the three LA component muscles. Embryology studies have also demonstrated that the puborectalis muscle is a portion of the LA muscle and shares a common primordium with the iliococcygeus and pubococcygeus muscles.

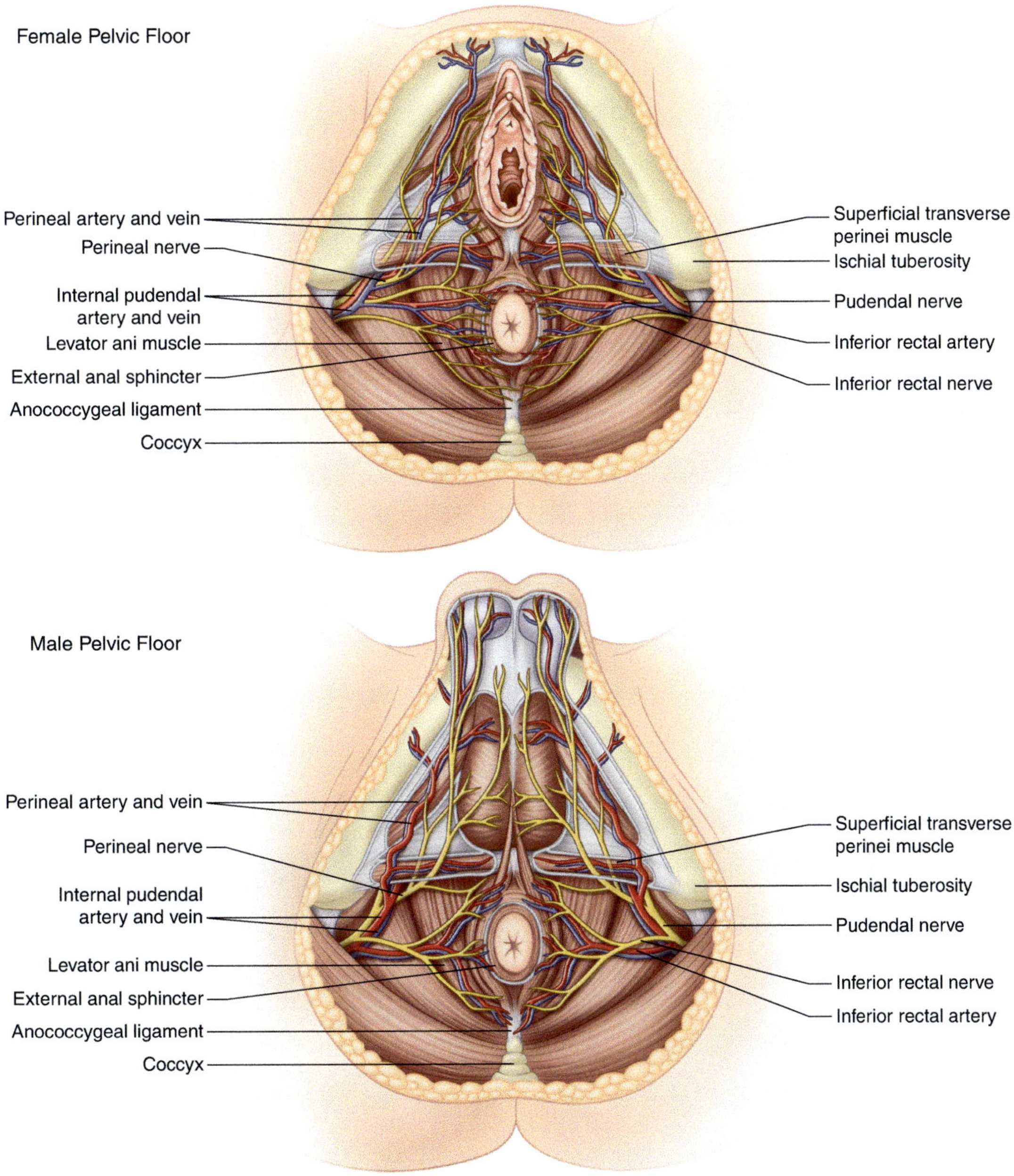

Fig. 1.3 Pelvic floor nerves and blood supply

- Contemporary cadaveric studies suggest that the LA muscles are innervated by the pudendal nerve branches: perineal nerve and inferior rectal nerve as well as direct sacral nerves S3 and/or S4 (i.e., levator ani nerve). The pubococcygeus muscle and puborectalis muscle are primarily innervated by the pudendal nerve branches, while the iliococcygeus muscle is primarily innervated by the direct sacral nerves S3 and/or S4 (Fig. 1.3).

Puborectalis Muscle

- The puborectalis muscle (PRM) fibers arise from the lower part of the symphysis pubis and from the superior fascia of the urogenital diaphragm and run alongside the anorectal junction. Posterior to the rectum, the fibers join forming a sling. The "anorectal ring" is composed of the upper borders of the internal anal sphincter and puborectalis muscle. Contraction of the PRM sling causes a horizontal force that closes the pelvic diaphragm and decreases the anorectal angle during squeeze. This is widely considered the most important contributing factor to gross fecal continence.

Iliococcygeus Muscle

- Iliococcygeus muscle (ICM) fibers arise from the ischial spines and posterior obturator fascia, pass inferior/posterior and medially, and insert into the distal sacrum, coccyx, and anococcygeal raphe. The ICM, along with the pubococcygeus muscle, contributes to "lifting" of the pelvic floor.

Pubococcygeus Muscle

- The pubococcygeus muscle (PCM) lies medial to the PRM. PCM fibers arise from the anterior half of the obturator fascia and the high posterior pubis. The PCM fibers intersect with fibers from the opposite side and form the anococcygeal raphe (or anococcygeal ligament). PCM fibers insert in the distal sacrum and tip of the coccyx, and portions contribute to the conjoined longitudinal muscle. The PCM forms the "levator hiatus" as it ellipses the lower rectum, urethra, and either the vagina in women or the dorsal vein of the penis in men. The levator hiatus is connected to the intrahiatal organs by a fascial condensation called the "hiatal ligament" (Fig. 1.4). The hiatal ligament arises circumferentially around the hiatal margin as a continuation of the fascia on the pelvic surface of the levator muscle. Enlargement of the levator hiatus has been implicated as a cause of female pelvic organ prolapse.

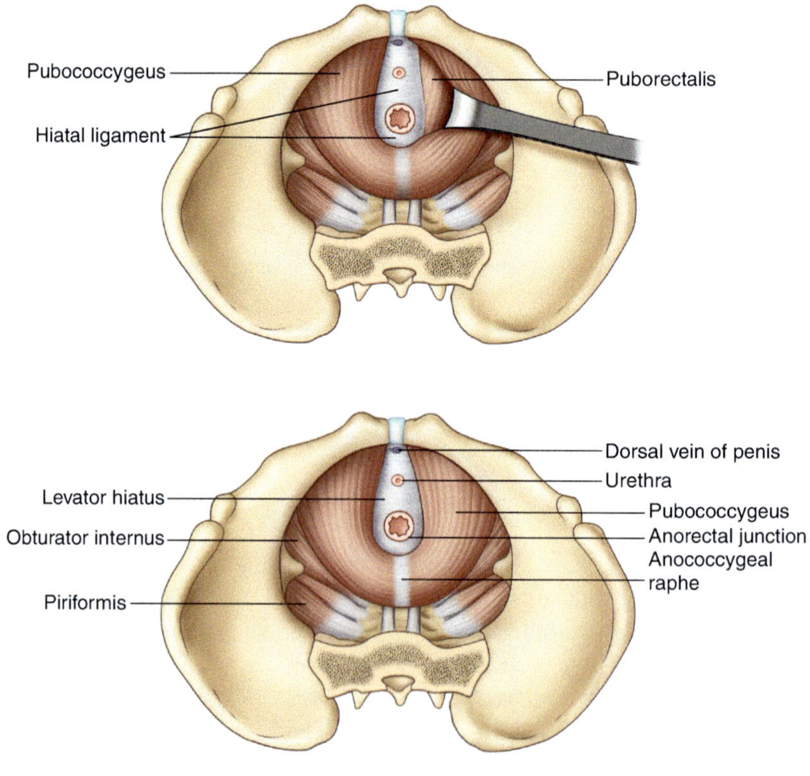

Fig. 1.4 Pelvic floor anatomy, abdominal view

Anatomy of the Rectum

- The rectum is of variable length but is commonly described as the upper (12–15 cm), middle (7–12 cm), and lower (0–<7 cm) rectum. While not anatomically distinct, the divisions are important when considering surgical treatment of rectal cancer. The upper rectum can be distinguished from the sigmoid colon by the absence of taenia coli and epiploic appendages.
- The majority of the rectum is extraperitoneal. Anteriorly and laterally the upper rectum is covered by a layer of visceral peritoneum down to the peritoneal reflection. The location of the anterior peritoneal reflection is highly variable but on average is 9 cm from the anal verge in females and 9.7 cm in males.

Mesorectum

- In anatomic terms, the prefix "meso" refers to two layers of peritoneum that suspend an organ, and the suffix applied indicates the target organ (e.g., mesocolon). Therefore the term mesorectum is a misnomer except in patients with a mobile suspended rectum as can be seen in rectal prolapse.
- The mesorectum is a term employed by surgeons to describe the fascial envelope of the rectum that is excised during surgical treatment of rectal cancer. Indeed, failure to completely excise this envelope intact has been associated with an increased incidence of local recurrence of rectal cancer. The mesorectum is contained within the fascia propria. The fascia propria is an upward projection of the parietal endopelvic fascia that lines the walls and floor of the pelvis. The fascia propria encloses the perirectal fat, lymphatics, blood vessels, and nerves.

Presacral Fascia

- The presacral fascia is a thickened portion of the parietal endopelvic fascia overlying the sacrum that covers the presacral veins and hypogastric nerves (Fig. 1.5). It extends laterally to cover the

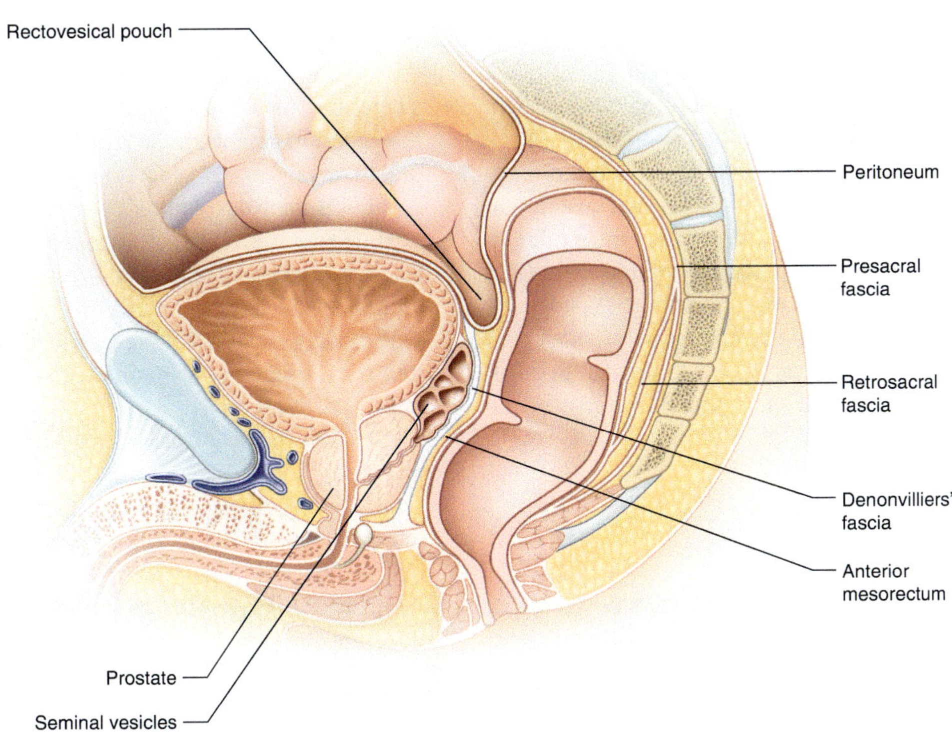

Fig. 1.5 Fascial relationships of the rectum

piriformis and upper coccyx. As the presacral fascia extends laterally, it becomes continuous with the fascia propria and contributes to the lateral ligaments of the rectum. Caudally, this fascia extends to the anorectal junction covering the anococcygeal ligament. During total mesorectal excision, the fascia propria is elevated sharply off the presacral fascia. Leaving the presacral fascia intact eliminates the possibility of causing substantial presacral bleeding.

Retrosacral Fascia

- The retrosacral fascia originates at the third and fourth portion of the sacrum and extends anteriorly to the posterior layer of the fascia propria 3–5 cm proximal to the anorectal junction. This tough fascia layer is surgically relevant as it must be sharply incised during total mesorectal excision. The space posterior to the retrosacral fascia is referred to as the supralevator or retrorectal space.

Waldeyer's Fascia

- There is significant confusion about what Waldeyer's fascia represents as the eponym has been used to describe the presacral fascia, the rectosacral fascia, or all fascia posterior to the rectum. In Waldeyer's original description of pelvic fascia, there was no particular emphasis on the presacral component. While the debate continues regarding "Waldeyer's fascia," it is important to simply understand that the phrase can have the potential to mean presacral fascia, retrosacral, or retrorectal fascia.

Denonvilliers' Fascia

- Denonvilliers' fascia arises from the fusion of the two walls of the embryological peritoneal cul-de-sac and extends from the deepest point of the rectovesical pouch to the pelvic floor. It was originally described by Denonvilliers in 1836 as a "prostatoperitoneal" membranous layer between the rectum and seminal vesicles.
- Denonvilliers' fascia is also present in females as part of the rectovaginal septum and is sometimes referred to as rectovaginal fascia. It is found immediately beneath the vaginal mucosa and is clearly what most would consider as part of the vaginal wall. It merges superiorly with the cardinal/uterosacral complex in females or the rectovesical pouch in males. It merges laterally with the endopelvic fascia overlying the levator muscle and distally with the perineal body. It contains collagen and some strands of smooth muscle and heavy elastin fibers.
- Microscopically, Denonvilliers' fascia has two layers, but they are not grossly discernable. In the anterior rectal plane, the mesorectum is contained by the fascia propria which lies dorsal to Denonvilliers' fascia.
- The cavernous nerves run in neurovascular bundles at the anterolateral border of Denonvilliers' fascia.

Lateral Ligaments

- There are two controversial points regarding the lateral ligaments of the rectum. Do the lateral ligaments exist? What do they contain?
- In his seminal description of abdominoperineal resection in 1908, William Ernest Miles refers to division of the lateral ligaments of the rectum.
- One modern cadaveric dissection study identified the presence of a middle rectal artery in only 22% of specimens.
- Total mesorectal excision, as popularized and described by Heald, involves sharp dissection along the fascia propria circumferentially to the pelvic floor. While acknowledging that the middle rectal vessels are "divided as far from the carcinoma as possible," Heald does not mention "lateral ligaments" of the rectum at all.
- One review of the anatomy of the lateral ligament states that it is a common misconception

that the lateral ligaments contain the middle rectal artery. It appears that the lateral ligaments comprise "primarily nerves and connective tissue" and their division without bleeding attests to the absence of a "significant accessory rectal artery in this location in the majority of patients."

- In another cadaveric study, the lateral ligaments of the rectum were identified as trapezoid structures originating from mesorectum and anchored to the endopelvic fascia at the level of the midrectum. It was recommended that, as lateral extensions of the mesorectum, the ligaments must be cut and included in the total mesorectal excision (TME) specimen. It was further noted that the lateral ligaments did not contain middle rectal arteries or nerve structures of importance. Other modern cadaveric investigations note the rarity of middle rectal arteries and the absence of clinically relevant neurovascular structures in the lateral ligaments.

Valves of Houston

- The rectum has been classically described to have three distinct, semicircular, inner folds called valves of Houston (Fig. 1.1) with the superior and inferior valves located on the left side of the rectum and the more prominent middle rectal valve on the right.
- Anatomic variation is common, with only 45.5% of patients having the classic "three valve anatomy"; 32.5% will have only two valves, and 10.25% will have four valves.

Anorectal Spaces

- Several anorectal spaces are created by the various myofascial relationships in the pelvis. They are important in understanding how anorectal sepsis can spread throughout the pelvis.

Perianal Space

- The perianal space contains external hemorrhoid cushions, thc subcutaneous external anal sphincter, and the distal internal anal sphincter. The perianal space is in communication with the intersphincteric space (Fig. 1.6). Its cephalad boundary is the dentate line, and its lateral boundaries are the subcutaneous fat of the buttocks. It is contained by fibers extending from the conjoined longitudinal muscle often referred to as *corrugator cutis ani* muscle fibers. Otherwise, the perianal space is contained by anoderm.

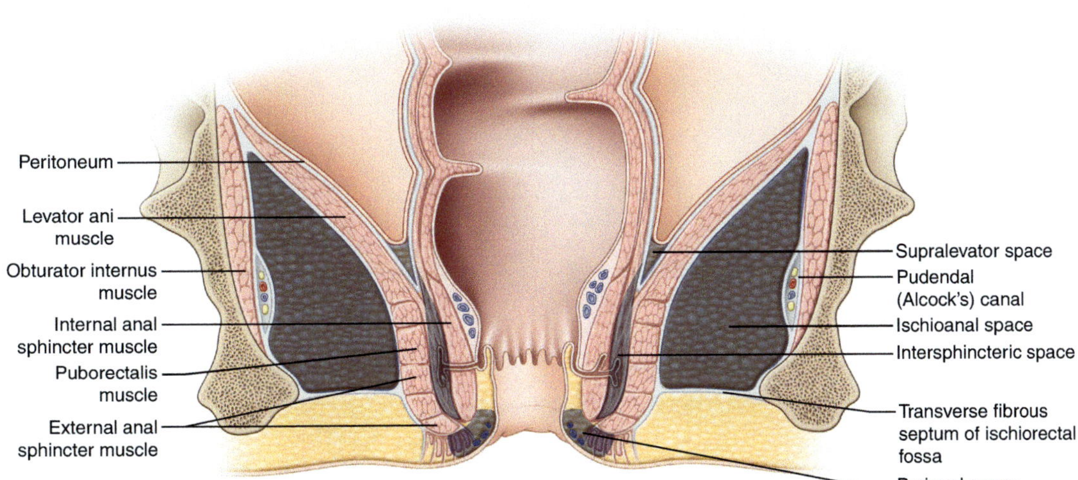

Fig. 1.6 Perianal and perirectal spaces, coronal view

Intersphincteric Space

- The intersphincteric space is the potential space that lies between the internal and external anal sphincters and is continuous with the perianal space. It is of clinical importance as cryptoglandular infections tend to begin in this area and expand elsewhere to create anal fistulas.

Submucous Space

- This space lies between the medial border of the internal anal sphincter and the anal mucosa proximal to the dentate line. It is continuous with the submucosa of the rectum. This area contains internal hemorrhoid vascular cushions.

Ischioanal/Ischiorectal Space

- The ischioanal (also referred to as ischiorectal) space is the largest anorectal space. It has been described as a pyramid shape with its apex at the levator muscle insertion into the obturator fascia. Its borders are as follows:
- Medial – the levator ani muscle and external anal sphincter
- Lateral – obturator internus muscle and obturator fascia
- Posterior – the lower border of the gluteus maximus muscle and the sacrotuberous ligament
- Anterior – the superficial and deep transverse perineal muscles
- Caudal – the skin of the perineum
- The ischioanal fossa contains the adipose tissue, pudendal nerve branches, and superficial branches of the internal pudendal vessels.
- The right and left ischioanal space communicate posteriorly through the deep postanal space between the levator ani muscle and anococcygeal ligament (Fig. 1.7). When the ischioanal and perianal spaces are regarded as a single space, it is referred to as the ischioanal fossa.

Supralevator Space

- The upper boundary of the supralevator space is the peritoneum, the lateral boundary is the pelvic wall, the medial boundary is the rectum, and the inferior boarder is the levator ani muscle (Fig. 1.8).

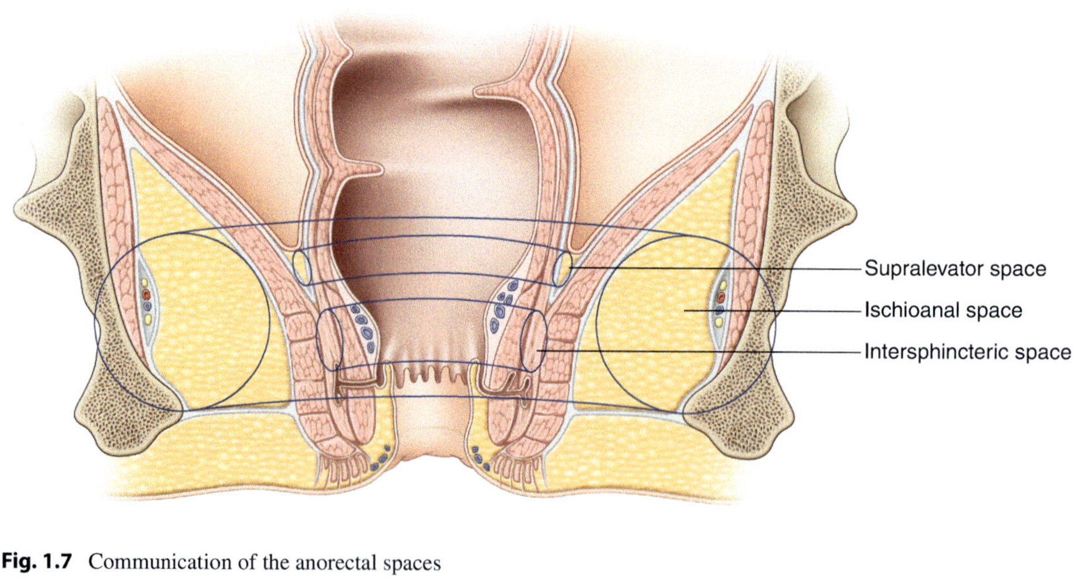

Fig. 1.7 Communication of the anorectal spaces

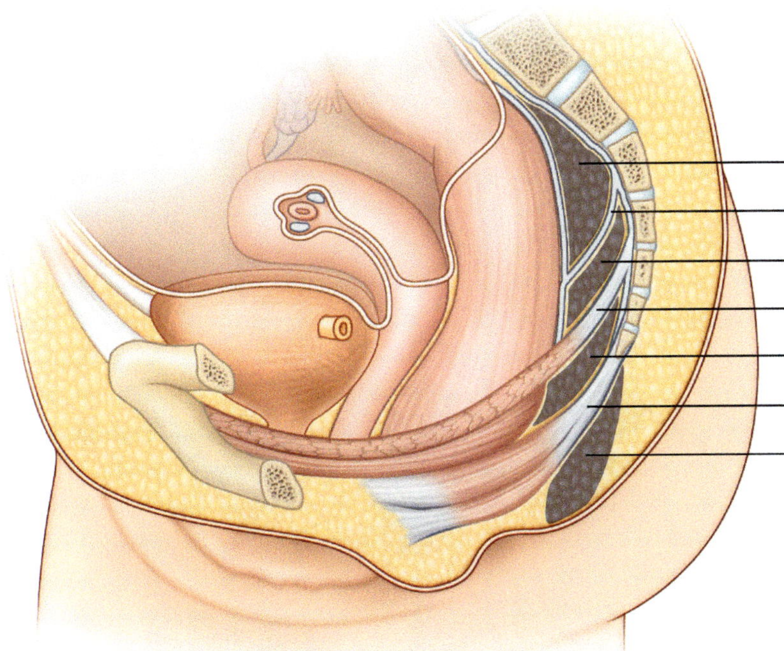

Fig. 1.8 Perianal and perirectal spaces, lateral view

Superficial and Deep Postanal Spaces

- These spaces are located posterior to the anus and inferior to the levator muscle. The superficial postanal space is more caudal and is located between the anococcygeal ligament and the skin. The superficial postanal space allows communication of perianal space sepsis.
- The deep postanal space (retrosphincteric space of Courtney) is located between the levator ani muscle and the anococcygeal raphe. This space allows ischioanal sepsis to track from one side to the other resulting in the so-called "horseshoe" abscess.

Retrorectal Space

- The retrorectal space is found between the presacral fascia and fascia propria. It contains no major blood vessels or nerves. It is limited laterally by the lateral ligaments of the piriformis fascia and inferiorly by the rectosacral fascia. The fascia propria and presacral fascia come together at the apex of this space.

Rectal Blood Supply

- The rectum is supplied by the superior, middle, and inferior rectal (hemorrhoidal) arteries (Fig. 1.9). Both the middle and inferior hemorrhoidal vessels are paired arteries, while the superior rectal artery is not.

Superior Rectal Artery

- The superior rectal artery (SRA) is the continuation of the inferior mesenteric artery as it crosses the left iliac vessels. The SRA gives off a rectosigmoid branch and an upper rectal branch and bifurcates into right and left terminal branches. On average, eight terminal branches of the SRA have been identified in the distal rectal wall.

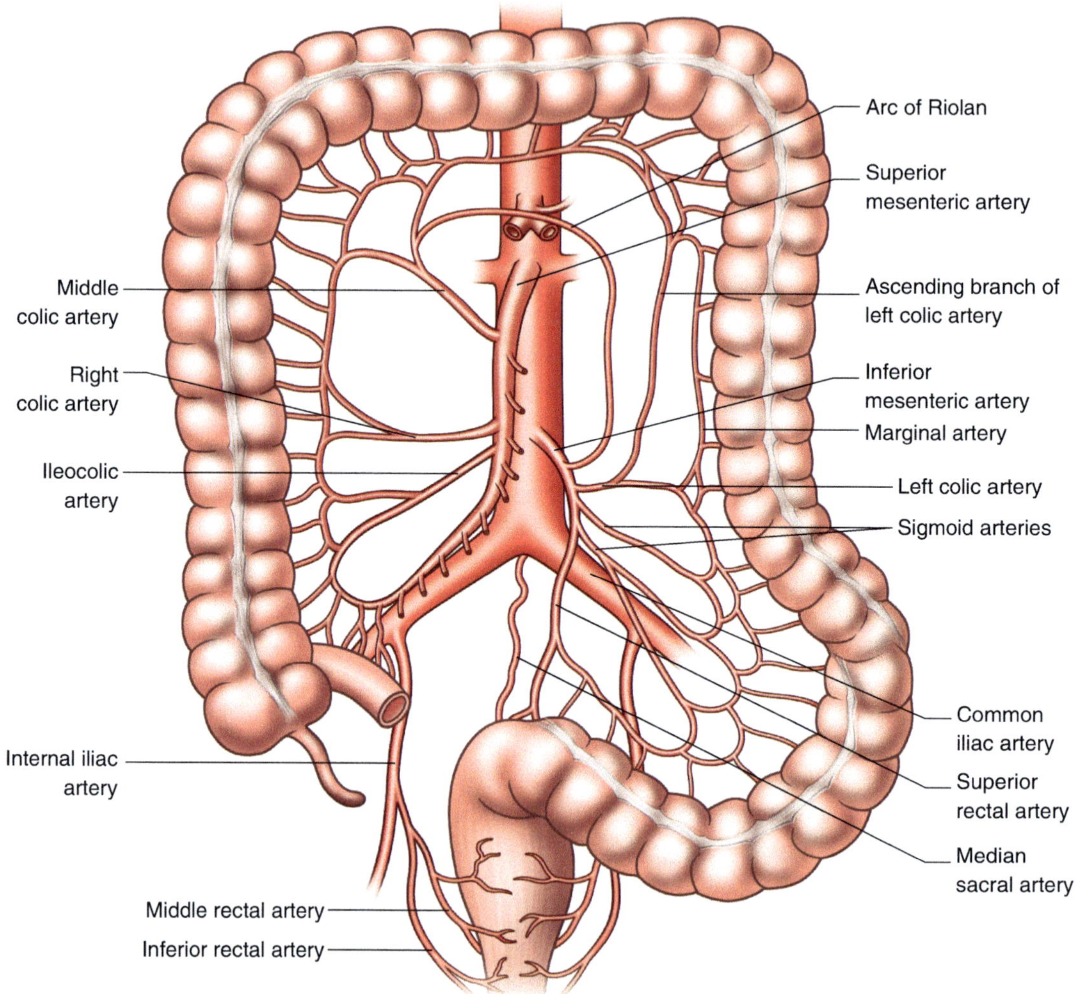

Fig. 1.9 Arterial anatomy of the colon and rectum

Middle Rectal Artery

- The middle rectal artery (MRA) has been variably noted in many studies. It may be found on one or both sides of the rectum and has been noted to be present 12–28% of the time. The MRA originates from the anterior division of the internal iliac or pudendal arteries.

Inferior Rectal Artery

- The inferior rectal arteries (IRA) are paired vessels that originate as branches of the internal pudendal artery that receives its blood supply from the internal iliac artery. The artery originates in the pudendal canal and is entirely extrapelvic (caudal to the levator ani) in its distribution. The IRA traverses the obturator fascia and the ischiorectal fossa and pierces the wall of the anal canal in the region of the external anal sphincter.

Venous and Lymphatic Drainage of the Rectum and Anus

- Venous drainage from the rectum and anus occurs via both the portal and systemic systems. Middle and inferior rectal veins drain to

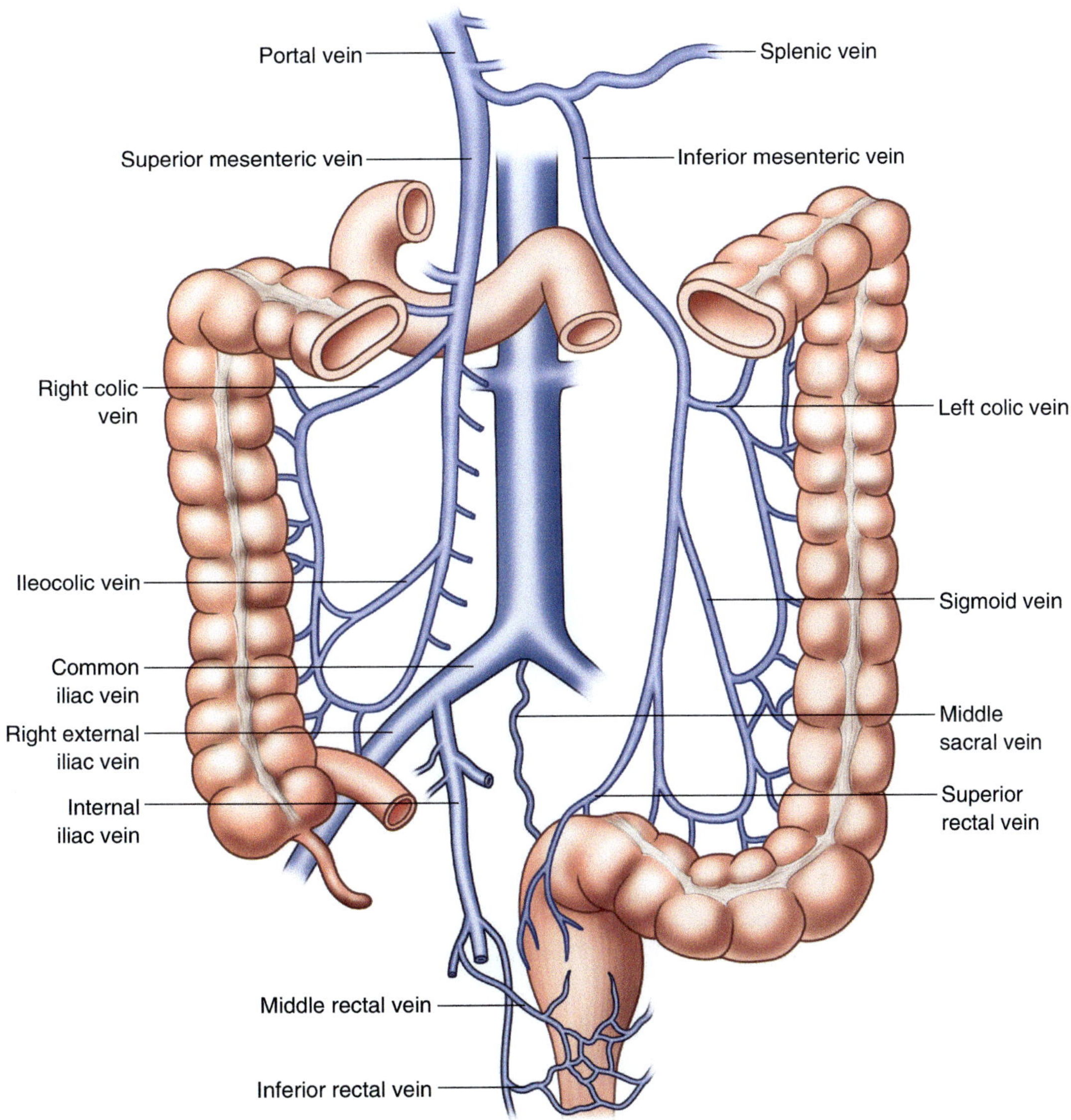

Fig. 1.10 Venous anatomy of the colon and rectum

the systemic systems via the internal iliac vein, while the superior rectal vein drains the rectum and upper anal canal into the portal system via the inferior mesenteric vein (Fig. 1.10).

- Lymphatics from the upper two-thirds of the rectum drain to the inferior mesenteric lymph nodes and then to the para-aortic lymph nodes.
- Lymphatic drainage from the lower third of the rectum occurs along the superior rectal artery and laterally along the middle rectal artery to the internal iliac lymph nodes.
- In the anal canal, lymphatic above the dentate drains to the inferior mesenteric and internal iliac lymph nodes. Below the dentate line, lymphatics drain along the inferior rectal lymphatics to the superficial inguinal nodes.

Innervation of the Rectum and Anus

- Sympathetic fibers arise from L1, L2, and L3 and pass through the sympathetic chains and join the preaortic plexus (Fig. 1.11). From there, they run adjacent and dorsal to the inferior mesenteric artery as the mesenteric plexus and innervate the upper rectum.
- The lower rectum is innervated by the presacral nerves from the hypogastric plexus. Two main hypogastric nerves, on either side of the rectum, carry sympathetic information from the hypogastric plexus to the pelvic plexus. The pelvic plexus lies on the lateral side of the pelvis at the level of the lower third of the rectum adjacent to the lateral stalks (described above).
- Parasympathetic fibers to the rectum and anal canal originate from S2, S3, and S4 to penetrate through the sacral foramen and are called the nervi erigentes. These nerves course laterally and anteriorly to join the sympathetic hypogastric nerves and form the pelvic plexus on the pelvic sidewall. Postganglionic mixed parasympathetic and sympathetic nerve fibers supply the rectum, genital organs, and anal canal.
- The periprostatic plexus is considered a subdivision of the pelvic plexus and supplies the prostate, seminal vesicles, corpora cavernosa,

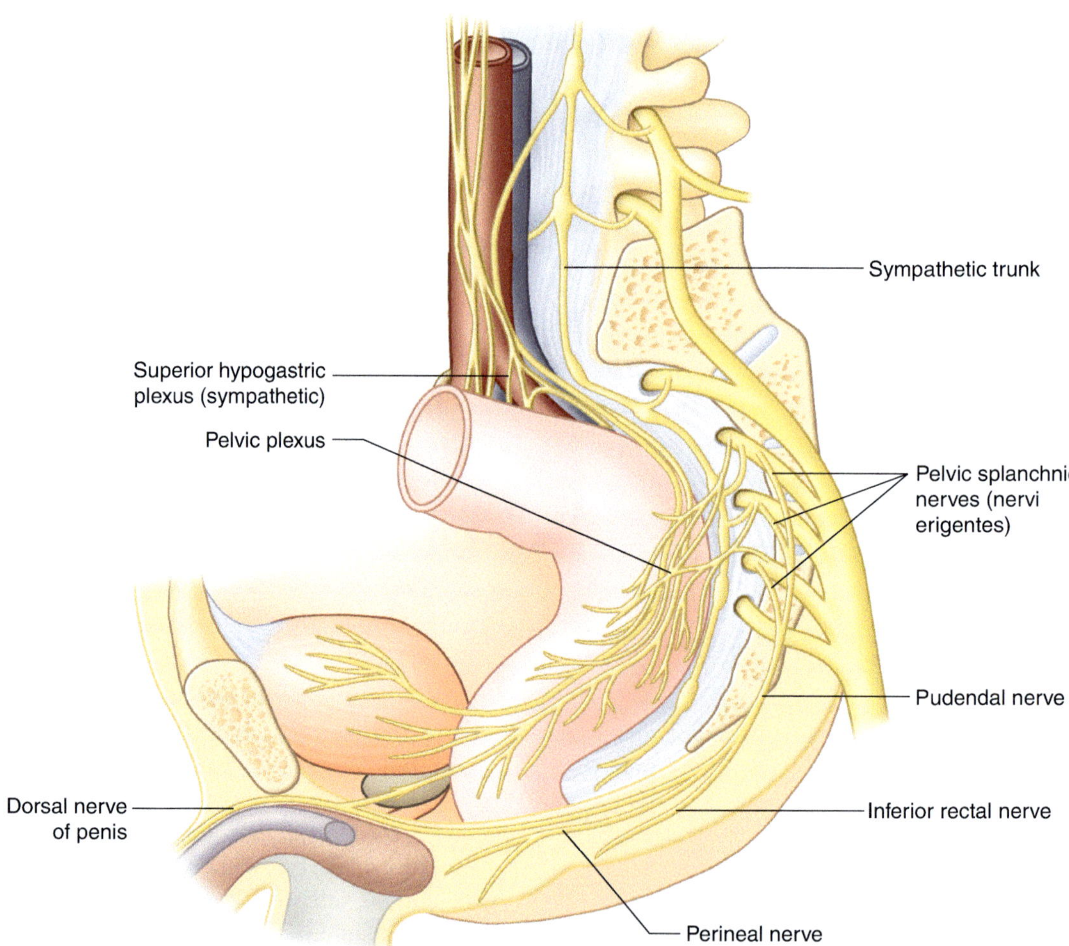

Fig. 1.11 Nerves of the rectum

vas deferens, urethra, ejaculatory ducts, and bulbourethral glands.

- The internal anal sphincter is innervated by sympathetic (L5) and parasympathetic (S2, S3, and S4) nerves following the same route as the nerves to the rectum as noted above.
- The external anal sphincter is innervated on each side by the inferior rectal branch of the internal pudendal nerve (S2 and S3) and by the perineal branch of S4.
- Anal sensation is mediated by the inferior rectal branch of the pudendal nerve.

Anatomy of the Colon

- The colon is a long tubular organ consisting of muscle and connective tissue with an inner mucosal layer. Its diameter differs depending by segment, generally decreasing from about 7 cm in the cecum to 2.5 cm in the sigmoid colon. The average length is about 150 cm.
- The right and left sides of the colon are fused to the posterior retroperitoneum (secondarily retroperitonealized), while the transverse colon and sigmoid colon are relatively free within the peritoneum. The transverse colon is held in position via its attachments to the hepatic and splenic flexures and is further fused to the omentum.
- The appendices epiploicae are non-mesenteric fat protruding from the serosal surface of the colon. They are likely residual from the antimesenteric fat of the embryologic intestine that dissipates (unlike the omentum on the stomach).
- The taenia coli are three thickened bands of outer, longitudinal muscle of the colon and are separately named: *taenia libera* to represent the anterior band, *taenia mesocolica* for the posteromedial band, and *taenia omentalis* for posterolateral band. They run along the full length of the colon but are not as long as the bowel wall. This difference in length results in outpouchings of the bowel wall between the taeniae referred to as haustra. The haustra are further septated by the plicae semilunares.

Cecum

- The proximal-most portion of the colon is termed the cecum, a sac-like segment of the colon below (proximal to) the ileocecal valve. At its base is the appendix, and terminating in the posteromedial area of the cecum is the terminal ileum (ileocecal valve).
- The ileocecal valve is a circular muscular sphincter which appears as a slit-like ("fish-mouth") opening noted on an endoscopic evaluation of the cecum. The valve is not competent in all patients, but when present, its competence leads to the urgency of a colon obstruction as it develops into a closed-loop obstruction. Regulation of ileal emptying into the colon appears to be the prime task in ileocecal valve function.

The Appendix

- The appendix is an elongated, true diverticulum arising from the base of the cecum and of variable length (2–20 cm). Its blood supply is via the appendiceal vessels contained within the mesoappendix. The most common location of the appendix is medial on the cecum toward the ileum, but it has great variability in its location including pelvic, retrocecal, preileal, retroileal, and subcecal.

Ascending Colon

- From its beginning at the ileocecal valve to its terminus at the hepatic flexure where it turns sharply medially to become the transverse colon, the ascending colon measures on average, about 15–18 cm.
- Its anterior surface is covered in the visceral peritoneum, while its posterior surface is fused with the retroperitoneum.
- The lateral peritoneal reflection can be seen as a thickened line termed the white line of Toldt, which can serve as a surgeon's guide for mobilization of the ascending colon off of its attachments to the retroperitoneum, most

notably the right kidney (Gerota's fascia) and the loop of the duodenum located posterior and superior to the ileocolic vessels.
- The right ureter and the right gonadal vessels pass posteriorly to the ascending mesocolon within the retroperitoneum.

Transverse Colon

- The transverse colon traverses the upper abdomen from the hepatic flexure on the right to the splenic flexure on the left. It is generally the longest section of colon (averaging 45–50 cm) and swoops inferiorly as it crosses the abdomen.
- The entire transverse colon is covered by visceral peritoneum, but the greater omentum is fused to the anterosuperior surface of the transverse colon. Superior to the transverse mesocolon, inferior to the stomach, and posterior to the omentum is the pocket of the peritoneal cavity termed the lesser sac, with the pancreas forming the posterior-most aspect.
- The splenic flexure is the sharp turn from the transversely oriented transverse colon to the longitudinally oriented descending colon. It can be adherent to the spleen and to the diaphragm via the phrenicocolic ligament.

Descending Colon

- The descending colon travels inferiorly from the splenic flexure for the course of about 25 cm. It is fused to the retroperitoneum (similarly to the ascending colon) and overlies the left kidney as well as the back/retroperitoneal musculature.
- Its anterior and lateral surfaces are covered with visceral peritoneum, and the lateral peritoneal reflection (white line of Toldt) is again present.

Sigmoid Colon

- The sigmoid colon is the most variable of the colon segments. It is generally 35–45 cm in length. It is covered by visceral peritoneum, thereby making it mobile. Its shape is considered "omega-shaped," but its configuration and attachments are variable.
- Its mesentery is of variable length but is fused to the pelvic walls in an inverted V shape creating a recess termed the intersigmoid fossa. Through this recess travel the left ureter, gonadal vessels, and often the left colic vessels.

Rectosigmoid Junction

- The end of the sigmoid colon and the beginning of the rectum is termed the rectosigmoid junction. It is noted by the confluence of the taenia coli and the end of appendices epiploicae.
- It is the narrowest portion of the large intestine, measuring 2–2.5 cm in diameter. Endoscopically, it is noted as a narrow and often sharply angulated area above the relatively capacious rectum and above the three rectal valves.
- A recent evaluation of the rectosigmoid junction utilizing anatomic and histologic studies as well as radiographic evaluation concluded that there was an anatomic sphincter at the rectosigmoid junction. [Microscopic evaluation of the area does reveal thickening of the circular muscle layer as it progresses toward the rectum. Though not identifiable externally, radiologic evaluation can identify the area as a narrow, contractile segment].

Blood Supply

- Although the blood supply of the colon is variable, it receives blood supply from two main sources, branches of the superior mesenteric artery (SMA) (cecum, ascending and transverse colon) and branches of the inferior mesenteric artery (IMA) (descending and sigmoid colon) (Fig. 1.9).
- Just proximal to the splenic flexure, the branches of the left branch of the middle colic artery anastomose with those of the left colic

artery. This watershed area represents the border of the embryologic midgut and hindgut.

- The cecum and right colon are supplied by the terminus of the SMA, the ileocolic artery. The right colic artery is less consistent. If present (absent in 20%), it either arises directly from the SMA, from the ileocolic, or from other sources.
- The transverse colon is supplied via the middle colic artery, which branches early to form right and left branches. The middle colic artery originates directly from the SMA. The left colon and sigmoid colon are supplied by branches of the IMA, namely, the left colic and a variable number of sigmoid branches.

Superior Mesenteric Artery

- The superior mesenteric artery (SMA) is the second, unpaired anterior branch off of the aorta (Fig. 1.9). It arises posterior to the upper edge of the pancreas (near the L1 vertebrae), courses posterior to the pancreas, and then crosses over the third portion of the duodenum to continue within the base of the mesentery.
- From its left side, the SMA gives rise to up to 20 small intestinal branches, while the colic branches (ileocolic, right colic, middle colic) originate from its right side.
- The most constant of the colic branches is the ileocolic vessel which courses through the ascending mesocolon where it divides into a superior (ascending) branch and an inferior (descending) branch.
- The middle colic artery arises from the SMA near the inferior border of the pancreas. It branches early to give off right and left branches. The right branch supplies the hepatic flexure and right half of the transverse colon. The left branch supplies the left half of the transverse colon to the splenic flexure. In up to 33% of patients, the left branch of the middle colic artery can be the sole supplier of the splenic flexure.

Inferior Mesenteric Artery

- The inferior mesenteric artery (IMA) (Fig. 1.9) is the third unpaired, anterior branch off of the aorta, originating 3–4 cm above the aortic bifurcation at the level of the L2–L3 vertebrae. As the IMA travels inferiorly and to the left, it gives off the left colic artery and several sigmoidal branches.
- After these branches, the IMA becomes the superior hemorrhoidal (rectal) artery as it crosses over the left common iliac artery. The left colic artery divides into an ascending branch (splenic flexure) and a descending branch (the descending colon). The sigmoidal branches form a fairly rich arcade within the sigmoid mesocolon (similar to that seen within the small bowel mesentery).

The Marginal Artery and Other Mesenteric Collaterals

- The major arteries noted above account for the main source of blood within the mesentery, but the anatomy of the mesenteric circulation and the collaterals within the mesentery remain less clear.
- The marginal artery (of Drummond) (Fig. 1.9) has been shown to be discontinuous or even absent in some patients, most notably at the splenic flexure (Griffiths' critical point), where it may be absent in up to 50% of patients. This area of potential ischemia is the embryologic connection between the midgut and hindgut.
- Another potential site of ischemia is at a discontinuous area of marginal artery located at the rectosigmoid junction termed Sudeck's critical point. This has been confirmed by a recent fluorescence study; however its clinical importance remains in doubt.

Venous Drainage

- Venous drainage of the colon largely follows the arterial supply with superior and inferior mesenteric veins draining both the right and left halves of the colon (Fig. 1.10). They ultimately meet at the portal vein to reach the intrahepatic system.
- The superior mesenteric vein (SMV) travels parallel and to the right of the artery.

- The inferior mesenteric vein (IMV) does not travel with the artery but rather takes a longer path superiorly to join the splenic vein. It separates from the artery within the left colon mesentery and runs along the base of the mesentery where it can be found just lateral to the ligament of Treitz and the duodenum before joining the splenic vein on the opposite (superior) side of the transverse mesocolon. Dissecting posterior to the IMV can allow for separation of the mesenteric structures from the retroperitoneal structures during a medial-to-lateral dissection.

Lymphatic Drainage

- The colon wall has a dense network of lymphatic plexuses. These lymphatics drain into extramural lymphatic channels that follow the vascular supply of the colon.
- Lymph nodes are plentiful and are typically divided into four main groups. The *epiploic* group lies adjacent to the bowel wall just below the peritoneum and in the epiploicae. The *paracolic* nodes are along the marginal artery and the vascular arcades. The *intermediate* nodes are situated on the primary colic vessels. The *main* or *principal* nodes are on the superior and inferior mesenteric vessels.
- Once the lymph leaves the main nodes, it drains into the cisterna chyli via the para-aortic chain.

Nervous Innervation

- The colon is innervated by the sympathetic and parasympathetic nervous systems and closely follows the arterial blood supply.
- The sympathetic innervation of the right half of the colon originates from the lower six thoracic splanchnic nerves which synapse within the celiac, preaortic, and superior mesenteric ganglia. The postganglionic fibers then follow the SMA to the right colon.
- The sympathetic innervation for the left half originates from L1, L2, and L3. Parasympathetic fibers to the right colon come from the posterior (right) branch of the vagus nerve and celiac plexus. They travel along the SMA to synapse with the nerves within the intrinsic autonomic plexuses of the bowel wall. On the left side, the parasympathetic innervation comes from S2, S3, and S4 via splanchnic nerves.

Embryology

Anus and Rectum

- The colon distal to the splenic flexure, including the rectum and the anal canal (proximal to the dentate line), is derived from the hindgut and therefore has vascular supply from the inferior mesenteric vessels (Fig. 1.9).
- The dentate line (Fig. 1.1) is the fusion plane between the endodermal and ectodermal tubes. The cloacal portion of the anal canal has both endodermal and ectodermal components that develop into the anal transitional zone. The terminal portion of the hindgut or cloaca fuses with the proctodeum (an ingrowth from the anal pit).
- The cloaca originates at the portion of the rectum below the pubococcygeal line, while the hindgut originates above it. Before the fifth week of development, the intestinal and urogenital tracts are joined at the level of the cloaca. By the eighth week, the urorectal septum migrates caudally to divide the cloacal closing plate into an anterior urogenital plate and a posterior anal plate. Anorectal rings result from a posterior displacement in the septum and the resultant smaller anal opening. By the tenth week, the anal tubercles fuse into a horseshoe-shaped structure dorsally and into the perineal body anteriorly. The external anal sphincter forms from the posterior aspects of the cloacal sphincter earlier than the development of the internal sphincter. The internal sphincter develops from enlarging fibers of the circular muscle layer of the rectum. The sphincters migrate during their development with the internal sphincter moving caudally, while the external sphincter enlarges cephalad. Meanwhile, the longitudinal muscle descends into the intersphincteric plane.

- In females, the female genital organs form from the Müllerian ducts and join the urogenital sinus by the 16th week of development.
- In males, the urogenital membrane obliterates with fusion of the genital folds, while the sinus develops into the urethra.

Colon and Small Intestine

- The endodermal roof of the yolk sac develops into the primitive gut tube. This initially straight tube is suspended upon a common mesentery. By week 3 of development, it has three discernible segments, namely, the foregut, midgut, and hindgut. The midgut starts below the pancreatic papilla to form the small intestine and the first half of the colon. The distal colon, rectum, and anal canal develop from the hindgut.
- There is a normal process by which the intestinal tract rotates (Fig. 1.12). The first stage is the physiologic herniation of the midgut, the second stage is its return to the

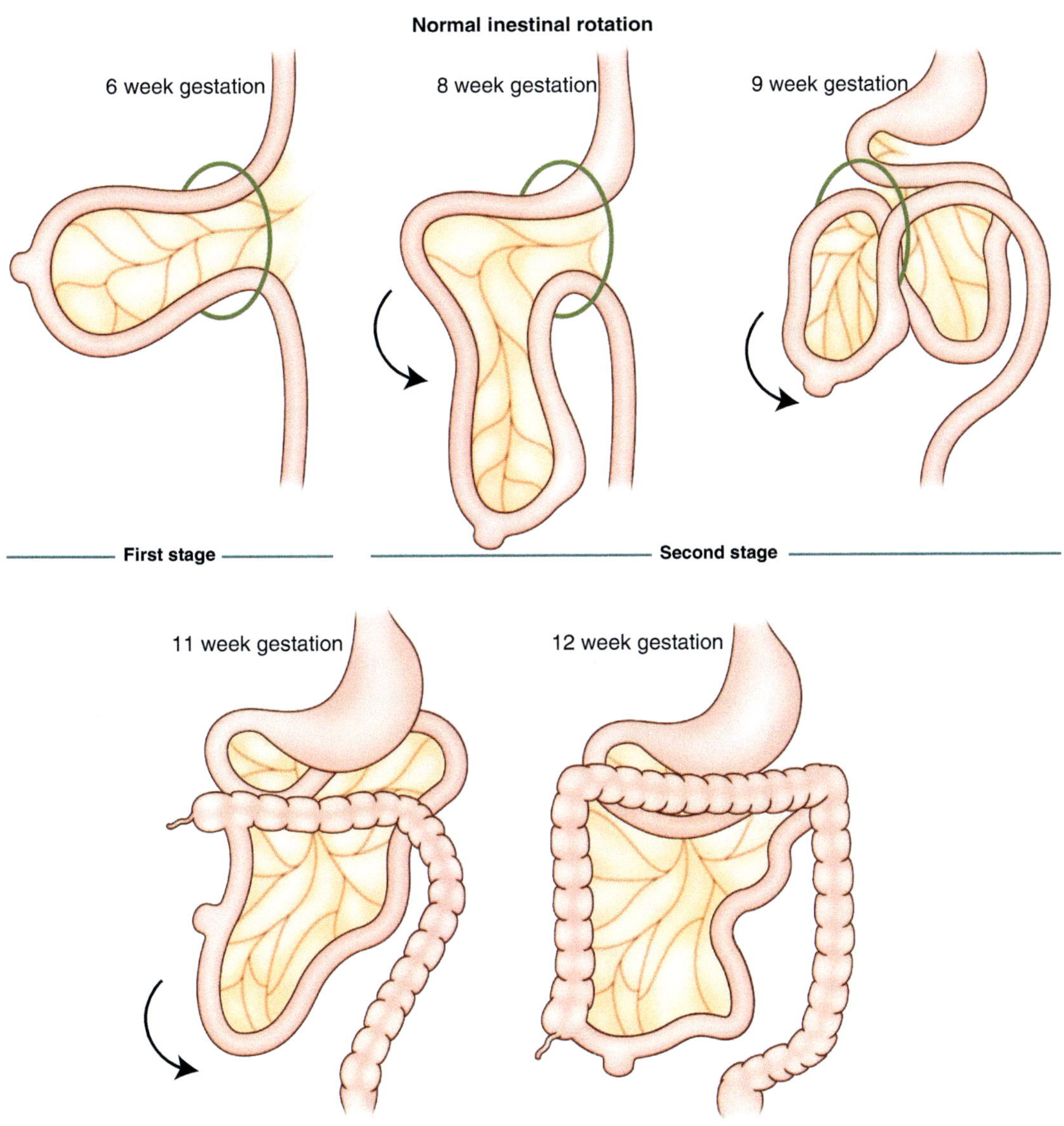

Fig. 1.12 Summary of normal intestinal rotation during development

abdomen, and the third stage is the fixation of the midgut. Abnormalities in this normal process lead to various malformations. The physiologic herniation (first stage) occurs between weeks 6 and 8 of development. The primitive gut tube elongates over the superior mesenteric artery and bulges out through the umbilical cord (Fig. 1.13). These contents move in a counterclockwise fashion, turning 90° from the sagittal to the horizontal plane (Fig. 1.14).

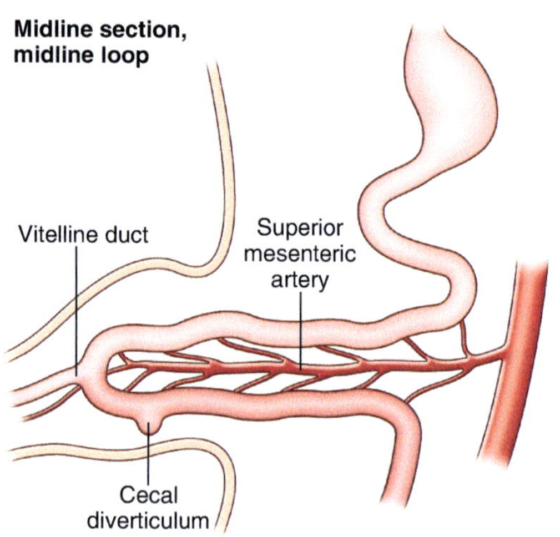

Fig. 1.13 Elongation of the midgut loop

- During the second stage, the midgut loops return to the peritoneal cavity and simultaneously rotate an additional 180° in the counterclockwise direction (Fig. 1.15). The pre-arterial portion of the duodenum returns to the abdomen first, followed by the counterclockwise rotation around the superior mesenteric vessels, resulting in the duodenum lying behind them. The colon returns after the rotation, resulting in their anterior location.
- The third stage (fixation of the midgut) begins once the intestines have returned to the peritoneal cavity and ends at birth. The cecum migrates to the right lower quadrant from its initial position in the upper abdomen (Fig. 1.16). After the completion of this 270° counterclockwise rotation, fusion begins, typically at weeks 12–13. This results in fusion of the duodenum as well as the ascending and descending colon (Fig. 1.17).

Major Anomalies of Rotation

Non-rotation

- The midgut returns to the peritoneum without any of the normal rotation. This results in the small intestine being on the right side of the abdomen and the colon on the left side

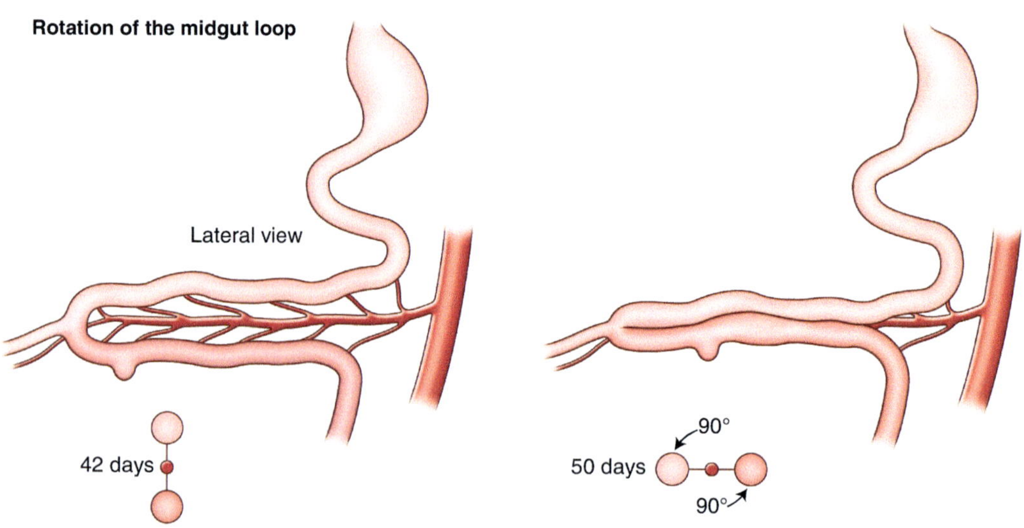

Fig. 1.14 Rotation of the midgut loop

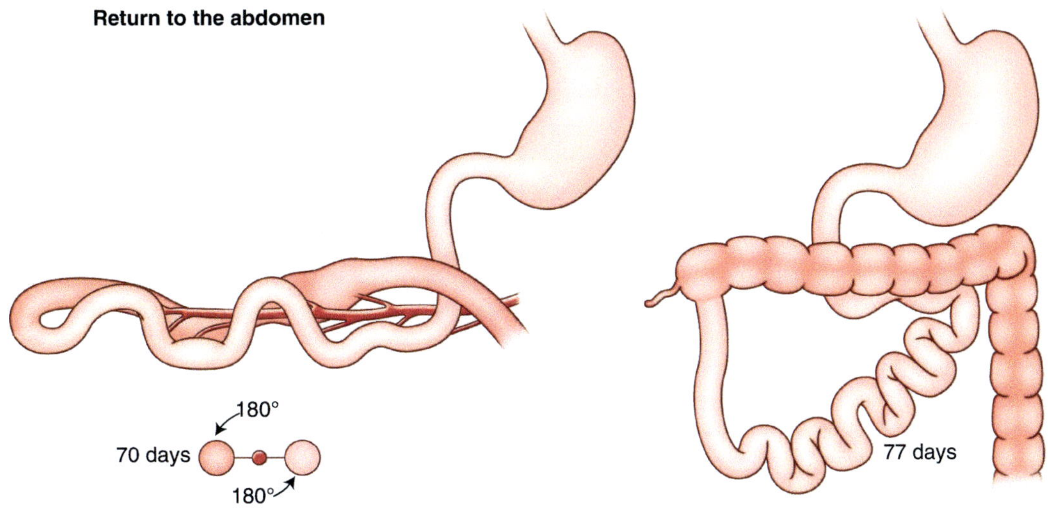

Fig. 1.15 Return of the intestinal loop to the abdomen

Fig. 1.16 Later fetal development

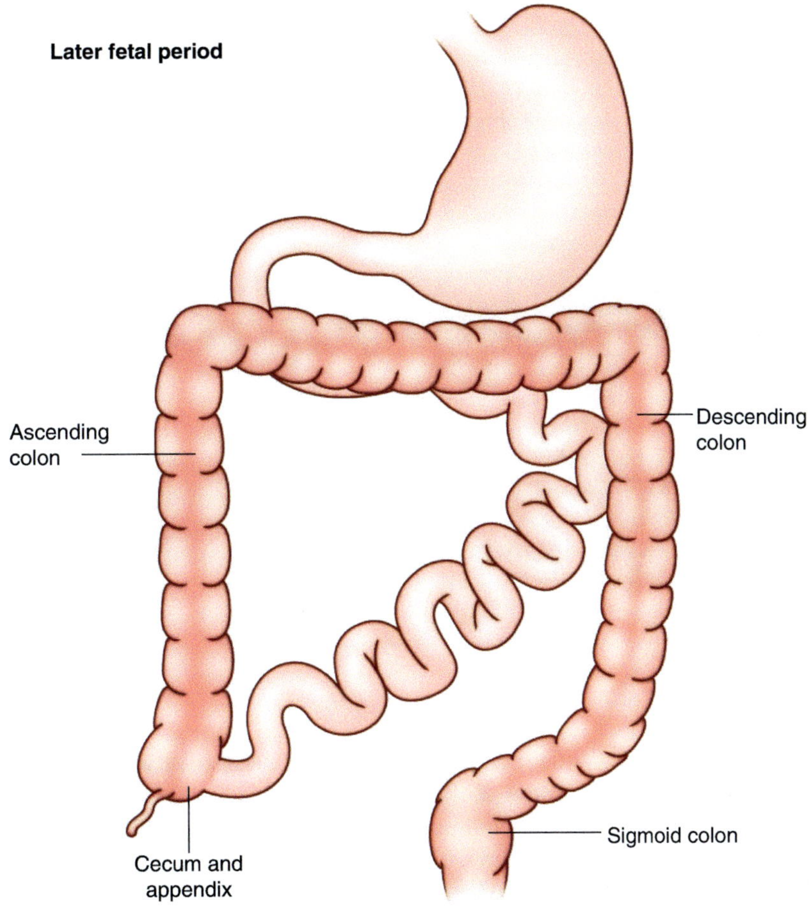

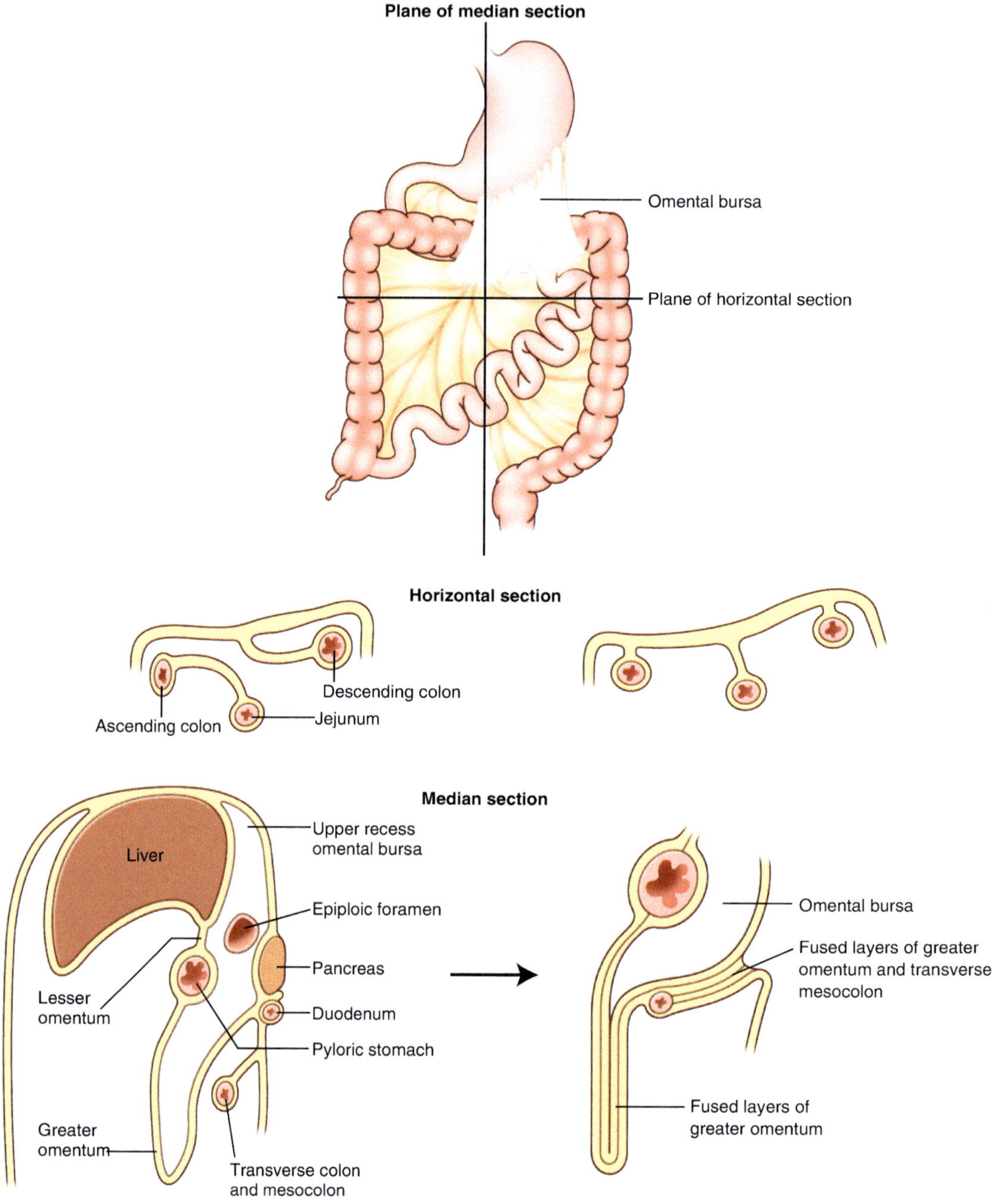

Fig. 1.17 Development of the mesentery and omental fusion

(Fig. 1.18). This condition can remain asymptomatic (a finding noted at laparoscopy or laparotomy) or result in volvulus affecting the entirety of the small intestine. The twist generally occurs at the duodenojejunal junction as well as the midtransverse colon.

Malrotation

- There is normal initial rotation, but the cecum fails to complete the normal 270° rotation around the mesentery. This results in the cecum being located in the mid-upper abdomen with lateral bands (Ladd's bands)

Fig. 1.18 Intestinal non-rotation

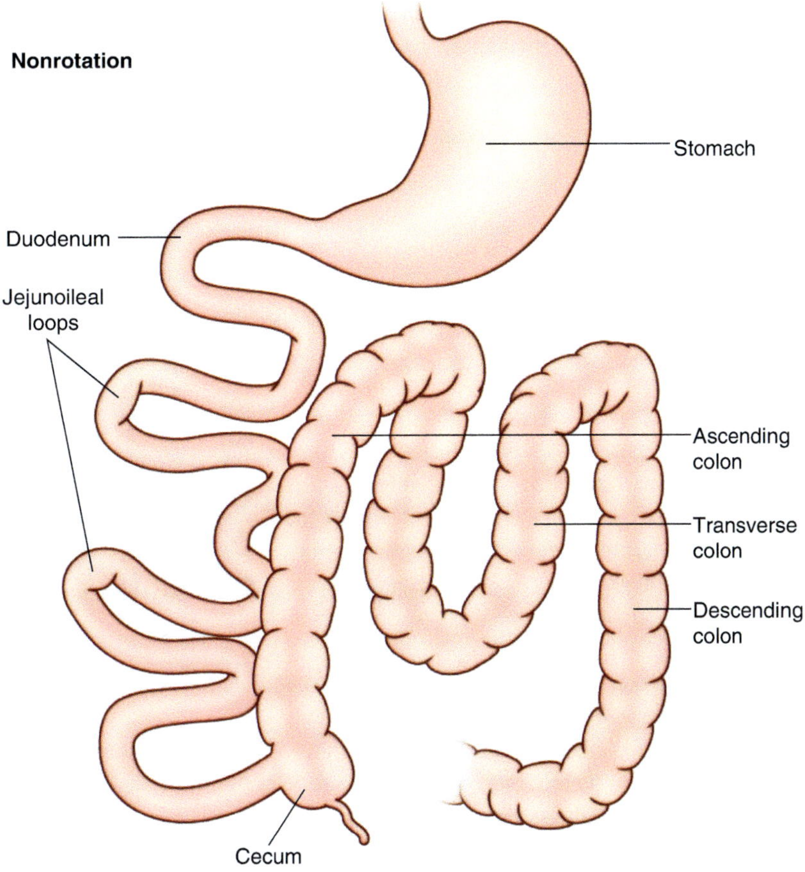

fixating it to the right abdominal wall (Fig. 1.19). These bands can result in extrinsic compression of the duodenum.

Reversed Rotation

- Clockwise (rather than counterclockwise) rotation of the midgut results in the transverse colon being posterior to the superior mesenteric artery, while the duodenum lies anterior to it.

Omphalocele

- An omphalocele is, basically, the retention of the midgut within the umbilical sac and its failure to return to the peritoneal cavity.

Internal Hernias

- Internal hernias, as well as congenital obstructive bands, can cause congenital bowel obstructions. These are considered failures of the

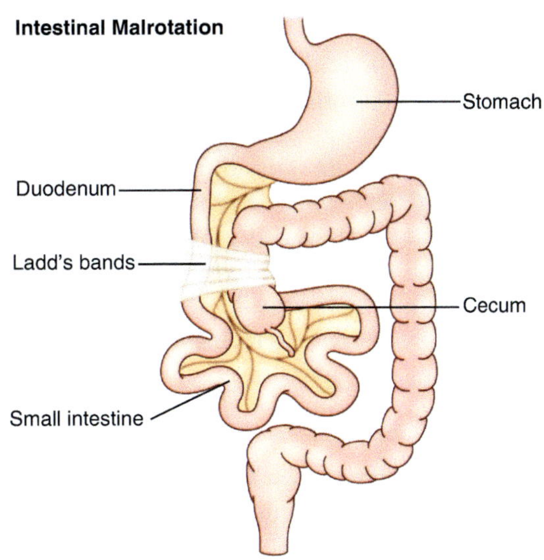

Fig. 1.19 Intestinal malrotation

process of fixation (the third stage of rotation). This can be the result of an incomplete fusion of the mesothelium or when structures are abnormally rotated. Retroperitoneal hernias can occur in various positions, most notably paraduodenal, paracecal, and intersigmoid.

Other Congenital Malformations of the Colon and Small Intestine

Proximal Colon Duplication

- There are three general types of colonic duplication: mesenteric cysts, diverticula, and long colon duplication. Mesenteric cysts are lined with intestinal epithelium and variable amounts of smooth muscle. They are found within the colonic mesentery or posterior to the rectum (within the mesorectum). They generally present as a mass or with intestinal obstruction as they enlarge.
- Diverticula can be found on the mesenteric or antimesenteric sides of the colon and are outpouchings of the bowel wall. They often contain heterotopic gastric or pancreatic tissue.
- Long colonic duplications of the colon are the rarest form of duplication. They usually run the entire length of the colon and rectum, and there is an association with other genitourinary abnormalities.

Meckel's Diverticulum

- A Meckel's diverticulum is the remnant of the vitelline or omphalomesenteric duct (Fig. 1.13). It arises from the antimesenteric aspect of the terminal ileum, most commonly within 50 cm of the ileocecal valve.
- They can be associated with a fibrous band connecting the diverticulum to the umbilicus (leading to obstruction), or it may contain ectopic gastric mucosa or pancreatic tissue (leading to bleeding or perforation) (Fig. 1.20).
- An indirect hernia containing a Meckel's diverticulum is termed a Littre's hernia.
- Meckel's diverticulum is generally asymptomatic and, per autopsy series, is found in up to 3% of the population.
- Surgical complications are more common in children than adults and include hemorrhage, obstruction, diverticulitis, perforation, and umbilical discharge.

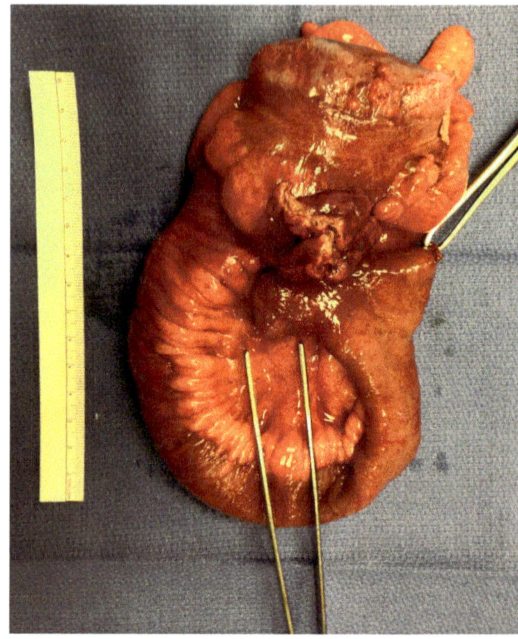

Fig. 1.20 Perforated Meckel's diverticulum with fistula to the ileum

Atresia of the Colon

- Colonic atresia, representing only 5% of all gastrointestinal atresias, is a rare cause of congenital obstruction. They are likely the result of vascular compromise during development. They vary in severity from a membranous diaphragm blocking the lumen to a fibrous cord-like remnant, on to a complete absence of a segment.

Hirschsprung's Disease

- This nonlethal anomaly, which is more common in males, results from the absence of ganglion cells within the myenteric plexus of the colon.
- It is caused by interruption of the normal migration of the neuroenteric cells from the neural crest before they reach the rectum. This results in dilation and hypertonicity of the proximal colon.
- The extent of the aganglionosis is variable, though the internal sphincter is always involved. Its severity is dependent upon the length of the involved segment.

Anorectal Malformations

- Abnormalities in the normal development of the anorectum can be attributed to "developmental arrest" at various stages of normal development. Skeletal and urinary anomalies are associated in up to 70%, while digestive tract anomalies (e.g., tracheoesophageal fistula or esophageal stenosis) and cardiac and abdominal wall abnormalities are also noted in patients with anorectal anomalies.

Anal Stenosis

- Twenty-five to twenty-nine percent of infants are born with anal stenosis, but only about 25% of these are symptomatic. The majority of these children undergo spontaneous dilation by 6 months of age.

Membranous Atresia

- This very rare condition is characterized by the presence of a thin membrane of the skin between the blind end of the anal canal and the surface. It is also termed the covered anus. It is more common in males.

Anal Agenesis

- The rectum develops below the puborectalis where it either ends in an ectopic opening (fistula) in the perineum, vulva, or urethra or it ends blindly (less commonly). The sphincter is present at its normal site.

Anorectal Agenesis

- Anorectal agenesis is the most common type of "imperforate anus." More common in males, the rectum ends well caudal to the surface, and the anus is represented by a dimple with the anal sphincter usually being normal in location. In most cases, there is a fistula to the urethra or vagina. High fistulae (to the vagina or urethra) with anorectal agenesis develop as early as the sixth or seventh week of gestation, while the low fistulae (perineal) or anal ectopia develop later, in the eighth or ninth week of development.

Rectal Atresia or "High Atresia"

- In rectal atresia, the rectum and the anal canal are separated from one another by an atretic portion. It is embryologically the distal-most type of colon atresia but is still considered an anorectal disorder clinically.

Persistent Cloaca

This rare condition, which only occurs in female infants, is the result of total failure of descent of the urorectal septum. It occurs at a very early stage of development.

Colonic Physiology

2

Joshua I. S. Bleier and Kirsten Bass Wilkins

Key Concepts

- Colonic innervation is supplied by both extrinsic and intrinsic pathways. The extrinsic pathways are derived from the autonomic nervous system including parasympathetic and sympathetic routes. Parasympathetic input is excitatory, while sympathetic input is inhibitory to colonic motor function. The intrinsic colonic nervous system consists of the myenteric plexus.
- Short-chain fatty acids are produced by the colon as a result of the fermentation of complex carbohydrates by colonic flora. The SCFA, butyrate, is the primary energy source of the colon.
- The colon absorbs sodium and water and secretes bicarbonate and potassium. Aldosterone mediates the process of active sodium absorption in the colon.
- Colonic contractile events are divided into (1) segmental contractions and (2) propagated contractions (including low-amplitude and high-amplitude propagating contractions, LAPC and HAPC, respectively). The main function of HAPC is to propagate colonic contents toward the anus.
- The interstitial cells of Cajal (ICC) are the primary pacemaker cells governing the function of the enteric nervous system.

J. I. S. Bleier (✉)
Clinical Surgery, University of Pennsylvania Health System, Perelman School of Medicine, Philadelphia, PA, USA

Department of Surgery, Hospital of the University of Pennsylvania/Pennsylvania Hospital, Philadelphia, PA, USA
e-mail: Joshua.bleier@uphs.upenn.edu

K. B. Wilkins
Department of Surgery, RWJ Barnabas Health, Edison, NY, USA

Colonic Anatomy

Introduction

- The colon is highly efficient at absorbing sodium chloride, water, and short-chain fatty acids.
- The colonic epithelium is a typical electrolyte-transporting layer that is capable of moving large quantities of water and salt from the lumen toward the blood.
- It is presented with between 1 and 2 liters of electrolyte-rich fluid per day, and nearly 90% of this fluid is absorbed resulting in the excretion of feces with a sodium concentration of approximately 30 mmol/liter and a potassium concentration of approximately 75 mmol/liter. Fecal and plasma osmolality are similar.
- The colonic epithelium secretes bicarbonate, potassium chloride, and mucus. Colonic epithelial cells are polarized and equipped with numerous ion channels, carriers, and pumps that are localized on both the luminal

S. R. Steele et al. (eds.), *The ASCRS Manual of Colon and Rectal Surgery*,
https://doi.org/10.1007/978-3-030-01165-9_2

Fig. 2.1 Normal colonic mucosa. H&E, 250x. The layers of the normal colonic wall are indicated by the brackets. (Courtesy of Julieta E. Barroeta, MD)

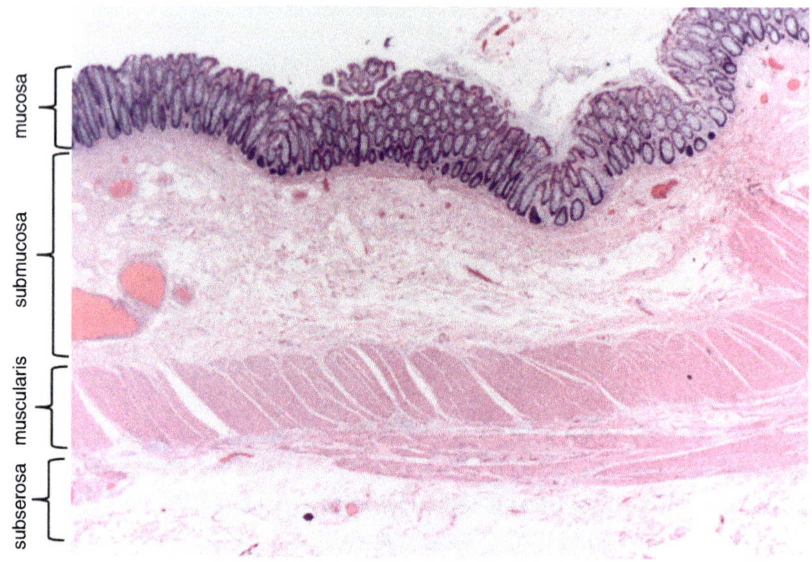

and basolateral membranes. Many transport proteins have been identified and their functions elucidated.

Colonic Wall Anatomy

- The luminal surface of the colon is lined by the epithelium. Deep to this is the submucosal layer, rich in vascular and lymphatic supply. This is surrounded by the continuous inner circular muscle layer and the outer longitudinal muscle layer which has three condensations known as taenia coli. The serosa, or outer layer of the colon, is surrounded by the visceral peritoneum.

Colonic Epithelial Cell Types

- Three main cell types are present in the colonic epithelium including columnar epithelial cells, goblet cells, and enterochromaffin cells. Columnar epithelial and goblet cells comprise nearly 95% of the cells in the colonic epithelium.
- Crypt epithelium is highly proliferative and relatively undifferentiated and secretes chloride. The surface epithelium in contrast has low proliferative activity, is well-differentiated, and is highly absorptive.
- Epithelial cells become increasingly differentiated the farther they are from the crypt base. The base of the crypts forms the source of continually regenerating epithelial cells (Figs. 2.1 and 2.2). Ion absorption and secretion occur at both the surface and crypt levels.
- The cells responsible for the enteric nervous system, the enteric ganglia, are located in the submucosa (Meissner's plexus). An additional layer of ganglia is located between the inner circular and outer longitudinal muscle layers known as Auerbach's plexus.
- The interstitial cells of Cajal (ICC), c-kit-positive cells that primarily serve as the pacemaker cell of the enteric nervous system, link the colonic submucosa electrochemically with the myenteric plexi. These are the cells of origin of GI stromal tumors (GISTs) which arise from the colonic wall rather than the mucosa.

Colonic Flora

Feces contain as many as 10^{11}–10^{12} bacteria/gram of stool (over 400 species) contributing to approximately 50% of fecal mass. The majority are anaerobes that feed on residual proteins and undigested carbohydrates. They contribute to the metabolic support of the colonocyte and gut- associated lymphoid tissue (GALT), which

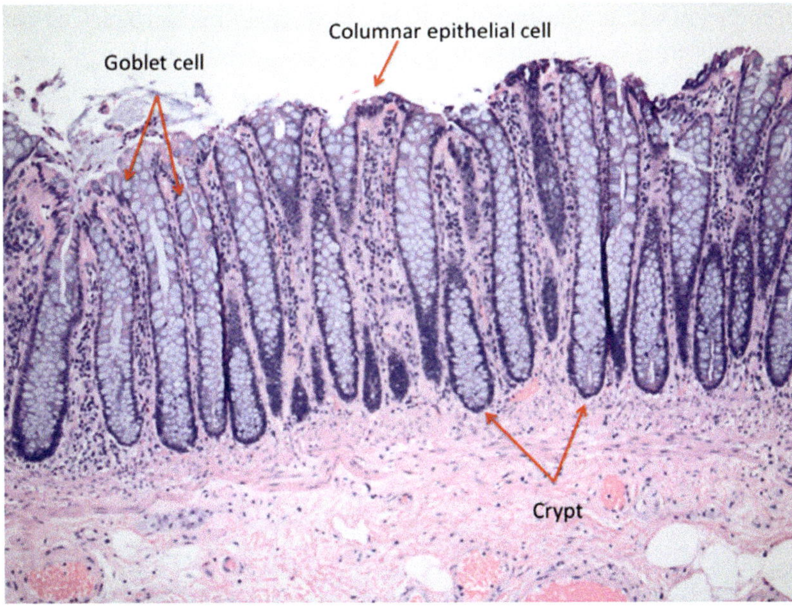

Fig. 2.2 Normal colonic mucosa. H&E, 1000x. Epithelial cells types are clearly visible including goblet cells and columnar epithelial cells. The crypts are the source of the continually regenerating mucosal cells. (Courtesy of Julieta E. Barroeta, MD)

contributes significantly to both innate and adaptive immunity.

- *Bacteroides* species are the predominant bacterial type throughout the colon and are responsible for almost 2/3 of the bacteria within the proximal colon. The other predominant species are facultative aerobes – *Escherichia*, *Klebsiella*, *Proteus*, *Lactobacillus*, and *Enterococci*.
- The colonic mucosa receives its nutrition from undigested dietary fiber which is metabolized by colonic bacteria through the process of *fermentation* and produces gas and short-chain fatty acids including butyrate – the main energy source for colonocytes.
- Cellulose is a partially fermented starch, which leaves behind bulk, whereas fruit pectins are completely metabolized.
- Several dietary complex carbohydrates, including lignin and psyllium, are not metabolized at all but remain as hydrophilic molecules in stool. These lead to water retention and stool bulking.
- Protein fermentation (*putrefaction*) results in the formation of potentially toxic metabolites including phenols, indoles, and amines. Toxic end products of bacterial metabolism may promote carcinogenesis.
- Increased stool bulk is felt to provide enhanced colonic transit resulting in decreased time of exposure of the colonic lumen to these toxins, as well as a decreased need for higher intracolonic pressures necessary for segmental motility, a process that may retard the development of diverticular disease. These aspects are the reason for many of the recommendations for dietary supplementation with indigestible fiber.

Electrolyte Regulation and Water Absorption

- A majority of sodium chloride absorption occurs in the proximal colon and is driven primarily through electroneutral absorption by tightly-coupled luminal Na+/H+ and Cl-/HCO3- exchange. Three types of Na+/H+ exchangers (NHE) have been identified in colonic epithelium. Similarly, several Cl- exchange mechanisms have been identified. The luminal Cl-/HCO3- exchange is represented by the anion exchanger type 1 (AE1). A separate Cl-/OH- exchange is represented by a protein called DRA (downregulated in colonic adenomas).
- Epithelial cells in the distal colon participate in electrogenic absorption of sodium. The

epithelial sodium channel (ENaC) mediates this absorption and is located on the luminal surface. Potassium is secreted on the luminal side and is driven by the electrogenic uptake of sodium.

- Chloride is absorbed through luminal cystic fibrosis transmembrane conductance regulator (CFTR) and other chloride channels. It is excreted on the basolateral side via multiple mechanisms including KCL cotransporter (KCC1), Cl- channels, and CL-/HCO3- anion exchangers. The net result is tight regulation of electrolyte secretion in excreted stool (Fig. 2.3).
- Changes in intracellular sodium concentration during sodium chloride absorption downregulates ENaC activity.
- Blood pressure and potassium levels also regulate sodium absorption via angiotensin II.
- Aldosterone targets the renal and colonic epithelium and increases activity of NHE3. Early- and late-phase aldosterone actions have

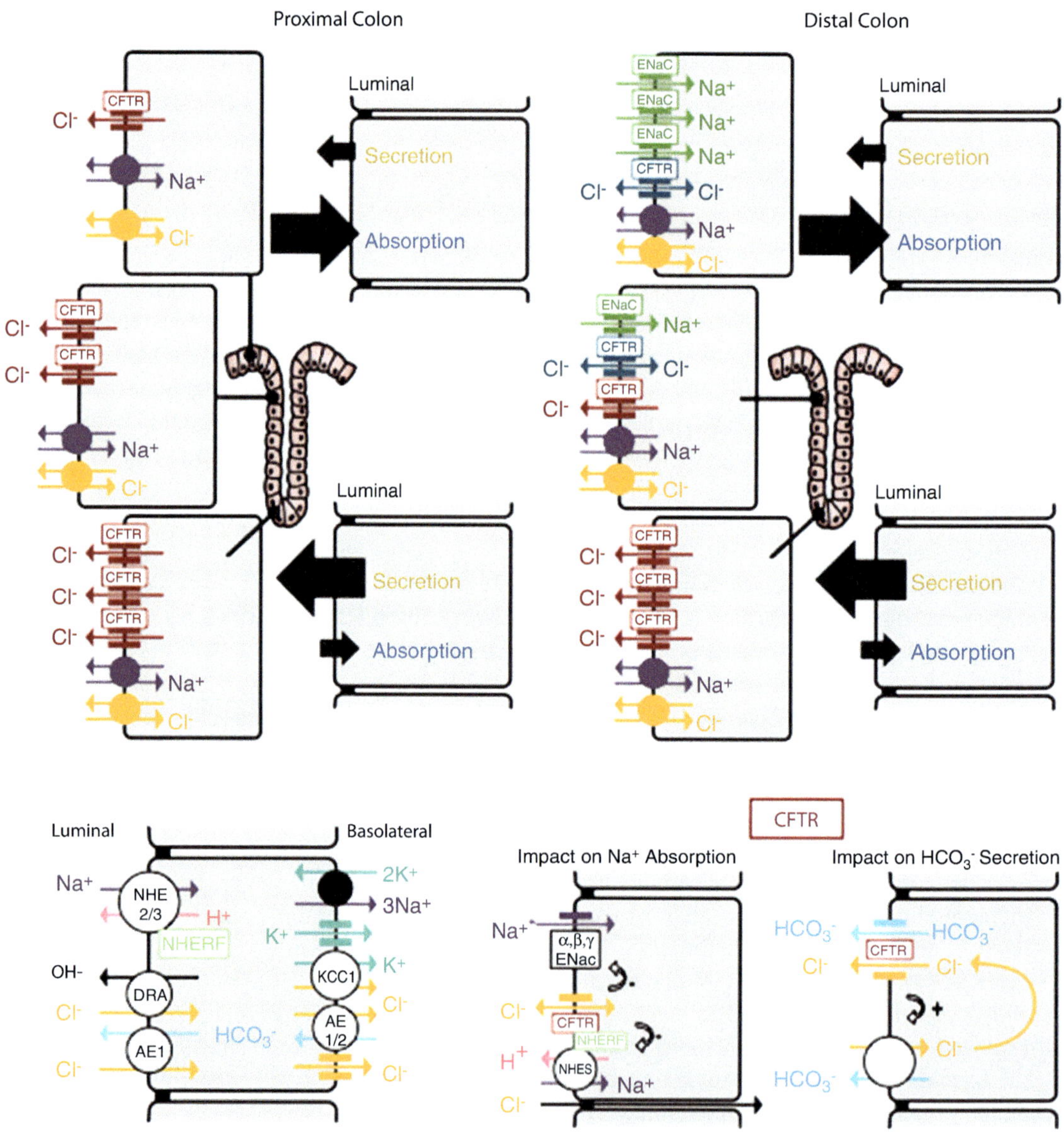

Fig. 2.3 Schematic of ion-transport channels in proximal and distal colonocytes. (Courtesy of Robin Noel)

been identified. In the first 1–6 h, aldosterone-induced proteins including serum and glucocorticoid-inducible kinase (Sgk), corticosteroid hormone-induced factor (CHIF), and K-Ras (KRAS) increase the posttranslational activation of existing ion channels and other proteins involved in ion transport such as ENaC. In the late phase (> 6 h), aldosterone acts via the upregulation of nuclear transcription of these receptors. In addition, electroneutral absorption is known to be regulated in response to some G protein-linked receptors, tyrosine kinase-coupled receptors, and protein kinases. For example, activation of protein kinase C and Ca2+/calmodulin-dependent kinase and increases in cAMP inhibit NHE3.

- ENaC, NHE3, and CFTR are coexpressed in colonic epithelial cells, and thus CFTR plays a role in both the electrogenic and electroneutral absorption of electrolytes. CFTR inhibits both electroneutral NaCl absorption and electrogenic Na+ absorption. In the crypts, CFTR is a cAMP-mediated chloride channel that is essential for chloride secretion. In patients with cystic fibrosis, mutations in CFTR result in both impaired chloride secretion and enhanced sodium absorption.
- Along with the kidneys, the colon assists with potassium homeostasis through the absorption and secretion of potassium. Active potassium absorption is restricted to the distal colon and is mediated by H+-K+-ATPase.
- Water is passively absorbed and can be transported by various pathways including through paracellular shunts and through transcellular flux potentially through aquaporin channels located on luminal and basolateral membrane surfaces.

Short-Chain Fatty Acid Absorption

- Short-chain fatty acids (SCFA) are produced during fermentation of dietary fibers by luminal bacteria and are absorbed by nonionic diffusion and paracellular absorption in the proximal colon. Butyrate plays a major role in the stimulation of sodium chloride absorption and inhibition of chloride secretion. Chloride absorption is also upregulated by increased HCO3- production and stimulation of the luminal Cl-/HCO3- exchanger. This HCO3- luminal secretion is paramount in regulating luminal intestinal pH. It has been proposed that antibiotic-associated diarrhea is secondary to decreased butyrate production resulting in net secretion of fluid.
- Butyrate stimulates cell proliferation in the crypts and reduces the number and size of aberrant crypt foci – the earliest precursors of colonic neoplasms. In colon cancer cell lines, butyrate induces apoptosis and cell cycle arrest. It also has an anti-inflammatory role via inhibition of nuclear factor kB (NF-kB). Butyrate stimulates the production of MUC2 mucin part of the colonic defense barrier. And it may decrease visceral sensitivity.
- Commercially available butyrate for oral administration is limited by its short half-life, poor palatability, and side effects such as nausea and anorexia. Rectal formulations are most commonly utilized at this time. Prebiotics and probiotics which produce butyrate are alternative methods of delivery. Prebiotics are nutrients (typically carbohydrates) that support the growth of probiotics bacteria. Probiotics are live bacteria that when consumed in sufficient quantities confer positive health benefits.

Secretory Role of the Colonic Epithelium

Electrolyte secretion helps transport mucus from the crypts and is activated by an increase in intracellular cAMP that parallels electrolyte secretion.

- Chloride secretion occurs predominantly in the crypt cells and is activated by cAMP-dependent stimulation of CFTR chloride channels.
- Additional Cl- channels have been identified in the colonic mucosa that belongs to a family of ClC Cl- channels. Lubiprostone accelerates

colonic transport through the activation of ClC-2 channels on the apical membrane of epithelial cells.
- Bicarbonate is also secreted to the luminal side of the epithelium and is responsible for the slightly alkaline pH of the colonic lumen.
- Mucus is secreted by goblet and crypt epithelial cells. An outer loose layer contains bacteria and lubricates feces and protects epithelial cells from abrasion and chemical insult. An inner layer is essentially sterile and is a dense gel that contains antimicrobial peptides, enzymes, and secretory immunoglobulin A (IgA) among other substances. Cholinergic stimulation releases preformed mucus, and intracellular cAMP induces mucus synthesis. Prostaglandins stimulate mucus secretion from columnar epithelial cells.

Regulation of Electrolyte and Water Absorption and Secretion

- There is a net absorption of sodium chloride and water.
- Under pathologic conditions, active Cl- secretion predisposes to the development of diarrhea.
- The major neuronal input is via the myenteric (Auerbach's) plexus and the submucosal (Meissner's) plexus. These plexi innervate epithelial as well as vascular smooth muscle cells and regulate colonic blood flow, absorption, and secretion.
- Food substances, bile acids, and bacterial or viral toxins may act as secretagogues.
- Secretory hormones and neurotransmitters include vasoactive intestinal polypeptide (VIP), acetylcholine (ACh), histamine, secretin, and serotonin.
- Substances that inhibit secretion include growth hormone, neuropeptide Y, somatostatin, opiates, and norepinephrine.
- Gasotransmitters play a role in colonic ion transport. Examples include nitric oxide, carbon monoxide, and hydrogen sulfide.

Colonic Innervation

Nerves supplying the colon serve to control and modulate colonic motor function and have a multitude of functions including the following: (1) afferent input via chemoreceptors and mechanoreceptors, (2) efferent output to smooth muscle cells that either stimulate or inhibit contraction by the release of neurotransmitters, (3) modulate the release of neurotransmitters through the release of neuromodulators, (4) control colonic sphincter activity for functions including defecation, and (5) generate signals for the initiation of propagating and nonpropagating motor complexes (see below).

- The extrinsic pathways originate from the central and autonomic nervous systems. Intrinsic innervation consists of the enteric nervous system.
- Autonomic pathways run along parasympathetic and sympathetic chains. Each of these pathways includes afferent (sensory) and efferent (motor) innervation.
- Vagal and pelvic nerves provide parasympathetic input to the colon. Vagal fibers reach the proximal colon along the posterior vagal trunk that follows the arterial blood supply along superior mesenteric arterial branches.
- The rectum and distal colon receive parasympathetic input from the sacral nerves (S2–S4) through the pelvic plexus. Parasympathetic stimulation stimulates motor activity of the circular and longitudinal muscle throughout the colon.
- The pelvic afferents contain pain fibers and thus convey visceral sensory input (Fig. 2.4).
- Acetylcholine is the major cholinergic parasympathetic neurotransmitter.
- Sympathetic fibers originate from several sources including the lumbar ventral roots (L2–L5), postganglionic hypogastric nerves, and the splanchnic nerves (T5–T12). The lumbar ventral nerve roots provide the main sympathetic supply to the colon and synapse on the inferior mesenteric ganglia.

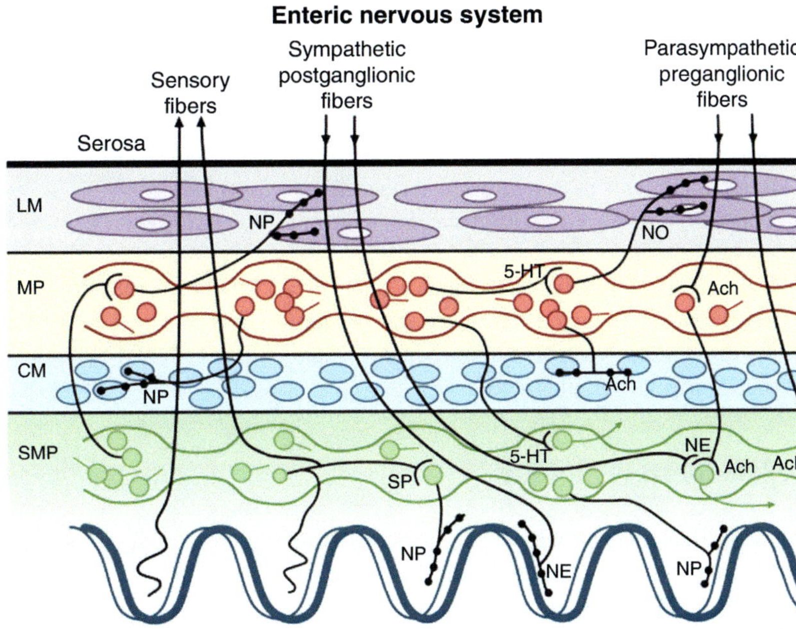

Fig. 2.4 Schematic representation of the components of the enteric nervous system. (Courtesy of Robin Noel)

- Postganglionic nerves course along the inferior mesenteric artery to synapse on the enteric ganglia.
- The postganglionic hypogastric nerves originate from the inferior mesenteric ganglia, join the pelvic plexus, and primarily innervate the anal sphincters.
- The splanchnic nerves reach the proximal colon as they course along the blood supply and innervate the proximal colon.
- Sympathetic innervation is inhibitory to the myenteric ganglia (inhibits colonic contractions) and excitatory to the sphincter muscle.

Norepinephrine acts as an inhibitory neurotransmitter via a-2 adrenergic receptors in the myenteric plexus.

- The intrinsic (enteric) nervous system of the colon can continue to function even when these circuits have been interrupted due to the complex system of 200–600 million ganglia of neural crest origin. This system consists of full reflex circuits comprised of sensory neurons, interneurons, and motor neurons regulated by a multitude of neurotransmitters and neuromodulators.

The myenteric or Auerbach's plexus is located between the longitudinal and circular smooth muscle layers and plays a crucial role in colonic smooth muscle function.

- The submucosal or Meissner's plexus regulates ion transport. The extreme importance of these is demonstrated in Hirschsprung's Disease where the ganglia of the myenteric and submucosal plexuses are congenitally absent resulting in segments that do not relax causing severe constipation.
- Nearly 20 types of enteric neurons have been identified, and every class of CNS neurotransmitters (as well as many endocrine and paracrine chemicals) has been identified in the enteric nervous system.
- Intrinsic primary afferent neurons (IPANs) are the neurons through which enteric reflexes are initiated by sensing changes in luminal chemistry (transepithelially) and pressure as well as colonic muscular tone. IPANs are present in the myenteric and submucosal plexi.
- Enterochromaffin (EC) cells represent a type of this sensory transducer cell and contain large quantities of serotonin.
- Serotonin can be excitatory or inhibitory depending on which type of serotonin receptor with which it interacts.

Colonic Motility

- Basic colonic motility requirements include slow net caudal propulsion, extensive mixing of semisolid stool, and uniform exposure of luminal contents to the mucosal surface.
- The colon also moves stool caudally during mass movements.
- Most colonic motility is involuntary and is primarily mediated by the enteric nervous system in association with autonomic parasympathetic and sympathetic input.

Cellular Basis of Motility

The muscular apparatus of the colon consists of smooth muscle cells arranged into circular and longitudinal layers and interconnected by gap junctions that allow electrical signals to spread in a coordinated fashion.

- Important to this function are the colonic pacemaker cells (interstitial cells of Cajal) which are of mesenchymal origin and (1) have electrical pacemaker activity and (2) serve as conduits for muscle innervation and may transmit sensory information.
- ICC density is able to be measured by c-Kit immunohistochemistry.

ICC occur in the submucosa (ICC-SM), generate electrical stimuli with an oscillatory pattern of 2–4 Hz, and are coupled to smooth muscle cells triggering large, slow repetitive depolarizations referred to as slow waves.

- Higher-frequency oscillations (17–18 Hz) are generated in the ICC of the myenteric border (ICC-MP).

Slow waves from the ICC-SM predominate.

Motility Patterns and Measurement

- Colonic motor activity is not rhythmic but is characterized by brief (phasic) and sustained (tonic) contractions.
- At least seven different patterns of human colonic phasic pressure activity have been identified. Nonpropagating pressure waves occur randomly for at least 30 s. Simultaneous pressure waves occur simultaneously at least 10 cm apart with an onset time of <1 s. Periodic colonic motor activity also manifests as discrete random bursts of phasic and tonic pressure waves with a frequency of >/= 3 per minute and a cycle duration of >/= 3 per minute.
- Similar discrete bursts of phasic and tonic pressure waves also occur in the rectosigmoid and occur predominantly at night and are referred to as periodic rectal motor activity (PRMA).
- The function of these nonpropagating waves may be as a means for local mixing of luminal contents and may allow for adequate mucosal sampling.
- Propagating pressure waves and contractions serve to propel the colonic contents in aborad and orad directions. Aborad pressure waves include propagating pressure waves that migrate aborad across >/= 10 cm at a velocity of 0.5 cm /sec and high-amplitude propagated contractions (HAPC) of pressures >/= 75 mmHg and that migrate aborad >/= 15 cm. HAPCs occur approximately six times a day and serve to move stool en masse across the colon. Frequently, but not always, these occur prior to defecation. There are also retrograde waves that migrate orad >/= 15 cm with a velocity of > 0.5 cm/sec.
- Phasic activity demonstrates diurnal variation with activity decreasing during sleep and increasing upon awakening.
- Phasic activity also increases within a few minutes after a meal and continues for up to 2.5 h depending on the nutrient composition and caloric content of the meal.
- Altered colonic motility may be manifested as constipation.
- Patients with slow transit constipation have a reduced frequency of HAPCs and lack the normal phasic response that is elicited by the intake of a meal. The diurnal variation of colonic motor activity also may be abnormal in patients with slow transit constipation. Loss and injury to the ICC have also been observed in patients with constipation. Taken together, slow transit constipation may be associated with both myopathic and neuropathic etiologies.

3 Anal Physiology: The Physiology of Continence and Defecation

Vitaliy Y. Poylin and Thomas E. Cataldo

Abbreviations

FI	Fecal incontinence
MR	Magnetic resonance
RAIR	Rectoanal inhibitory reflex
SNS	Sacral nerve stimulation

Key Concepts

- The innervation of the anal sphincter complex is a mixed sympathetic and parasympathetic crossed-over system that provides redundant safeguards to continence.
- Normal continence and defecation require intact sensation and motor control and reflexes to sense, retain, and voluntarily expect the rectal contents at a socially appropriate time and place.
- The normal physiology of the anus can be disturbed in a variety of ways resulting in lack of control, inability to expel, or chronic pelvic pain.
- The process of childbirth can contribute significantly to alteration in anorectal anatomy and physiology resulting in a variety of disorders of defecation and/or incontinence.

Electronic Supplementary Material The online version of this chapter (https://doi.org/10.1007/978-3-030-01165-9_3) contains supplementary material, which is available to authorized users.

V. Y. Poylin · T. E. Cataldo (✉)
Division of Colon and Rectal Surgery, Department of Surgery, Beth Israel Deaconess Medical Center, Harvard Medical School, Boston, MA, USA
e-mail: tcatald1@bidmc.harvard.edu

Introduction

- The physiology of the anus and its surrounding structures is the physiology of continence and controlled defecation.
- Normal continence requires a balance between the pressure inside the rectum and the combined tone of the internal and external sphincters.
- Defecation and the controlled passage of gas or stool at socially appropriate circumstances required very fine sensation and ability to discern the rectal contents. It requires the balance to tip in favor of the rectal pressure and contraction with simultaneous coordinated relaxation of the pelvic floor and internal and external sphincters.
- Disturbance in any part of this complex balance can result in incontinence either through reduced anal tone, excess rectal contraction, reduced sensation, or the inability to differentiate the consistency of the rectal contents.
- Disorders tipping in the opposite direction may result in inability to properly or completely empty the rectum.
- More proximal conditions resulting in chronic diarrhea or constipation may tip the balance. Forces even higher can contribute to the behavioral and psychosocial aspects of ordered and disordered function of the rectum and anal canal.

S. R. Steele et al. (eds.), *The ASCRS Manual of Colon and Rectal Surgery*,
https://doi.org/10.1007/978-3-030-01165-9_3

Normal Anatomy and Physiology

- The internal sphincter begins as a condensation of the inner circular involuntary smooth muscle of the GI tract at the top of the surgical anal canal, as the top of the anorectal ring. It extends downward to just proximal to the end of the external sphincter.
- The length of the normal internal sphincter is 2–4 cm. It appears as a hypoechoic band 2–3 mm in diameter on transanal ultrasound imaging.
- The internal sphincter is chronically contracting and contributes approximately 50–75% of the resting tone of the anus.
- The external sphincter is a cylinder of striated muscle that extends downward from the levator ani muscle to the distal anoderm.
- It exists in a chronically contracting state, but when stimulated under voluntary control, it more than doubles the tone of the anus above the resting state.

Innervation of the Anus and Pelvic Floor

- The parasympathetic fibers to the rectum and anal canal emerge from the sacral foramina at the S2, S3, and S4 levels. They join the sympathetic hypogastric nerves in the pelvic plexus. From there mixed postganglionic fibers extend to the lower rectum and anal canal.
- The internal sphincter is innervated by L5–S4 mixed autonomic function in crossed fashion so that unilateral injury still results in preserved function.
- The external sphincter is similarly innervated from branches of S2–S3 via the inferior rectal branch of the pudendal nerve and the perineal branch of S4. This nervous distribution also carries the nerves of sensation and contributes to the functional aspects of continence.
- The upper anal canal contains a high density of free and organized sensory nerve endings including Meissner's corpuscles (touch), Krause's bulbs (cold), Golgi-Mazzoni bodies (pressure), and genital corpuscles (friction).

Normal Continence

Rectal Capacity

- Normal continence first requires a location to temporarily hold and assess the contents and expel them under control. The empty rectum is a low-pressure vessel with the capacity to receive stool from the sigmoid and to accommodate stool under pressure.
- Patients with diminished rectal capacity will suffer from fecal frequency and urgency and frequently may contribute to incontinence.

Pressure and Motility

- Baseline pressure in the rectum is low, about 5 mmHg with frequent low amplitude contractions every 6–12 s. Occasional high-pressure waves up to 100 mmHg have been demonstrated.
- Pressure in the anal canal ranges 10–14 times that of the rectum.
- Motor activity is more frequent, and contractile waves are of higher amplitude in the rectum than in the sigmoid producing a reverse gradient that resists the forward motion of stool.
- Slow waves are observed in the anal canal with increasing frequency distally and help maintain continence by propelling the contents back into the rectum.

Rectoanal Sensation and Sampling

- The conscious sensation of the need to defecate lives in the levators and the anal canal. Distention of the rectum triggers contraction of the external anal sphincter and significant internal anal sphincter relaxation – the rectoanal inhibitory reflex (RAIR).
- It allows the highly innervated sensitive epithelial lining of the upper anal canal to sample the contents of the distal rectum to determine its quality and consistency.
- Impaired anal sensation has been associated with childbirth, perineal descent, and mucosectomy.

Structural Considerations

- In addition to the baseline resultant tone provided by the anal sphincter complex and the puborectalis sling, the entire structure is held close by the angulation created by the puborectalis in its chronically contracted unstimulated state.
- This angle between the axis of the anus and the axis of the rectum is between 80° and 90° and is responsible for the majority of gross fecal continence. It may increase normally above 90 while sitting and will extend beyond 110° during normal defecation.
- The flap valve theory advocated by Parks suggests the anterior rectal mucosa constitutes a flap that lies over the upper end of the anal canal. Increased inter-abdominal pressure not associated with defecation increased the angulation and closes flap more firmly over the upper anal canal. The flap is opened when the perineum descends and the anorectal angle is straightened.

Role of Hemorrhoids in Normal Continence

- It has been postulated that the normal function of the hemorrhoids is as an additional important component of normal continence. These vascular cushions have the ability to expand as needed to create a seal above the anus creating the fine-tuning of continence.

Sensation and Innervation

- The rectum has a mixed sympathetic and parasympathetic innervation derived from the hypogastric nerves and the sacral parasympathetic nerves through the pelvic plexi.
- Extrapelvic innervation comes to the anus from the pudendal nerve derived from S2 to S4 via the inferior rectal nerve and ultimately spreads around the anus from both sides entering at lateral to slightly anterior positions.
- There is significant crossover innervation around the anus as a complete disruption of either pudendal nerve does not result in asymmetric sphincter atrophy or fecal incontinence.
- Sensory innervation within the rectum is sensitive only to stretch, resulting in vague sensation to visceral pelvic pain.
- Distal rectal stretch or distention can result in significant parasympathetic stimulation of the vagus nerve, thereby resulting in bradycardia and hypotension.
- Somatic sensory innervation begins in the anal transitional zone proximal to the dentate line for a short variable distance of 0.3–1.5 cm. Within this zone, there is a dense collection of nerve endings for pain, touch, pressure, and temperature. These fibers are derived from the pudendal branches, and complete anesthesia to this area can be provided by bilateral anal nerve blockade.

Normal Defecation

- Normal defecation is a complicated mechanism that relies on a close interaction between the somatic and autonomic nervous systems and includes the conscious and unconscious control of both sensory input and muscle contraction.
- Stool arrives in the rectum and is sampled. If it is not an appropriate time for defecation, the anal sphincter will contract, and rectum will start to distend.
- This process continues with progressive distention of the rectum without a person's full awareness, but conscious sampling is also present.
- As the rectum continues to expand, a person becomes aware, and there is an urge to defecate that usually lasts for a few seconds and can be controlled by further contraction of the external anal sphincter (efferent nerve endings end in lumbosacral spine which is under higher control that allows conscious suppression of the urge).
- When it becomes socially appropriate to proceed, the defecation process again relies on both conscious and unconscious responses.

- The process starts with contraction of abdominal musculature (Valsalva), which is also associated with contraction of the sigmoid colon to move stool forward.
- A combination of relaxation of the puborectalis (releases sling around anorectal junction) and levator muscle allows the pelvic floor to descend slightly and straighten the anorectal angle.
- The rectum itself starts to contract, and both internal and external sphincters relax, and at this point pressure in the rectum exceeds pressure in the anal canal, and defecation will occur.
- This process can also be aided by assuming the squatting position, which increases the intra-abdominal pressure and straightens the rectum further.
- Once begun a number of patterns can occur. There may be a single evacuation of the rectal contents accompanied by mass peristalsis of the left and sigmoid colon clearing the bowel in one continuous movement or the passage of smaller volumes of stool individually over a short time requiring recurrent efforts and straining.
- If a large volume of stool is delivered quickly to the rectum, normal rectal compliance and accommodation may be insufficient. In this case the patient with normal sensation and function will have a sense of acute urgency and can forestall defecation for 40–60 se with the use of voluntary contraction of the external sphincter to allow accommodation or move to a socially appropriate location to evacuate.

Physiology of Tibial Nerve and Sacral Nerve Root Stimulation in Fecal Continence (FI)

- Chronic electrical stimulation of nerves entering the pelvis has effects of visceral function and activity.
- Unilateral stimulation of the S3 or S4 nerve as it exits the foramen has been used for urinary incontinence for over 30 years, during which time benefits for fecal incontinence were recognized as well – though the mechanism of how sacral nerve stimulation (SNS) creates its effect remains unclear.
- Similarly, intermittent stimulation of the posterior tibial nerve has a beneficial effect on fecal incontinence through a mechanism that is not fully understood.
- The following is a summary of findings related to SNS:
  - SNS has no demonstrable effect of rectal compliance or motility.
  - It seems to reduce hypersensitivity in those with reduced capacity and hypersensitivity while increasing sensitivity in those patients with reduced sensitivity.
  - It increases mucosal blood flow when on and returns to baseline when off, and there are higher levels of the neuropeptide substance P identified in rectal biopsies of those undergoing stimulation, which reverses after it is discontinued.
  - Forty studies have examined changes in anal sphincter function through the use of anorectal manometry. Fourteen studies reported a significant increase in voluntary anal squeeze, with eight of these also reporting an increase in resting pressure.

Spinal Cord Injuries and Defecation

- Patients with spinal cord injuries are a very heterogeneous group of patients with degrees of injury that can vary significantly from patient to patient.
- High spinal cord injuries (above T7) interrupt higher control and sensation of the abdominal and pelvic floor musculature as well as the colon in the rectum resulting in lower tone in the colon and rectum. Constipation in these patients is multifactorial: (1) slowed transit due to decreased propulsive ability of the colon, (2) inability to generate adequate intra-abdominal pressure or take squatting position to aid defecation, (3) unopposed stimulation of the lower neurons that increase contraction and spasticity of the pelvic floor, and (4) impaired

sensation. They often rely on a strict bowel program, which is a combination of laxatives, rectal stimulation, and manual disimpaction. Rectal stimulation can allow some patients to have decreased anal sphincter pressure.

- Patients with low spinal cord injuries such as cauda equina syndrome often have impaired afferent fibers that results in loss of tone in the internal and external sphincter muscle as well as impaired sensation. This can result in significant incontinence since any generation of intra-abdominal pressure may result in bowel movement.

Obstructed Defecation

- Obstructed defecation is a poorly understood group of disorders resulting from an alteration in sensation, muscle relaxation, or both. Some causes of abnormal sensation can be fairly evident in patients such as those with significant proctitis (infectious or inflammatory) or those after anorectal injury/surgery.
- Dysfunction may be associated with conscious/subconscious inhibition of the need to defecate during childhood. According to this theory, repeated delays in defecation result in altered sensation that eventually leads to dyscoordination between the anorectal and pelvic floor musculatures. Changes in sensation cause an increase in stimulation of lower (lumbosacral) neuronal loop (the relaxing effects of the upper parts of the nervous system), which are insufficient to overpower the abnormal stimulation. Once this occurs, and pelvic floor musculature such as puborectalis and sphincter complex fail to relax appropriately, increasingly higher intra-abdominal pressure is needed to overpower the rectal/anal pressure to evacuate.
- Over time there is damage to the sensory pathways which eventually affect the structural integrity of the pelvic floor. Obstructed defecation disorders include intussusception, rectocele, non-relaxing puborectalis/levator muscle spasm, dyssynergic puborectalis, as well enterocele and rectal prolapse.
- Intussusception is mucosal descent causing blockage of the lower rectum/anal canal. It is possible that it is a primary process in some patients arising from redundancy of mucosa, poor tone, and pelvic floor descent (either primary structural problems or as a result of childbirth and muscle/nerve damage in women). In most patients it is likely a secondary process resulting from increased pushing and decreased relaxation. Once developed, intussusception itself generates mechanical blockage to defecation and further attempts to generate more pressure to evacuate stool.
- Rectocele is defined as greater than 2 cm of rectal wall outpouching or bowing anteriorly while straining. Rectoceles are caused by abnormal relaxation of the pelvic floor/sphincter complex or structural defects in the rectal wall created during childbirth. During evacuation generated pressure delivers stool anteriorly toward the weakened portion of the wall that is not contracting appropriately causing a sensation of bulge and incomplete evacuation (Fig. 3.1). Most symptomatic patients likely have a combination of a weaker rectal wall as well as dyssynergy of the sphincters or puborectalis.
- Pelvic floor dyssynergy (pelvic outlet obstruction) results from a failure of the puborectalis and/or sphincter complex to relax or abnormal

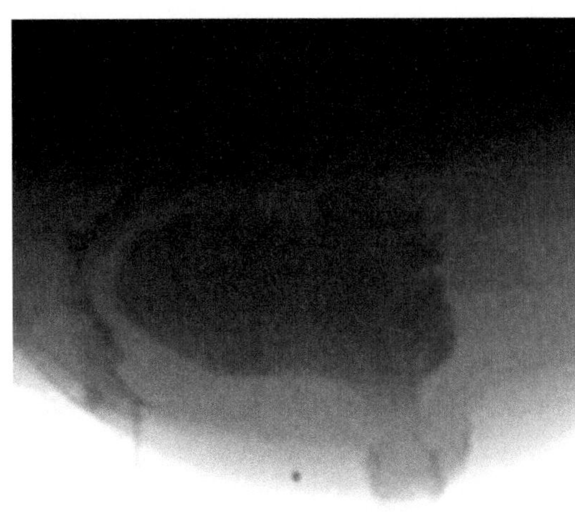

Fig. 3.1 Defecography still image of a rectocele

contraction. During attempts to evacuate, the anorectal angle may not increase or may even become sharper. A patient's natural response is to generate higher pressures in which only further worsens the symptoms. Over time, these changes likely cause more damage to the musculature and nerves. Similar to the rest of the disorders in this group, rectal sensation is also impaired, but whether it is a result of long-term damage or from an inciting event is unclear.

Functional Anorectal Pain

- There is a small group of pain disorders that are related to more functional rather than structural problems.
- Levator ani syndrome (levator spasm, puborectalis syndrome) is often described as a dull pain high in the rectum that is often made worse with sitting. Some episodes may be triggered by difficult defecation. Alternations in sensation or behavioral factors (deferring defecation, damage with hard stool) contribute to its development. Prolonged muscle contraction may result in compression of vasculature and relative ischemia leading to activation of nociceptors in the muscle (bradykinin, substance P).
- Proctalgia fugax is a sudden severe anal pain of unknown etiology, lasting seconds to minutes, that disappears completely. It is associated in some patients with a thickened internal sphincter muscle. Some studies suggest smooth muscle contraction is responsible for this pain.

Pathophysiology of Obstetric-Related Problems

- One of the worrisome potential sequelae of pregnancy and delivery is fecal incontinence which may develop as a result of direct disruption of the anal sphincter, muscle, and connective tissue or pudendal nerve injury.
- Progesterone released during pregnancy causes decreased gut motility and diminished tonic contraction of anal sphincters.
- Androgen, progesterone, and estrogen receptors are found in the squamous epithelium of the anal canal, indirectly supporting possible effects of this hormone on the sphincters.
- Progesterone causes ligamentous laxity that, when combined with increased intra-abdominal pressure, contributes to stretching of the pelvic floor musculature, widening of the levator hiatus, and potentially pudendal nerve injury. Pudendal nerve injury can affect the anal sphincters by de-innervating them and causing muscle atrophy as well as by affecting sensory components and altering RAIR. Evidence of neuropathy in the pelvic floor musculature has been found after delivery as well as in idiopathic FI and constipation.
- Labor further complicates issues of continence with further muscle stretching or even evulsion and pudendal nerve injury. A longer second stage of labor (pushing) is associated with higher rates of FI later in life.
- Use of additional devices to aid labor such as forceps and vacuum is associated with increased incidence of FI.
- Tearing and episiotomy are additional risk factors for FI and related to direct damage to the sphincter complex.
- Cesarean section is associated with lower incidences of flatus and stool incontinence, but this difference is smaller when comparing emergent cesarean sections and vaginal deliveries.
- Emergent cesarean is often initiated after failure of labor to progress following significant pushing.

Urogynecological Considerations and Pelvic Pain

- The pelvic floor is anatomically a very small area that includes the pelvic musculature and its corresponding nerves responsible for maintenance of continence and normal defecation as

well as normal urinary gynecologic function. Dysfunction in any single system is common, but more than one system is frequently affected.
- Physiologic and muscular changes associated with pregnancy and labor which affect the posterior compartment often have similar effects on middle and anterior compartment structures as well.
- Uterine prolapse and urinary problems are more common in multiparous women than nulliparous ones. The mechanism for these issues is a combination of hormonal effects as well as direct damage to the pelvic floor muscle, nerves, and sphincters.
- Widening of the levator hiatus has been shown to affect middle and anterior compartments as well as posterior one. This can result in uterine and bladder prolapse in addition to rectal prolapse, intussusception, and rectocele.
- Pregnancy and delivery effects on anal sphincters can affect urinary sphincters as well, and it is common for women presenting with urinary incontinence to report fecal incontinence as well.
- Urogynecologists see and treat a number of patients with anorectal problems, and treatments available are similar between specialties (e.g., pelvic floor physical therapy, sacral nerve stimulation).
- Pelvic floor prolapse problems may contribute to obstructed defecation. Failure to diagnose concomitant middle and anterior compartment problems may compromise success of treatment of posterior compartment dysfunction.

Endoscopy

4

Kurt Davis and Michael A. Valente

Key Concepts

- The endoscopic examination is critical for patients with colorectal complaints and is a key component of the complete colorectal examination.
- The anoscopic examination is the best way to adequately evaluate the anoderm and dentate line and evaluate for internal and external hemorrhoids and anal masses.
- Multiple bowel preparation regimens exist, but regardless which prep is chosen, splitting the timing into the half the day prior to and half the day of the procedure results in a better prep.
- There is no ideal sedation medication, but the endoscopist must be familiar with the side effect profile of any medications being used and be prepared and comfortable with any reversal agents.
- Adjunctive maneuvers employed with endoscopy serve as the markers between seasoned experts and novices: these include abdominal pressure, adjusting position, torqueing, and dithering.
- PillCam endoscopy allows the clinician to evaluate the small bowel for occult gastrointestinal bleeding, insipient tumors, polyposis syndromes, or Crohn's disease.

Introduction

- Endoscopic evaluation of the patient with colorectal complaints allows the physician to visually assess the intestinal tract and is key in the diagnosis, treatment, and monitoring of the effectiveness of any therapy.

The Complete Anorectal Examination

- While performing any examination, an anxiety-free and modest environment must be created. This can be accomplished by effective communication, keeping the patient covered as much as possible, keeping ancillary personnel in the room to a minimum, and not rushing through the examination.
- The local examination is an important precursor to any endoscopic examination and consists of proper patient positioning, visual inspection, and manual palpation of the anorectal region followed by the digital rectal examination.

K. Davis (✉)
Department of Surgery, Lousiana State University Health School of Medicine, New Orleans, LA, USA

M. A. Valente
Department of Colorectal Surgery, Digestive Disease Institute, Cleveland Clinic, Cleveland, OH, USA

S. R. Steele et al. (eds.), *The ASCRS Manual of Colon and Rectal Surgery*, https://doi.org/10.1007/978-3-030-01165-9_4

Patient Position

- The choice of patient position may depend on several variables including available equipment, patient age and comorbid status, and physician preference.

Prone Jackknife

- The prone jackknife position (knee-chest), performed with the aid of a specialized proctoscopic table, is commonly employed and allows for excellent visualization of the entire anus and perianal and perineal region, as well as the sacrococcygeal region (Fig. 4.1). The table is angled forward gradually so that the patient's buttocks and perineum are superior, while the head and feet are inferior.

Left Lateral

- The left lateral recumbent (Sims') position is if a specialty bed is not readily available (Fig. 4.2) and is well suited for elderly or debilitated patients. The patient lies on their left side, the thighs are flexed as to form a 90-degree angle with the trunk, and the buttocks project slightly beyond the edge of the examining table.

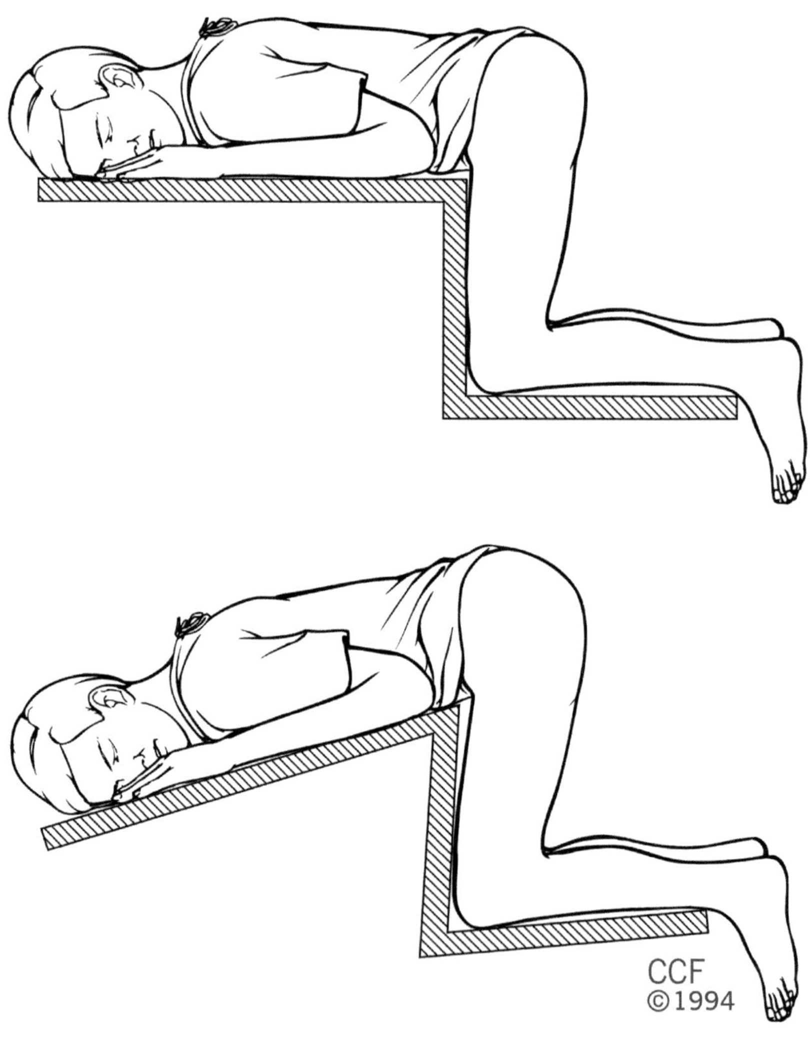

Fig. 4.1 Prone jackknife position. (Reprinted with permission, Cleveland Clinic Center for Medical Art & Photography ©2015. All Rights Reserved)

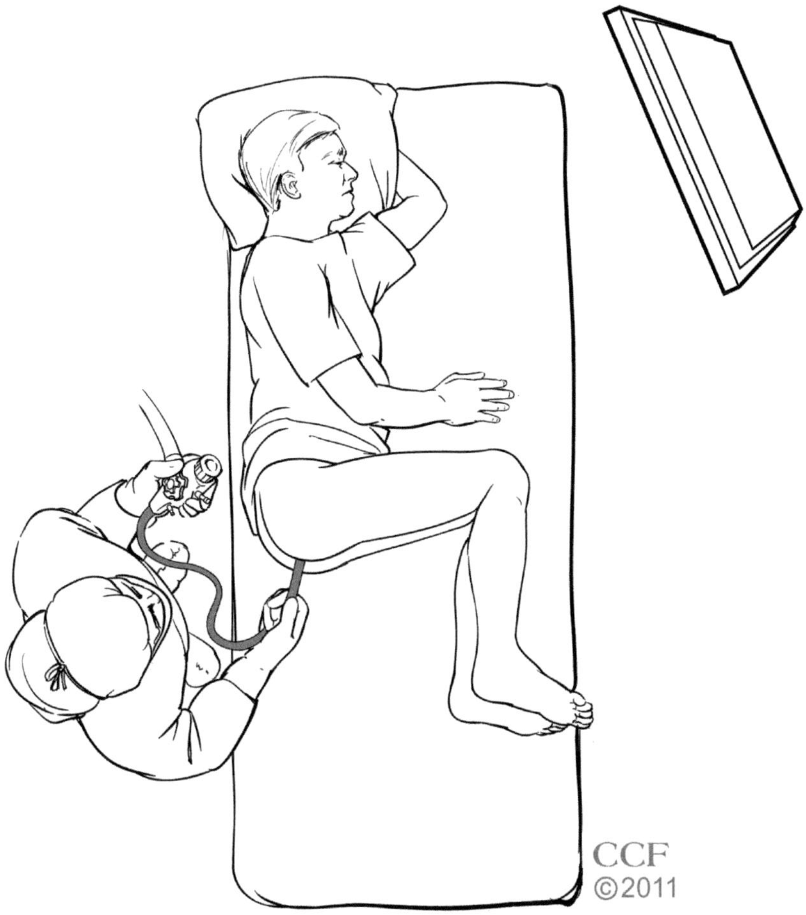

Fig. 4.2 Left lateral (Sims') position. (Reprinted with permission, Cleveland Clinic Center for Medical Art & Photography ©2015. All Rights Reserved)

Inspection and Palpation

- Proper stepwise visual inspection of the perineum, anal canal, rectum, and vagina should precede any other examination. Proper lighting is essential. It is more proper to delineate – exam findings should be described using anatomical location using the cardinal quadrants (i.e., left lateral, right anterior, right posterior) as opposed to a clockface description.
- A great deal of information can be gained from visualization, and gentle spreading of the buttocks provides proper exposure.
- The patient is asked to strain (Valsalva maneuver) to help determine and assess for perineal descent and uterine, vaginal, bladder, or rectal prolapse.
- Palpation of the anorectal region also gives the examiner a great detail of information. Gently touching the anal verge will elicit the anocutaneous reflex (anal wink), which is indicative of an intact pudendal nerve.

Spreading of the anus will help elicit an anal fissure or ulceration. Palpation of the gluteal region can help identify an abscess, external opening of a fistulous tract, or possibly a mass.

Digital Rectal Examination

- Digital rectal examination (DRE) provides information regarding potential pathology of the anal canal, distal rectum, and adjacent organs, as well as an assessment of the neurological function of the muscles of fecal continence.

- There are relative contraindications to performing this portion of the exam such as painful lesions.
- The keys to a successful DRE can be summarized by simple rules: adequate lubrication, gentleness, and attention to detail.
- After proper communication with the patient, a well-lubricated index finger is placed across the anus to lubricate the general area. The fingertip is then gently inserted into the anal opening. If the patient's response is an involuntary spasm of the internal sphincter, the examiner should withdraw their fingertip and gently try again. Ask the patient to bear down as to pass a stool, which causes relaxation of the entire sphincter complex and should facilitate an easy digital insertion.
- The distal rectum and anal canal along with surrounding structures should be investigated in an organized and stepwise fashion. Resting anal tone followed by squeeze tone should be assessed. Assessment should be made of the entire circumference of the lumen by gently sweeping around the entire anus and distal rectum.
- Anteriorly in a male, the prostate should be palpated.
- In the female, anteriorly palpate for a rectocele.
- Posteriorly, the presence of a presacral (retrorectal) mass may be palpated.
- Redundant rectal mucosa may be palpated as well as a stricture or narrowing. Induration or a fibrous cord, representing an internal fistulous opening, may also be felt on DRE. The patient should be asked to perform a Valsalva maneuver to potentially bring any lesions of the upper rectum or the rectosigmoid into the examiners reach.
- If a mass is palpated, it's size, position, characteristics (sessile, polypoid, ulcerated), mobility (mobile, tethered, fixed), and relationship to other structures (distance from the anal verge, distance for the anorectal ring) must be accurately recorded.
- The levator ani/puborectalis muscles can also be assessed on DRE with evaluation of both the strength and function of these muscles, along with any tenderness on direct palpation. When a patient with good sphincter function is asked to squeeze these muscles, the examiner's finger will feel the muscle tighten.
- Additionally, when the examiner pulls posteriorly on these muscles, the anal opening should gape and then return to normal, representing an intact reflex pathway to the thoracolumbar spinal cord.
- Immediately prior to any of the endoscopic procedures described below, a DRE should be performed.

Anoscopy/Proctoscopy

- The anorectal examination may be followed with some component of an endoscopic investigation to complete the workup. This may include anoscopy, proctoscopy, or flexible endoscopy.
- It should be noted that the term proctoscopy will be used as to describe the rigid scope implemented to evaluate the rectum and the distal sigmoid colon. Therefore, "rigid proctosigmoidoscope" or "proctosigmoidoscopy" will be referred to as "rigid proctoscopy" or "proctoscopy." Sigmoidoscopy refers to the use of the flexible sigmoidoscope.

Anoscopy

- Anoscopy is the best way to adequately evaluate the anoderm, dentate line, internal and external hemorrhoids, papillae, fissures, anal masses, and distal rectal mucosa.
- The anoscope is a relatively simple instrument consisting of an obturator, the scope itself, and a light source (Fig. 4.3).
- The anoscope (with obturator in place) is liberally lubricated and gently and gradually advanced until the instrument is fully inserted along the anterior-posterior axis of the anus.
- After successful insertion, the obturator is removed and examination of the anorectum undertaken. The obturator should then be reinserted while the scope still in the anus, and the

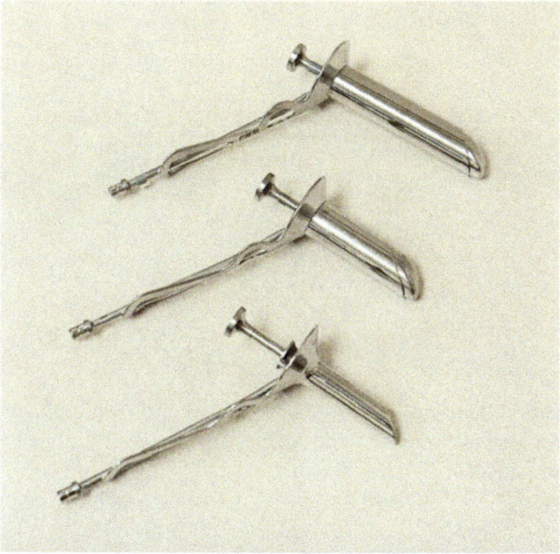

Fig. 4.3 Various beveled anoscopes. From top to bottom: large Hirschman (short bevel), Buie-Hirschman anoscope (long bevel), small (pediatric) Hirschman anoscope

anoscope is gently rotated to examine a new area.

- During the examination, the patient is asked to strain while the anoscope is withdrawn to visualize any prolapsing anorectal mucosa or hemorrhoidal tissue.
- During the anoscopic examination, hemorrhoids may be banded, or biopsies of any suspicious lesions may be obtained.
- Complications of anoscopy are rare but may include occasional bleeding from hemorrhoids or inadvertently tearing the anoderm.

Proctoscopy

- Rigid proctoscopy is suitable to examine the rectum, and in some patients, the distal sigmoid colon may also be evaluated. The patient should receive an enema preparation prior to the procedure.
- The proctoscope consists of an obturator, the scope itself, and a light source. A lens is attached to the external orifice of the scope after the obturator is removed. A bellows is attached to the scope allowing for insufflation of air to gain better visualization and negotiation of the scope proximally through the rectum. A suction device or cotton-tipped swabs can be used to remove any endoluminal debris or fluid or to enhance visualization (Fig. 4.4).
- Proctoscopes are 25 cm in length with three available luminal diameters (Fig. 4.5).
  - Disposable plastic and self-lighted proctoscopes are available.
- The procedure can be performed in either the prone jackknife or left lateral position as previously described. Pain may occur with stretching of the rectosigmoid mesentery due to over insufflation of air or the scope hitting the rectal wall.
- Proctoscopy use has declined but is still used in the identification and precise localization of rectal lesions or in the evaluation of rectal bleeding. Contraindications are

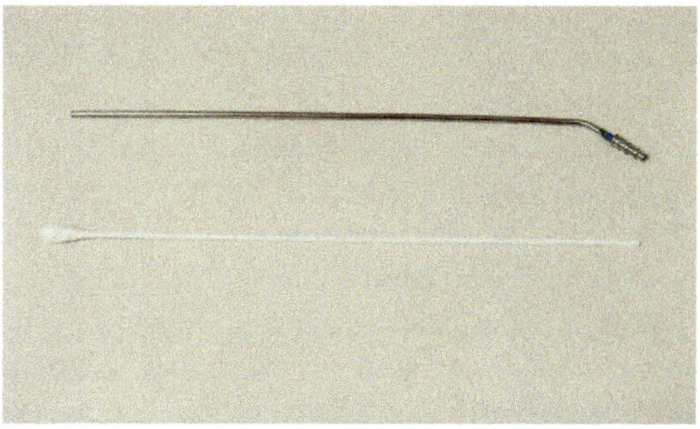

Fig. 4.4 Proctoscopy suction catheter and long cotton-tipped applicators for clearing small amounts of fecal debris. The cotton-tipped swabs are also used for manipulating the rectal and anal mucosa during anoscopy and proctoscopy

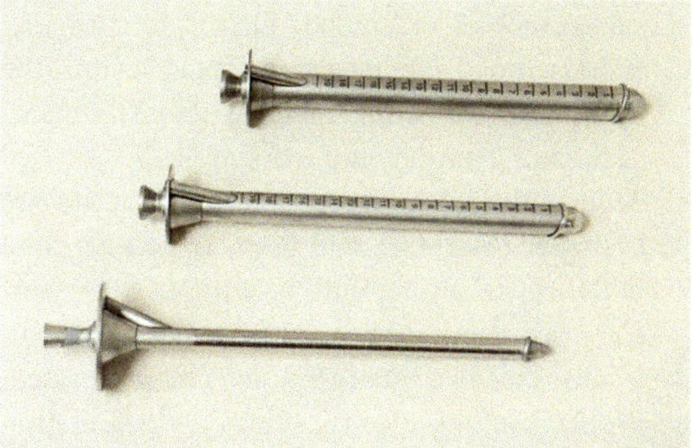

Fig. 4.5 Proctoscopes. From top to bottom: large proctoscope, length 25 cm, diameter 19 mm; standard proctoscope, length 25 cm, diameter 15 mm; pediatric proctoscope, length 25 cm, diameter 11 mm

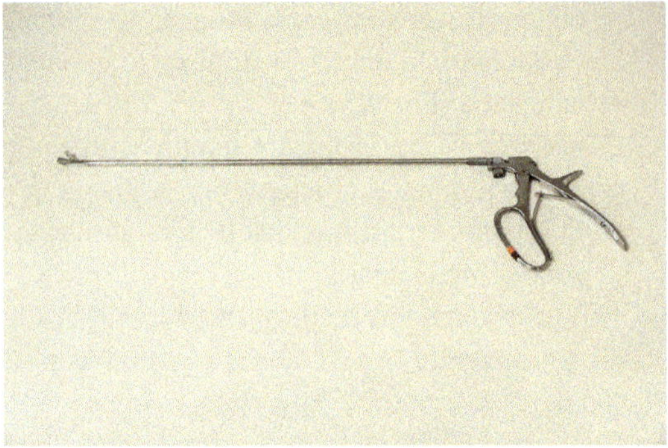

Fig. 4.6 Turrell-angulated biopsy forceps. A curved upper jaw allows for 360-degree rotation. A variety of jaw sizes and types are available

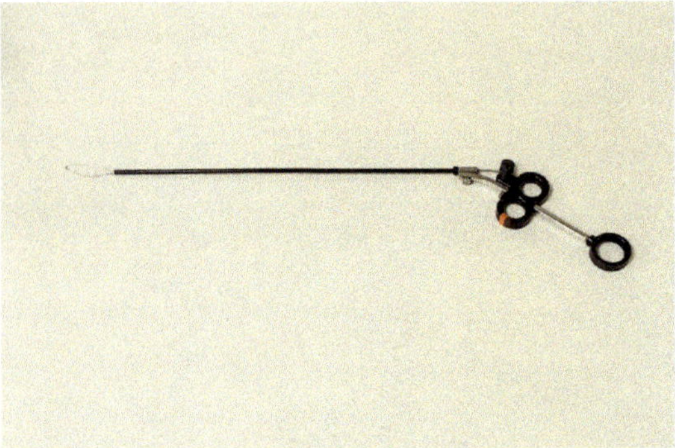

Fig. 4.7 Rigid-wire (Frankfelt) snare. This snare allows for polypectomy or tumor debulking via the anoscope or proctoscope

similar to anoscopy and include painful anorectal conditions.

- After adequate lubrication, while the obturator is held in place with the right thumb, the instrument is gently inserted into the anal canal and advanced approximately 4–5 cm in the general direction of the umbilicus. The scope is then aimed toward the sacrum and advanced for an additional 4–5 cm. The obturator is then removed, and the viewing lens is placed. Minimal air insufflation is used in order to open the bowel lumen, and gently withdrawing and advancing the scope to straighten out angulations proximally aid in achieving successful navigation.
- The proximal extent reached on proctoscopic examinations averages approximately 17–20 cm and very rarely can the scope be inserted to its full length.
- The proctoscope is withdrawn and the mucosal surface is examined. Description of any lesions found includes size of the lesion, the exact distance from the anal verge, appearance, and location on the bowel wall.
- Several different types of biopsy forceps are available (Fig. 4.6), and biopsies can be done in the office setting with or without the use of electrocautery. Additionally, polyps or small lesions can be snared (Fig. 4.7) or fulgurated. Proper suction, electrocautery, and irrigation devices should be readily available in the examining room for these purposes (Fig. 4.8).
- Serious complications during rigid proctoscopy are rare and include bleeding and perforation.

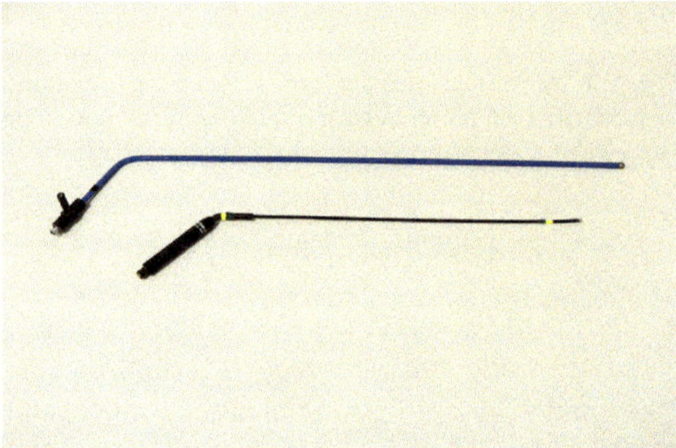

Fig. 4.8 Suction catheter/electrocoagulation catheter. From top to bottom: an insulated catheter for combining suction and electrocautery and an electrocoagulation catheter

Anal and Rectal Ultrasound

- Endoanal ultrasonography (EUS) is an imaging modality that provides information on the anatomy and function of pelvic floor structures, anorectal disease processes, and anorectal tumors.
- Advantages of EUS include the relatively inexpensive cost to perform and its widespread availability. A disadvantage of EUS is that it is an operator-dependent test.
- Circumferential assessment of the anal canal and distal rectum is made possible by a 360-degree rotating transducer that is either a 7 or 10 megahertz (MHz) probe for two-dimensional (2D) units or a 13 MHz probe for three-dimensional (3D) units (Fig. 4.9).

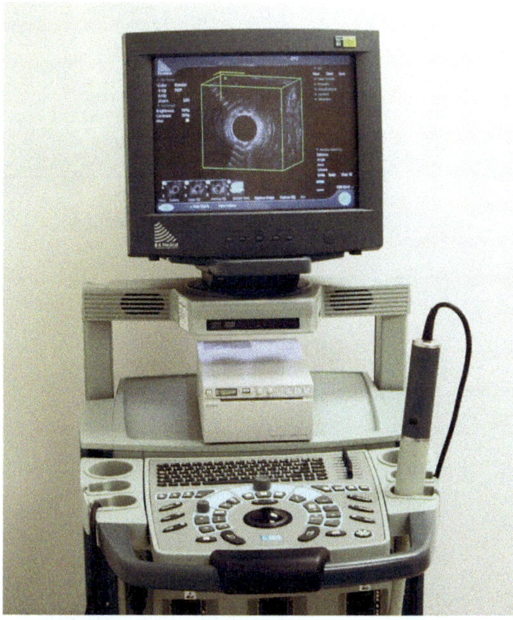

Fig. 4.9 B-K Medical (Herlev, Denmark) three-dimensional anorectal ultrasound equipment

- Patients receive an enema prior to testing which is most commonly performed with the patient in the left lateral recumbent position.
- The well-lubricated ultrasound probe is inserted and slowly advanced and then withdrawn to view the entire area of the anal canal/rectum (in modern systems, a crystal moves up and down along the transducer to acquire images while the probe is held stationarily).
- The anal canal is divided into three levels on EUS.
- The upper anal canal is defined by the U-shaped puborectalis muscle.
- The middle canal has both EAS and IAS muscles visible (this is also where the IAS is at maximum width).
- The lower anal canal has only the most distal external sphincter fibers (Figs. 4.10, 4.11, and 4.12).
- Highly reflective tissue on EUS reveals a hyperechoic (white) image, while poorly reflective tissues are hypoechoic (black).

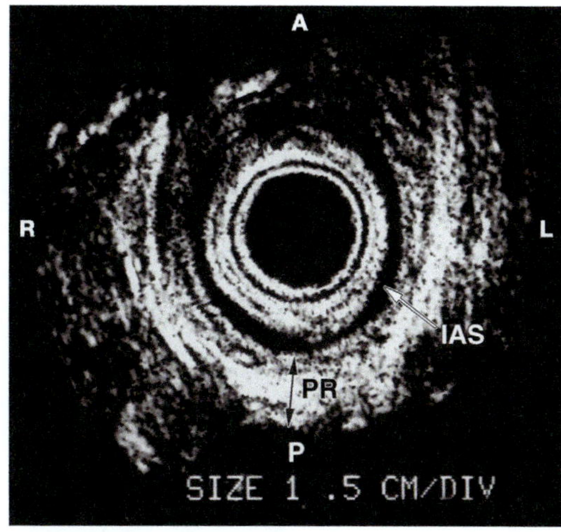

Fig. 4.10 Two-dimensional endoanal ultrasound view of the U-shaped puborectalis muscle (PR). *IAS* internal anal sphincter

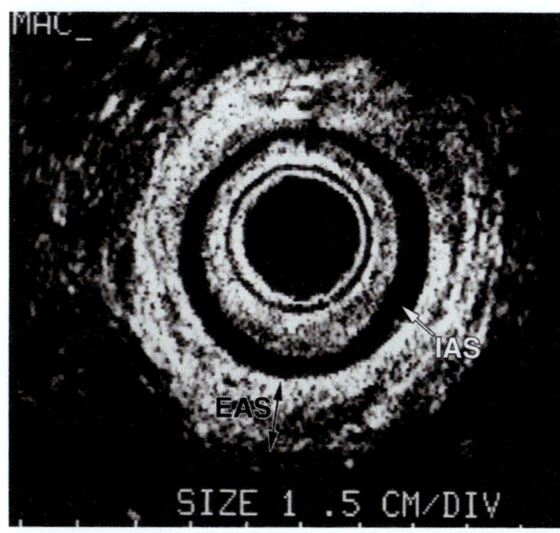

Fig. 4.11 Two-dimensional ultrasound from the mid-anal canal. This ultrasound image represents normal, intact internal anal sphincter (IAS) (hypoechoic) and external anal sphincter (EAS) (hyperechoic)

- The smooth muscle-based IAS, which has higher water content, shows up black on EUS. In post-obstetrical sphincter injuries, the defect is usually located anteriorly and encompasses the EAS and may involve the IAS as well (Fig. 4.13).
- The accuracy of EUS compared to surgical findings has been reported to be as high as 90%–100%.

Fig. 4.12 Three-dimensional coronal view of the upper, middle, and lower anal canal. *EAS* external anal sphincter, *IAS* internal anal sphincter

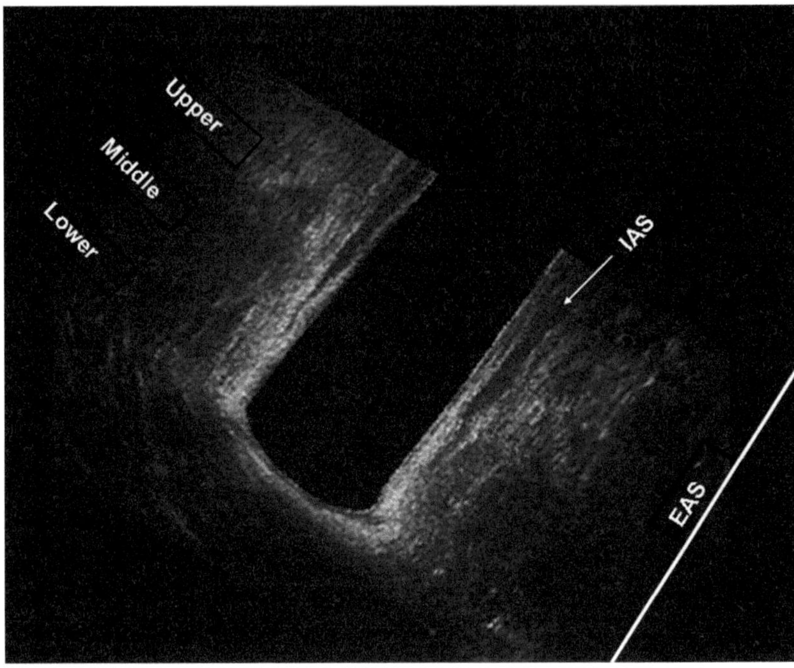

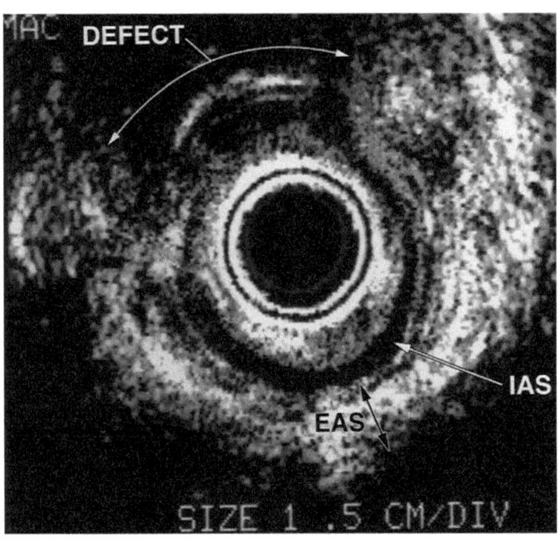

Fig. 4.13 Anteriorly located defect of both the EAS and IAS in the mid-anal canal

Flexible Endoscopy

Flexible Endoscopic Insertion Techniques

- The techniques described here are generalizations and guidelines to help navigate the flexible endoscope to its completion.

Torque

- The twisting motion applied to the shaft of the scope by the endoscopist's right hand is called torque (Fig. 4.14). Torque is an essential technique that allows for a stiffening of the scope and alters the direction in which the tip deflection controls the work.

Tip Deflection

- The tip of the endoscope should always be kept in the middle of the bowel lumen. The techniques of torque, pull/push, and dithering-jiggle will tend to move the tip in several directions. The endoscopist should bring the tip back by controlling both the outer and inner controls with their left hand. With practice, the endoscopist should be able to control and use both tip deflection control knobs in different directions with only the thumb of the left hand.

Dithering/Jiggle

- The rapid up-and-down, side-to-side, and to-and-fro movements of the shaft of the scope

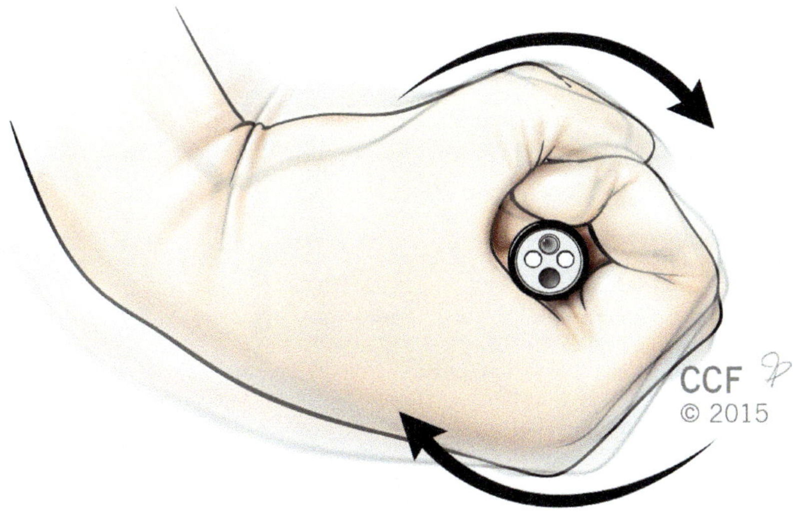

Fig. 4.14 Torque – a twisting motion of the endoscopist's right hand to the left (counterclockwise) or right (clockwise). (Reprinted with permission, Cleveland Clinic Center for Medical Art & Photography ©2015. All Rights Reserved)

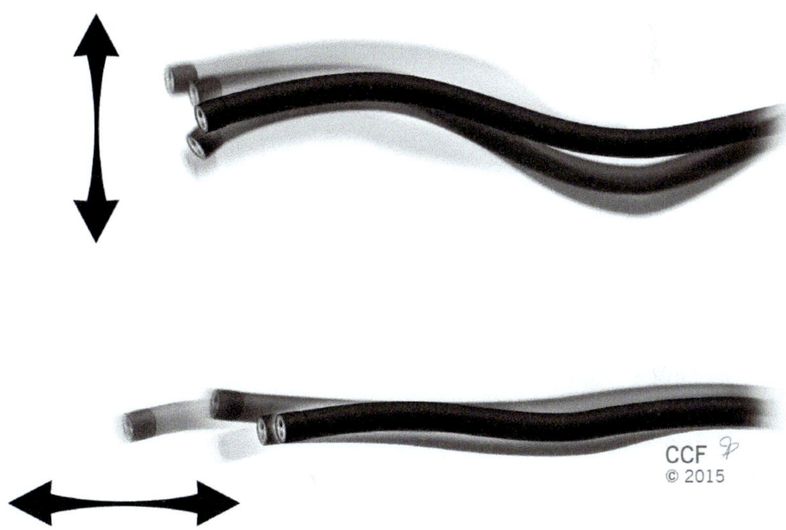

Fig. 4.15 Jiggle (dithering) – rapid side-to-side, up-and-down, and to-and-fro movements of the endoscope in order to pleat or "accordion" the colon onto the scope's shaft. (Reprinted with permission, Cleveland Clinic Center for Medical Art & Photography ©2015. All Rights Reserved)

are referred to as dithering or jiggle (Fig. 4.15). This technique can be combined with torqueing as well as in and out movements of the scope. The object of this important maneuver is to pleat the colon onto the shaft of the endoscope in order to shorten the colon and to keep the scope straight.

Aspiration of Air and Breath Holding

- As insufflation of air accumulates during the procedure, the colon becomes distended and elongates. The judicious and cautious use of air is important during the examination, but thoughtful and calculated aspiration/suction of air is an important adjunct insertion technique.
- Another technique to help the scope around the flexure is the "breath-hold" maneuver. While negotiating difficult turns and bends (especially the hepatic and splenic flexure), have the patient take a deep breath in and hold it. This causes the diaphragm to drop and pushes the flexures over the scope and thereby allows the scope to pass.

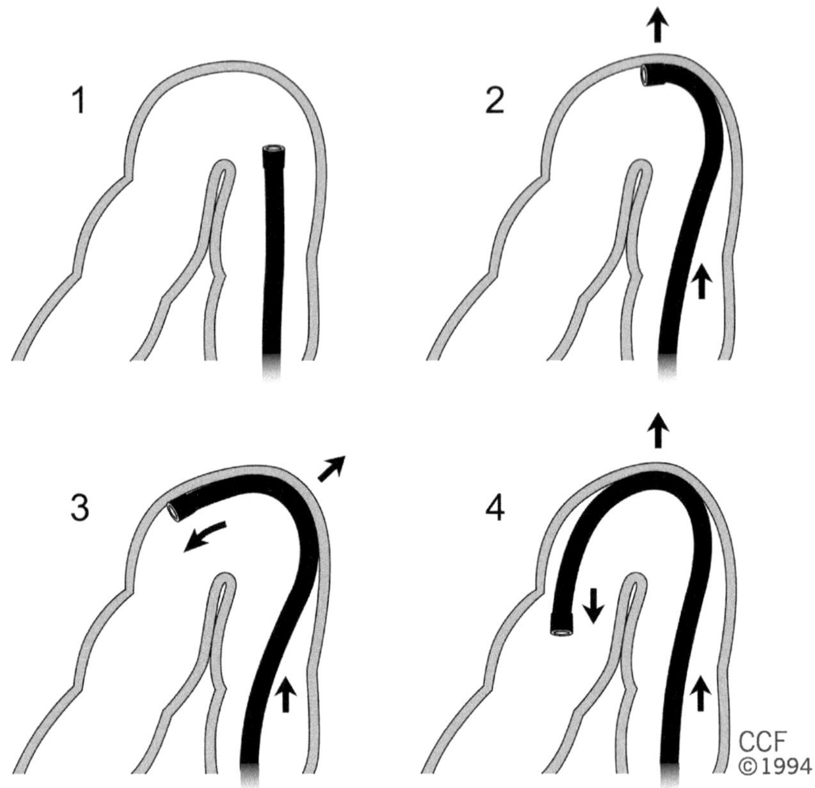

Fig. 4.16 Slide-by technique. The colonoscope is blindly pushed around a bend, guided by the curve of the scope and the curvature of the bowel wall. Slide-by should be terminated with excessive patient pain or blanching of the mucosa occurs. This technique should be avoided in diseased bowel or in the presence of diverticuli. (Reprinted with permission, Cleveland Clinic Center for Medical Art & Photography ©2015. All Rights Reserved)

Slide-By

- The technique of pushing blindly into a turn or bend with maximum tip deflection and without full visualization of the colon lumen to guide the scope along the curvature of the bowel wall to advance the scope past the turn is termed a slide-by technique. This controversial technique should never be used by unsupervised trainees or novice endoscopists due to the risk of perforation. It should be terminated if there is resistance to forward advancement or the mucosa becomes blanched at the tip of the scope (Fig. 4.16).

Adjunctive Maneuvers for More Difficult Examinations

- The adjunctive maneuvers employed with endoscopy often serve as the markers between seasoned experts and novices. There are several different maneuvers including abdominal pressure and other external manipulations provided by an assistant under the direct supervision of the endoscopist. In addition it is possible to adjust the position of the patient to either the supine or prone positions. There are also commercially produced overtubes, which are seldom required now with the advent of adjustable stiffness endoscopes. All of these adjunctive maneuvers are designed to reduce the loop formation of the endoscope or to prevent it from reforming once it has been reduced. In one study evaluating the use of ancillary techniques, directed abdominal pressure was used in 56% of colonoscopies, while turning to the left and right was performed in 17 and 23% of exams, respectively. (7) Like all techniques, however, they are best learned under the supervision of a seasoned endoscopist.
- The most likely cause of a difficult examination is the formation of a loop, which makes further advancement of the scope impossible,

painful, and potentially harmful. It should be remembered that when facing a difficult to negotiate area of the colon, a different technique must be employed to facilitate success. It is the authors' opinion that once a technique has failed twice, a new technique should be employed. The technique of withdrawing the scope all the way back to the rectosigmoid and starting the procedure over is a valuable maneuver and again should not be overlooked. It may be necessary during a difficult examination to "take a few steps backwards in order to move forward."

Patient Position

- The procedure starts with the patient on their left side, but transitioning to a supine position may ease the navigation of the sigmoid, sigmoid/descending, splenic flexure, and hepatic flexure.
- While the patient is being moved with the assistance of the endoscopy team, the endoscopist should keep their eye on the screen and attempt to maintain the scope in the middle of the lumen.
- Turning the patient to their right side is a technique that is especially useful when the examination has reached the ascending colon and it cannot be advanced into the cecum.

Abdominal Pressure

- The technique of splinting certain redundant areas of the colon with external pressure via the abdominal wall may help reduction in loop formation. Initial attempts at "blind pressure" should be from superior and right of the umbilicus directed toward the left lower quadrant in order to stabilize the sigmoid colon. However, pressure may need to be applied to different areas of the abdomen in order to successfully reduce the loop. Pressure should be applied gradually to avoid rapid changes in intra-abdominal pressure which may increase the risk of aspiration in deeply sedated patients.

Turning the Scope

- During the navigation of a very difficult or acute turn, it may help to change the entire angle of approach of the scope. This is accomplished by torqueing the shaft 180 degrees while keeping the tip of the scope stabilized in the middle with the help of the deflection knobs (Fig. 4.17).

Sigmoidoscopy

- The use of the flexible sigmoidoscopy (FS) in the office setting has increased due to its ease of use and high yield of findings over conventional rigid proctoscopy.

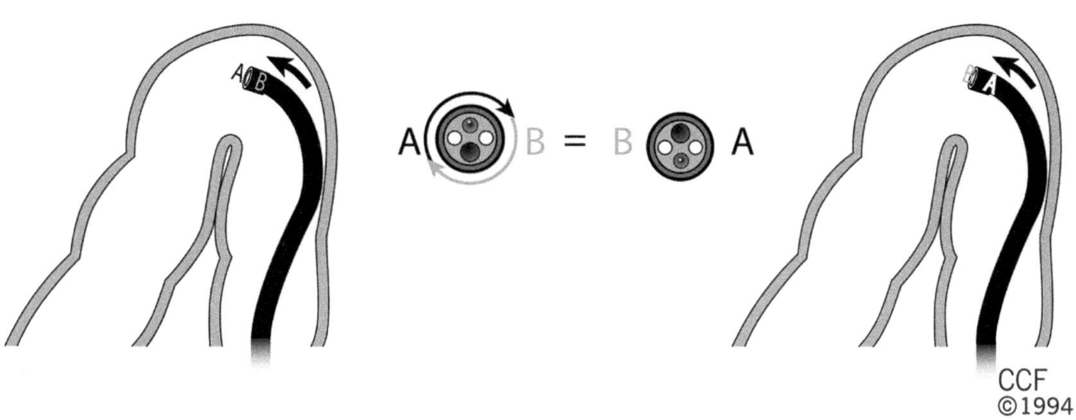

Fig. 4.17 Turning the scope. This maneuver allows the examiner to change the angle of approach to a turn. Scope torque of 180 degrees is accomplished, while the deflection controls keep the tip centered in the lumen. (Reprinted with permission, Cleveland Clinic Center for Medical Art & Photography ©2015. All Rights Reserved)

- While the scope can reach the splenic flexure, evaluation of the entire sigmoid colon is obtained in up to 85% of patients.
- The flexible sigmoidoscope offers a three- to sixfold increase in the yield of findings, especially neoplasms, in the rectum and sigmoid colon compared to rigid proctoscopy.
- The flexible sigmoidoscope is available from various companies, but in general the channel size ranges between 2.6 and 3.8 mm, the diameter of the scope ranges between 12 and 14 mm, and the length varies from 60 to 71 cm (Fig. 4.18).
- The indications for FS in the office setting are broad but include bright-red rectal bleeding, diarrhea, surveillance of rectal neoplasia, and postoperative anastomosis evaluation.
- Patients are typically given one to two enemas prior to the procedure. The position that offers the easiest approach is the left lateral recumbent, but the prone jackknife position can also be used. Sedation is not typically necessary in the vast majority of patients.
- The well-lubricated scope is inserted "side first" rather than "end on" which allows for the edge of the endoscope to act as a leading point and avoids pushing the blunt end "en face" against the anal sphincter with subsequent trauma and pain (Fig. 4.19). After

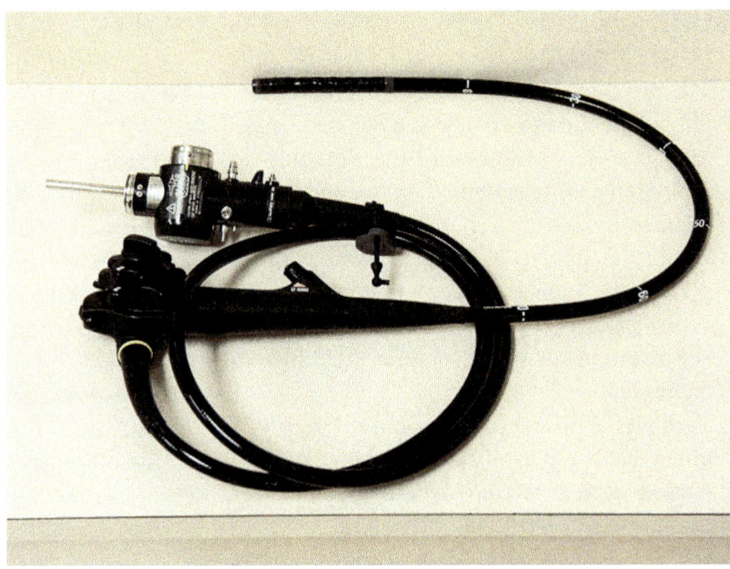

Fig. 4.18 Flexible sigmoidoscope

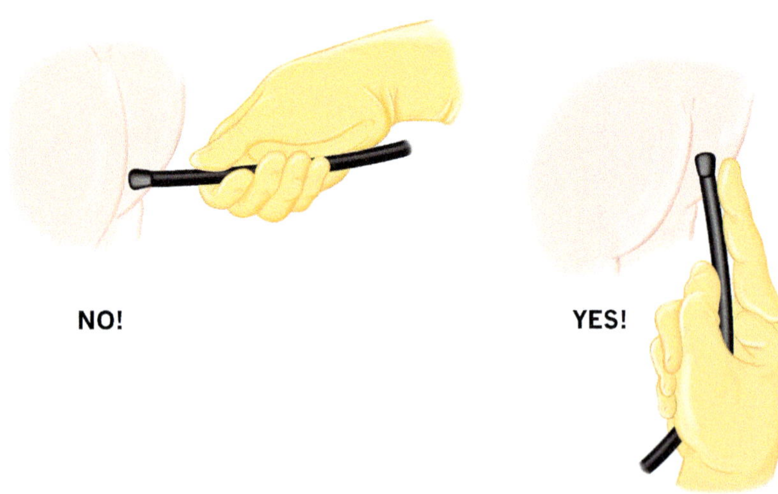

Fig. 4.19 The flexible endoscope should be inserted "side first" for less painful passage through the anal canal. (Reprinted with permission, Cleveland Clinic Center for Medical Art & Photography ©2015. All Rights Reserved)

proper insertion of the scope, gentle air insufflation is achieved, and the scope is advanced under direct visualization to approximately 10–12 centimeters. The instrument is then passed into the sigmoid colon by a combination of the abovementioned techniques.

- The mucosal surface is examined on withdrawal of the scope, and lesions can be biopsied. Larger polyp removal may be best suited during a subsequent colonoscopy when a full-bowel preparation has been achieved.
- Complications of FS are uncommon and include abdominal pain and perforation. Electrocoagulation should be avoided or used very judiciously in biopsies or snare techniques unless the patient has received a full mechanical bowel preparation to reduce the risk of explosion due to the presence of hydrogen and methane gas within the bowel lumen.

Colonoscopy

- A thorough colonoscopy allows the physician to completely evaluate the mucosa of the terminal ileum, colon, and rectum and obtain biopsies or photo-documentation of any abnormalities identified.
- Over 90% of colon and rectal surgeons reported performing colonoscopies as part of their regular practice.

Indications and Contraindications

- The specific indications for performing a colonoscopy are multiple. And there is debate regarding the appropriateness of performing the procedure in varying clinical scenarios.
- The European Panel on the Appropriateness of Gastrointestinal Endoscopy was revised to serve as a guide for referring physicians to determine if colonoscopy is appropriate to a given clinical situation and is available online at http://www.epage.ch/.
- There are numerous publications demonstrating that a significant number (13-30%) of colonoscopies are inappropriate when compared to indications by national guidelines.
- The only absolute contraindication for performing a colonoscopy is in a patient who requires immediate operative intervention. All other contraindications are relative and are at the discretion of the endoscopist.
- Patients with active colitis or those with a recent intestinal anastomosis are at a higher risk for complications, but a careful endoscopic examination can be safely conducted in these patients.

Bowel Preparation

- The bowel prep is of critical importance in order to be able to adequately examine the entire colon, with inadequate cleaning reported in up to 27% of patients.
- Although a great deal of research has gone into making it more effective and the process more palatable for the patient, the optimal regimen has yet to be determined.
- The choice of bowel prep is somewhat practice-dependent, but more practitioners use PEG-based preparations in their practices than the osmotic agents.
- Osmotic agents (sodium phosphate and magnesium citrate) increase the passage of extracellular fluid across the bowel wall.
- Following the FDA alert regarding renal damage associated with oral sodium phosphate, its use declined precipitously in the United States. The potential side effects associated with its use include nephropathy and renal insufficiency resulting from the tubular deposition of phosphate.
- Stimulants such as senna and bisacodyl increase bowel wall smooth muscle activity and are primarily used as adjuncts.
- Evidence to suggests that regardless which agent is chosen, splitting the timing into the half-day prior to and half-day of the procedure results in an overall better cleansing.
- At least one meta-analysis demonstrates that a 4 L split-dose PEG is superior to other preparation strategies.
- It is also critical that the instructions that are given to the patient are understood.

- Reporting of the quality of the bowel prep is both an important part of documentation of the procedure and a standard of quality.
- An adequate bowel preparation should be achieved and documented in greater than 85% of procedures.
- There are numerous scales for grading the adequacy of the bowel prep, all of which are subjective.
- The Aronchick scale grades the overall quality on a scale of 5 (excellent) to 0 (inadequate).
- The Ottawa (31), Boston (32), and Chicago (33) scales grade the preparation quality in different anatomic areas of the colon adding them together to form a total score.
- The easiest and therefore the most commonly employed is the 4-point scale of excellent, good, fair, and poor.

Special Considerations

The Difficult-to-Prep Patient

- It is recommend that patients undergo early repeat colonoscopy when the bowel preparation quality is deemed inadequate, defined as the inability to detect polyps smaller than 5 mm.
- There are no prospective studies dealing with this patient population, and the practices are individualized. Strategies include increasing the amount of liquid diet by 1 day, adding an osmotic or cathartic agent, and prescribing antiemetics or anxiolytics.
- In hospitalized patients, it has also been demonstrated that the prep can be administered via a gastroscope the day prior to colonoscopy.

The Patient Requiring Antibiotics

- Antibiotic prophylaxis against infective endocarditis is not routinely recommended for colonoscopy.
- The ASGE guidelines were published in 2003 and revised in 2008 (Table 4.1).
- Even high-risk patients are not required to have antimicrobial prophylaxis prior to endoscopic procedures, but a discussion with the patient's cardiologist or infectious disease specialist may be warranted.

Table 4.1 Antibiotic prophylaxis for elective colonoscopy +/− biopsy

Conditions	Patient risk	Antibiotics
Prosthetic heart valves	High-risk patients	Prophylaxis is optional
History of endocarditis		
Systemic-pulmonary shunt		
Complex cyanotic congenital heart disease		
Cardiac transplant with valvulopathy		
Other congenital cardiac abnormalities	Moderate-risk patients	Prophylaxis is not recommended
Mitral valve prolapse with regurgitation		
Rheumatic heart disease		
Hypertrophic cardiomyopathy		
CABG	Low-risk patients	Prophylaxis is not recommended
Defibrillators		
Pacemakers		
Repaired septal defect or PDA		
Physiologic heart murmurs		
Mitral valve prolapse without regurgitation		
Prosthetic joints <6 mo	Patients to consider prophylaxis	Consider prophylaxis
Peritoneal dialysis		
Vascular grafts	Insufficient data	Consider prophylaxis

The Anticoagulated Patient

- The anticoagulated patient poses a dilemma for the endoscopist. A diagnostic colonoscopy poses little bleeding risk; however the possibility of biopsies or polypectomy must be considered.
- The endoscopist must weigh the risk of possible thrombotic events if any medication is withdrawn against those of bleeding. This must often be done prior to the procedure, when knowledge of any pathology or whether any biopsy or polypectomy does not exist.
- According to the 2005 ASGE guidelines, a diagnostic colonoscopy and a colonoscopy with biopsy are considered low-risk procedures for causing hemorrhage. A polypectomy however is considered to be a high-risk procedure, and any anticoagulant medications should be adjusted according to the medication that is being taken (Table 4.2).
- Assessment of the thrombotic risk may require coordination with the physician monitoring the anticoagulant.
- The incidence of post-polypectomy hemorrhage peaks at 4–6 days, and this risk extends to at least 14 days. In general, the morbidity of a thromboembolic event is greater than that of hemorrhage; therefore, resuming anticoagulation as soon as possible and treating hemorrhagic complications as they occur seem to be the most prudent management strategy.

Table 4.2 Management of anticoagulation medications for elective lower GI endoscopy

↑ Risk procedures			↓ Risk procedures
Polypectomy >1 cm			Diagnostic endoscopy
Endoscopic dilatation			Flexible sigmoidoscopy/ colonoscopy +/– biopsy
			Stent placement without dilation
Medications			
Medication	Risk	Medication instructions	Medication restart
Warfarin		Hold 3–5 days prior	
A-fib		Hold warfarin and start UFH or LMWH when INR < _2.0	
A-fib with history of embolic event		Hold warfarin and start UFH or LMWH when INR < _2.0	
Mechanical valvular heart disease			
Low-molecular-weight heparin (LMWH)	↓	No medication adjustment necessary	
	↑	D/C 8 hr. prior to procedure	Re-starting medication individualized
Bridging LMWH: To replace heparin window		Consider 1 mg/kg q 12 hour	D/C as above
D/C warfarin 3–5 days prior to procedure			
Thienopyridines Clopidogrel/ ticlopidine	↓	No change necessary	
	↑	D/C 7–10 days prior to procedure, consider continuing aspirin if on dual therapy	Re-starting individualized
Dipridamole	↓	If no pre-existing bleeding disorder, no change necessary	
	↑	Unknown	
GIIb/IIIa inhibitor		Medication not usually used in patients undergoing elective procedures. Consult with prescribing physician or cardiology	

Incomplete Colonoscopy

- A complete colonoscopy examination to the cecum should be achieved in >95% for screening cases and is considered a major benchmark of quality. The slight decrease in colorectal cancer incidence over the past several decades is attributed in part to early detection and removal of colorectal polyps with greater benefit for left-sided lesions vs right-sided lesions.
- Rates of incomplete colonoscopy range from 5% to 25%.
- Patients who had an incomplete colonoscopy due to an unsatisfactory prep should undergo additional and/or alternative bowel preparation and a repeat colonoscopy.
- In patients in whom the procedure was terminated secondary to tortuosity or pain, a repeat colonoscopy under alternate analgesia or a repeat colonoscopy with a more experienced endoscopist may be appropriate.
- Alternatively, CT colonoscopy (virtual colonoscopy) may also be performed. It should be noted that any lesion >6 millimeters found on CT colonoscopy will require a standard colonoscopy as follow-up.
- Double-contrast barium enema can be considered; however a recent large population-based study showed a cancer miss rate of 22%, which makes this a very poor second test to either standard or CT colonoscopy.
- In patients in whom the colonoscopy was incomplete secondary to stricture or an obstructing lesion, options include on-table colonoscopy at the time of resection, preoperative CT colonoscopy, or postoperative colonoscopy.

Procedure

The Endoscopy Suite

- The endoscopy suite should provide an adequate amount of space for the necessary equipment personnel.
- It is imperative to have a designated person, whose primary responsibility is to monitor the patient throughout the procedure.
- Most colonoscopies in the United States are performed with sedation, and there is a consensus statement that patients who are having their procedure performed under moderate or deep sedation "must have continuous monitoring before, during, and after the administration of sedatives."
- Standard monitoring of sedated patients undergoing GI endoscopic procedures includes recording the heart rate, blood pressure, respiratory rate, and oxygen saturation but does not replace a well-trained and vigilant assistant.

Instruments

- Colonoscopes vary from 130 to 168 cm in length and in diameter from 11.3 mm (pediatric) to 12.8 mm.
- The basic colonoscope consists of variable stiffness controls in addition to a suction channel, an air/water channel, and fiber-optic bundles for light transmission, along with a biopsy port, which is connected into the suction channel (Fig. 4.20a, b).

Sedation

- While there is literature demonstrating that colonoscopy can be performed adequately and safely on the un-sedated patient, the practice in the United States is rare. The most common sedation regimen is a combination of midazolam and fentanyl, but several alternatives have been evaluated.

Nitrous Oxide

- Some studies show that nitrous oxide is not an effective substitution for intravenous sedation and analgesics.
- In a review of seven randomized trials using nitrous oxide for colonoscopy, four showed that nitrous oxide is as good at controlling pain as conventional methods, while another showed that sedation was actually improved. It is not widely used in clinical practice.

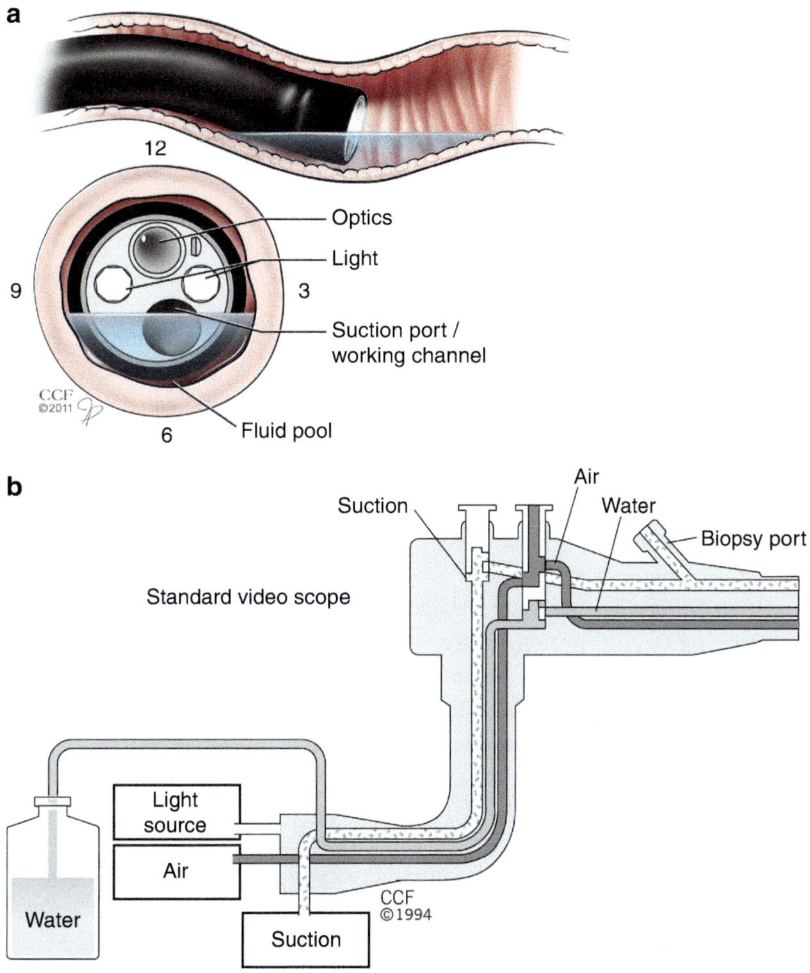

Fig. 4.20 (**a**) End-on view of the endoscopic tip, showing suction/biopsy channel, air/water channel, lens, and light source. (**b**) Basic endoscope design. (Reprinted with permission, Cleveland Clinic Center for Medical Art & Photography ©2015. All Rights Reserved)

Ketamine

- In one study, the addition of low-dose ketamine to a standard sedation regimen resulted in more rapid and better quality of sedation with stable hemodynamic status and similar recovery times.

Propofol

- Propofol use for colonoscopy has increased recently.
- Cochrane review demonstrated that, compared to standard sedation, propofol results in shorter time to recovery and discharge and greater patient satisfaction.
- An anesthesia provider is typically required to administer the agent (thereby increasing the cost associated with the procedure) though the medication can be delivered in a patient-controlled setting or by a nurse under the supervision of the endoscopist.

Colonoscopy Technique

- The act of negotiating a 5 to 6 foot flexible tube through a tortuous colon painlessly and efficiently while performing detailed surveillance and therapeutic maneuvers is a difficult task. This section will describe successful navigation to the full extent of the colonoscopy relying on the principles mentioned prior.

Anal Intubation

- The well-lubricated colonoscope is inserted as previously described for sigmoidoscopy.
- The examiner must make sure that the scope is brought over to the patient straight without any twists or loops from the endoscopy tower.

The Rectum and Rectosigmoid

- Once the endoscope is placed into the anus, it is advanced into the rectum while insufflating. Negotiating through the rectum is usually not difficult (Fig. 4.21).
- The rectosigmoid can pose extreme difficulty and is often one of the more challenging areas of the colonoscopy.
- If the patient has undergone prior pelvic surgery, especially hysterectomy, the sigmoid may become fixed and adherent which makes negotiation of the turn difficult, and a combination of all the basic maneuvers discussed should be employed.
- This portion of the exam requires adequate patient sedation and relaxation, and multiple small advancing steps toward getting the tip of the scope past the angle with tip deflection and torque are needed. Slide-by maneuvers should not be routinely performed. Tip deflection and some torque will help reduce any loops.

Sigmoid Colon

- The sigmoid colon is the most tortuous segment of the colon with associated high muscular tone, spasm, and a higher incidence of diverticulosis (Fig. 4.22). The sigmoid colon is not fixed and can be very redundant and elongated resulting in significant looping. Use of insertion-pull back, jiggle, and a variable amount of torque (usually clockwise), allows the sigmoid to "accordion" over the scope producing efficient advancement and preventing subsequent loop formation.
- Diverticula, when present, can be of various sizes, and the larger ones can be dangerous as they can be mistaken for the true bowel lumen.

Sigmoid-Descending Junction

- The junction of the sigmoid and descending colon can be difficult if a sigmoid loop is present. Short advances using the previously

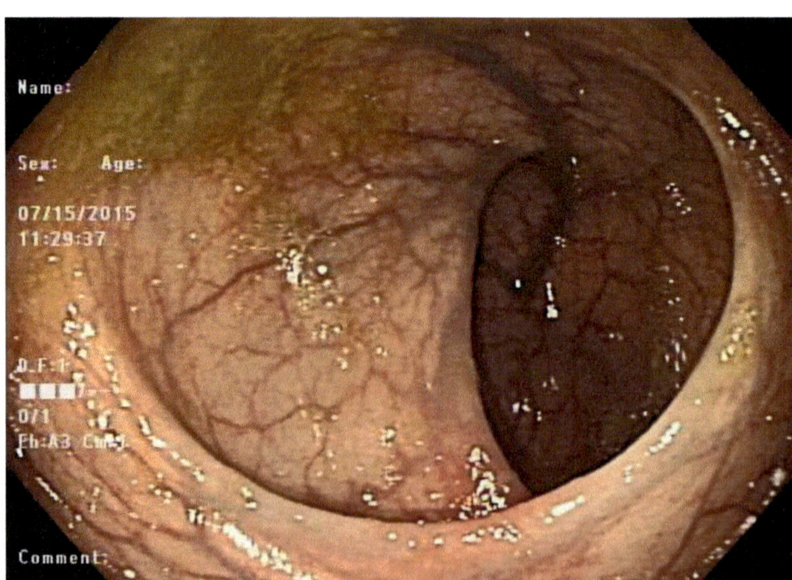

Fig. 4.21 The first and second rectal valves of Houston. Note the large submucosal venous plexus

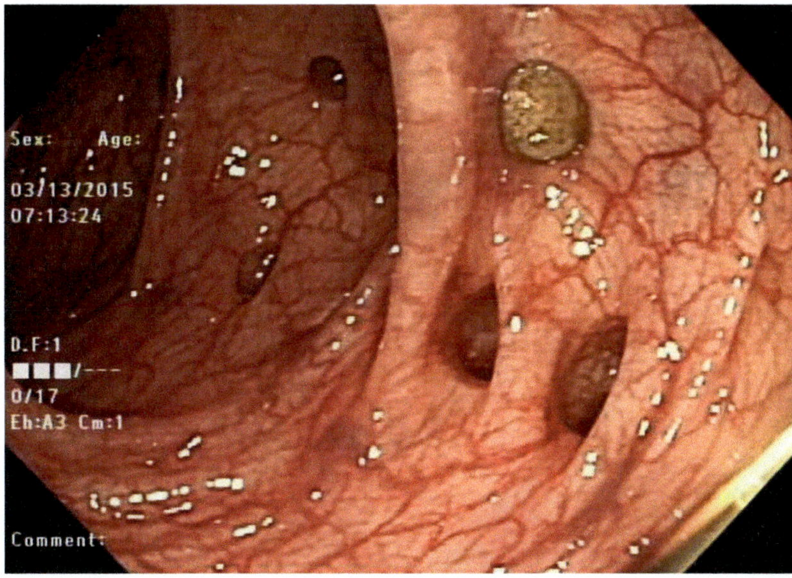

Fig. 4.22 The sigmoid colon has variable degrees of tortuosity, spasm, diverticular disease, and muscular tone

described techniques, abdominal pressure, or changes in patient position assist in attempts to advance into the descending colon.

Descending Colon

- The descending colon is usually straighter and less muscular than the sigmoid colon. It should be noted that even though this segment of the colon is easier to advance, jiggle, torque, air suction, and push and pullback techniques should still be employed to pleat the colon over the scope.

Splenic Flexure

- The splenic flexure is identified by the strong cardiac pulsations often seen and occasionally the blue shadow from the spleen itself. The splenic flexure may be a series of turns and twists in multiple planes that should be treated as already described using tip deflection, torque, and push and pull techniques.

Transverse Colon

- The transverse colon is characterized by the triangular appearance formed by the taenia coli (Fig. 4.23). If no proximal loop has been formed, the scope will advance readily through this segment. Loop reduction is performed as previously described.

Hepatic Flexure

The hepatic flexure is often recognized by the large blue shadow from the liver (especially in thin patients) (Fig. 4.24).

If the flexure turn is very acute, the novice endoscopist often mistakes this "fools cecum" for the true one, believing that they are at the end of the colon. Often, one can gently push through a loop and get into the ascending colon and then reduce the loop.

Ascending Colon and Ileocecal Valve

- As the scope advances past the hepatic flexure into the ascending colon, prevention of a new loop is critical, as any proximal loop at this point will make further advancement of the scope extremely difficult.
- Pushing through a loop in the ascending colon is not as successful as it is on the left side of the colon since there are many bowel loops to accommodate before push pressure is transmitted to the end of the scope.
- It can be very common to have the entire length of the scope inserted, and there is still

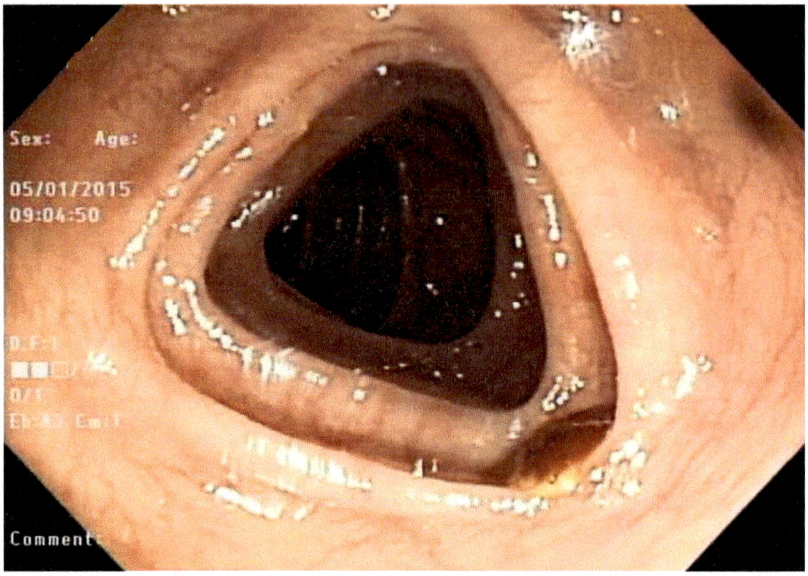

Fig. 4.23 Transverse colon: note the common triangular appearance of the lumen

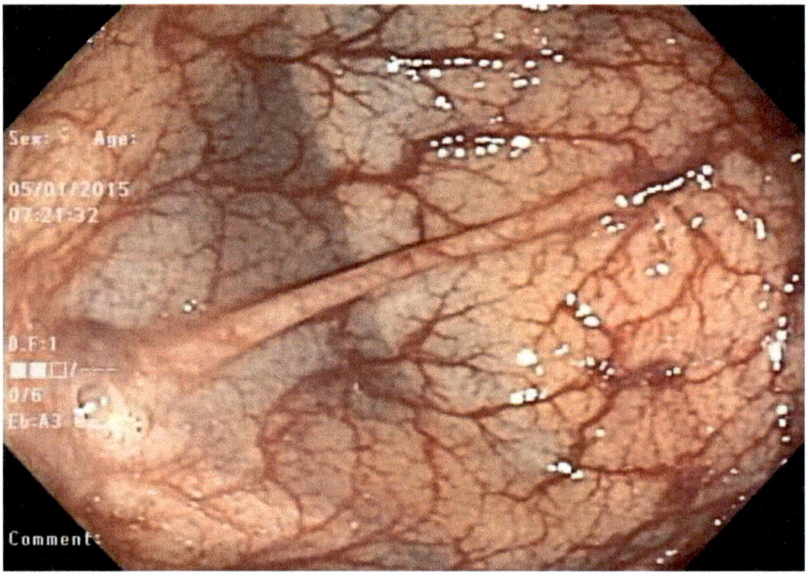

Fig. 4.24 Hepatic flexure: note the blue shadow from the liver. There is usually a sharp turn which can be quite difficult to negotiate

additional colon to traverse, due to inappropriate or minimal pleating techniques and the presence of loops.

- A change in patient position to either supine, right lateral, or prone coupled with the basic insertion techniques will prove to be extremely important in these situations and help advance the scope to the cecum.
- The ileocecal valve is a fold at the base of the ascending colon that may appear as an obvious polypoid-like yellowish mass or can be totally hidden (Fig. 4.25a, b).

Cecum

- The complete colonoscopic examination is ensured when the cecum has been reached. This blind sac is characterized by the "crow's foot" which is made up of the muscular arrangement of the colonic wall and the crescent or circular-shaped appendicle orifice (Fig. 4.26a, b). These landmarks are extremely important in quality assurance of a complete examination, and photo-documentation is mandatory.

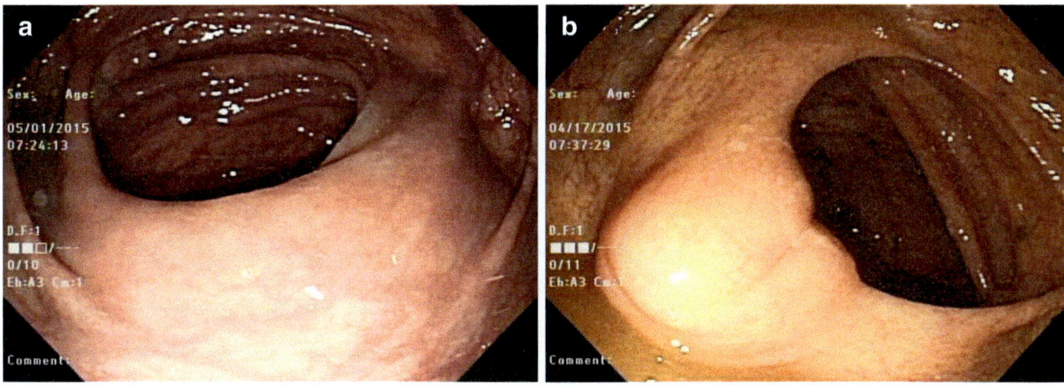

Fig. 4.25 Different appearances of the ileocecal valve: (**a**) Flat and invisible. (**b**) Polypoid and obvious

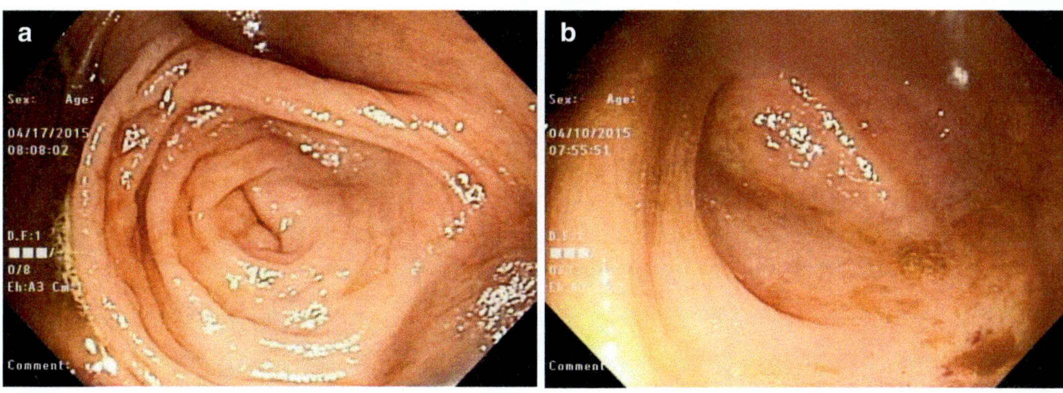

Fig. 4.26 Reaching and proper identification of the cecum is compulsory for a complete examination. (**a**) Round appendiceal orifice with associated crow's foot. (**b**) Crescent-shaped appendiceal orifice

- Careful and detailed examination of the entire cecum is important due to the fact that many cecal lesions, including serrated adenomas, are flat or recessed and can be quite deceptive and easily missed with a casual examination.

Ileocecal Valve Intubation

- It is common for some endoscopists to routinely advance the endoscope into the terminal ileum, and it is considered a critical assessment when performing either an initial evaluation or follow-up for Crohn's disease or in a search for lower gastrointestinal bleeding.
- The technique involves first removing any loops from the colonoscope. The edge of the ileocecal valve is hooked with the curved endoscope, and the scope is then gently inserted into the ileum when the lumen is visualized (Fig. 4.27).
- The addition of routine ileoscopy to screening colonoscopy has been demonstrated to detect asymptomatic small bowel carcinoid tumors and has led some to argue that this should be considered part of the endoscopic examination.
- However in a study at the Mayo Clinic, terminal ileum intubation showed gross abnormalities in only 1% of the patients, and pathologic abnormalities were identified for only 0.3% of the patients. These authors concluded that intubation of the terminal ileum should not be a required part of screening colonoscopy.

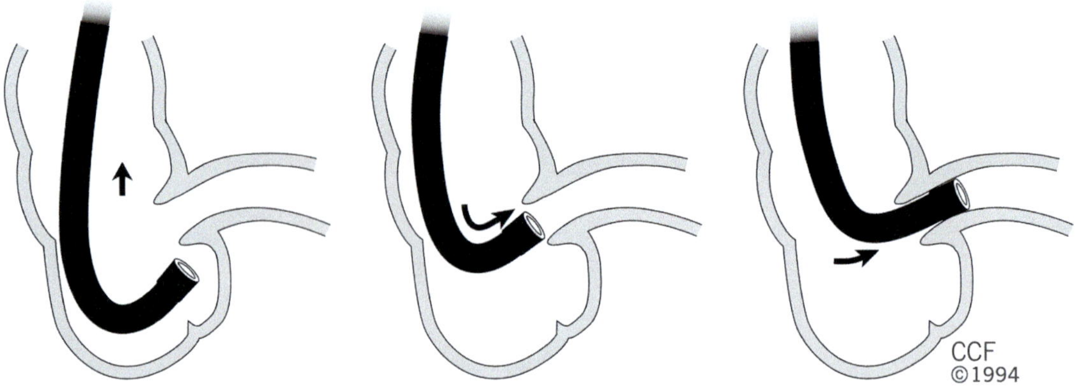

Fig. 4.27 Intubation of the ileocecal valve: identification of the orifice, impacting the scope while giving air insufflation and then waiting for the bowel to relax before advancement into the terminal ileum. (Reprinted with permission, Cleveland Clinic Center for Medical Art & Photography ©2015. All Rights Reserved)

Terminal Ileum

- If the endoscopist chooses to intubate the ileum, it is easily recognizable by noting its granular appearance (Fig. 4.28). Quite often in younger patients, there will be innumerable lymphoid follicles that may resemble small polyps.

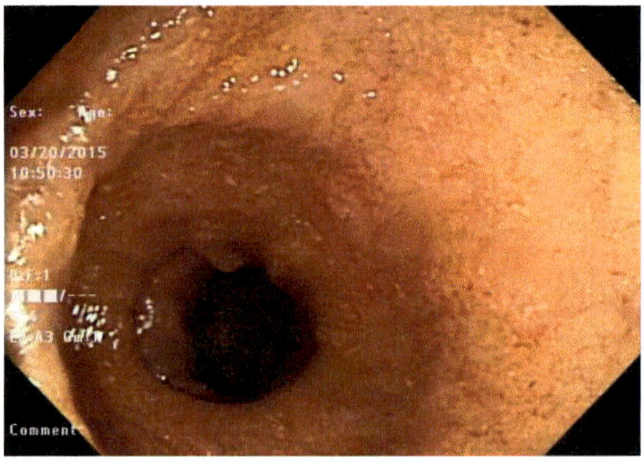

Fig. 4.28 Terminal ileum: note the granular mucosa and the fine muscular folds

Alternate Techniques

CO2 Insufflation

- Two alternatives to traditional air infusion colonoscopy are water-assisted colonoscopy and insufflation with carbon dioxide.
- CO2 is more rapidly diffused than air, and therefore it is expected that there will be less pain. Some evaluations have been consistent with this hypothesis, while others have not shared these findings.

Water Insufflation

- It has been demonstrated in limited studies that the use of water-assisted colonoscopy has a positive effect on patients, predominantly with lower levels of pain during the procedure. In a meta-analysis of nine studies, warm water infusion was demonstrated to be less painful than standard air insufflation while reducing the need for sedation or analgesia during the procedure.

Chromocolonoscopy (Chromoendoscopy)

- Chromocolonoscopy involves the use of dye with spray catheters to spray coat the colonic mucosa in an attempt to improve the visualization abnormalities of the mucosa. There has been some demonstrated benefit with this technology in high-risk populations such as those with inflammatory bowel disease or those with known genetic disorders.

High-Definition/NBI Endoscopy

- High-definition endoscopes with wider-angle viewing capability have the ability to increase the magnification and the visualization in endoscopy but have not proven superior in the ability to detect additional colon neoplasms.

- Narrow-band imaging (NBI) uses a filter to narrow the blue and green wave light and eliminates the red wavelength from standard white light which leads to an accentuation of the microvasculature and improved visualization of pathology. In some studies, NBI has resulted in an increase in the number of adenomatous polyps detected and assists in better prediction of histology. This may play a role in the future resection and discarding of diminutive polyps.

Full-Spectrum Endoscopy

- Full-spectrum endoscopy uses three cameras, with the two additional cameras located adjacent to the scopes tip. The endoscopist has simultaneous viewing images from all three cameras. To date there is no proven benefit regarding increased adenoma detection.

Retroflexion

- Many endoscopists routinely perform retroflexion in the rectum.
- There is sparse data on either the benefits or the risks associated with the routine use of retroflexion of the endoscope in the rectum. In one study of over 450 patients, retroflexion resulted finding pathology in only 9 additional cases – predominantly hyperplastic polyps.
- In another study of over 1500 patients, only 7 polyps were visualized solely by retroflexion. Six of these were hyperplastic, and one was a 4 mm sessile tubular adenoma. A higher rectal perforation rate has been reported with the technique.
- One study evaluating routine retroflexion in the right colon showed that it could be safely achieved in the majority of patients undergoing screening colonoscopy.
- Retroflexion identified additional polyps, predominantly adenomas, increasing the polyp yield as well as the adenoma detection rate in one study. Due to the concerns regarding missed lesions in the right colon, retroflexion in patients with polyps identified on initial forward viewing should be considered.

Complications

- Possible complications should be discussed with the patient frankly and documented prior to the procedure.
- The complications can be broadly grouped into those relating directly form the procedure such as bleeding and perforation and those relating to the sedation involved with the procedure – primarily cardiac and pulmonary complications.
- The exact incidence of all complications varies widely in the literature, from 4.0 for 10,000 colonoscopies to 17.8 per 1000 procedures. The incidence of serious complications (hospital admission within 30 days of the procedure) occurs with a rate of 1 per 1000 to 5.0 per 1000 exams.

Sedation Complications

- The primary concerns regarding the administration of sedation revolve around the cardiac and pulmonary complications associated with these medicines.

Vasovagal/Cardiac Arrhythmia

- A vasovagal reaction is a slowing of the heart rate, often accompanied by a drop in blood pressure, and is believed to reflect the stimulation of the vagus nerve. It occurs in up to 16% of colonoscopies and likely results from the distension of the bowel.
- These episodes are typically self-limited but should be addressed by colonoscopic aspiration of air and/or reduction of loops.
- True cardiac arrhythmias are uncommon in association with colonoscopy occurring in approximately 2% of patients undergoing endoscopic procedures.
- The administration of sedative medications, particularly midazolam, causes transient hypotension in 20% of patients, with ST-segment depression in 7%.
- When comparing patients not having a colonoscopy, the incidence of myocardial infarction

or stroke is similar to patients undergoing colonoscopy.
- Colonoscopy in patients with a recent myocardial infarction is associated with a higher rate of minor, transient, and primarily cardiovascular complications compared with control patients but is infrequently associated with major complications.

Pulmonary

- The incidence of pulmonary complications is even less common than for cardiac events. Patients over 80 have higher rates of pulmonary complications.
- There are reports of aspiration following the administration of sedative medications for colonoscopy which is more common with deeper sedation.
- Pneumothorax or pneumomediastinum following a colonoscopy should prompt investigation for an intra-abdominal perforation.

Procedural Complications

Splenic Injury

- The incidence of splenic injury in association with a colonoscopy is uncommon.
- A comprehensive literature search identified just over 100 patients worldwide with this complication.
- It is believed that the etiology of this injury is from traction and subsequent tearing of the splenocolic ligament during the procedure, with subcapsular hematoma the most common injury pattern seen.
- Splenic rupture at colonoscopy usually presents with abdominal pain developing within the first 24 h.
- The majority of patients described in the literature have required splenectomy.

Perforation

1. A perforation of the colon during a colonoscopy can be a devastating complication that can result in serious morbidity or mortality. The incidence of perforation is reported to be between 0.012% and 0.016% in large studies.
2. There are three mechanisms responsible for colonoscopic perforation:
    - Mechanical perforation resulting from direct trauma from the colonoscope which occurs more commonly in the sigmoid colon
    - Barotrauma from air insufflation which occurs more commonly in the ascending colon or cecum, which would be the most susceptible to this mechanism
    - Therapeutic procedures such as polypectomy (thermal injury or full-thickness excision) or the dilation of strictures
3. Management of perforations depends on its etiology and the condition of the patient.
4. If the patient presents acutely and has peritonitis, the management is relatively clear, and the patient warrants an emergent laparotomy.
5. If the patient had a therapeutic endoscopy and is clinically stable, then an attempt at non-operative management (IV antibiotics, bowel rest) is acceptable.
6. Perforations from a diagnostic colonoscopy are likely larger and are less successfully managed with non-operative treatment unless the perforation is immediately recognized and repaired endoscopically.
7. If the patient requires surgical intervention, primary repair or resection with a primary anastomosis has proven to be an effective management strategy.
8. One emerging technology is the use of clips to manage a perforation that is either identified endoscopically or as prophylaxis when the endoscopist feels that the depth of resection from a polypectomy makes perforation likely.
9. A literature review of perforations managed with this technology shows that if the clips were placed for a perforation during therapeutic colonoscopy, it is successful in 69–93% of cases.
10. This technology has a place in the endoscopist's armamentarium but should also be employed with surgical consultation, so that early decisions regarding operative management can be made.

Post-polypectomy Syndrome

- Post-polypectomy syndrome is a spectrum of symptoms including abdominal pain, fever, leukocytosis, peritoneal tenderness, and guarding, following a colonoscopic polypectomy.
- It is believed to be the result of an electrocoagulation injury to the colonic wall, thereby creating a transmural burn with localized peritoneal inflammation, but without evidence of perforation. Patients present up to several days following a colonoscopy with fever, localized abdominal pain, and leukocytosis and may have localized peritoneal signs on physical examination. The majority of these patients do not require surgical treatment and are usually adequately managed with bowel rest, intravenous hydration, and broad-spectrum parenteral antibiotics until symptoms resolution.

Bleeding

- Bleeding following a polypectomy is the most common serious complication following a colonoscopy (3% of cases).
- Patients should be given specific written instructions regarding the actions they should take if it should occur.
- Immediate bleeding is dealt with by the endoscopist at the time of the procedure. Clinically significant post-polypectomy hemorrhage typically manifests itself 4–6 days following the procedure but may occur up to 14 days post-procedure.
- Risks for post-polypectomy bleeding include difficult procedures with procedural bleeding, patients on anticoagulation, hypertension, right-sided polyps, larger polyps, and pedunculated polyps with a thicker stalk. Factors which don't impart an increased risk of bleeding include aspirin, NSAIDs, or polyp morphology (sessile vs pedunculated)
- The initial management of a patient with post-polypectomy bleeding is identical to any patient with intestinal bleeding and includes measurement of coagulation parameters and resuscitation based upon hemodynamic parameters.
- Most patients can be managed with a repeat endoscopy if there is evidence of ongoing hemorrhage. Commonly employed hemostatic techniques are hemostatic clips, epinephrine injection, and electrocautery.
- Angiographic embolization has been demonstrated to be effective in the management of post-polypectomy bleeding.
- Endoscopic clipping has been demonstrated beneficial in patients at increased risk for post-polypectomy hemorrhage. One study demonstrated a significantly decreased rate of post-procedure bleeding for polyps >2 cm when the site was prophylactically clipped. Another report showed clipping to be beneficial in anticoagulated patients with lesions larger than 1 cm who were able to undergo successful polypectomy without interrupting the anticoagulation or antiplatelet medications.

Infectious Complications

- The endoscopist should have a basic understanding of the process involved in the cleaning of the endoscopes and endoscopic equipment, as the majority of the rare infectious complications result from breaches in cleaning procedures.
- *Salmonella*, *Pseudomonas*, and *Mycobacterium* species are the most commonly transmitted organisms associated with endoscopic equipment, and the ability of these bacteria to form biofilms on the inner channel surfaces is believed to contribute to their ability to survive the decontamination process.
- The endoscopist should always be vigilant regarding the equipment used and ensure that proper protocols are in place and are being followed.

Training and the Use of Simulation

- The criteria of what constitutes adequate training to perform colonoscopy is controversial.
- There are differences in the way gastroenterologists and surgeons educate and evaluate their trainees in performing procedures.

- Most of the literature on the topic involves gastroenterology fellows and tends to focus on the number of procedures necessary in order to achieve competency. In evaluating gastroenterology fellows, it was found that the ability to intubate the cecum successfully improved and reached the requisite standard of competence – defined as completing the task greater than 90% of the time and within 20 min after 150 procedures had been performed. An independent completion rate of 90% was not obtained until after 500 colonoscopies were performed. As with the ability to technically perform the procedure, quality metrics of trainees also improve with experience as well.
- In one of the few comparisons between gastroenterology and surgery trainees, there was a disparity in endoscopic performance between trainees favoring the gastroenterology trainees although a separate study showed that following the use of endoscopy simulation, surgery residents were capable of performing colonoscopy equivalent to their gastroenterology counterparts using quality metrics as the benchmark.

Simulation

- The practice of endoscopy lends itself well to simulation, yet it has not been fully embraced. The improvement of trainees using simulation is most noticeable during the beginning of their endoscopic experience. Following a 6-h colonoscopy simulation, trainees were noted to significantly outperform those who did not have the training, but these advantages are negligible after approximately 30 procedures on patients.

Documentation and Quality

Documentation

- After completion of the procedure, it is important to adequately document any findings as well as any adjunctive procedures that were performed at the time.
- It is imperative to photo-document any lesions or that were biopsied and describe their size and morphology, location, completeness of removal and the endoscopists interpretation of these lesions.
- A Multi-Society Task Force on Colorectal Cancer developed a consensus-based set of data points that reflected what should be included in any colonoscopy report (Table 4.3). There are numerous commercially available software programs that allow rapid and accurate documentation, and these guidelines will look familiar to any provider who has utilized these systems. Attention to detail is required to enter accurate information that will be relayed to the patient and any other treating physicians.

Quality

- There is increasing attention to quantifiable measures of quality in medicine, and colonoscopy lends itself well to metric analysis, and therefore there has been a great deal of attention paid to these performance measures.
- The five most frequently cited quality measures are cecal intubation rate, adherence to recommended screening and surveillance interval, adenoma detection rate, quality of bowel preparation, and colonoscopy withdrawal time.

PillCam Endoscopy

- The advent of PillCam endoscopy (PCE) has revolutionized the evaluation of the small intestine. It allows the clinician to evaluate this portion of the intestine that was previously relegated to inaccurate or uncomfortable studies such as small bowel radiographic series or enteroclysis.
- The procedure is most commonly used in patients with occult gastrointestinal bleeding or in the search for other small bowel pathologies, such as insipient tumors, polyposis syndromes, or Crohn's disease.

Table 4.3 Recommended elements in standard colonoscopy report

Documentation of informed consent
Facility where endoscopy performed
Patient demographics and history
Age/sex
Receiving anticoagulation: if yes, document management plan
Need for antibiotic prophylaxis: if yes, document reason and management plan
Assessment of patient risk and comorbidity
ASA classification
Indication(s) for procedure:
Procedure: technical description
Procedure date and time
Procedure performed with additional qualifiers (CPT codes, polypectomy, etc.)
Sedation: medications given and by the type of provider responsible
Level of sedation (conscious, deep, general anesthesia)
Extent of examination by anatomic segment: cecum, ascending colon, etc.
If cecum is not reached, provide reason
Method of documentation: i.e., photo of ileocecal valve and/or appendiceal orifice
Time of examination: scope was inserted, withdrawal started, when withdrawn from patient
Retroflexion in rectum (yes/no)
Bowel prep: type of preparation, quality, adequate, or inadequate to detect polyps >5 mm
Technical performance: not technically difficult or examination difficult
Patient discomfort/looping/need for special maneuvers including turning patient
Type of instrument used: model and instrument number
Colonoscopic findings
Colonic masses or polyp(s)
Anatomic location: length/size, mm
Descriptors: pedunculated/sessile/flat/obstructive (% of lumen reduced)/ulcerated
Biopsy obtained: hot/cold or snare/tattoo (if performed)
Fulguration or ablation with cautery
Completely removed (yes/no)/retrieved (yes/no)/sent to pathology (yes/no)
Mucosal abnormality:
Suspected diagnosis: ulcerative colitis, Crohn's, ischemia, infection
Anatomic location/extent/pathology obtained (yes/no)
Other findings:
Diverticulosis/arteriovenous malformations/hemorrhoids
Assessment:
Follow-up plan:
Immediate follow-up/further tests, referrals/medication changes
Follow-up appointments and recommendation for follow-up colonoscopy and tests
Documentation of communication directly to the patient and referring physician
Pathology:
Pathology results reviewed, communicated with referring provider with recommendation for follow-up and communicated with patient

Adapted from Lieberman D, Nadel M et al. Standardized colonoscopy reporting and data system: report of the Quality Assurance Task Group of the National Colorectal Cancer Roundtable. Gastrointest Endosc 2007 May;65(6):757–66. (17)

- It is typically performed after an upper and lower endoscopic examination has already been completed. However it can complement them as well, as in at least one study, 28% of abnormalities identified on PCE were within the area normally covered by an endoscopic exam.
- Capsule endoscopy does not require a bowel preparation, but most patients are instructed to remain either NPO or on a clear liquid diet for

10–12 h prior to the procedure. The patient swallows the disposable capsule, which then transmits images wirelessly to a recorder, and the clinician can review the images at a time when it is convenient to spend the 15–60 min, on average, for image viewing and documentation.

- While there are concerns for evaluating patients with stricturing Crohn's disease, as the capsule can be retained at the location of a stricture, this is typically less of a concern for a surgeon contemplating operative management and can serve as a marker of stricture location enabling the procedure to be performed with minimally invasive techniques. PCE has resulted in medication changes in up to 60% of patients in some studies and has proven superior to other imaging modalities in identifying obscure sources of intestinal bleeding and is beneficial in the localization of small bowel neoplasms.

Endoscopic Management of Polyps, Polypectomy, and Combined Endoscopic and Laparoscopic Surgery

5

Kelly A. Garrett and Sang W. Lee

Key Concepts

- Colonoscopic polypectomy is the treatment of choice for diagnosing and removing most colon polyps.
- Operator variability influences the quality of colonoscopy for both detection and resection.
- Multiple questions remain about best practice techniques for colonoscopic polypectomy.
- EMR of colorectal lesions is safe and effective but results in piecemeal resection that may prevent accurate histological diagnosis. Colonoscopy surveillance is required to assess for and manage local recurrence of neoplasia.
- ESD is able to resect superficial lesions en bloc regardless of tumor size, location, and fibrosis. These advantages come at a cost of an increased risk of perforation, bleeding, and a longer procedure time as compared with EMR.
- Combined endo-laparoscopic surgery is an adjunct to endoscopic polypectomy that may help to avoid colectomy.

Electronic Supplementary Material The online version of this chapter (https://doi.org/10.1007/978-3-030-01165-9_5) contains supplementary material, which is available to authorized users.

K. A. Garrett
Department of General Surgery, Section of Colon and Rectal Surgery, Weill Cornell Medical College, New York Presbyterian Hospital, New York, NY, USA

S. W. Lee (✉)
University of Southern California, Los Angeles, CA, USA
e-mail: sangwl@med.usc.edu

Introduction

- Colon cancer is the third most common cause of cancer-related mortality in the United States.
- In 2015 there were estimated 93,090 new cases of colon cancer with almost 50,000 deaths due to colon cancer.
- There has been a steady decline in the colorectal cancer incidence since the mid-1980s which is partially attributed to the introduction of colorectal cancer screening.
- There has even been a more rapid decline in recent years (4% or greater per year from 2008 to 2011) which may be multifactorial but likely reflects the increased use of screening colonoscopy. Among adults aged 50–75 years, colonoscopy use increased from 19.1% in 2000 to 54.5% in 2013.
- Colonoscopic polypectomy is the treatment of choice for diagnosing and removing most colon polyps.
- Large polyps or polyps in an anatomically difficult location can be challenging to remove endoscopically. Traditionally the most common recommendation for these patients has been to undergo a colon resection.

S. R. Steele et al. (eds.), *The ASCRS Manual of Colon and Rectal Surgery*,
https://doi.org/10.1007/978-3-030-01165-9_5

Identification of Polyps

- Indicators of quality colonoscopy include cecal intubation, withdrawal time, and polyp detection rate.
- Low cecal intubation rates have been associated with higher rates of interval proximal colon cancers.
- Colonoscopy studies in screening patients in the United States have reported cecal intubation rates of 97% or higher.
- The US Multi-Society Task Force on Colorectal Cancer recommended a withdrawal time (defined as the time from cecal intubation to the time the colonoscope is withdrawn out of the anus) of at least 6 min as an indicator of quality colonoscopy.
- A correlation between longer withdrawal time and an increased rate in the detection of adenomas has been demonstrated.
- The American Society for Gastrointestinal Endoscopy (ASGE) and the American College of Gastroenterology (ACG) recommend a minimum target for overall adenoma detection rate (ADR) of at least 25% based on the observation that higher ADRs were associated with a reduced risk of both proximal and distal cancers.

Criteria for Polypectomy

- Polyps should be removed as any adenomatous tissue visualized should be assumed to carry some malignant potential.
- More than 95% of colorectal cancers arise from adenomatous polyps (adenoma to carcinoma sequence) in a process that may take many years.
- Polyps are characterized by their size and morphology (pedunculated or sessile).
- An advanced adenoma is one that is ≥1 cm in size or contains high-grade dysplasia or appreciable villous tissue.
- The prevalence of advanced adenomas is 6–9% for average-risk screening colonoscopy.
- The malignant potential of adenomas <0.5 cm is not as well studied.
- A retrospective study analyzed 7590 adenomatous polyps. Size was the strongest predictor of advanced pathologic features (high-grade dysplasia or invasive cancer). The percentages of adenomas with advanced pathologic features were 3.4%, 13.5%, and 38.5% for adenomas <0.5 cm, 0.5–1.0 cm, and >1 cm, respectively. Villous change, left-sided location, and age ≥ 60 were also associated with advanced pathologic features.
- If there are characteristics suspicious for malignancy (induration, mucosal irregularity, vascular pattern on narrow band imaging, ulceration or central umbilication, large size, failure to lift with submucosal injection), a polypectomy should not be performed.
- Large polyp size (without other concerning features) may be a reason to defer polypectomy due to higher risk of perforation during resection.
- A polypectomy should not be performed if the risks outweigh the benefits, for example, short life expectancy or significant comorbidites.

Polypectomy Techniques

- The principles of polypectomy are to remove all visible adenomatous tissue, but there are many different techniques that are used which create a wide variability in practice.
- Polypectomy is best performed with the polyp in the 5–7 o'clock position.
- Cold biopsy forceps is the simplest method of polypectomy and is frequently used for diminutive lesions (polyps <5 mm). The biopsy forceps is passed through the biopsy channel of the colonoscope, and the jaws are positioned over the polyp which is grasped, removed, and retrieved. More than one bite may be needed to remove all polypoid tissue. Minor bleeding may occur and there is an insignificant risk of perforation. Residual polyp tissue is present in 29–38% of specimens.
- Comparison of jumbo forceps (jaw volume 12.44 mm^3) to standard forceps (jaw volume 7.22 mm^3) showed a higher complete

histologic eradication with the jumbo forceps, but this did not reach statistical significance.

- Removing small polyps with the application of electrocautery to the forceps (hot biopsy forceps) during tissue removal fulgurates the base of the polyp while the specimen is protected in the jaws.
- Risks of this technique include architectural distortion from thermal energy and delayed bleeding or perforation in the right colon. The risk of persistent viable polyp is up to 17% of polypectomy. Some guidelines recommend avoidance of hot biopsy forceps for polyps >5 mm and those in the right colon.
- Snare polypectomy is a common technique. The device is passed through the working channel of the scope, and the snare is extended from a plastic sheath and passed around the base of the polyp. The snare is closed while simultaneously the sheath tip is advanced to the base of the polyp. The base is transected either with or without electrocautery.
- Cold snare produces a resection margin of 1–2 mm. Bleeding is typically not significant. Randomized trials have shown that bleeding is similar between cold and hot snare polypectomies in lesions up to 8 mm.
- Electrocautery with snare polypectomy is more common for larger polyps (>8 mm) and pedunculated polyps.
- The polyp should optimally be in the 5–7 o'clock position. For pedunculated polyps, consider repositioning the patient, so the base of the polyp is not in a dependent position to make post-polypectomy bleeding easier to control.
- Techniques to decrease bowel injury for hot snare are the following: (1) The polyp should be tented toward the center of the lumen to stretch the submucosa away from the muscularis propria and serosa. (2) The duration of energy delivery should be minimized to prevent injury to the wall of the colon.
- For pedunculated polyps, the snare should be closed at a third or halfway from the base of the polyp to ensure a sufficient stump to regrasp if there is immediate bleeding.
- There are many different snare devices available, but there are no trials to establish the advantage of one device over another.

Endoscopic Mucosal Resection

- Large polyps, those involving more than one third of the circumference of the colon or two haustral folds or those with a flat or depressed morphology, are more challenging to remove with the standard polypectomy technique.
- Endoscopic mucosal resection (EMR) is a technique of removal of these lesions and was originally described and popularized in Japan for the treatment of gastric and esophageal tumors. EMR tends to result in piecemeal excision of polyps which can cause difficulty with histologic diagnosis, staging, and evaluation of margins, and is associated with higher rates of complications (e.g., perforation) than standard colonoscopy.
- A solution is injected into the submucosa beneath the lesion to elevate the mucosal layer on a submucosal fluid cushion providing a safety zone for snare resection. Many different solutions have been used for injection. Once the lesion is raised, snare polypectomy is performed. For large lesions, piecemeal polypectomy is invariably required.
- The cap-assisted technique (EMRC) is another method used which involves a cap with a lip on the distal end. A snare is positioned around the lip of the cap, and then the target mucosa is suctioned into the cap. Once the tissue is aspirated, the snare is then closed around the tissue (Figs. 5.1 and 5.2).
- EMR is limited by the difficulty in determining which lesions are likely to be confined to the mucosa. In a prospective, multicenter cohort, risk factors for submucosal invasion were Paris classification 0-IIa+c morphology, nongranular surface morphology, and Kudo pit pattern type V (Tables 5.1 and 5.2). The presence of multiple risk factors magnified the risk of submucosal invasion. EMR was attempted on

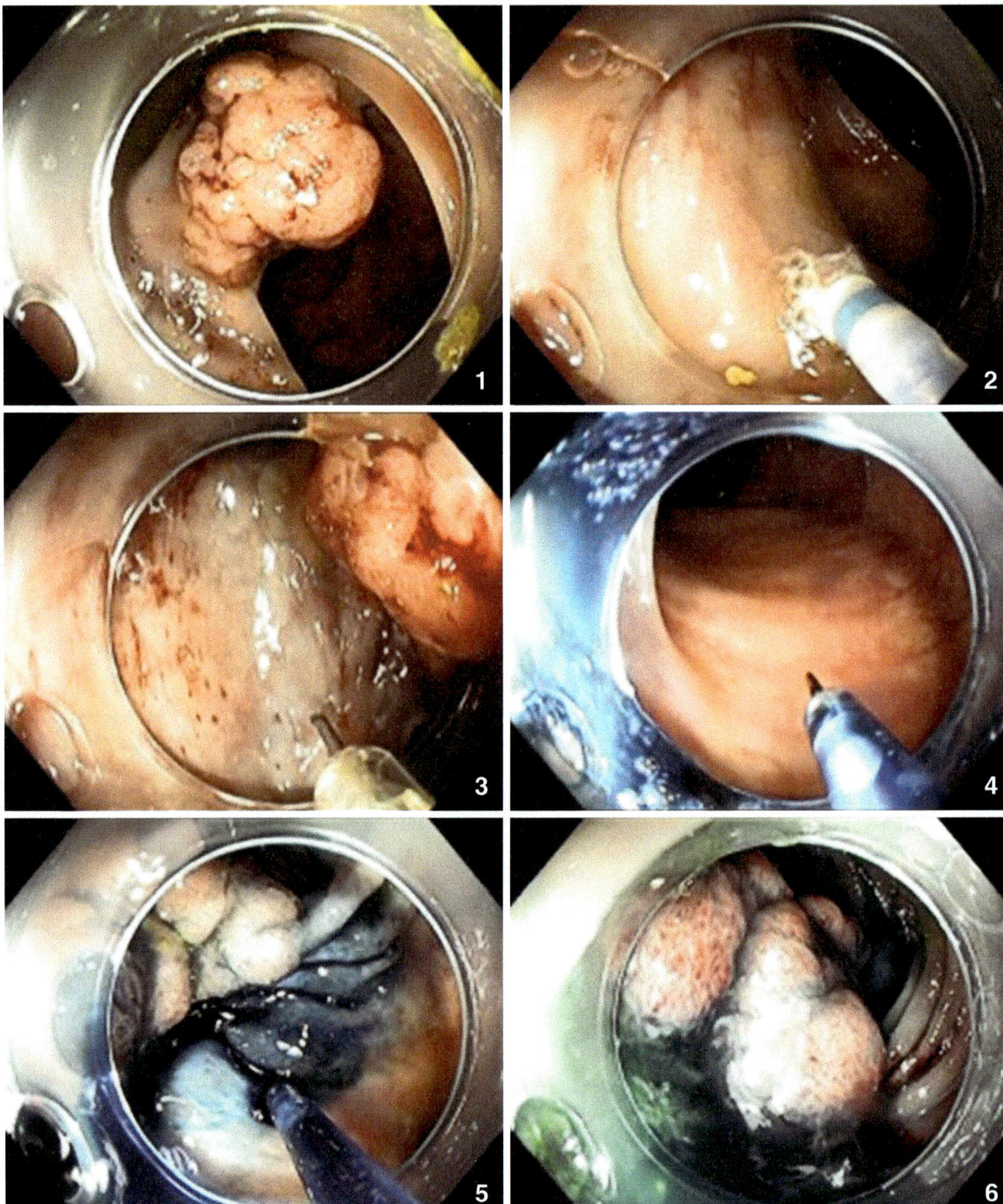

Fig. 5.1 Illustration of piecemeal endoscopic mucosal resection. (1–6) Mucosal lift by submucosal injection of Indigo carmine

464 patients and successful in 89% of patients, and risk factors for failure included a prior attempt at difficult position and ileocecal valve involvement.

- EMR is effective and practical with good outcomes (Table 5.3). When performed by experts, greater than 90% of referred polyps are removed endoscopically with

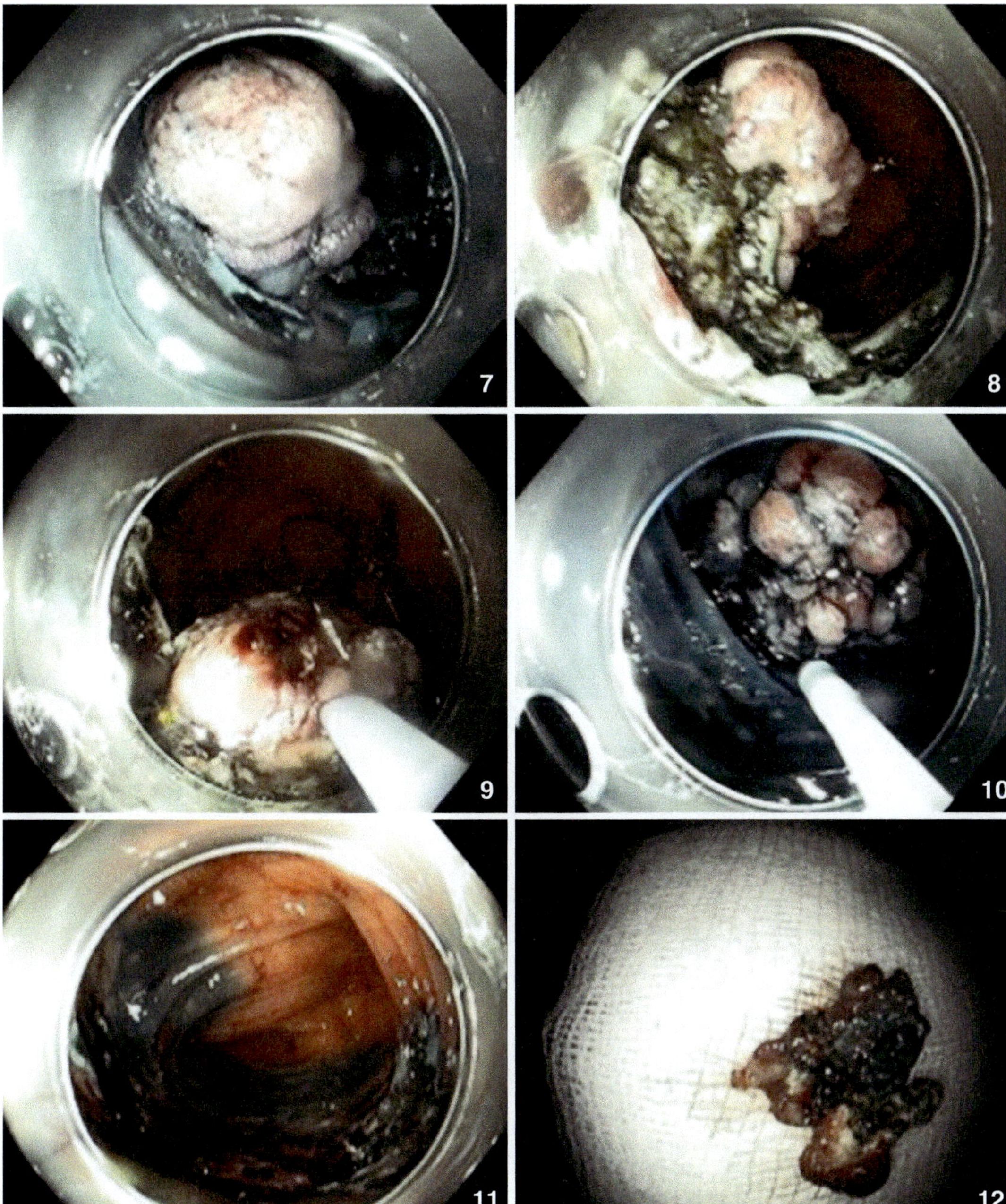

Fig. 5.2 Illustration of piecemeal endoscopic mucosal resection. (7–10) Piecemeal hot snare polypectomy. (11) Intact muscularis. (12) Removed specimen

approximately 44% of lesions are removed en bloc.

- Intraprocedural bleeding occurs in about 8% of patients, post-procedural bleeding in 0–1%, and perforation in 1–2%.
- Local recurrence after EMR is variable and reported in up to 27% of cases and can be managed endoscopically in 93% of cases.
- Risk factors for recurrence are lesion size >4 cm, use of argon plasma coagulation to

Table 5.1 Paris classification

Pedunculated	Ip
Subpedunculated	Isp
Sessile, higher than height of closed forceps (2.5 mm)	Is
Slightly elevated, below height of closed forceps (2.5 mm)	IIa
Completely flat lesion, does not protrude above mucosal surface	IIb
Slightly depressed, lower than mucosa but depth <1.2 mm	IIc
Excavated/ulcerated, deep ulcer below mucosa below 1.2 mm	III

Table 5.2 Kudo pit pattern

Pit pattern type	Characteristics
I	Round pits
II	Stellar or papillary pits
III S	Small tubular or round pits (smaller than type I pits)
III L	Large tubular or round pits (larger than type I pits)
IV	Branch-like or gyrus-like pits
V	Irregular or nonstructured pits (absence of pit pattern)

ablate adenomatous tissue, intraprocedural bleeding, granular appearance, distal rectal location, lesion, and distal rectal lesions.

- Incomplete resection and resections with deep positive margins should be considered for surgery.

Endoscopic Submucosal Dissection

- The technique of endoscopic submucosal dissection (ESD) developed for en bloc resection for large and ulcerative lesions in the stomach has been widely accepted in Japan for the treatment of early gastric cancer.
- Compared with EMR, ESD has the advantage of permitting an en bloc and, therefore, histologically complete resection with fewer limitations on size, location, and fibrosis. These advantages come at the cost of an increased risk of perforation, bleeding, and a longer procedure time as compared with EMR.
- A major difference between surgical resection and endoscopic resection is the absence of lymph node dissection; therefore endoscopic resection should only be considered in lesions that have an insignificant risk of lymph node metastasis.
- This technique is indicated when an en bloc resection cannot be done with EMR or polyps with intramucosal to shallow submucosal invasion. Experience with ESD outside of Japan is still limited.
- The technique of ESD is similar to EMR in that it involves a single channel scope and submucosal injection. The border of the lesion may first be marked out by injecting dye or scoring the mucosa with electrocautery. A variety of solutions have been used for submucosal injection, but the most common are normal saline, glycerol, and hyaluronic acid.
- Once the lesion is lifted, specialized endoscopic knives help to dissect out the lesion (Fig. 5.3). There are a variety of electrocautery knives available, but the two traditional types are needle knives and insulated-tip knives. Management of bleeding is important for the procedure to be successful and is accomplished using either monopolar or bipolar coagulation forceps.
- ESD has a long learning curve.
- Compared with gastric lesions, ESD in the colon and rectum is more difficult due to anatomic features (thin wall, peristalsis, folds), and the position of the endoscope is less stable especially outside of the rectum.
- Successful en bloc resection may be as low as 60% in initial cases but increases up to 88–97% with experience. Similarly, R0 resection rate improves with experience and is reported as high as 96%.
- Bleeding occurs in 1.5–7.9% and perforation in up to 10.7% of cases (Table 5.4).
- Frequently, complications are successfully treated with endoscopic clipping.

Surveillance after ESD is case dependent but aims to detect residual disease or recurrent disease early.

Table 5.3 Endoscopic mucosal resection

Author	Year	Polyps	Polyp size, cm	Macroscopic classification	Operating time, min	En bloc resection, %	LOS, day	Leakage/ fistula, %	Postoperative bleeding %	Cancer %	Depth	Recurrence %
Gomez	2014	131	3.3	NA	NA	27	NA	3	2.3	7.6	Unknown	17
Maguire	2014	269	2.8	NA	NA	0	NA	1.3	3	16	Tis, 6.3%; T1, 9.3%	24
Knabe	2013	252	>2.0	Paris	NA	12	NA	1.6	1.6	3.2	Unknown	22
Buchner	2012	315	2.3	Paris	NA	54	<1	0.4	7.2	4.4	Unknown	27
Conio	2004	139	2.0	NA	NA	0	NA	0	0	12.2	Tis, 6; T1, 3; T2, 1	21.9
Stergiou	2002	68	>3.0	Sessile/ pedunculated	NA	38	NA	0	4	10	Unknown	29

LOS length of stay, *Tis* carcinoma in situ, *NA* not available

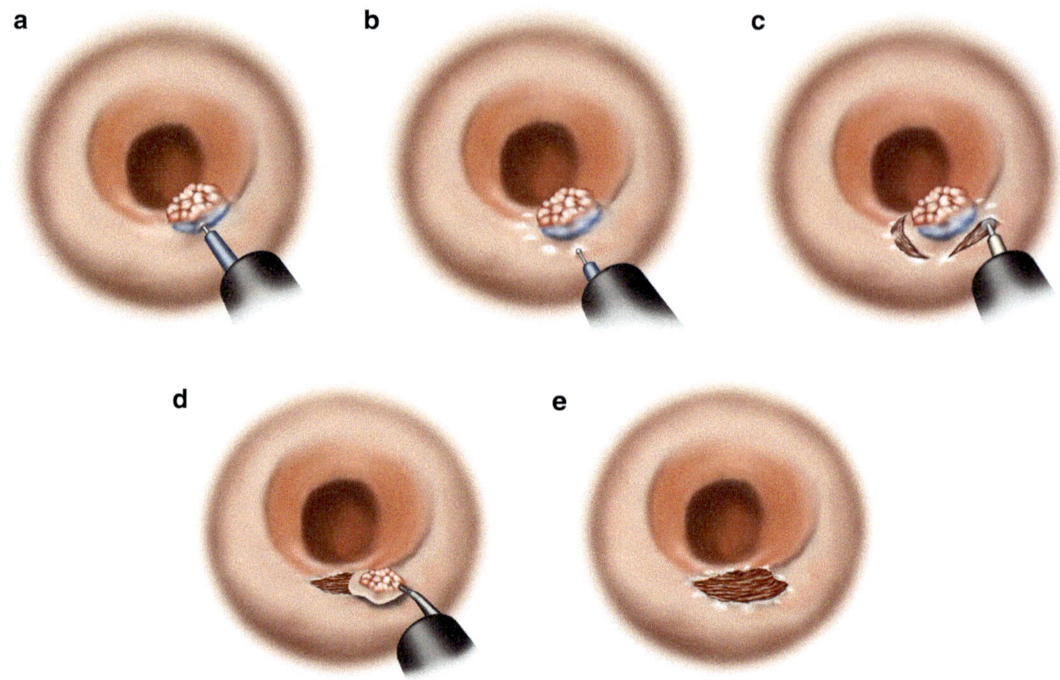

Fig. 5.3 Steps of endoscopic submucosal dissection. (**a**) Submucosal injection. (**b**) Marking of the resection margin. (**c**) Submucosal dissection using a needle knife. (**d**) Extraction of specimen. (**e**) Intact muscularis

Combined Endo-Laparoscopic Surgery (CELS)

- As previously discussed, large polyps or polyps within or behind a haustral fold can be very challenging to remove endoscopically. Although EMR and ESD are performed for these polyps, these techniques are not widely available and require a high level of technical skill. Traditionally, the most common recommendation for these patients has been segmental colectomy – an oncologic resection. Although the laparoscopic approach can minimize the morbidity associated with colectomy, only a minority of the colon resections performed in the United States are being done laparoscopically. Furthermore, even if a minimally invasive approach is used, it still entails a major abdominal operation with associated morbidities. Combined endo-laparoscopic surgery (CELS) has been described as an alternative to bowel resection in select patients.
- Laparoscopic-assisted polypectomy was first described in 1993, and larger retrospective studies have since been published.
- There are several ways in which laparoscopic assistance during colonoscopic polypectomy can be helpful: (1) the underlying colon can be invaginated to assist in snaring of a flat polyp, (2) laparoscopic mobilization of flexures and angulated colon can provide better access and exposure, and (3) full-thickness injury to the colon can be detected and repaired laparoscopically.
- Simultaneous performance of laparoscopy and colonoscopy can often present a technical challenge, but the use of carbon dioxide (CO_2) for insufflation during colonoscopy has been shown to be safe and can remedy this issue since CO_2 gas is absorbed approximately 150 times faster than room air.
- Several published studies have similarly addressed this combined technique, considering it a safe and effective method to avoid colectomy and remove difficult polyps in many cases (Table 5.5). One of the largest

Table 5.4 Endoscopic submucosal dissection

Author	Year	Polyps	Polyp size, cm	Macroscopic classification	Operating time, min	En bloc resection	LOS, day	Perforation, %	Postoperative bleeding %	R0 resection rate, %	Cancer %	Depth	Recurrence %
Saito	2014	900	3.7	Paris	60	91	NA	2.7	1.7	87	74	Unknown	NA
Toyonaga	2014	468	3	NA	60	99	NA	1.5	1.5	NA	66	Tis: 49%; T1: 17%; T2: 0.4%	NA
Lee	2013	874	2.7	Sessile/ pedunculated	54	97	3.5	5.3	0.5	91.2	43	Tis: 28%; T1: 15%; T2: 0.2%	0.4
Yoshida	2013	530	3.1	Protruding/ superficial	93	91	NA	4.1	2.3	NA	54	Tis: 41%; T1: 12%	NA
Nakamura	2014	300	3.0	LST/ non- LST	90	91.7	5	1.7	5	91	99	M-SM-s: 92%; SM-d: 7%	NA

LOS length of stay, *NA* not available, *Tis* carcinoma in situ, *M-SM-s* mucosal or shallow submucosal invasion <1000 mcm from the muscularis mucosae, *SM-d* >1000 mcm of submucosal invasion

Table 5.5 Combined endo-laparoscopic surgery

Author	Year	Patients	Polyps	Polyp size, cm	Frozen section	Operating time, min	Intraoperative complications %	Postoperative complications, %	Mortality, %	LOS (days)	Tis, %	Submucosal cancer, %	Successful endoscopic resection, %	Conversion to open surgery, %	Prognosis, m = months
Goh	2014	30	30	1.4	–	105 (75–125)	0	13.3	0	2.0	HGD 26.7	6.7	73	0	No recurrence at 20 m
SW Lee	2013	75	75	3 (1–7)	If needed	145 (50–249)	0	9.2	0	1	HGD 9.3	6.7	74	3	10% recurrence at 65 m
Wood	2011	13	16	3 (2 – 5)	All	NA	0	15	0	2	7.7		77	0	NA
Grunhagen	2011	11	12	2 (0.6–4.5)	–	45 (15–80)	0	18.1	0	1	9	0	82	0	No recurrences at 11 m
Cruz	2011	25	25	2.4 (1–4)	–	92.7 (60–145)	0	8	0	1.5	8	4	76	0	NA
Agrawal	2010	19	19	0.6–6	All	35.3–37	0	5.6	0	0–14	5.3		58	NA	No recurrences at 3 m
Wilhelm	2009	146	154	NA	–	100 (40–272)	1	25	0.7	8	11		73	5	Local recurrence of adenoma 0.9% at 35 m
Franklin	2009	176	251	3.7 (2–6)	All	96.5	0	10	0	1.1	10.2		91	0	No recurrences at 65 m

NA not available, *HGD* high-grade dysplasia, *Tis* carcinoma in situ, *LOS* length of stay studies to date was reported by Franklin and Portillo describing the technique of laparoscopic-monitored colonoscopic polypectomy in 176 patients with excision of 251 polyps. The procedure was performed successfully in all but four patients (97.8%). This study was an update of two previous publications from their group in 2000 and 2007. In their practice, all specimens were sent for frozen section, and ultimately, 18 (10.2%) patients required colectomy for cancer.

- Overall, technical success rates for CELS are consistently reported between 74% and 97%. Postoperative complications are typically minor and less than 5%. Recurrence rates are low, reported in 10–15%, and can typically be approached endoscopically or with CELS.

Preoperative Assessment of Colorectal Patients

6

Jennifer S. Davids and Justin A. Maykel

Key Concepts

- A thorough history and physical exam performed by the surgeon is the single best preoperative "test."
- Complex surgical patients with multiple comorbidities need careful preoperative assessment in order to minimize risk of perioperative complications.
- Preoperative laboratory studies should be ordered on a selective basis, as "routine" preoperative labs on otherwise asymptomatic, healthy patients have low diagnostic yield.
- Depending on patient's risk factors, a preoperative cardiac risk assessment should be made and appropriate testing obtained. Cardiac medications should be continued, although beta-blockers should not be initiated in the preoperative setting. Cardiac interventions should be performed for standard indications, independent of the need for abdominal surgery.
- Smoking cessation should be strongly encouraged prior to elective surgery.
- The surgeon should carefully review the patient's medication list, paying particular attention to anticoagulants, immunosuppressants, and chemotherapy agents.

Evaluation of the Routine Colorectal Patient

In Office by Surgeon

- The in-office surgical consultation includes a detailed history, review of the patient's medical record, medications, and physical exam.
- It is essential to communicate with specialists who are the primary managers of any comorbid conditions. The task of coordinating these patients' preoperative care can be enormously time-consuming for the busy surgeon; however, it is incredibly important to communicate and exchange vital information prior to elective surgery, in order to minimize risk of perioperative complications.

Major Abdominal Surgery

- The history should make sure to include a detailed list of active medications, including blood thinners and over-the-counter drugs or supplements.
- Personal and/or family history of clotting or bleeding disorders (or bleeding complications from prior surgery) should be obtained.

J. S. Davids
Department of Surgery, University of Massachusetts Memorial Medical Center, Worcester, MA, USA

J. A. Maykel (✉)
Division of Colon and Rectal Surgery, University of Massachusetts Memorial Medical Center, Worcester, MA, USA
e-mail: Justin.maykel@umassmemorial.org

S. Steele et al. (eds.), *The ASCRS Manual of Colon and Rectal Surgery*,
https://doi.org/10.1007/978-3-030-01165-9_6

- The surgeon should ask about activity level, in order to estimate exercise capacity. Poor baseline exercise capacity has been shown to correlate with increased risk of perioperative cardiac complications.
- Can the patient walk up a flight of stairs, do heavy housework, or walk up a hill? "Yes" to these questions indicates that the patient can perform at least four METs (metabolic equivalents), and if otherwise healthy, the patient does not need a preoperative cardiac workup.

Anorectal Surgery

- Anorectal surgical procedures are considered low acuity and do not trigger the major physiologic changes associated with major abdominal surgery. Accordingly, it is not necessary to obtain any additional preoperative workup for healthy patients undergoing elective anorectal procedures.

Preoperative Testing

Laboratory Studies

- Multiple studies have demonstrated that routine preoperative labs are very low yield in identifying abnormalities that require a change in management in healthy, asymptomatic patients. A selective approach to preoperative laboratory studies should be taken.
- When laboratory tests are indicated, lab values from the 4-month timeframe prior to surgery may be used, unless there has been a change in clinical status.
- *Hemoglobin* is recommended for all patients age 65 or older who are undergoing abdominal surgery. Younger patients should be tested if there is potential for major blood loss or if the history is suggestive of anemia.
- *White blood cell count* as a screening test is of limited utility, but is certainly relevant in cases where recent infection has been treated or in the setting of immunosuppression.
- *Platelet counts* should be checked if the patient will undergo spinal or epidural anesthesia. *Coagulation studies and bleeding time* are not needed in patients with no personal or family history of bleeding disorders.
- Pre-transfusion testing, consisting of *ABO and Rh typing* ("type and screen"), should be performed preoperatively in all patients undergoing major abdominal surgery, including bowel resection. This is particularly important for patients who have a significant transfusion history, who may have multiple alloantibodies.
- Serum *creatinine* should be checked in patients 50 years or older, as elevated creatinine is an independent predictor of increased postoperative cardiac complications as well as mortality in elective non-cardiac surgery. Some anesthetics require dose adjustments for patients with impaired renal function.
- Routine *electrolytes* are not required unless the patient has a history of prior electrolyte abnormalities, chronic kidney disease, or diuretic use.
- Routine blood *glucose* measurements are not indicated in nondiabetic patients, as the incidence of asymptomatic hyperglycemia is low.
- *Liver function tests* should not be routinely ordered in a healthy, asymptomatic patient.
- Routine *urinalysis* does not need to be performed in healthy, asymptomatic patients.
- *Pregnancy tests* should be performed on all women of childbearing age, if the results would alter management.

Electrocardiogram

- In asymptomatic patients undergoing low-risk surgery, ECG is unlikely to identify abnormalities that result in a change in management. According to the ACC/AHA guidelines, preoperative ECG should be performed on patients with known heart disease, peripheral arterial disease, or cerebrovascular disease.

Chest X-ray

- CXR are low yield in identifying clinically significant abnormalities that alter management. However, the American College of Physicians recommends obtaining chest x-ray (CXR) for patients with known cardiopulmonary disease, as well as all patients 50 years or older who require major abdominal surgery.

Patients with Specific Comorbidities

Assessment of Cardiac Risk

- It is essential to identify patients who may be at increased risk for perioperative cardiac complications A large study of high-risk patients undergoing non-cardiac surgery demonstrated that postoperative myocardial infarction is associated with high 30-day mortality (11.6%), and the majority (65%) were not associated with ischemic symptoms.

Initial Workup

- Patients should be asked about exercise tolerance (can they climb two flights of stairs and/or walk four city blocks?) and specific symptoms: palpitations, chest pain, syncope, dyspnea, and orthopnea.
- Patients should be queried about a history of cardiac disease and diseases associated with an increased risk of coronary artery disease.
- There are several validated models that can be used by the clinician to predict risk of perioperative cardiac adverse events including the Revised Goldman Cardiac Risk Index (RCRI) (Table 6.1) and the American College of Surgeons National Surgical Quality Improvement Program (ACS-NSQIP) risk calculator. The calculator is online and accessible at http://riskcalculator.facs.org.

Who Needs Additional Testing?

- The extent of preoperative workup is based on the patient's estimated risk according to these models. Patients whose risk is 1% or more are likely to have a known history of recent myocardial infarction, unstable angina, heart failure, valvular disease, or arrhythmias. These patients should be evaluated preoperatively by their cardiologist. Generally, additional testing is not usually performed beyond what is ordinarily needed if the patient was not undergoing surgery, as this has not been shown to improve perioperative outcomes in non-cardiac, nonvascular surgery.

Preoperative "Optimization"

- Once the preoperative cardiac assessment has been completed, the managing physician may institute treatment that optimally limits the risk of a perioperative cardiac adverse event. While long-standing beta-blockers should be continued, beta-blockers should *not* be initiated in the preoperative setting.
- Antihypertensive medications can be adjusted to avoid perioperative hypotension, targeting a systolic blood pressure of 116–130 mmHg and heart rate of 60–70 beats per minute.
- Dysrhythmias can be controlled with anti-arrhythmic agents.
- Decompensated heart failure increases perioperative risk, and this risk may be mitigated by

Table 6.1 Revised Goldman Cardiac Risk Index (RCRI)

Six independent predictors of major cardiac complications
High-risk type of surgery (examples include vascular surgery and any open intraperitoneal or intrathoracic procedures) History of ischemic heart disease (history of myocardial infarction (MI) or a positive exercise test, current complaint of chest pain considered to be secondary to myocardial ischemia, use of nitrate therapy, or ECG with pathological Q waves does not count prior to coronary revascularization procedure unless one of the other criteria for ischemic heart disease is present) History of heart failure (HF) History of cerebrovascular disease Diabetes mellitus requiring treatment with insulin Preoperative serum creatinine <2.0 mg/dL (177 μmol/L)
Rate of cardiac death, nonfatal myocardial infarction, and nonfatal cardiac arrest according to the number of predictors (2)
No risk factors – 0.4% (95% CI: 0.1–0.8)
One risk factor – 1.0% (95% CI: 0.5–1.4)
Two risk factors – 2.4% (95% CI: 1.3–3.5)
Three or more risk factors – 5.4% (95% CI: 2.8–7.9)

treatment with ACE inhibitors, aldosterone antagonists, and digoxin for at least 1 week preoperatively.
- Cardiac catheterization should be reserved for patients with high-risk features on noninvasive testing.
- Revascularization (operative or endoluminal) should be reserved for those patients who meet the criteria for cardiac intervention regardless of the need for non-cardiac surgery, and the timing should be chosen based on the indication for and urgency associated with the colorectal resection.

Coronary Stent Management

- For patients with either a bare-metal stent (BMS) or drug-eluting stent (DES), the current recommendation is to continue dual antiplatelet therapy (aspirin plus an oral antiplatelet agent such as clopidogrel) for at least 12 months. For patients who need to undergo non-emergent non-cardiac surgery, the recommendation is to complete at least 1 month dual antiplatelet therapy preoperatively for BMS and at least 6 months for DES.
- The RECO study is a prospective multicenter observational cohort study of 1134 consecutive patients with coronary stents which sought to quantify risk of major adverse cardiac and cerebrovascular events (MACCEs) and major bleeding. 54.9% had bare-metal stents (BMS) only, and 32.4% had drug-eluting stents (DES). Overall, there was a 10.9% rate of MACCEs and a 9.5% rate of hemorrhagic complications. Risk factors for major bleeding included hemoglobin <10 g/dl, creatinine clearance 30–60 ml/min, duration from stent implantation to surgery <3 months, and high-risk surgery. This study highlights the importance of delaying elective surgery >3 months after stent placement if possible, as well as the need to maintain oral antiplatelet agents through the perioperative period in order to minimize risk for major adverse cardiac and cerebrovascular events.
- Not infrequently colon and rectal surgeons are presented with patients who require urgent abdominal surgery and who also have recently implanted DES. Patients on oral antiplatelet agents for recently implanted drug-eluting coronary stents can be safely "bridged" with IV infusions of shorter-acting antiplatelet agents.
- A pilot study of 30 patients with recently implanted DES undergoing major surgery had clopidogrel withheld 5 days preoperatively and were bridged with tirofiban. There were no adverse cardiac events during the index hospitalization, and 28 patients (93%) did not experience significant postoperative bleeding. One of the two patients had an anastomotic bleeding after partial colectomy that occurred 4 days after restarting clopidogrel; this was controlled with endoscopic clip placement. This study demonstrates the importance of careful coordination with the inpatient cardiologist in order to optimize outcomes for these complex patients who require urgent abdominal surgery while on antiplatelet therapy for a recently placed coronary stent.

AICD/Pacemaker Management

- It is important to determine if the patient is pacemaker-dependent. For patients who are not pacemaker-dependent, the anesthesiologist should place a magnet over the device, which will prevent inappropriate delivery of shocks. For patients who are pacemaker-dependent, the device may need to be reprogrammed intraoperatively. All AICD patients should have an external defibrillator and transcutaneous pacer immediately available, and the pads should be affixed to the patient at the start of the case.
- AICD activity can be affected by monopolar cautery, causing electromagnetic interference. Intent to use monopolar cautery should be clearly communicated to the anesthesia team prior to the case.

Assessment of Pulmonary Risk

COPD

- Patients with chronic obstructive pulmonary disorder (COPD) are at high risk of perioperative pulmonary complications.

- Bronchodilators should be continued perioperatively.
- Glucocorticoid use must be balanced against potential for increased risk of surgical complications.
- A randomized controlled trial of 48 high-risk pulmonary patients demonstrated significant decrease in postoperative pulmonary complications in the group receiving aggressive pulmonary care.

Obstructive Sleep Apnea (OSA)

- Obstructive sleep apnea (OSA) is the most common sleep disorder and is characterized by upper airway obstruction, causing apneic episodes.
- OSA is a risk factor for perioperative cardiopulmonary complications and is associated with unplanned ICU admission.
- Patients undergoing major abdominal surgery should be screened for OSA, and there are several simple and efficient clinical screening tools available, including the STOP-Bang questionnaire (Table 6.2). Patients with high scores who are undergoing major abdominal surgery should be referred to a pulmonologist for a formal workup. A randomized controlled trial of patients with OSA demonstrated that patients who used auto-titrated continuous positive airway pressure (APAP) perioperatively had significantly decreased rates of hypoxia and apnea.

Diabetes

- Diabetic patients represent a complex subset of surgical patients, who often have long-term complications of their disease and comorbidities such as chronic renal insufficiency and cardiovascular disease. Diabetic patients undergoing major abdominal surgery should have the following as part of their preoperative workup: ECG, CXR, serum creatinine, serum glucose, and an AIC level (within 4–6 weeks preoperatively).
- Elevated A1C levels have been shown in cardiac surgery to be associated with increased risk of surgical complications, including infections, myocardial infarction, and death.

Table 6.2 STOP-Bang questionnaire

☐ Yes	☐ No	**Snoring?** Do you **snore loudly** (loud enough to be heard through closed doors or your bed-partner elbows you for snoring at night)?
☐ Yes	☐ No	**Tired?** Do you often feel **tired**, **fatigued**, **or sleepy** during the daytime (such as falling asleep during driving)?
☐ Yes	☐ No	**Observed?** Has anyone **observed** you **stop breathing** or **choking/gasping** during your sleep?
☐ Yes	☐ No	**Pressure?** Do you have or are being treated for **high blood pressure**?
☐ Yes	☐ No	**Body mass index more than 35 kg/m^2?**
☐ Yes	☐ No	**Age older than 50 years old?**
☐ Yes	☐ No	**Neck size large? (measured around Adam's apple)** For male, is your shirt collar 17 inches or larger? For female, is your shirt collar 16 inches or larger?
☐ Yes	☐ No	**Gender = male?**
Scoring criteria*:		
Low risk of OSA: Yes to 0 to 2 questions		
Intermediate risk of OSA: Yes to 3 to 4 questions		
High risk of OSA: Yes to 5 to 8 questions		

OSA = obstructive sleep apnea

Obesity

- Obesity is defined as having body mass index (BMI) of 30 or more, and super-obese is a BMI of 40 or more. BMI is calculated as the patient's weight (in kilograms) divided by square of the height (in meters). An online BMI calculator is available at the CDC website (http://www.cdc.gov/healthyweight/assessing/bmi/adult_BMI/english_bmi_calculator/bmi_calculator.html).
- A prospective multicenter study of over 100,000 patients undergoing non-bariatric surgery demonstrated that overweight and obese patients had a significantly lower postoperative *mortality* which can be explained by increased nutritional stores, as well as the chronic inflammatory state of obesity that may prime these patients for the inflammatory surge of surgery.
- Obese patients undergoing non-bariatric abdominal surgery have been shown to have increased risk of perioperative venous thromboembolism and superficial site infection.
- Obese patients pose significant intraoperative challenges, some of which can be mitigated with appropriate preoperative planning. If a stoma may be needed, marking on the thinner upper abdomen will be helpful. Laparoscopic surgery has the advantage to the patient of smaller incisions and improved visualization for the surgeon. Avoiding incisions which incorporate a large pannus minimizes wound-related complications.
- Clear communication with the operating room staff prior to the case is essential, to ensure availability of long instruments, deep retractors, appropriate beds, and equipment such as blood pressure cuffs and large pneumatic compression boots.

Malnutrition

- Nutritional risk tends to be a reflection of the patient's overall health and has been correlated with the Eastern Cooperative Oncology Group score and the presence of anorexia or fatigue.
- Poor nutrition is associated with increased postoperative complications, longer length of stay, and higher mortality following elective surgery.
- Nutritional support can be delivered in the preoperative or postoperative setting and can be administered via the enteral and parenteral routes. While most studies are limited by heterogeneity when delivered appropriately, the malnourished colorectal patient realizes several benefits from perioperative nutritional support including fewer postoperative complications, shorter hospital length of stay, and lower mortality.
- Most patients will complain of some degree of intolerance of oral intake as a result of poor appetite, nausea, abdominal bloating, abdominal pain, weakness, and recent weight loss. Physical examination will typically show muscle wasting and loose skin. These variables can be objectified using grading systems such as the relatively intuitive subjective global assessment (SGA) to classify patients as well nourished, moderately malnourished, or severely malnourished. The subjective global assessment (SGA) utilizes five features of the history (weight loss over 6 months, dietary intake change, gastrointestinal symptoms, functional capacity, and the impact of disease on nutritional requirements) and four features of the clinical exam (loss of subcutaneous fat, muscle wasting, ankle edema, sacral edema, ascites) to elicit a SGA rank based on subjective weighting.
- Serum albumin level of <3.0 g/dL defines the "malnourished state," but its reliability is limited because fluctuation of levels is multifactoral. Other short turnover proteins such as prealbumin, transferrin, and retinol binding protein have similar limitations as nutritional markers although all of them can be useful when followed as trends over time.
- Patients with inflammatory bowel disease, intestinal obstruction, large tumors, fistulizing diseases, and diarrhea are often unable to

sustain themselves orally and limits the ability to intervene using the enteral route.
- Total parenteral nutrition (TPN) can be used as long as central intravenous access is obtained, an appropriate formula is prescribed (1.5 grams protein per kilogram and 25 kcal per kilogram), and tight glycemic control is maintained (serum blood sugars <150 g/dL).
- The use of preoperative nutrition has not been well studied in the malnourished GI surgery patient populations, but three studies that evaluated preoperative parenteral nutrition showed a significant reduction in postoperative complications, predominantly in malnourished patients.

Solid Organ Transplant Recipients

- Over 150,000 patients in the USA are living with functional kidney transplants, and this number is on the rise, and the majority of these patients are maintained on chronic immunosuppressive regimens.
- These agents are generally continued throughout the perioperative and early postoperative period to minimize risk of rejection.
- The newer immunosuppressive agents, sirolimus and everolimus, which belong to the drug class known as inhibitors of the mammalian target of rapamycin (mTOR), have been shown to negatively impact healing of surgical wounds. A prospective trial of patients randomized to receive either sirolimus or tacrolimus on postoperative day 4 after kidney transplant found a significantly higher rate of wound-related complications in the sirolimus cohort. This data has prompted clinicians to replace mTOR inhibitors with tacrolimus for 6 weeks prior to elective surgery.

Substance Abuse

- All surgical patients should be asked about their use of tobacco, alcohol, and street drugs.
- In one study 7.6% of Americans had a substance abuse disorder within the year prior to surgery.

Alcohol

- Alcoholism has been shown to be associated with a number of different perioperative complications in a dose-dependent manner.
- The AUDIT-C questionnaire is a validated screening tool that can be used by the clinician to identify patients at high risk for perioperative complications (Table 6.3).
- A randomized controlled trial that studied patients with alcoholism undergoing elective colorectal surgery demonstrated that abstinence 1 month preoperatively was associated with fewer cardiac complications as well as overall decreased complication rate.

Tobacco

- Smoking has been shown in multiple studies to increase perioperative pulmonary risk, as well as risk of wound infections, neurologic complications, and ICU admission. The best way to minimize this risk is to encourage patients to quit smoking prior to elective surgery. Prior data suggested that smoking cessation less than

Table 6.3 AUDIT-C questionnaire

Question # 1: How often did you have a drink containing alcohol in the past year?	
Never	(0 points)
Monthly or less	(1 point)
Two to four times a month	(2 points)
Two to three times per week	(3 points)
Four or more times a week	(4 points)
Question # 2: How many drinks did you have on a typical day when you were drinking in the past year?	
1 or 2	(0 points)
3 or 4	(1 point)
5 or 6	(2 points)
7 to 9	(3 points)
10 or more	(4 points)
Question # 3: How often did you have six or more drinks one occasion in the past year?	
Never	(0 points)
Less than monthly	(1 point)
Monthly	(2 points)
Weekly	(3 points)
Daily or almost daily	(4 points)

The AUDIT-C score on a scale of 0–12 (scores of 0 reflect no alcohol use). In men, a score of 4 or more is considered positive; in women, a score of 3 or more is considered positive

8 weeks preoperatively was associated with a paradoxical increase in pulmonary complications, but this has been disproven in multiple large studies. The recommendation is smoking cessation, regardless of the timing of surgery, although ideally surgery can be planned for at least 4 weeks from the "quit date."

Opioids

- For all patients on narcotics, the surgeon should always ask preoperatively what is the indication, how long have they been taking it, what are the side effects (such as constipation), if there is a plan to wean off the drug, as well as who has been prescribing it?
- Opioid dependency will result in increased narcotic requirements perioperatively.
- The acute pain management service should be involved preoperatively. A clear plan should be made with the patient and the clinician who has been prescribing chronic opioids regarding postoperative pain management following hospital discharge, particularly who will be prescribing, and for how long.
- Nonnarcotic adjunct therapies can be considered, including thoracic epidural catheters and transversus abdominis plane (TAP) blocks, as well as drugs such as ketorolac (Toradol), acetaminophen, and gabapentin (Neurontin).

Medications

- In the era of polypharmacy, it is essential for the colorectal surgeon to carefully assess the patient's current medication list. Decisions on holding or continuing medications in the perioperative period should be made in consultation with the prescribing physician and a full consideration of the risks and benefits of these medications.

Anticoagulation

- Several novel oral anticoagulants are commercially available and are widely used in patients with atrial fibrillation or history of stroke, as well as in patients with coronary or endovascular stents. When determining how to manage anticoagulation perioperatively, risk of bleeding must be balanced against the risk of thromboembolic complications. Additionally, it should be determined whether "bridging" with a short-acting anticoagulant is necessary. Although there are evidence-based guidelines, these decisions should be made on a case-by-case basis and should closely involve the patient's cardiologist and/or hematologist. The patient should be educated upfront about the potential risks involved and to recognize that the ability to restart the medication postoperatively relates to the extent of surgery and associated bleeding risk.
- *Clopidogrel (Plavix)* is a member of the platelet receptor PY12 blocker drug class and is used in patients with history of myocardial infarction or stroke, as well as recent coronary or peripheral vascular stent placement.
- For most patients, the maintenance dose is 75 mg orally per day.
- If the decision has been made to discontinue clopidogrel prior to elective surgery, it should be discontinued 5–7 days preoperatively and resumed as soon as possible after surgery.
- *Warfarin (Coumadin)* is an inhibitor of vitamin K-dependent clotting factor synthesis, and the half-life of warfarin is 36–42 h.
- Therapeutic dose range is measured by the prothrombin time (PT), which is generally maintained at a goal of INR (international normalized ratio) 2.0–3.0 for most conditions except prosthetic cardiac valves.
- For elective surgery, warfarin should be discontinued 5 days preoperatively. Most abdominal surgery is safe to perform when INR is </=1.4(60).
- For urgent surgery (within 1–2 days), warfarin can be reversed with vitamin K (2.5–5 mg oral or intravenous).
- For emergency surgery, warfarin can be rapidly reversed with fresh frozen plasma (FFP), which contains the necessary clotting factors.
- Provided that there was adequate hemostasis during surgery, warfarin may be restarted (at the preoperative dose) as early as 12–24 h postoperatively.
- *Heparin* binds to and inactivates antithrombin III and has a half-life of 45 min. Unfractionated

heparin is administered as an IV infusion, using a weight-based nomogram to titrate the dose. Compared to low molecular weight heparin, unfractionated heparin is less costly, is easier and faster to reverse, and is preferable in patients with renal insufficiency (the dose is not affected by creatinine clearance). IV unfractionated heparin should be held 6 h prior to surgery.

- *Enoxaparin (Lovenox)* is a low molecular weight heparin that has comparable efficacy to unfractionated heparin but has many advantages. It is easier to use, is administered as a subcutaneous injection (and therefore can be given in the outpatient setting), and does not require monitoring. Its half-life is 3–5 h.
- In preparation for surgery, if twice-daily dosing is used, the evening dose should be held on the night prior to surgery; if once-daily dosing is being used, a half-dose should be given the morning prior to surgery.
- Patients on any heparin derivative need to be monitored for heparin-induced thrombocytopenia (HIT), although this risk is less significant with low molecular weight heparin.
- Heparin products can be reversed with protamine sulfate.
- *Apixaban (Eliquis)* is an oral factor Xa inhibitor that is commonly used in patients with atrial fibrillation, as well as for both prophylaxis and treatment of venous thromboembolism.
- The major advantage of apixaban over Coumadin is that drug levels do not need to be checked routinely.
- The dose must be decreased for Cr>/=1.5, as well as for age > 80 and body weight </=60 kg.
- Apixaban should typically be discontinued for a minimum of 48 h prior to abdominal or anorectal surgery.
- There is a boxed warning regarding the use of neuraxial anesthesia and risk of spinal or epidural hematoma (which could result in temporary or permanent paralysis), as the optimal interval from drug discontinuation to intervention is not well-defined. Therefore we recommend not using this drug for perioperative anticoagulation if an epidural catheter or spinal anesthesia is planned. There are currently no specific reversal agents for this drug.
- *Aspirin* impairs platelet function primarily by downstream effects of irreversibly inhibiting cyclooxygenase-1 (COX-1). Its antiplatelet effects start as soon as 30 min after ingestion and last throughout the platelet life span, which ranges from 8 to 10 days.
- Perioperative continuation of low-dose (81 mg) aspirin in low-risk patients (for primary prevention of thrombotic cardiovascular events) undergoing abdominal surgery has not been shown to be associated with an increase in major postoperative bleeding complications. Very few studies specifically evaluate the perioperative risk of high-dose (325 mg) aspirin.
- In our practice, we do not discontinue low-dose "baby" aspirin perioperatively for anorectal or abdominal cases, regardless of the indication for its use. For patients on high-dose (325 mg) aspirin, the decision is more individualized and requires input of the patient's cardiologist and/or vascular surgeon. If the decision is made to discontinue aspirin preoperatively, it should be held for 7 days prior to surgery.

Immunosuppressive Agents

- *Corticosteroids* have been shown to impair wound healing in both animal models and clinical studies.
- Clinical studies have also demonstrated a higher rate of anastomotic complications in patients on chronic steroids.
- A meta-analysis evaluating the risk of corticosteroids on colorectal anastomotic integrity demonstrated an overall leak rate of 6.77% compared to 3.26% in the non-corticosteroid group.
- In addition, corticosteroids impact wound healing, are a risk factor for the development of superficial and deep surgical site infections, and have even been shown to impact postoperative mortality.
- *Immunomodulators*, including azathioprine and 6-mercaptopurine, are used in both Crohn's disease and ulcerative colitis to maintain steroid-induced remission. These drugs often take 3–4 months until clinical benefit is apparent and

have infrequent but serious side effects such as leucopenia, liver function abnormalities, pancreatitis, and lymphoma. A retrospective study of 417 operations involving bowel anastomoses for Crohn's disease demonstrated no difference in the rate of anastomotic complications for patients on immunomodulators.

- *Biologic agents* include infliximab (Remicade), a chimeric monoclonal antibody that targets tumor necrosis factor, a pro-inflammatory cytokine that has been shown to be elevated in inflamed tissue of IBD patients. Biologics including infliximab have been demonstrated to induce remission and control symptoms in patients with moderate-to-severe Crohn's and ulcerative colitis. Overall the existing literature is limited and controversial, but biologic agents are thought to impact wound healing, and most surgeons prefer to hold these agents for 4–6 weeks if possible prior to major abdominal surgery.

Chemotherapy

- Through a myriad of mechanisms, the final common pathway of cytotoxic chemotherapy is induction of cell death. Ideally this effect is minimized in non-tumor cells, including healing anastomoses. Large studies have attempted to evaluate the overall effect of neoadjuvant and adjuvant chemotherapy on the rate of anastomotic leak, and there have been conflicting results.
- *Bevacizumab* (Avastin) is a humanized monoclonal antibody, which targets vascular endothelial growth factor A (VEGF-A), and is thought to work in solid tumors by restricting neoangiogenesis, which is necessary for tumor growth. It is the first of the antiangiogenic drugs to be approved for first-line treatment of metastatic colorectal cancer and is also used for other solid tumors including breast, kidney, ovarian, and lung cancer. Bevacizumab is associated with increased incidence of postoperative complications, including impaired wound healing and anastomotic leak. Bevacizumab has also been associated with late anastomotic complications. Other newer antiangiogenic drugs have also been implicated in the development of anastomotic leak, including pazopanib and aflibercept in small series and case reports. As with most chemotherapy agents, these agents are held for 6 weeks before major surgery, when possible.

7 Optimizing Outcomes with Enhanced Recovery

Conor P. Delaney and Raul Martin Bosio

Key Concepts

- Enhanced recovery pathways (ERPs) include measures for preoperative management, intraoperative care, postoperative recovery, and pathway quality evaluation.
- ERP improves the quality of patient care by establishing standardized care paths based on evidence-based literature and current practice guidelines.
- A modified frailty index (MFI) allows for preoperative risk stratification and identifies patients that will require extra healthcare resources.
- A combination of oral antibiotics administered during the preoperative phase combined with intravenous antibiotics administered within 1 h of surgery appears to be the most efficacious strategy to decrease SSI.
- Measurement of ERP compliance is necessary to make sure the individual stated pathway items are being accomplished.

C. P. Delaney (✉)
Department of Colorectal Surgery, Digestive Disease Institute, Cleveland Clinic, Cleveland, OH, USA
e-mail: DELANEC@ccf.org

R. M. Bosio
ProMedica Physicians General Surgery, Sylvania, OH, USA

Introduction

- Delivering high-quality patient-centered care while maintaining a low procedure-specific morbidity and readmission rate is important in the era of bundled payment, "pay for performance," and ongoing cuts in healthcare reimbursement.
- Minimally invasive techniques have had a major impact on postoperative recovery, contributing to a reduction in length of stay (LOS) and cost.
- Optimizing patient recovery goes beyond a particular technical approach and requires a multidisciplinary approach.
- Standardization of perioperative care measures combined with minimally invasive colorectal surgery can decrease length of stay without adversely affecting readmission rate.

What Is an Enhanced Recovery Pathway (ERP)?

- Traditionally, pre-, intra-, and postoperative management has varied (depending on individuals' practice preferences of the various members of the healthcare team involved) which increases complications and healthcare cost as patients are not necessarily managed according to current recommendations.

S. Steele et al. (eds.), *The ASCRS Manual of Colon and Rectal Surgery*,
https://doi.org/10.1007/978-3-030-01165-9_7

Table 7.1 Quality measures between patients managed within or outside an established enhanced recovery pathway (ERP)

Author	Within ERP	Outside ERP	Morbidity (ERP vs. non-ERP)	LOS (days) (ERP vs. non-ERP)	Readmission rates (ERPs vs. non-ERP)
Bradshaw et al. (1998)	36	36	8 vs. 11%	4.9 vs. 6	3 vs. 3%
Basse et al. (2002)	130	130	25 vs. 55%	3.3 vs. 10	21 vs. 12%
Anderson et al. (2003)	14	11	28 vs. 45%	3.9 vs. 6.9[a]	0 vs. 0%
Raue et al. (2004)	23	29	17 vs. 24%	4 vs. 7	4 vs. 7
Delaney et al. (2003)	33	31	22 vs. 30%	5.2 vs. 5.8[a]	9.7 vs. 18.2%
Gatt et al. (2005)	19	20	47 vs. 75%	6.6 vs. 9[a]	5.3 vs. 20%
Khoo et al. (2007)	35	35	25 vs. 51%	5 vs. 7[a]	9 vs. 3%
Serclova et al. (2009)	52	51	21 vs. 48%	7.4 vs. 10.4[a]	0 vs. 0%
Muller et al. (2009)	75	76	21 vs. 49%	6.7 vs. 10.3[a]	3.9 vs. 2.6%
LAFA (2011) laparoscopic	100	109	34 vs. 37%	5 vs. 6	6 vs. 6.4%
LAFA (2011) open	93	98	43 vs. 41%	6 vs. 7	7.4 vs. 7.1

Data obtained and combined into current table from Wind et al., Vlug et al., and Adamina et al.
[a]Mean length of stay (LOS)

- ERPs seek to create specific evidence-based protocols or pathways where the various components of pre-, intra-, and postoperative care are standardized, thus minimizing variability among providers.
- As patients progress through a healthcare intervention, specialty-specific order sets clearly outline patients' management at any given point in time, from the preoperative encounter until care is completed, generally at the time of hospital discharge.
- The consequences of the application of specialty-specific pathways are well documented and include a reduction in morbidity, mortality, and LOS (Table 7.1).

Where Does the Pathway Start?

- From a surgeons' perspective, an ERP starts with a surgeon implementing a specialty-specific order set.
- As the use of ERP is applicable to most specialties across the board, and affects hospitals' expenditure and therefore profit margins, more advanced setups require the participation of multiple teams (surgery, anesthesia, nursing, etc.).
- Institutional support facilitates their introduction and use.
- Creation of specialty-/department-specific committees allows for input from these teams to be incorporated into the ERP. Teams usually include but are not limited to surgeons, nursing staff, physical therapist, information technology, residents, respiratory therapist, and ostomy team members.

Components of an ERP

- From a practical standpoint, ERP can be divided in four parts: (a) preoperative management, (b) intraoperative care, (c) postoperative recovery, and (d) quality pathway evaluation measures.

Preoperative Management

Preoperative Evaluation: Frailty Score and Prehabilitation

- Patient factors can negatively affect outcome after elective colorectal surgery including nutritional status.
- Several tools can be used to evaluate nutritional status. The subjective global assessment (SGA) tool allows patients to be stratified in well, moderate, and severely malnourished (SGA-A, SGA-B, and SGA-C, respectively).

- Postoperative complications and LOS after colorectal surgery correlate with nutritional status, and preoperative nutritional support may improve nutrition within 2–3 weeks and decrease complications.
- Frailty, defined as a decrease in physiologic reserve and multisystem impairment independent of the normal aging process, is also a marker of increased postoperative morbidity and mortality.
- A modified frailty index (MFI) allows for preoperative risk stratification and may allow to identify patients that will require extra healthcare resources early on and to plan in accordance. Eleven variables are considered, and some of them can be optimized preoperatively, such as chronic obstructive pulmonary disease or congestive heart failure.
- Published data has demonstrated a correlation with LOS.
- Preoperative optimization is recommended when possible, and certain measures such as stopping alcohol or smoking 4 weeks prior to surgery are associated with improved outcomes.
- Prehabilitation, a term that refers to a structured process aim to improve patients' capacity to respond to surgical stress and decreased postoperative complications, is currently an area of research within ERP protocols.

Fasting Prior to Surgery, Mechanical Bowel Preparation, and Preoperative Antibiotics Usage

- Classic preoperative management teaching had focus on limitation of oral intake prior to surgery, the role of mechanical bowel preparation, and antibiotics usage.
- Traditionally, patients are asked to fast from midnight onward prior to surgery. Several studies have evaluated the role of carbohydrate loading prior to elective surgery which appears to be of some benefit in terms of decreasing postoperative insulin resistance, LOS, and patient satisfaction.
- The level of evidence is low, and further studies are required to determine how it may affect patient recovery.
- Independent of potential benefits, reducing fasting times and the usage of preoperative carbohydrate drinks up to 2 h prior to surgery is safe as there is no increased risk of anesthesia complications.
- Mechanical bowel preparation prior to colorectal surgery has been a topic of debate, with a large body of literature showing that there is no difference in outcomes whether mechanical preparation is used or not.
- A Cochrane review demonstrated no difference in wound infection, anastomotic leakage, intra-abdominal infectious complications, or need for reoperation independently of whether a mechanical bowel preparation was used or not.
- Colonic manipulation during laparoscopic surgery is easier when a mechanical bowel preparation is used.
- A long-term follow-up data from one study found a change in cancer-specific survival in favor of mechanical bowel preparation although a separate study found no difference in survival among groups (bowel preparation versus none).
- The authors use mechanical bowel preparation when a patient will be diverted, for left colon and rectal resections, when an intracorporeal anastomosis is planned, and in those cases that may require an intraoperative colonoscopy.
- The third component of the preoperative management includes the usage of antibiotics prior to surgery.
- Adequate coverage should include both aerobic and anaerobic flora.
- Meta-analyses have shown that there is a decreased in surgical wound infection (SSI) when antibiotics usage is compared to placebo.
- Surgeons currently administer antibiotics routinely within 1 h of the surgical starting time.
- The ideal regimen should not only control SSI but also consider cost and adverse effects of a selected regimen.

- Continuation of antibiotics beyond 24 h after elective surgery offers no benefit, and it is not recommended under current guidelines.
- It is the authors' practice to give oral antibiotics the day prior to surgery during the bowel preparation, followed by one dose in the operating room. Re-dosing varies depending on the antibiotic used half-life and the length of the case.

Patient Education

- From a surgeon-patient interaction perspective, an ERP starts in the first office visit because managing patients' expectations is important.
- Patient education is a key component of an ERP, and patients should be actively engaged in the recovery process.
- These goals and expectations can be discussed during the preoperative encounter and reinforced by written educational material.
- From a patient's perspective, being discharged home on postoperative day 2 or 3 after a major abdominal may be perceived as a daunting scenario. Easy accessibility to the healthcare team through healthcare extenders helps develop trust in the system and contributes to improve patient satisfaction.

Intraoperative Pathway

Minimally Invasive Colorectal Surgery

- Current data shows that only 50–70% of colorectal resections in the United States are performed in a minimally invasive fashion.
- The national average LOS after colorectal surgery reported by Medicare is approximately 9 days.
- LOS of 2–3 days is common after laparoscopic colorectal resections.
- The average cost per inpatient day in the United States varies between $1625 and $2025 (2010 data). This difference in LOS represents gross savings of approximately $9750 per patient per hospital stay.
- Early hospital discharge has been associated with readmission rates comparable to patients being managed outside an ERP.
- ERP can be successfully applied for patients undergoing open colorectal procedures, with data supporting a decreased in morbidity and LOS compared to non-pathway patients.

Intraoperative Fluid Administration

- Fluid administration during surgery is an area of ongoing debate.
- As fluid homeostasis is affected by changes in several hormones during the postoperative period, the amount of fluid given during the surgery itself varies significantly based on individual practices.
- Historically, fluid resuscitation tends to overestimate requirements which translate into early postoperative weight gain secondary to fluid retention and third spacing.
- Studies using restrictive fluid resuscitation strategies have shown a decrease in cardiopulmonary complications and LOS without an adverse effect in anastomotic leakage or surgical specific complications.
- The data is not clear regarding the optimal strategy. Studies used different regimens, with variations in the type of fluid used and variations in the parameters used to guide fluid resuscitation (intraoperative clinical parameters or measurement of intraoperative "real-time" volume status transesophageal Doppler or transcutaneous monitors).
- Currently, intraoperative restrictive fluid administration appears to be superior to traditional intraoperative fluid resuscitation protocols, and a standardized anesthesia protocol should be established as part of an ERP.
- Further studies are necessary to determine the role of goal-directed therapy, independently of whether intraoperative transesophageal Doppler monitoring or finger-probe monitoring is used, as there may be a subset of patients that could benefit from this technology.

Analgesia

- Pain control starts prior to surgery and continues during the procedure and the hospital stay and is adequately maintained based on specific patient needs after discharge.
- Adequate pain controlled is of paramount importance after surgery, as patients are more likely to ambulate and resume some routine daily activities sooner when postoperative pain is well managed.
- There is no ideal pain regimen as analgesia requirements vary from patient to patient.
- Ideally, the selected analgesia regimen will control patients' pain while minimizing the development of adverse effects, such as PONV, POI, hypotension, or kidney injury, among others.
- Blocking nociceptor activation prior to a painful stimulus, a term described as "preemptive" analgesia. High-quality data to support its usage is scarce.
- Preemptive analgesia includes multiple interventions, from oral analgesic administration starting the day prior to surgery to placement of epidural catheters or spinal analgesia prior to the beginning of the procedure or local infiltration of the surgical sites in the case of laparoscopy. Nonsteroidal anti-inflammatory drugs (NSAIDS) such as ibuprofen or diclofenac are usually incorporated into the ERP and administered starting 24 hours prior or the day of surgery.
- Gabapentin, a central acting agent, can also be started in the preoperative stage, and it is part of the ERP protocol used by the authors.
- Intraoperatively, local infiltration of the surgical port sites has not shown to decrease postoperative pain requirements. Liposomal bupivacaine may be used; however there is yet no evidence to support its use.
- Peripheral nerve blocks such as a transverse abdominis muscle plane (TAP) block have shown to decrease postoperative opioid usage. It is a technically simple, low-cost procedure that can easily be performed under laparoscopic or ultrasound guidance.
- Postoperative analgesia has also been subject to extensive debate. The use of epidural analgesia versus a combination of intravenous opioids delivered using patient controlled analgesia (PCA) equipment and scheduled intravenous NSAIDS and/or paracetamol appears to be similar in controlling pain in most cases. Although the use of epidurals catheters may improve pain scores initially, overall pain control, LOS, and patient satisfaction appear to favor the latter.
- The combination of an opioid PCA and intravenous ketorolac or acetaminophen in the initial postoperative phase (postoperative day 0 or 1) followed by a combination of these medications by mouth as soon as patients start oral intake is favor by the author and is part of the standard ERP protocol and the electronic order sets.
- A combination of epidural analgesia administered and intravenous opioids and NSAIDS is an alternative that should be considered in chronic opioid users. Epidurals analgesia may be limited to the administration of a local anesthetic or to a combination of a local anesthetic and opioids.
- A one-time intrathecal administration of an opioid and local anesthetic (0.5% bupivacaine) followed by a combination of a narcotics PCA and NSAIDS may be superior than both of the abovementioned options. However it is an invasive procedure, and further data is required to determine its real impact on LOS. It is not currently part of the authors' ERP.

Venous Thromboembolism (VTE) Prophylaxis

- SCIP guidelines require starting venous thromboembolism prophylaxis within 24 h of surgery which is commonly built in as part of the mandatory electronic admission order sets.
- This allows for variability in the usage of the medication, as surgeons may opt to administer it prior to the surgical procedure itself or within the 24 h period.

- Data supporting the use of either unfractionated heparin or low molecular weight heparin shows very little difference between these prophylactic agents.
- A Cochrane meta-analysis that included four randomized trials demonstrated a reduction in VTE from 1.7% to 0.2% when prophylaxis was maintained for 4 weeks.
- However, a database review of more than 52,000 patients found that the prevalence of postoperative symptomatic VTE after only inpatient prophylaxis was 0.67%.
- A recently published randomized controlled trial of 1 vs. 4 weeks of pharmacological VTE prophylaxis specifically after colorectal laparoscopic surgery showed that VTE occurred in 9.7% vs. 0.9%, respectively. Symptoms of VTE were present in only two and one patient, respectively. No episodes of pulmonary embolism occurred in either group. Guidelines indicated that prophylaxis should be continued for 4 weeks, especially in oncologic patients.
- In our practice patients with limited mobility, being discharge to a skilled nursing facility, with morbid obesity, with advanced malignancies, with coagulation disorders, or with prior history of VTE or PE are usually discharged on a 4-week course.

Postoperative Recovery

Analgesia

- Pain control should continue during the inpatient stay and continue after discharge, but a gradual decrease in medications usage is expected.
- Medication (both opioids and NSAIDS) should be prescribed keeping this in mind and considering the potential for abuse associated with narcotics usage.
- The amount of narcotics usage in the United States is significantly higher when compared to the rest of the world, and efforts are being implemented at a government level to monitor opioid usage. A fine line is required to maintain adequate pain controlled and patients' satisfaction while preventing abuse.

Intravenous Fluid Management

- ERP have demonstrated the safety of initiating early oral intake, thus being able to decrease intravenous fluid requirements.
- Published data indicate that restricting intravenous fluids to less than <2 l/d versus >3 l/day is associated with increased gastric emptying, faster recovery of gastrointestinal function, and overall decreased morbidity and LOS.

Early Oral Feeding, Ambulation, and Role of Nasogastric Tube

- A large body of literature has shown that early introduction of oral intake within 24 hours of surgery is safely tolerated in 70–90% of patients.
- A Cochrane review and a meta-analysis fail to show a reduction in LOS when early feeding is introduced.
- Numerous single institution reports over the last 10 years or more have reported average LOS of just over 2 days, and restarting oral intake within the first day of surgery has been an integral part of their ERPs.
- Early feeding increases the risk of vomiting, but the risk of aspiration pneumonia remains the same whether feeding is started early on or after return of bowel function.
- Encouraging and facilitating early ambulation through the aid of ancillary staff while the patient is still in the hospital is key to achieve the goal of a short LOS. Early ambulation helps decrease muscle waste and helps prevent a reduction in gastrointestinal motility associated with an increased time in bed.

Prevention of Postoperative Nausea and Vomiting (PONV) and Postoperative Ileus (POI): Role of Nasogastric Tube and Motility Agents

- ERP routinely includes medications that try to decrease PONV and prevent the development of POI. Several classes of antiemetics are available, and each class has been shown to be superior to placebo in the management of PONV. A combination of two or more drugs decreases even further the incidence of PONV.
- A single dose of intravenous dexamethasone during surgery combined with ondansetron (serotonergic 5-HT3 receptor antagonists) appears to be the most adequate strategy to prevent PONV.
- Ondansetron is continued during the postoperative period at a dose of 4 mg every 6–8 h as needed.
- For patients at increased risk of developing PONV, a combination of a transdermal scopolamine patch and ondansetron can be used with studies suggesting increased efficacy when compared to ondansetron alone.
- Postoperative ileus (POI) refers to a transient impairment in gastrointestinal motility that prevents oral intake.
- Classically, it has described as a delay to restart oral intake for more than 3 days after laparoscopic surgery or to more than 5 days after open procedures.
- Senagore et al. proposed an alternative classification by describing POI as any situation that requires a return to "nil per os" or the insertion of a nasogastric (NG) tube. He further defines ileus as primary or secondary based on whether it is associated (secondary) or not to any other complications (i.e., anastomotic leakage).
- Primary POI causes not only patient discomfort and delays hospital discharge; it is a significant cause of healthcare expenditure, accounting for approximately $750 million per year.
- Alvimopan, a peripheral acting mu-opioid receptor antagonist, has been shown to decrease the time required for return of gastrointestinal function and decrease POI and LOS after open and laparoscopic colorectal surgery.
- Its role after laparoscopic colorectal surgery and an established ERP is less clear.
- Delaney et al. described a reduction in POI from 4% to 12% when comparing two matched laparoscopic colectomy groups when alvimopan was used. However, LOS (3.6 vs. 3.7 days) and hospital readmission rates (4% vs. 4.2%) were the same in both groups (134–141).
- Oral magnesium oxide was described to facilitate return of bowel function after colonic surgery and as part of an ERP protocol. However, the data available is small and has not been validated in further studies.
- Bisacodyl, either orally or as a suppository, facilitates return of bowel function; however LOS is unchanged and the amount of data available is limited.
- Chewing sugarless gum postoperatively has also been associated with a decrease time to return of bowel function and decreased LOS. The level of evidence is very robust, and its associated cost and reported adverse effects (i.e., bloating) are minimal.
- Nasogastric tube decompression has been shown to have no role as a preemptive measure to prevent PONV or POI. Furthermore, it delays return of bowel function and hospital discharge. Therapeutic NG decompression still has a role in the treatment of POI; however its usage is required in less than 10% of patients.

Venous Thromboembolism (VTE) Prophylaxis

- VTE prophylaxis should be initiated within 24 h per SCIP guidelines. This topic has been addressed earlier on the chapter while discussing intraoperative management; however addressing VTE prophylaxis is mandatory during the postoperative period under current practice parameters.

Discharge Planning, Follow-Up, and Coordination of Care

- Discharge planning, follow-up, and coordination of care with other healthcare teams should be initiated early on during hospital stay.
- Incorporation of ancillary support staff such as nurse practitioners, stoma therapists, social workers, and physical therapists as member of the ERP team allows for active education, planning, and early identification of patients that may need home care or to be discharged to physical rehabilitation or extended care facilities and decreased unnecessary hospital stay secondary to poor planning or administrative delays such as insurance approval.

Quality Pathway Evaluation Measures

Electronic Order Sets Creation and Updates to Comply with Best Practice Parameters Guidelines and Evidence-Based Literature

- Creation of specialty-specific order sets requires the participation of the various members that contribute on a daily basis to patient care and application of the ERP.
- Data have shown that the initial cost of implementing an ERP is offset by the reduction in morbidity and LOS achieved with the subsequent pathway implementation.
- Regular meetings are required to ensure that the ERP and the associated order sets remain in compliance with changes in practice parameters, evidence-based guidelines, and government and insurance policies.

Implementation and Monitoring of Pathway Application

- Compliance and application of the numerous components of an ERP have been shown to vary within members of any given colorectal group.
- Changes in members of the ERP can impact the way ERPs are implemented, and morbidity and LOS may change accordingly. Mobile Internet-based applications currently exist and are being used in high-volume centers to monitor in real-time ERP pathway compliance and to identify variables that can affect its application, such as individual surgeon's preferences or a lack of support personnel.

Quality Improvement Measures

- Since the beginning of the century and secondary to high morbidity and mortality rates and a constant increase in healthcare cost, numerous programs have been developed to try to standardize care.
- With the objective of improving quality by decreasing variability among healthcare providers and containing cost, programs such as SCIP and National Surgical Quality Improvement Program (NSQIP) were developed. Over time, regional initiatives supported by private funding also developed as the opportunity to change individuals' practice styles toward an evidence-based and best practice guidance model was seen as a way to achieve those goals.
- Compliance with SCIP measures is becoming part of everyday practice. However, some of the standardize measures have failed to significantly improve quality.
- Internal practice monitoring and benchmarking them to national standards, as long as confounding variables can be included (i.e., tertiary center patients' complexity and postoperative morbidity), may allow physicians and hospitals to modify practice parameters and improve outcomes.

- An easy to apply metric to evaluate for quality in colorectal surgery was described by the senior author of this chapter. The HARM score takes into consideration hospital stay, readmission, and mortality rates. The score is calculated by giving each patient discharge a value from 1 to 10. As the mean hospital HARM score increases from <2, to 2–3, to 3–4, and more than 4, an increase in complication rates after elective colorectal surgery is seen, ranging from 23% to 30.7%, to 39.5%, and 47.9%, respectively. This metric provides surgeons a low-cost tool to compare quality and may allow for identification of true-outlier performers.

8 Postoperative Complications

Andrew Russ and Gregory D. Kennedy

Key Concepts

- Thorough preoperative evaluation including assessment of social situation, cognitive status, and comorbidities contributes to safe postoperative recovery.
- Laparoscopic approach to colorectal surgery is associated with a decreased risk for postoperative complications.
- Risk for mortality after major postoperative complications is a reflection of surgeon as well as the system in which the surgeon operates.
- Meticulous operative technique with particular attention to hemostasis will lead to improved postoperative outcomes.
- Postoperative management with an enhanced recovery after surgery protocol leads to decreased postoperative complications.
- Bowel preparation with oral antibiotics correlates with a decreased risk of superficial surgical site infection.

A. Russ (✉)
Department of Surgery, University Colon and Rectal Surgery, University of Tennessee Medical Center, Knoxville, TN, USA
e-mail: ARuss@utmck.edu

G. D. Kennedy
Department of Surgery, University of Alabama-Birmingham, Birmingham, AL, USA

Introduction

- Postoperative complications are common in colorectal surgery with an incidence as high as 40%.

Preoperative Considerations and Prediction of Postoperative Complications

- Much current work focuses on prevention of complications.
- Many authors have used the American College of Surgeons National Surgical Quality Improvement Program (NSQIP) to characterize postoperative complications.
- One of the most significant developments is the ACS NSQIP Surgical Risk Calculator which uses procedure-specific information to provide an accurate prediction of risk for complications and length of stay.
- The ACS NSQIP calculator provides risk stratification that allows the patient to see their risk in the context of other more average-risk patients. Figure 8.1a and b is example reports.
- This type of informed consent allows surgeons to consider the outcomes that are most important to patients so they can make decisions that align with their goals of life.
- Risk prediction is dependent upon the accuracy of the data entered into the model, and

S. R. Steele et al. (eds.), *The ASCRS Manual of Colon and Rectal Surgery*,
https://doi.org/10.1007/978-3-030-01165-9_8

a

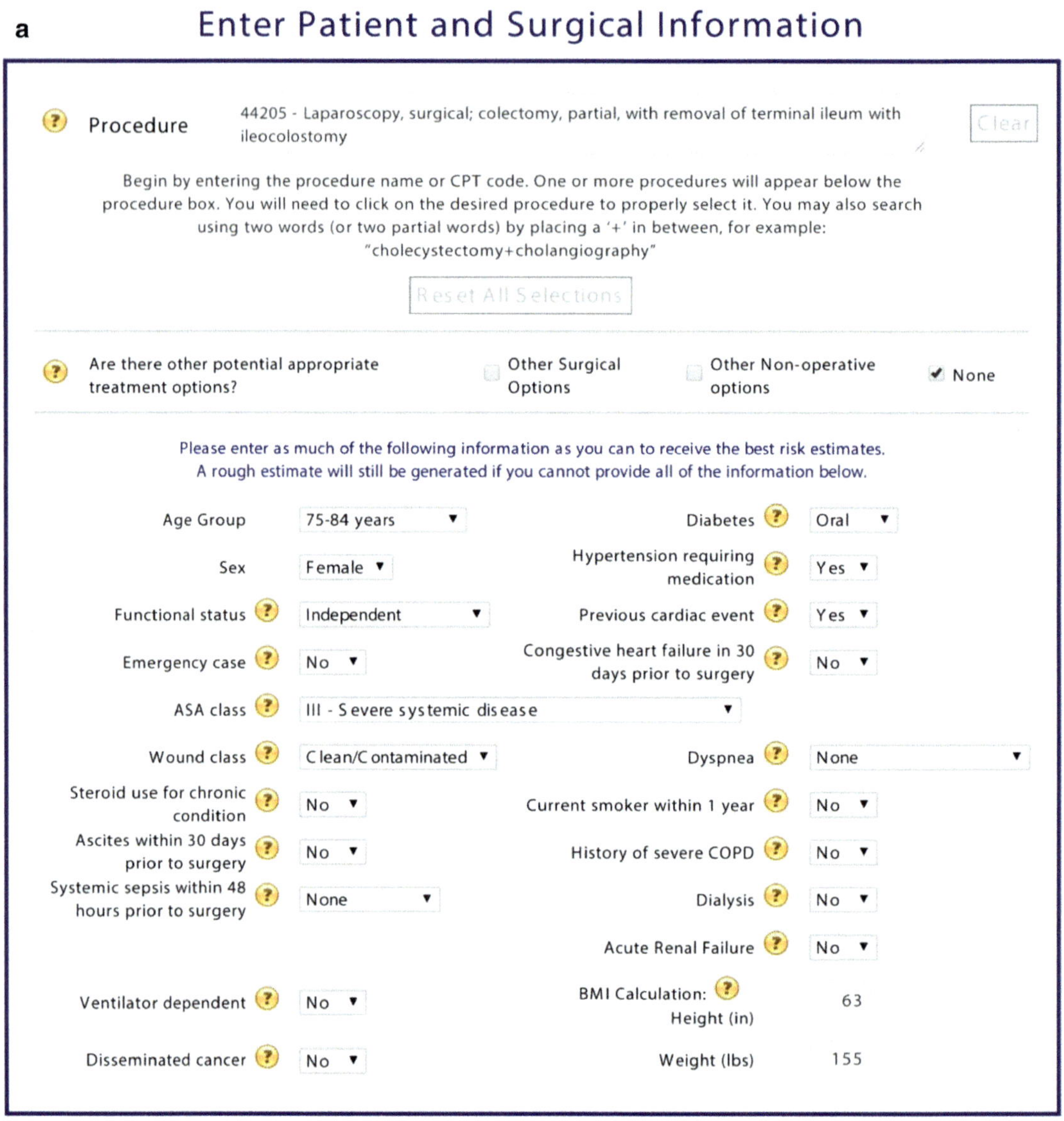

Fig. 8.1 A sample of the American College of Surgeons Risk Calculator is shown. The calculator was found at http://riskcalculator.facs.org/, and details of a made-up patient were inserted according to the instructions. (**a**) In this example, a 77-year-old female patient will undergo a laparoscopic right hemicolectomy. Her made-up comorbidities were inserted, and the risk calculator was run. (**b**) Results of the risk calculation were obtained and shown here. This sample patient was found to be of average risk for serious complication and slightly higher than average risk for any complication. Risks for specific complications are shown. (© American College of Surgeons, used with permission)

b

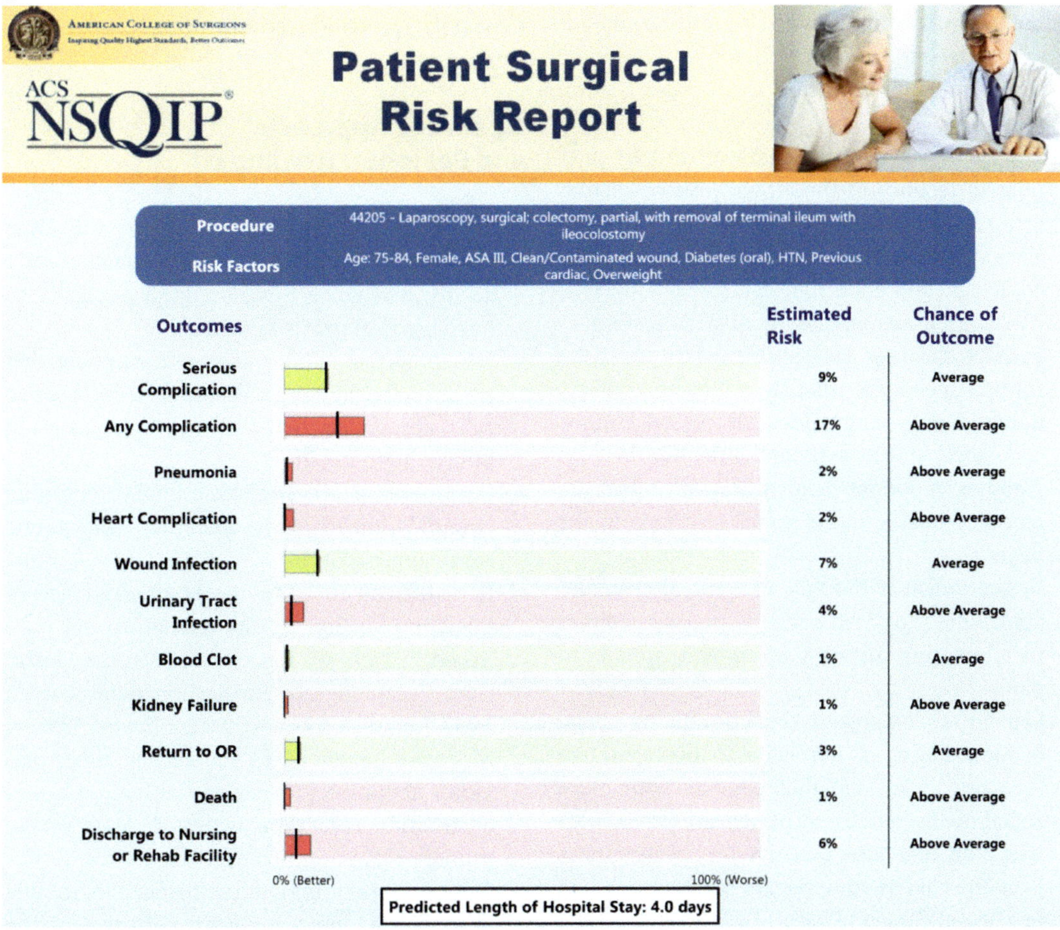

Fig. 8.1 (continued)

factors exist that impact the outcomes that cannot be measured by any specific model.

- Patient comorbidity clearly impacts risk for postoperative complications.
- As patients with surgical problems age, surgeons must be able to address issues that are specific to the older adult population such as frailty, cognitive impairment, and social support which impact patient outcomes.
- These variables are largely neglected by any current predictive nomogram, but it is clear that these factors contribute to postoperative outcomes.
- Cognitive impairment has been shown to correlate with discharge to a higher level of care in the older adult population.
- In one study, 41% of patients with a score ≤ 14 on the Mini-Mental Status Examination (MMSE) were discharged to a higher-level care facility compared to only 11% of patients who scored >14. Others have also found that preoperative cognitive impairment correlated with a higher risk for postoperative complications, longer length of stay, and higher 6-month mortality.
- Cognitive impairment also correlated with longer length of stay and higher 6-month

mortality. Taken together, the data indicate that cognitive impairment should be considered an important predictor of outcome when dealing with the older adult population.

- Frailty is a syndrome characterized by age-related declines in functional reserves across an array of physiologic systems.
- The syndrome is highly prevalent in older adults and confers a high risk for falls, disability, hospitalization, and institutionalization.
- Perhaps the best measurement is termed the frailty phenotype that is characterized by unintentional weight loss, decreased energy, and decrease in activity and strength.
- Another important factor likely to impact the recovery course is the social structure of the patient.
- In general, it is thought that social structure contributes to postoperative recovery either in alleviating anxiety, pain, or response to pain.
- One group examined the concept of social connectedness as it relates to postoperative recovery and found that patients with more social connectedness experienced less subjective pain and less perceived unpleasantness from the pain as compared to patients who had less social connectedness.
- It is not understood if connectedness contributes to recovery after suffering a major complication or if the concept of connectedness contributes to a patient's underlying risk for suffering a postoperative complication.
- Quality measures, including outcomes related to safety, effectiveness, and patient centeredness, are already included in many facets of clinical practice such as credentialing and reimbursement. Therefore, it is imperative that all surgeons embrace these measures, become more comfortable with the details, and strive to improve outcomes.
- Future work will focus on enhancing the scoring systems as well as understanding how a surgeon can modify the approach to improve surgical outcomes.

Intraoperative Factors that Contribute to Postoperative Outcomes

Operative Approach and Postoperative Impact

- Laparoscopy for colon surgery was first reported in a small case series in the early 1990s, and since then, multiple publications have highlighted its benefits.
- It is important to consider those endpoints that are affected by surgical approach in order to fully appreciate the benefit of laparoscopy in improving outcomes.
- Postoperative bowel obstruction is a common complication of many abdominal and pelvic surgical procedures.
- It is difficult to know the exact incidence of this complication, but a landmark paper published in 1999 by Beck et al. used the Health Care Financing Administration dataset from 1993 found that between 12.4% and 17% of Medicare beneficiaries undergoing either pelvic or abdominal operations suffered a bowel obstruction sometime within 2 years of the primary operation.
- Others have found the incidence of bowel obstruction due to adhesive disease to be less than 3% and to be dependent upon the cavity in which the operation was performed.
- The evidence regarding the impact of laparoscopy on the development of postoperative bowel obstruction is mixed.
- In summary, the use of laparoscopy may decrease adhesion formation, which likely will result in lower rates of adhesive postoperative bowel obstruction.
- The impact of laparoscopy on other complications and outcomes is clearer.
- The prospective randomized controlled trial reported by the Clinical Outcomes of Surgical Therapy Study Group (COST) found that perioperative recovery was faster in subjects randomized to laparoscopy compared to those undergoing open procedures.

  - Rates of intraoperative complications, 30-day mortality, complications at discharge and at 60 days, hospital readmission, and reoperation were similar between groups.
- Results from the MRC CLASICC trial demonstrated shorter length of stay for patients treated with a laparoscopic approach, with no difference in 30-day or 3-month complications.
- Comparative effectiveness studies looking at the issue of laparoscopic versus open approach to colon surgery in general have found that minimally invasive techniques are correlated with improved short-term outcomes.
- These studies report at least a 50% reduction in superficial surgical site infections, a 50% reduction in deep wound infection, and a significant reduction in postoperative length of stay in patients who have a laparoscopic operation.
- These studies have generally reported similar mortality associated with the two approaches.

Luminal Organ Injuries and Postoperative Impact

- In 2003, the Agency for Healthcare Research and Quality (AHRQ) proposed a set of patient safety indicators (PSIs) intended to reflect the quality of care delivered in hospitals.
- Several PSIs are included in the current CMS pay for performance plan, directly affecting reimbursement, and are presumed to be preventable by provider or system changes and include iatrogenic events such as accidental puncture or laceration (APL) during a procedure.
- In over 2 million Veterans Health Administration admissions, 7023 were flagged for APL including serosal tears, enterotomy, and injury to the ureter, bladder, spleen, and blood vessels. Of these, 27% were minor injuries such as small serosal tears with no clinically significant impact.
- Evidence from the Cleveland Clinic group found that accidental puncture laceration was more correlated with complexity of the operation and largely had no impact on postoperative recovery.
- Since the rate of APL is publicly available and used in pay for performance models, it is important we fully understand the limitations of this PSI. These data suggest that the utility of APL is limited and better measures of safety are necessary if we are to compare organizations in a fair and non-biased fashion.

Vascular Injury and Failure of Hemostatic Devices

- Blood loss has been shown in many studies to correlate with outcomes across various different types of operations.
- Using the NSQIP PUF database, Greenblatt et al. found intraoperative blood transfusion to be significantly associated with postoperative complications in patients undergoing surgery for rectal cancer.
- These results are consistent with those found in the single-institution study published by Gu and others examining outcomes in patients undergoing ileal pouch-anal anastomosis.
- Halabi et al. demonstrated a dose-dependent effect of blood transfusion, with worse outcomes in patients receiving more than 3 or more units of blood compared to those receiving only 1–2 units of blood.
- These data indicate that careful attention to hemostasis is not only consistent with good operative technique but also contributes to decreased postoperative morbidity.
- The exact incidence of major vascular injury during colorectal surgery is unclear but relatively rare.
- Others have examined the rate of trocar injuries to the vasculature at the time of laparoscopy. Larobina and Nottle found a rate of 0.04% in a literature review which included over 760,000 patients and concluded that vascular injuries at the time of trocar insertion are rare and can be eliminated by an open, Hassan access technique.

- There are a myriad of minimally invasive and open instruments available for hemostasis during colorectal procedures.
- A Cochrane review looked at various commercially available instruments used for laparoscopic colectomy and found significantly less blood loss in studies using ultrasonic coagulating shears (UCS) compared to monopolar electrocautery scissors (MES).
  - Hemostatic control was found to be improved in UCS and electrothermal bipolar vessel sealers (EBVS) over MES.
  - This review also found that laparoscopic staples/clips used for pedicle ligation in colectomy were associated with more failures in vessel ligation and cost more when compared to EBVS.
- A randomized clinical trial comparing the cost and effectiveness of bipolar sealers versus clip and vascular staples for laparoscopic colorectal resection found that bipolar sealers reduced both the time spent and the cost of disposable instruments for achieving vascular control.
- Another prospective randomized trial by Marcello and colleagues found increased failure rates in cases where vascular staplers and clips were used for pedicle ligation, but the amount of blood loss associated with device failure was higher in those using EBVS for pedicle ligation.
- There are now multiple instruments capable of 7 mm vessel sealing with various other capabilities.
- Based on the current available literature, electrothermal bipolar vessel sealing allows for faster operating times, less blood loss, and less sealing failure.
- It is the authors' practice to take vascular pedicles with an electrothermal bipolar vessel sealing device. For device failure or inadequate seal, we favor the use of clips or alternatively an endoloop, as blindly sealing vessels in a crimson field is often fraught with complication.
- In the setting of a known atherosclerotic vessel, the application of a vascular stapler should be considered.

Urologic Injuries and Their Management

Ureteral Injury

- Iatrogenic ureteral injury has a documented incidence of 0.3–1.5%.
- Risk factors for ureteral injury include the presence of rectal cancer, adhesions, metastatic cancer, weight loss/malnutrition, and teaching hospitals.
- Palaniappa et al. found a significantly higher rate of ureteral injury associated with laparoscopic colectomy compared to open (0.66% vs. 0.15%, $P < 0.05$). Female sex, increased operative blood loss, and reoperation conferred an increased risk of iatrogenic injury. Ureteral injuries were associated with higher morbidity and mortality, longer length of stay, and higher hospital charges by over $30,000.
- Preoperative or intraoperative ureteral catheterization is sometimes used to aid in identification of the ureters and subsequent injury.
- Most data suggest that placement of ureteral stents neither reduces the incidence of injury nor ensures intraoperative identification of injury.
- In a NSQIP analysis, there was an increasing trend of ureteral stent use over time from 1.1% to 4.4% from 2005 to 2011. There were no statistically significant differences in any primary or secondary endpoints (including overall renal complications), but there was a significant increase in length of stay with stent utilization.
- Early identification of injury is paramount in minimizing morbidity and preserving renal function.
- Diagnosis of a suspected injury can be confirmed with an on-table intravenous pyelogram (IVP), retrograde injection of methylene blue, intravenous administration of methylene blue or indigo carmine, or ureteral catheter contrast administration.
- Transection and laceration are repaired based on location of injury.
- General principles include use of absorbable suture, tension-free spatulated anastomosis

over an indwelling stent, and placement of a closed suction drain.

- For those injuries in the proximal one-third (2% of injuries), repair depends on length of the damaged segment: (1) simple spatulated ureteroureterostomy (U-U) is the preferred method of repair; (2) for mobilization, a nephropexy can be performed with fixation to the psoas tendon; and (3) bowel interposition can be utilized for long segment damage.
- The preferred method of injuries to the middle third account (7% of injuries) repair is via ureteroureterostomy for short segment injury with a psoas hitch or Boari flap if a tension-free anastomosis is not possible. A less desirable option is transureteroureterostomy (TUU) (anastomosis to the contralateral uninjured ureter).
- Injuries to the distal one-third of the ureter are preferentially repaired with ureteroneocystostomy with psoas hitch or Boari flap used if adequate length is not present. Foley catheter should be left in place for 7–14 days with stent removal 4–6 weeks after surgery.

Bladder Injury

- Bladder injury can present in a delayed fashion or at the time of initial surgery.
- Risk factors include previous operations, radiation treatment, malignant infiltration, chronic infection, and inflammatory conditions.
- Radiographic diagnosis can be obtained with CT cystogram or fluoroscopic cystogram.
- Primary repair (cystorrhaphy) with placement of closed suction drains is the preferred approach when injury is immediately recognized.
- Small extraperitoneal injuries can be effectively treated with 7–14 days of Foley catheter decompression.
- For injuries to the ventral bladder, dome, or posterior bladder away from ureteral orifices, the bladder can be repaired primarily with 2-layer mucosal and seromuscular closure using absorbable suture.
- Permanent suture must be avoided to prevent the long-term development of bladder stones.
- For injuries involving the posterior bladder or trigone, near the ureteral orifices, inspection for ureteral injury is mandatory and can be accomplished via cystotomy.
- Indigo carmine can then be administered intravenously to aid in identification of ureteral orifices. Posterior repair is then performed through this anterior cystotomy.
- Delayed diagnosis of urine leak from the bladder is often managed with percutaneous drainage of an urinoma and continued Foley catheter decompression.
- Consider consultation with specialized services when faced with these injuries.

Urethral Injury

- The least frequent intraoperative urologic injury involves those to the urethra.
- The most common urethral injury during colon and rectal surgery is related to traumatic Foley catheter placement.
- Direct injuries also occur during extirpative surgery.
- Many of these patients have a history of radiation therapy and are prone to fistula formation.
- The most common presentation of a urethral injury is postoperatively by virtue of fistula formation.
- Cystoscopy, retrograde urethrogram, exam under anesthesia, and CT scan with both oral and rectal contrast help to delineate the location of injury.
- Primary repair at the time of injury in two layers with absorbable suture is the preferred method. An omental flap or local tissue flap can reduce the risk of postoperative fistula formation.
- In the case of extensive urethral loss recognized at the time of surgery, local tissue flaps may be used to aid in reconstruction. If repair is not feasible, a suprapubic catheter should be placed, and repair can be performed after several months.
- Injuries recognized postoperatively are staged according to location, size, and history of radiation treatment.

- Stage 1 – low (<4 cm from anal verge, non-irradiated)
- Stage 2 – high (>4 cm from anal verge, non-irradiated)
- Stage 3 – small (<2 cm diameter irradiated)
- Stage 4 – large (>2 cm diameter irradiated)
- Stage 5 – large (ischial decubitus fistula)

- Principles of repair include transection and closure of fistulas and placement of interposed local or regional tissue flaps or grafts.
- Fecal diversion is recommended for stages 3 through 5.
- A suprapubic catheter is recommended in addition to a Foley catheter for adequate decompression and drainage.
- Trans-anal advancement flap alone can be performed for stage 1 fistulas or in combination with other techniques for higher stage fistulas.
- Perineal or transsphincteric approaches have also been described.
- Other approaches include interposition of regional myofascial flaps alone or in combination with abdominoperineal pull-through with resection of the fistula and hand-sewn colo-anal anastomosis.

Postoperative Management Decisions that Contribute to Postoperative Complications

IV Fluid Management

- Improper administration of intravenous fluids contributes to postoperative complications.
- In one study 20 patients were randomly allocated to either standard fluid management or a restricted fluid protocol. Restricted fluid patients had earlier return of bowel function, shorter length of stay, and lower rates of complications.
- A meta-analysis of randomized controlled trials found that length of stay was reduced by an average of 2.5 days and postoperative morbidity was 50% lower in patients managed on an ERAS protocol (including fluid restriction) compared to those receiving standard postoperative care.
- Outside of an ERAS protocol, the management of fluids should be tailored to each individual patient.
- In general, the data indicate that fluid restriction is a critical part of an ERAS protocol and that patients have improved outcomes when managed on these types of regimented pathways.

Wound Management

- There are some general recommendations that may lead to lower rates of postoperative superficial surgical site infections (SSI).
- Dressings are considered a standard of care in the management of surgical wounds, but there has been no standardization.
- A recent Cochrane review on the topic of wound dressings and their effect on wound infection found no evidence that one type of wound dressing decreased incidence of SSI over any other type.
- Table 8.1 lists features of an ideal wound dressing.
- The utility of a negative pressure wound dressing on primarily closed wounds for the prevention of wound infections has been examined, and in general, the work with negative pressure units are filled with bias, and the

Table 8.1 Features of an ideal wound dressing

1. The ability of the dressing to absorb and contain exudate without leakage or strike-through
2. Lack of particulate contaminants left in the wound by the dressing
3. Thermal insulation
4. Impermeability to water and bacteria
5. Suitability of the dressing for use with different skin closures (sutures, staples)
6. Avoidance of wound trauma on dressing removal
7. Frequency with which the dressing needs to be changed
8. Provision of pain relief
9. Cosmesis and comfort
10. Effect on formation of scar tissue

role for this technology for the prevention of wound infections remains to be seen.

- The etiology of a wound infection is largely unknown.
- Contamination at the time of surgery contributes to risk for infection, but it is also possible that wound hematoma or seroma may be the inciting event.
- Towfigh and others randomized 76 patients with high-risk wounds to either daily wound probing or standard wound management and showed that patients treated with daily wound probing had lower rates of SSI (3% vs. 19%). These results have never been reproduced or expanded to a larger population in general or colorectal surgery.

Bladder Management

- Urinary tract infection (UTI) and catheter-associated UTI (CAUTI) are frequently encountered postoperative complications related to colorectal surgery procedures.
- A study from the NSQIP PUF (participant use file) found the rate of UTI after colorectal resection to be 4.1% compared to 1.8% after other general surgery operations.
- Factors that correlated with an increased risk for developing a postoperative UTI included female sex, ASA class >2, procedure of a total colectomy, proctocolectomy, or APR, functional status of partially or totally dependent, and age greater than 75.
- Other significant factors such as presence of indwelling catheter, number of catheter days, and incidence of postoperative urinary retention are known to strongly associate with risk for UTI, but are unfortunately not included in the NSQIP database.
- In 2008 the Centers for Medicare and Medicaid Services (CMS) implemented a policy whereby they would reduce payment for hospitalizations that included a preventable complication. Included among these hospital-acquired conditions is the surveillance measure of catheter-associated urinary tract infection (CAUTI).
- Best practices and care bundles have been widely published in attempts to decrease the rates of CAUTI.
- The question facing surgeons is how to effectively do this while still managing the patient according to a standard of care.
- For example, if all catheters are discontinued upon completion of an operation, we will certainly reduce the rate of CAUTI in our patient population, but Kwaan et al. have found that early removal of the urinary catheter increases rates of urinary retention in patients undergoing pelvic surgery – resulting in increased rates of catheter reinsertion.
- These high rates of urinary retention lead to increased catheter reinsertion, which likely contributes to an increased rate of urinary tract infection in patients who suffer postoperative urinary retention (POUR).
- Therefore, before a policy of early catheter removal can be instituted for all patients undergoing colorectal surgery, we must better understand the problem of POUR and implement effective methods to deal with this complex problem.

Pain Management

- Perioperative pain is a potent trigger for the stress response that can activate the autonomic nervous system and may contribute to adverse postoperative outcomes.
- While there is very little evidence that poor pain control itself contributes to worse postoperative outcomes, one study found that hospitals with low patient satisfaction scores related to pain control had higher rates of postoperative mortality compared to similar hospitals.
- While it is not clear if poor pain control contributes to complications, very few surgeons will argue against the principle of good pain control in order to ensure humane, high-quality postoperative care of all patients.
- Because of the many obvious negative implications of poor pain control, many studies have assessed the best route of analgesic delivery.

- Many studies have examined intravenous versus epidural delivery of pain medications and have, in general, found that epidural delivery results in improved postoperative pain control, whereas other studies have found no real differences between epidural and patient-controlled intravenously delivered analgesia.
- Randomized controlled trials of laparoscopic versus open colectomy have found pain scores to be generally decreased in patients undergoing laparoscopic colectomy.
- A meta-analysis recently published found that although pain control was improved by the use of an epidural in patients undergoing laparoscopic colectomy, there was no difference in return of bowel function and no impact on length of stay.
- Enhanced recovery after surgery protocols has largely adopted non-opioid-based pain regimens, and more work is focusing on local blocks, such as the transversus abdominis plane (TAP) block, to enhance pain control.
- Regardless, it is clear that adequate pain control improves the overall patient experience.

Impact of Hospital Structure on Postoperative Complications

Academic Medical Center

- The impact of resident training on patient outcome has long been debated in both the academic and lay press.
- Kiran et al. found a correlation between increased rates of complications and resident involvement in patient care but also found that resident participation was associated with a lower rate of failure to rescue.
- Englesbe et al. examined the rate of complications according to the time of year using the NSQIP dataset and found that patients treated later in the academic year had lower rates of mortality and morbidity.
- Summarizing the available data is not entirely clear that trainee presence is independently associated with postoperative complications. Furthermore, mortality rates after major complications seem to be lower in hospitals that have training programs.

Surgical Volume and Postoperative Complications

- Much has been written on the effect of surgical volume on complications.
- There may be a very complex interplay between the volume of the surgeon and the volume of the institution.
- This interplay can be seen quite nicely in two papers written by Dr. Birkemeyer and colleagues, which described a relationship between hospital volume and postoperative mortality for specific complicated operations.
  - They found that the rate of mortality after all resections, including proctectomy, decreased as the volume of the procedure increased at the hospital.
  - The group then expanded this work and looked at the impact of provider volume on these mortality rates and found that provider volume could mitigate some of the effect of the institutional volume for some operations.
  - The end result is a complex relationship between provider and institutional volume suggesting that the system in which a patient undergoes an operation contributes to outcomes. This type of work has been demonstrated multiple times using many different datasets over the years although little has been accomplished in understanding the mechanism behind this complex observation.

Prevention and Management of Specific Complications

Wound Complications

- Wound complications and, specifically, surgical site infections (SSIs) are among the most common source of nosocomial morbidity for patients undergoing surgical procedures.
- SSIs are associated with increased hospital length of stay, increased risk of mortality, and decreased health-related quality of life.
- Wound infections are commonly thought of as occurring in the superficial tissues, deep tissues, or in the organ space.

- It has been estimated that a SSI adds between $10,000 and $25,000 to the care of a patient depending on extent of infection.
- Preoperative, perioperative, and postoperative interventions have been implemented in an attempt to decrease the rates of wound infections in all patients.

Preoperative Considerations

- There are a myriad of patient-specific factors that predispose to an increased risk of perioperative complications.
- Elevated BMI has been a validated risk factor for SSIs, with some reporting SSI rate as high as 60% among obese patients. However, BMI does not account for all of the obesity-associated risk with wound infection, and there has been recent interest in the role of waist circumference (WC) and waist-to-hip ratio (WHR) on the development of perioperative outcomes.
- To evaluate the effect of WC and WHR on surgical complications, a prospective, multicenter, international study of 1349 patients undergoing elective colorectal surgery was performed. Increased WHR was identified as an independent predictor of intraoperative complications, conversion, medical complications, and re-interventions, whereas increased BMI was a risk factor only for abdominal wall complications.
- Another well-established risk factor for SSI is administration of allogeneic blood transfusion.

Perioperative Interventions

- The role of mechanical bowel preparation in the prevention of SSIs has been extensively studied and debated. The data are conflicting, and often times, the arguments for or against bowel preparation relate more to personal preference than to evidence. There have been three recent meta-analyses of RCTs evaluating the need for mechanical bowel prep prior to surgery.
- One study evaluating nine RCTs demonstrated a significant increase in the percentage of anastomotic leak in prepared patients (6.2% vs. 3.2% [OR 2.03]). An update of this analysis failed to detect significant differences in anastomotic leakage or SSI between those patients receiving and not receiving bowel preps. A second meta-analysis similarly found no difference in anastomotic leakage rates; however, analysis of secondary outcomes yielded a significant difference in SSI, favoring no MBP.
- Despite these results, the majority of colorectal surgeons still favor the use of mechanical bowel prep. Reasons for this include improved handling of a prepared colon and reduction of stool burden proximal to a fresh anastomosis. A large retrospective review of nearly 10,000 patients did not find any difference in SSI between those with and without MBP. However, the use of oral antibiotics alone was associated with a 67% decrease in SSI, and oral antibiotics plus mechanical bowel prep was associated with a 57% decreased in SSI.
- Various skin prep techniques and products are available for colorectal procedures, but clear evidence supporting one over another is lacking.
- In one randomized controlled trial, the use of chlorhexidine-alcohol rather than povidone-iodine was shown to significantly reduce both superficial surgical site infections and deep incisional infections.

Another group performed a sequential implementation study in which different skin preparation agents were serially used over the course of a defined time period and found the lowest rates of SSI in the time frame that used iodine povacrylex in isopropyl alcohol.

- Another relatively straightforward intervention at the time of operation that may prevent superficial SSI is the use of a wound protector.
- While there are conflicting data regarding the utility of these devices in preventing wound infections in abdominal surgery, a recent randomized study and a meta-analysis found that the use of a wound protector was significantly associated with reduced incidence of incisional SSI.

- A meta-analysis of prospective randomized trials of supranormal levels of oxygen during anesthesia demonstrated a significant decrease in SSI with the use of 80% FI02 in the perioperative setting, favoring the use of perioperative hyperoxia.
- In contrast, a recent multicenter study [PROXI] that randomized patients to receive 80% FI02 intraoperatively and 2 h postoperatively versus 30% FI02 in a similar fashion found no difference in outcomes.
- None of these studies reported any adverse events attributable to the administration of supranormal levels of oxygen.
- Another readily available intervention that has been shown to reduce SSI in colorectal surgery patients involves the application of an active warming strategy perioperatively.
- Multiple reports have demonstrated the utility of closing the midline wound with a suture length-to-wound length ratio of at least 4. This technique mandates taking either >10 mm fascial bites at greater intervals than previously recommended or alternatively smaller bites of the fascial edge (5–8 mm) in closer intervals. These techniques were compared in a randomized controlled trial which demonstrated a significant increase in SSI and incisional hernia when utilizing the former approach.
- Specific to colorectal surgery, ileostomy closure poses a unique challenge with regard to infection. In this setting, purse-string closure of ileostomy wounds has been significantly associated with reduced SSI rate in a meta-analysis of three RCTs.
- In summary, multiple low-risk perioperative interventions can be taken together (bundled) which may contribute to improved outcomes.

Management of Superficial Surgical Site Infection

- Regardless of the interventions taken to prevent these hospital-acquired infections, it seems the most efficient method involves standardizing the practice to include a bundle of care that is included for every operation.
- Monitoring of compliance with the care bundle is also critically important as compliance with all parts of a bundle correlates with a lower risk of wound infection (2.5% in those hospitals with 100% compliance compared to 17.5% in those hospitals that were the most noncompliant).
- The adoption of bundled care ensures all members of the surgical team are focused on the safety of the patient and gives the team a template from which to work.
- Despite all attempts to prevent surgical site infections in colorectal surgery, the average institution will continue to see rates of infections near 10%.
- For an uncomplicated superficial surgical site infection, the standard treatment is drainage of the infection and local wound care without the routine use of antibiotics.
- If patients exhibit signs and symptoms of shock, one must suspect the presence of a deeper infection (including organ space), and aggressive interventional therapy or reoperation may be required.

Cardiovascular and Respiratory Complications

- In the previously mentioned study of 1349 patients, which identified elevated waist/hip ratio (WHR) as a predictor for postoperative complications, the incidence of stroke, deep venous thrombosis, myocardial infarction, congestive heart failure, and pulmonary embolism were all less than 1%.
- Postoperative venous thromboembolism carries a current prevalence of 1.4–2.4% in colorectal surgery patients and is one of the most important potentially preventable conditions leading to increases in morbidity, mortality, hospitalization length, and hospital charges.
- Risk-adjusted factors associated with DVT included age greater than 70, African-American race, ASA score >2, hypoalbuminemia, disseminated cancer, steroid used, and obesity. Other risks include open colorectal

procedures, emergently admitted patients, ulcerative colitis, and anesthesia length greater than 150 min.

- The majority of VTE and PE events occurred during the first week after surgery; however, 34.6% and 29.3% of patients diagnosed with VTE and PE, respectively, are diagnosed after discharge.
- These data underscore a possible role for anticoagulating after discharge.
- It is the authors' practice to administer 5000 units of unfractionated heparin (UFH) prior to skin incision and to immediately implement additional prophylaxis to include UFH or LWMH, on postoperative day 1. They do not routinely anticoagulate after discharge; however this practice should be considered as we evaluate the most recent literature.
- A recent randomized prospective analysis evaluating 1 week versus 4 week prophylaxis in patients undergoing laparoscopic colorectal surgery for colorectal cancer found a significant reduction in rates of VTE among those undergoing 4-week prophylaxis with LMWH with similar rates of bleeding between the two groups.

Mortality and Failure to Rescue

- Postoperative mortality is uncommon after elective colorectal surgery and even in the oldest patient populations undergoing elective colectomy for colon cancer, the rate of mortality is at most 4% in hospitals participating in the NSQIP program.
- In general, mortality after elective surgery does not occur in isolation but rather follows another major complication.
- The Agency for Healthcare Research and Quality (AHRQ) has defined death rate among surgical inpatients with serious treatable complications as a patient safety indicator in order to track this metric across institutions.
- Failure to rescue is considered a measure of system of care and is defined as death per 1000 surgical discharges among patients aged 18–89 with serious treatable complications such as deep vein thrombosis/pulmonary embolism, pneumonia, sepsis, shock/cardiac arrest, or gastrointestinal hemorrhage/acute ulcer.
- System-related factors such as number of hospital beds, teaching status, nurse-to-patient ratio, and high technology utilization correlate with low failure to rescue rates.

Long-Term Complications

- Many colorectal surgery interventions result in long-term physiological changes for patients. Effective management and patient counseling requires a thorough understanding of potential long-term complications and their natural history.

Genitourinary Complications

- Bladder dysfunction following colorectal surgery is most commonly related to extirpative procedures in the region of the autonomic pelvic plexus.
- Abdominoperineal resection and low anterior resection have incidences of postoperative bladder dysfunction of nearly 50% and 15–25%, respectively.
- The most common sequel of autonomic nerve damage during colorectal surgery is parasympathetic detrusor denervation, resulting in impaired contractility of the bladder. A majority of patients will regain the ability to empty the bladder; however this can take up to 6 months.
- If careful bladder care is neglected, deleterious effects such as hydronephrosis, urinary reflux, pyelonephritis, and declining renal function may ensue.

Fertility Complications

- Female patients undergoing pelvic procedures should be engaged in a thoughtful discussion preoperatively of the potential risk for fertility problems.

- A meta-analysis found a postoperative infertility rate of 48% after restorative proctocolectomy for ulcerative colitis, compared to 15% preoperatively.
- Some authors contend that this is more likely related to the disease process itself, rather than the type of surgery performed, and a cross-sectional study of FAP patients found no association between fertility problems and type of surgery but did report an increased risk of fertility difficulty in women undergoing surgical procedures earlier in life.

Bowel Dysfunction

- Pelvic surgery that includes restoration of bowel continuity is not only technically complicated but introduces new physiology to the life of the patients.
- Low anterior resection syndrome includes a variety of symptoms, including fecal incontinence, urgency, frequent bowel movements, and clustering of bowel movements.
- When undergoing a procedure for rectal cancer, it is often assumed that restorative and sphincter-sparing techniques afford patients a quality of life, which is superior to that of a permanent.
- A recent Cochrane review did not find evidence that the Qol after anterior resection is superior to that of patients who had undergone abdominoperineal resection or Hartmann's procedure.
- 50–90% of patients undergoing sphincter-sparing low anterior resection have some degree of bowel dysfunction postoperatively.
- Using a validated LARS score, Juul et al. found that the quality of life after rectal cancer surgery is closely associated with the severity of the low anterior resection syndrome.
- The etiology of the symptoms constituting LAR syndrome is unknown.
- The severity of symptoms also seems to correlate with tumor height, total mesorectal excision, and patients treated with radiotherapy.
- While previous reports have assumed that the quality of life with restorative and sphincter-sparing procedures is greater than the quality of life with a permanent stoma, this is not always the case, and therefore when counseling a patient with rectal cancer, specifically one who qualifies for neoadjuvant treatment, an earnest conversation must be had regarding postoperative functional outcomes.

Impact of Postoperative Complications on Oncologic Outcomes

- It is clear that postoperative complications carry implications for short-term quality of life and negatively impact the cost of care, and there is evidence of negative impacts on long-term oncologic outcomes.
- Postoperative complications result in either delay in receiving or complete omission of chemotherapy in patients with clear indications for systemic treatment.
- Tevis and colleagues found that postoperative complications independently correlated with decreased overall survival even in patients who received chemotherapy.
- While no single study has definitively answered the question, most have found similar negative correlations between postoperative complications and long-term survival, suggesting that there is a relationship between the two.

Anastomotic Construction

9

Steven R. Hunt and Matthew L. Silviera

Key Concepts

- Benign effluent from a peri-anastomotic drain does not rule out anastomotic leak or abscess.
- It is safe practice to leave the mesenteric defect open after constructing an ileocolic anastomosis.
- Fecal diversion reduces septic complications in patients with coloanal anastomoses.
- Diverting loop ileostomy and loop colostomy have similar complication rates.
- Leak testing should be performed on anastomoses to the rectum.

Introduction

- This chapter will focus on the most common techniques and the problems associated with construction of anastomoses.
- Various clinical situations and differing anatomy make it important to be familiar with multiple approaches to the same type of anastomosis.

Electronic Supplementary Material The online version of this chapter (https://doi.org/10.1007/978-3-030-01165-9_9) contains supplementary material, which is available to authorized users.

S. R. Hunt (✉) · M. L. Silviera
Division of General Surgery, Section of Colon and Rectal Surgery, Department of Surgery, Barnes Jewish Hospital, Washington University School of Medicine, St. Louis, MO, USA
e-mail: hunts@wudosis.wustl.edu

- No matter how well planned the creation of an anastomosis, problems may arise during execution, and the ability to salvage an anastomosis is a skill every colorectal surgeon must master.

General Principles of Anastomoses

Surgical Staplers

- Rudimentary surgical staplers first appeared in the early 1900s. They improved dramatically in the 1970s with preloaded disposable cartridges of multiple staggered staple lines. Titanium staples have replaced stainless steel. A variety of staple heights are available to match tissue thickness.
- The simplest linear stapler (TA or thoracoabdominal) applies two rows of staples in a staggered configuration.
- The linear cutting stapler (GIA or gastrointestinal anastomosis) applies four rows of staggered staples and cuts between the middle two rows of staples.
- Circular staplers (e.g., EEA: end-to-end anastomosis) have a detachable anvil. Once the anvil and head are coupled together, two circular rows of staggered staples are applied as a circular blade cuts out the interior tissue, allowing communication of the two lumens.

S. R. Steele et al. (eds.), *The ASCRS Manual of Colon and Rectal Surgery*,
https://doi.org/10.1007/978-3-030-01165-9_9

Handsewn Anastomoses

- Gastrointestinal anastomoses have been performed by various handsewn techniques.
- No difference in anastomotic leak rates has been shown between single-layer and double-layer anastomoses, interrupted and continuous suture techniques, or type of suture material (absorbable monofilament vs absorbable braided)

Compression Anastomoses

- A compression anastomosis (first reported in the 1800s) is created when two ends of bowel are held together for a period of time by physical forces during which anastomotic healing takes place. The compressed tissue necroses and the device separates and is passed. The anastomosis is held together by the adhesions that form between the tissues adjacent to the area of necrosis.
- In the 1980s the biofragmentable anastomotic ring (BAR) was developed and studied extensively. Despite the encouraging clinical data, several reports of intraoperative problems with the BAR emerged, and the device never gained widespread acceptance.
- A more recent device utilizes a smart metal (Nitinol) that is a temperature-dependent, shape-memory alloy. Two compression rings are mounted on an instrument that is very similar to a conventional EEA stapler (ColonRing).
- There is no prospective randomized data on ColonRing, and it has been taken off the market in the United States.

Tension

- One of the tenants of anastomotic creation is that it must be tension-free. This can be a significant problem with the pelvic colorectal anastomosis.
- In order to gain adequate length of the descending colon so that it may reach down into the pelvis, three maneuvers may be employed: (1) high ligation of the IMA, (2) ligation of the IMV at the inferior border of the pancreas, and (3) complete mobilization of the splenic flexure with division of the distal transverse colon mesentery back to the middle colic vessels.

Blood Supply

- Adequate blood supply to the ends of the bowel is another tenant of anastomoses.
- Visual confirmation of bowel viability is not entirely sufficient.
- Pulsatile, bright red bleeding from the marginal artery at the cut edge of the proximal portion of bowel to be anastomosed confirms excellent perfusion.
- Very dark or even black blood from the marginal artery often indicates a problem with the venous outflow and requires a change in the level of the planned anastomosis.
- Another method of intraoperative perfusion assessment uses near-infrared indocyanine green (ICG)-induced fluorescence angiography.
- A prospective, multicenter, clinical trial studied the utility of fluorescence angiography on colorectal anastomoses with the mean level of anastomosis 10 cm from the anal verge. The overall anastomotic leak rate was 1.4%. In the 8% of patients who had a change in their anastomotic plan due to findings from the perfusion assessment, none of the patients had an anastomotic leak.

Prophylactic Drainage

- The prophylactic use of drains to avoid anastomotic complications is controversial and varies among surgeons.
- Multiple studies have been conducted with varying results.
- Open or passive drains are made of synthetic material and act to provide a route of egress for fluids.
- Closed suction drains consist of a soft, hollow tube that is placed under negative pressure to actively evacuate fluids.

- Advocates of drainage maintain that drains will prevent the accumulation of fluid or blood around the anastomosis, permit early detection of a leak, mitigate the consequences of a leak, and provide a "window into the abdomen."
- Critics assert that drains provide the surgeon with a false sense of security, that they may cause a leak secondary to negative pressure, or that they may provide an avenue for the introduction of infection.
- Meta-analyses of prophylactic drainage includes a heterogenous group of studies with regard to the type of drain used and the location of the anastomoses and do not show a difference in clinical anastomotic leak, radiographic anastomotic leak, wound infection, reoperation, and mortality.
- The largest randomized controlled trail of closed suction drainage had both intraperitoneal and extraperitoneal colonic anastomoses and found no difference between groups.
- A more recent systematic review of observational studies looking strictly at extraperitoneal colorectal anastomoses showed that there was a difference in the rate of anastomotic leakage favoring the drained group.
- While there is scant data to support routine prophylactic drainage, there is no evidence that drains cause adverse events.
- Benign appearing effluent in the drain does not rule out an anastomotic leak or abscess.

Treatment of Mesenteric Defects

- For open colon resections, routine closure of the mesenteric defect was considered essential to avoid internal herniation leading to obstruction or strangulation.
- While the catastrophic consequences of an open mesenteric defect have been discussed in case reports, studies that have looked at this question specifically have shown that it is safe to leave the defect open after creating an ileocolic anastomosis.
- With ileorectal and ileal pouch anal anastomoses, there is the risk of axial torsion of the small bowel around the free edge of the mesentery. Some surgeons choose to close this defect by securing the free edge of the small bowel mesentery to the preaortic retroperitoneal fascia however there is no evidence to support this practice.

Diversion

- For an in-depth discussion on diversion, see Chap. 55.
- Fecal diversion has a role in protecting distal anastomoses that are at high risk for leakage.
- Any anastomosis within 5 cm of anal verge should be considered for diversion as they have a five- to six-fold increase in the rate of clinical anastomotic leakage compared to more proximal anastomoses.
- Defunctioning stomas can also be used to divert more proximal anastomoses at risk for leakage. Diversion in these settings should be used judiciously, as proximal diversion itself is not a license to create an anastomosis regardless of the clinical situation.
- Diversion mitigates the consequences of anastomotic leaks, but the difficulty lies in predicting which patients are most likely to leak.
- Diverting stomas and the procedure to reverse them have their own attendant morbidity.
- In theory, proximal diversion decreases the load of contamination in an anastomotic leak and may allow the body to seal off a leak – diminishing clinical consequences. Multiple studies demonstrate that diverted anastomoses have a decreased rate of fecal peritonitis, sepsis, and reoperation.
- Both loop colostomies (Fig. 9.1) and loop ileostomies have advantages and disadvantages.
- Ileostomies are associated with peristomal dermatitis, pouching difficulties, dehydration, and acute renal failure.
- Diverting colostomies are more prone to prolapse and are more difficult to close through a peristomal incision and increase the risk of disrupting the marginal blood supply to the colon.

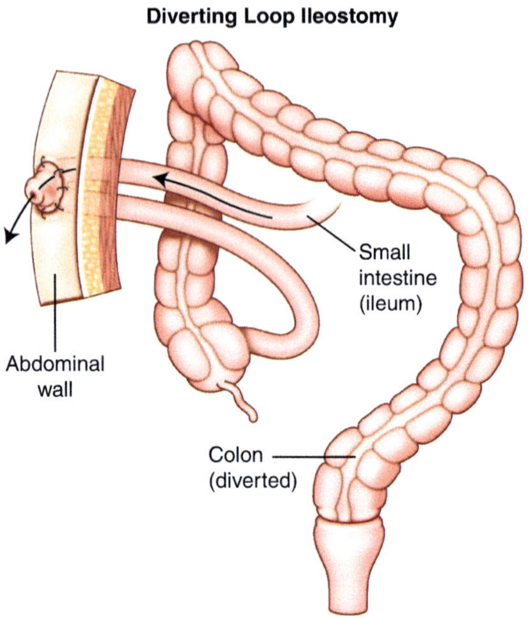

Fig. 9.1 Diverting loop ileostomy

- Meta-analysis of randomized controlled trials comparing diverting loop colostomies to loop ileostomies shows no difference between the two groups in complications related to the stoma or in time to ostomy closure.

High-Risk Anastomoses

- There are certain clinical situations in which clinical judgment precludes the creation of an anastomosis, even with proximal diversion. Some factors to consider include severe malnutrition, significant immunosuppression, gross or longstanding fecal contamination, and the risk of developing hemodynamic instability in the postoperative period.

Abdominal Anastomoses

Small Bowel Anastomoses

- Both stapled and handsewn techniques can be used to complete small bowel anastomosis.
- In creating a stapled side-to-side anastomosis, the bowel is divided proximally and distally with a linear stapler with the staple line oriented along the axis from the mesentery to the antimesenteric border of the bowel and beveled from the mesenteric side away from the specimen. The antimesenteric corners of the transverse staple line are removed, and the limbs of the GIA stapler are introduced. As the stapler is closed, the mesentery of each limb of bowel should be pulled laterally to ensure that it is not included in the staple line. The common enterotomy is closed with a stapler or handsewn.
- A meta-analysis by Leung et al. failed to show any differences between surgical techniques for ileostomy reversal; however, there was a trend toward less postoperative bowel obstruction with stapled small bowel anastomoses.

Ileocolic Anastomoses

- Ileocolic anastomoses are frequently created after an ileocolic resection for Crohn's disease or a right hemicolectomy for cancer.
- A recent Cochrane review compared the techniques of stapled side-to-side anastomoses with handsewn anastomoses. The overall leak rate was significantly lower for stapled anastomoses (2.5%) compared with handsewn anastomoses (6%).
  - When creating a stapled side-to-side (functional end-to-end) anastomosis, up to four linear stapler firings may be needed to construct the anastomosis. Cost can be contained and overlapping staple lines avoided by creating a "Barcelona" anastomosis (Fig. 9.2a–d). In this technique, after the mesentery of the bowel has been divided up to the points of proximal and distal resection, two enterotomies are created on the antimesenteric border of the bowel. The limbs of a GIA stapler are advanced into these openings and fired along the antimesenteric border of the bowel. The common enterotomy is then closed and the specimen transected with a second firing of a linear stapler.
- Another technique for an ileocolic anastomosis is the stapled end-to-side technique in

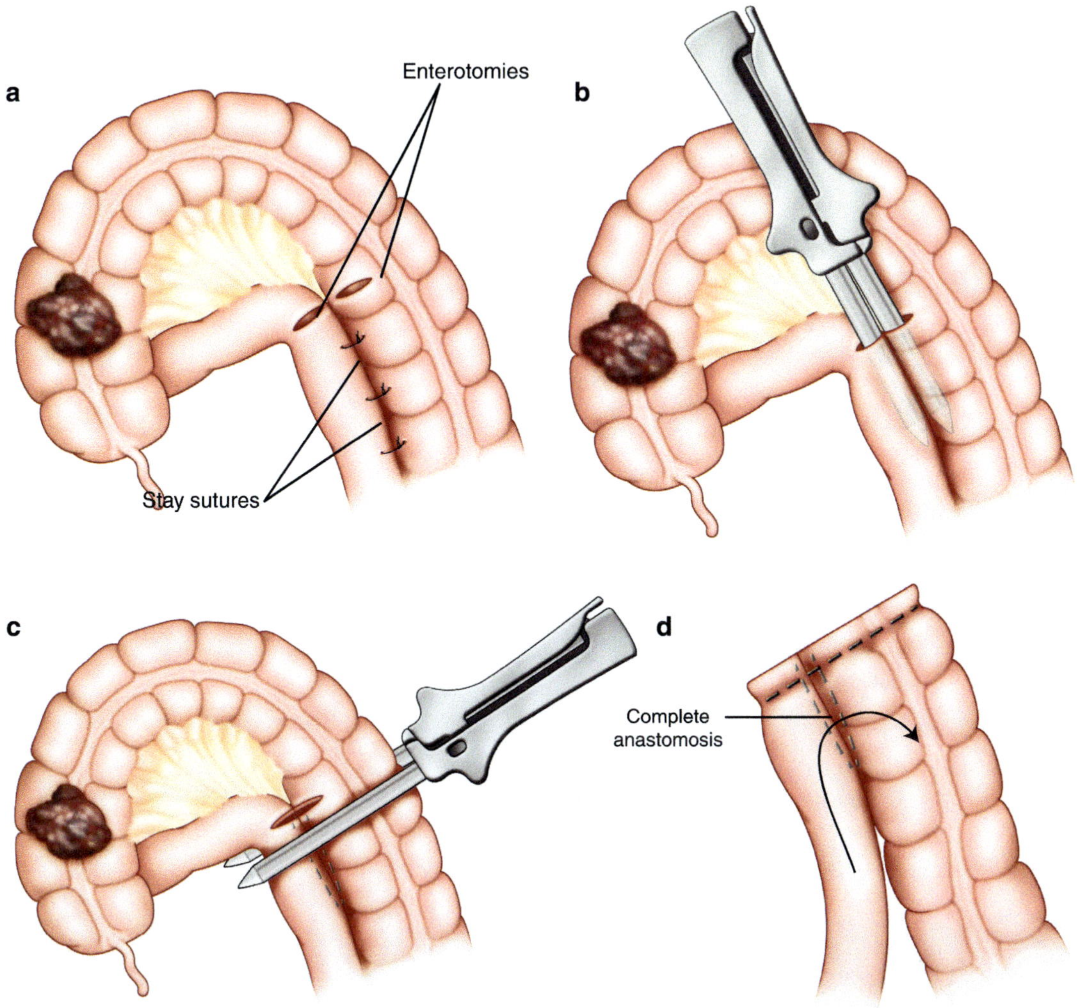

Fig. 9.2 (**a–d**) Barcelona anastomosis. (**a**) Stay sutures are placed and two antimesenteric enterotomies are made. (**b**) A linear stapler is used to construct the common wall. (**c**) An additional firing of the linear stapler is used to complete the anastomosis and resect the specimen. (**d**) Completed anastomosis

which an EEA stapler (25–29 mm) is used (Fig. 9.3a–d). The terminal ileum is divided, a purse-string suture is placed, and the EEA anvil is secured in the end of the ileum. A colotomy is created within the specimen, and the EEA stapler is advanced through the colotomy in an antegrade fashion to the antimesenteric border of the colon several centimeters distal to the intended margin of transection. The spike is brought out through the antimesenteric wall of the colon, and the anvil within the ileum is connected. The stapler is then closed and fired. The colon is divided with a linear stapler a few centimeters proximal to the EEA anastomosis to ensure that the anastomosis and blind end of the colon is well perfused.

- For laparoscopic ileocolic resections and right hemicolectomies the anastomosis is typically created extracorporeally through a small periumbilical incision. In recent years, totally laparoscopic right hemicolectomy with intracorporeal anastomosis has gained popularity. The most common technique for performing an intracorporeal anastomosis is to create a stapled side-to-side (functional end-to-end)

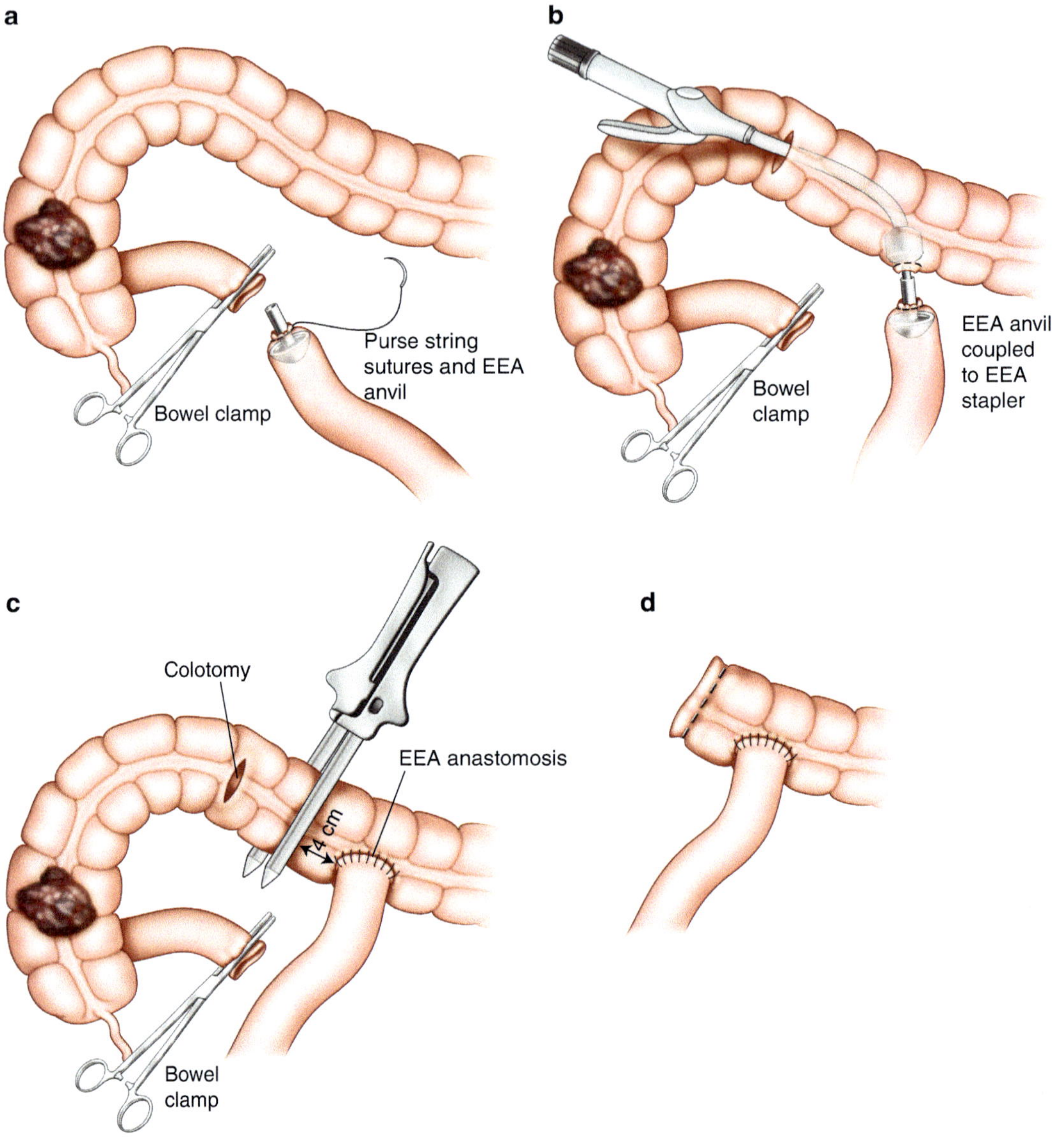

Fig. 9.3 (**a–d**) End-to-side ileocolic anastomosis. (**a**) An EEA anvil is placed into the end of small bowel through a purse string after dividing the bowel. (**b**) A colostomy is made and the EEA stapler is passed and coupled the spike to the EEA anvil. (**c**) Following the EEA anastomosis, a linear stapler is used to close the colon defect. (**d**) Completed anastomosis

anastomosis using laparoscopic linear staplers. The resultant common enterotomy can then be stapled or sewn closed.

- A meta-analysis of non-randomized comparative studies looking at intracorporeal anastomosis vs extracorporeal anastomosis for laparoscopic right hemicolectomies shows no difference in the rate of anastomotic leak.

Pelvic Anastomoses

Basic Principles of Pelvic Anastomoses

- Studies have documented that low pelvic anastomoses have a higher rate of leakage than more proximal anastomoses (Fig. 9.4).

- Tension is a concern with all anastomoses, but significantly more so in the pelvis, where anatomic factors can make it a significant challenge to create a tension-free anastomosis.

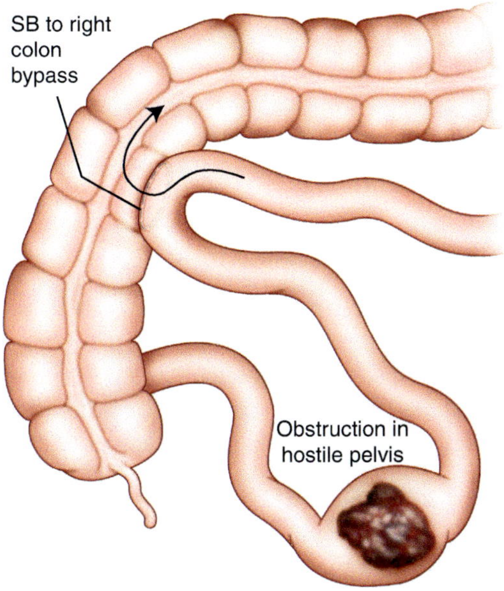

Fig. 9.4 Intestinal bypass

- Adequate visualization during dissection and creation of the anastomosis is extremely important and includes optimal lighting.
- When creating a pelvic anastomosis, extraneous structures can be incorporated in the anastomosis. One must be diligent in ensuring that the vagina is out of harm's way during the dissection, rectal division, and anastomotic construction.
- There are several reasons the descending colon should be used preferentially to the sigmoid colon when creating the colorectal anastomosis. (1) In a resection for cancer, the inferior mesenteric artery should be divided at its origin for an adequate lymphadenectomy, possibly resulting in insufficient blood supply to the sigmoid colon. (2) The sigmoid colon's thick muscular wall and diverticulosis makes this segment a poor substrate to use in creating what is already a precarious anastomosis.

Stapled Colorectal Anastomoses

- With wide availability of circular EEA staplers, the stapled colorectal anastomosis has gained favor among surgeons (Fig. 9.5). Both

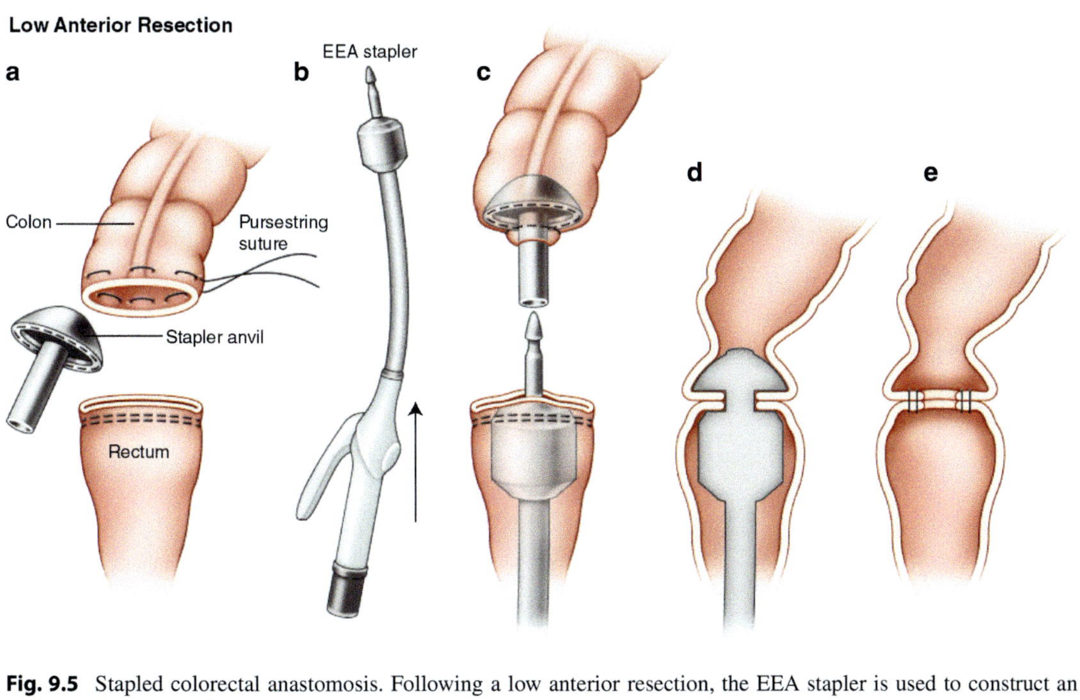

Fig. 9.5 Stapled colorectal anastomosis. Following a low anterior resection, the EEA stapler is used to construct an end-to-end anastomosis

single-stapled and double-stapled techniques will be described.

- The stapler anvil is secured in the proximal colon with a purse string. The pre-anastomotic colon falls easily into the pelvis, aligned in a straight course to the left of the ligament of Treitz. Evaluate the colon blood flow. The EEA stapler is introduced through the anal canal and remaining rectum to the transverse rectal staple line.
- The stapler spike is advanced slowly under close scrutiny of the abdominal operator and should be delivered near the midpoint of the transverse staple line. The anvil is secured to the spike, and the stapler is closed under direct visualization – inspection for alignment is repeated. The stapler is fired and then opened and removed per manufacturer's instructions.
- The single-stapled technique differs from the double-stapled technique in that there is no transverse staple line on the rectal pouch. Instead, the rectum is divided sharply, and a purse string is also placed around the open rectal stump prior to placing the stapler in the rectum.
- Rarely, advancing the EEA stapler to the apex of the rectal stump can prove to be extremely difficult. Circumferential mobilization of the rectum in the mesorectal fascial plane will often eliminate the kinks or folds that inhibit stapler introduction. If this fails, the anastomosis can be created in an end-to-side fashion on the anterior wall of the rectum, several centimeters below the transverse staple line.

Handsewn Colorectal Anastomosis

- In the upper and mid-rectum, it is possible to create a handsewn colorectal anastomosis (Fig. 9.6a–d). The evidence suggests that

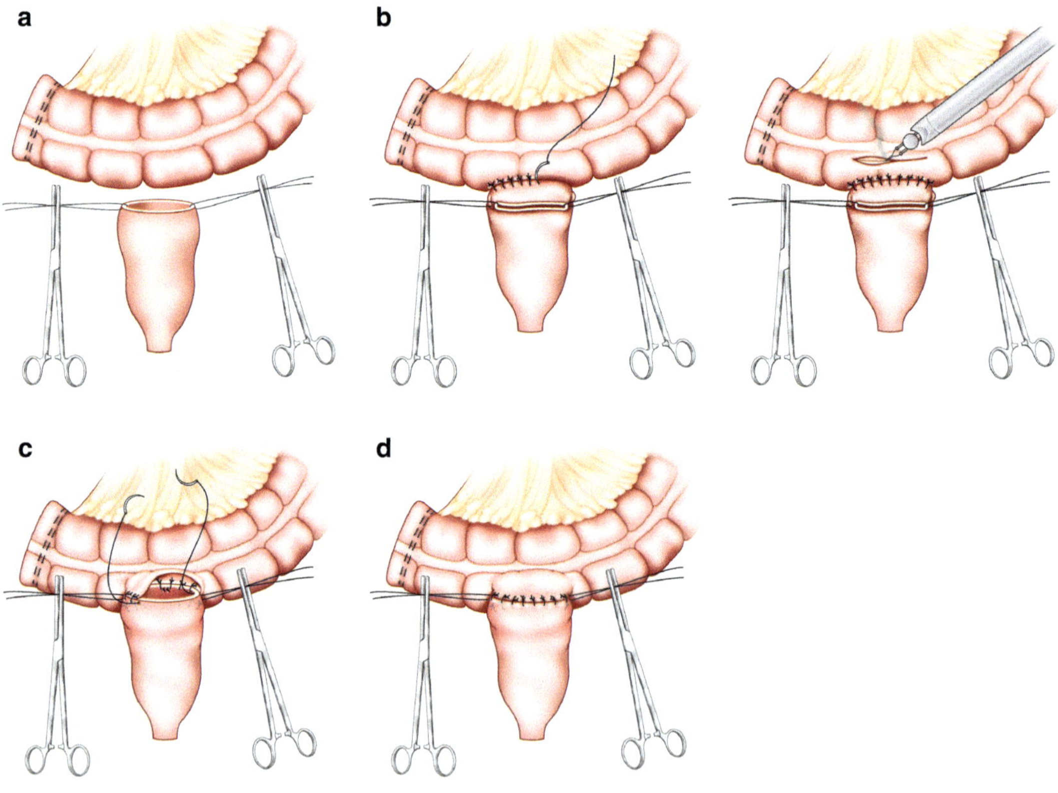

Fig. 9.6 (**a–d**) Handsewn colorectal anastomosis. (**a**) The distal end of the colon is closed, and stay sutures are placed on the rectum. (**b**) A posterior layer of sutures are placed (left) and a colotomy is made (right) to match the size of the opening on the rectal stump. (**c**) The anastomosis is constructed using two continuous running sutures. (**d**) The anterior suture line is oversewed with interrupted sutures

handsewn and stapled colorectal anastomoses are equivalent in leak rate.

- If a handsewn anastomosis is selected, there is no proven advantage of double-layer over single-layer anastomosis. We will describe a two-layer colorectal anastomosis, but the techniques to create a single-layer anastomosis are similar.
- The fatty mesentery of the colon and rectum makes a handsewn end-to-end anastomosis difficult to perform. Baker described a side-to-end colon to rectal anastomosis that is created several centimeters proximal to this closed end of the colon. A posterior layer of interrupted Lembert sutures is placed, and then a longitudinal antimesenteric colotomy is created. A running layer absorbable monofilament suture is started at the midpoint of the posterior wall and advanced posterior inner layer. As the sutures proceed onto the anterior aspect of the anastomosis, a Connell suture is used to create the anterior inner layer closure. The anterior suture line is then oversewn with interrupted Lembert sutures.

Ileorectal Anastomosis

- The ileorectal anastomosis after an abdominal colectomy is performed in the same fashion and following the same precautions as the colorectal anastomosis. Often, the small caliber of the ileum will not accommodate the use of the larger EEA stapler, and a smaller 25 mm stapler diameter is required.

Ultralow Colorectal and Coloanal Anastomoses

- The techniques involved in creating the low anastomoses in the pelvis remain the same as the upper rectal anastomoses. However, in addition to the technical challenges inherent in creating a low anastomosis, the surgeon must be mindful of the functional consequences of resecting the majority of the rectal reservoir.

Neorectal Reservoirs

- Using techniques developed for restorative proctocolectomy, Lazorthes and Parc both proposed the creation of a colonic reservoir in order to decrease the functional consequences of a low anastomosis.
- Over the ensuing years, multiple studies demonstrate that the colonic J-pouch is superior to the straight coloanal anastomosis in terms of frequency, incontinence, and quality of life and long-term results show that these functional advantages are durable out to 5 years.
- Several trials evaluating smaller (5–6 cm) colonic pouches found them to be superior to larger pouches.
- Creation of the colonic J-pouch first requires confirmation that the colon is adequately mobilized and that the intended apex of the pouch will reach the cuff without tension (Fig. 9.7a–d). An antimesenteric colotomy is then created 5–6 cm from the divided end of the colon. A linear cutting stapler is inserted through this colotomy, with one limb of the stapler inserted into the blind end and the other limb delivered up the proximal limb (avoid including the mesentery in the staple line) of the colon the pouch is created by firing the stapler. If a stapled anastomosis is to be created, a purse-string suture is then placed around the apical colotomy, and the anvil is secured in the pouch. The anastomosis is then created similarly to other colorectal anastomoses.
- Some studies showed a significant decrease in the anastomotic leak rate for the colonic J-pouch when compared to a straight coloanal anastomosis.
- Reservoirs anastomosed more than 5–6 cm above the anal verge may actually create problems emptying.
- Patients with a small pelvis, fatty mesentery, extensive diverticulosis, mucosectomy, or insufficient colonic length are not good candidates for J-pouch creation.
- Z'graggen was the first to describe the transverse coloplasty as an alternative to the colonic J-pouch.
- An 8 cm longitudinal incision is made on the antimesenteric colon with the distal end of the

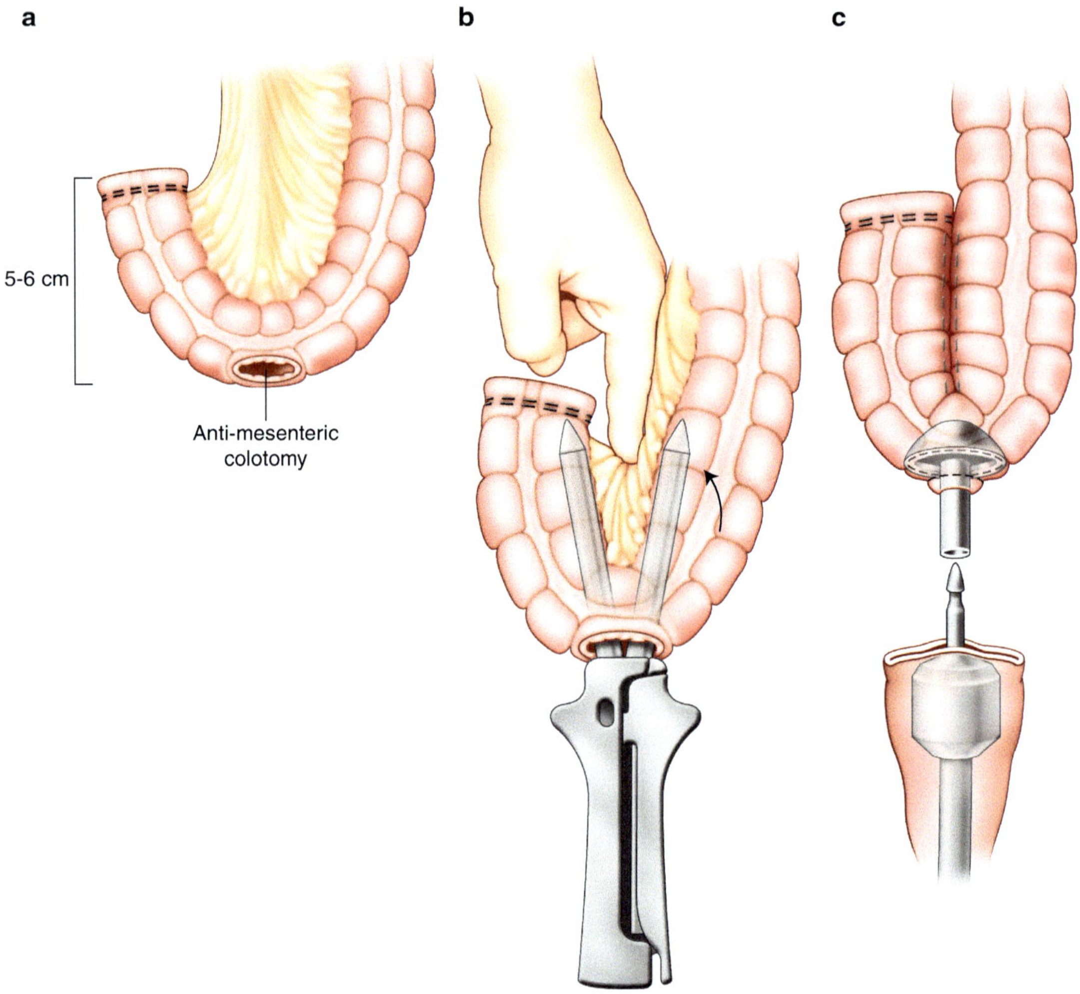

Fig. 9.7 (**a–c**) Colonic J-pouch. (**a**) A 5–6 cm colonic J-pouch is formed, and a colotomy is made on the antimesenteric portion of the bowel wall. (**b**) The pouch is formed using a linear stapler with 1–2 loads ensuring the colon mesentery is pulled out of the staple line. (**c**) The colorectal anastomosis is constructed using an EEA stapler

incision approximately 4 cm proximal to the stapler anvil, and the colotomy is closed transversely (Fig. 9.8a–d).

- A large, multicenter randomized controlled trial compared the colonic J-pouch to the transverse coloplasty (and comparing coloplasty to straight coloanal anastomosis for patients in whom a J-pouch was not technically possible). At 2 years, the colonic J-pouch proved superior to the transverse coloplasty in frequency, clustering, soilage, and continence. Although the sample sizes were smaller, the transverse coloplasty showed no improvement in any functional assessment compared to the straight coloanal anastomosis.
- Huber et al. proposed the side-to-end anastomosis (Fig. 9.9a, b). A randomized controlled trial compared side-to-end anastomosis with colonic J-pouch and showed that the techniques had similar frequency, continence, and functional scores. At 2 years neorectal volumes were 40% higher in the colonic J-pouch group.
- A systematic review comparing the side-to-end anastomosis to the colonic J-pouch did not show any difference in function between these two techniques.
- The physiologic basis for the improved function of neorectal reservoirs is not completely understood, but the increased volume reservoir

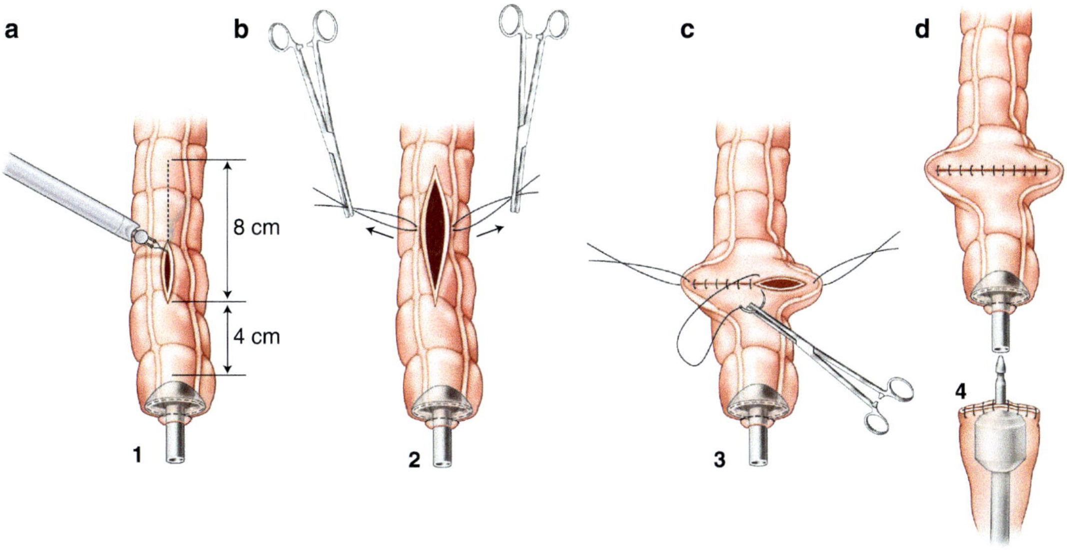

Fig. 9.8 (**a**–**d**) Transverse coloplasty. (**a**) An 8 cm linear colostomy is made 4 cm from the distal end of the colon (panel 1). (**b**) The anvil is placed in the end and stay sutures are placed at the midpoint on each side of the colotomy (panel 2). (**c**) The longitudinal colotomy is closed in a transverse fashion (panel 3). (**d**) An end-to-end anastomosis is performed (panel 4)

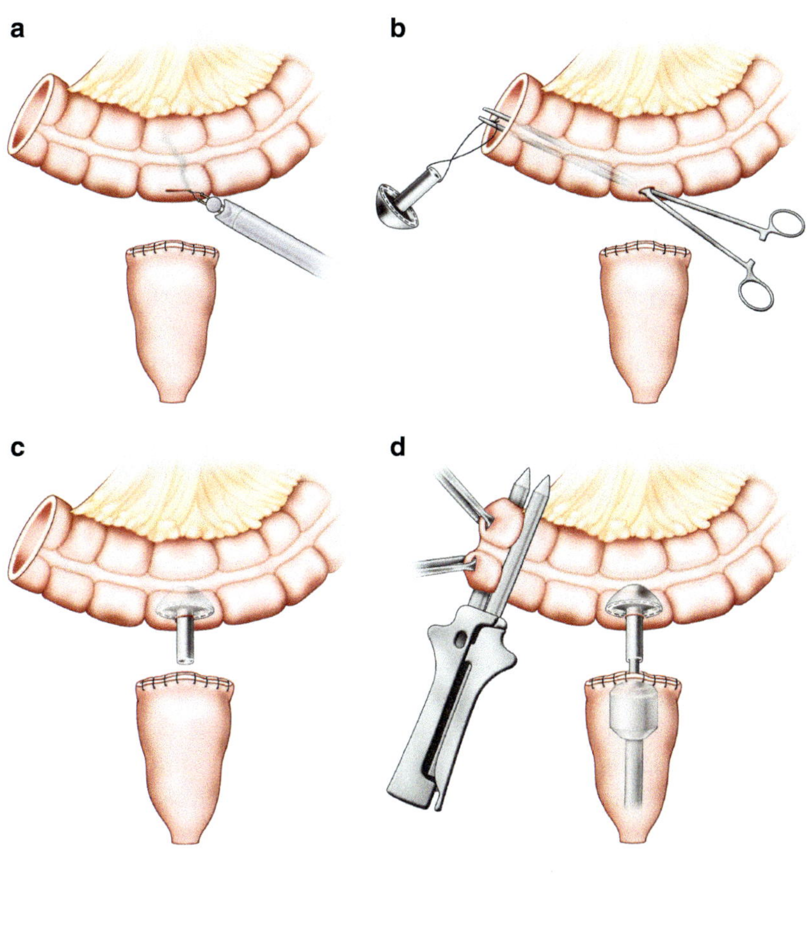

Fig. 9.9 (**a**–**b**) Side-to-end coloanal anastomosis. (**a**) A colotomy is made proximal to the open end of the colon (left), and the EEA anvil is passed through this opening (right). (**b**) The colonic opening is closed using a linear stapler (left), and the anastomosis is performed using an EEA stapler (right)

is one explanation. Ho et al. showed the function of the J-pouch was superior (J-pouch vs straight) but the neorectal capacity was similar for both groups. Furst et al. reached the same conclusion and suggested that the pouch works by decreasing forward propulsive motility in the J segment.

- Ho et al., using radioactive isotopes, found that solid stool transport through the colon was the same for both techniques and that the J-pouch had significantly better retention of liquid stools in the distal colon above the pouch.
- In summary, for low colorectal or coloanal anastomoses, the colonic J-pouch may give the best functional results, but the long-term durability of this benefit is unclear. When the J-pouch is not feasible, the transverse coloplasty or the straight coloanal anastomosis appear to offer similar functional results. The role of the side-to-end coloanal anastomosis is still undefined.

Handsewn Coloanal Anastomosis

- There are circumstances in which a handsewn coloanal anastomosis is the only option to avoid an ostomy.
- In order to perform a handsewn anastomosis, the surgeon must have good visualization of the cut edge of the anal canal. This is accomplished through a combination of sutures or self-retaining retractors (for exposure) and lighting.
- The transanal dissection, either intersphincteric dissection or mucosectomy, should be performed as appropriate for the pathology.
- The orientation of the colon mesentery should be confirmed after it is passed through the anal canal. A simple full-thickness suture is then placed in each quadrant of the anal canal. The anastomosis is then completed by placing intervening sutures in the remaining gaps.
- Baik et al. reported on a case series of patients that had straight handsewn coloanal anastomoses, 31% of patients had anal incontinence at 6 months. The percentage of patients with incontinence decreased to 14% at 1 year. Twenty percent of patients reported more than 6 bowel movements a day at 1 year.
- In the only randomized controlled trial comparing handsewn to stapled coloanal J-pouch anastomoses (total 37 pts), Laurent et al. reported that functionally the two groups appeared equivalent.

Assessment of Pelvic Anastomosis

- Some form of intraoperative anastomotic assessment should be performed at the time of creation. Mechanical tests of anastomoses demonstrate intraoperative leaks in 5–25% of anastomoses.
- The air insufflation test is the simplest to perform, and multiple studies show it reduces postoperative anastomotic leak rates. In addition to allowing for an air-leak test, intraoperative flexible endoscopic assessment of the anastomosis allows for visualization of the anastomosis.
- There is no definitive confirmation that intraoperative endoscopy is more effective than a simple air-leak test.
- The bowel several centimeters proximal to the anastomosis should be occluded manually or with a bowel clamp. Saline is added to the pelvis to cover the anastomosis, and air is insufflated into the rectum. The anastomosis should be manipulated in all directions to confirm that a small leak is not being hidden or occluded by extraneous tissue. If there is bubbling, the saline should be slowly removed with suction down to the level of the anastomosis in order to localize the leak.
- When an intraoperative leak is discovered, options include suture repair, proximal diversion, or takedown and refashioning of the anastomosis. For small leaks, suture repair is often adequate.
- Larger leaks, circumferential leaks, and leaks that cannot be visualized or adequately repaired require takedown and refashioning of the anastomosis.

Troubleshooting Problems with Pelvic Anastomoses

Unanticipated Pelvic Anastomosis

- Situations arise in which the surgeon must create an unplanned pelvic anastomosis and the patient is positioned so that access to the perineum is not possible. One option is repositioning that allows for the standard double-stapled anastomosis.
- It is not always necessary or possible to reposition the patient. A handsewn anastomosis remains an option, but becomes more difficult lower in the pelvis.
- It is also possible to create a stapled side-to-end anastomosis similar to the Baker anastomosis with the patient in supine or even lateral position. In this technique the anvil for the circular stapler is secured in the rectum and the stapler introduced into the colon via a colotomy. (Fig. 9.10a–d)

Inadequate Colonic Length

- For a left colectomy, adequate reach is usually achieved by performing basic maneuvers including splenic flexure mobilization, division of the inferior mesenteric artery at its origin,

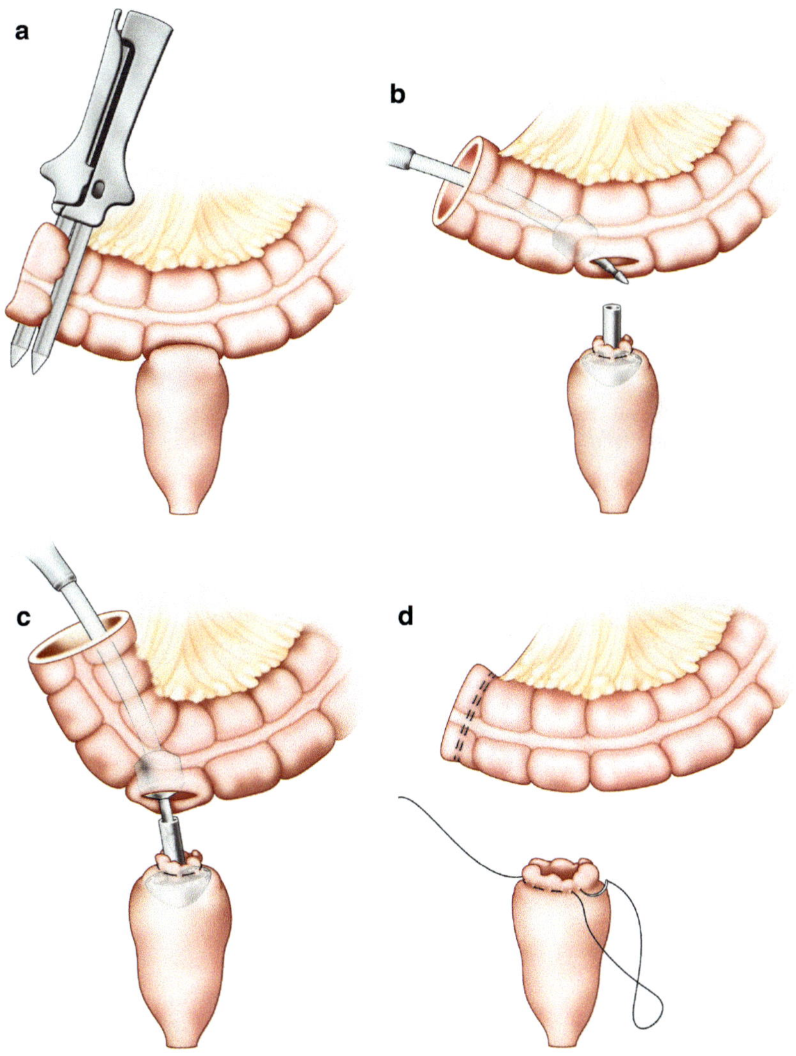

Fig. 9.10 (**a**–**d**) Unexpected colorectal anastomosis. (**a**) A purse string is sewn into the open end of the rectum. (**b**) The EEA anvil is placed through the rectal stump, and the EEA stapler is passed retrograde through the open end of the colon. (**c**) The anastomosis is completed with firing of the EEA stapler. (**d**) A liner stapler is used to close the open end of the colon

and division of the inferior mesenteric vein at the inferior border of the pancreas cephalad to the vein branch to the splenic flexure.

- Complete mobilization is accomplished by division of the peritoneal attachments in the left upper quadrant, separation of the omento-colic attachments to the distal transverse colon, deliberate division of the renocolic attachments of the mesentery to Gerota's fascia of the left kidney, and lysis of the gastro-colic attachments between the posterior gastric wall and the transverse colon mesentery.
- Resection of the splenic flexure as part of an extended left hemicolectomy often presents a challenge in obtaining adequate colonic length.
- Serial ligation of the middle colic vessels proceeding from left to right provides more length. Unfortunately, adequate blood supply and adequate reach sometimes find themselves at odds.
- If, after division of the middle colic pedicles, there is compromise of the blood flow to the pre-anastomotic colon, it should be resected back to the point where there is good arterial inflow and satisfactory venous drainage.
- If the colon will not reach the pelvis in the typical course to the left of the ligament of Treitz, one opion is to create a window in the terminal ileal mesentery that allows passage of the colon through this retroileal opening (Fig. 9.11a, b). The window is created in the space between the ileocolic artery and the distal superior mesenteric artery.
- Another option is mobilization of the hepatic flexure and counter-clockwise rotation of the colon (Deloyers' procedure) (Fig. 9.12a–d).

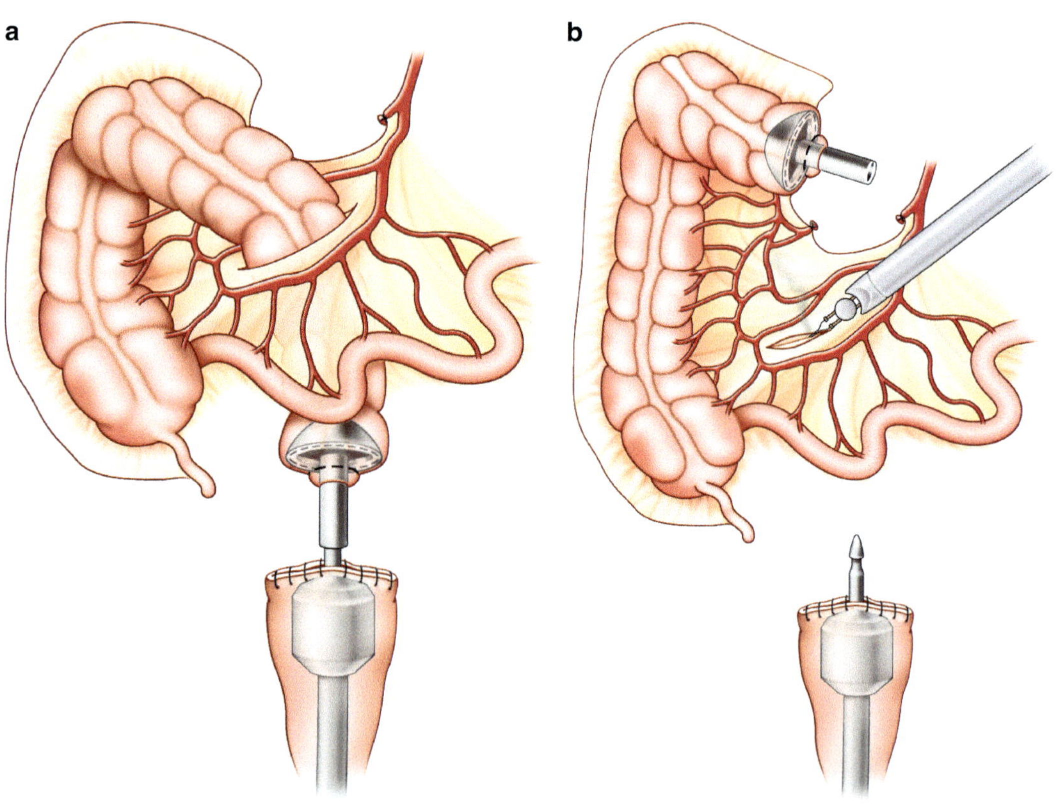

Fig. 9.11 (**a** and **b**) Retroileal pull-through. (**a**) A window is made on the superior aspect of the ileocolic pedicle after the terminal ileum is mobilized from the retroperitoneum. (**b**) The colon is passed through this window and into the pelvis to perform the end-to-end anastomosis

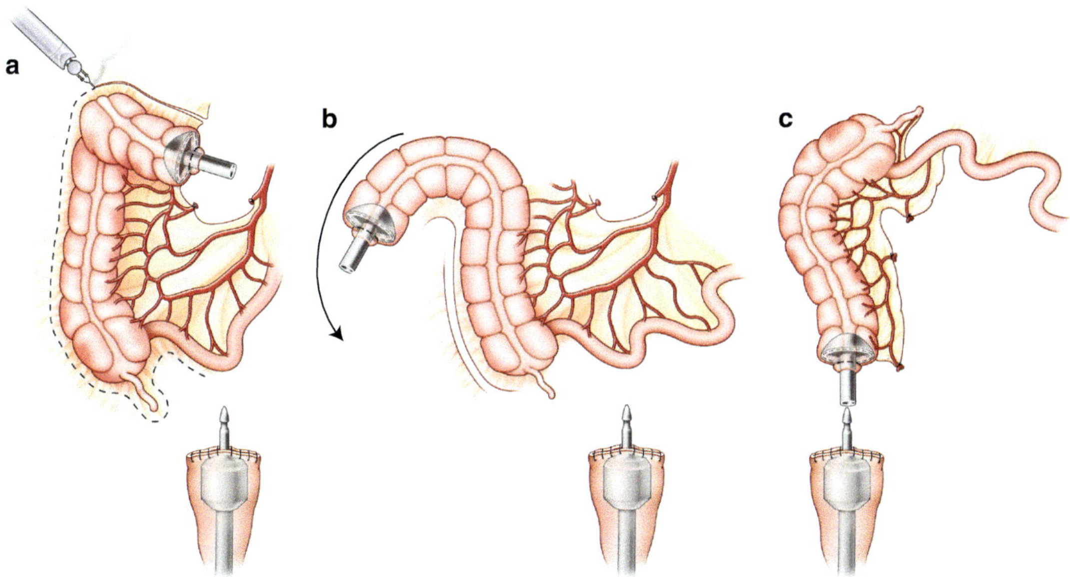

Fig. 9.12 (**a–c**) Deloyer's technique. (**a**) The hepatic flexure and right colon are mobilized laterally along with the terminal ileum from the retroperitoneum. (**b**) The colon is rotated in a counter-clockwise direction and delivered to the pelvis. (**c**) The anastomosis is constructed

- If all salvage maneuvers fail to allow a tension-free colorectal anastomosis with adequate blood supply, remaining options include a completion colectomy with an ileorectal anastomosis or an end colostomy.

Intraoperative Anastomotic Failure

- Failed anastomoses are inevitable in pelvic surgery.
- When a pelvic anastomosis fails, an attempt should be made to resect below the anastomosis and recreate it in standard fashion.
- If it is impossible to place the transverse stapler below a failed anastomosis, the anastomosis should be excised and a purse string placed around the open rectum. The circular stapler is then passed through the anal canal and delivered to the point just below the open end of the rectum and purse string. The stapler spike is advanced through the open rectal cuff, and the purse string is tied around the spike and inspected to confirm that the purse string is complete. A standard stapled anastomosis to the pre-anastomotic colon is then performed and assessed.

Anastomotic Complications

10

Konstantin Umanskiy and Neil Hyman

Key Concepts

- Patients who develop diffuse peritonitis after intestinal resection with anastomosis should undergo prompt exploratory laparotomy.
- Colorectal anastomoses should be routinely tested prior to abdominal closure.
- Hemodynamically unstable patients who develop a leak after sigmoid resection should undergo a Hartmann procedure.
- Late anastomotic leaks commonly present with subtle and insidious symptoms such as failure to thrive.
- Endoscopic balloon dilation is the procedure of choice for short anastomotic strictures.
- Most cases of anastomotic bleeding resolve with conservative measures.
- Persistent anastomotic bleeding should be treated by colonoscopy with epinephrine injection and/or endoscopic clips.

K. Umanskiy
Department of Surgery, University of Chicago, Chicago, IL, USA

N. Hyman (✉)
Section of Colon and Rectal Surgery, University of Chicago Medicine, Chicago, IL, USA
e-mail: nhyman@surgery.bsd.uchicago.edu

Anastomotic Leak

Overview

- Anastomotic leak is perhaps the most feared and dreaded complication after bowel resection and typically necessitates a lengthy hospitalization with considerable morbidity and cost.
- The cause of leak in any particular patient is frequently unknown although many risk factor have been identified.
- The pathophysiology of this potentially devastating problem is poorly understood.
- Avoiding tension on the anastomosis and assuring adequate perfusion to the two ends of the intestine to be joined remain valid and fundamental surgical principles.
- Optimization of comorbid conditions and suspected risk factors is also of value.
- Leaks often occur when no technical error, defect in surgical judgment, or patient- specific factor can be readily identified.
- In short, it seems clear that our present concepts regarding the causes and prevention of anastomotic leak are lacking.

Scope of the Problem

- The reported incidence of anastomotic leakage after bowel resection varies from 1 to more than 20% (5–8% most commonly),

S. R. Steele et al. (eds.), *The ASCRS Manual of Colon and Rectal Surgery*,
https://doi.org/10.1007/978-3-030-01165-9_10

based on the definitions used, location of the anastomosis, and length of follow-up.

- Small bowel anastomoses have the lowest leak rate, and low colorectal or coloanal anastomoses carry the highest risk.
- The definition of a leak varies. In a systematic review, Bruce noted that there were 56 different definitions of "leak" used in the 97 constituent studies of gastrointestinal anastomoses.
- "Anastomotic leak" can signify anything from an apparently trivial, clinically meaningless radiologic finding to a profound septic insult causing a rapid decline, multiorgan failure, and death.
- The spectrum of clinical entities with distinct clinical consequences that can complicate low pelvic anastomoses include "free" leaks, anastomotic sinuses, peri-anastomotic abscesses, and fistulas.
- Patients with "simple" fluid alone in the pelvis on a CT scan without any other evidence of a leak appeared to have impaired long-term function.
- Anastomotic infectious complications may be divided into leak, surgical site infection (SSI) organ space, and SSI deep.

Consequences

- An anastomotic leak is a life-threatening complication, with a mortality of 10–15% range from sepsis to progressive multiorgan failure.
- Timely diagnosis and treatment prior to the onset of advanced organ dysfunction has been emphasized as a key factor in reducing the mortality rate.
- Patients with a more indolent course may also succumb to venous thromboembolic or other indirect complications owing to the prolonged hospital stay, limited mobility, and persistent inflammatory state.
- Patients with an anastomotic leak often require difficult and complicated reoperations in a hostile local environment, with considerable additional postoperative morbidity.
- Functional, physical, emotional, and psychological recovery is often measured in months or even years.
- Prolonged wound care, ventral hernias, bowel obstructions, and management challenges associated with gastrointestinal adaptation to the altered anatomy may continue to be active considerations for long periods of time.
- Local sepsis may lead to an impaired functional result, especially after low pelvic anastomosis.
- There is an adverse relationship between anastomotic leak and local recurrence after rectal resection for cancer.

Prevention

- Because we still do not know why most anastomotic leaks occur, we remain limited in our ability to prevent many of them.
- Even among high-volume surgeons, significant differences may be found in leak rates, suggesting that technical and/or judgment errors play a causative role in at least some leaks.
- Many patient- and surgeon-specific factors have been associated with an increased risk of an anastomotic leak (Table 10.1).
- Many patient factors are simply markers for a sicker patient, and it is unclear which of the factors on this list are simply associated with a leak versus actually contributory.
- Attention to controlling certain risk factors (smoking, nutritional status, weight) does seem worthwhile.
  - A systematic review documented an impressive reduction in anastomotic complications when the anastomosis was tested during surgery.
- When a leak is identified intraoperatively, the options are to (1) repair a well-defined defect, (2) redo the anastomosis, (3) proximally divert, or (4) a combination of the above.
- Intriguing work regarding the relationship of the microbiome and anastomotic leak has been reported by Alverdy and coworkers.

Table 10.1 Reported risk factors for anastomotic leak

Patient factors	
	Overall physiological status
	Steroids
	Need for low rectal/anal anastomosis
	Immunomodulators
	Malnutrition/weight loss
	Emergency surgery
	Obesity
	Male gender
	Advanced age
	Alcohol use
	COPD
	Cigarette smoking
	Previous radiation
	Prior abdominal surgery
	Right vs. left colon (left increased)
	Primary disease (e.g., Crohn's disease, diverticulitis)
Surgeon factors	
	Length of surgery
	Blood loss
	Use of pelvic drain
	Bowel preparation
	Use of vasopressors
	Proximal diversion
	Blood supply

- Specific bacteria that produce locally destructive collagenolytic proteins (e.g., certain *Enterococcus, Pseudomonas*, or *Serratia* species) may be an important cause of anastomotic leaks, and perioperative suppression/eradication of these microbes may reduce leak rates.

Diagnosis

- The diagnosis is simple in patients who present in the first few days after surgery with excruciating abdominal pain, hemodynamic instability, diffuse peritonitis, and/or a rapid and dramatic change in their clinical course.
- The diagnosis of anastomotic leak is not always straightforward or clinically obvious as many leaks present in a subtle and insidious manner.
- One study reviewed the clinical course of 452 consecutive patients who had a bowel resection with anastomosis. The predictive value for abnormal vital signs or leukocytosis ranged from only 4 to 11%.
- Radiologic findings are often ambiguous and equivocal requiring careful and considered correlation with the clinical picture.
- The sensitivity for contrast radiography and CT scan in the setting of a leak has been reported to be in the range of 50%; therefore, a high index of suspicion must be maintained even when the imaging study appears to be negative.
- There is broad overlap of radiologic findings in postoperative patients with or without a leak. For example, free air was seen on CT scan up to 9 days after surgery and localized extraluminal air up to 26 days postoperatively in patients without a leak.
- Of the radiologic findings that are often considered to be indicative of a leak, only loculated fluid with air (Fig. 10.1) was observed more commonly in patients with an anastomotic leak.
- In a review of patients undergoing an intestinal anastomosis, the leak rate was 2.7%. 14/33 leaks were only diagnosed upon readmission to the hospital, and 12% were identified more than 30 days after surgery.
- The positive predictive value of CT scan was 89.5% versus 40% for contrast enema, but these studies were used in different clinical settings.

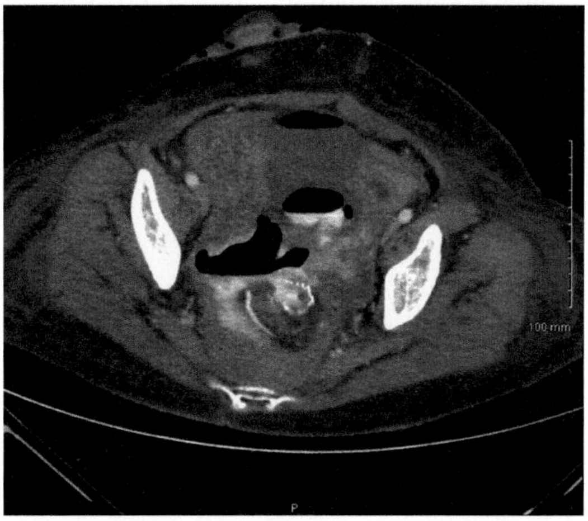

Fig. 10.1 CT scan in a patient with anastomotic leak after low anterior resection

Treatment

- Factors to be considered when deciding on the appropriate management for a patient with an anastomotic leak include patient-specific factors (hemodynamic derangement, physiologic reserve, nutritional status, comorbid complications, initial surgical indications/goals) and features of the leak (location, size of the defect, presence of concomitant tissue ischemia).
- Perhaps the most useful classification in outlining the principles of management is early versus late presentation.
- Patients with an early leak classically present in the first week after surgery with signs and symptoms of peritonitis, organ dysfunction associated with sepsis, and hemodynamic instability.
- In this clinical setting, prompt return to the operating room is required (Fig. 10.2).
- Patients with an anastomotic leak often present with signs and symptoms that lead the surgeon astray and suggest other serious postoperative complications (e.g., pulmonary embolism, myocardial ischemia).
- If the diagnosis is established in the first few days after the initial surgery, most patients will require operative exploration.
- Intravenous antibiotics and close observation may be appropriate in a few highly selected patients with small, contained leaks that otherwise appear reasonably well (low colorectal anastomosis, especially if they have a proximal diversion).
- At re-operative surgery, the peritoneal cavity is thoroughly irrigated and appropriate cultures obtained.
- In general, patients with a small bowel to small bowel or ileocolic anastomosis are best treated with resection and repeat anastomosis.
- Patients who are hemodynamically unstable may be treated with an ileostomy and end-loop stoma, where the distal end is brought out through the same aperture as the ileostomy (Fig. 10.3a–c).
- Anastomosis with proximal loop ileostomy is another alternative to address this situation where primary anastomosis alone is deemed unwise.
- When a colocolic anastomosis breaks down, dividing the anastomosis and creating an end colostomy is usually the most appropriate option.
- Resection with anastomosis and proximal loop ileostomy is an option for hemodynamically stable patients.
- Leak after low anterior resection creates challenging management decisions. If the anastomosis is divided and a colostomy created, then subsequent attempts for another low pelvic anastomosis may be a formidable endeavor.
- When there is no ischemia and the leak is relatively small and contained, loop ileostomy and drainage of the anastomosis are usually most appropriate.
- In stable patients with major disruptions, resection with anastomosis and proximal diversion may also be an option.
- The management of anastomotic leaks diagnosed beyond the first week to 10 days postoperatively usually differs in many important regards from its earlier counterpart.
- Careful imaging including a CT scan of the abdomen and pelvis with intravenous and enteric (including rectal) contrast is typically the key to diagnosis and treatment planning.
- Re-operative surgery is usually unnecessary and will quite often make things worse.

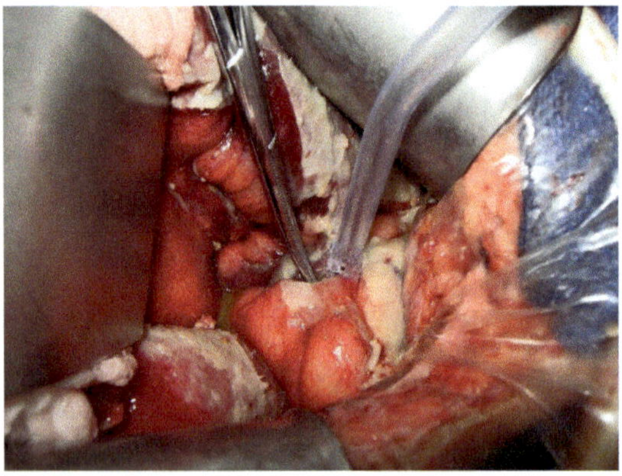

Fig. 10.2 Diffuse peritonitis after major anastomotic disruption

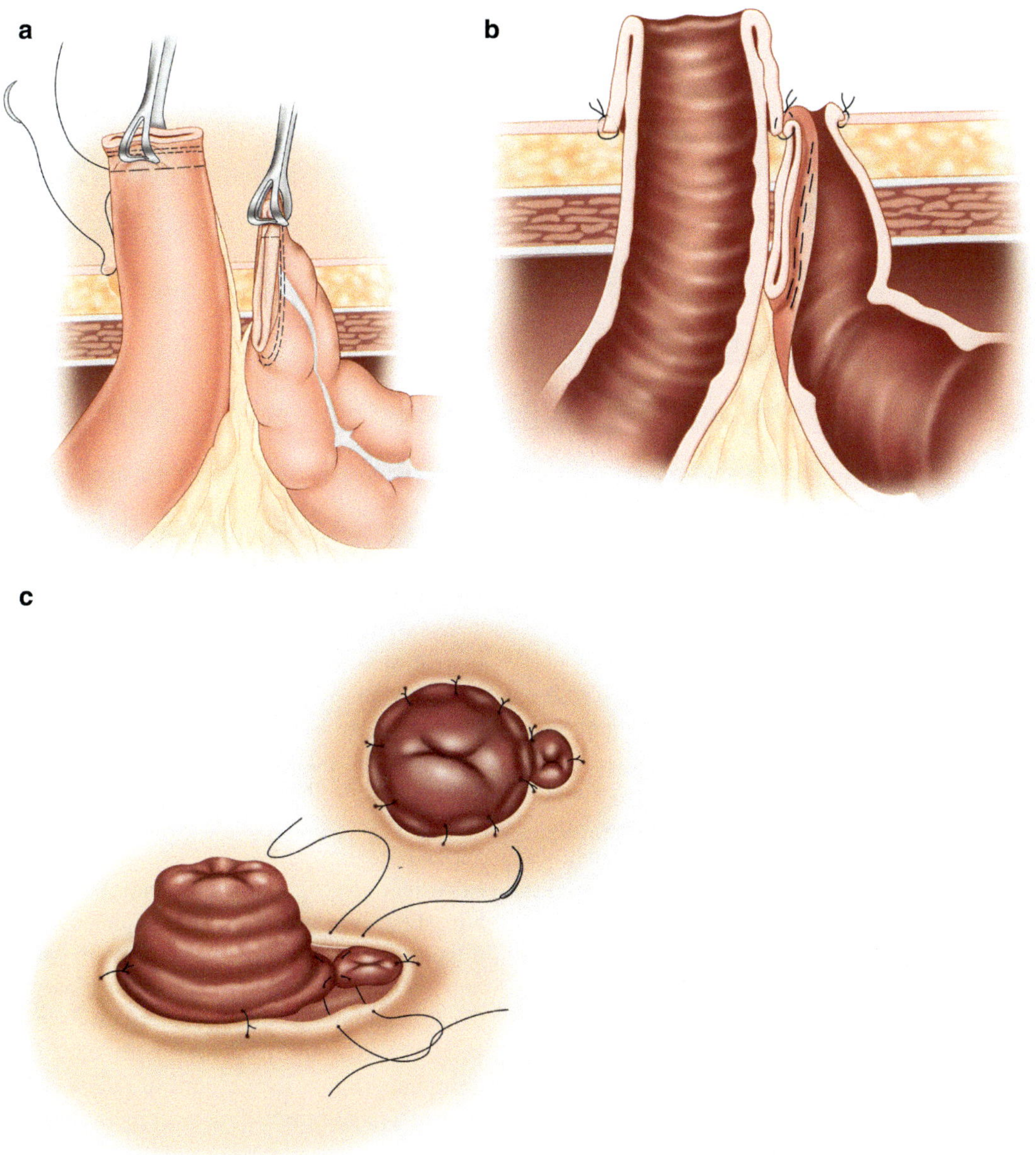

Fig. 10.3 End-loop stoma. (**a**) The bowel is divided, and each end is brought up through the opening. (**b**) The proximal portion is completely matured, while the distal end has only a corner matured. (**c**) Side and top view of the matured stoma

- Most patients with late presentations are most often best managed by patience, antibiotics, and percutaneous drainage.
- Both covered stents and vacuum-assisted devices have been used with anecdotal success.
- Nutritional support, using the enteral route whenever possible, should not be neglected.

Anastomotic Stricture

- Anastomotic stricture is a relatively common complication of colorectal or pouch-anal anastomosis, occurring in 3% to 30% of cases.
- The exact pathophysiology underlying anastomotic strictures remains unknown, but

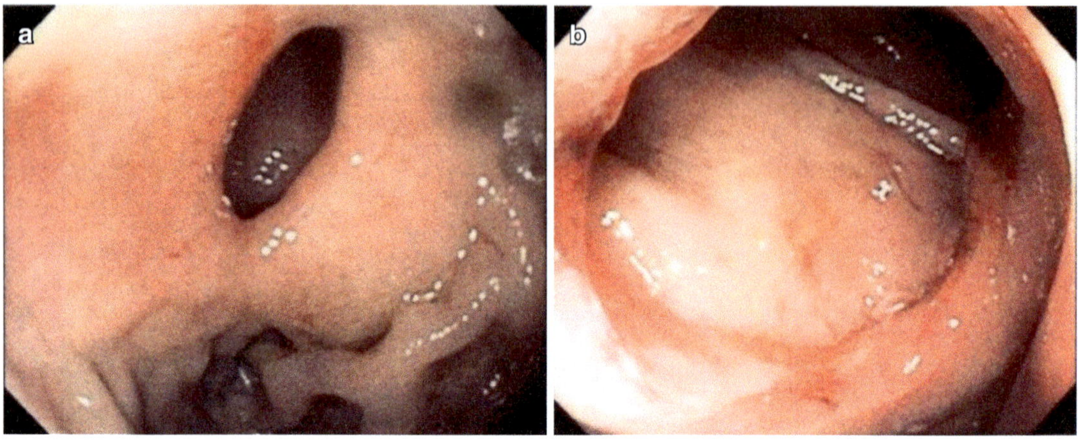

Fig. 10.4 (**a**) Colorectal anastomotic stricture, before dilation. (**b**) Anastomosis after through the scope balloon dilation

ischemia, incomplete "doughnuts" from stapled anastomotic reconstruction, anastomotic leakage, hemorrhage, and radiotherapy are probably contributing factors.

- Symptoms most commonly associated with rectal strictures are increasing constipation and partial large bowel obstruction.
- Asymptomatic patients with a stricture and diverting stoma can be identified based on digital rectal examination or upon radiographic or endoscopic evaluation prior to stoma reversal.
- Diagnosis is typically made by imaging (i.e., contrast enema) or endoscopically—the inability to pass a 12-mm-diameter sigmoidoscope through the anastomotic narrowing.
- Luchtefeld found that stenosis was diagnosed at 1–6 months after surgery in 54% of patients and at more than 6 months after surgery in 14%.
- Recurrent cancer must be considered as a cause of stricture prior to deciding on the treatment approach.
- Short strictures in low colorectal, coloanal, and ileoanal pouch anastomoses can be treated by simple digital dilation or Hegar dilators with a low rate of restenosis.
- Endoscopic balloon dilatation is the most commonly used method for treatment of short (<1 cm) colonic and colorectal anastomotic strictures (Fig. 10.4a, b) with success rates that range from 86% to 97%.
- A less frequently used method of bougie dilation of anastomotic stricture is accomplished by the radial vector of an axially directed force.
- In a case study, Pietropaolo found balloon dilation more effective than bougie dilation with respect to the proportion of patients successfully treated in a single session (76.9% vs. 51.8%).
- Recurrent cicatricle strictures may be treated with the combination of incision plus balloon dilation or endoscopic stricturotomy with neodymium-yttrium aluminum garnet laser.
- Complications of electrocautery and laser strictureplasty are very low, with only one group reporting a 2.7% technical failure rate.
- Alternatively, transanal endoscopic microsurgical approach (TEM) strictureplasty with electrocautery or laser can be used.
- Anastomotic strictures that are irregular, markedly angulated, fixed, or longer than 1–2 cm in length may not be amenable to endoscopic treatment.
- Re-operative rectal dissection in the presence of scarring from previous operations or from ongoing local sepsis is technically demanding and should not be underestimated.
- Shleigel reported a series of 27 patients who underwent surgical correction of anastomotic

stenosis (7 colorectal anastomoses for upper rectal anastomotic strictures and 20 coloanal anastomoses for middle and lower rectal strictures). Intestinal continuity was restored in all cases.

- In long segment distal rectal strictures or after failure of local therapy, immediate or delayed coloanal anastomosis through a combined abdominal and perineal approach is recommended.
- A less invasive technique using an end-to-end anastomosis (EEA) stapler may be applied to correct mid- to proximal rectal strictures with or without laparotomy. Prior to stapling, the rectal anastomotic stricture is dilated and assessed by rigid sigmoidoscopy. Long-term results following this technique of stricture resection have been reported as 89–100% return to normal bowel function with a mean follow-up of 12–49 months.
- Self-expanding metallic stents (SEMS) have been considered for medium-term symptom relief for recalcitrant benign colorectal strictures in patients who are otherwise unfit for surgery. They associated with a delayed complication rate of 38% of cases.
- Diverting ileostomy or colostomy may be the only available treatment option in some cases.

Anastomotic Bleeding

- Anastomotic bleeding following stapled colorectal, colonic, or intestinal anastomosis is usually self-limited complication occurring in up to 5% of anastomoses.
- The risk of postoperative bleeding can be decreased by avoiding the inclusion of mesocolon into the staple line.
- We recommend intraoperative assessment of colorectal anastomoses with intraoperative flexible sigmoidoscopy where an actively bleeding vessel can be visualized and immediate hemostasis achieved by placement sutures under direct inspection, endoscopic injection of 1:200,000 epinephrine, or careful coagulation.
- The optimal treatment choices depend on the site of bleeding, patient factors, and skill of the surgeon or endoscopist.
- Postoperative anastomotic bleeding usually occurs in the first 9 days.
- Initial management includes correction of any associated coagulopathy and transfusion of blood and blood products if necessary.
- Between 2 and 10 units of packed red blood cells may be required in the nonoperative treatment of anastomotic bleeding, and hypothermia should be avoided.
- For persistent bleeding, colonoscopy allows for direct inspection of the anastomosis and potentially for treatment.
- Submucosal peri-anastomotic injection of up to 10 ml of 1:200000 epinephrine in saline has been shown to result in control of anastomotic bleeding.
- Cirocco reported the successful use of electrocoagulation (anastomotic fistula that developed in one of six cases may have been related to this technique).
- Endoscopic application of clips is an excellent alternative to coagulation and has been shown to be safe and effective in control of anastomotic bleeding.
- Briskly bleeding anastomoses may be amenable to angiographic localization and embolization but with the risk of bowel ischemia or infarction by interrupting the distal arterial blood supply.
- Although extremely rare, significant anastomotic bleeding after large bowel resection can be severe enough to require reoperation with surgical revision or reconstruction of anastomosis.

Part II

Anorectal Disease

11 Approach to Anal Pain

Amir L. Bastawrous

Key Concepts

- A careful history should direct the diagnosis for patients with anal pain.
- A considerate yet thorough physical exam will usually establish the diagnosis by visualizing pathology or by palpating abnormalities. If not possible in the office, then an exam under anesthesia should be performed.
- Imaging is rarely needed to determine the etiology.
- An anal fissure will typically cause sharp anal pain during and after a hard bowel movement.
- The anal pain associated with a thrombosed external hemorrhoid is usually constant and accompanied by a palpable swelling but without systemic signs of infection.
- Cancer should always be included in the differential diagnosis.

Introduction

- Anal and rectal pathologies can be inconvenient and are commonly debilitating.
- Anal pain is a symptom which encompasses a broad spectrum of diagnoses from the benign and self-limited to the neoplastic and life-threatening.

A. L. Bastawrous (✉)
Swedish Cancer Institute, Swedish Colon and Rectal Clinic, Seattle, WA, USA
e-mail: amir.bastawrous@swedish.org

Patient History

- An experienced colorectal surgeon can often surmise the patient's diagnosis prior to any examination just by listening to key descriptions by the patient.
- Pain characteristics are important [duration, location (intra-anal, external), character (burning, sharp, dull), causative agents (bowel movement, diarrhea, hard stool, exercise, fecal incontinence, drainage), associated signs and symptoms (fever, chills, weight loss, change in bowel habits), and items that provide any relief (warm water bath, bowel movement, topical creams)].
- Elements of the patient history can provide some guidance:
  - Diabetes may suggest an anal abscess or Fournier's gangrene.
  - Inflammatory bowel disease may hint at an anal fissures, fistulae, or abscess.
  - Infliximab or etanercept use may point to psoriasis as a cause for pruritus.
  - Family history of colorectal cancer may lead to consideration to rule out rectal cancer.
  - Anoreceptive intercourse may raise the concern about sexually communicable infectious diseases, anal dysplasia, or anal cancer.

S. R. Steele et al. (eds.), *The ASCRS Manual of Colon and Rectal Surgery*,
https://doi.org/10.1007/978-3-030-01165-9_11

- Finally, one should not be misled by either the patient's or referring physician's working diagnosis, which is often inaccurate.

Anal Fissure (Fig. 11.1)

- Patients typically describe sharp, "knifelike," during and immediately after a bowel movement.
- The pain may last for minutes or hours after passing stool.
- Spotting of blood on the toilet paper after wiping or dripping into the bowl is common.

Acutely Thrombosed External Hemorrhoid (Figs. 11.2 and 11.3)

- Patients describe sharp, constant pain following straining (either with a bowel movement (loose or constipated) or lifting something heavy).
- The pain will coincide with a "bulge" they feel near the anal opening.
- The pain will last all day, usually increasing gradually, and then decrease over the week.

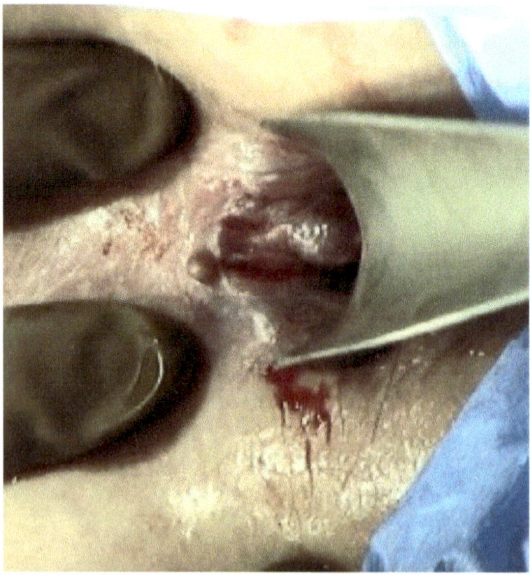

Fig. 11.1 Anal fissure

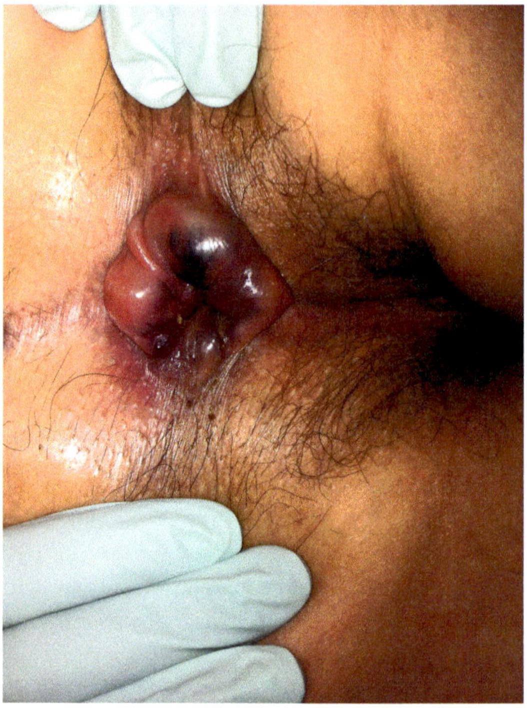

Fig. 11.2 Acutely thrombosed external hemorrhoid

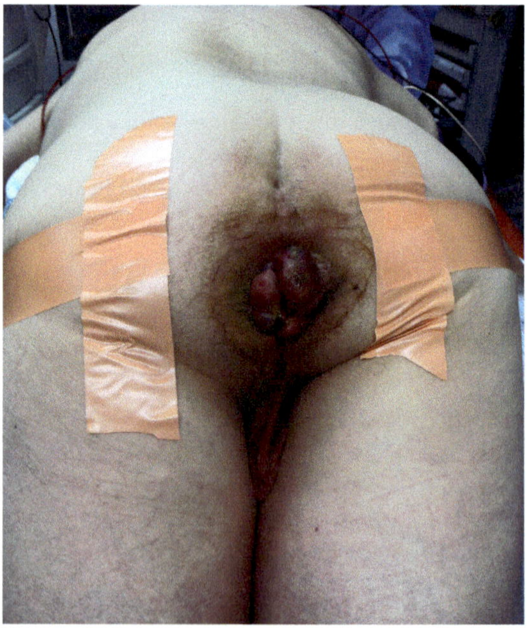

Fig. 11.3 Hemorrhoidal crisis

Perianal, Perirectal, or Ischiorectal Abscess (Fig. 11.4)

- Their history is one of the gradually worsening pressures and pain.
- The pain is constant but worse before and during a bowel movement.
- They will typically describe fever and chills.
- These patients often refuse to sit due to the pain.
- There can be some similarity of symptoms with patients who have a thrombosed external hemorrhoid, but the primary difference in presenting symptoms is the presence of systemic symptoms of infection.
- Inability to urinate is a rarely associated complaint, seen most commonly with large abscesses.

Pruritus Ani (Fig. 11.5)

- The pain can be described as pain but is often clarified to be burning or itching, with some overlap.
- The irritation is nearly universally chronic in nature, occurring in flares and cycles.

Levator Syndrome

- A lack of fitting into a typical pain pattern often makes the diagnosis challenging.
- The pain may be sharp, dull, burning, or achy.

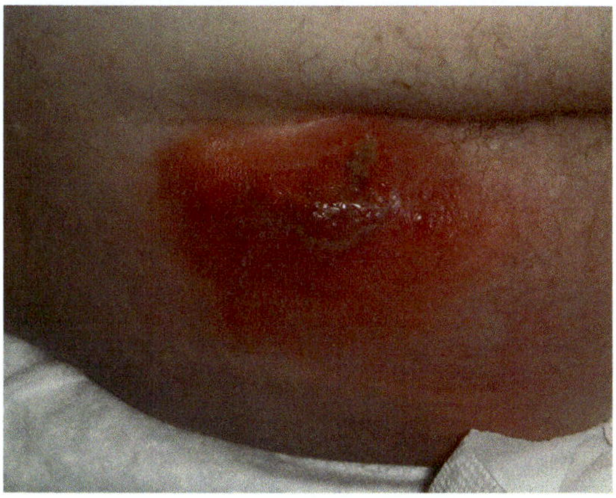

Fig. 11.4 Perianal abscess

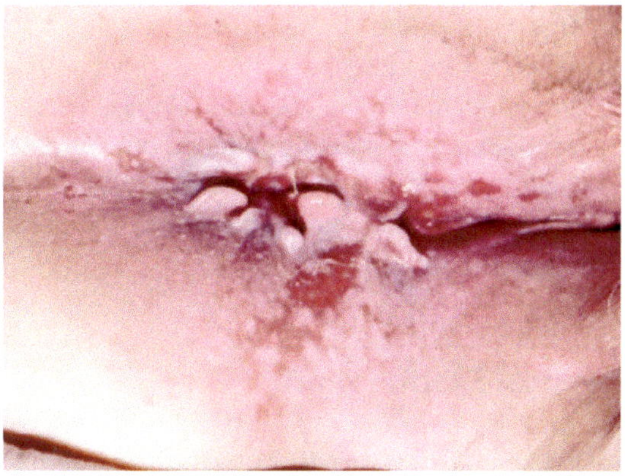

Fig. 11.5 Pruritus ani

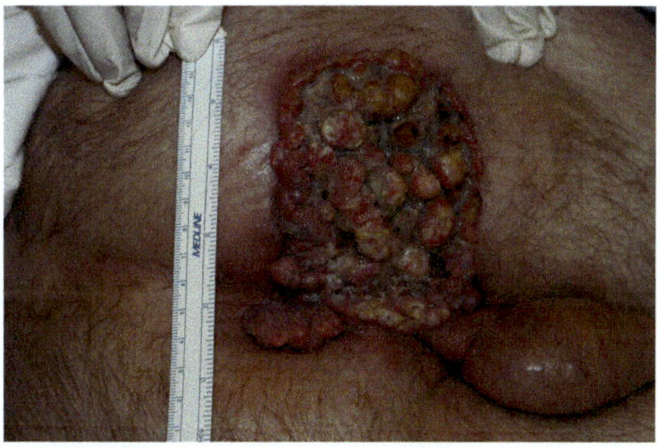

Fig. 11.6 Anal squamous cell carcinoma

- It may be intermittent or constant, may improve with warm water baths, or may be worsened or improved with bowel movement.
- Often the pain is chronic and worse late in the day.
- Some will complain of difficulty with evacuation of stools.

Anal or Rectal Cancer (Fig. 11.6)

- The majority of patients who present with anal pain have benign processes; however, the alert physician will always consider cancer within the differential diagnosis.
- Anal and rectal cancers can present with pain, often with concurrent bleeding and/or change in bowel habits.

- Anal cancer can present more subtly with symptoms overlapping with those of anal fissure with pain during and after a bowel movement along with spotting of blood on the toilet paper.
- There may or may not be an associated mass felt by the patient.

Physical Examination

- The regional high yield focus of the examination includes the abdomen; inguinal, perianal skin and soft tissue; buttocks and gluteal cleft; and anal canal and rectum.

Abdominal Examination

- Anal pathology can on occasion manifest with abdominal findings.
- An obstructing cancer can cause distention or alteration of bowel sounds.
- Metastases can present with hepatomegaly.
- Crohn's disease patients may be very thin and cachectic if they have both anal disease and bowel manifestations.

Inguinal Examination

- The inguinal examination may identify adenopathy in the setting of low rectal adenocarcinoma or anal canal and anal margin squamous cell carcinomas.
- This exam finding has implications for radiotherapy mapping and surveillance of disease regression or recurrence.

Perianal, Gluteal, and Intergluteal Examination

- Patients will appreciate a careful description of the exam as it is performed and an explanation of findings along the way.

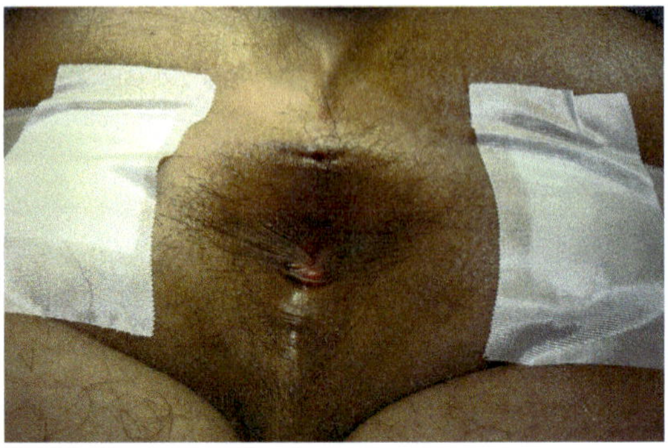

Fig. 11.7 Anal fistula

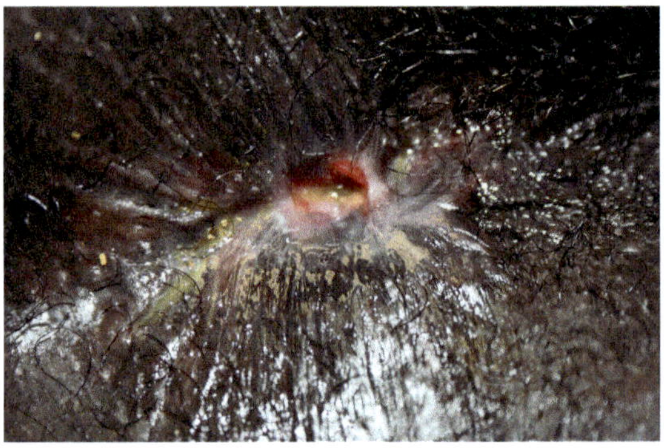

Fig. 11.8 Anal stricture

- Visual examination of the perianal skin includes color, scaly skin, thickened folds, masses, secondary openings of fistula-*in-ano* (Fig. 11.7), evidence of abscess with swelling or redness, skin tags, and external hemorrhoid enlargement.
- Anal fissure can be diagnosed by visualizing the anoderm with gentle retraction of the buttocks to evert the anoderm and expose the fissure.
- In the intergluteal cleft, look for sinuses, abscess, and pilonidal pits.
- Anal stenosis can be seen in some patients after anal surgery (Fig. 11.8).
- The rare subcutaneous mass may be benign or malignant; an assessment of size, fixation, character, firmness, and tenderness is sometimes helpful in establishing the diagnosis (Fig. 11.9).

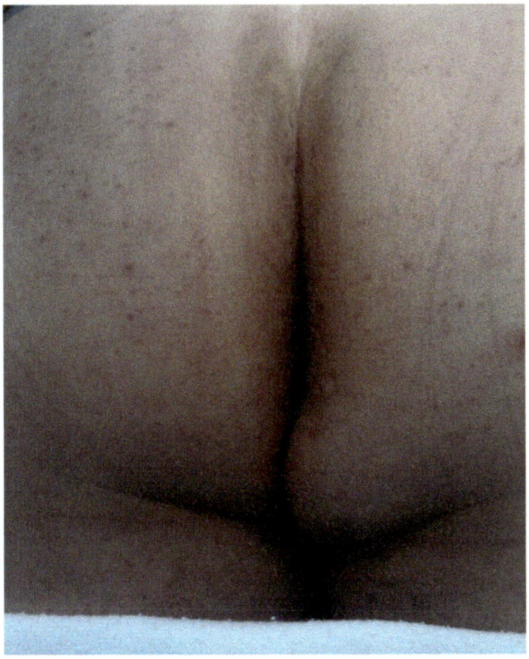

Fig. 11.9 Solitary fibrous tumor

Digital Rectal Examination

- One should feel for any abnormal anal or distal rectal masses and anal tone:
  - If low resting tone, stool seepage may be a cause for pruritus pain.
  - If tone is high and there is twitching of the anal sphincter, even if there is no visible fissure, a diagnosis of anal fissure disease is likely.
- The tightness of levator muscles should be assessed bilaterally starting at the coccyx; this will often reproduce the pain or pressure of levator spasm.
- The sacral hollow should be examined for presacral masses or cysts.
- The coccyx should be distracted/palpated to assess for coccydynia.
- The prostate should be palpated since prostatitis may be the cause of anal pain.
- If the pain is too intense and the patient cannot tolerate the exam in the office setting, an examination under anesthesia should be scheduled in the proper clinical circumstances.

Anorectal Inspection, Anoscopy, and Sigmoidoscopy

- An anoscopic examination should be performed to identify intra-anal lesions.
- A sigmoidoscopic should be performed to identify rectal lesions.
- Lesions including hemorrhoids, polyps, masses, mucosal inflammation, and rare anal melanoma may be seen (Fig. 11.10).

Imaging and Diagnostic Testing

- Following the history and examination, one may need to gather additional diagnostic imaging studies:
  - CT of the pelvis (mass, pain, or abscess)
  - Cine-videodefecogram or dynamic MRI of the pelvis (proctalgia fugax or other pelvic floor disorders)

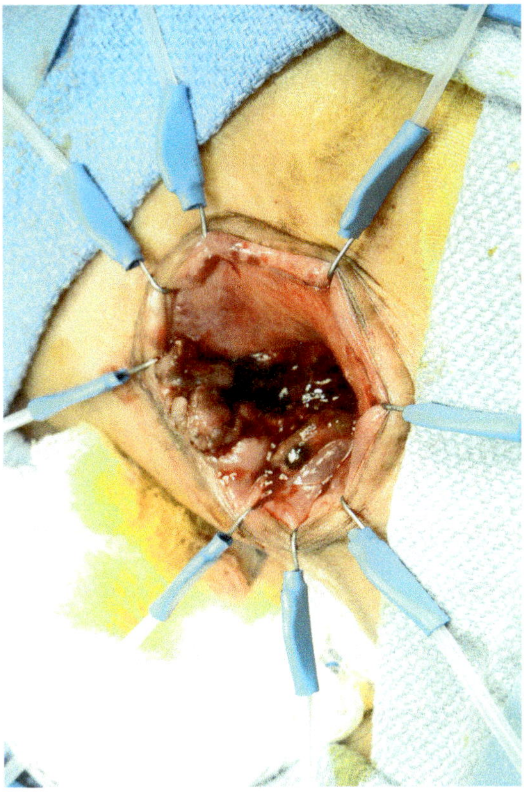

Fig. 11.10 Anal melanoma

 – Anorectal manometry and balloon expulsion (outlet obstruction, constipation)
 – Staging ultrasound or MRI (anal or rectal cancer)
 – A pelvic radiograph (foreign bodies) (Fig. 11.11)

Conclusion

- A systematic approach to anal pain will ensure efficient diagnosis and initiation of effective treatments (Fig. 11.12).

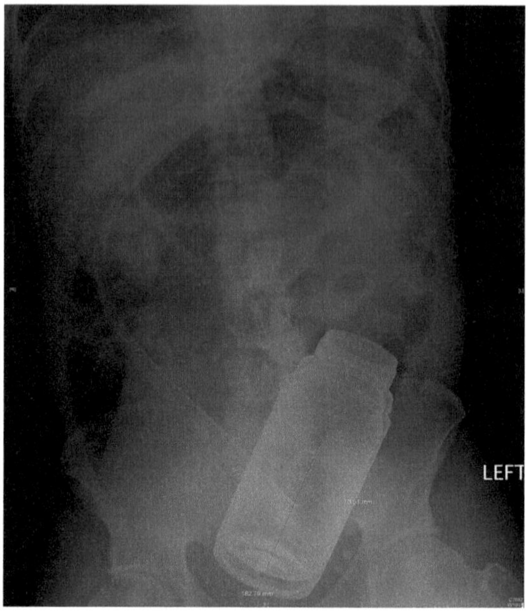

Fig. 11.11 Foreign body

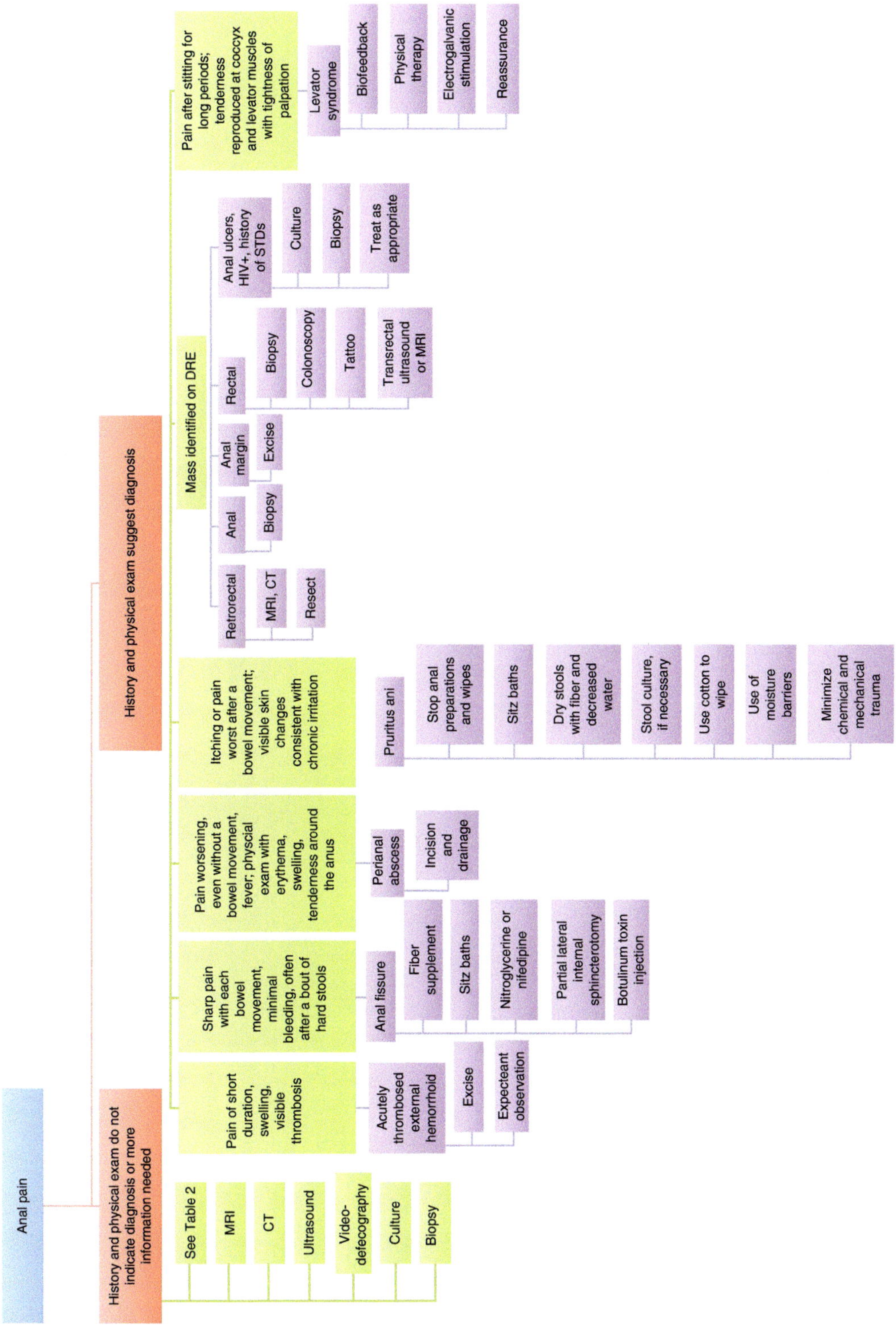

Fig. 11.12 Systematic approach to anal pain. (With permission from Billingham R. Chronic anal pain. In: Steele, S.R., Maykel, J.A., Champagne, B.J., Orangio, G.R. (Eds). Complexities in Colorectal Surgery. Decision-Making and Management. Springer, New York, 2014. © Springer)

Hemorrhoids

12

Martin Luchtefeld and Rebecca E. Hoedema

Key Concepts

- Hemorrhoids are one of the most common ailments that will be seen by a colon and rectal surgeon.
- The classification system of hemorrhoidal disease is based on the degree of clinical prolapse seen on the physical examination.
- Medical therapy for hemorrhoidal symptoms should be the initial treatment recommendation and can include dietary changes, increased water intake, fiber supplementations, and ointment therapy.
- Office-based procedures are offered mainly for internal hemorrhoidal disease with the most common procedure being rubber band ligation.
- Injection sclerotherapy may be performed on an anticoagulated patient due to the fibrotic reaction with almost no increased risk of bleeding.
- Excisional hemorrhoidectomy is the gold standard by which all surgical procedures are compared.
- Postoperative bleeding can occur at one of two different times, right after the procedure itself and delayed hemorrhage occurring 7–10 days post procedure.
- Urgent hemorrhoid surgery is usually reserved for the patient with strangulated, incarcerated, gangrenous hemorrhoids.

Anatomy

- Hemorrhoids are a normal part of the anal canal.
- Anatomically the three main "vascular cushions" of submucosa filled with blood vessels and muscle fibers are located in the left lateral, right anterior, and right posterior positions.
  - The muscle fibers arise from the internal sphincter and from the conjoined longitudinal muscle.
  - The arterial blood supply to hemorrhoids is primarily from the terminal branches of the superior hemorrhoidal artery.
  - Venous outflow is from the superior, middle, and inferior hemorrhoidal veins (Fig. 12.1).

Electronic Supplementary Material The online version of this chapter (https://doi.org/10.1007/978-3-030-01165-9_12) contains supplementary material, which is available to authorized users.

M. Luchtefeld (✉) · R. E. Hoedema
Department of Colon and Rectal Surgery, Spectrum Health/Ferguson Clinic, Grand Rapids, MI, USA
e-mail: Martin.Luchtefeld@spectrumhealth.org

S. R. Steele et al. (eds.), *The ASCRS Manual of Colon and Rectal Surgery*,
https://doi.org/10.1007/978-3-030-01165-9_12

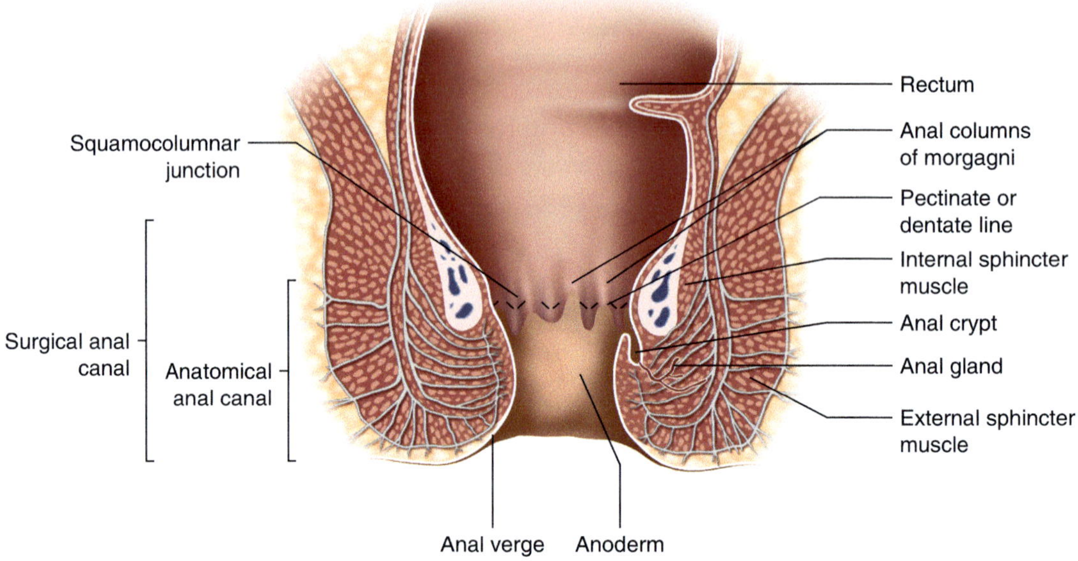

Fig. 12.1 Hemorrhoid anatomy

Etiology

- There are numerous possible reasons why hemorrhoids become symptomatic.
- During straining, the vascular cushions engorged to prevent the escape of fecal material or gas.
- With the passage of time, the anatomic structures supporting the muscular submucosa weaken, allowing the hemorrhoidal tissue to slip or prolapse.
  - Matrix metalloproteinases (MMP) are enzymes present in the extracellular space and can degrade collagen, elastin, and fibronectin.
  - MMP-9 has been found to be overexpressed in hemorrhoid tissue in association with breakdown of elastic fibers.
  - Once the hemorrhoids start to prolapse, the internal sphincter can slow the rate of venous return and increase the hemorrhoid engorgement.
- Increased vascular supply and neovascularization may play a role in making hemorrhoids more symptomatic.
  - Terminal branches of the superior hemorrhoidal artery are larger in diameter, had greater flow, and higher peak velocity and acceleration velocity in patients with hemorrhoids.
  - Microvascular density has also been found to be increased in hemorrhoids.
  - Endoglin (CD105) (binding site for TGF-B and is a proliferative marker for neovascularity) and higher expression of vascular endothelial growth factor (VEGF) (angiogenesis-related protein) have been found in hemorrhoidal specimens.
- Other possible causes include pregnancy, chronic cough, pelvic floor dysfunction, and simply being erect.
- Despite the many theories that have been proposed, most of these are very speculative, and almost certainly hemorrhoidal symptoms result from a combination of multiple different factors.

Epidemiology

- It is difficult to know the true incidence of hemorrhoids.
- One study done in 1990 suggested that the prevalence in the United States was 4.4% with the highest rate being in Caucasian patients

between 45 and 65 years of age and elevated social economic status.

- In 2004, the National Institutes of Health noted that the diagnosis of hemorrhoids was associated with 3.2 million ambulatory care visits, 306,000 hospitalizations, and 2 million prescriptions in the United States.

Classification

- Hemorrhoids are generally classified as internal, external, or mixed.
  - Internal hemorrhoids are those located above the dentate line.
  - External hemorrhoids are located below the dentate line.
- In addition, there is a classification system of the internal hemorrhoids based on the degree of clinical prolapse (Fig. 12.2).

Clinical Presentation

- Bleeding, pain, and protrusion are the most common symptoms associated with hemorrhoids.
- When internal hemorrhoids are the primary source of the problem, the main symptoms are a combination of rectal bleeding and prolapse.
  - Pain is very rarely associated with internal hemorrhoids.
  - The bleeding is typically bright red, ranges in frequency, and is seen on the toilet paper or in the toilet water.
  - Bleeding can be enough bleeding to lead to anemia.
  - Another common symptom of internal hemorrhoids is prolapse. This can reduce after each bowel movement or can be chronically prolapsed.

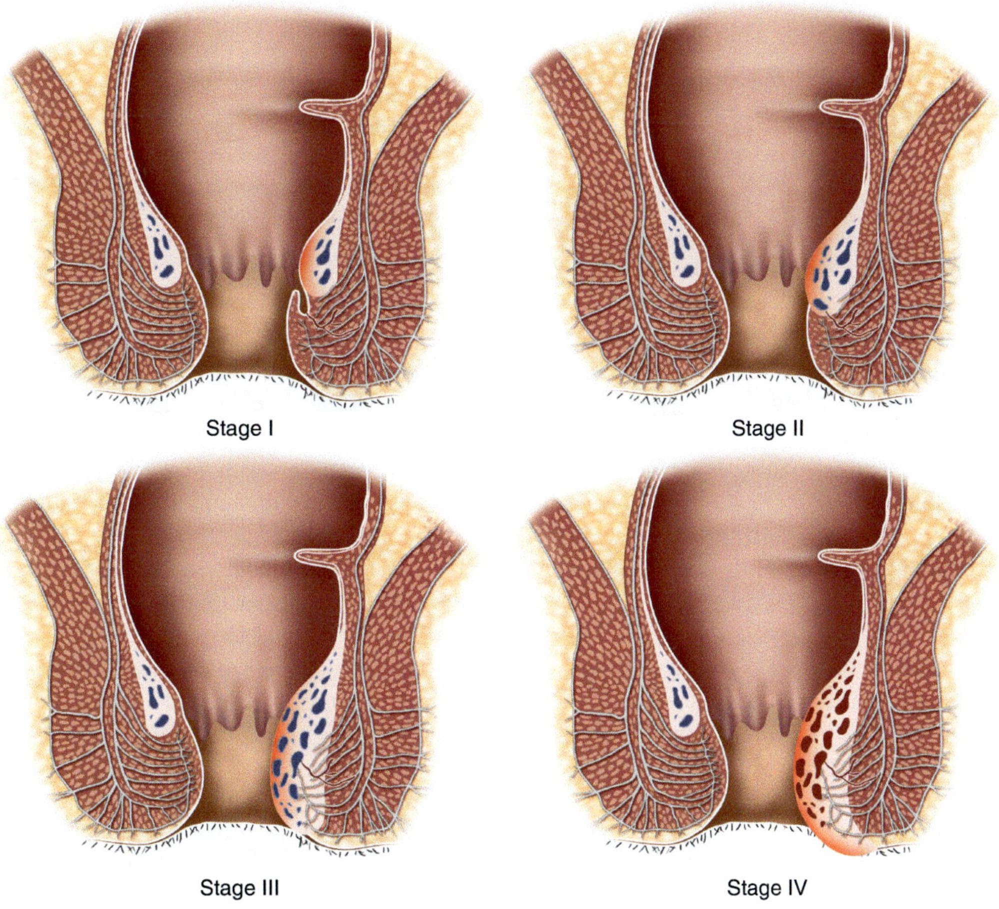

Fig. 12.2 Hemorrhoid classification table/grading system

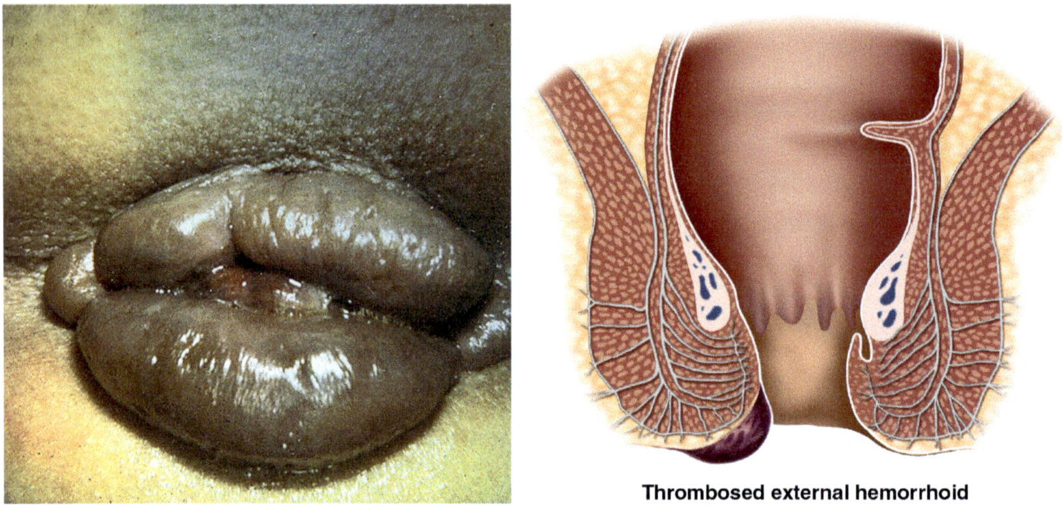

Fig. 12.3 Thrombosed external hemorrhoid. Courtesy of Richard Billingham

- External hemorrhoids are more likely to be associated with pain from engorgement and edema.
  - Patients typically complain of tags which swell, itch, and make hygiene difficult.
- Mixed hemorrhoids result in the intra-anal prolapsing out of the anal canal along with the internal hemorrhoid.
- A patient with a thrombosed hemorrhoid will describe a sudden onset of pain and swelling in the perianal region (Fig. 12.3).
  - The swelling will usually last at least days if not weeks.
  - The pain can vary greatly in severity but is typically constant and unrelenting.
  - Thrombosed hemorrhoids typically occur in the external component but in severe cases can go on to involve the internal hemorrhoids as well.
- It is important to keep in mind the wide differential diagnosis in patients presenting with anorectal complaints (Table 12.1).

Table 12.1 Hemorrhoid symptoms

Hemorrhoid symptoms
Rectal bleeding
Bright red blood in stool
Dripping in toilet
On wiping after defecation
Pain during bowel movements
Anal itching
Rectal prolapse (while walking, lifting weights)
Thrombus
Extreme pain, bleeding, and occasional signs of systemic illness in case of strangulation

Evaluation and Physical Examination

History

- The history should include the patient's bowel habits, presence of pain, bleeding, and tissue protrusion.

Physical Examination

- Examination position includes the supine, prone jackknife, or left lateral (Sims) position (Fig. 12.4).
- It is important to be as reassuring as possible during this examination as it is inherently embarrassing and uncomfortable.
- The examination begins by inspection, gently spreading the buttocks and inspecting the skin, perineum, and the external anal opening.
- A digital rectal exam is then performed to assess for masses, pain, and sphincter tone.
- Anoscopy is required to fully assess the anal canal (see Fig. 4.3).
  - Asking the patient to bear down with the anoscope in place can give a better assessment of the severity of the hemorrhoidal problems and specifically the degree of prolapse.

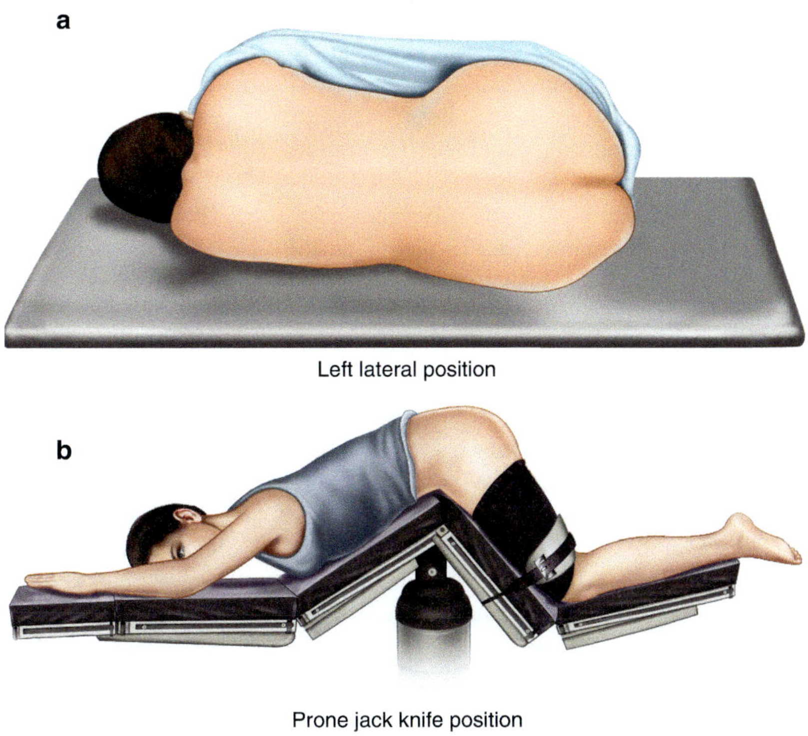

Fig. 12.4 Patient positioning. (**a**) Left lateral position. (**b**) Prone jackknife position

- Many patients should also undergo a rigid proctoscopy to rule out malignancies or inflammatory conditions that could be mimicking hemorrhoids.
- The patient who presents with rectal bleeding should always be considered for colonoscopy.
  - The young patient with typical hemorrhoidal bleeding that responds to treatment and with no family history of colon cancer likely does not need further evaluation.
    - In a large series of classic "outlet" bleeding, colonoscopy revealed adenomas in less than 2% and no cancers in patients less than 50 years of age.
    - When considering all age groups, 6.7% of the patients had a significant lesion (e.g., cancer, large polyps, or carcinoma in situ).

Treatment

- The options for the treatment of hemorrhoids can be categorized into medical management, office-based treatments, and operative therapies.
- Treatment aggressiveness is determined by the degree of symptoms and patient preference.

Medical Management

Dietary

- The main components of dietary management are geared toward minimizing constipation and consist of a high-fiber diet accompanied by an adequate fluid intake.
  - The recommended dose of dietary fiber is 25 g (for women) to 38 g (for men) per day.
  - Many patients find that attempting to reach the maximum amount of fiber leads to bloating and excessive gas and this can be a limiting factor.
  - Along with the increased fiber, patients should also drink at least 64 ounces of fluid per day.
  - The desired outcome of the increased fiber and fluid is a soft but formed bowel movement that can be expelled with minimal effort.

- Stool softeners are simple and safe and can be very helpful for patients that have exceptionally hard bowel movements.
- Hyperosmolar laxatives such as polyethylene glycol are a good choice for those patients that do not do well with fiber supplements.
- For the occasional patient with diarrhea, evaluation must be carried out to determine the etiology.
- Loperamide can be very useful to minimize diarrhea in patients with irritable bowel syndrome.
- In many patients, the hemorrhoidal symptoms are tied into their toileting habits, and time spent on the toilet should be minimized.
- Sitz baths are often used as part of the treatment for hemorrhoids to decrease pain, burning, and itching following a bowel movement.
- They can also aid in hygiene as well as decrease anal canal pressures.
- Excessive use can lead to macerated skin and even more discomfort; soaking time should be limited to 10–15 min two to three times per day.

Topical Therapies

- There is a vast array of over-the-counter hemorrhoidal treatments, combining a barrier protectant with some other active ingredients including vasoconstriction agents, local anesthetics, anti-inflammatory agents, and astringents.
- There is very little science to support the use of these agents; however, some patients do claim to get relief from these products, and there appears to be little or no harm in their use.
- Topical nitrates such as calcium channel blockers can decrease internal sphincter tone and have been shown to be beneficial in patients with high sphincter tone and hemorrhoids.
- Suppositories are difficult to maintain in the correct anatomic location and do not cure hemorrhoids, yet some patients do get relief with their use.

Oral Therapy

- Flavonoids are a type of plant-based phlebotonics that increase vascular tone, reduce venous capacity, decrease papillary permeability, increase lymphatic drainage, and have anti-inflammatory effects.
- They have been shown to decrease bleeding, pain, and itching with their use.

Office-Based Treatments

- The relative lack of somatic innervation of the internal hemorrhoids allows such treatments to be performed in the office.

Rubber Band Ligation

- Barron first described rubber band ligation of internal hemorrhoids in 1963.
- By applying a rubber band at the apex of the internal hemorrhoid, the hemorrhoid is fixed high in the anal canal, correcting the prolapse, and by decreasing the blood flow caudally, the hemorrhoids shrink in size.
- The technique of rubber band ligation is straightforward (Fig. 12.5).
  - The patient is placed in either the prone jackknife or left lateral decubitus position.
  - Anoscopy is then done to determine which hemorrhoids will be banded.
  - There are a number of different banders available (Fig. 12.6); some banders utilize a grasp, while others use suction to pull the internal hemorrhoid into the banding instrument.
  - Once the bander is in place, the rubber band is deployed to place it at the base of the internal hemorrhoid.
  - It is important to place the band at least 1–2 cm above the dentate line to minimize significant pain.
  - Anywhere from one to three bands can be done at the same setting; application of multiple bands can increase pain, urinary retention, and vasovagal reactions.
- Patients should be warned that there can be a show of blood 5–7 days following the ligation.
- An office appointment should be made in 4 weeks to evaluate the success of the banding, and serial banding can be performed.
- Complications following banding are unusual and include delayed rectal bleeding (1%), thrombosis, abscess, or urinary dysfunction.

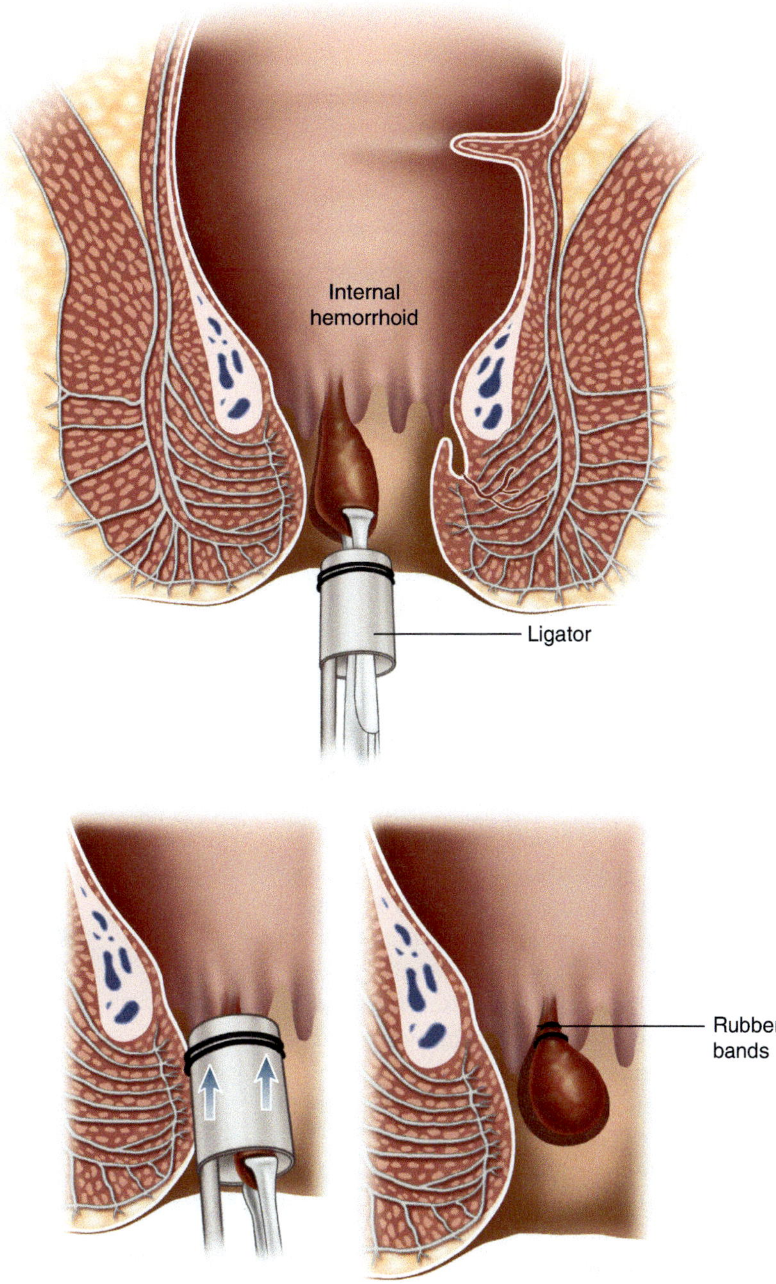

Fig. 12.5 Hemorrhoid banding technique

- A potentially devastating yet rare complication is pelvic sepsis.
  - Patient presents with the triad of symptoms: increasing pain, fever, and urinary retention.
  - Clinicians should be aware of this potential complication and be ready to treat it aggressively if it does occur.
  - CT scan of the pelvis may illustrate air outside the rectum and/or inflammation.

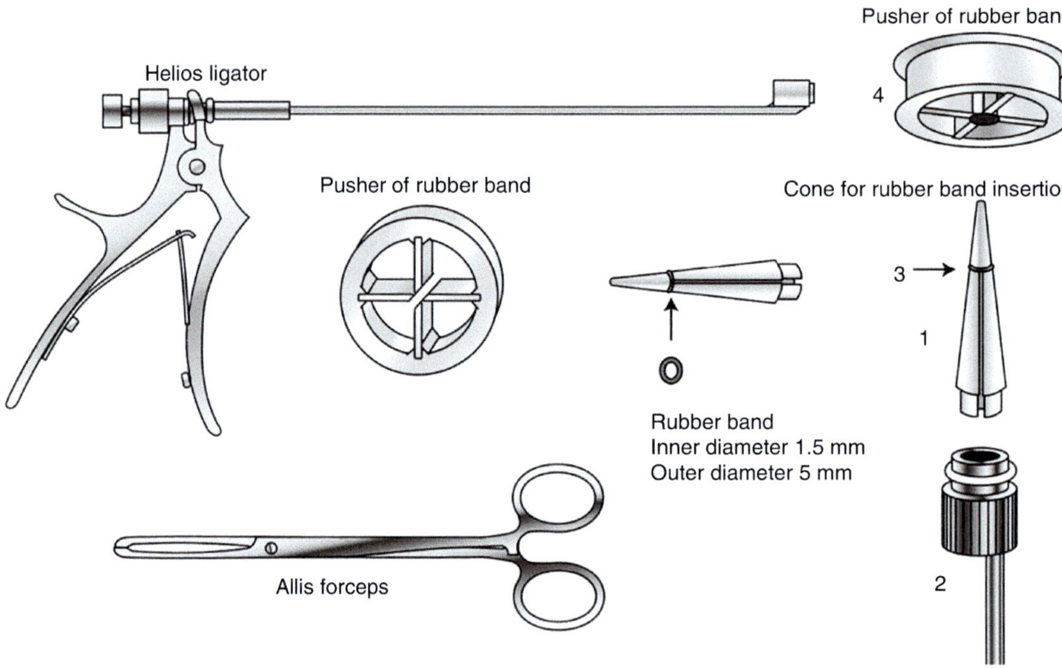

Fig. 12.6 Hemorrhoid bander. Helio's product is easy to mount a rubber band. It uses a rubber band mounting cone (1), inserts rubber band at the end of cone (2), and pushes the rubber band to the bottom of the cone (3) using a rubber band pusher (4). (With permission from Hyung Kyu Yang, Nonsurgical treatment of hemorrhoids. In: Hyung Kyu Yang, ed. Hemorrhoids. Springer, New York, 2014; pp: 47–63.© 2014 Springer)

  - The diagnosis can also be made in the operating room with an exam under anesthesia.
  - Treatment includes debridement of the wound with intravenous antibiotics that may suffice and, in more severe cases, laparotomy with diverting colostomy and pelvic drainage.
- Rubber band ligation is very effective for the treatment of grade 1–3 hemorrhoids.
- 18–32% of patients require repeat treatments when followed in the long term.

Infrared Photocoagulation

- Energy ablation can be used to treat internal hemorrhoids; these options include infrared photocoagulation, bipolar diathermy, and direct current electrotherapy (Fig. 12.7).
- Ischemia of the internal hemorrhoidal vascular complex leads to scarring and fibrosis in the normal anatomic location.

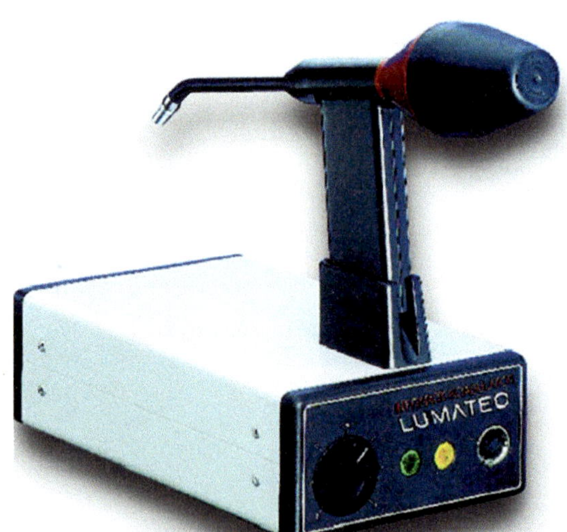

Fig. 12.7 Infrared photocoagulation machine. (With permission from Hyung Kyu Yang, Nonsurgical treatment of hemorrhoids. In: Hyung Kyu Yang, ed. Hemorrhoids. Springer, New York, 2014; pp: 47–63. ©2014 Springer)

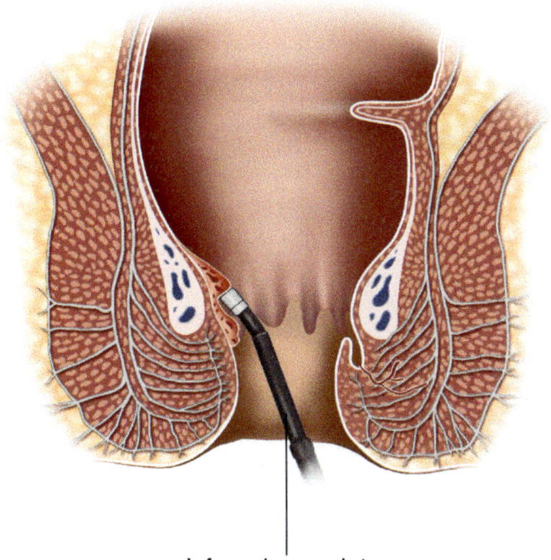

Fig. 12.8 Infrared photocoagulation technique

- Infrared radiation generates heat that penetrates approximately 3 mm and leads to heat necrosis that causes tissue destruction and eventually fibrosis and scarring.
  - Once the patient is positioned, the tip of the infrared coagulator is used three to four times at the apex of each internal hemorrhoid.
  - Each application of the photocoagulation is done for 1–1.5 s (although the device allows a range of 0.1–3 s) (Fig. 12.8).
  - There is usually minimal discomfort once the treatment is complete, and all three hemorrhoid complexes can be treated at the same session.
- Infrared coagulation is most effective for the treatment of bleeding; it is less useful for treating significant prolapse of hemorrhoids and may be less painful than hemorrhoidal banding.
- Complications are rare following infrared photocoagulation and consist primarily of pain and bleeding due to excessive application of energy.
- Bipolar diathermy and direct current electrotherapy are not as popular as infrared coagulation as patients require subsequent operative therapy.

Sclerotherapy

- A sclerotherapy solution is injected at the apex of the internal hemorrhoid complex which leads to scarring and fibrosis and fixation of the internal hemorrhoidal complex.
- Many different agents have been tried including phenol, carbolic acid, quinine in urea, sodium morrhuate, and sodium tetradecyl.
- A spinal needle is used to place approximately 1–1.5 mL of the agent in a submucosal fashion at the apex of the internal hemorrhoid (Fig. 12.9).
- Placement too superficially can cause mucosal sloughing, while placing it too deep leads to more risk of infection, abscess, or significant pain.
- Urinary retention and impotence postinjection sclerotherapy have also been reported.
- Sclerotherapy is reported to be highly successful but is still not quite as effective as rubber band ligation especially for grade 3 hemorrhoids.
- The best role for sclerotherapy may be in patients that require anticoagulation since the risk of bleeding is minimal with this technique.
- Multiple repeat attempts should be avoided due to the cumulative risk of stricture.

Operative Management of Hemorrhoids

- Patients who have failed medical management or have recurrent, persistent symptoms despite undergoing some of the internal hemorrhoidal treatments mentioned above.
- Typically, only 5–10% of patients with hemorrhoidal complaints require operative hemorrhoidectomy.
- In the acute setting, patients with extensive thrombosed hemorrhoids or strangulated, gangrenous hemorrhoids need immediate attention and operative intervention (Fig. 12.10).
- Excisional hemorrhoidectomy has excellent results, minimal recurrence rates, and few complications yet is associated with significant postoperative pain.

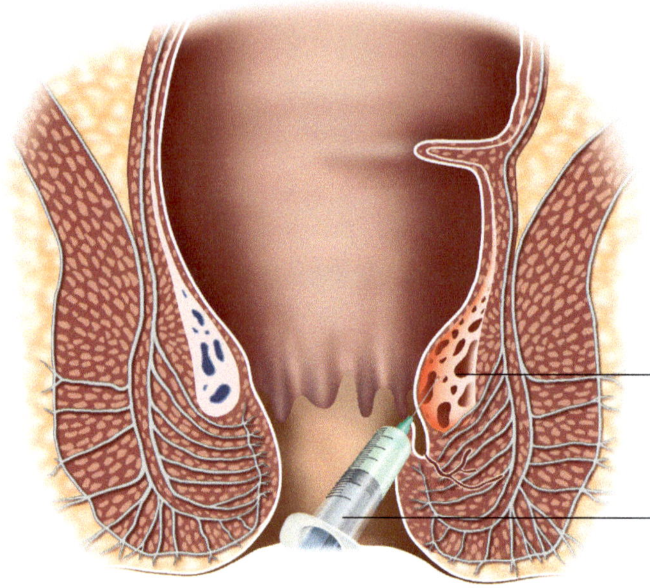

Fig. 12.9 Sclerotherapy technique

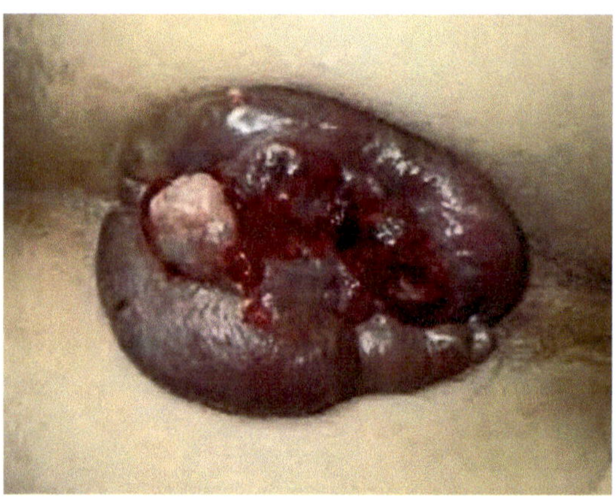

Fig. 12.10 Strangulated, gangrenous hemorrhoids

Excisional Hemorrhoidectomy-Closed Technique

- Dr. Lynn Ferguson of the Ferguson Clinic first described the closed hemorrhoidectomy technique in the early 1950s.
- Anesthesia can be tailored to the patient and can range from something as simple as local anesthesia plus intravenous sedation to a full general anesthesia with intubation.
- Positioning is per surgeon preference and includes the options of lithotomy, prone jackknife, and left lateral decubitus.
- The operation starts with a digital exam followed by anoscopy to help clearly define which hemorrhoid complexes should be excised (Fig. 12.11).
- Injecting the perianal skin and hemorrhoids with local anesthetic combined with epinephrine 1:200,000 can help to decrease bleeding during the procedure.
- An elliptical incision is made around the hemorrhoid starting at the perianal margin, and a proportional incision should be made so that the length of the incision is approximately three to four times longer than its breadth.
- The hemorrhoid is then elevated off the underlying sphincter muscle fibers.
- At the apex of the hemorrhoid, the vascular pedicle is then clamped and then the hemorrhoid excised.
- The vascular pedicle is then suture ligated with an absorbable suture; the same suture is then used to reapproximate the tissue.
- When multiple hemorrhoids are removed, it is important to maintain adequate skin and tissue bridges between the excision sites to minimize the risk of postoperative anal stenosis.

Fig. 12.11 Closed hemorrhoidectomy

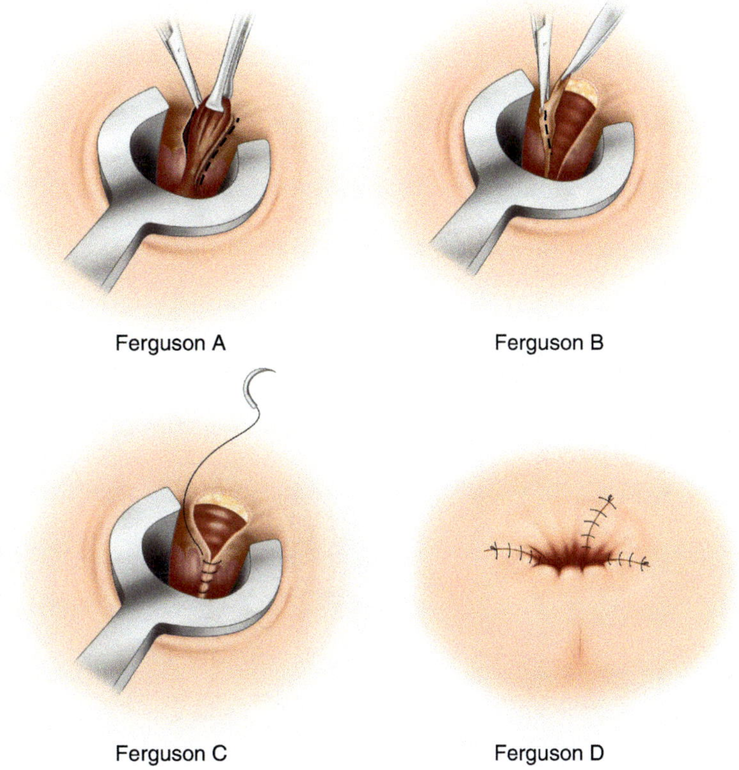

- A notable variation on the technique is the use of energy devices such as the LigaSure bipolar device or the harmonic device which both can be used to perform the excisional hemorrhoidectomy with reports that there may be less postoperative discomfort.

Excisional Hemorrhoidectomy Open Technique (Milligan-Morgan)

- The open technique of excisional hemorrhoidectomy is very popular in the United Kingdom.
- This technique results in a very similar excision as the Ferguson technique except that the wounds are not closed other than suture ligating the vascular pedicle (Fig. 12.12).

Excisional Hemorrhoidectomy (Circumferential or Whitehead)

- A circumferential incision is made at the level of the dentate line, and then the submucosal and subdermal hemorrhoidal tissues are dissected out and removed.
- Any redundant rectal mucosa is excised and then the remaining proximal rectal mucosa sutured down to the anoderm.
- This operation is not in common use at this time due to the complication of a whitehead deformity (Fig. 12.13).

Results of Hemorrhoidectomy

- Excisional hemorrhoidectomy remains the gold standard for the long-term relief of hemorrhoidal symptoms.

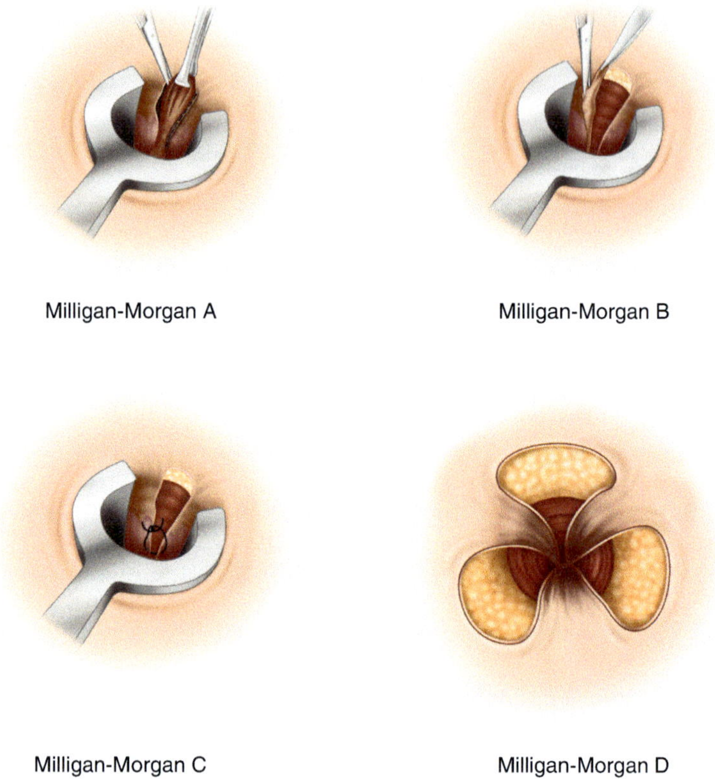

Fig. 12.12 Open hemorrhoidectomy

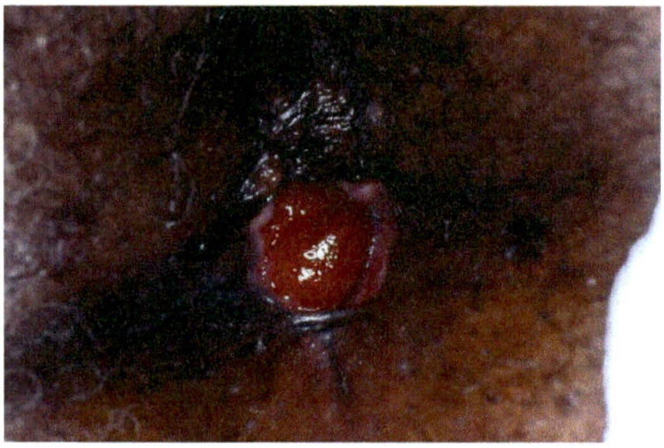

Fig. 12.13 Whitehead deformity. Courtesy of the American Society of Colon and Rectal Surgeons

- Although there has been considerable controversy over the relative merits of opened versus closed techniques, there is very little difference between the two techniques.
- Energy sources such as the harmonic scalpel or the LigaSure have been compared to excisional hemorrhoidectomy.
  - Studies suggest less pain and faster operative time.
  - Long-term follow-up data is not yet available.
- Less postoperative pain has been suggested with use of simultaneous lateral internal sphincterotomy, topical nitroglycerin, and both oral and topical metronidazole.

Complications of Hemorrhoidectomy

Urinary Retention

- Urinary retention is one of the most common complications following hemorrhoidectomy.

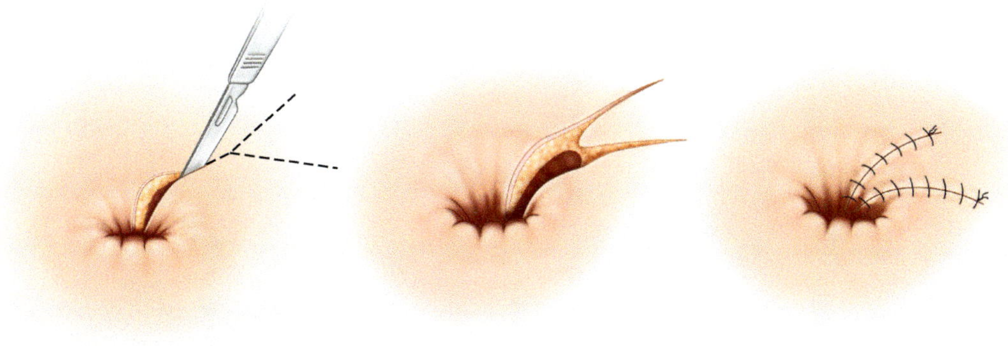

Fig. 12.14 Y-V anoplasty

- The number of quadrants excised and analgesia requirements were both important risk factors.
- Fluid restriction and pain control in the perioperative period are important to prevent this complication.

Postoperative Hemorrhage

- Postoperative hemorrhage risk is still relatively low.
- In 1% of cases, the bleeding will occur in the immediate postoperative period (technical error).
- Delayed hemorrhage can occur in up to 5.4% of patients and will typically occur 7–10 days after surgery.
  - Observation, packing of the anal canal or tamponade with a Foley balloon.
  - If the bleeding does not stop, then an exam under anesthesia may be warranted.

Anal Stenosis

- Anal stenosis is rare but can occur if excessive anoderm is removed at the time of the hemorrhoidectomy.
- The most common setting for anal stentosis to occur is an emergency hemorrhoidectomy for prolapsed thrombosed hemorrhoids. Care should be taken to avoid resecting too much anoderm.
- Treatment can be as simple as the use of bulk laxatives but may require dilation and or anoplasty (Fig. 12.14).

Postoperative Infection

- Postoperative infections are surprisingly uncommon (less than 1%).

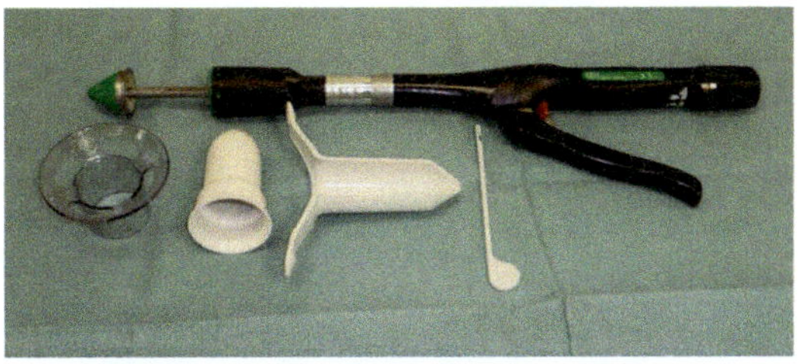

Fig. 12.15 Stapled hemorrhoidectomy (PPH) (With permission from Schwandner O. Procedure for Prolapse and Hemorrhoids (PPH; Stapled Hemorrhoidopexy). In: Wexner SD, Fleshman JW. Colon and Rectal Surgery: Anorectal Operations. Wolter Kluwers, 2011. © Copyright Wolters Kluwer 2011)

- Prophylactic antibiotic therapy is not indicated for elective hemorrhoid surgery.
- If abscess or cellulitis occurs, it may require antibiotics and/or operative drainage.

Fecal Incontinence

- Fecal soiling or incontinence following hemorrhoidectomy is rather unusual.
  - Sphincter stretch
  - Direct injury to the sphincter complex
  - Loss of the hemorrhoidal piles (thought to contribute approximately 10–15% of continence)

Stapled Hemorrhoidopexy

- Developed as a procedure for prolapse using a hemorrhoidopexy technique (Fig. 12.15).
- End-to-end circular stapler is used to excise a circumferential ring of internal hemorrhoids,

including the mucosa and submucosa above the dentate line (Fig. 12.16).

- The remaining hemorrhoids are pulled up into the anal canal and fixed in place.
- Some of the blood supply to the remaining hemorrhoids is also interrupted so that there is less engorgement of the remaining hemorrhoids.

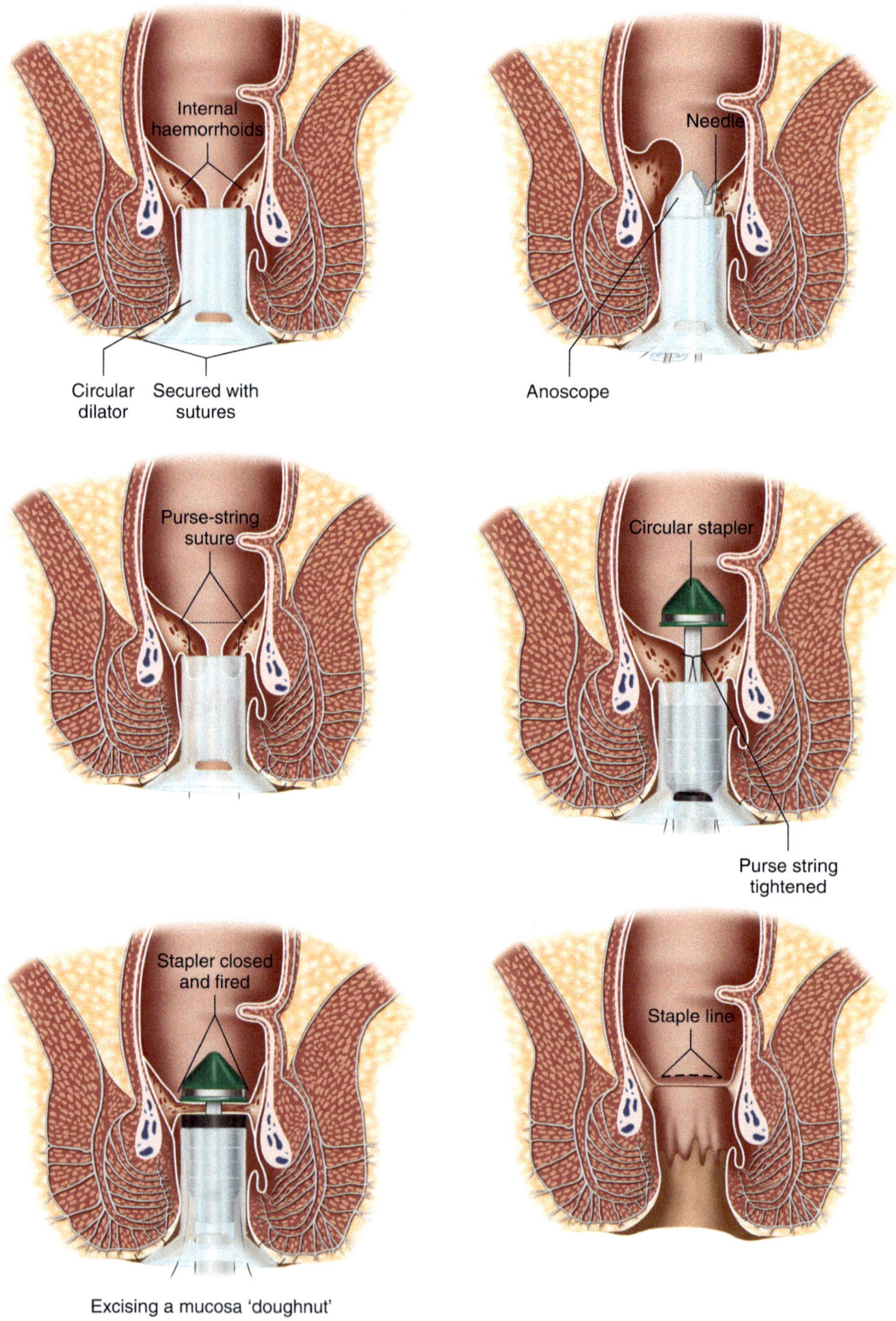

Fig. 12.16 Stapled hemorrhoidectomy technique

- Indications for stapled hemorrhoidopexy include patients with second- or third-degree hemorrhoids.
- Because the operation occurs above the dentate line, there has been reported less postoperative pain compared to a hemorrhoidectomy.
- Procedure
  - With the anoscope in place, a purse-string suture is placed in a circumferential fashion into the submucosa approximately 2 cm above the transitional zone.
  - The head of the stapler (similar to an EEA, but the head is not detachable) is then introduced into the rectum past the purse-string suture.
  - The purse string is tied down around the stapler, and then the anvil is very slowly closed while giving gentle traction on the purse-string suture externally.
  - Once closed, the stapler is fired and then removed along with the excised tissue.
  - The staple line should be inspected carefully for bleeding and may require suture ligation.
- Outcomes
  - Randomized controlled studies confirmed there was significantly less postoperative pain compared to excisional hemorrhoidectomy and with equal relief of hemorrhoidal symptoms.
  - Compared to excisional hemorrhoidectomy, patients undergoing excisional hemorrhoidectomy had fewer recurrences of prolapse and fewer symptoms than those undergoing stapled hemorrhoidopexy.
  - Some unique complications that have been reported with this procedure include rectal perforation, persistent rectal pain, retroperitoneal sepsis, rectal obstruction, and rectovaginal fistula.

Transanal Hemorrhoidal Dearterialization

- Transanal hemorrhoidal dearterialization (THD) is a relatively new technique first described by Morinaga in 1995 (Fig. 12.17).
- Doppler is used to guide ligation of the arterial inflow to the hemorrhoids.

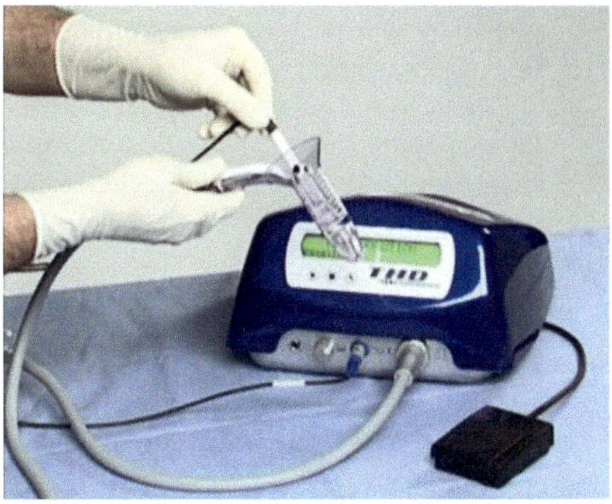

Fig. 12.17 Transanal hemorrhoidal dearterialization device

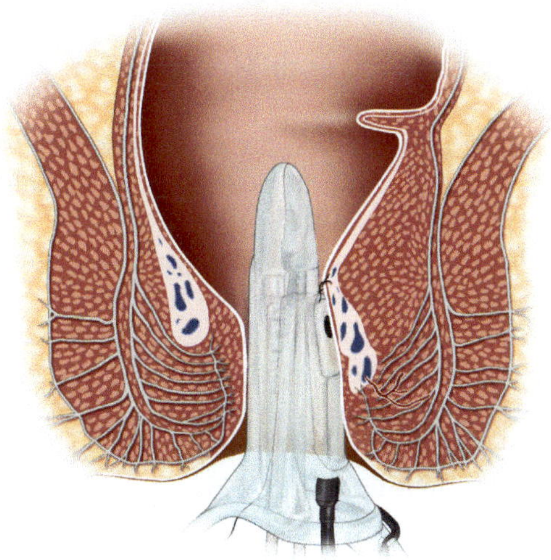

Fig. 12.18 Transanal hemorrhoidal dearterialization technique

- Although not initially described, suture rectopexy can be done at the same setting to minimize prolapse.
- Procedure
  - A specialized anoscope with a Doppler is introduced into the anal canal (Fig. 12.18).
  - The Doppler is used as the anoscope is rotated until one of the feeding arteries is identified and suture ligated.
  - The anoscope is rotated until all of the significant arteries are identified and ligated

(generally four to six arteries, but this can be quite variable).
  - Depending on the need to correct the prolapse, a suture mucopexy can be performed immediately following the ligation using the same stitch.
- Outcomes
  - The arterial ligation and mucopexy are all done above the dentate line; data suggests less painful than a hemorrhoidectomy.
  - It appears to be a safe alternative with a recurrence rate of 10.8% for prolapse, 9.7% for bleeding, and 8.7% for pain at defecation at follow-up of 1 year or more.

Special Clinical Scenarios

Thrombosed External Hemorrhoid

- Patient presents with the acute onset of anal pain along with a hard lump in the perianal region (Fig. 12.3).
- The perianal pain and discomfort are constant and can be worse around day 3 or 4.
- The thrombosis can sometimes cause pressure ulceration and eventually skin necrosis leading to a spontaneous evacuation of the clot.
- The aggressiveness of the treatment is primarily driven by the patient's symptoms.
  - If the patient is relatively comfortable, it is best to allow the thrombosis to resolve on its own.
  - If the patient presents with severe, unrelenting pain, excision of the thrombus can be very helpful (Fig. 12.19).
- In the office setting, local anesthesia can be used at the level of the thrombosed hemorrhoid.
- The skin should be excised overlying the thrombosis to allow clot removal.
- Bleeding is usually not troublesome and can be controlled with pressure, silver nitrate, cautery, and suture ligation (see Video 12.1).

Strangulated (Thrombosed Prolapsed) Hemorrhoids (Fig. 12.10)

- Acute episode of pain and protrusion that is no longer reducible.
- May also complain of urinary retention and referred pain.
- A significant amount of edema may be present and, if left untreated, may progress to ulceration, necrosis, and eventually gangrene.
- Treatment usually consists of an urgent excisional hemorrhoidectomy in the operating room.
- An alternative treatment option, if the patient does not want surgery hemorrhoid, may be reduced using local anesthetic, applying pressure and/or massage to decrease the edema in the tissues, and then using a combination of rubber band ligations and thrombectomies. This will provide immediate relief for the patient and will not usually require a future surgical hemorrhoidectomy.

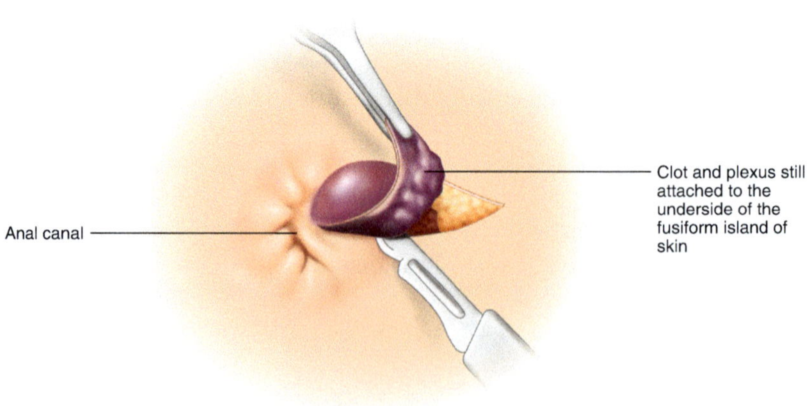

Fig. 12.19 Enucleation of the thrombosed hemorrhoid

Portal Hypertension and Hemorrhoids

- Rectal varices in patients with portal hypertension are a distinct entity.
- Rectal varices in patients with portal hypertension provide collateral circulation from the portal system into the systemic venous circulation.
- Fortunately, anorectal varices rarely bleed.
- Treatment recommendations include:
  – Medical management of the portal pressures, sclerotherapy, suture ligation, stapled anopexy, and, lastly, TIPS and portosystemic shunts

Pregnancy

- Hemorrhoid symptoms present during pregnancy usually resolve after delivery and rarely need intervention.
- Surgical intervention is not warranted unless strangulated, gangrenous hemorrhoids (approximately 2% incidence).

Crohn's Disease

- Any anorectal surgical intervention must be performed with caution in patients with Crohn's disease due to prolonged wound healing and ulcerations.
- Crohn's disease is not an absolute contraindication to surgical intervention when disease is controlled medically as the rate of prolonged healing and associated complications is much less.
- Hemorrhoidectomy, however, should not be performed in those patients with anorectal Crohn's disease or Crohn's proctitis.

Immunocompromised Patients

- Similar to the Crohn's disease population, extreme caution should be exercised when considering surgical therapies due to risk of poor wound healing and infectious complications.
- The HIV/AIDS population does suffer a higher degree of complications post hemorrhoidectomy.
- Patients who are neutropenic should be offered non-operative therapies first although the mortality rate in this patient population who undergoes a hemorrhoidectomy is not higher.

Figure 12.20 shows a treatment algorithm for symptomatic hemorrhoids.

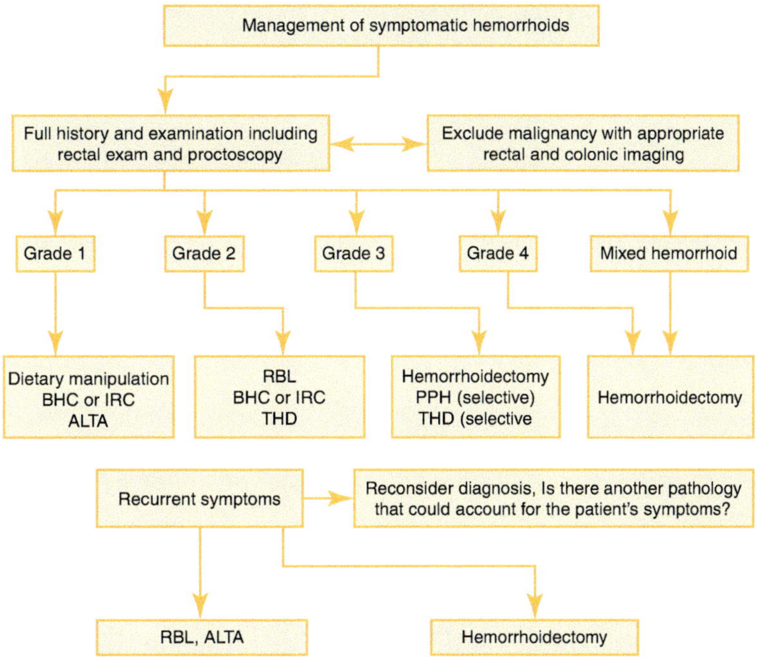

Fig. 12.20 Treatment algorithm for symptomatic emorrhoids. *RBL* rubber band ligation; *IRC* infrared coagulation; *THD* transanal hemorrhoidal dearterialization; *PPH* procedure for prolapsing hemorrhoids; *BHC* bipolar hyperthermic coagulation; *ALTA* Aluminum potassium sulfate and tannic acid (sclerotherapy)

13 Anal Fissure

Kim C. Lu and Daniel O. Herzig

Key Concepts

- An acute anal fissure (symptoms <6 weeks) is likely to heal (87%) with dietary modification and supportive care.
- In a chronic anal fissure (symptoms >6 weeks), topical nitroglycerin or calcium channel blockers are slightly better than placebo in inducing healing.
- Injection of botulinum toxin into the internal anal sphincter can heal fissures refractory to topical ointments, though this is not as effective as lateral internal anal sphincterotomy.
- Lateral internal anal sphincterotomy is the most effective therapy in healing fissures; there is an increased risk, however, of fecal incontinence.
- For anal fissures associated with decreased anal sphincter tone, a dermal advancement flap is a reasonable option.

Electronic Supplementary Material The online version of this chapter (https://doi.org/10.1007/978-3-030-01165-9_13) contains supplementary material, which is available to authorized users.

K. C. Lu (✉)
Division of Gastrointestinal and General Surgery, Department of Surgery, Oregon Health & Science University, Portland, OR, USA
e-mail: luk@ohsu.edu

D. O. Herzig
Division of Gastroenterology and General Surgery, Department of Surgery, Oregon Health and Science University, Portland, OR, USA

Definition/Clinical Presentation

- An anal fissure is a tear in the epithelial lining of the distal anal canal.
- Extremely common condition.
- Fissures can be classified as acute vs. chronic and typical vs. atypical.
  - Acute fissures (<6 weeks)
    - Bright red bleeding with bowel movements.
    - Sharp, burning, tearing anal pain or spasm.
    - Can last for hours after the bowel movement.
    - Physical findings: linear separation of the anoderm, visible with just separation of the buttocks (Fig. 13.1).
    - Posterior midline: the site of up to 90% of typical anal fissures.
    - Remaining minority of typical fissures are found in the anterior midline.
  - Chronic fissures (>6 weeks)
    - Additional physical findings of an external sentinel tag at the external apex, exposed internal sphincter muscle, and a hypertrophied anal papilla at the internal apex (Fig. 13.2)
  - Typical fissures
    - Located in the posterior or anterior midline
    - Not associated with other diseases

S. R. Steele et al. (eds.), *The ASCRS Manual of Colon and Rectal Surgery*,
https://doi.org/10.1007/978-3-030-01165-9_13

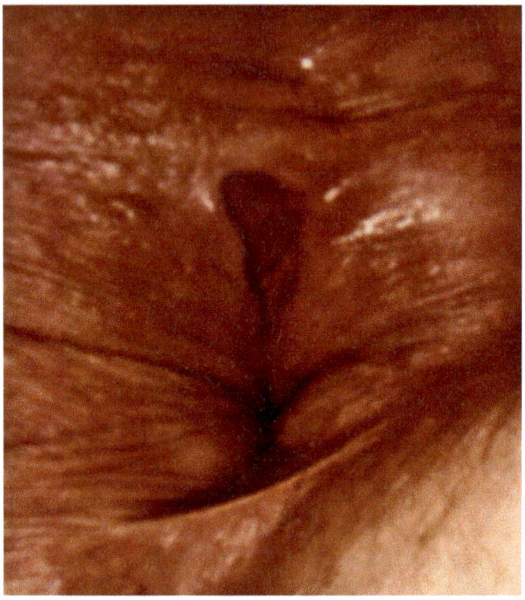

Fig. 13.1 Chronic fissure with external sentinel tag, internal hypertrophied papilla, and thickened internal anal sphincter muscle

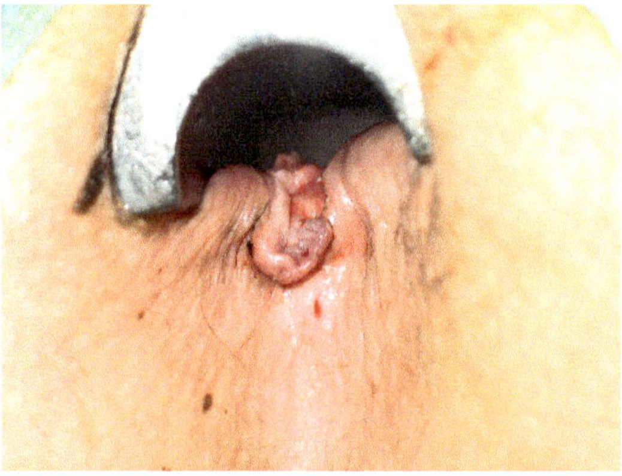

Fig. 13.2 Acute fissure with clear edges and no signs of chronicity of sphincter hypertrophy. (Courtesy of Richard P. Billingham, MD)

- Atypical fissures
  - Can occur anywhere in the anal canal (Fig. 13.3)
  - Tend to be associated with other diseases, including malignancy, Crohn's disease, human immunodeficiency virus (HIV) infection, syphilis, and tuberculosis (Fig. 13.4)

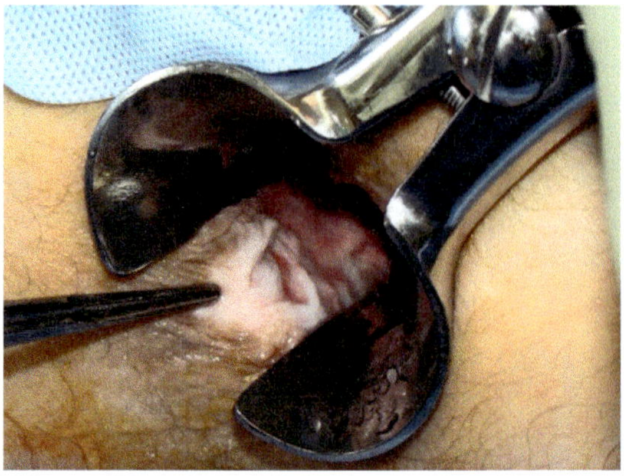

Fig. 13.3 Atypical fissure with skin changes, broad base, and lateral location. (Courtesy of Sam Atallah, MD)

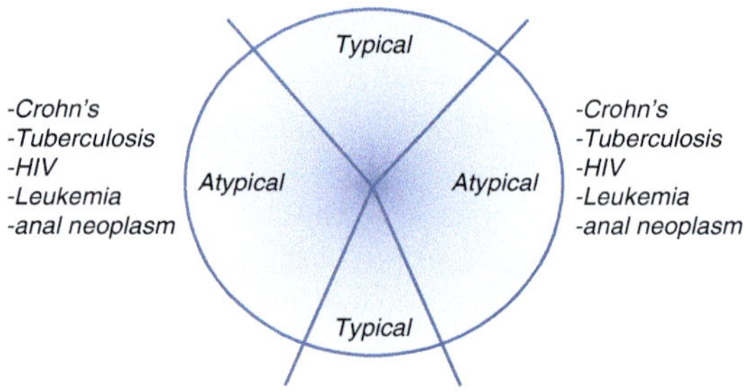

Fig. 13.4 Type of fissure by location

Pathogenesis

- The exact etiology remains uncertain.
- Typically occur after the passage of a large, hard stool or anal trauma.
- Fissures can occur in the absence of any trauma or constipation.
- Theories:
  - Mechanical theory – the anorectal angle creates the greatest stress posteriorly.
  - Sphincter hypertonicity – it is documented by manometry in multiple studies, undetermined if the cause of the disease or an effect.
  - Ischemia – the posterior midline is relatively ischemic by both arteriographic studies and laser Doppler.

Non-operative Treatment

Healing Rates in Acute Anal Fissure

- Safe, few side effects, and should usually be the first step in therapy
- Up to 90% with acute anal fissure when prescribed 10 g of unprocessed bran twice daily and use of a warm sitz bath for 15 min twice daily and after bowel movements

Healing Rates in Chronic Anal Fissure

- Spontaneous healing rates are likely to be seen in only a minority of patients.
- Cochrane Review of the non-operative treatment of chronic anal fissure (over 70 randomized trials): healing rate in the combined placebo group was 35.5%.
- Because internal anal sphincter hypertonicity is related to anal fissure, initial non-operative treatment is targeted to alleviate internal anal sphincter activity through two topical agents, nitroglycerin and diltiazem, and one injectable agent, botulinum toxin A.

Topical

Nitroglycerin

- Nitric oxide is the neurotransmitter mediating relaxation of the internal anal sphincter.
- Topical application of 0.2% glyceryl trinitrate (GTN) ointment relaxes the anal sphincter by manometric studies.
- A landmark randomized trial was reported in 1997 that showed a healing rate of 68% with GTN treatment, compared with 8% in the placebo group (15).
- Cochrane analysis of 18 trials, however, showed a healing rate of 48.9% with GTN treatment, compared to 35.5% in the placebo or control group.
- With longer-term follow-up, recurrence varied from 51% to 67%.
- Most common side effect of topical GTN treatment is headache (27–50%).
- A second potential drawback is tachyphylaxis, which does not respond to escalations in dose or frequency.
- In 2011, the FDA approved Rectiv: 0.4% nitroglycerin applied endoanally bid for 6–8 weeks. At 24-week follow-up, there was a 77% healing rate.

Calcium Channel Blockers

- Both diltiazem and nifedipine have been described either orally or topically to cause relaxation of the smooth muscle of the internal anal sphincter.
  - Oral and topical nifedipine have been shown to lower mean resting anal pressure. Diltiazem has been shown to decrease mean resting anal pressure, although the effect is greater with topical diltiazem.
- Multiple small trials suggest healing rates equivalent to GTN with fewer side effects.
- Neither diltiazem nor nifedipine are FDA-approved for the treatment of anal fissure. There is no topical formulation available in the United States, so a compounding pharmacy is needed.

Botulinum Toxin Type A

- Botulinum toxins are a family of neuroparalytics synthesized by *Clostridium botulinum.*
- They inhibit the release of acetylcholine at the neuromuscular junction.
- They have also been used off-label in other disorders, including chronic anal fissures. There is no uniformly recommended dose or site of injection.
- Botulinum toxin type A is supplied as a powder in 100-unit single-patient use vials. Relaxation of the muscle occurs within days and lasts for 2–4 months.
- This has the theoretical advantage of allowing fissure healing while avoiding permanent fecal incontinence.
- Various methods of injection, including injection into the internal or external sphincter, at

single or multiple sites, and in various doses, have been described.

- Comparative trials
  - Botulinum toxin injections vs. placebo, botulinum toxin A injection superior to nitroglycerin ointment
    - Healing rate: 73% after nitroglycerine, 13% with placebo ($p = 0.003$).
  - Botulinum toxin injection vs. lateral internal sphincterotomy
    - 92.5% for the lateral internal sphincterotomy, 45% botulinum toxin.
    - Meta-analysis of seven randomized controlled trials; the healing and recurrence rates were worse with botulinum toxin compared to LIAS.
- There is limited data regarding the long-term effectiveness of botulinum toxin.

Operative Treatment

Anal Dilation

- Dilation is not more effective than sphincterotomy and has a higher rate of incontinence
- Balloon dilation is a more standardized and objective method of anal stretch, with lower incontinence rates.

Anal Sphincterotomy (Technique)

- Posterior internal sphincterotomy at the site of the fissure led to a posterior midline "gutter" or "keyhole" deformity, leading to fecal soiling in 30–40% of patients.
- Lateral sphincterotomy laterally eliminated this problem and has become the main surgical intervention for failure of medical management.
- The variations currently include open vs. closed technique and conservative vs. traditional sphincterotomy.
  - Closed technique is performed by inserting the scalpel blade in the intersphincteric groove and then turning it medially to break the fibers of the internal sphincter (Fig. 13.5).
  - Open technique is done through a radial incision overlying the intersphincteric groove, and the distal internal anal sphincter is divided under direct vision (Fig. 13.6).
  - Division was originally described to the dentate line, but recent reports describe a more conservative approach, either with division of the muscle to the fissure apex or with division just until the band of hypertrophied muscle is released.

Outcomes Between Closed and Open Anal Sphincterotomy

Cochrane Review: no difference in either persistence of fissure or incontinence with the two techniques

Postoperative endoanal ultrasounds showed that open sphincterotomy is associated with a significantly higher proportion of complete sphincterotomies.

Extent of Sphincterotomy

- Controversial topic: excessive division increases the risk of incontinence, yet inadequate division increases the risk of persistence or recurrence.
- Lateral internal sphincterotomy to the dentate line vs. to the apex of the fissure:
  - Mentes et al. prospectively randomized 76 patients with chronic anal fissure.
    - Treatment failure was zero in the traditional group and 13% in the conservative group after 1 year of follow-up.
    - No statistically significant difference in the postoperative incontinence scores.
  - Elsebae et al. prospectively randomized 92 patients.
    - Treatment failure was 0 in the traditional group and 4% in the conservative group (p = NS).
    - Persistent incontinence was 4% in the traditional group and 0% in the conservative group (p = NS).
- Magdy et al. randomized 150 patients to traditional sphincterotomy, V-Y advancement flap, or conservative sphincterotomy + V-Y advancement flap.

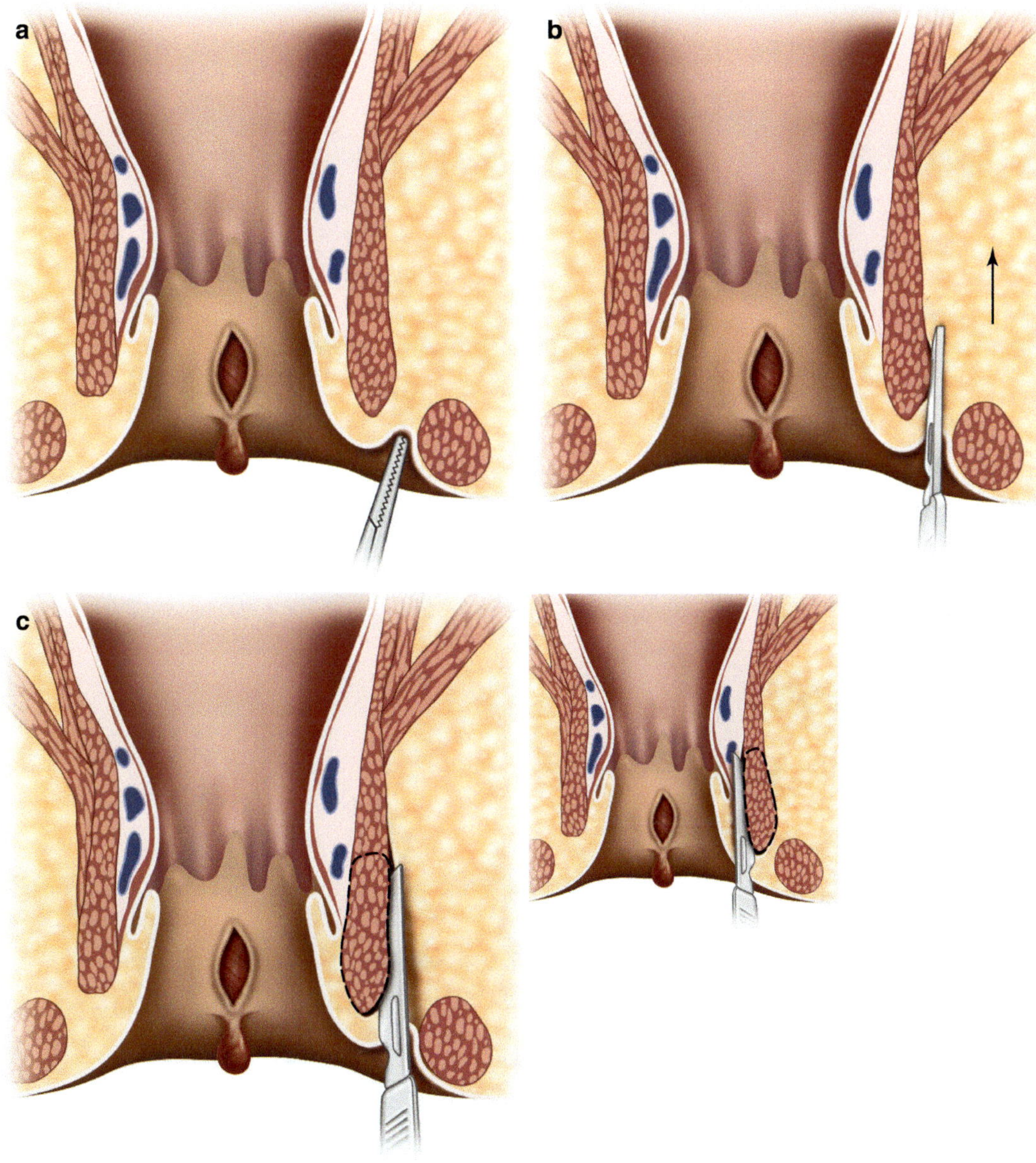

Fig. 13.5 Closed lateral sphincterotomy. (**a**) Location of the intersphincteric groove. (**b**) Insertion of the knife blade in the intersphincteric plane. (**c**) Lateral to medial division of the internal anal sphincter (*inset:* medial to lateral division of the muscle)

- The healing rates were 84% in the traditional group and 94% in the conservative division/advancement flap group.
- The incontinence rates were 14% vs. 2%, respectively.

Fissurectomy

The hallmark of chronic fissure is the triad of a hypertrophied internal sphincter, a hypertrophied anal papilla, and an external sentinel tag.

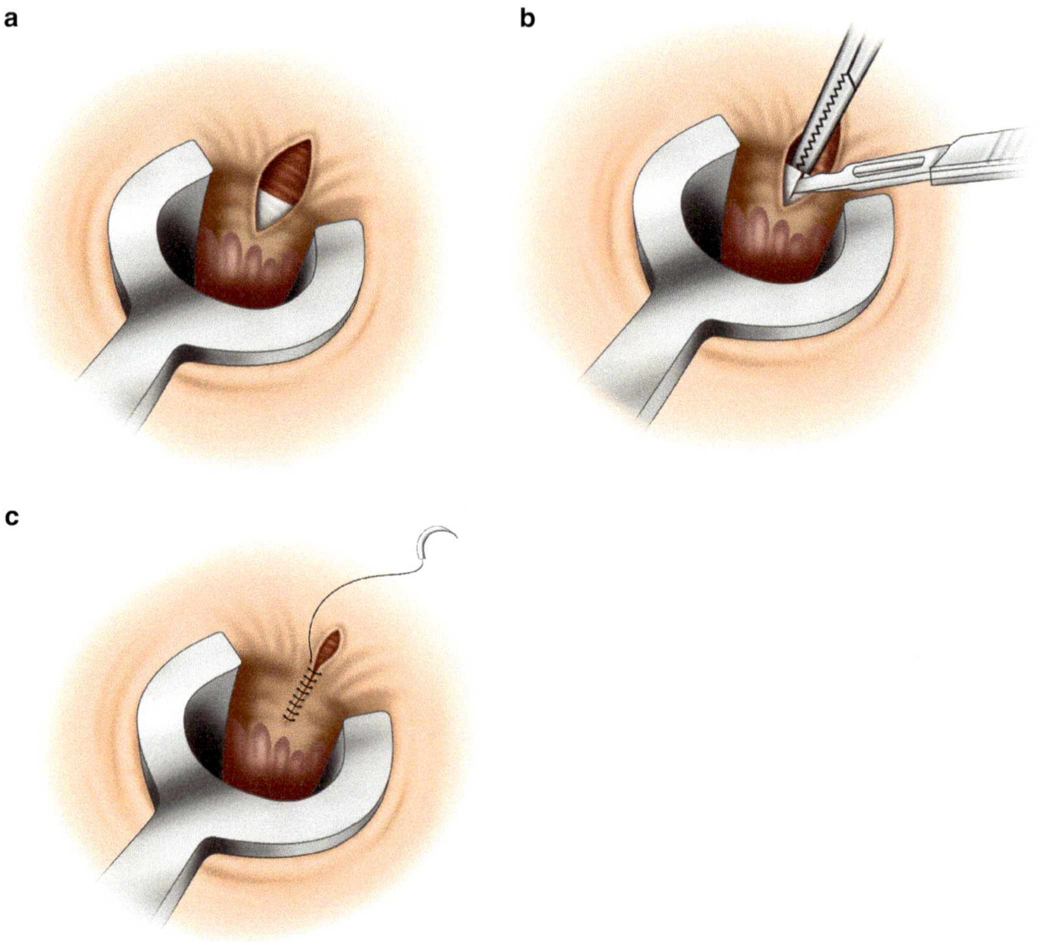

Fig. 13.6 Open lateral internal sphincterotomy. (**a**) Radial skin incision distal to the dentate line exposing the intersphincteric groove. (**b**) Elevation and division of the internal sphincter. (**c**) Primary wound closure

Results of Sphincterotomy

- A myriad of additional nonrandomized reports are available, describing a wide range of results from lateral internal sphincterotomy.
- While most reports cite low rates of treatment failure, the incontinence rate is widely variable and is as high as 30–40%.
- The disease, however, is largely measured by the subjective experience of the patient, who is ultimately the best judge of which treatment is worth pursuing and which risks are worth taking.
- With multiple options available to patients, the ultimate time to healing is prolonged, but 72% of patients can avoid operative treatment, and 97% of patients can be healed.
- The low rate of sphincterotomy comes at the price of increased recurrences before complete healing and a longer time spent in treatment.

Fissures Without Anal Hypertonicity

- A subset of patients with fissure will not demonstrate hypertonicity.
- Giordano et al.: simple cutaneous advancement flap in 51 patients over a 6-year period

for all patients, regardless of anal tone, 98% treatment success rate.

- Nyam et al.: island advancement flap in 21 patients with fissures and below-normal anal pressure resulted in complete healing and no incontinence in all patients.
- While this technique may be useful for all patients with refractory fissures, it holds particular promise in addressing the fissure in the setting of a hypotonic anus. Video 13.1 demonstrates the technique of an anal flap.

Crohn's Disease

- Fissures are commonly seen in people with Crohn's disease, affecting approximately 30% of patients.
- Tend to be in more atypical locations, deeper, and associated with other pathology, especially fistula.
- Some authors have reported acceptable outcomes from interventions in these patients, but caution should be the rule, and sphincter salvage is prudent.
- Appropriate medical management of the disease may lead to resolution of the anorectal disorders in 50% or more of these cases.

Human Immunodeficiency Virus

- HIV-related anal disease includes both typical fissures and anorectal ulcers, which can appear as deep, broad-based, or cavitating lesions.
- Small studies have reported successful treatment of typical fissures, and the medical treatment of HIV continues to improve.
- Concerns about delayed wound healing and increased infectious complications, however, remain.

Conclusions

- A suggested treatment algorithm is provided in Fig. 13.7.

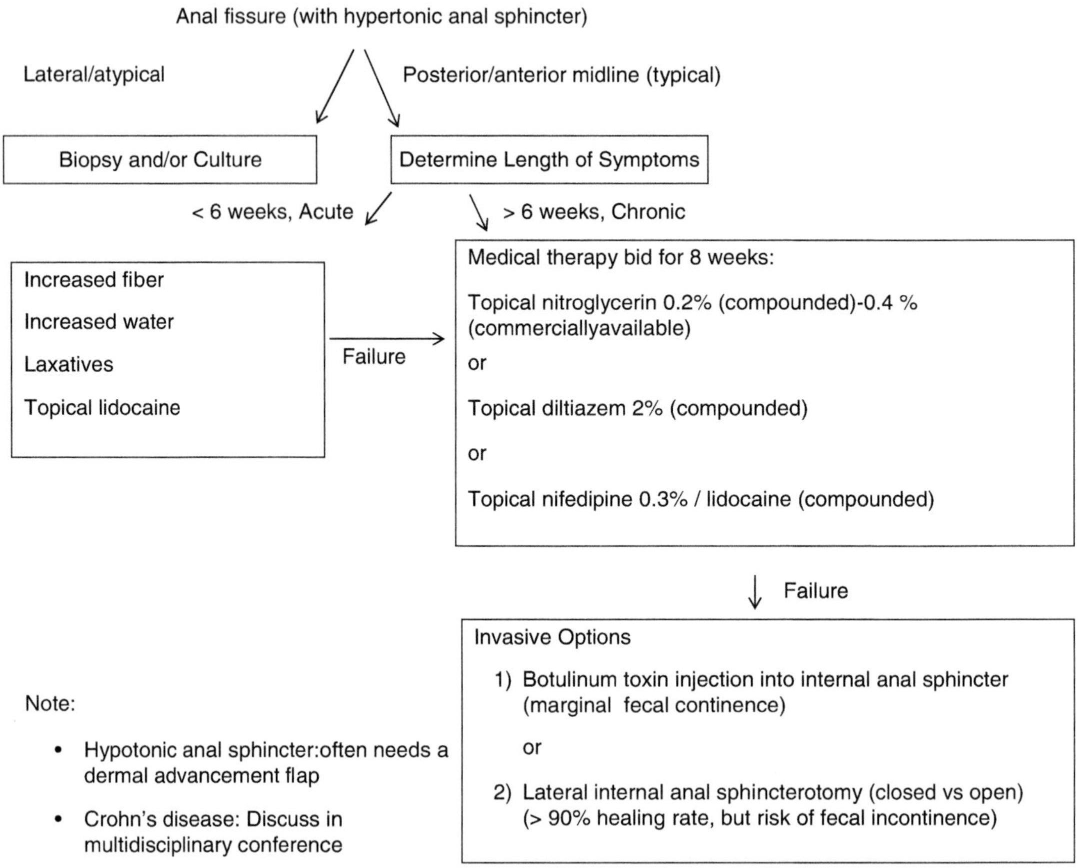

Fig. 13.7 Treatment algorithm for anal fissure

Anorectal Abscess and Fistula

14

Bradley R. Davis and Kevin R. Kasten

Key Concepts

- Successful management of anorectal abscesses requires an in-depth knowledge of pelvic floor anatomy and potential spaces through which sepsis can spread.
- The spaces occupying the anus and their anatomic landmarks will define the nomenclature of abscesses – perianal, perirectal, supralevator, and postanal space.
- Drainage of most abscesses can be performed in the office without drains or setons. If a fistula is encountered, it should only be addressed if the anatomy in relationship to the sphincters is clearly identified.
- Necrotizing soft tissue infections are life-threatening emergencies that require aggressive surgical debridement and management of the offending anal gland.
- Fistulas will complicate a significant proportion of perirectal abscesses and are classified based on their relationship with the anal sphincter complex.
- Physical examination is often the only modality needed to determine the fistula track and selection of treatment, and preoperative imaging (MRI, US) is typically unnecessary except for patients with multiple external openings, when the internal opening cannot be identified or for recurrent cases.
- Goodsall's rule, while being helpful, is accurate in about 60% of cases and is more accurate for posterior fistulas.
- Fistulotomy is the most successful of the surgical treatments but is also associated with the highest rates of continence disturbances – several non-cutting techniques have been described – all of which have limitations and varying degrees of success.

Introduction and Epidemiology

- Delay in diagnosis, mismanagement of the disease, or failure to recognize the diagnoses can result in multiple procedures, increased cost, and protracted suffering.
- Although the true incidence and prevalence is elusive, the incidence of abscess is reportedly between 0.4% and 5% of patients undergoing operative management, yielding between 68,000 and 96,000 cases of anorectal abscess each year in the United States.
- Patients are males at a 3:1 ratio.
- Mean age of 40 years (range 20–60 years).

B. R. Davis (✉) . K. R. Kasten
Department of Surgery, Section of Colorectal Surgery, Atrium Health, Carolinas Medical Center, Charlotte, NC, USA
e-mail: bradley.davis@uc.edu

S. R. Steele et al. (eds.), *The ASCRS Manual of Colon and Rectal Surgery*,
https://doi.org/10.1007/978-3-030-01165-9_14

Pathophysiology

Anatomy

- Between the columns of Morgagni, which number between 6 and 14, are unevenly distributed anal crypts whereby anal ducts empty.
- Importantly, ducts may extend into the internal sphincter, the intersphincteric space, or through the internal sphincter into the external sphincter.
- As a consequence of these extensions, select anorectal spaces are at risk for transmission of bacteria with subsequent formation of abscess.
- The perianal space (Fig. 14.1a) lies immediately around the anal verge, with medial extension to the dentate line and lateral extension to the subcutaneous fat of the buttocks. The ischiorectal/ischioanal fossa is a pyramidal-shaped potential space between the perineum and levator ani (Fig. 14.1b).

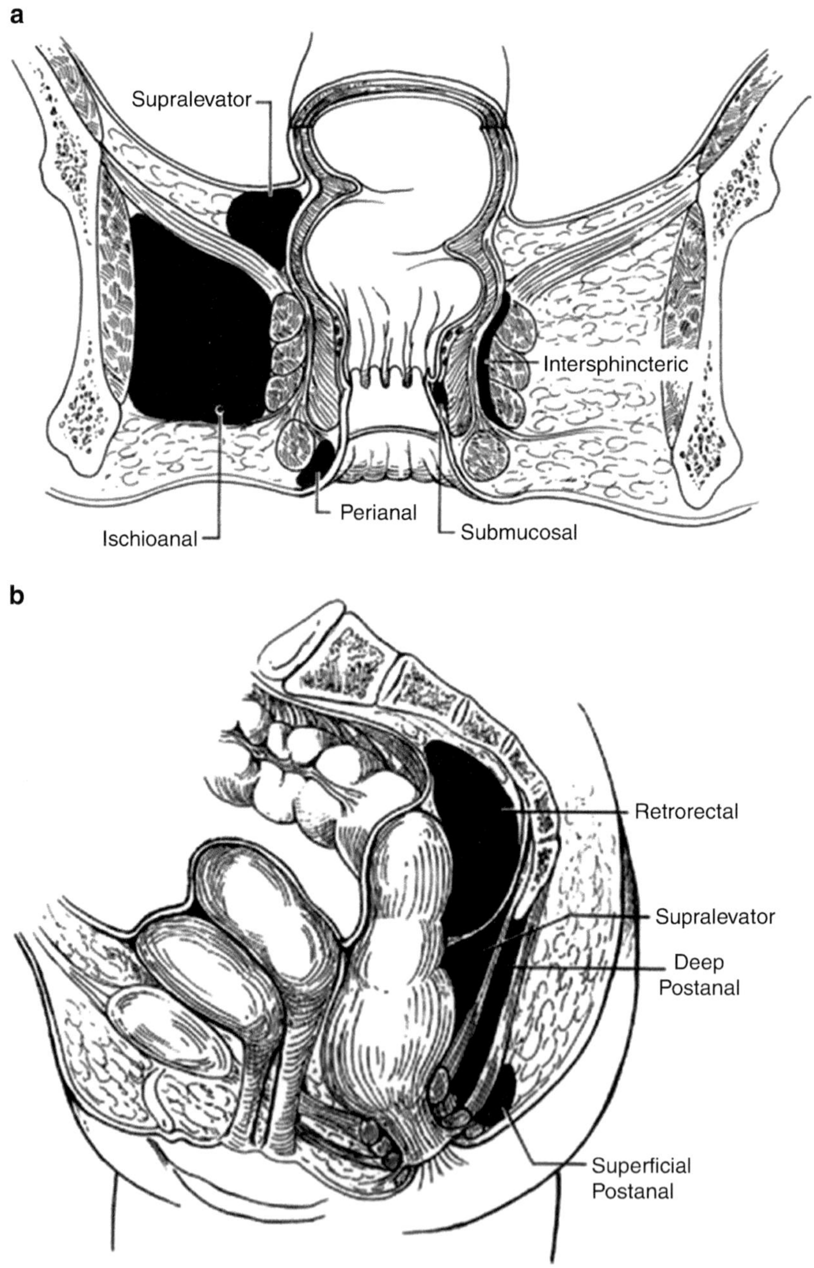

Fig. 14.1 Anorectal spaces: (**a**), coronal section; (**b**), sagittal section. Vasilevsky CA. Anorectal abscess and fistula-in-ano. ((168) © 1997 David Beck, MD, with permission)

- Above the anococcygeal ligament and below the levator ani, these fossae are continuous with the deep posterior anal space.
- Above the levator ani, between the pelvic wall and rectum, lies the supralevator space.
  - Because this space is superiorly bordered by the peritoneum, abscesses may form from intersphincteric sources that track superiorly or abdominal sources that track from the peritoneal cavity.

Etiology

- Anal crypts are considered the primary source for development of perianal abscesses.
- The cryptoglandular theory hypothesized that obstruction of a crypt by foreign body or perianal debris led to abscess formation due to stasis within the ducts.
- Predisposing factors include liquid stool entering the anal duct, trauma, tobacco abuse, and cystic dilation of the duct resulting in poor emptying.
- The remaining 10% are the result of specific disorders such as inflammatory bowel disease (IBD), trauma, and malignancy (Table 14.1).

Classification

- Each anorectal abscess is classified based upon the potential space it inhabits (Fig. 14.2).
- Perianal and ischiorectal abscesses are the most common, accounting for over 80% of all diagnoses.

Table 14.1 Etiology of anorectal abscess

Nonspecific
Cryptoglandular
Specific
Inflammatory bowel disease
Crohn's disease
Ulcerative colitis
Infection
Tuberculosis
Actinomycosis
Lymphogranuloma venereum
Trauma
Impalement
Foreign body
Surgery
Episiotomy
Hemorrhoidectomy
Prostatectomy
Malignancy
Carcinoma
Leukemia
Lymphoma
Radiation

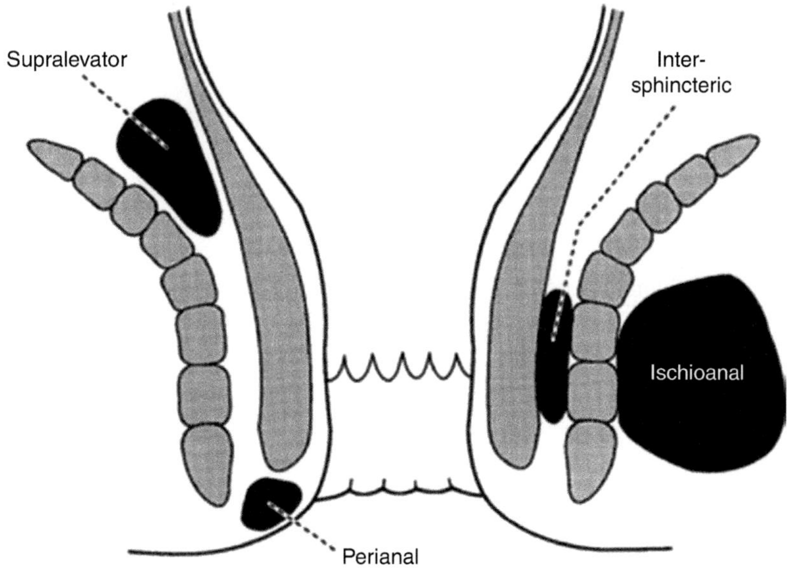

Fig. 14.2 Classification of anorectal abscesses. ((169) © 1997 David Beck, MD, with permission)

- Supralevator abscesses are the least common.
- The "horseshoe abscess" describes a process whereby bilateral disease occurs via connection through the intersphincteric, supralevator, or ischiorectal spaces.

Evaluation

History and Symptoms

- The patient with an anorectal abscess presents most commonly with acute pain in the perianal or perirectal region.
- The pain is usually worsened with sitting and defecation.
- Associated symptoms of urinary dysfunction may distinguish the abscess as supralevator.
- Other symptoms include fever, chills, swelling, erythema, spontaneous drainage, and malaise.
- Past medical history can alert the clinician to other possible causes of rectal pain including fissure, hemorrhoids, levator spasm, sexually transmitted infections, tuberculosis, HIV, IBD, malignancy, and trauma.
- Given the possibility of surgical intervention, determining sphincter function and any history of fecal incontinence is important in these patients.

Physical Examination

- External evaluation will reveal classic signs of infection including erythema, induration, fluctuance, pain, and spontaneous drainage.
- For patients with an intersphincteric or supralevator abscess, external review is unlikely to reveal definitive signs; however, upon digital rectal exam, fluctuance or extreme discomfort should alert the clinician to this diagnosis.
- Unfortunately, pain oftentimes precludes an adequate rectal exam.
- When the diagnosis is in doubt, consideration should be given to performance of an exam under anesthesia with anoscopy and possible flexible sigmoidoscopy.
- Suspicion for supralevator abscess, or in patients with complicated medical history, further imaging may be warranted.

Imaging

Computed Tomography (CT)

- Indicated in any patient:
  - When the diagnosis of anorectal abscess is unclear
  - With complex suppurative anorectal conditions
  - With significant comorbidities in which missing the diagnosis would prove harmful
  - As a possible substitution for surgical evaluation
- Can also be considered in patients with perianal Crohn's disease to assist delineation of rectal inflammation from anorectal abscess.
- Triple contrast is often required (Fig. 14.3 a–c).

Magnetic Resonance Imaging (MRI)

- MRI for evaluation of anorectal abscess is uncommon, occurring more frequently in chronic, complex fistula-in-ano disease.
- Best for any recurrent of incompletely drained abscess to assist identification of horseshoe/postanal, supralevator, and other complex abscesses.

Endoanal Ultrasound (EAUS)

- Familiar to most colorectal surgeons, endoanal ultrasound utilizes a probe with 2D or 3D capabilities at a frequency of 5–16 MHz.
- Similar in discomfort to anoscopy, this technology allows effective characterization of abscesses and fistulas with reported accuracy of 85%.

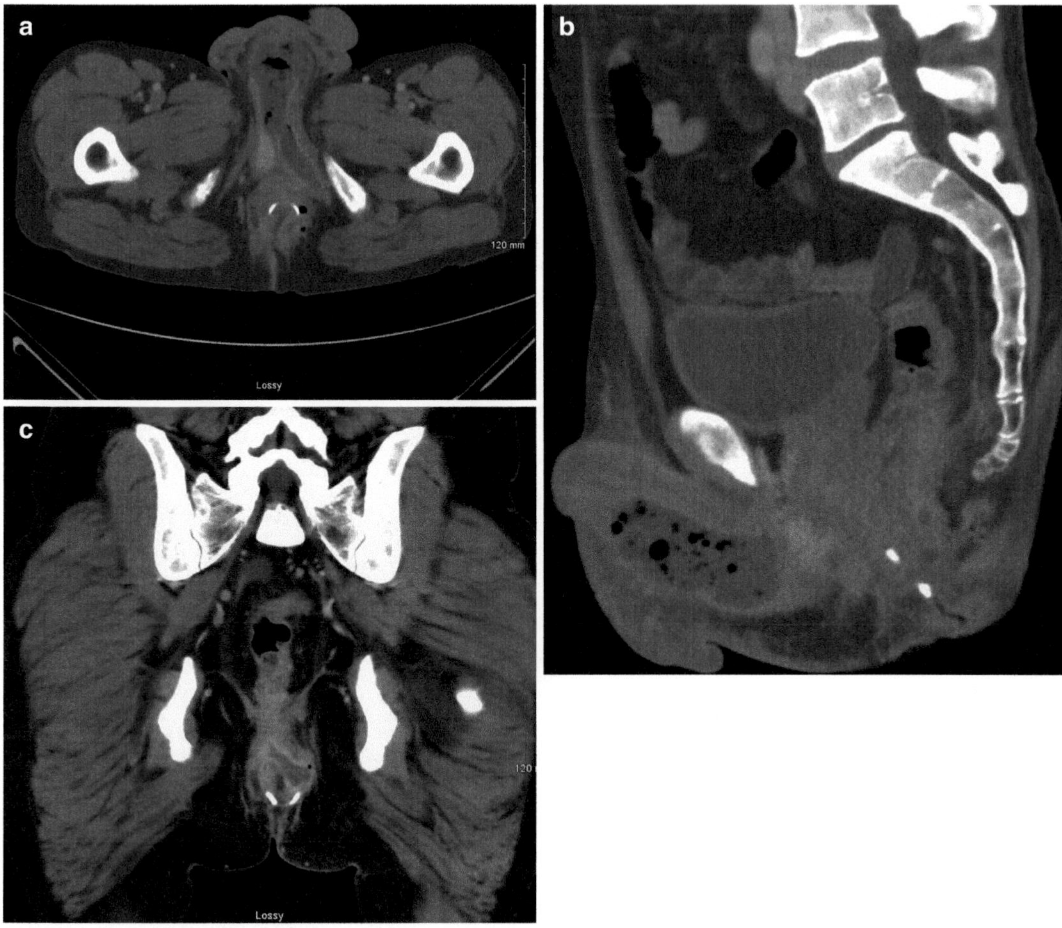

Fig. 14.3 Computed tomography of complex anorectal abscess extending anteriorly toward the scrotum. Axial images (**a**), coronal image (**b**), sagittal image (**c**)

Transperineal Sonography (TP-US)

- A lesser-known technique in the colorectal field, TP-US can be quite accurate in diagnosis of fluid collections, internal opening, and even existence and course of a fistulous track.
- Most importantly, in experienced hands it distinguishes perianal from perirectal abscess and sepsis.
- In a comparison of TP-US and MRI, the former was more accurate for superficial fluid collections, while the latter was more accurate for perirectal infection.

Treatment

Role of Antibiotics

- The surgical principles for management of abscesses hold true with prompt drainage and debridement being the cornerstone.
- Antibiotics are indicated when:
  - Associated cellulitis is present.
  - Patients who fail to improve following appropriate drainage.
  - Immunosuppressed patients.

- Coverage is directed toward *Escherichia coli*, *Enterococcus species*, and *Bacteroides fragilis* in immunocompetent patients and *Neisseria gonorrhoeae, Chlamydia trachomatis,* cytomegalovirus, and herpes simplex virus in immunocompromised patients.
- Consider wound culture only in high-risk patient populations and individuals with recurrent or non-healing disease.
- Risk of fistula formation was unrelated to antibiotic usage.
- Fistula formation is related to location of the abscess with an eight times higher risk associated with ischiorectal location and a three times higher risk with intersphincteric compared to the perianal location.

Incision and Drainage

- Simple, superficial perianal or ischiorectal abscesses requiring external drainage at the skin level are amenable to bedside drainage in the office, emergency room, or hospital ward.
- A simple rule of thumb recommends "outward" drainage whenever an abscess enters, or passes through, skeletal muscle (i.e., levator ani, external sphincter).
- All others should be drained internally through the rectum/anus.
- The choice of elliptical incision, or cruciate incision combined with excision of skin flaps, prevents early closure and recurrence (Fig. 14.4).
- When possible, the incision is made as near the anal verge as possible to limit the length of any potential fistula. Packing is not required in this scenario, and its absence yields quicker healing with less pain.
- Patients requiring internal drainage, those with recurrent or bilateral disease, and those with large abscesses at risk for inadequate bedside drainage, should undergo operative drainage.
- For abscesses of significant size, consider multiple counter incisions with interposition of setons or penrose drains to accelerate healing.

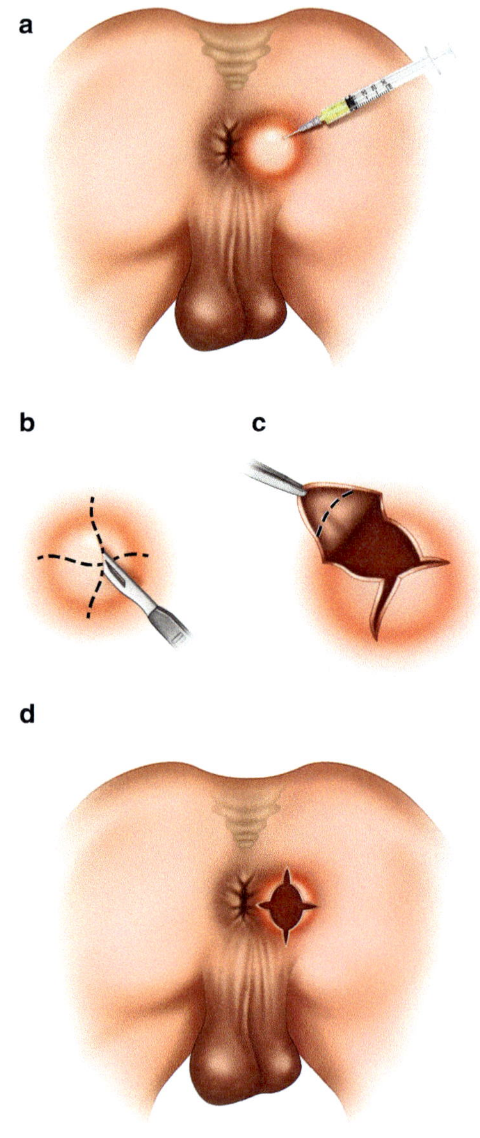

Fig. 14.4 Drainage of abscess: (**a**) injection of local anesthesia, (**b**) cruciate incision, (**c**) excision of skin, (**d**) drainage cavity

- Drains are removed at 2–3 weeks postoperatively when the base of the cavity has granulated and shrunk.
- Further candidates for internal drainage include:
  1. Submucosal abscess
  2. Intersphincteric abscess
  3. Supralevator abscess from intersphincteric fistula

4. Supralevator abscess from pelvic disease

- The diagnosis of intersphincteric fistula should be entertained in patients with pain out of proportion to exam findings.
- Definitive management involves incision of the internal sphincter along the length of abscess, with or without marsupialization of the wound edges.
- Supralevator abscesses require delineation of the track by imaging before surgical correction is undertaken.
- Transrectal drainage is indicated in most scenarios.
- Abdominal drainage can be considered depending upon ease of access and directionality of the abscess cavity.
- When the source is intra-abdominal, percutaneous management may prevent creation of a fistulous track through the levator plate via improper ischiorectal drainage and is often more successful than transrectal drainage.
- The scenario of supralevator extension from ischiorectal abscess due to a transsphincteric fistula requires ischiorectal drainage.
  - For instances where a supralevator abscess forms as an upward extension of an intersphincteric fistula, internal drainage via incision of the internal sphincter is best (Fig. 14.5).
- Bilateral abscess disease, or "horseshoe" abscess, requires operative drainage to delineate and control the source.
- This difficult-to-treat entity most commonly arises from a deep postanal space abscess.
- Options for management include the Hanley or modified Hanley procedures, consisting of open posterior drainage through the anococcygeal ligament, posterior midline incision of the internal sphincter and inciting anal duct, and open drainage of bilateral ischiorectal fossae to control lateral tracks (Fig. 14.6).

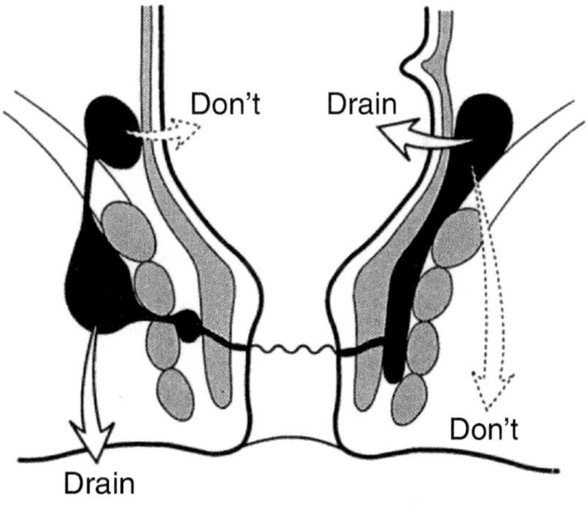

Fig. 14.5 Drainage of a supralevator abscess

Fig. 14.6 Drainage of a horseshoe abscess

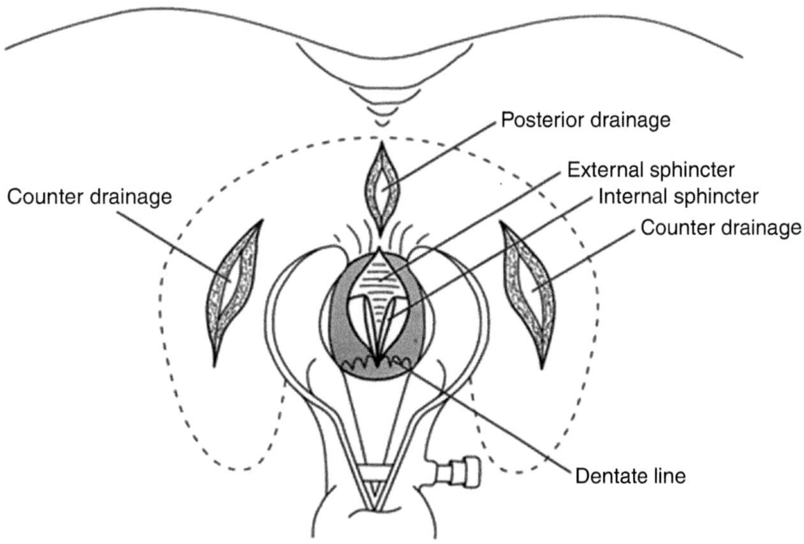

- If necessary, a seton (cutting or non-cutting) is placed in the posterior midline, with subsequent definitive management taking place at a later time (Fig. 14.7).

Catheter Drainage

- Appropriate size and external fixation of catheter is necessary to ensure adequate drainage.
- A mushroom tip catheter (e.g., de Pezzer, Malecot, Cook Medical) between 10 and 14 Fr is inserted to full cavity depth and secured to the skin (Fig. 14.8).
- Recommendations differ with regards to duration of treatment, ranging from 3 to 21 days.

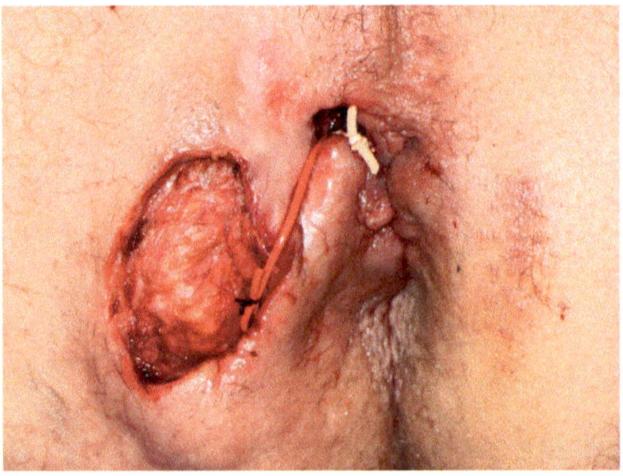

Fig. 14.7 Horseshoe fistula managed with drainage and seton

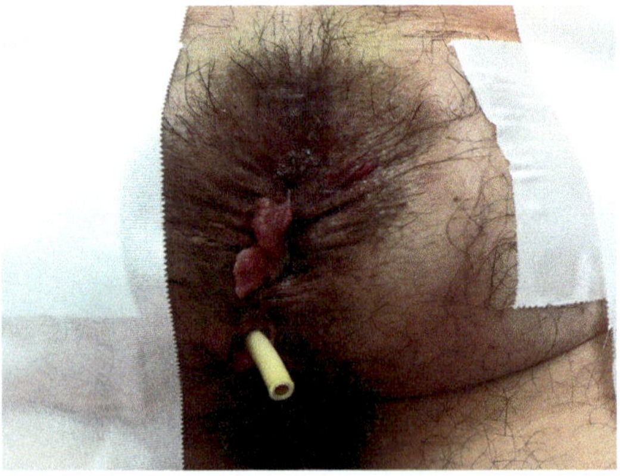

Fig. 14.8 Pezzer catheter in an ischiorectal fossa abscess

Drainage with Primary Fistulotomy

- Historically, primary fistulotomy was performed when draining the abscess for source control, thereby increasing the rate of healing without need for subsequent procedure.
- The acute setting inflammation may inhibit clear determination of muscle involvement, thereby increasing the risk of excessive muscle incision; placement of seton may be indicated preventing the unintended consequence of incontinence.
- Reports indicate a high rate of spontaneous healing following effective abscess drainage alone with the incidence of recurrent abscess reported to be 30% and subsequent fistula formation between 26% and 50%.
- Localizing the offending duct is difficult, and misidentification leads to complications; alternative methods are available.
  - Manual pressure on the abscess cavity while looking for purulent extrusion
  - Identification of inflammation indicating the culprit duct
  - Simple blind probing
  - Injection of 2 cc of 2% hydrogen peroxide combined with 1–2 drops of methylene blue into the abscess cavity
- Unfortunately, there is no clear answer to the question of primary fistulotomy at time of abscess drainage.
- Superficial and low transsphincteric (less than 30–40% external sphincter involvement) fistulas with minimal sphincter involvement provide the best opportunity for successful fistulotomy at the time of abscess drainage.

Postoperative Management

- Local wound care involves sitz baths 2–3 times daily followed by wound coverage using gauze.
- Packing is not necessary and should be avoided.

- There is no data to support the use of topical antibiotics.
- Endpoint for removal of catheters is cessation of purulent drainage from the drain.
- Patients are followed until complete healing of the wound or cavity, especially since recurrence and fistula formation is associated with delay/lack of surgical follow-up.
- Antibiotics are not warranted in the postoperative setting unless cellulitis is present or in the immunocompromised patient.

Complications

Immediate Postoperative Period

- Complications related to abscess drainage and fistulotomy include bleeding (1–2%) and urinary retention (2–6%).
- Universal risk factors for urinary retention in anorectal procedures include age over 50, female sex, and intravenous fluid (IVF) greater than 1 L perioperatively.

Abscess Recurrence and Fistula Formation

- Rates of abscess recurrence following drainage are estimated at 4–31%, with a median of 13%.
- Rates of recurrence are higher in those undergoing management more than 7 days after onset of symptoms.
- Early recurrence is usually the result of inappropriate technique, early skin apposition, and reformation of the abscess.
- Insufficient drainage leads to continued inflammation, prolonged healing, and fistula formation.
- Reasons for semi-acute recurrence include missed loculations, prior intervention with associated scarring, and destruction of natural barriers to infection.
- Horseshoe abscesses recur more frequently with a reported incidence between 18% and 50%, usually requiring multiple operations before healing occurs.

Misdiagnosis

- Pilonidal disease, hidradenitis suppurativa, tuberculosis, herpes simplex virus, HIV, and inflammatory bowel disease (specifically, Crohn's disease) must be part of the differential diagnosis.

Special Considerations

Necrotizing Anorectal Infection (Fournier's Gangrene)

- Necrotizing anorectal infections are rare.
- Medical risk factors commonly associated with necrotizing soft tissue infections include diabetes, hypertension, elderly age, obesity, immunosuppression (especially when due to malnutrition, liver disease, malignancies), drug use, and recent surgery.
- Long-standing or inappropriately managed perianal disease predates an episode of necrotizing fasciitis, and 50–60% had underlying anorectal abscess as their inciting source.

Diagnosis

- Presenting symptoms include severe pain out of proportion to exam, fever, chills, erythema, and induration at the site (Fig. 14.9).
- In polymicrobial and clostridial infections, crepitance is often noted.
- As necrotizing soft tissue infections progress along fascial planes, the extent of disease is easily underestimated.
- White blood cell count, creatinine kinase, and lactate are most helpful in estimating severity of infection and confirming the diagnosis.
- When the diagnosis is unclear, imaging is recommended using CT abdomen/pelvis to identify the source and extent of infection.

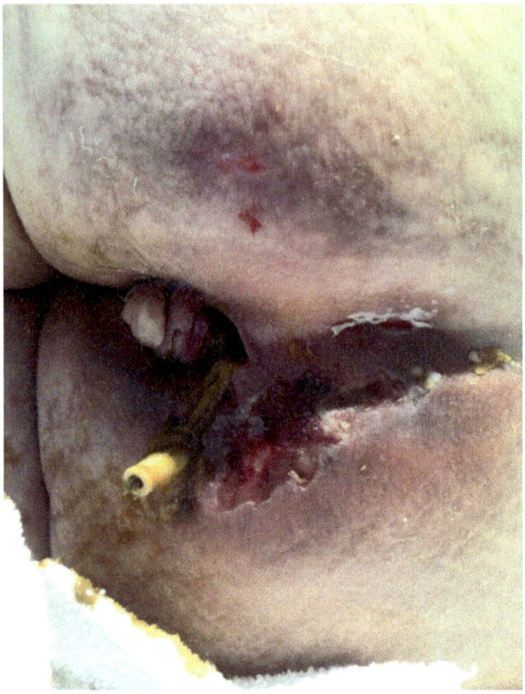

Fig. 14.9 Necrotizing soft tissue infection in a patient with a supralevator fistula and abscess inadequately drained

Treatment

- Prompt diagnosis and treatment is necessary to maximize survival.
- Treatment involves aggressive fluid resuscitation and initiation of broad-spectrum antibiotics (penicillin g, metronidazole, third-generation cephalosporin, gentamicin).
- Next, the patient undergoes surgical intervention with wide local excision of affected tissue (Fig. 14.10).
- Due to rapid spread, surgical excision should extend beyond visibly infected tissues.
- It is common to return to the operating room within 24–48 h to re-excise margins and to ensure appropriate source control. A useful adjunct when anorectal abscess incites necrotizing fasciitis involves the loose-seton technique, where multiple radial incisions are made in the external sphincter at its outer margins.

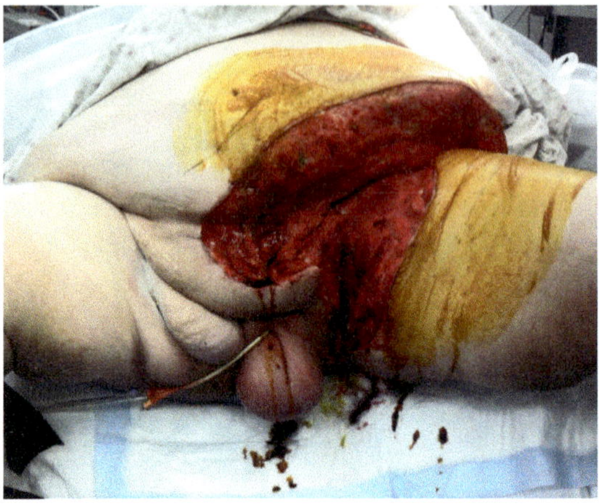

Fig. 14.10 Extensive soft tissue debridement of necrotizing soft tissue infection starting as an anorectal abscess

- Some advocate creation of a colostomy to help with wound care after extensive dissection.

Outcomes

- Necrotizing fasciitis remains a lethal disease, despite significant advances in diagnosis, surgical care, and supportive management.
- Mortality rates in the literature span 4–80%; however, most large studies demonstrate a consistent range of 7–10%.
- Death is usually the result of sepsis and sequelae of multi-organ system failure.
- The Fournier's gangrene severity index (FGSI) predicts mortality.

Anorectal Infections in Immunosuppressed Patients

Hematologic Abnormalities in Immunosuppression

- In patients with hematologic malignancies, or those treated with myelosuppressive regimens, immunosuppression and low neutrophil count produce an incidence of anorectal sepsis approaching 10%.
- Diagnosis is often difficult and delayed due to low neutrophil counts, whereby non-fluctuant

induration with minimal erythema evades untrained eyes.

- However, systemic complications of sepsis are more likely in this patient population, including death, with mortality approaches 60% when untreated.
- Antibiotics are standard of care, aimed at coverage of standard gastrointestinal flora using a local antibiogram.
- For patients with absolute neutrophil count (ANC) < 1000/mm^3, antibiotics are first-line therapy with rates of resolution between 30% and 90%.
- Patients with higher neutrophil counts will demonstrate an abscess, which requires incision and drainage.
- Physical exam is limited in these patients, so imaging studies are indicated for delineation of size, extent, and involved structures.
  - CT scans are rapid, easily obtained, and demonstrate supralevator components with high degree of accuracy.
  - MRI with T1- and T2-weighted images provides superior imaging for diagnosis, particularly for possible necrotizing infection.
- The decision on timing of surgical intervention is not always clear-cut.
- Patients with neutropenia suffer higher rates of morbidity following surgery, and mortality was upwards of 45% in one study versus 9% in those treated only with antibiotics.
- Rates of antibiotic failure in neutropenic patients range between 30% and 37%.
- Surgical debridement is indicated for abscess formation, lack of improvement, or development of necrotizing infection.

Human Immunodeficiency Virus (HIV)

- There is little distinction between the management of HIV patients and otherwise healthy individuals with anorectal abscess.
- In this patient population, alternative diagnoses including sexually transmitted infections and CMV are also common.

Anal Fistula

Etiology

- A fistula is defined as an abnormal connection between two epithelial-lined surfaces such as a set of organs or vessels, which do not normally connect, e.g., the connection between the distal alimentary tract and the integument.
- The incidence is believed to be 2 per 10,000/year, while the prevalence is not truly known.
- The etiology of anal fistula is cryptoglandular in 90% of cases, postoperative or traumatic in 3%, inflammatory bowel disease 3%, as a result of anal fissure 3%, and tuberculosis related in less than 1% of cases.
- Cryptoglandular origin.
  - 100 anatomical specimens, anal glands in 55% of specimens; in 33% the ducts penetrated the internal sphincter.
  - 6–10 mucous-producing glands originating from the anal crypts.
  - Glands terminate variably into the submucosa, internal sphincter, or intersphincteric groove.
  - Free channel for infection to pass from the anal lumen deep into the sphincter muscles.
  - Anal crypts become blocked by inspissated debris or stool.
  - Infection develops at the anal glands, which extends in a path of least resistance, forming an abscess in the intersphincteric space leading to the development of a fistula (36–66% risk).
    - Age less than 40, BMI exceeding 25 kg/m^2, prior diabetes, hyperlipidemia, dermatosis, sedentary lifestyle, regular alcohol intake, smoking, nonfistula anorectal surgery, prolonged sitting on the toilet for defecation, and a previous history of enteritis were independently correlated with a risk of anal fistula.

Classification

- Anal fistula can be characterized as simple or complex (50%).
- The definition of a "complex" fistula is not standardized.
  - Any fistula that is high transsphincteric or when a fistulotomy would result in incontinence should be considered complex.
  - Includes suprasphincteric, extrasphincteric, all anterior transsphincteric fistulas in women.
  - Fistulas caused by Crohn's disease, malignancy, surgery, and trauma.
- Anal fistulas are also classified based on their relationship to the anal sphincter complex. Parks et al. (Table 14.2) based on his analysis of 400 cases of treated anal fistula over a 15-year period.
- He anchored his classification system on the external sphincter due to the importance it played in the surgical management (Fig. 14.11 a–d).

1. An intersphincteric fistula (Fig. 14.11a):
   - 20–45% of cases
   - Does not penetrate the external sphincter
   - High blind track subtype, which has an extension in the intersphincteric groove cephalad toward the rectum

Table 14.2 Classification of fistula-in-ano

Intersphincteric
Simple low intersphincteric
High blind tract
High tract with an opening in the rectum
High tract with rectal opening, no perineal opening
Extra-rectal extension
Secondary to pelvic disease
Transsphincteric
Uncomplicated
High blind tract
Suprasphincteric
Uncomplicated
Horseshoe extension
Extrasphincteric
Secondary to anal fistula
Trauma related
Pelvic inflammation
Inflammatory bowel disease or other anal disease

2. A transsphincteric fistula (Fig. 14.11b):
   - 30–60% of cases
   - Penetrates the external sphincter below the level of the puborectalis muscle exiting into varying levels within the ischiorectal fossa.
   - A high blind track can end at the apex of the ischiorectal fossa or alternatively pass through the levator plate into the true pelvic cavity.
   - Care should be taken *not* to iatrogenically perforate the rectum, or an extrasphincteric fistula will be the result (Fig. 14.12).
3. A suprasphincteric fistula (Fig. 14.11c):
   - 20% of cases in the series by Parks et al. has been reported at a much lower frequency by other authors (<2%).
   - Track is over the top of the puborectalis and then downward again through the levator plate to the ischiorectal fossa and finally the skin.
   - Abscess formation in this space can result in a horseshoe extension around the rectum.
4. Extrasphincteric fistula (Fig. 14.11d):
   - 2–5% of cases
   - Passes from the perineal skin through the ischiorectal fat and levator muscles into the rectum.
   - It is outside the external sphincter complex altogether.
   - May result from a transsphincteric fistula with a high blind tract that penetrates through the levator plate.
   - May be due to trauma, inflammatory bowel disease, malignancy, or pelvic inflammation that necessitates through the levators to the perineal skin (ruptured appendicitis, terminal ileal Crohn's disease, or diverticulitis are the most common causes).

Diagnosis

- Fistula that results from cryptoglandular disease will usually be preceded by a history of an anorectal abscess that was drained (either purposefully or spontaneously).

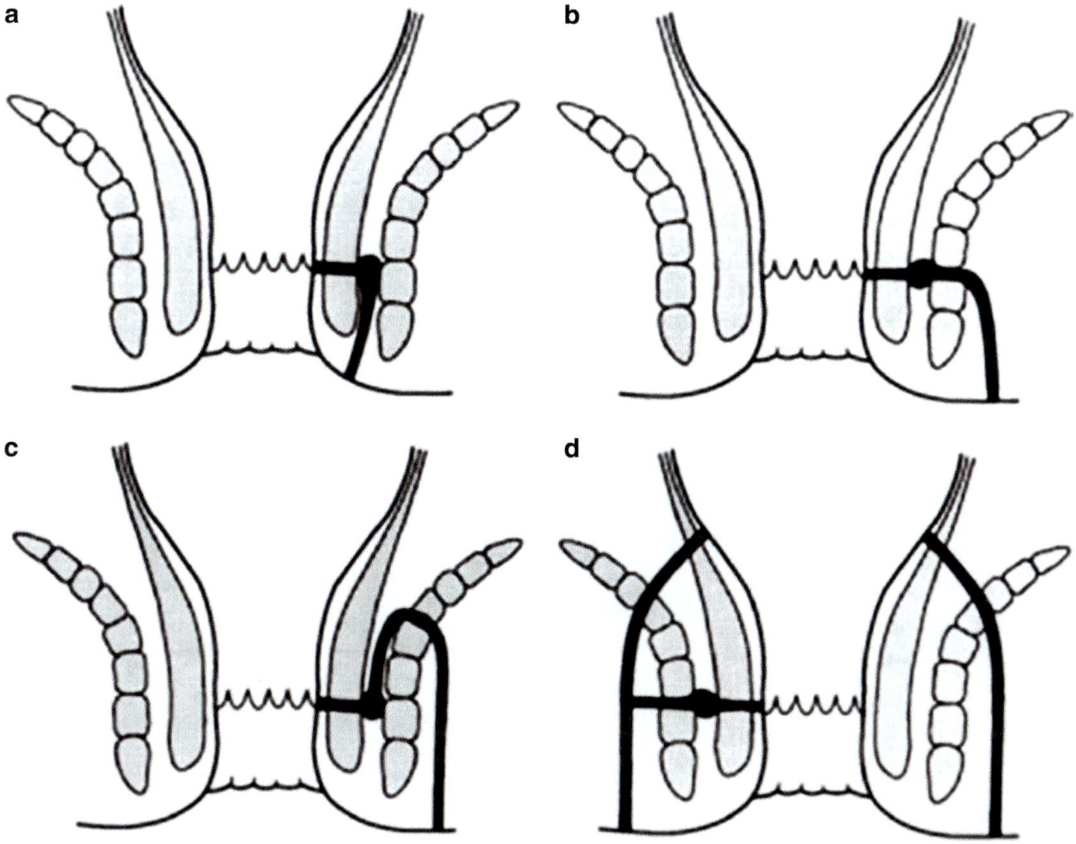

Fig. 14.11 Classification of anal fistula. (**a**) intersphincteric, (**b**) transsphincteric, (**c**) suprasphincteric, (**d**) extrasphincteric

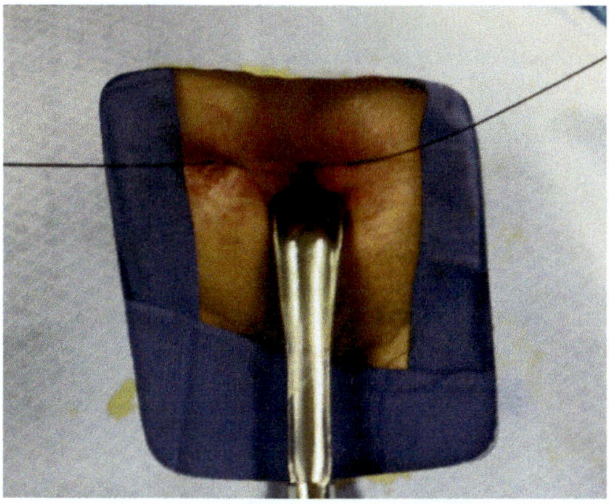

Fig. 14.12 Flexible glide wire to delineate a transsphincteric fistula with a high blind extension

- Bleeding is common due to the hypergranulation tissue that forms on the external opening.
- Irritation of the anal margin skin ensues from chronic moisture or from fecal contact.
- Pain may be a feature for patients with chronic infection or ongoing inflammation and is often cyclical as a result of spontaneous abscess formation and drainage.
- Physical exam findings are usually pathognomonic for an anal fistula with an opening on the anal margin skin with heaped-up granulation tissue that is tender and often draining (Fig. 14.13).
- The nature of the drainage can vary and may be serous, purulent, or feculent depending on the fistula.
- Low transsphincteric fistulas have been shown to occur more often in the anterior location and are less likely to be preceded by an abscess.
- External openings in the ischiorectal fossa are usually the result of transsphincteric or suprasphincteric fistula, and the examiner should

suspect that the external sphincter muscle will be involved.

- Goodsall's rule can be applied to help locate the internal opening.
  - The transverse anal line is of importance as external openings.
  - Fistulas that are located anteriorly are postulated to drain to an internal opening radially situated.
  - Posterior external openings drain to the posterior midline.
  - The positive predictive value of Goodsall's rule (Fig. 14.14) has been estimated to be 59% and is more accurate for posteriorly located fistulas.

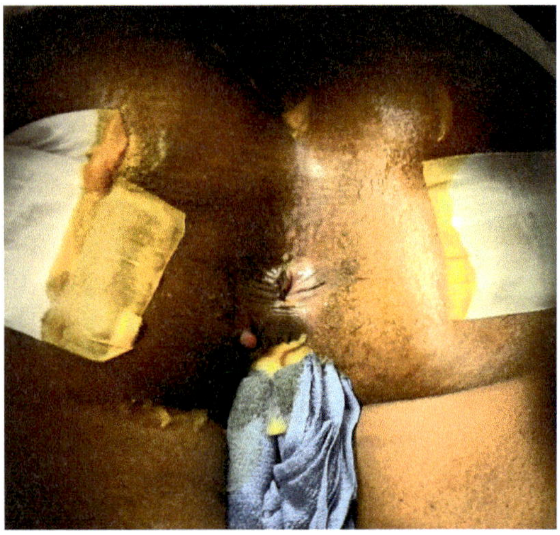

Fig. 14.13 External opening noted left anterolateral with heaped-up edge

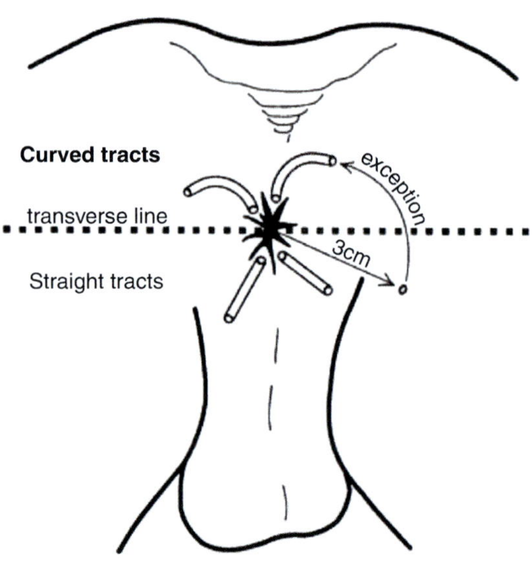

Fig. 14.14 Goodsall's rule for anal fistula

- Palpation of the anal canal using the pad of an experienced finger can frequently determine the location of the internal opening by subtle changes in the anoderm.
- Anoscopy is helpful to exclude inflammatory conditions of the anal canal or other potential causes of the fistula, but the internal opening is rarely seen unless pus is draining from it.
- Preoperative imaging (CT or MRI) is reserved for:
  - Patients with multiple external openings
  - Those in which an internal opening cannot be identified on physical exam either preoperatively or intraoperative
  - In cases of recurrence following surgical procedures

Fistulography

- Water-soluble contrast injected into the external opening under fluoroscopy using a small feeding tube (Fig. 14.15).
- Due to the limitation of plain film imaging, more recent attempts at fistulography have incorporated CT imaging in combination with contrast injection.
- Limited value given the alternatives available in modern radiology suites or colorectal offices.

Endoanal Ultrasound

- Characterize complex fistula and their relationship to the sphincter complex.
- Fistulas appear as a hypoechoic track, which can be enhanced by the instillation of hydro-

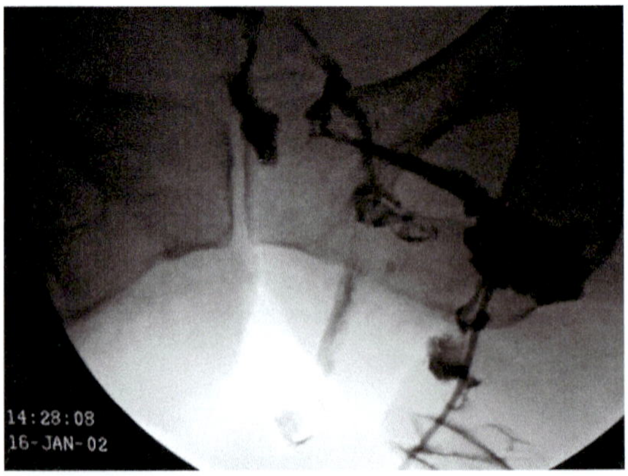

Fig. 14.15 Fistulography of complex anal fistula (arrow on fistula tract)

gen peroxide or a Levovist™ into the external opening.
- Can also help determine the presence of secondary tracts as well as horseshoe extensions.
- Conflicting data regarding any advantage compared to intraoperative assessment/findings.
- The results of these studies are influenced by the expertise and experience of the endosonographer and results may not be reproducible in all surgeons' hands.

Magnetic Resonance Imaging

- The introduction of the 1.5 Tesla (T) and 3.0 T magnets in the acquisition of images has negated the need for the endoanal coil in the evaluation of anal and rectal disease.
- Magnetic resonance imaging (MRI) of the sphincter complex has some advantages in diagnosing anal fistulas.
  - No instrumentation of the anus is required, and the exam is not operator dependent.
  - Able to demonstrate hidden areas of sepsis and secondary extensions, both of which contribute to the high rate of recurrence after surgery.
  - MR imaging can be used to define the anatomic relationships of the fistula to predict the likelihood of postoperative fecal incontinence.
- Taken together, multiple studies confirm that MR imaging is an accurate modality for evaluation of perianal fistulas and associated complications. T.
- The most cost-effective algorithm for managing all patients with anal fistula has yet to be established.
- Preoperative imaging should be considered when recurrent fistula are encountered following treatment, in cases in which multiple external openings exist and when the anatomy is unclear either in the office or at the time of surgery.

Treatment

- The goals however of surgical treatment:
  1. Elimination of sepsis
  2. Closure of the fistula track
  3. Preservation of patient's fecal continence and sphincter function
  4. Minimizing recurrence
- Identification of the external and internal opening is critical.
  - Physical examination in the operating room is quite reliable.
  - Inject either methylene blue or hydrogen peroxide into the external opening (83% success) 83% of cases.
  - A gently curved probe inserted into the external opening is an alternative technique for finding the internal opening (Fig. 14.16).
  - Care must be taken not to create a false passage.
    - Chronic tracks will have granulation tissue within them and its absence should raise the suspicion that a false track was created following a fistulotomy.
  - The ultimate choice of treatment will depend on the amount of sphincter involved in the fistula track.
    - Cutting procedures more likely for intersphincteric and low transsphincteric fistula
    - Non-cutting techniques for all others

Lay-Open Technique (Fistulotomy)

- For simple and most distal or intersphincteric fistula (Table 14.3).

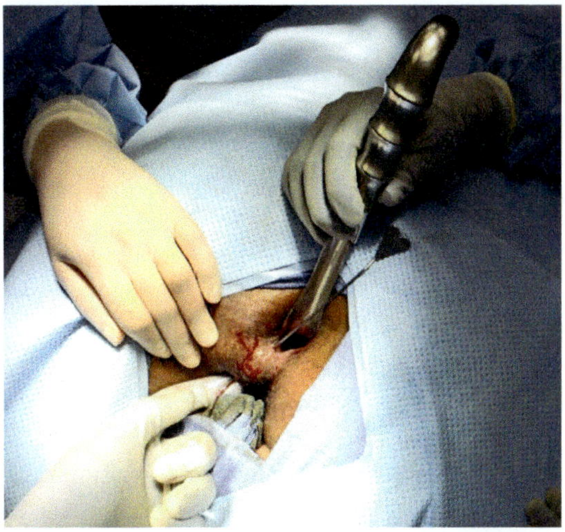

Fig. 14.16 Probe through the external and internal opening of the anal fistula

Table 14.3 Experience with fistulotomy in treating anal fistula

Author	Year	Surgical procedure	# patients	Outcome	Follow-up
Kronborg	1985	Fistulotomy	26	Recurrence 11%	12 months
Hebjorn	1987	Incision and drainage with fistula surgery	20	Recurrence 10% Minor incontinence 8.3%	12 months
Schouten	1991	Incision and drainage with fistula surgery	36	Recurrence 3% Minor incontinence 39%	42.5 months
Tang	1996	Incision and drainage with fistula surgery	24	Recurrence 0% Minor incontinence 0%	12 months
Ho Y	1997	Incision and drainage with fistula surgery	24	Recurrence 0% Minor incontinence 0%	15.5 months
Ho	1998	Fistulotomy	52	Healing time 10 weeks Minor incontinence 11%	9 weeks
Belmonte Montes	1999	Fistulotomy	24	Incontinence 5%	12 months
Oliver	2003	Incision and drainage with fistula surgery	100	Recurrence 5% Minor incontinence 6%	12 months
Pescatori	2006	Fistulotomy	52	Minor incontinence 8.3% Recurrence 8.3%	10 months
Atkin	2011	Fistulotomy	180		
Tozer	2013	Fistulotomy	50	Recurrence 7% Minor incontinence 20%	11 months
Hall	2014	Fistulotomy	146	Recurrence 6%	3 months

- Fistulotomy wounds typically heal after 4–6 weeks, which may be shortened by marsupializing the wound edges.
- Recurrence and incontinence are the most significant complication and rates vary widely.
  - 4% of patients with intersphincteric fistula
  - 7% with transsphincteric fistula
  - 33% for suprasphincteric and extrasphincteric fistulas
- Incontinence increased with the complexity of the fistula (up to 34%).
- Lowest for intersphincteric fistula (37%) and highest for extrasphincteric fistula (83%).
- Factors associated with recurrence included type and extension of the fistula, lack of identification or lateral location of the internal opening, previous fistula surgery, and the surgeon experience.
- Incontinence was associated to female sex, high anal fistula, type of surgery, and previous fistula surgery.
- Most complex anal fistulas and fistulas associated with Crohn's disease are specific examples in which a lay-open technique would have significant or complete impairment of fecal continence or when healing of the subsequent wound would not be expected to occur (Fig. 14.17).

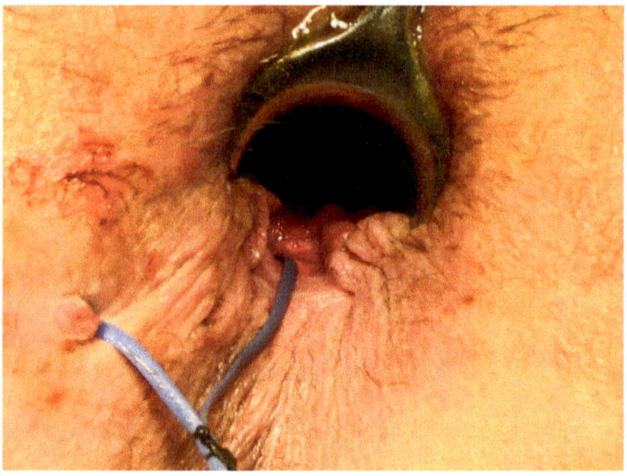

Fig. 14.17 Seton in anal fistula

Setons

- A variety of materials have been described for use as setons including wire, non-absorbable suture such as silk, vessel loops, and silastic catheters.
- Placed loosely in an effort to promote drainage and fibrosis of the fistula track either as a bridge to a non-cutting repair or as definitive treatment.
- Alternatively they may be tightened sequentially over time as a cutting seton in an effort to slowly divide the sphincter muscle over days to weeks and preserve continence by

allowing a scar to form between the cut ends of the sphincter complex.
  - Recurrence rates between 3% and 5%
  - Fecal incontinence rates 5.6–25.2%
- Non-cutting or draining setons.
  - Bridge for definitive treatment in an effort to promote fibrosis decreases the inflammatory response and aids in identifying the internal opening at the time of the secondary procedure.
  - Can be left in place to prevent recurrent abscess formation in patients with Crohn's disease or in patients who are not deemed candidates for additional surgery.

Advancement Flap

- Endorectal advancement flap (ERAF) has been advocated as an effective treatment for high transsphincteric or suprasphincteric fistulas.

  Essential operative elements include:
  - Debridement or excision of the fistula tract
  - Mobilization of a vascularized, tension-free mucosal flap
  - Coverage of the internal opening with absorbable suture

Technique

1. With the patient in prone jackknife position or in lithotomy position, the internal opening of the fistula is exposed – this can be accomplished by everting the anal canal with the Lone Star® retractor system (Fig. 14.18a).
2. The internal opening is identified and the crypt-bearing tissue excised.
3. A small rim of the anoderm, below the internal opening, is excised to create a neo-dentate line.
4. The defect in the internal anal sphincter is closed with absorbable sutures (2-0 Vicryl, Ethicon Inc., Somerville, NJ) (Fig. 14.18b).
5. A curvilinear incision is made at the level of the internal opening extending laterally to create a wide tissue flap.
6. Dissection is performed in the submucosal plane consisting of mucosa, submucosa, and few superficial fibers of the internal anal sphincter and then mobilized over a distance of 4–6 cm proximally.
7. The fistulous tract is alternatively curetted or cored out, and the defect in the internal anal sphincter is closed with absorbable sutures.
8. The flap is advanced and sutured over the top of the internal opening with absorbable sutures (Fig. 14.18c).
9. Vascular supply of the flap is maintained through the submucosal plexus.

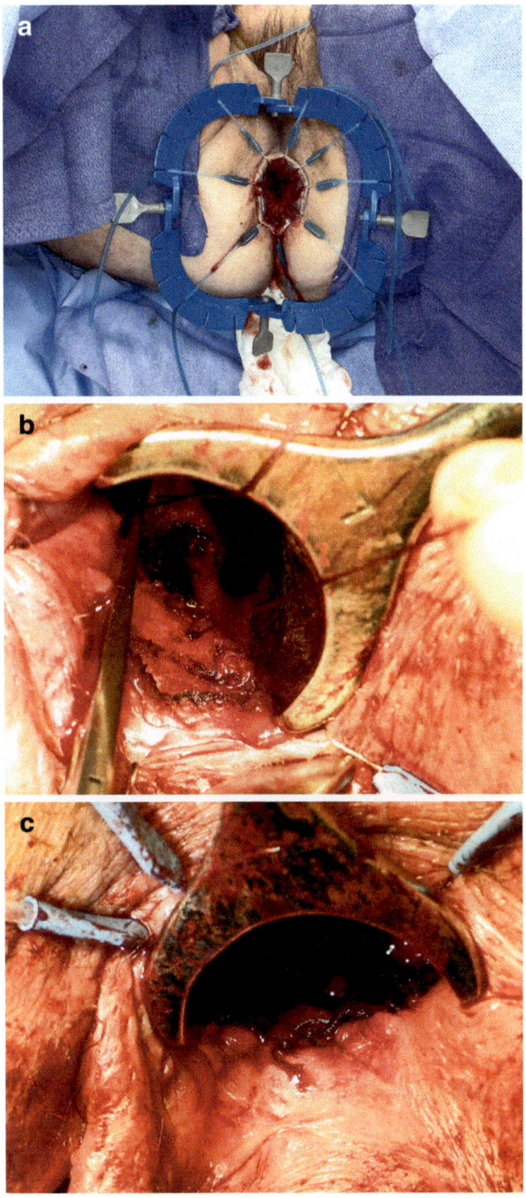

Fig. 14.18 (**a**) Lone Star to evert the anal canal. (**b**) Closing the internal opening. (**c**) Securing the flap

- The reported healing rates after flap repair vary between 60% and 100%.
- Patient, disease, and technical factors appear to be associated with either improved or worse outcomes following ERAF repair of complex anal fistula.
  - No difference in outcome seen:
    - Fistula tract "core out" found no difference in recurrence.
    - The location of the internal opening (posterior vs. anterior) has no impact on outcomes.
    - Preoperative seton placement did not impact outcomes of flap repairs.
    - Medically induced bowel confinement has not been shown to improve outcomes.
  - Difference in outcome seen:
    - Repeat anorectal advancement flap after recurrence has been shown to be feasible but has been shown to be a risk factor for failure; success of flap advancement was inversely correlated with the number of prior attempts (0–1; 87% vs. 2 or more; 50%).
    - The combination of fibrin glue with advancement flap repair has also been associated with worse outcomes when compared to just flap repairs alone.
    - Full-thickness flaps have been shown to be superior to partial thickness flaps in several studies (recurrence was 35% and 5%, respectively).
    - Patient smoking, which both decreases the mucosal blood flow, negatively impacts success of flap repairs.
    - Obesity negatively impacted advancement flap repairs.
    - Crohn's disease has also been shown to be a risk factor for failure.
- Reports have demonstrated some degree of fecal incontinence following surgery, with reductions in maximum resting and squeeze pressures.

Ligation of Intersphincteric Fistula

- Appropriate for all patients with high trans-sphincteric fistulas assuming that a well-formed fistula track has been established (Table 14.4)

Technique

1. Identify the internal opening by injecting peroxide or saline through the external opening.
2. Incise circumanally in the intersphincteric plane at the site of fistula using a 3–4-cm curvilinear incision.
3. Identify the intersphincteric tract using a soft catheter or Lockhart–Mummery and lacrimal probes.
4. Dissect around the intersphincteric portion of the fistula tract being careful not to injure or disrupt the tract. A right-angle probe can be used for this purpose. Using narrow malleable retractors can facilitate exposure of the intersphincteric plane. A Lone Star retractor can also facilitate this exposure.
5. Hook the intersphincteric tract using a small right-angle clamp.
6. Doubly ligate the tract close to the internal and external sphincter with 2-0 Vicryl (Ethicon Inc., Somerville, NJ), and transect it between the sutures. Some surgeons prefer a transfixation suture.
7. Inject the external opening to confirm that the tract was divided completely.
8. Curette the external portion of the fistula tract.
9. Drain the external opening.
10. Re-approximate the intersphincteric incision wound loosely with an interrupted 3-0 Vicryl (Ethicon Inc., Somerville, NJ).

- Variations in this technique include:
  - Orienting the incision in a radial fashion and performing a partial fistulotomy up to the external sphincter.
  - Unroofing the fistula from the internal opening to intersphincteric groove, ligating the fistula tract, but preserving the external sphincter.
  - Inserting a biologic mesh in the intersphincteric groove or as a plug in the external tract.

Table 14.4 Experience with LIFT procedure

Author	Year	# patients	Procedure	Follow-up (weeks)	Percent healed (%)	Type of study
Rojanasakul et al.	2007	18	LIFT	4	94	Prospective observational
Shanwani et al.	2010	45	LIFT	7	82	Prospective observational
Ellis et al.	2010	31	bioLIFT	6	94	Retrospective
Bleier et al.	2010	39	LIFT	10	57	Retrospective
Ooi et al.	2011	25	LIFT	6	96	Prospective observational
Tan et al.	2011	93	LIFT	4	92	Retrospective review
Steiner et al.		18	LIFT	6	83	Retrospective
Aboulian et al.	2011	25	LIFT	24	68	Retrospective review
Mushaya et al.	2012	25	LIFT	4	68	Prospective randomized
Abcarian et al.	2012	50	LIFT	15	74	Retrospective
Lo et al.	2012	25	LIFT	2	98	Retrospective
Van Onkelen et al.	2012	42	LIFT	12	51	Prospective
Chen et al.	2012	10	LIFT	6	100	Retrospective
Lehmann et al.	2013	17	LIFT	4	47	Prospective
Liu et al.	2013	38	LIFT	26	61	Retrospective
Madbouly et al.	2014	35	LIFT	56	74	Prospective randomized
Ye, F et al.	2015	43	mLIFT	60	87	Retrospective
Bastawrous, A. et al.	2015	66	mLIFT	21	71	Retrospective

- There is not enough evidence that variants in the surgical technique achieve better outcomes (Bio-LIFT, LIFT-Plug, LIFT-Plus).
- Results
  - Single-site studies show 74–79% success at 3 months.
  - Hospitals that performed more LIFT procedures had higher rates of healing.
  - Meta-analysis looking at the success of the LIFT procedure 18 studies was reviewed including 592 patients (65% male).
    - The mean healing rate reported was 74.6%.
    - The risk factors for failure were obesity, smoking, multiple previous surgeries, and the length of the fistula tract.
    - The median length of fistula tract was shorter in the healed group compared with the failed group (4 cm vs. 6 cm, P = 0.004).
    - The mean healing time was 5.5 weeks.
    - The patient satisfaction rates ranged from 72% to 100%.
    - No de novo incontinence developed secondary to the LIFT procedure.
- When the LIFT procedure fails, simple fistulas can be managed with fistulotomy or local wound care.

Fibrin Glue

- The advantages of fibrin glue are its simple and repeatable with no significant learning curve and no division of the sphincter muscle.
- The glue is infused into the fistulous tract with the idea that collagen formation within the tract will stimulate healing.
- It also stimulates the migration and proliferation of fibroblasts and pluripotent endothelial cells to heal the fistula.
- Between 7 and 14 days postoperatively, plasmin that is present in the surrounding tissue

lyses the fibrin clot as the tract is replaced by synthesized collagen.

Technique

1. The patient is placed in the prone jackknife position, and anesthesia is introduced (spinal, general, or locoregional).
2. Both openings of the fistula track are identified and mechanically curetted and irrigated with normal saline or hydrogen peroxide.
3. If extensive side branching or undrained abscess is encountered, the procedure is aborted and a seton is placed.
4. A double-barreled syringe, containing the two components of the glue, is inserted into the external opening until the tip is seen at the internal opening (Fig. 14.19).
5. At this point the internal opening can be variably sutured closed or left opening depending on the surgeon's preference – there is no significant advantage of one technique over the other.
6. The syringe is depressed, which mixes the two components as they are injected into the canal while withdrawing the syringe. The tract is filled completely until a bead of glue is seen at the external opening.
7. The glue is allowed to set for 30–60 s to form its stable clot.

- The efficacy of fibrin glue injection as a curative procedure remains in question.
- Success rates vary greatly depending on the etiology and complexity of the fistulas, type of fibrin glue used, and the length of patient follow-up. (Table 14.5).
- Cintron et al. have reported the largest series of patients with perianal fistulas treated with fibrin glue.
  - Non-randomized prospective study.
  - Three different types of fibrin glue: autologous, Viguard-FS (V. I. Technologies, Inc., New York, NY), and Tisseel VB (Baxter, Deerfield, IL).

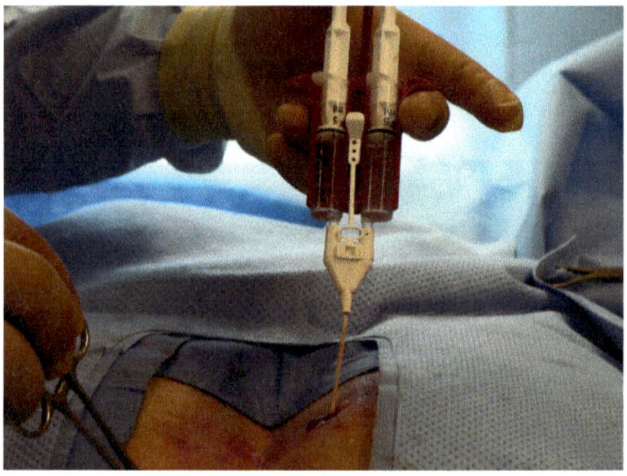

Fig. 14.19 Fibrin glue injection into an anal fistula

Table 14.5 Experience with fibrin glue

Author	Year	# patients	Success rate (%)	Follow-up (months)
Cintron et al.	1999	26	81	3.5
Cintron et al.	2000	79	61	18
Patrlj et al.	2000	69	74	28
Park et al.	2000	29	68	6
Sentovich	2001	20	85	10
Lindsey et al.	2002	42	63	4
Sentovich	2003	48	69	22
Loungnarath et al.	2004	39	31	26
Zmora et al.	2005	60	53	6
Gisbertz et al.	2005	27	33	7
Singer et al.	2005	75	21a	27
Maralcan et al.	2006	36	83	12
Ellis and Clark	2006	28	54	22
Dietz	2006	39	31	23
Witte et al.	2007	34	55	7
Adams et al.	2008	36	61	3
de Parades et al.	2010	30	50	12

- The majority of fistulas were transsphincteric, and 8% were secondary to Crohn's disease. The overall success rate was 66%, with a mean follow-up of 1 year.
- Healing rates correlated with fistula complexity: intersphincteric 82%, transsphincteric 62%, and Crohn's-related 33%.
- The type of glue used did not affect success rates.
- The average time to fistula recurrence was 3.3 months while the latest was seen at 11 months.

- Meta-analysis of 12 published studies of 378 patients with complex anal fistula overall healing rate was 53% with a wide variation between studies (10–78%).
- The only factor that was found to account for this diversity was fistula complexity, with series including a high proportion of complex fistulas reporting worse outcomes.
- No impact on continence.
- The heterogeneity of published data regarding the success of this treatment makes it difficult to recommend as a first-line therapy of complex anal fistula.

Anal Fistula Plug

- Surgisis® (Cook Surgical, Inc., Bloomington, IN), a bioabsorbable xenograft, made of lyophilized porcine intestinal submucosa, acts as a tissue scaffold for host fibroblasts to promote healing and ingrowth of tissue into the fistula track (Fig. 14.20).

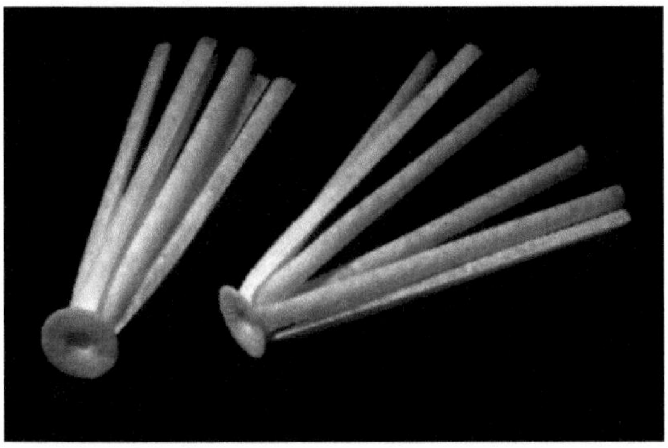

Fig. 14.20 Bio A absorbable fistula plug (W.L. GORE & Associates, Newark, DE, Courtesy of Michael Stamos, MD, with permission)

Technique

1. The patient is placed in the prone jackknife position, and anesthesia is introduced (spinal, general, or locoregional).
2. Both openings of the fistula track are identified and irrigated with normal saline or hydrogen peroxide.
3. The plug is rehydrated, usually in a 0.9% normal saline solution for 3–5 min, before insertion.
4. The tapered end of the fistula plug is then tied to the anal side of the seton or silk suture and pulled into the fistula tract through the primary opening until it fitted snugly.
5. The plug is then trimmed flush with the primary opening. A 2-0 Vicryl (Ethicon Inc., Somerville, NJ) suture is used to anchor the plug to the mucosa/submucosa and internal sphincter at the primary opening with a figure-of-eight stitch, completely covering it with mucosa at the completion of the stitch.
6. The excess plug protruding from the external opening is trimmed such that the external opening is partially open to allow drainage and prevent infection.

- Since introduction of the AFP, success rates have varied widely between 14% and 87% (Table 14.6).
  - The plug extrusion rate was 8.7%.
  - The proportion of non-Crohn's patients achieving fistula closure varies widely between studies, ranging from 0.2 to 0.
  - The proportion of patients achieving fistula closure in patients with non-Crohn's fistula-in-ano is 0.54.
  - Factors ascribed to the failures include:
    - The absence of preoperative seton placement
    - Overly aggressive curetting of the fistula track resulting in widening of the track
    - Inadequate fixation of the plug into the internal opening
    - Presence of multiple tracks
    - Increased tract length, because fistulas longer than 4 cm were nearly 3 times more likely to heal compared with shorter fistulas

Table 14.6 Experience with anal fistula plug

Author	Year	Type of study	# patients	Success rate (%)	Follow-up (months)
Johnson et al.	2006	Prospective	25	87	3
Champagne et al.	2006	Prospective	46	83	12
O'Connor et al.	2006	Prospective	20	80	10
Ellis	2007	Retrospective	13	92	6
Ky et al.	2008	Prospective	45	55	6.5
Christoforidis et al.	2008	Retrospective	47	43	6.5
Safar et al.	2009	Retrospective	36	14	4.2
Ortiz et al.	2009	Prospective randomized	15	20	12
El-Gazzaz et al.	2010	Retrospective	33	25	7.4
van Koperen et al.	2011	Prospective	31	29	11
Chan et al.	2012	Prospective	44	50	10.5
Cintron et al.	2013	Prospective	73	42	15
Tan et al.	2013	Retrospective	26	13	15
Adamina et al.	2014	Prospective	46	43.5	68

Novel Techniques

- Laser probe [Fistula laser closure (FiLaC™), Biolitec, Germany], which destroys the fistula epithelium and simultaneously obliterates the remaining fistula tract.
  - Includes closure of the internal opening by means of an anorectal flap.
  - Pilot study, 11 patients with cryptoglandular fistula, underwent FiLaC™ procedure with an overall success of 81%.
- Adipose-derived stem cells (ADSC) to treat complex anal fistula mostly in patients with Crohn's disease.
  - Autologous ADSC obtained with liposuction with minimal adverse effects on the patient.
  - In a multicenter randomized controlled trial, Garcia-Olmo et al. used ADSC to treat complex cryptoglandular, rectovaginal, and Crohn's-related fistulas.
  - Initially they achieved a 71% success rate with ADSC, compared with 16% in the control group (fibrin glue only).
  - At 1 year this had decreased to 62.5 and to 33% at 3 years.
- Injectable form of Permacol (Tissue Science Laboratories, Covington, GA), a type of porcine acellular collagen matrix, was modified by centrifugation to form a paste and has been used to inject anal fistula in combination with an ERAF.
  - Studies are limited, but success rates in non-Crohn's patients have been reported as high as 82%.(167)

15 Complex Anorectal Fistulas

Giulio A. Santoro and Maher A. Abbas

Key Concepts

- The history and physical examination are the mandatory first step, providing in most cases the appropriate information to classify a fistula as "simple" or "complex." Anal continence should be evaluated using a validated incontinence score such as the Cleveland Clinic Florida Fecal Incontinence Score (CCF-FIS) grading system.
- *Imaging procedures include (in order of authors' preference)* two- and three-dimensional endoanal ultrasound (2D/3D EAUS), pelvic magnetic resonance imaging (MRI), computed tomography (CT), and fistulography. Imaging can provide invaluable information on the anatomy of the fistula, including the primary track, internal opening, horseshoe extension, secondary cavities or extensions, and associated sphincter lesions, and is a useful guide in surgical management.
- Complex anal fistula is challenging to treat due to the risk of postoperative anal incontinence and the high rate of recurrence. Three factors determine the outcome of surgical treatment: patient-related factors, fistula characteristics, and the surgeon choice of operation inclusive of its technical conduct.
- Each surgical procedure has advantages and disadvantages, and the choice of operative intervention should be individualized based on patient-related factors and fistula characteristics taking into account success rate as well as impact on patient anal continence.
- Rectourethral fistula is often the result of prostate cancer treatment whether surgical or radiotherapy-based. A multidisciplinary approach involving a urologist and a colorectal surgeon is essential. Small distal fistulas and those not radiation-induced can be amenable to a local anal repair such as an endorectal advancement flap. Large fistulas, those induced by radiation, or persistent/recurrent fistulas are best approached by a transperineal approach with a gracilis interposition flap or in select cases by a transabdominal approach with rectal excision. Due to its rarity, rectourethral fistula is best managed in tertiary or quaternary centers with experience managing this condition.
- Ileal-pouch fistula is uncommon and can be extremely challenging to manage due to the

Electronic Supplementary Material The online version of this chapter (https://doi.org/10.1007/978-3-030-01165-9_15) contains supplementary material, which is available to authorized users.

G. A. Santoro
Treviso Regional Hospital Italy, Treviso, Italy

M. A. Abbas (✉)
Al Azhra Hospital Dubai, Dubai, UAE
e-mail: abbasm@clevelandclinicabudhabi.ae

S. R. Steele et al. (eds.), *The ASCRS Manual of Colon and Rectal Surgery*,
https://doi.org/10.1007/978-3-030-01165-9_15

morbidity associated with any intervention, failure rate of various surgical options, and long-term consequences to the patient. Simple procedures should be attempted first before more complex procedures are considered. Due to the low incidence of this condition, few centers worldwide have accumulated enough experience with ileal-pouch fistula management. Early referral to such centers is advisable.

Introduction

- Anal fistula may be termed "complex" when one or more of the following findings are present:
  - The tract crosses more than 30% of the external anal sphincter (high transsphincteric with or without a high blind tract, suprasphincteric, and extrasphincteric).
  - Horseshoe configuration.
  - Anterior location in a female.
  - Multiple tracts, recurrent.
  - In the setting of Crohn's disease.
  - Prior radiotherapy.
  - Baseline incontinence.
  - Rectovaginal fistula, rectourethral fistula, anastomotic fistula following colorectal surgery, post-traumatic fistula, and malignant fistula.
- Rectovaginal fistula and Crohn's-related fistula are not covered in this chapter but dealt with in other parts of this textbook.

Complex or Recurrent Cryptoglandular Fistulas

Definition, Classification, and Pathophysiology

- The aim of anal fistula treatment is to eradicate the fistulous tract, prevent recurrence, minimize postoperative septic complications, and minimally impact anal continence.

Clinical Assessment and Diagnostic Evaluation

- The history should include the type of prior anal operations, obstetrical history in females, the presence of gastrointestinal disorders such as inflammatory bowel disease, medical comorbidities such as diabetes, prior radiation therapy to the pelvis, current smoking status, and inquiry about the patient's bowel habits using a validated score such as the Cleveland Clinic Florida Fecal Incontinence score (CCF-FIS) grading system (Fig. 15.1).
- Physical examination can be helpful in delineating the fistula anatomy and reaches a very good accuracy in identifying superficial (100%) and transsphincteric (100%) tracts, but it appears inadequate for supralevator (63.6%) and intersphincteric (33.3%) tracts.
- Considering the limitation of physical examination, it may perform imaging procedures (two- and three-dimensional endoanal ultrasound (2D and 3D EAUS), pelvic MRI, CT scan, and fistulography).
  - Information on the anatomy of the fistula, including the primary tract, internal opening, horseshoe extension, secondary cavities or extensions, and associated sphincter lesions.
  - Clear delineation of the fistula anatomy to guide operative intervention can be helpful for surgical planning and may impact surgical outcome.
  - The difficulty in comparing these modalities is related to the ability to define a true reference standard for fistula-in-ano due to the following potential sources of bias.
- In addition to imaging, baseline assessment of sphincter function with anorectal manometry can be helpful in select patients (Fig. 15.2a, b).

Surgical Treatment

- The goal to eradicate the fistula should be balanced with the aim to preserve as much of the sphincter integrity to avoid impairment of continence.

Fig. 15.1 Cleveland Clinic Florida Fecal Incontinence Score (CCF-FIS). Scale: 0, complete continence; 20, complete incontinence

Type of incontinence	Never	Rarely <1/mo	Sometimes <1/week >1/month	Usually <1/day >1/week	Always >1/day
Solid	0	1	2	3	4
Liquid	0	1	2	3	4
Gas	0	1	2	3	4
Wears pad	0	1	2	3	4
Lifestyle alteration	0	1	2	3	4

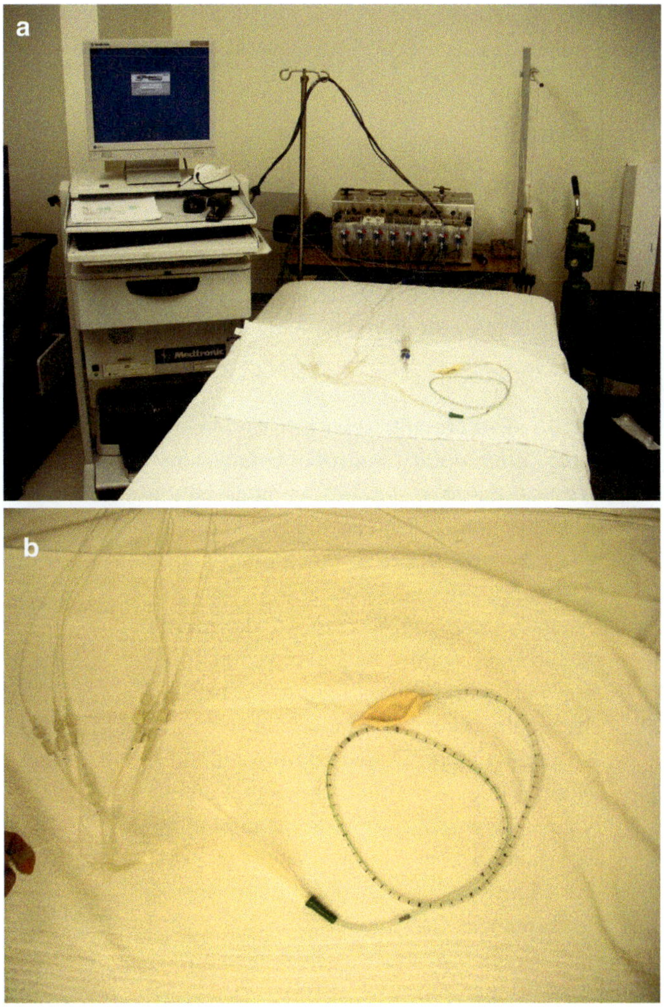

Fig. 15.2 (**a**) Low-compliance water perfusion anorectal manometry system. (**b**) Anorectal manometry catheter

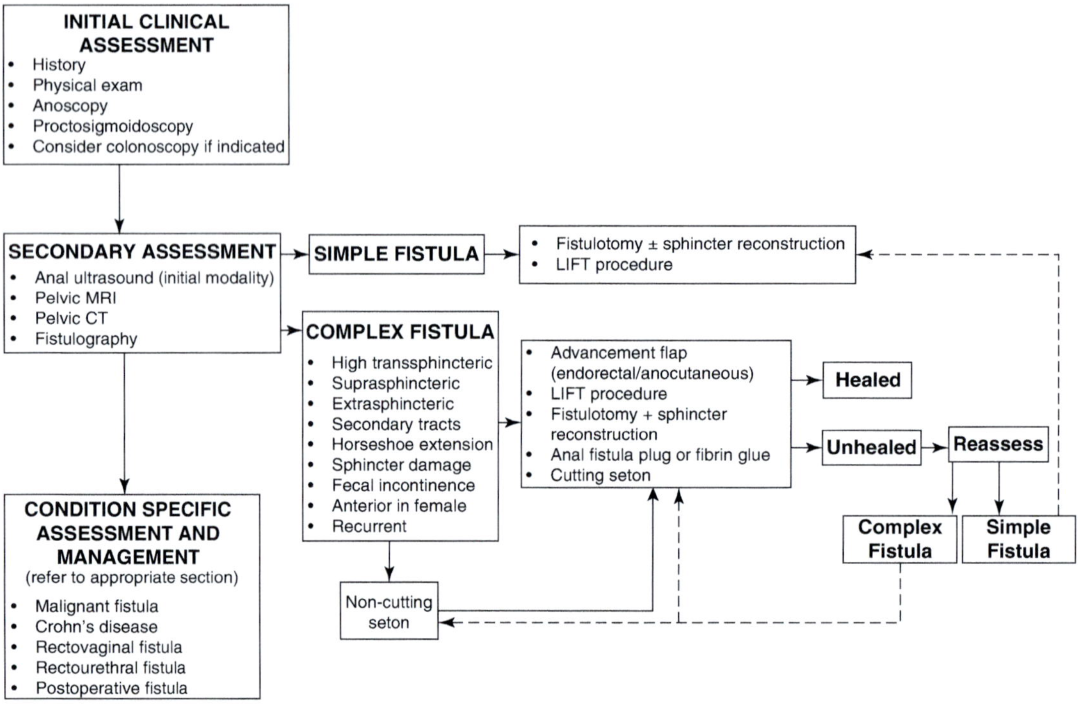

Fig. 15.3 Carepath for evaluation and treatment of complex anal fistula secondary to cryptoglandular disease

- Figure 15.3 provides a comprehensive carepath for a structured approach to guide the care of patients with anorectal fistula.

Seton

- Seton is an important treatment option that can provide temporary control of fistula symptoms or can serve as a definitive intervention to control or eradicate a chronic fistula.
  - A variety of materials including suture material (Ethibond, silk, nylon, polypropylene, suture size #2.0 to #2, depending on the tract width), vascular vessel loop, Penrose drain, rubber band, cable tie, and chemically impregnated material.
  - A draining seton is tied loosely around a fistulous tract to promote drainage, to minimize acute abscess formation, and to allow for scarring of the fistulous tract (Figs. 15.4 and 15.5).
    - Permanent solution
    - Temporary measure as the patient awaits additional definitive fistula surgery (12 or more weeks)

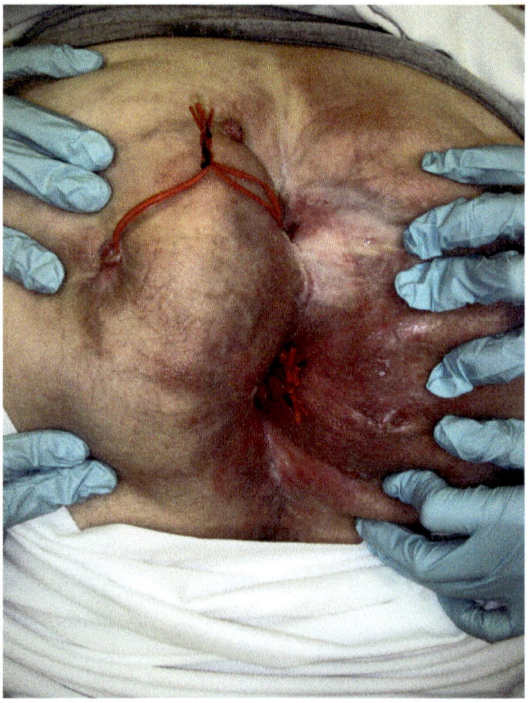

Fig. 15.4 Draining setons in a patient with multiple complex anorectal fistulas and prior radiation therapy to the pelvis

- A cutting seton is the second type of seton (Fig. 15.6a).
  - The patient gradually pulls the seton through the muscular portion of the tract (Fig. 15.6b).
  - Progressive cutting by the seton produces a slow fistulotomy, which allows for scarring of the divided tract minimizing wide separation of the divided muscle.
  - An alternative variation of the cutting seton is the multiple seton technique, and at various time intervals, each suture is tightened progressively after taking out the previously tightened suture which becomes loose.

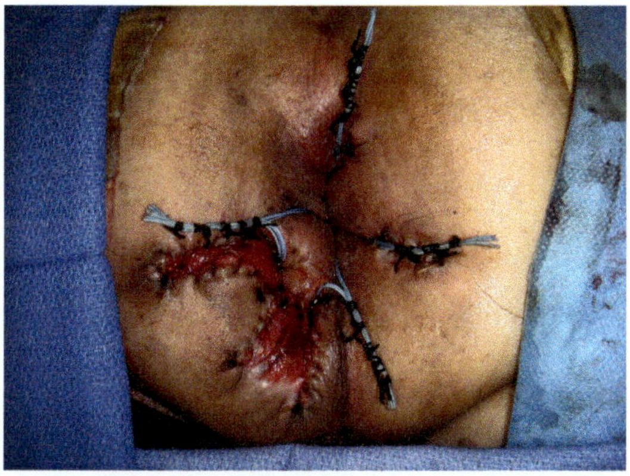

Fig. 15.5 Draining setons in a patient with long-standing history of multiple fistulas emanating from different internal openings in all four anal quadrants

Anal Flap

- The endorectal advancement flap is our preferred method to treat most complex anal fistula secondary to cryptoglandular disease, except for posterior-based horseshoe fistula.
- There are two types of anal flaps: transanal endorectal advancement flap and anocutaneous flap.
- Usually a non-cutting draining seton is placed for 12 or more weeks to allow for fibrosis of the fistulous tract.

1. The tract is irrigated with hydrogen peroxide, and the tract is traced with a fistula probe.
2. The planned flap is outlined and infiltrated with 1% lidocaine with 1:100,000 epinephrine for hemostasis (Fig. 15.7a, b).
3. The subcutaneous portion of the external opening is excised, and the fistula is debrided with a curette (Fig. 15.7c).
4. A curvilinear incision is made approximately 1 cm distal to the internal opening, and a partial- or full-thickness broad-based (3–4-cm-wide) endorectal flap is raised (Fig. 15.7d).
5. It is important to avoid a mucosa-only based flap as it is associated with a higher failure rate due to ischemia.
6. Once the flap is raised, the intramuscular portion of the internal opening is closed with interrupted 3-0 Vicryl suture (Fig. 15.7e).

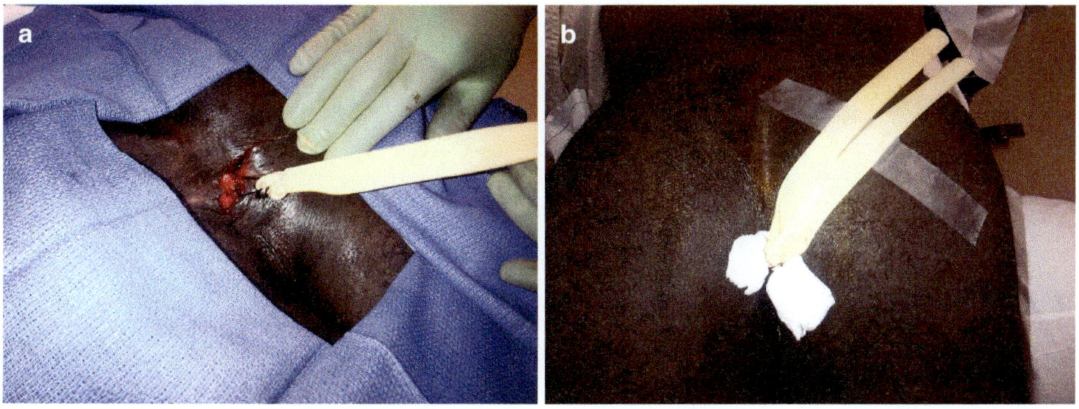

Fig. 15.6 (**a**) Cutting seton in a patient with suprasphincteric fistula. The skin and subcutaneous portion of the tract are divided before tightening the seton. (**b**) The cutting seton is connected to a Penrose drain to allow the patient to gradually pull through the fistula

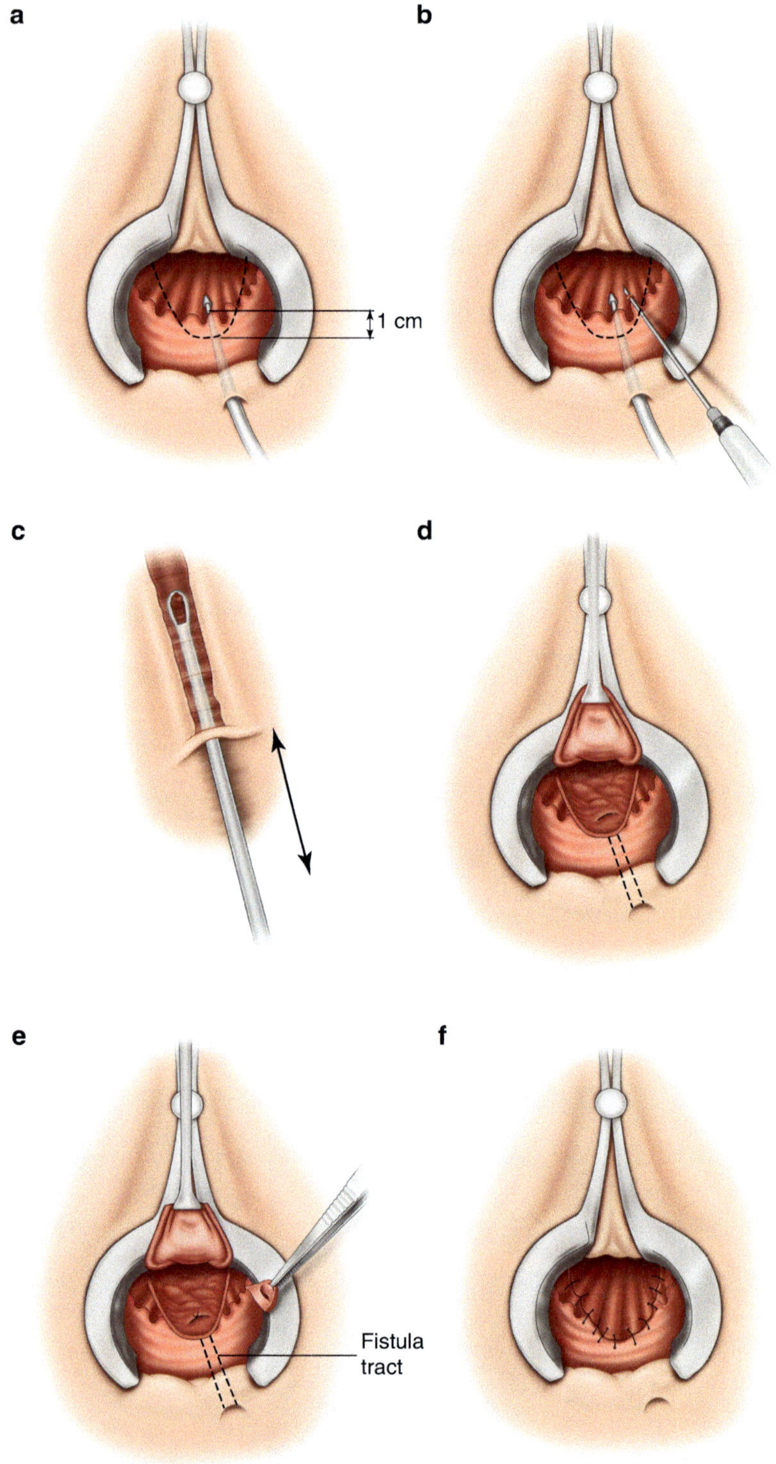

Fig. 15.7 (a–f) Technical steps of endorectal advancement flap

7. The distal portion of the flap containing the mucosal portion of the internal opening is trimmed.
8. The flap is matured over its muscular bed using 3-0 Vicryl single interrupted sutures (Fig. 15.7f).
9. Upon completion of the flap, an antibiotic-impregnated gelfoam is placed inside the anal canal.

Ligation of the Intersphincteric Fistula Tract

1. Described in 2007 by Rojanasakul and colleagues from Thailand (Videos 15.1, 15.2, 15.3, 15.4, 15.5, 15.6, 15.7, and 15.8).
2. Division and ligation of the fistulous tract in the intersphincteric plane.
3. Suprasphincteric and horseshoe fistulas can pose technical challenges and in general are not suitable candidates for the LIFT procedure.
4. Wet fistulas with copious drainage and those associated with a cavity can benefit from a draining seton prior to the LIFT procedure.
5. Procedure:
   - A metallic probe is inserted into the external opening and passed gently through the tract to exit through the internal opening (Fig. 15.8a, b).
   - The intersphincteric groove is identified externally, and a small circumanal skin incision overlying the fistula is performed to enter the intersphincteric space between the internal and the external sphincter muscles.
   - The dissection in the intersphincteric plane is continued until the fistulous tract is reached and encircled (Fig. 15.8c).
   - The fistula tract is then encircled by using a right-angle clamp, and two absorbable sutures (2-0 Vicryl) are used to ligate the fistula tract medially and laterally leaving a space in between to sharply divide the fistula (Fig. 15.8d).
   - Care is taken not to dislodge the tied sutures (Fig. 15.8e).
   - The intersphincteric plane is closed in two layers (muscle approximation and the skin) by using single interrupted 3-0 Vicryl (Fig. 15.8f).
   - Both the internal and external openings are left opened to allow drainage.
6. Variations to the conventional LIFT procedure:
   - BioLIFT procedure: a bioprosthetic porcine graft interposed between the internal and external sphincter muscles to overlap 1–2 cm area of the ligated and divided fistulous tract.
   - LIFT-PLUS procedure which adds a partial fistulectomy of the subcutaneous portion of the tract from the skin to the external sphincter muscle.
   - LIFT procedure combined with endorectal advancement flap.

Fistulotomy with Sphincter Reconstruction

1. Fistulotomy with sphincter reconstruction is a suitable technique for complex or recurrent fistulas in incontinent patients or in patients who are at risk for incontinence.
2. Procedure:
   - If a draining seton has been previously placed, it is removed, and a fistula probe is introduced through the external opening and guided through the tract until it protrudes out of the internal opening (Fig. 15.9a).
   - The fistula tract is completely divided using electrocautery (Fig. 15.9b).
   - Curettage of the tract and any associated cavities is performed to ensure that all granulation tissue is debrided.
   - Excision of the fibrous tract can be performed taking care not to excise any muscle, or alternatively the fibrous tract is left in situ.
   - An end-to-end primary sphincteroplasty is performed using a series of horizontal mattress sutures using 2-0 Vicryl or PDS sutures (Fig. 15.9c).

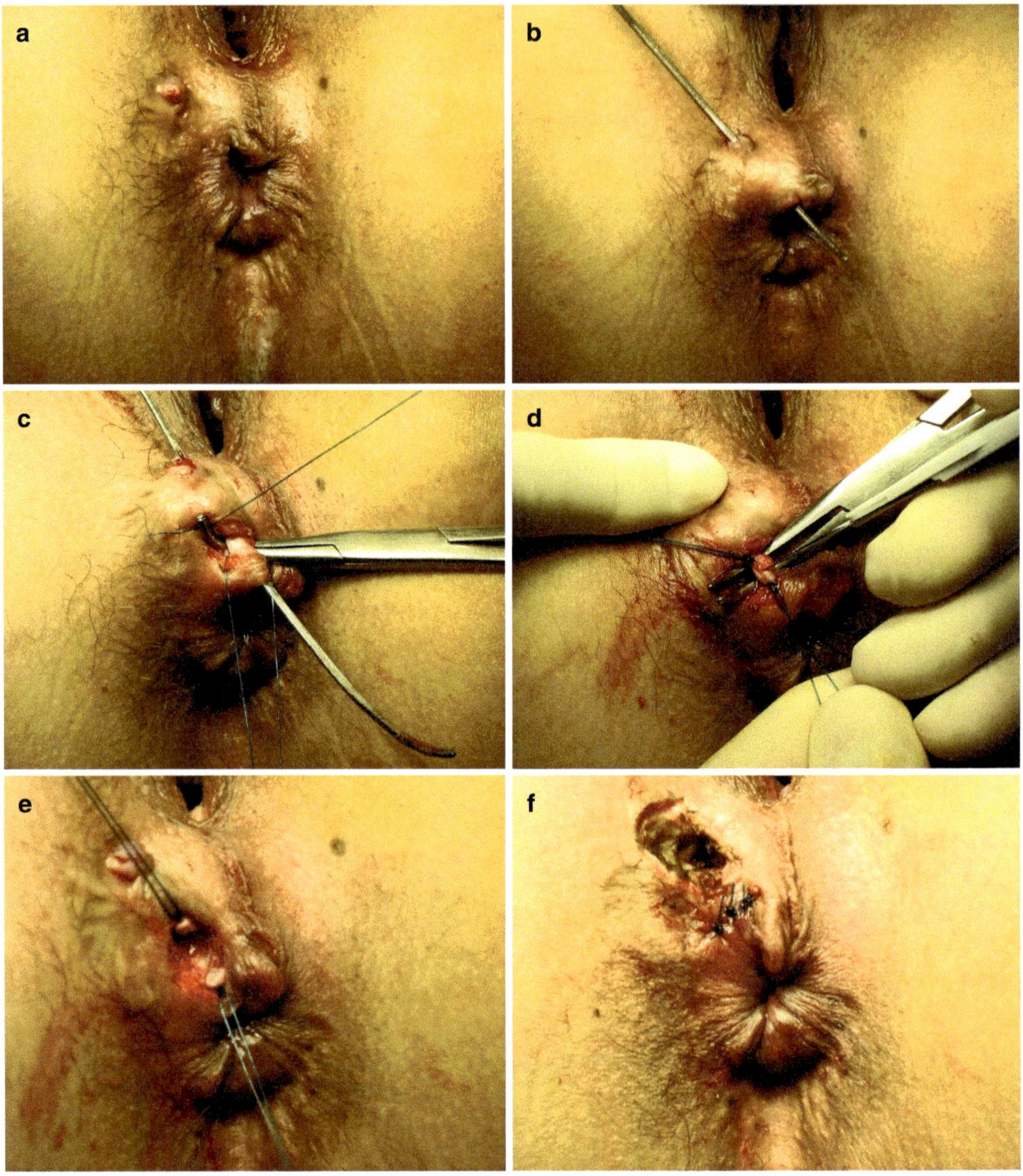

Fig. 15.8 (**a–f**) Intraoperative demonstration of the LIFT procedure

- The fistula bed of the divided fistulous tract is incorporated in the suturing to completely obliterate any potential space behind the muscle reconstruction.
- The edges of the open wound are finally marsupialized by tacking the divided mucosal and submucosal layer to the muscle repair (Fig. 15.9d) keeping the most superficial aspect of the wound open to allow for drainage.

Anal Fistula Plug

1. The anal fistula plug is used to close the primary internal opening and serves as a matrix for the obliteration of the fistulous tract.
2. Procedure:
   - The tract is traversed with a fistula probe and then curetted.
   - A 2-0 silk suture is tied to the tapered end of the plug and then pulled through the internal opening using the fistula probe

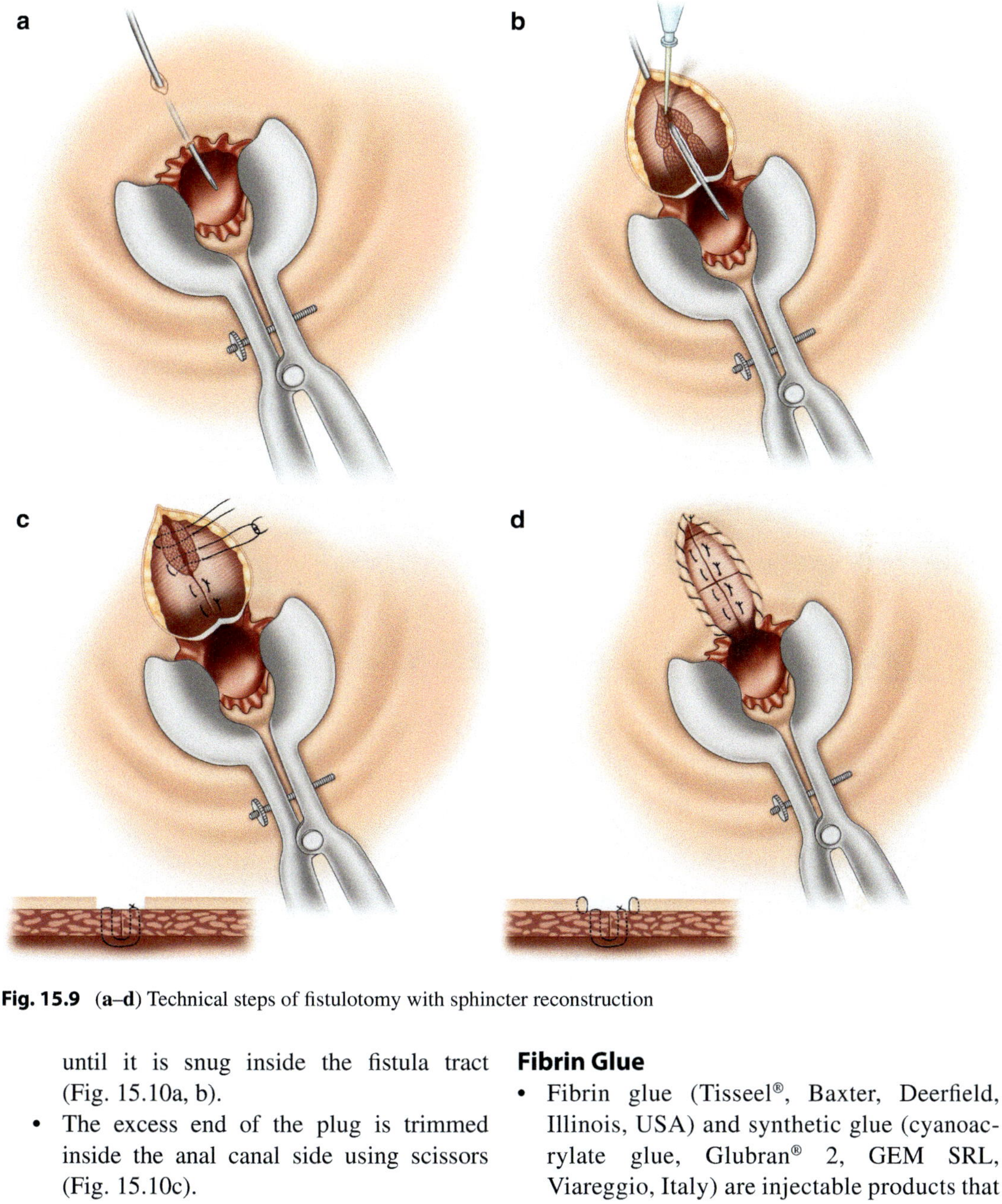

Fig. 15.9 (**a**–**d**) Technical steps of fistulotomy with sphincter reconstruction

until it is snug inside the fistula tract (Fig. 15.10a, b).

- The excess end of the plug is trimmed inside the anal canal side using scissors (Fig. 15.10c).
- The trimmed portion of the plug is fixed to the internal opening and internal anal sphincter muscle using 3-0 Vicryl suture (Fig. 15.10d).
- The mucosal/submucosal opening at the internal fistula opening is approximated with the same suture.
- The external opening of the fistula is left open to drain after trimming the tapered end of the plug (Fig. 15.10e).

Fibrin Glue

- Fibrin glue (Tisseel®, Baxter, Deerfield, Illinois, USA) and synthetic glue (cyanoacrylate glue, Glubran® 2, GEM SRL, Viareggio, Italy) are injectable products that can be used in the treatment of anorectal fistulas.
- They act as tissue sealants and are believed to stimulate the growth of fibroblasts and pluripotent endothelial cells into the fistulous tract.
- This physiologic response triggers collagen deposition and wound healing. Fibrin glue treatment is simple and repeatable and may be a good initial option in patients with high fistulas.

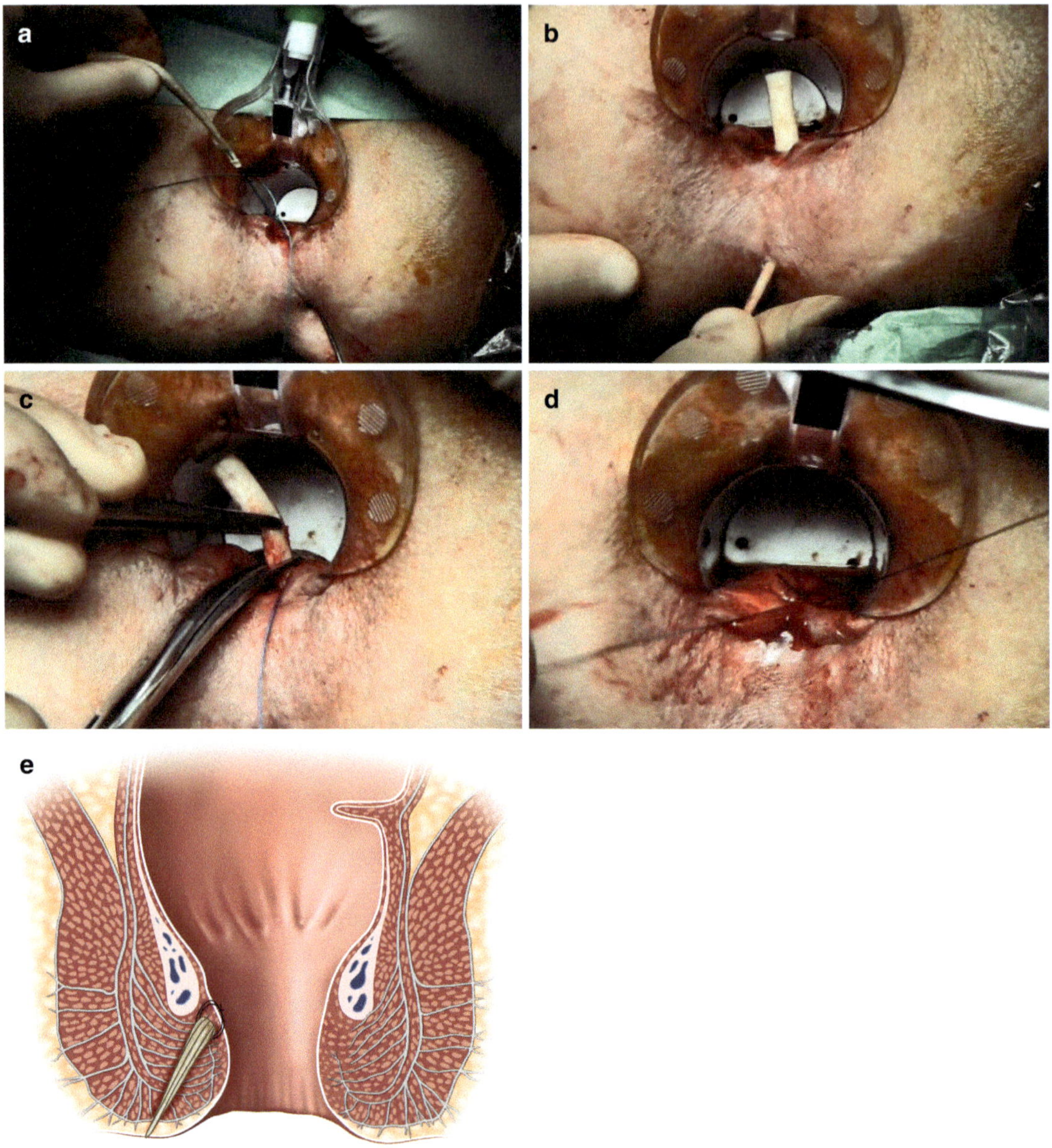

Fig. 15.10 (**a–d**) Intraoperative demonstration of the anal fistula plug (Surgisis® AFP) procedure in a patient with high transsphincteric fistula. (**e**) Anatomical view of obliterated fistula tract following placement of anal fistula plug (Surgisis® AFP)

- Associated with an overall low success rate.
- The procedure starts by identifying the external fistula opening, followed by the curettage of the fistula tract. Approximately 5 ml of reconstituted fibrin glue is injected through the external opening (Fig. 15.11a) until it extrudes from the internal opening area (Fig. 15.11b). The internal opening is closed with 3-0 Vicryl suture.

Newer and Evolving Technologies: VAAFT, FiLaC™, and Stem Cell

1. New technologies:
    - Video-assisted anal fistula treatment (VAAFT)
    - Fistula laser closure (FiLaC™)
    - Stem cell therapy
2. At this stage of development, it is premature to tell what long-term roles these evolving

technologies will play in the field of anorectal fistula surgery.

3. The video-assisted anal fistula treatment (VAAFT):
   - The kit includes a rigid fistuloscope (Karl Storz, Tuttlingen, Germany) (Fig. 15.12), an obturator, a unipolar electrical diathermy probe, an endobrush, an endoscopic grasper, and a synthetic cyanoacrylate glue.
   - The fistuloscope video equipment is an 8-degree angled endoscope with an optical working channel to introduce the instruments and an irrigation channel.
   - In the diagnostic phase, the fistuloscope is inserted through the external opening and advanced by the irrigation of the glycine-mannitol 1% which expands the fistula tract.
   - Primary and secondary openings and tracts are explored via the fistuloscope.
   - During the operative phase, the aim is to destroy the fistula tract from the inside by curetting the tract, obliterating it, and closing the internal opening.
   - Through the working channel of the fistuloscope, the fistula tract is cauterized, and necrotic material is removed using an endobrush and irrigation.
   - Finally, the internal opening is closed by either suturing or stapling with a linear or semicircular stapler or alternatively by advancing an anal flap.

- The fistula laser closure is a novel sphincter-saving technique that uses a radially emitting laser probe [FiLaC™, Biolitec, Germany] to destroy the fistula epithelium and simultaneously obliterate the remaining fistula tract.
- FiLaC™ eliminates fistula epithelium and granulation tissue in a circular manner causing shrinkage and obliteration of the tract.
  - The fistula tract is debrided with a curette, and a plastic hollow 14 French catheter is inserted using a guidewire.

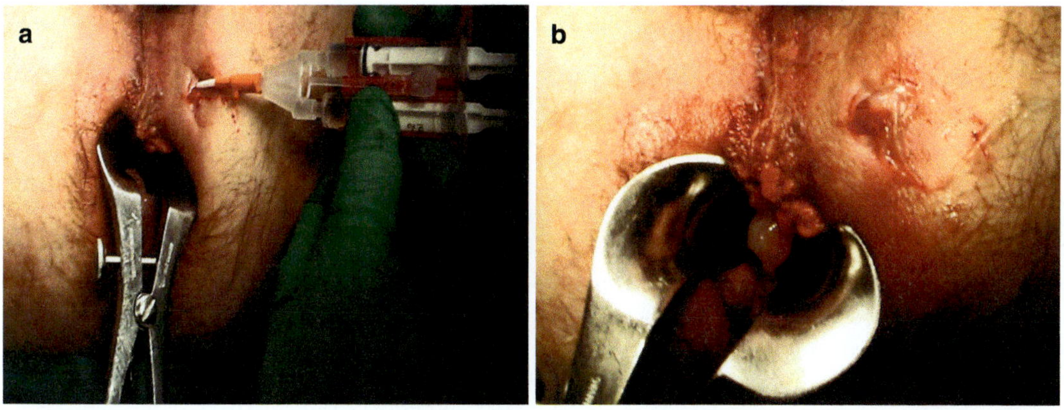

Fig. 15.11 (**a**) Fibrin glue injection of a high transsphincteric fistula through the external fistulous opening. (**b**) Fistula tract sealed with the fibrin glue. Note the fibrin glue extruding from the internal opening inside the anal canal

Fig. 15.12 Anal fistuloscope (Karl Storz, Tuttlingen, Germany)

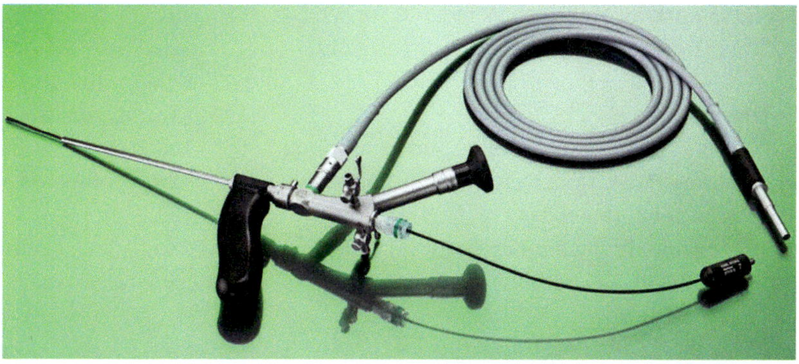

  - A 400 micron radial-emitting disposable laser fiber is inserted into the catheter with its tip emerging at the internal orifice. The fiber delivers laser energy homogenously at 360°, and by applying continuous energy, the tract is closed while withdrawing it at a speed of 1 mm per second.
  - The procedure includes the closure of the internal opening by means of an anorectal flap. When some scar tissue prevents that, either a mucosal or anodermal flap is used for closure of the internal opening.
- Application of autologous expanded adipose-derived stem cells (ASCs) represents a novel approach for enhancing regeneration of damaged tissues.
  - ASCs are obtained from subcutaneous fat by liposuction, and this process yields 100 times more stem cells than bone marrow aspirates.
  - Following curettage of the fistula tract and suture closure of the internal opening, ASC solution is injected into the tract and into the walls of the fistula.
  - The tract is subsequently sealed with fibrin glue.

Outcomes

- Complex fistulous disease challenges even the most experienced surgeons.
- Success rate in patients with complex or recurrent anorectal fistulas is lower than in patients with simple anal fistulas.
- Often more than one procedure is needed to eradicate the fistula.
- Risk for incontinence is usually higher due to the complexity of the fistula, recurrent or persistent disease, and/or prior failed interventions.

Seton

- Non-cutting seton is usually used as a bridge to additional surgical intervention and typically is not curative.
- A high rate of incontinence (38%) has been reported with cutting seton.
  - Typically reserved for patients with high complex fistulas who failed multiple prior interventions or in fistulas not amenable to other techniques such as high posterior-based fistulas in patients with deep buttock cleft.
  - Overall the fecal incontinence was 5.6% when the internal anal sphincter was preserved compared to 25.2% when it was divided.
  - Women with prior vaginal deliveries experienced significant incontinence leading the authors to advice against the use of cutting seton in this subgroup of patients especially in the setting of an anterior fistula.
  - Frequent gas incontinence developed postoperatively in 9.5% of the patients, and 21.4% developed occasional gas incontinence.

Advancement Flap

- Endorectal flap has demonstrated a success rate of between 60% and 93%, and it has been advocated as the treatment of choice for complex fistula-in-ano.
- It can be technically challenging especially in posterior-based fistula in males and in patients with deep buttock cleft.
- Postoperative incontinence rate has been reported between 7% and 38%.
- Prior drainage with a non-cutting seton is believed to increase success rate.
- Patients who fail an initial flap can be considered for a repeat procedure.
  - Primary healing occurred in 72% of patients, and secondary healing (following a second flap after initial failure) occurred in 57% of cases yielding an overall healing rate 93%.
- The flap technique can impact success rate.
  - Overall recurrence rate was 24% and was much lower in the full thickness subgroup (5%) compared to the mucosal subgroup (35.3%).
- Smoking has been associated with a lower success rate.

  - During a median time of 14 months, healing rate was 60% in smokers compared to 79% in nonsmokers.

Ligation of the Intersphincteric Fistula Tract

- LIFT procedure appears to be an effective sphincter-conserving approach for the treatment of complex fistula-in-ano. The initial reported success rate of the LIFT procedure was 94%.
- Subsequent studies with longer follow-up have shown a wider range of success rate from 40% to 95%, mean 76% (Table 15.1).
- In those patients with recurrence, the LIFT technique can transform a complex fistula into a simple intersphincteric fistula that could be effectively treated by subsequent intersphincteric fistulotomy.
- Minor continence disturbance was observed in 0–6% of cases.
- A recent prospective randomized trial comparing the LIFT procedure with mucosal advancement flap in patients with high trans-sphincteric fistula found similar long-term healing rate, recurrence rate, continence, and quality of life.
- BioLIFT procedure success rate is 63–94%.
- LIFT-PLUS procedure success rate is 85%.

Anal Fistula Plug

- Several studies have reported variable results with this minimally invasive procedure; success rate in various studies have ranged from 13.9% to 87% (Table 15.2).
- The postoperative abscess/sepsis rate has ranged from 4% to 29%.
- Failures have been related to technical issues, plug extrusion, and infection.
- In a systematic review (22 studies included, 488 patients) of the anal fistula plug, fistula closure was achieved in 54% of cases.
- Tract length and number of tracts are predictors of outcome with longer fistula tracts carrying higher success rate.
- Ortiz and colleagues conducted a randomized clinic trial comparing the Surgisis® AFP with the endorectal advancement flap in patients with high cryptoglandular fistula-in-ano.
  - The trial was closed prematurely due to a high failure rate of the plug (80%) compared to the flap (12.5%).
- The GORE® BIO-A® Fistula Plug was the second plug introduced in the field of fistula surgery but is no longer commercially available.

Fibrin Glue

- The use of fibrin sealant injection initially demonstrated promising results with high success rates between 60% and 80%.

Table 15.1 Results of LIFT procedure

	Year	No. of patients	Follow-up (months)	Success (%)	Incontinence (%)
Rojanaskul et al.	2007	18	6.5	94	0
Ellis (24)	2010	31	15	94	0
Shanwani et al.	2010	45	9	82	0
Aboulian et al.	2011	25	6	68	0
Tan et al.	2011	93	5.8	85	0
Abcarian et al.	2012	40	4.5	74	0
Mushaya et al.	2012	39	16	92	0
Ooi et al.	2012	25	5.5	68	0
Wallin et al.	2012	93	19	40	31
Han et al.	2013	21	14	95	5
van Onkelen et al.	2013	22	19.5	82	0
Lehmann et al.	2013	17	13.5	65	0
Sirikurnpiboon et al.	2013	41	4.8	83	0
Sileri et al.	2014	26	16	73	0

Table 15.2 Results of the anal fistula plug

	Year	No. of patients	Follow-up (months)	Success (%)	Extrusion (%)
Johnson et al.	2006	15	3.5	87	N.R.
Champagne et al.	2006	46	12	83	4
Schwandner et al.	2008	18	9	61	2
Christoforidis et al.	2008	47	5	38	14
Theckkinkattil et al.	2008	36	11	50	10
Starck et al.	2008	32	12	59	N.R.
Lawes et al.	2008	20	7.4	24	N.R.
Safar et al.	2009	35	4.2	13.9	9.7
Ortiz et al.	2009	15	12	20	15
Wang et al	2009	29	9	34	N.R.
McGee et al.	2010	41	24	44	5
Anyadike et al.	2010	33	14	73	N.R.
Van Koperen et al.	2011	31	11	29	13
Ommer et al.	2012	40	12	57.5	N.R.
O'Riordan et al.	2012	488	3–24.5	54	8.7

Table 15.3 Results of fistulotomy with sphincter reconstruction

	Year	No. of patients	Follow-up (months)	Success (%)	Incontinence (%)
Parkash et al.	1985	120	6–60	83.3	3.7
Christiansen and Ronholt	1995	14	12–48	85.7	21.4
Perez et al.	2006	35	32	92.9	12.5
Roig et al.	2010	75	13	89.4	18.3
Kraemer and Picke	2011	38	N.R.	97.4	9.4
Arroyo et al.	2012	70	81	91.4	16.6
Ratto et al.	2013	72	29.4	95.8	11.6

- Subsequent studies with longer follow-up have reported lower success rates of 32% to 54%.
- The high failure rate associated with fibrin glue injection has been attributed to the difficulty in ensuring the glue remains in the fistula tract, failure of closure of the internal opening, and lack of autologous tissue ingrowth to seal the tract.
- A Cochrane database systematic review analyzed ten randomized controlled trials.
  - There was no significant difference in recurrence rate or incontinence rate in any of the studied operation except in the case of advancement flap which carried higher success rate.
  - A higher recurrence rate was noted when fibrin glue injection was added to an endorectal advancement flap, favoring a flap-only technique.
  - Both fibrin glue injection and advancement flap had low incontinence.

Fistulotomy with Sphincter Reconstruction

- Patients with baseline incontinence, those at risk for incontinence (such as patients with previous childbirth, anterior fistula in females, existing sphincter defect from prior anal surgery), and patients with recurrent disease can be suitable candidates for this technique.
- Overall healing rates range from 83.3% to 97.4%, and the incontinence rates between 3.7% and 21.4% (Table 15.3).

Newer and Evolving Technologies: VAAFT, FiLaC™, and Stem Cell

- Using the VAAFT procedure:
  - Meinero and Mori achieved an overall success rate of 73.5% in 136 patients with non-Crohn's disease-related anal fistula, and recurrence rate was 26.5% within 2–3 months of follow-up.

- Kochhar and colleagues found the recurrence rate to be 15.8%.
- Due to the limited data on VAAFT, it is premature to draw any firm conclusion about its long-term efficacy, additional benefits, and limitations compared to the existing surgical options.

FiLaC™ procedure:

- The FiLaC™ procedure remains investigational at this stage, and additional data is needed prior to making firm recommendations for its use.
- Recommend the placement of a draining seton prior to the procedure to help create a more homogenous tract caliber and may contribute to the closure of secondary tracts.
- So far it appears not to impact continence level; however long-term success rate is unknown.
- Autologous adipose-derived stem cells:
  - Novel approach for the management of complex anal fistula, limited data.
  - A phase III multicenter, randomized, single-blind, add-on clinical trial was performed to investigate the safety and efficacy.
  - In treatment of complex anal fistula, a dose of 20 or 60 million adipose-derived stem cells alone or in combination with fibrin glue was considered a safe treatment, achieving healing rates of approximately 40% at 6 months and of more than 50% at 1-year follow-up.

Rectourethral Fistulas

Definition, Classification, and Pathophysiology

- Rectourethral fistula (RUF) is uncommon and can be congenital or acquired, resulting from surgery, radiation, inflammatory bowel disease, malignant neoplasm, pelvic infections, or trauma.
- In the Western world, the most common mechanism of RUF is a multimodality treatment for prostate cancer, including surgery, external beam radiation therapy (EBRT), or brachytherapy, with an incidence of 0.1–3% in patients who received these therapies.
- Fifty percent of patients with RUF have a history of irradiation, leading to microvascular injuries and mucosal ischemia.
- The mean time from the last radiotherapy session and the diagnosis of RUF ranged from 14 months to as long as 14 years.
- Rectal injury during radical prostatectomy is uncommon with a reported overall incidence ranging from 0.12% to 9% (0.47–2% of laparoscopic cases).

Clinical Assessment and Diagnostic Evaluation

- Symptoms of RUF include fecaluria, pneumaturia, hematuria, recturia, rectal bleeding, urinary tract infection, and severe rectal or pelvic pain.
- Physical examination (inspection, palpation, digital rectal examination) is performed to determine the size and location of the fistula in relationship to anal verge.
- Diagnostic modalities include cystoscopy (Fig. 15.13), colonoscopy or flexible sigmoidoscopy (Fig. 15.14), voiding cystography, retrograde urethrography, gastrografin enema (Fig. 15.15), computed tomography scan, and magnetic resonance imaging.
- If feasible, urodynamic evaluation can be performed for the preoperative assessment of urinary function as those with total urinary incontinence or severe voiding dysfunction may be treated with a permanent urinary diversion.

Surgical Treatment

- A multidisciplinary team approach involving a colorectal surgeon, a urologist, and in some

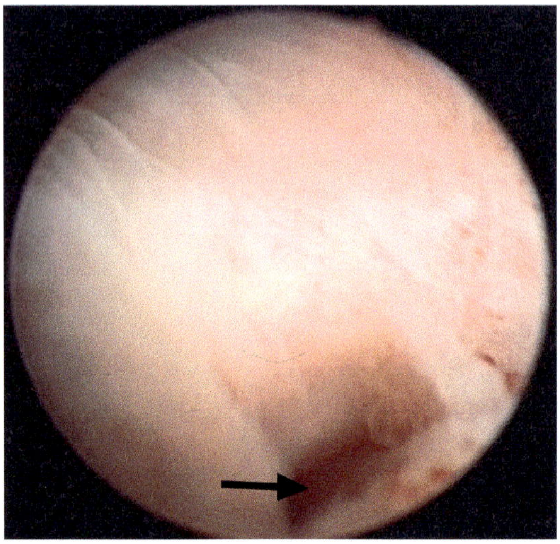

Fig. 15.13 Cystoscopic view of external beam radiation-induced rectourethral fistula

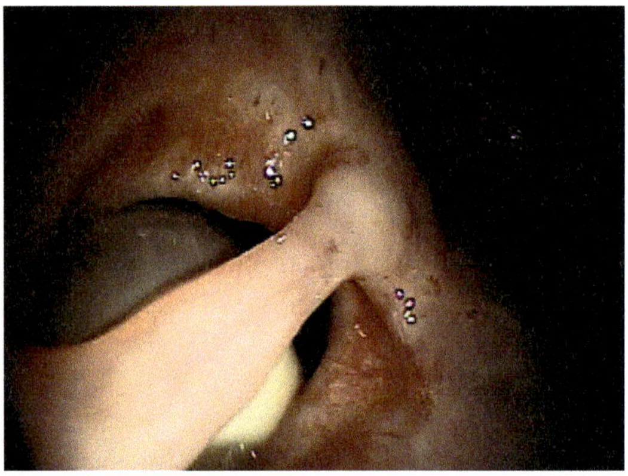

Fig. 15.14 Reflex view during flexible sigmoidoscopy demonstrates post-radical prostatectomy rectourethral fistula. Note the urethral catheter on the bladder side

instances a reconstructive surgeon is needed for optimal management.

- The management of RUF has not been standardized, and large variations in treatment approaches exist.
- Figure 15.16 provides the carepath algorithm.
- Small, minimally symptomatic, non-irradiated RUF can be managed initially with a urethral catheter and if needed suprapubic catheter drainage.
- Cases do sometimes heal spontaneously without fecal diversion (60%).

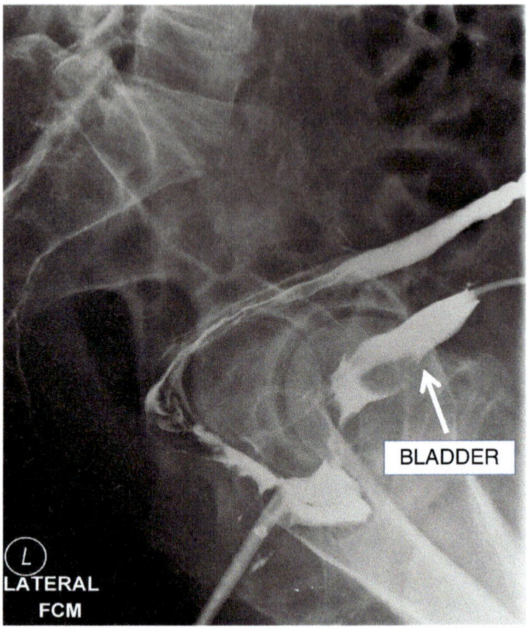

Fig. 15.15 Gastrografin enema reveals a rectourethral fistula secondary to laparoscopic radical prostatectomy. Note the contrast flow into the bladder [white arrow]

- If RUF remains unhealed for 2 or more months, surgical intervention is usually warranted.
- Local transanal flap repair is a good option for small non-irradiated RUF.
- If RUF remains unhealed following local flap repair, a diverting stoma followed by additional local flap repair or transperineal repair with gracilis interposition flap or dartos flap would be the next step.
- Patients with large RUF (> 1 cm), prior radiation or cryotherapy, significant symptoms, severe urethral stricture, or prior failed repair require fecal diversion with suprapubic catheter drainage.
- After 3 months of fecal diversion, the RUF should be reassessed.
  - If healed, the patient can then undergo stoma closure.
  - It is important to reassess the patient with a minimum of two diagnostic studies [endoscopic or imaging] from the bladder and rectal side to confirm complete healing prior to closing the stoma.

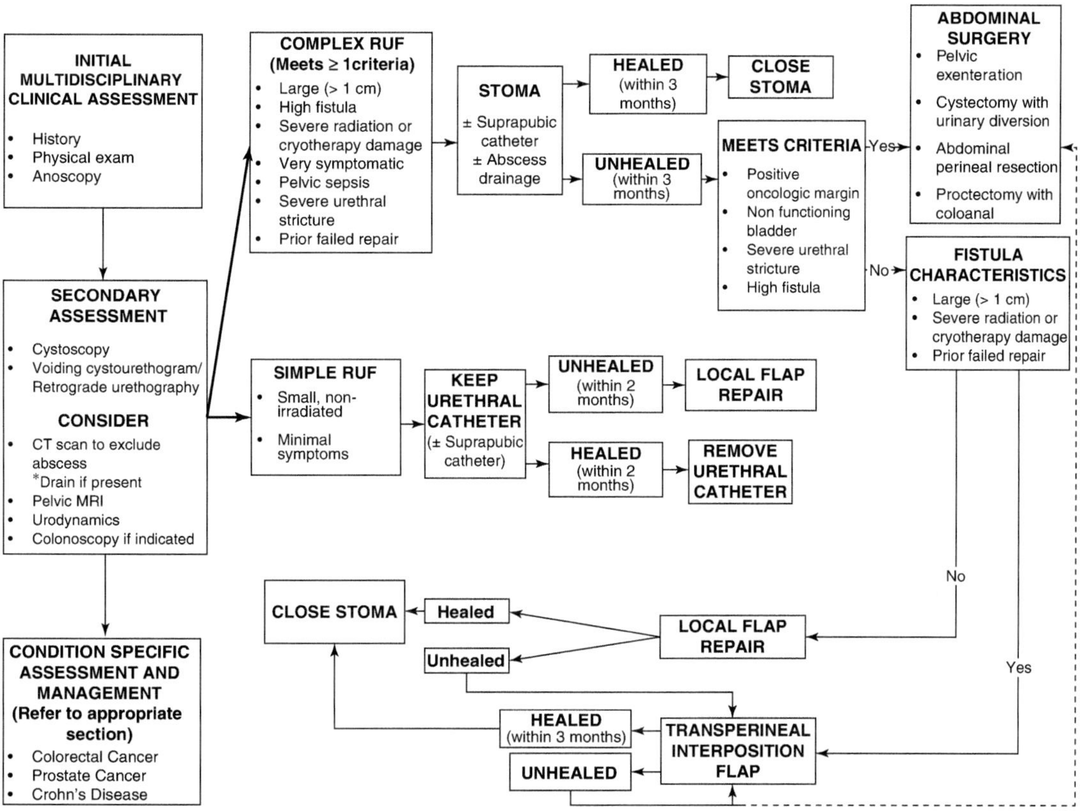

Fig. 15.16 An algorithm-based approach to the management of rectourethral fistula

- Patients who desire definitive repair can be approached via a transabdominal [proctectomy with coloanal with or without omental flap, pelvic exenteration with or without sphincter preservation], transanal, transperineal [gracilis flap interposition or dartos flap], transsphincteric, or trans-sacral technique.
- Urethral reconstruction can be achieved with a buccal mucosal flap or biologic mesh.

Transanal Approach

- For a non-irradiated small RUF, a transanal approach with rectal advancement flap is a good option in patients without anal stricture.
- The addition of biologic material can be helpful in a patient with larger defect and good vascularized tissue which can facilitate tissue ingrowth.
- A urethral catheter is kept for 4–6 weeks postoperatively before assessing fistula healing.

Posterior Approach

- High RUF can be approached via a posterior approach either through a York-Mason transsphincteric dissection or a Kraske approach.
  - York-Mason technique involves posterior sagittal division of the anal sphincter and levator muscles as well as the posterior wall of the rectum to gain access to the fistula.
  - Kraske approach entails resection of the coccyx and division of the tissues between the coccyx and the sphincters to provide access to the posterior wall of the rectum, which is then opened to provide access to the fistula.
- The use of a transsphincteric approach has decreased significantly over the past years, because of the risk of fecal incontinence.

Transperineal Approach

- The transperineal approach is the preferred method for most mid to low RUFs that require

Table 15.4 Outcome of patients with rectourethral fistula in various series

	Year	No. of patients	Procedure	Follow-up	Closure (%)
Youssef et al	1999	12	Dartos flap	9–42 months	69
Garofalo et al	2003	14	Rectal flap	31 months	68
Lane et al.	2006	22	Transabdominal (68%)	29 months	88
Wexner et al.	2008	36	Gracilis flap	N.R.	78
Ghoneim et al.	2008	25	Gracilis flap	28 months	100
Gupta et al.	2008	10	Gracilis flap	24 months	100
Ulrich et al.	2009	26	Gracilis flap	22 months	100
Kasraeian et al.	2009	12	Transsphincteric	22 months	75
Vanni et al.	2010	74	Gracilis flap + tissue rectal flap	20 months	92
Samplaski et al.	2011	13	Gracilis flap	2.5 months	92
Hechenbleikner et al.	2013	416	Gracilis flap (72%)	N.R.	87.5
Keller et al.[a]	2015	30	Transperineal (54%) Transanal (31%) Transabdominal (15%)	72 months	90

[a]43% required definitive fistula repair

interposition of healthy and well-vascularized tissue.

- Tissue interposition can be provided with a dartos flap or gracilis muscle.

Transabdominal Approach

- Patients with postoperative RUF following prostate or rectal surgery and positive oncologic margins can be offered a transabdominal approach.
- Additional indications include:
  - High RUF not accessible to a transanal or transperineal approach
  - Patients with nonfunctioning irradiated bladder or severely stricture urethra which requires excision with urinary diversion
  - Patients with prior failed repairs
- The type of abdominal operation include:
  - Cystectomy with urinary diversion
  - Proctectomy with coloanal anastomosis
  - Abdominoperineal resection
  - Pelvic exenteration
- An omental flap or rectus abdominis flap interposition can be used if needed.

Outcome

- The outcome of RUF treatment is difficult to evaluate because published studies with large number of patients are scarce.
- Significant heterogeneity exists in the various reports due to differences in patient populations and operative techniques.
- Table 15.4 summarizes the results of several large series.
- The reported success rate following definitive operative intervention ranges from 68% to 100%. A spontaneous closure rate of 14%–46.5% has been reported after fecal diversion, and some patients can heal small RUF with urethral catheter drainage alone.
- The overall permanent urinary diversion rate was 8.3% and was significantly higher in irradiated patients (42.5%) compared to non-irradiated patients (4%).
- The transanal approach with rectal advancement flap is safe and effective in the absence of prior radiation therapy with reported 85% closure rate.
- The gracilis muscle interposition is currently the most commonly used method for treating complex, large, recurrent, and/or irradiated RUF.

Postoperative Fistulas

Definition, Classification, and Pathophysiology

- Ileal-pouch fistula can be classified as pouch-anal, pouch-vaginal, and pouch-perineal.

  - Fistula is defined as complex if there are multiple tracts and/or the internal opening is at or above the IPAA (high fistula).
- Perianal fistula may occur as a postoperative complication after ultralow anterior resection, coloanal anastomosis, Hartmann reversal procedure, abdominoperineal resection, or transanal endoscopic microsurgery for distal rectal cancer.
- Major risk factors associated with development of postoperative fistulas include elderly age, diabetes, vasculopathy, smoking, preoperative/postoperative radiotherapy, operative technique, and postoperative pelvic sepsis.

Clinical Assessment and Diagnostic Evaluation

- Fistulas often present with pelvic and perianal sepsis or drainage and pain.
- Patients with an inadequate clinical assessment should undergo examination under anesthesia.
- Preoperative imaging to evaluate the anatomy of the fistula tract includes endoanal ultrasound, pelvic MR imaging, CT scan, pouchography, and fistulography.

Surgical Treatment

- The guiding principles are to control pelvic and perianal sepsis and eliminate the fistulous tract.
- An acute abscess should be drained, and when necessary, a non-cutting seton may be placed to control anorectal infection.
- Operative techniques include gracilis muscle interposition, lay-open fistulotomy, collagen plug insertion, ileal advancement flap, transvaginal advancement flap, fibrin glue, transperineal repair, Martius (i.e., bulbocavernosus) flap, pouch excision, or redo pouch.
- Simple procedures should be attempted first, if there is a chance of success, before more complex procedures are considered.
- Temporary diverting ileostomy, permanent end ileostomy with/without pouch excision, and redo-RPC should be considered in patients with ileal-pouch fistulas.
- Temporary diverting colostomy with/without coloanal/colorectal anastomoses or permanent end colostomy with/without anastomoses removal or completion proctectomy should be considered in rectal cancer patients.
- Complex perineal fistula occurring after APR or pelvic exenteration can be treated by the use of an omentoplasty or rectus abdominis musculocutaneous flap to fill the dead space of the pelvis with well-vascularized tissue.
- Medical treatment including anti-TNF agents should be the first-line therapy for patients who present delayed onset of pouch fistula and a suspicion for Crohn's fistula.

Outcome

- Mallick and colleagues reviewed the Cleveland Clinic Experience with pouch-vaginal fistulas.
  - Fistula occurred in 102 females: 59 at ≤12 months (early fistula) and 43 at >12 months (late-onset fistula).
  - Local repair was performed in 77.3% of patients (ileal pouch advancement flap in 49.5% of cases and transvaginal repair in 27.8% of cases).
    - The healing rate after ileal pouch advancement flap was 42% when performed as a primary procedure and 66% when performed secondarily after a different procedure.
    - The healing rate for transvaginal repair was 55% when done as a primary procedure and 40% when performed secondarily.
  - Nineteen patients underwent redo ileal pouch construction, with an overall pouch retention rate of 40%.
  - At median follow-up of 83 months, 57.7% of the 102 patients had healed the pouch-vaginal fistula; pouch failure occurred in 34 women (35%, 12 early onset and 22 late onset).

Rectovaginal Fistula

16

Jamie A. Cannon

Key Concepts

- Rectovaginal fistulas (RVFs) are abnormal communications between the anus or rectum and the vagina.
- Repair of rectovaginal fistulas should be tailored to the individual patient based on the anatomy of the fistula and associated conditions.
- Perianal sepsis must be controlled prior to attempting a definitive repair.
- Patients with RVFs from obstetric trauma should be evaluated for concomitant sphincter defects.
- Patients who have a Crohn's-related RVF should have their disease medically optimized prior to repair of the fistula.
- Introduction of healthy, well-vascularized tissue such as a Martius flap or gracilis interposition should be considered in patients who have attenuated tissues or have undergone multiple previous unsuccessful repairs.
- Patients may present with stool per vagina resulting in frank incontinence or gas or drainage per vagina.
- Anatomically, there is little muscle in the thin rectovaginal septum, which may make it more difficult for this region to heal.
- Fistulotomy, the most successful surgery for managing perianal fistulas, is contraindicated as it invariably results in some degree of incontinence.
- There is not an ideal operation with a uniformly high success rate.
- Preoperative fecal diversion has not been shown consistently to lead to better outcomes, but this may represent selection bias in those patients chosen for diversion.

J. A. Cannon (✉)
Division of Gastrointestinal Surgery, Department of Surgery, University of Alabama at Birmingham, Birmingham, AL, USA
e-mail: jacannon@uab.edu

S. R. Steele et al. (eds.), *The ASCRS Manual of Colon and Rectal Surgery*,
https://doi.org/10.1007/978-3-030-01165-9_16

Etiology of Rectovaginal Fistulas

- Rectovaginal fistulas can be the result of obstetric injuries, cryptoglandular disease, or Crohn's disease, malignancy, radiation therapy, or leaks from a colorectal, coloanal, or ileal pouch-anal anastomosis.

Obstetric Injury

- Obstetric injury is the most common cause of RVFs.
- Rectovaginal fistulas are reported to occur following 0.1–0.5% of all vaginal deliveries.
- Obstetric fistulas can arise from a fourth-degree tear in which the repair has broken down.
  - This type of fistula will generally become clinically apparent 1–2 weeks after delivery and is most often located at the level of the anal sphincters.
- Prolonged labor resulting in compression of the rectovaginal septum by the infant's head can lead to necrosis of the RV septum and cause a rectovaginal fistula that presents in a more delayed fashion.
- Traumatic injury from an instrumented delivery may result in an immediately apparent fistula.
- Repairs of RVFs caused by obstetric injury tend to be more successful than repairs of fistulas from other causes.
- Halverson et al. reported on 15 patients with obstetric-related RVFs; all fistulas were eventually able to be repaired for an overall success rate of 100% but required a total of 23 procedures for a per-procedure success rate of 65%.

Cryptoglandular Disease

- This occurs when an anteriorly located anal gland or its associated duct becomes occluded; the resulting abscess may form in the rectovaginal septum and decompress into the vagina.
- Generally located at the level of the dentate line on the rectal side and course through the anal sphincters to the low vagina or introitus.

Crohn's Disease

- They are the result of transmural inflammation from the anorectum; they are frequently associated with perianal sepsis, branching fistula tracts, additional rectocutaneous fistulas, and scarring and stricturing of the anorectum.
- Approximately 10% of women with Crohn's disease will develop a rectovaginal fistula, and they are more common in those who suffer from colonic Crohn's disease.
- Surgical repair of rectovaginal fistulas caused by Crohn's disease is not as successful as repair of fistulas of obstetric or cryptoglandular origin.
- Prior to attempting any repair, control of perianal sepsis is required by abscess drainage and seton placement.
- A discrete, epithelialized tract should be present before attempting repair, which is best achieved with initial seton placement.
- Multiple fistula tracts, a watering can perineum, or active inflammation of the rectal mucosa are contraindications to repair, Fig. 16.1.
- Repair should not be undertaken in the presence of active inflammation of the rectum as the repair is unlikely to heal.
  - Should be managed either medically, with a seton, or with a proctectomy
- The use of infliximab has been shown to lead to spontaneous healing of fistulas in Crohn's disease.
  - Kraemer et al. reported healing of symptomatic fistulas in 8 of 19 patients with Crohn's-associated anorectal fistulas treated with infliximab prior to surgery.
  - If the fistula does not close spontaneously, reducing the amount of associated inflammation will likely improve the chance of success with surgical repair.
  - ACCENT II trial studied infliximab in patients with fistulizing Crohn's disease;

29 patients in this trial had rectovaginal fistulas and at week 14 of treatment, 13 of those patients (44.8%) were found to have healed fistulas, Table 16.1.

- Successful surgical treatment of Crohn's-related RVF varies in the literature, with success rates ranging from 30% to 70%.
- Patients most likely to have a successful repair are those with an isolated RVF without other perianal disease and in whom their Crohn's disease is quiescent.
- Luffler et al.
  - Forty-five patients with Crohn's-related RVFs.
  - Underwent a total of 95 interventions, averaging 2.1 interventions per patient.

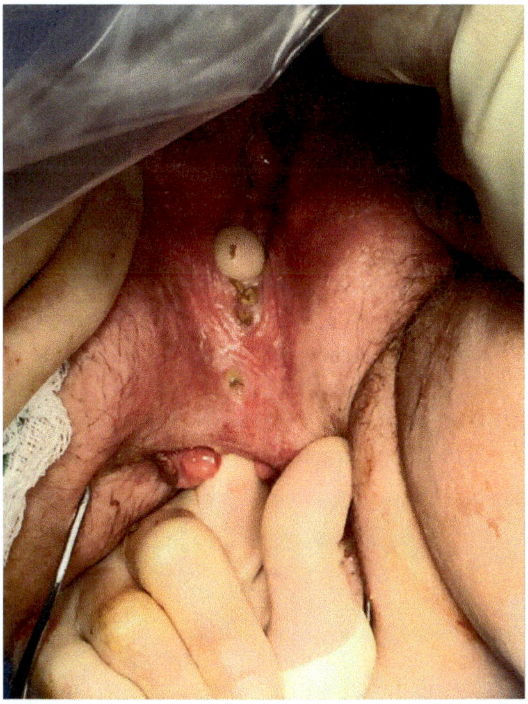

Fig. 16.1 Large Crohn's-related rectovaginal fistula with multiple external openings in the perineum

  - Their long-term success rate was 53%.
  - Ten patients (22.2%) required proctectomy.
  - Levatorplasty and endorectal advancement flaps – similar rates of success at approximately 50%.
- Hull and Fazio reported:
  - Forty-eight Crohn's patients with RVF.
  - Nine required proctectomy and five were treated with a seton only.
  - Of the 35 who underwent attempted definitive repair, 19 were successful (54%).
    - Five of the failures underwent subsequent successful procedures for an overall success rate of 24/35 (69%).
  - Success was more likely among the patients who had fecal stream diversion, with 8/9 diverted patients having successful repairs.
- El-Gazzaz et al.
  - Sixty-five women with Crohn's disease who underwent RVF repair
  - Thirty successes (46.2%)
  - Noted that many of the failures were late failures and thus recommended long-term follow-up

Evaluation of a Patient with a Rectovaginal Fistula

- The etiology of the fistula can often be determined from the patient's history.
- On digital rectal examination, the condition of the perineal body and rectovaginal septum should be noted.
- Care should be taken to assess the quality and strength of the anal sphincters.
- Careful palpation of the entire rectovaginal septum between the fingers of each hand may reveal the presence of a small fistula.

Table 16.1 Medical therapy for Crohn's-related RVFs

Author	Year of publication	Drug utilized	No. of patients	No. of successful closures (%)
Present	1980	6-MP	6	2 (33.3)
Ricart	2001	Infliximab	15	5 (33.3)
Bodegraven	2002	Infliximab	4	0 (0)
Sands	2004	Infliximab	29	13 (44.8)
Parsi	2004	Infliximab	14	2 (14.2)

- Note should also be made of any strictures or scarring of the anal canal.
- The location of the fistula relative to the sphincter muscles and pelvic floor should be determined as this can affect the type of repair chosen.
- Differential:
  - Colovaginal fistula, rather than a rectovaginal fistula, from diverticulitis is a more common condition.
  - Very small or high RVFs may not be palpable on exam.
- Imaging options include gastrograffin enema and vaginography.
  - Low yield, however, and are rarely successful in imaging distal fistulas.
  - They rely on occlusion of the anal canal or vaginal introitus in order to generate enough pressure to show passage of contrast through the fistula, and balloon placement may occlude the fistulous opening itself.
  - Figure 16.2 shows a RVF on gastrograffin enema.

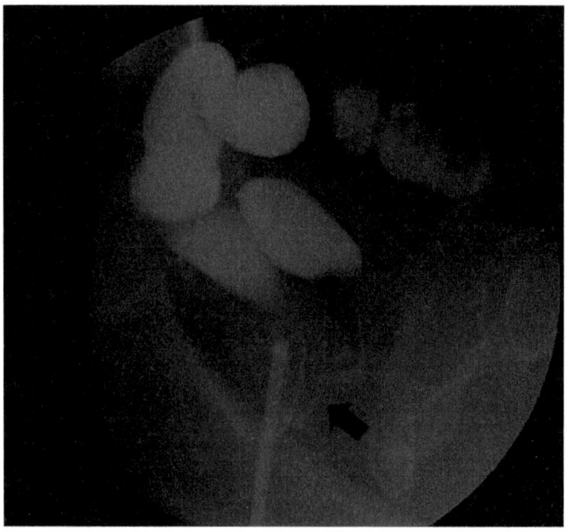

Fig. 16.2 Gastrograffin enema showing contrast passing through a rectovaginal fistula. © 2015 Kobayashi and Sugihara; licensee Springer. This is an Open Access article distributed under the terms of the Creative Commons Attribution License (http://creativecommons.org/licenses/by/4.0), which permits unrestricted use, distribution, and reproduction in any medium, provided the original work is properly credited

- Endoanal ultrasound and MRI are the most useful imaging studies to identify a fistula.
  - Figure 16.3 shows the appearance of a RVF on MRI.
  - Endoanal ultrasound has been reported to identify the tract in 73% of patients.
    - Injection of hydrogen peroxide through the tract may aid in identification.
    - Ultrasound is also useful in that it enables assessment of the anal sphincters; following obstetric trauma, it can evaluate sphincter damage.
- Patients with Crohn's disease should undergo a complete evaluation of their Crohn's disease, to include colonoscopy and CT or MR enterography.
  - While the fistula itself is rarely seen on colonoscopy, colonoscopy allows for identification of active disease and other Crohn's-related complications. Figure 16.4 demonstrates the appearance of an internal opening on colonoscopy.
- The best option for identifying an occult RVF is an examination under anesthesia.
  - This allows for probing of the rectovaginal septum with a fistula probe to elucidate the location (Fig. 16.5).
  - It also allows for inspection of the anal canal and rectal and vaginal mucosa to identify areas of inflammation or dimpling for more targeted inspection.

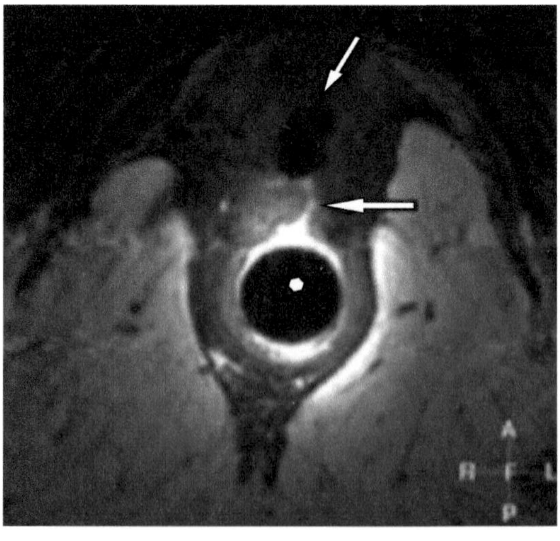

Fig. 16.3 Rectovaginal fistula as seen on MRI

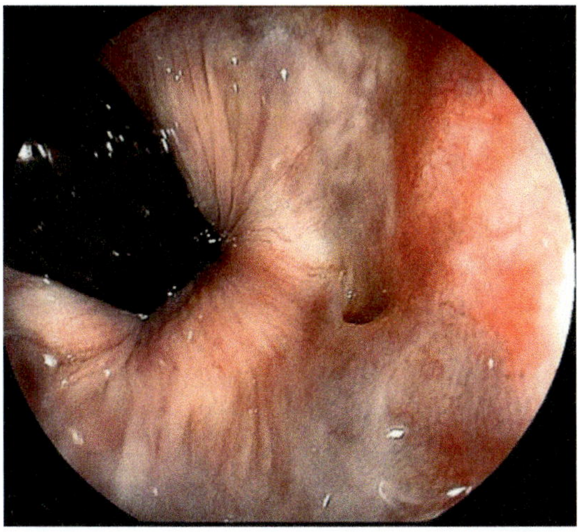

Fig. 16.4 Rectovaginal fistula on retroflexed view on colonoscopy.

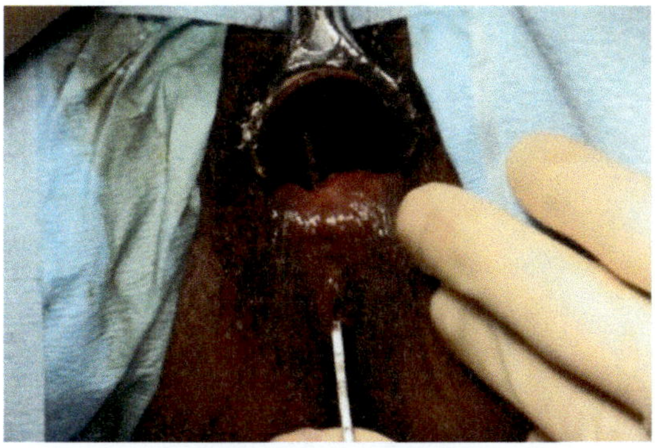

Fig. 16.5 Fistula probe passing through a rectovaginal fistula

- The vagina can be filled with saline, while the rectum is insufflated with air (Fig. 16.6).
- Alternatively, a tampon or operative sponge may be placed in the vagina, and saline with methylene blue dye can be introduced into the rectum, and blue staining on the gauze within the vagina confirms that a fistula is present.

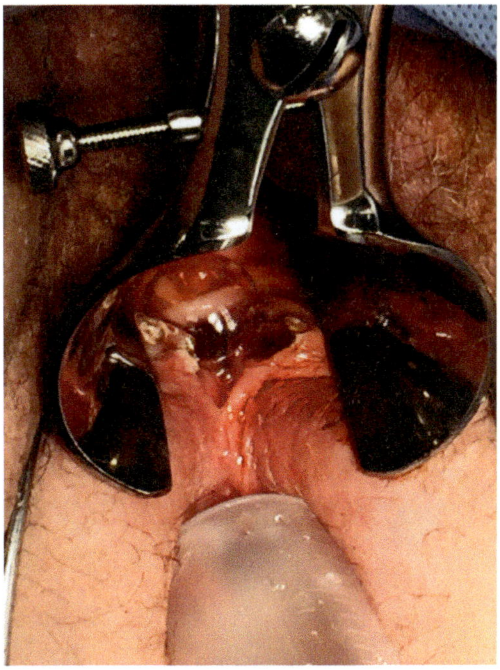

Fig. 16.6 With the patient in Trendelenburg position, saline is placed in the vagina. An Asepto syringe is used to inject air in the rectum. Bubbling in the vagina reveals the location of the rectovaginal fistula

Surgical Approaches to Repair of Rectovaginal Fistulas

- For many patients, more than one attempt at repair is necessary.
- For simple rectovaginal fistulas (located in the mid or lower vagina and without Crohn's disease), 74% healing.
- For recurrent fistulas of various etiologies, healing 79–87%.
- For patients with Crohn's, healing is only 44.2% per procedure, but 78% of patients were eventually healed.
  - Tobacco use was identified as a risk factor for recurrence.

Endorectal Repairs

- Endorectal advancement flaps are the most commonly performed procedure for the management of a rectovaginal fistula.

- The procedure as described by Rothenberger et al., in 1982, Fig. 16.7:
    1. The patient is placed in the jackknife prone position.
    2. A Pratt bivalve anoscope is used to expose the anterior rectal wall.
    3. Distal to the location of the fistula, an incision is made through the mucosa, submucosa, and down to the internal sphincter.
    4. A flap including mucosa, submucosa, and fibers of the circular muscle (internal sphincter) is raised in the rectum proximally.
    5. The flap is raised for a distance 4 cm proximal to the location of the fistula in order to allow for a tension-free anastomosis.
    6. Once the flap has been raised, the fistula itself is closed by approximating the fibers of the internal sphincter.
    7. The distal most portion of the flap that contains the fistula is excised.
    8. The healthy flap is brought down to cover the fistula opening and secured in place.

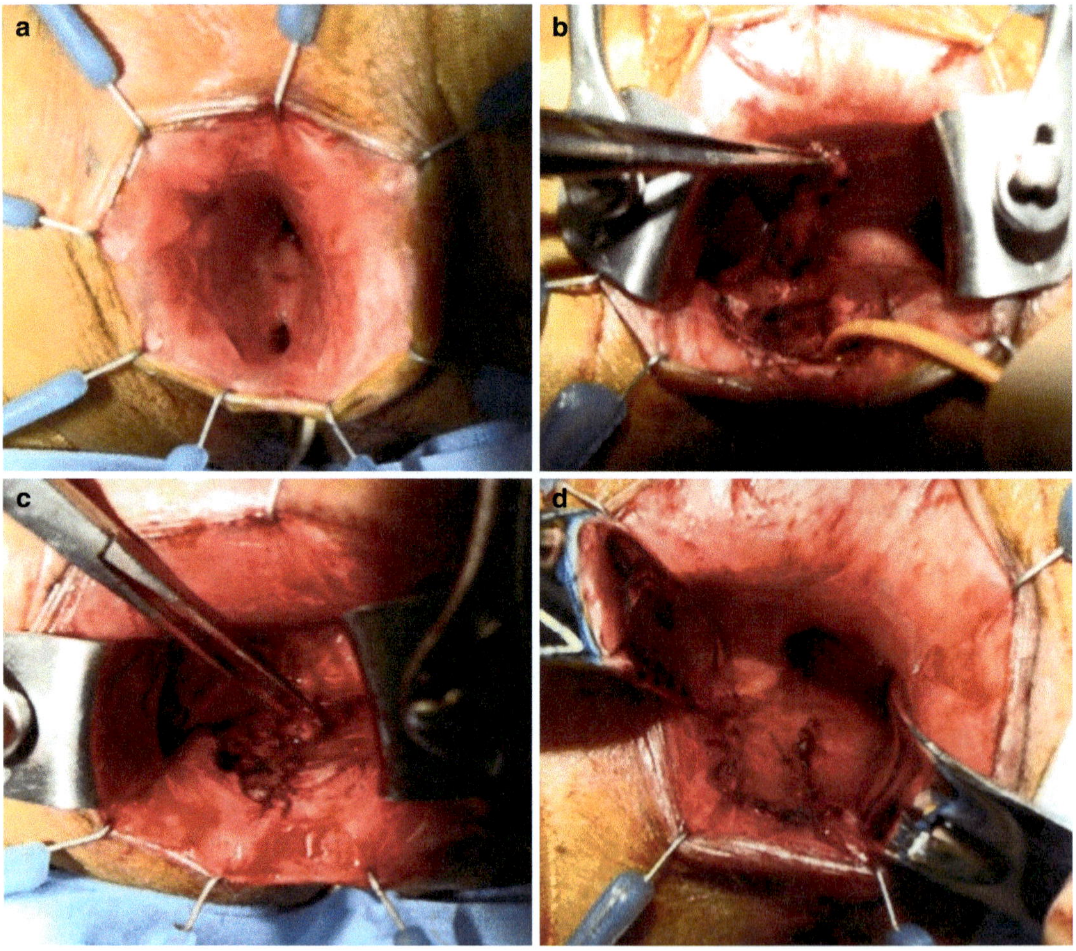

Fig. 16.7 Endorectal advancement flap for rectovaginal fistula. Rectovaginal fistula is seen from the anus (**a**). The flap of mucosa, submucosa, and circular muscle is raised (**b**). Circular muscle is sutured by horizontal mattress manner (**c**). The flap is advanced over the repaired area (**d**). The flap is sutured in place at its apex and along its sides.

Table 16.2 Endorectal advancement flaps

Author	Year of publication	No. of patients	No. of successful closures (%)
Rothenberger	1982	35	30(86)
Jones	1987	23	16 (70)
Lowry	1988	44	56 (78)
Watson	1995	12	7 (58)
Sonoda	2002	37	16 (43)
Ellis	2008	44	29 (66)
Hull	2011	37	23(62)

- The most common cause for failure is thought to be flap retraction or necrosis.
  - The base of the flap should be at least twice the width of the apex of the flap in order to ensure adequate blood supply.
- Rothenberger and Lowry reported overall good success of 86–88%.
- Ellis reported a 66% success rate in 44 patients.
- Sonoda et al. reported success in 16/37 (43.2%).
- Hull and colleagues in 23/37 (62%).
- Available data on endorectal advancement flaps is summarized in Table 16.2.
- Of note, the likelihood of a successful repair with an endorectal advancement flap decreases if patients have undergone previous repairs (30–55%).

Transperineal Repairs

- A number of variations in technique exist including episioproctotomy with layered closure, transperineal repair with levatorplasty, the LIFT procedure, and sphincteroplasty.
- These procedures all begin with an incision in the perineum that may be circumlinear around the anus, transverse, or vertical.
- Dissection continues cephalad along the rectovaginal septum.
- The rectum and vagina are separated from one another and the fistula tract divided, as seen in Fig. 16.8.
- The incision is closed in layers. Ideally, some tissue, preferentially muscle, is interposed between the rectum and vagina.

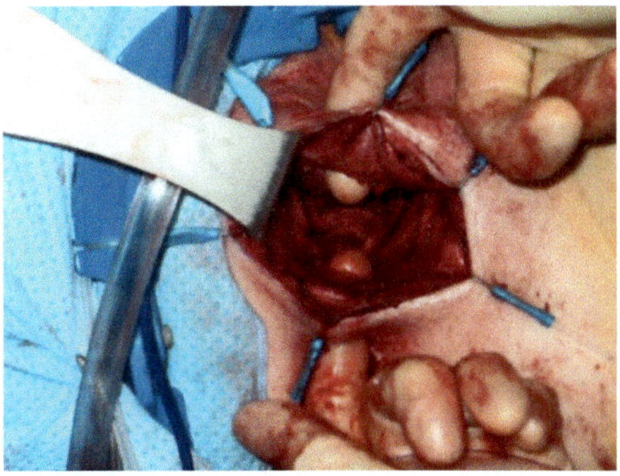

Fig. 16.8 Transperineal repair where the rectum and vagina have been separated and the defects in each are visible

- This may be done via levatorplasty or sphincteroplasty.
- The repaired areas of rectum and vagina can also be imbricated.
- A rectal advancement flap can be added to the procedure.
- Athanasiadis and colleagues reported good success with this technique in a Crohn's population with 14/20 (70%) undergoing successful repairs.
- Lowry had success in 22 of 25 patients who underwent a combined sphincteroplasty and endorectal advancement flap (88%), which was an improvement over the 78% success with advancement flap alone.
- Hull and associates reported success in 39/50 patients who underwent a transperineal repair (78%).
- The available data for transperineal repairs is summarized in Table 16.3.
- A transperineal repair with sphincteroplasty is the most appropriate type of repair in women

Table 16.3 Transperineal repairs

Author	Year of publication	No. of patients	No. of successful closures (%)
Athanasiadis	2007	20	14 (70)
Hull	2011	50	39(78)
Wiskind	1992	21	21(100)

who have a sphincter defect (most often from obstetrical injury), as this is addressed simultaneously.

Tissue Transposition Repairs

- Tissue transposition repairs offer the advantage of interposing healthy, well-perfused tissue between the rectum and vagina.
  - Add bulk and physically increase the distance between the rectum
  - Bring their own blood supply may aid in healing
  - Highest success rate of all transperineal repairs
- Fecal diversion is generally performed prior to or at the time of surgery.
- The labial fat pads with bulbocavernosus muscle (Martius flap) or gracilis muscle transposition are the most commonly used tissues.
- Use of other muscles including the sartorius and gluteal muscle has also been described.

Martius Flap

The Martius flap uses the bulbocavernosus muscle and labial fat pad for transposition.

1. The initial incision is made in the vaginal introitus distal to the fistula opening in order to expose the rectovaginal septum.
2. Dissection continues in the rectovaginal septum cephalad to the fistula (Fig. 16.9).
3. The fistula tract is curetted and closed primarily on the rectal side.
4. The vaginal portion of the fistula is excised from the vaginal flap.
5. In order to harvest the donor tissue, a vertical incision is made in the labia majora (Fig. 16.10).
6. The labial fat pad and underlying bulbocavernosus muscle are dissected out from the surrounding tissues.

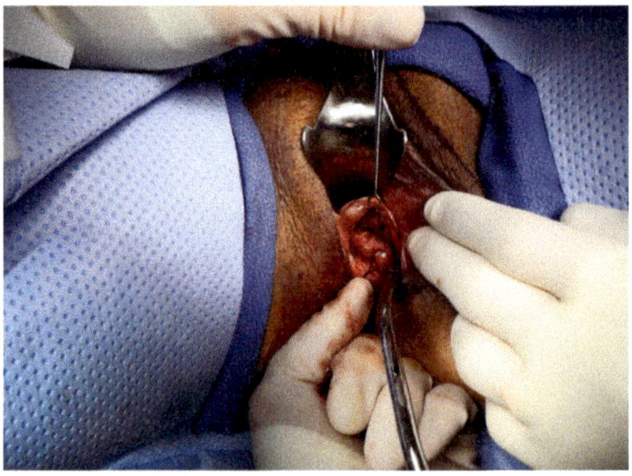

Fig. 16.9 Martius flap repair. The vaginal flap has been raised revealing the rectovaginal fistula. (Courtesy of Drs. Eric Johnson and Scott Steele)

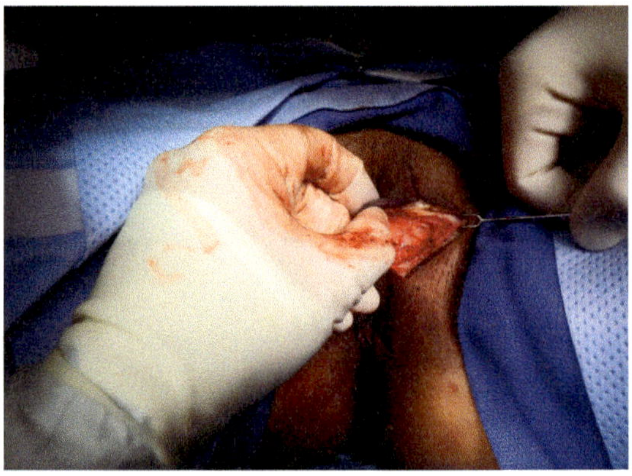

Fig. 16.10 Martius flap repair. Incision over the left labia majora to expose the fat pad and bulbocavernosus. (Courtesy of Drs. Eric Johnson and Scott Steele)

7. The blood supply to the flap comes in inferiorly and posteriorly from the posterior labial vessels.
8. The flap is transected superiorly and tunneled to the rectovaginal septum. It should be rotated carefully so as not to kink the blood supply (Figs. 16.11 and 16.12).
9. The flap is laid within the RV septum and the vaginal flap sutured over the Martius flap (Fig. 16.13).

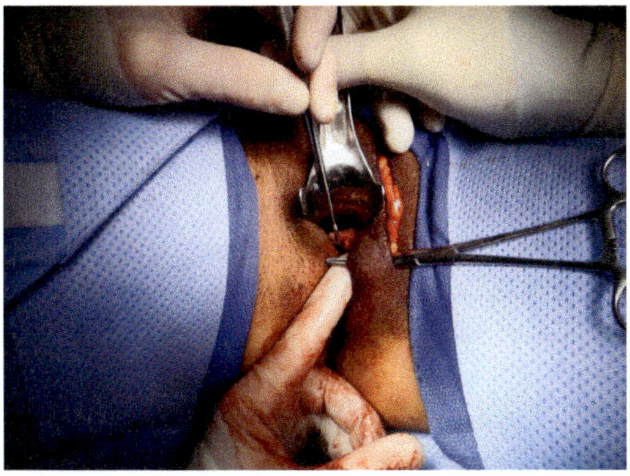

Fig. 16.11 Martius flap. A tunnel is created from the origin of the bulbocavernosus to the vaginal incision. (Courtesy of Drs. Eric Johnson and Scott Steele)

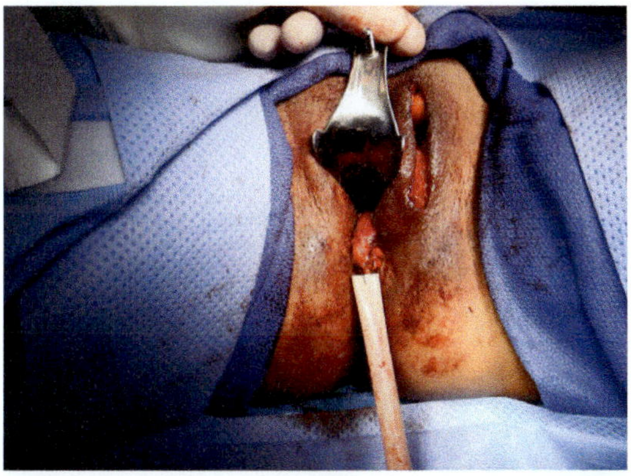

Fig. 16.12 Martius flap. The donor tissue has been brought into the rectovaginal septum. (Courtesy of Drs. Eric Johnson and Scott Steele)

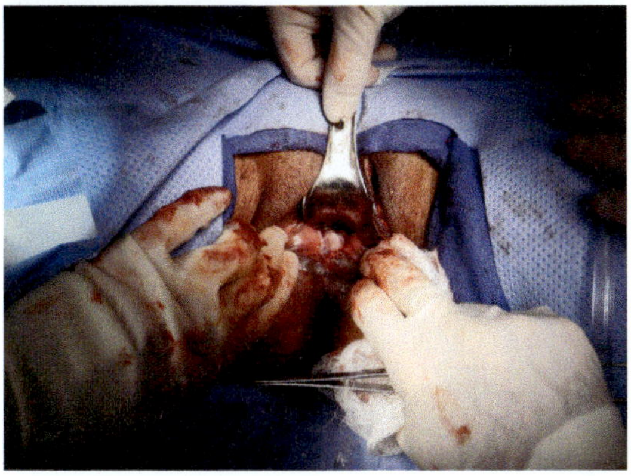

Fig. 16.13 Martius flap. The vaginal incision has been closed over the Martius flap. (Courtesy of Drs. Eric Johnson and Scott Steele)

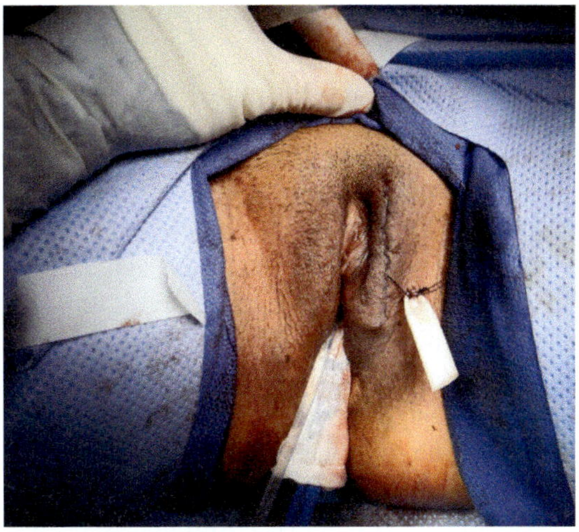

Fig. 16.14 Appearance after the Martius flap. (Courtesy of Drs. Eric Johnson and Scott Steele)

Table 16.4 Martius flap

Author	Year of publication	No. of patients	No. of successful closures (%)
White	1982	14	13(93)
Aartsen	1988	14	13(93)
McNevin	2007	16	15(94)
Sogne	2007	14	13(93)
Pitel	2011	23	15(65)
Kniery	2015	5	3 (60)

10. Figure 16.14 shows the postoperative appearance.
    - The largest case series using the Martius flap was published by Pitel et al., in 2011.
      - They reported a 65% success rate in 23 patients.
    - The available data is summarized in Table 16.4.

Gracilis Muscle Transposition

- Advantage of providing a large bulk of well-vascularized muscle to separate the vagina and rectum.
- Higher morbidity due to the mobilization and transposition of this large muscle.
- Fecal diversion is generally performed prior to or at the time of the procedure.

The operation involves:

1. Transperineal incision (Fig. 16.15), in which the rectum and vagina are separated. The fistula is divided and both the rectum and vagina are closed primarily.
2. Dissection should continue cephalad to the fistula until healthy tissue is reached.
3. An endorectal advancement flap can be added to the procedure as well.
4. The gracilis muscle is then harvested with either a long incision of the length of the gracilis or with separate smaller incisions near the muscle's origin and insertion.
5. The muscle is mobilized with division of the perforating vessels.
6. It is divided just above its insertion.
7. It is tunneled from the proximal most portion of the incision to the perineal incision, as seen in Fig. 16.16.
8. The muscle is secured to the apex of the rectovaginal dissection and the transperineal incision closed, as seen in Fig. 16.17.
   - Reported success rates range from 47%[(36)] to 92%; Table 16.5 summarizes the available data.

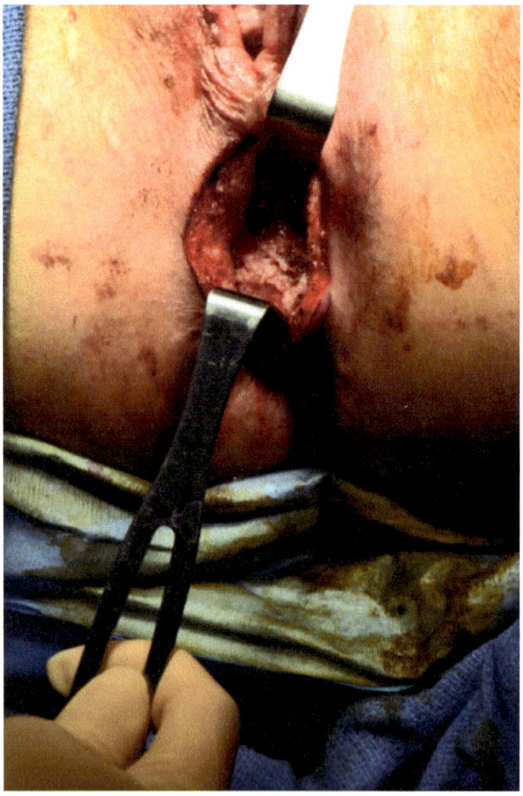

Fig. 16.15 Gracilis transposition. A transperineal incision is made to separate the rectum and the vagina. (Courtesy of Drs. Jamie Cannon, Andre Levesque, and James Long)

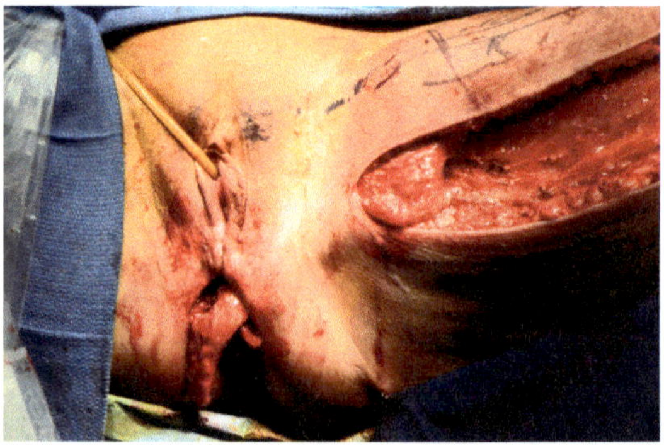

Fig. 16.16 Gracilis transposition. The gracilis muscle has been tunneled from the left thigh to the transperineal incision. (Courtesy of Drs. Jamie Cannon, Andre Levesque, and James Long)

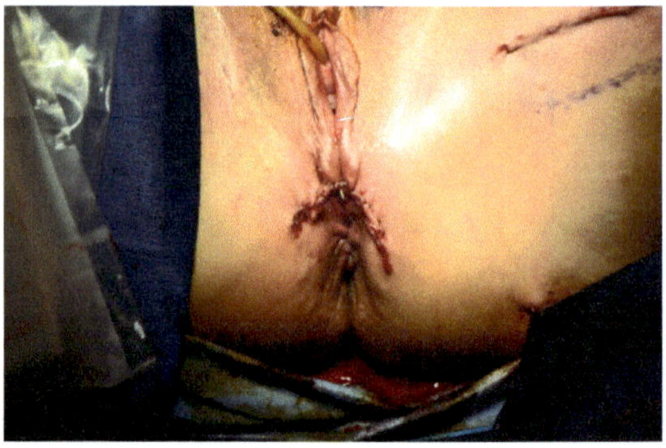

Fig. 16.17 Gracilis transposition. Postoperative appearance. (Courtesy of Drs. Jamie Cannon, Andre Levesque, and James Long)

Table 16.5 Gracilis muscle transposition

Author	Year of publication	No. of patients	No. of successful closures (%)
Furst	2008	12	11 (92)
Wexner	2008	17	9 (53)
Lefevre	2009	8	6 (75)
Pinto	2010	24	19 (79)

Transvaginal Repairs

- Transvaginal repairs are usually found more often in the gynecologic literature.
- Relative ease and better exposure gained through the vagina as compared to the anus.
- The rectum is the higher-pressure side of the fistula, so transvaginal repairs should involve closure of the rectum and not just of the vagina.
- Sher et al. report on the use of a transvaginal flap for Crohn's-related RVF.
  - All patients had fecal diversion.
  - 13/14 patients healed (93%).

Transabdominal Repair

- Generally reserved for fistulas that are located in the mid rectum with an internal opening at the fornix of the vagina.
- Involves a low anterior resection, where the segment of the rectum containing the fistula is resected and a colorectal or coloanal anastomosis performed.
- The vaginal side of the defect can be closed primarily.
- Van der Hagen and colleagues reported laparoscopically separating the rectum and vagina and repairing each primarily.
  - Omentum was mobilized and laid in-between the rectum and the vagina.
  - Reported successful repair in 38/40 patients.

Alternate Repairs

- Fistula plug has been described but should be limited to those with a long-tract RVF.
  - The plug is brought from the rectal to vaginal side, excess length on the plug is trimmed, and it is sutured in place with absorbable suture.
  - 44–86% success.
- Injection of fat into the tissue surrounding the fistula.
- Transanal endoscopic microsurgical (TEMS) approach.

Choice of Technique for Repair

- In deciding on a surgical approach, the surgeon should evaluate the patient for continuing inflammation or ongoing pelvic sepsis.
  - These must be controlled prior to surgical repair, or the chance of success is dismal.
    - Abscess drainage, antibiotics, and seton placement until resolved
  - Treatment with anti-TNF agents should be considered preoperatively in all patients with Crohn's disease.
    - Not all patients with Crohn's disease and RVF will be candidates for repair.
    - If this is not possible, non-cutting seton placement can be a long-term method of controlling symptoms.
    - Proctectomy is considered for those with severe disease.
- The surgeon must also decide whether preoperative diversion is indicated.
  - Has not been shown to decrease the rate of fistula recurrence, although this may well be because the patients that undergo fecal diversion have more complicated disease.
  - When low rates of success are anticipated (e.g., multiple prior repairs, poor tissue compliance), preoperative fecal diversion should be considered.
  - Patients undergoing major transabdominal resections, or muscle transposition procedures, should have fecal diversion.
- The anatomic location of the fistula will dictate a local repair versus a transabdominal approach (mid rectum and upper vagina).
- For local repairs, the quality of the patient's tissue should be assessed.
  - If the patient's tissues are healthy, have normal compliance, and lack scarring, an endorectal advancement flap is an appropriate first approach.
  - If the RVF is secondary to obstetric injury and a sphincter defect is also present, a transperineal repair with sphincteroplasty is performed.
  - A transperineal approach should be considered in those who have failed previous endoanal advancement flaps.

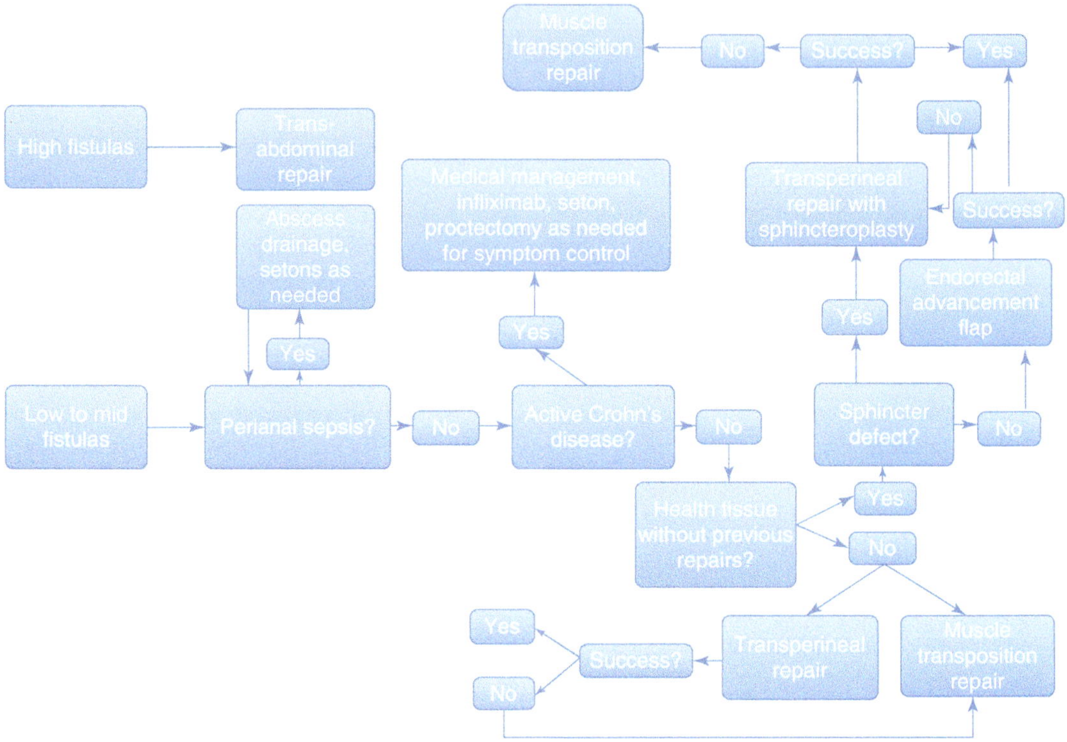

Fig. 16.18 Algorithm for management of rectovaginal fistulas

- For either endoanal advancement flaps or transperineal repairs, the surgeon may also consider the use of biologic grafts to reinforce the repair.
- If the local tissues are not adequate for repair, then transposition of healthy tissue should be considered.

- The most common tissues used for transposition are the Martius flap or gracilis muscle. Figure 16.18 provides an algorithm that summarizes the above recommendations.

Pilonidal Disease and Hidradenitis Suppurativa

17

Eric K. Johnson

Key Concepts

- Pilonidal disease presents with a wide range of symptoms, and multiple treatment options exist. Treatment should be tailored to the severity of disease, anatomy of disease, and patient expectations.
- Because of the wide array of available surgical options, the surgeon treating pilonidal disease should master 3–4 approaches that are applicable to a wide range of disease presentations.
- Treatments applied to both pilonidal disease and hidradenitis suppurativa should not be more disabling for the patient than the disease itself.
- There are numerous medical options available to treat hidradenitis suppurativa. They should be investigated and attempted prior to aggressive radical surgical management.
- Radical excision of hidradenitis suppurativa with surgical reconstruction offers the best hope to avoid disease recurrence.

Electronic Supplementary Material The online version of this chapter (https://doi.org/10.1007/978-3-030-01165-9_17) contains supplementary material, which is available to authorized users.

E. K. Johnson (✉)
Department of Colorectal Surgery, Cleveland Clinic, Cleveland, OH, USA

Background

The term “pilonidal” is derived from the root words “pilus” (a hair) and “nidus” (nest).

Etiology

- There has been considerable debate over whether PD is congenital or acquired, but most would currently agree that it is an acquired disease.
- It is generally believed that the initiating event is traumatization of the skin and surrounding hair follicles in the natal cleft.
- This occurs secondary to trapping of hairs, not necessarily those arising locally in the natal cleft.
- The local anatomy creates an unfavorable environment where friction, warmth, moisture, and perhaps local hypoxia lead to local trauma secondary to the barbed texture of the hair.
- A granulomatous foreign body-type reaction results.
- There is even some histological and immunohistochemical evidence that PD may represent a unilocalized type of hidradenitis suppurativa.
- Disease typically begins as a small sinus that may drain fluid but then can progress to numerous sinuses with associated cystic dilation and potential abscess formation.

S. R. Steele et al. (eds.), *The ASCRS Manual of Colon and Rectal Surgery*,
https://doi.org/10.1007/978-3-030-01165-9_17

- In some cases, unless the process is interrupted, it can become more widespread leading to worsening symptoms.
- Disease can range from the asymptomatic single sinus found incidentally up to a severe locally destructive process associated with significant disability.
- PD is not limited to the natal cleft area, and there are several reports of disease occurring in the interdigital areas in hair dressers and the umbilicus.
- Affect males more commonly than females, at 1.9 and 1.7 per 1000 person-years respectively.
- Several risk factors that have been implicated in the development of PD include positive family history of disease, elevated body mass index (BMI > 25), poor hygiene, hirsutism, deep natal cleft anatomy, occupation that requires prolonged sitting, and excessive sweating.
- A positive family history may not only predispose to disease occurrence but may also be associated with increased recurrence rates after surgery as well as earlier onset of disease.

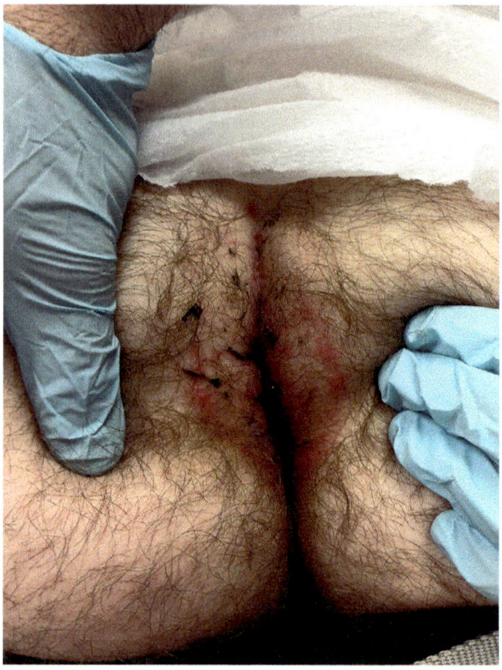

Fig. 17.1 This image shows a hirsute individual with midline "pits" that could go unnoticed. Note the poor hygiene

Clinical Presentation/Diagnosis

- Commonly encountered presentations:
  - Acute pilonidal abscess that requires drainage
  - Office visit to discuss definitive surgical therapy after either acute abscess drainage or persistent disease of moderate severity
- Simple history taking and a physical exam will in most cases solidify the diagnosis.
  - Patients will often complain of pain over the sacrococcygeal area with drainage of clear fluid or bleeding.
  - Physical exam will reveal "pits" in the midline. There may be one or several pits (Fig. 17.1).
  - In more significant cases, there may be open wounds that can have a large range in size (Fig 17.2a–c).
  - Acute abscess is typically associated with overlying erythema, fluctuance, and severe local tenderness (Fig. 17.3).

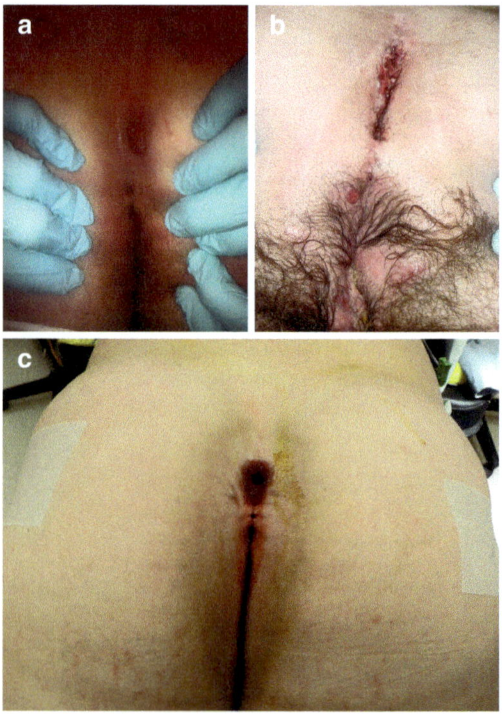

Fig. 17.2 (**a–c**) These images show a range of open wounds that may be seen with pilonidal disease

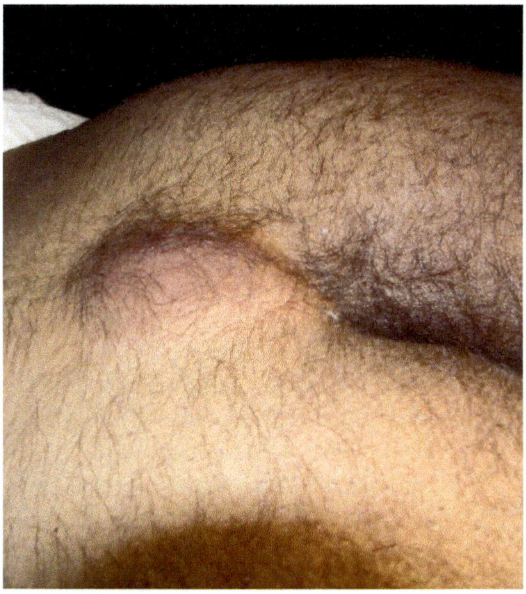

Fig. 17.3 This image depicts an acute pilonidal abscess

- Recurrent disease in the patient who has already undergone surgical excision is another commonly encountered scenario (Fig. 17.4).
  - Early recurrence is often actually persistence of an open wound that never healed after surgery, non-healing midline sacrococcygeal wound.
  - Recurrence presents similarly to primary PD and may be related to poor surgical technique, patient non-compliance, or failure to modify the pre-existing risk factors that led to disease in the first place.

Treatment

- Treatment should be tailored to the patient's expectations, disease anatomy, and disease severity.
- Options range from non-operative therapies up to wide local excision with local flap reconstruction.
- The debate of open wound management versus closed management remains.

Non-operative Management

- If the patient is asymptomatic, and physical examination reveals no concerning findings, they require no operative management.

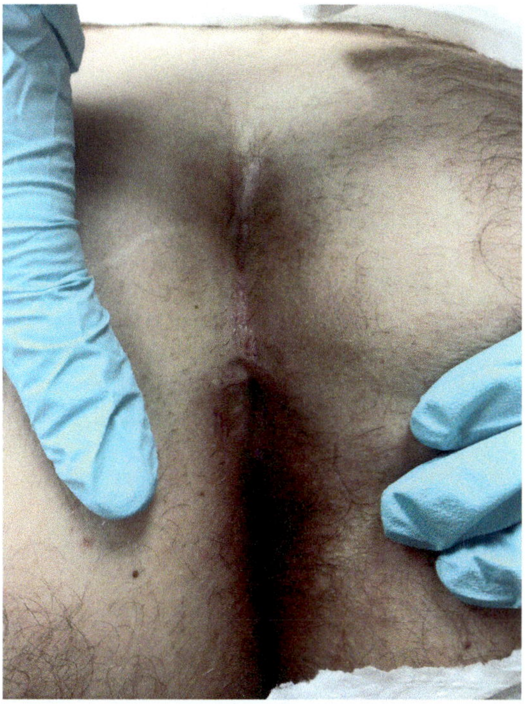

Fig. 17.4 This image shows a patient who developed recurrence after an attempt at a cleft lift procedure. Incorrect performance of the distal portion of the procedure may have led to this recurrence

- Risk factor modification such as weight loss, avoidance of prolonged sitting at work, improved hygiene, and weekly clipping of hair in and adjacent to the natal cleft may reduce the chance that a patient will develop symptoms related to PD.
- Laser hair removal has been advocated as a long-lasting alternative for the conservative management of PD that may reduce recurrence rates.
  - Treatments are performed over 3–11 sessions at 6–8-week intervals and can be quite costly.
- Although not necessarily considered non-operative (maybe non-excisional) therapy, methods employing the use of phenol or fibrin glue injection to ablate sinus tracts have been investigated in small series.
  - The potential advantages of these therapies over excisional methods are more rapid recovery and less post-procedural pain.

– These techniques often employ tract curettage, debridement, and hair removal, which contribute significantly to success.
– Use of phenol as an ablative agent has been associated with success rates of 60–95%.
– Fibrin glue injection combined with a variety of techniques has shown success in the range of 90–100%.
– A video-assisted ablative technique has also been described using a 4 mm rigid hysteroscope with a 5 French working for irrigation and hair removal, and the cavity and tracts are ablated using a bipolar electrode.

Operative/Excisional Management

- There are numerous methods available for the operative management of PD.
- Essentially, it is possible to find evidence to support whatever procedure one prefers to perform.

Basic Procedures

1. Laying open of the cyst and all sinus tracts: "unroofing" of disease.
   - Often, unroofing was combined with marsupialization of the wound.
   - Recurrence rates of 15–35%.
2. Wide local excision of all disease down to the post-sacral fascia.
   - Higher volume of excised specimen is associated with a higher surgical site infection rate and likely a higher risk of recurrent disease.
3. Simple tract unroofing and curettage are particularly helpful in the setting of minor disease affecting the perianal area (often mistaken as an anal fistula).
   - It is important to ensure that as much of the surgical wound as possible be kept off the midline, as midline wounds tend to have some difficulty with healing (Fig. 17.5a–c).
4. Primary closure has been combined with drainage in some settings with a wide variation in results.
   - The use of a drain has not been shown to result in improved results as far as patient satisfaction, healing, or infection.
   - A recent randomized controlled trial comparing the laying open method to wide excision with primary closure showed that healing occurred faster in the primary closure group with no differences in the groups noted at 1 year of follow-up.
5. Primary closure augmented by the placement of gentamicin-impregnated collagen in the

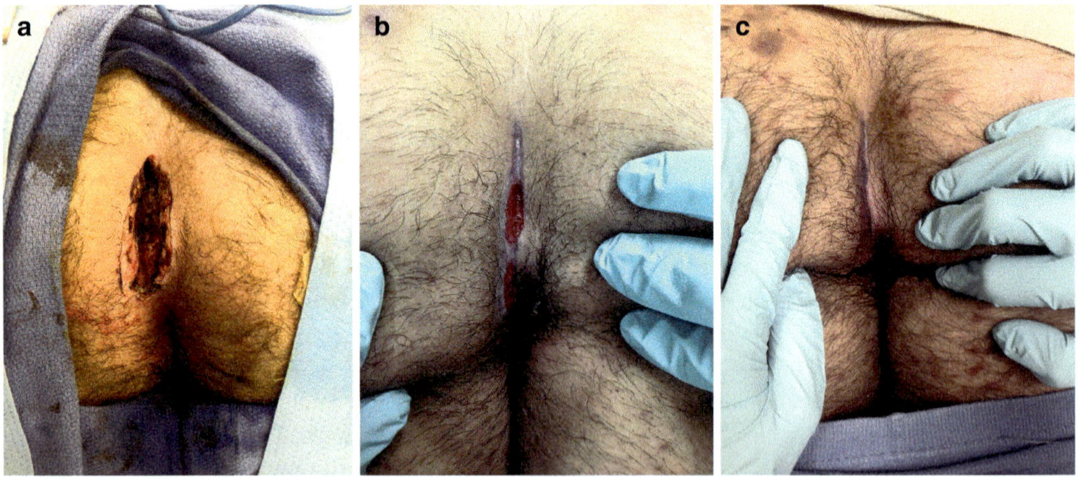

Fig. 17.5 (a–c) These images show yet another patient who presented with what was thought to be an anal fistula. Midline pits were noted, and the disease was treated with a lay-open technique, which resulted in rapid healing. Of note, this could potentially represent hidradenitis suppurativa

base of the wound with overlying tissue closure.
  - The results showed improved healing at 4 weeks, improved postoperative pain, and lower cost in the primary closure group.
  - Recurrence rates were no different at 5 years.
6. Primary closure with hydrogen peroxide irrigation or wide local excision with hydrogen peroxide irrigation.
  - The wide local excision combined with peroxide irrigation group showed the lowest recurrence rate and the fastest time to healing.
  - The investigators attributed this to the ability to clearly delineate all tracts and disease with peroxide irrigation, allowing them to perform a more precise and low-volume excision.
7. "Pit picking" procedures.
  - Relatively minor in terms of the amount of tissue excised, they result in small wounds and may be ideal for those suffering with mild-to-moderate levels of disease.
  - The basic premise of this method is that the central pits are excised with minimal surrounding tissue, hair and debris are removed, the old adjacent abscess cavity or "cyst" is excised through a lateral incision using an undermining technique, the pit excision sites are closed primarily, and the lateral incision is closed partially to allow for drainage (Fig. 17.6).
  - This results in a good cosmetic result with minimal pain, early return to work, and rapid healing.

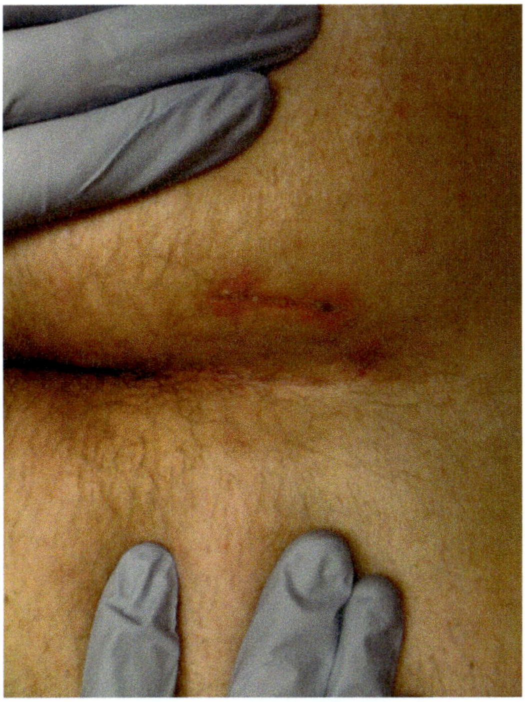

Fig. 17.6 This image shows a patient 2 weeks after a simple Bascom or "pit picking" operation

Complex Procedures

- The common thread among all "complex" procedures is the mobilization of adjacent tissue to achieve primary wound closure – in effect, the creation of a local flap.
- Some of these procedures combine wide local excision of diseased tissue with flap reconstruction, while others preserve as much local tissue as possible.
- Include the Karydakis flap, the Bascom cleft lift procedure, the rhomboid or Limberg flap procedure, Z-plasty, V-Y advancement flap, and other rotational flap techniques.
- It is possible that these procedures are more effective in curing disease, because they result in a flattening of the natal cleft anatomy.

Karydakis Flap

- Excision of the affected tissue in the midline, typically leaving an elliptical defect.
- A beveled skin flap is then created and mobilized across the midline to facilitate a primary closure that is lateral of midline (Fig. 17.7).
- A closed suction drain may be used or omitted.
- The purported advantages of this procedure are the tension free closure that is out of the midline coupled with some flattening of the natal cleft.
- Has been shown to be superior to simple primary midline closure in terms of patient satisfaction, recurrence rate, and rate of postoperative complications.

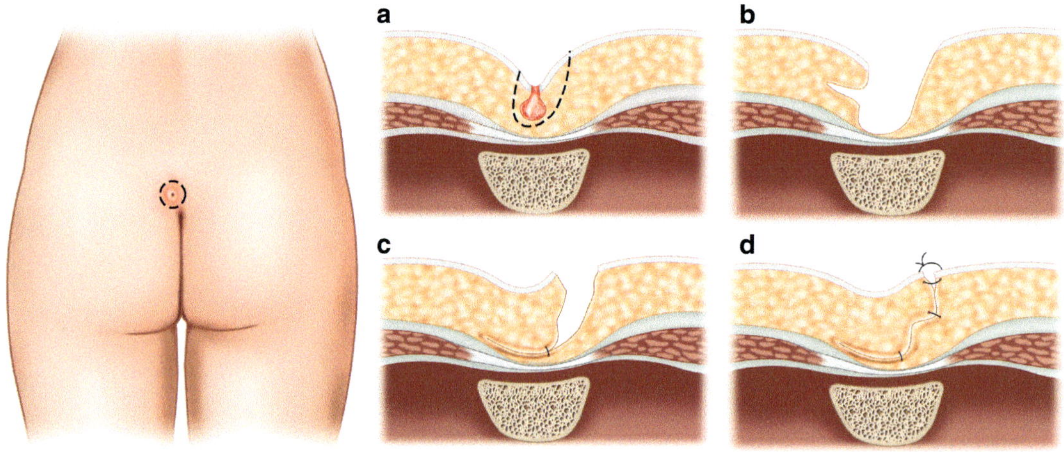

Fig. 17.7 This drawing depicts one method of performing a Karydakis flap

Cleft Lift Procedure (See Video 17.1)

Bascom cleft lift

- This is a simple but intricate procedure that is designed to "lift" the natal cleft and results in an incision that is closed off the midline.
- Interestingly, wide excision is not required. In fact, the only tissue that is excised is the overlying skin on one side of the natal cleft.
- This procedure requires that the patient be marked prior to incision to establish a "safe zone," beyond which no dissection is performed.
- Outcomes reveal excellent healing rates (97%) and low recurrence rates (2.5%).
- There is little question that this technique is easier to perform, takes less time, and removes less tissue than the more complex flap procedures such as the rhomboid flap.
- It results in flattening of the natal cleft, which is likely desirable.
- Unfortunately, not every patient with PD is a candidate for this procedure; those with complex recurrent disease and large open wounds and disease that is very close to the anus may not be ideal candidates and may require more extensive flap procedures.

Rhomboid/Limberg Flap (See Video 17.2)

- The rhomboid flap is a useful but more complex procedure that can be used in any setting of PD but is typically reserved for more severe cases.

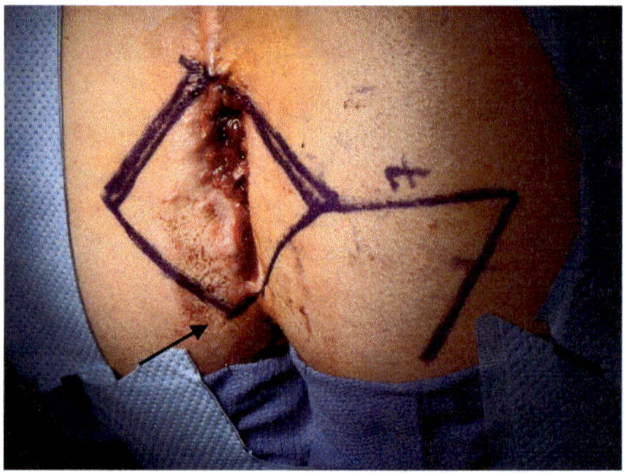

Fig. 17.8 This image shows the planned lines of incision for the rhomboid flap. Note that the caudal tip is *not* located directly over the anus. This modification results in a wound that does not come to a point at the location of highest risk

- The procedure involves a "diamond"- or rhombus-shaped area of wide excision encompassing all disease in the midline (Fig. 17.8).
- One must ensure that the thickness of the mobilized lipocutaneous flap approximates the thickness of the tissue that is excised.
- This technique works particularly well in the setting of complex recurrent disease.
- In some cases, the disease spans a very large area over the sacrum extending from the perianal area for a long distance cephalad.

  - When this is the case, the technique can still be used but may be modified.
  - The most difficult area in which to achieve healing is the caudal midline.
  - An excision can be performed, and flap created such that the caudal midline is covered leaving an open wound cephalad (Fig. 17.9).
  - The remaining wound can be managed in a variety of ways, but the use of a negative pressure wound therapy device makes this management easy (Fig. 17.10a, b).
- Potential surgical site-related postoperative complications include wound dehiscence, flap necrosis, hematoma, wound infection, and seroma (4%, 0–2%, 1%, 3–5%, and 3%, respectively).
- Recurrence can be seen in approximately 4%.
- The evidence indicates that the LF or MLF is associated with faster return to work, lower rates of surgical site infection, lower recurrence, and lower rates of wound dehiscence.

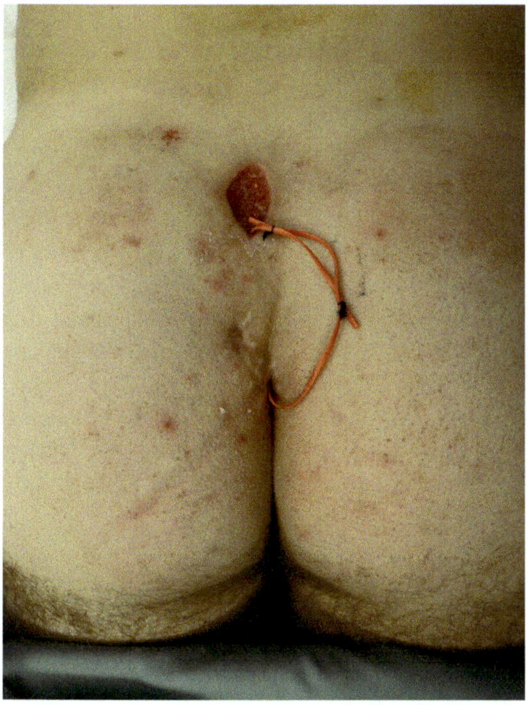

Fig. 17.9 This image shows a patient with recurrent disease that resulted in a large abscess that was drained superiorly and required some tissue debridement. This resulted in a large area of disease to be addressed

Disease Recurrence

- Familial history of disease, increased sinus number, larger cavity diameter, and primary wound closure have been shown to be associated with higher rates of recurrence. Recurrence has been shown to be lower in those that undergo surgical incision and drainage prior to definitive surgery as compared to those who have spontaneous abscess rupture.
- Surgery performed in the "after-hours" and potentially emergent setting has been associated with higher recurrence rates.
- Recurrences up to 20 years after surgery are seen, so studies investigating long-term outcomes should have at least 5 years of follow-up.

Hidradenitis Suppurativa

- The disease is a chronic inflammatory disorder involving the skin of apocrine gland-bearing areas, typically the perineum, inguinal, inframammary, and axillary regions.
- Individuals afflicted with HS suffer a tremendous impact upon their quality of life with effects on both their physical and mental health.
- The prevalence of HS is estimated to be 127.8 per 100,000 or 0.13%, with a higher prevalence among women.
- This translates to fewer than 200,000 affected patients in the United States.
- The reported mean age of onset is between 20 and 24 years of age, with less than 8% of affected individuals developing disease earlier than 13 years of age.
- Early-onset disease seems to be correlated with family history of disease.

Etiology/Presentation/Diagnosis

- It was once thought purely to be secondary to infection of the apocrine sweat glands, but there is now general agreement that this is not true.

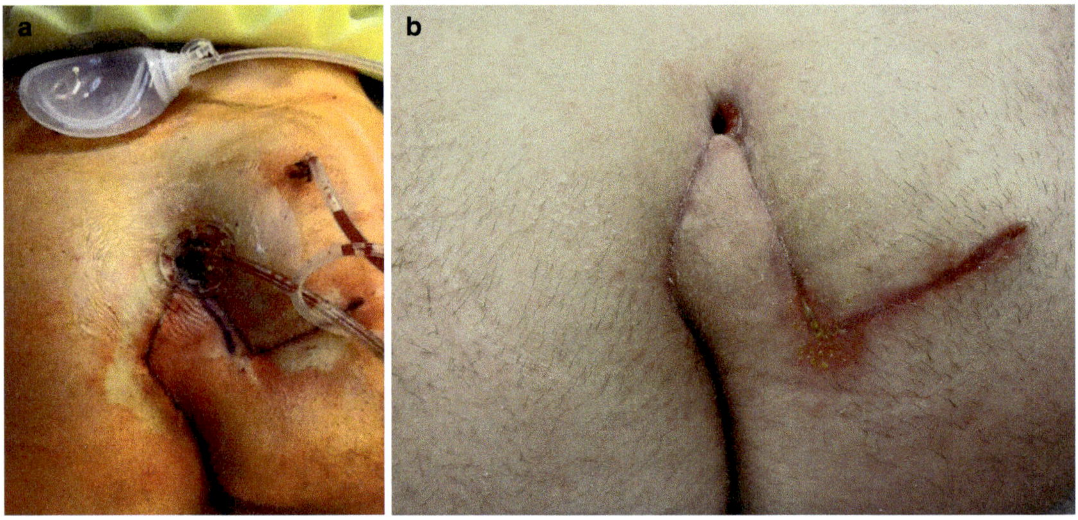

Fig. 17.10 (**a**, **b**) This image shows a patient similar to that in Fig. 17.9. The flap was created and closed leaving an open wound superiorly that was treated with negative pressure wound therapy and healed easily

- The disease is characterized by chronic follicular occlusion resulting in secondary inflammation of the apocrine glands.
- The initial inciting event is believed to be hyperkeratosis that leads to follicular occlusion.
- Others have proposed that the follicular occlusion occurs as a result of a defect in the follicular support system.
- In any case, there is ultimate dysfunction in the entire folliculopilosebaceous unit (FPSU) that leads to follicular rupture and secondary bacterial infection involving the apocrine glands.
- Disease manifests initially as open comedones, typically with a few "heads," and tender subcutaneous papules.
- In many this leads to a chronic and progressive worsening of symptoms in which additional nodules form, rupture, and drain a thick mucopurulent foul-smelling liquid. Over time this leads to sinus tract formation, fibrotic subcutaneous scarring, and potentially disabling contractures of the affected limb.
- There are a number of variables that have been identified as risk factors for disease.
  - Tobacco smoking and obesity have been associated with both the presence of disease and with lower remission rates.
  - Weight loss has been shown to be temporally associated with remission.
  - Sweating, shaving, deodorant use, and friction have also been implicated as potential exacerbating factors.
  - It is also believed that there may be dietary triggers that worsen disease (high carbohydrate diet, milk consumption).
- Diagnosis is typically made based on common physical exam findings including skin thickening, induration, abscess formation, the presence of draining sinuses, and contractures in the regions of the body considered at risk.
- There are several other diagnoses in the differential that should be considered (Table 17.1).
- There have been two classification or staging systems proposed to grade disease, the Hurley system and the Sartorius system (Tables 17.2 and 17.3).
- French group have introduced a latent classification system, which better groups HS patients into three distinct phenotypes (Table 17.4).
- Hurley system seems to be most useful to physicians making treatment recommendations for affected individuals.
- There is a well-established link between HS and acne, pilonidal disease, inflammatory

Table 17.1 A list of diagnoses that should be considered in the differential diagnosis of hidradenitis suppurative

Diseases to be considered in the differential diagnosis
Acne
Actinomycosis
Anal fistula
Carbuncles
Cat scratch disease
Cellulitis
Crohn's disease
Cutaneous blastomycosis
Dermoid cyst
Granuloma inguinale
Erysipelas
Furuncles
Inflamed epidermoid cyst
Lymphadenopathy
Lymphogranuloma venereum
Nocardia infection
Noduloulcerative syphilis
Perirectal abscess
Pilonidal disease
Tuberculous abscess
Tularemia

Table 17.2 Description of the Hurley classification of hidradenitis suppurativa, likely the most useful in the clinical setting

Hurley staging system of hidradenitis suppurativa	
Stage I	Abscess formation, single or multiple, without scarring or sinus tracts
Stage II	Recurrent abscesses with tract formation and scarring, single or multiple, with widely separated lesions
Stage III	Multiple interconnected tracts and abscesses throughout an entire region

Table 17.3 The Sartorius scoring or staging system. Some have modified the system by adding value to the presence of pain, drainage, or odor. This may be a more useful system in the research setting to quantify severity of disease

Sartorius staging system/Sartorius score	
Involvement in specific body areas	3 points for each area involved
Nodules	2 points for each
Fistulas	4 points
Scars	1 point
Other findings	1 point
Longest distance between two lesions	2–4 points
If lesions are separated by normal skin	Yes-0 points, no-6 points

Table 17.4 Latent or phenotypic classification proposed by Canoui-Poitrine et al.

Latent classification	Phenotype	Affected region
LC1	Axillary-mammary	Axilla, breast, perineum, inguinal
LC2	Follicular	Ears, chest, back, legs, axillary, breast
LC3	Gluteal	Gluteal fold

bowel disease (particularly Crohn's disease), spondyloarthropathy, genetic keratin disorders, and squamous cell carcinoma.

Treatment

- The best way to achieve the lowest recurrence rate is to aggressively remove all apocrine gland-bearing tissue in the affected area, which will often require a complex reconstructive approach.

Medical Therapy

- It appears that treatment is most successful when used in combined fashion as opposed to monotherapy.
- Forms of medical therapy include antibacterial washes, topical antibiotics, systemic antibiotics, topical and systemic retinoids, antiandrogens, intralesional and systemic corticosteroids, immunosuppressives, and oral metformin.
- While bacterial infection may be a secondary event in HS, it is clear from published research that persistence of bacterial colonization, likely in the form of biofilms, plays some role in the progression of disease.
- Retinoids are likely beneficial secondary to their effect on normalization of epithelial cell proliferation and differentiation, which in turn may reduce the occurrence of follicular occlusion.
- Evidence to support the use of antiandrogen therapy (estrogen/progestin combinations, finasteride, spironolactone) is fairly weak.
- Other treatment options include tumor necrosis alpha (TNF alpha) inhibitors (infliximab), photodynamic therapy, intense pulsed light therapy, and lasers.

Surgical/Excisional Therapy

- Excisional therapy is based on the premise that wide excision of all apocrine gland-bearing tissue in the affected region is the best method to sustain low recurrence rates.
- All affected skin and subcutaneous fat are excised down to the fascial level.
- This will often result in a very large defect that cannot be addressed through simple primary closure.
  - Local flap closure or split thickness skin grafting (Fig. 17.11) are commonly necessary to achieve adequate tissue coverage of the wound.
  - This may require the involvement of a plastic surgeon.
- Attempts at simple unroofing of sinus tracts seem to be associated with higher rates of recurrence.
- A technique referred to as STEEP (skin tissue-sparing excision with electrosurgical peeling) has been proposed as a "tissue sparing" option that leads to faster healing with improved outcomes.
- Vacuum-assisted closure devices can also be helpful in wounds that are too large to close primarily, but may not require more complex reconstructive options.
- In cases where skin grafting may be used, a two-stage approach has been described. It can potentially lead to improved outcomes.

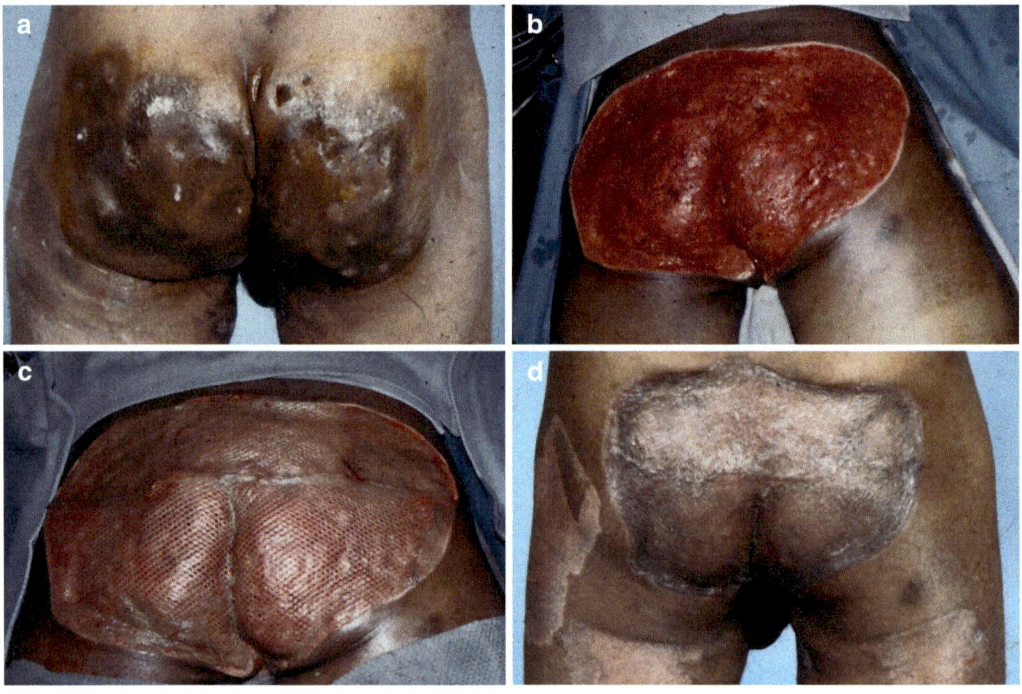

Fig. 17.11 (**a–d**) This series of images shows a patient with Hurley stage III disease who underwent radical excision and closure with split thickness skin grafting

Dermatology and Pruritus Ani

18

Wolfgang B. Gaertner and Genevieve B. Melton

Key Concepts

- Pruritus ani is a dermatologic condition characterized by itching or burning at the perianal area.
- Pruritus ani can be either primary (idiopathic) or secondary.
- Primary pruritus ani is the most common form of pruritus ani. The most common causes of secondary pruritus ani are local irritants and common anorectal conditions.
- All chronic perianal dermatoses require a detailed history and physical exam, including all past diagnostic tests and forms of treatment.
- The single most valuable diagnostic test in patients with recurrent or ongoing pruritus ani is skin biopsy.
- Treatment options for pruritus ani are numerous. Management should focus on the underlying or suspected etiology, following an evidenced-based stepwise diagnostic and treatment algorithm.

Introduction

- Dermatologic diseases of the anus are a group of inflammatory, infectious, and neoplastic conditions.
- Patients presenting with anal dermatologic disease are often seen by a diverse group of providers, including general practitioners, gastroenterologists, dermatologists, and colorectal surgeons.
- Pruritus ani is defined as a dermatologic condition characterized by persistent and unpleasant itching or burning sensation in the perianal region.
- The incidence is estimated to range from 1% to 5% in the general population.
  - Men being affected more than women in a 4:1 ratio
  - Most commonly diagnosed in the fourth to sixth decades of life
- Pruritus ani can be classified into primary or idiopathic (accounting for 50–90% of cases) and secondary.
- It may be caused by a wide spectrum of conditions, among which perianal eczema is probably the most common.
- Most patients have symptoms for many years, as well as a long list of prescribed or over-the-counter treatments.

W. B. Gaertner
Department of Colon & Rectal Surgery, University of Minnesota, Minneapolis, MN, USA

G. B. Melton (✉)
Division of Colon & Rectal Surgery, Department of Surgery, University of Minnesota Medical Center, Minneapolis, MN, USA
e-mail: gmelton@umn.edu

S. R. Steele et al. (eds.), *The ASCRS Manual of Colon and Rectal Surgery*,
https://doi.org/10.1007/978-3-030-01165-9_18

Pathophysiology of Perianal Signs and Symptoms

- The sensation of itch is elicited as a surface phenomenon mediated by non-myelinated C-fibers in the epidermis and subdermis and can be also classified as pruritoceptive (C-fiber mediated), neuropathic (i.e., after herpes zoster infection), and central or neurogenic.
- Biochemically, histamine, kallikrein, bradykinin, papain, and trypsin can experimentally and individually produce itching.
  - This may explain the lack of effectiveness of antihistamine medications against itching.
- While multiple itch mediators have been identified, the antagonism of these mediators produces varied clinical results (Table 18.1).
- This strongly suggests that specific neuronal pathways are involved at both peripheral and central levels in mediating itch.
- Scratching is thought to produce inadequate feedback to inhibit further itching.

Table 18.1 Itch mediators and corresponding antipruritic agents

Itch mediator	Antipruritic agent
Histamine	Antihistamines
Acetylcholine	Doxepin (mainly antihistaminic mechanism)
Serotonin	Paroxetine, fluoxetine (SSRIs) Mirtazipine (serotonin inverse agonist) Ondansetron (5HT3 antagonist)
Opioids	Naloxone, naltrexone, (μ-receptor antagonists) Nalfurafine, butorphanol (kappa-receptor agonists)
Leukotrienes	Zafirlukast, zileuton
Prostaglandins	NSAIDs
Substance P	Aprepitant
TRPV1	Capsaicin
TRPM8	Menthol
TNF-alpha	Thalidomide
GABA	Gabapentin, pregabalin

SSRI selective serotonin reuptake inhibitor, *TRPV1* transient receptor potential vanilloid 1, *TRPM8* transient receptor potential melastatin 8, *TNF* tumor necrosis factor, *GABA* gamma-amino butyric acid, *NSAIDs* nonsteroidal anti-inflammatory drugs, *5HT* 5-hydroxytryptamine

  - Persistent scratching causes skin trauma, which is an additional stimulus for itching and additional scratching; therefore, this can lead to a chronic vicious cycle.
  - Substituting scratching for other stimuli such as heat, cold, pain, or stinging by applying alcohol or pepper extract (capsaicin) may cause inhibitory feedback and then can decrease the urge to scratch.
- Itching associated with healing is also common after the inflammatory response caused by common anorectal conditions (i.e., fissure and hemorrhoids), as well as after anorectal operations and trauma.
  - The release of histamine and various kinins and prostaglandins is a contributing factor in this situation; therefore, antihistamines, topical anti-inflammatory agents (steroids), and topical anesthetics have shown beneficial effects in these patients.

Etiology and Contributing Factors

- Proposed etiologies of primary or idiopathic pruritus ani include a variety of associated factors, including anatomic, dietary, hygienic, psychogenic, local irritants and medications (Table 18.2).
- The causes of secondary pruritus ani can be divided into several broad categories: infectious, dermatologic, systemic disease and anorectal causes (Table 18.3).
- In the absence of a primary cutaneous disorder, pruritus ani is thought to have two probable causes:
  1. Irritation from mucus, fecal material, or other perineal moisture (such as urine in an elderly patient with urinary incontinence)
  2. Nerve impingement in the sacral region that causes a neuropathic itch or notalgia paresthetica
- Anal leakage alone is frequently associated with anal pruritus, and this has been correlated with a pronounced anal inhibitory reflex in patients with pruritus ani.

Table 18.2 Proposed etiologies of primary or idiopathic pruritus ani

Anatomic factors	Obesity, deep clefts, hirsutism, tight clothing
Diet	Coffee (including decaffeinated), chocolate, spicy and heavily condimented foods, citrus fruits, tomatoes, beer, dairy products, vitamin A and D deficiencies, fat substitutes, consumption of large volumes of liquids
Personal hygiene	Poor cleansing habits, excessive perianal hygiene causing trauma
Local irritants	Fecal contamination, moisture, soaps, perfumes, topical medications, toilet paper, wet wipes, alcohol, witch hazel
Drugs	Quinidine, colchicine, IV steroids
Psychogenic	Anxiety, neurosis, psychosis, neurodermatitis, neuropathy, "itch syndromes"

Modified from Stamos MJ, Hicks TC, Pruritus ani: diagnosis and treatment. In: Perspectives in Colon and Rectal Surgery, 1998;11(1):1–20. Thieme Medical Publishers

- Anxiety, stress, and fatigue, as well as personality, coping skills, and obsessive-compulsive disorders, probably play a role in the exacerbation of pruritus ani.

Irritants

- Pruritus ani can result from several products including lanolin, neomycin, parabens, topical anesthetics from the "caine" family, and certain toilet papers.
- The enzymes responsible for perianal skin irritation from fecal contamination include lipase, elastase, and chymotrypsin.
- Further skin irritation is often exacerbated by multiple and diverse treatment attempts and excessive hygiene measures, allowing for sensitization of the perianal area, which may then be followed by allergic contact dermatitis or perianal eczema.
- There are six common foods that often are associated with and thought to cause perianal irritation and pruritus: coffee, tea, cola, beer, chocolate, and tomato (ketchup).

Table 18.3 Causes of secondary pruritus ani

Infectious
Bacterial
Fungal/yeast
Viral
Parasitic
Dermatologic
Psoriasis
Lichen planus, lichen simplex chronicus
Lichen sclerosus
Contact dermatitis
Atopic dermatitis
Local malignancy (squamous cell carcinoma, Paget's and Bowen's disease)
Systemic disease
Diabetes mellitus
Leukemia, lymphoma, polycythemia vera
Liver disease (jaundice)
Chronic renal failure
Thyroid disorders
Colorectal and anal causes
Hemorrhoids (internal and external)
Rectal prolapse (mucosal and full-thickness)
Fissure
Fistula-in-ano
Diarrhea (infectious, inflammatory bowel disease, irritable bowel syndrome)
Secreting villous tumors
Other
Radiation dermatitis
Fecal incontinence and anal leakage
Gynecologic conditions (pruritus vulvae, vaginosis, vaginal discharge)

  - In some cases, total elimination will result in remission of itching in 2 weeks.
  - After a 2-week elimination period, foods may be reintroduced to determine the association and potentially the threshold exposure with the appearance of symptoms.

Steroid-Inducing Itching

- Although anogenital itching has been reported with both topical and systemic steroids, it commonly occurs as a rebound phenomenon after withdrawal of steroids.
- The potency and dosing of steroids should be tapered in a planned fashion with the goal of

eliminating steroids altogether from a maintenance regimen.
- Allergic contact dermatitis to topically applied steroids has been well documented and is class-specific.
- Switching to desoximetasone (a less commonly used agent in steroid class) may be a solution, but the ideal solution would be elimination of all steroids.
- Calcineurin inhibitors (tacrolimus and pimecrolimus) offer excellent anti-inflammatory effect without many of these steroidal side effects.

Infectious

- Perianal infections associated with pruritus can be bacterial, viral, fungal, or parasitic in origin.
- Common bacterial causes include beta-hemolytic streptococci, *Staphylococcus aureus*, and *Corynebacterium minutissimum*.
  - Beta-hemolytic streptococcus being the leading cause of perianal dermatitis in children.
  - *Staphylococcus aureus* perianal infections are more commonly reported in the adult population and typically present as a refractory and prolonged dermatitis.
  - Erythrasma, a superficial infection of the intertriginous skin caused by *Corynebacterium minutissimum*, has been reported to cause up to 18% of cases of pruritus ani in warm climates.
- Fungal infections may account for 10–43% of secondary infectious pruritus ani cases.
  - *Candida albicans* is the most common fungi identified in patients with pruritus ani.
  - Dermatophytes can cause pruritus ani less frequently but should be considered pathogenic and treated appropriately when found in patients with pruritus ani.
- Several viral and sexually transmitted diseases (STD) including herpes syndromes, syphilis, gonorrhea, molluscum contagiosum, and condyloma accuminata can present as pruritus ani.
  - Condyloma accuminata, which is associated with human papillomavirus infection, is a common cause of itching (Fig. 18.1).
  - Herpes syndromes are typically characterized by pain and burning with red macules that progress to vesicles that rupture, ulcerate, and may become secondarily infected.
  - Common perianal parasites include *Enterobius vermicularis* (pinworms), *Sarcoptes scabiei*, and *Pediculosis pubis*.
    - Pinworms, in particular, are a common cause of nocturnal and post-defecation pruritus ani, especially in children.

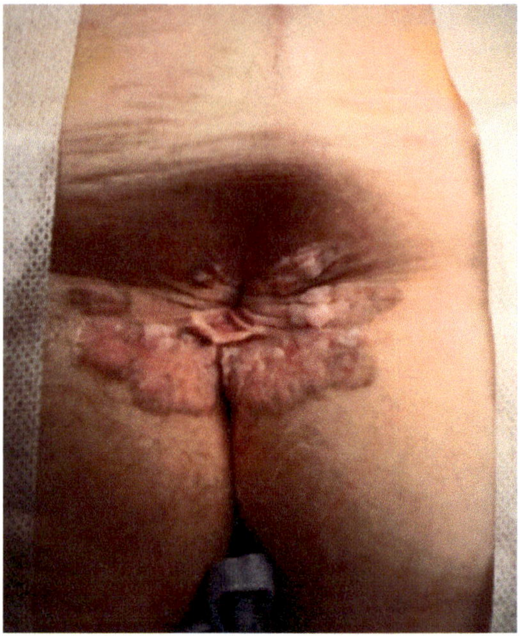

Fig. 18.1 Patient with external anal condyloma acuminata and perianal fungal infection that presented with anal pruritus. Condyloma fulguration and antifungal treatment were effective at resolving pruritus

Dermatologic

- Several dermatologic conditions may present as pruritus ani including psoriasis, seborrheic dermatitis, atopic dermatitis, contact dermatitis, lichen planus, lichen sclerosus, lichen simplex chronicus, and local malignancies.

- Anal eczema, probably the most common dermatologic cause of pruritus ani, is generally considered to primarily represent contact dermatitis to chemicals and medications that are applied to the anal area.
  - These substances are used by up to 57% of patients with anogenital complaints and include popular hemorrhoid ointments that contain potent sensitizers (local anesthetics, myroxylon pereirae, bufexamac), dyes and perfumes used in scented toilet paper and soaps, feminine hygiene sprays and deodorants, and medicated talcum powders and skin cleansers.
  - Patients with anal eczema are also more likely to have asthma and hay fever.
  - Most studies evaluating the role of specific allergens causing anal eczema have identified local anesthetics, aminoglycoside antibiotics, and thimerosal as the most common causative agents.
  - It is also important to test the patients' own products, as some studies have found these to be common and clinically relevant allergens.
  - The role of dry, moist, or recycled toilet paper has been looked at, and well-designed studies have not shown toxic effects of its components.
- Atopic dermatitis may be the most common hereditary cause of pruritus ani, with a frequency of 15–20% of the population.
  - Caused by disruption of the epidermal barrier function.
  - Filaggrin, the cement of the epidermis, is defective or absent in patients with atopic dermatitis because of mutations of the filaggrin gene.
  - Complete loss of the filaggrin gene is seen in ichthyosis vulgaris, a common keratinizing disorder frequently associated with atopic dermatitis and seen at the buttocks and perianal skin.
- Psoriasis affects 1–3% of the general population and is an important etiology of secondary pruritus ani, with reports varying from 5.5% to 55%.
- Seborrheic dermatitis is an uncommon cause of pruritus ani, characterized by extensive, moist erythema in the perineum.
- Lichen planus is a relatively common inflammatory disease that affects the skin and mucous membranes and is thought to be caused by an altered, cell-mediated immune response.
  - Commonly seen in patients with other disease processes, such as ulcerative colitis, primary biliary cirrhosis, hepatitis C infection, and myasthenia gravis
  - Typically self-limited, resolving after 8–12 months
- Lichen sclerosus is a disease of unknown cause.
  - Seen more frequently in women and involves the vulva extending posteriorly to the perianal region.
  - When it occurs on the penis, it is termed balanitis xerotica obliterans.
- Lichen simplex chronicus, also known as neurodermatitis, is a secondary skin manifestation that develops in an area of repetitive trauma from scratching or rubbing.
  - A primary etiology may not be found in many cases, and the pruritus is typically intermittent and worsens at night or when a patient is quiet or still.

Neoplasms

- Although uncommon, pruritus ani can be a presenting symptom of dermatologic neoplasms, such as condylomata, Paget's disease, and Bowen's disease.
- Although pruritus has not been well studied in large studies evaluating patients with AIN, it is commonly identified in patients with a history of anal warts (Fig. 18.2).
- Extra-mammary Paget's disease (cutaneous adenocarcinoma in situ).
  - Perianal region is the most commonly involved extra-mammary site, and pruritus is a common presenting symptom.

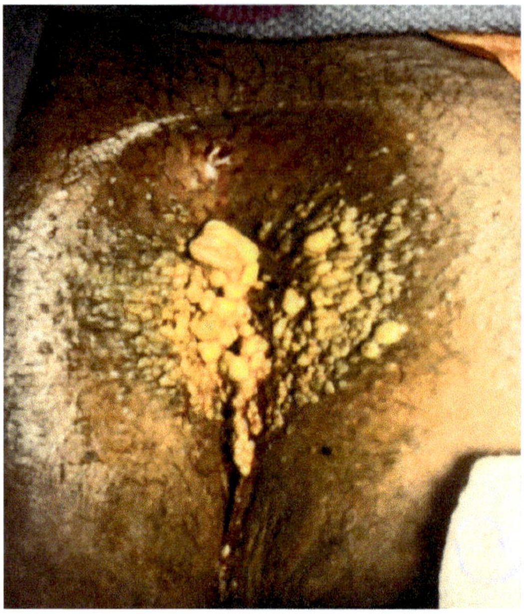

Fig. 18.2 External anal condylomata acuminata presenting with perianal pruritus. Condyloma fulguration was effective at resolving pruritus

  - May be indicative of and associated with an underlying apocrine or eccrine carcinoma.
    - Rate of anorectal malignancy associated with perianal Paget's disease ranges from 33% to 86%.
    - Therefore, investigations of the gastrointestinal, urinary, and gynecologic systems should be performed for a potential associated malignancy.
- Intraepithelial squamous cell carcinoma in situ, also known as Bowen's disease, of the anus is also rare but frequently presents with pruritus as the main symptom.

Anorectal Conditions

- Hemorrhoidal disease, skin tags, and chronic anal fissure-in-ano are commonly seen pathologies in patients with pruritus ani.
  - Associated with varying degrees of leakage, prolapse, and soiling.
  - Correcting these disorders in patients with pruritus ani is typically warranted.
  - In general it is difficult to know whether anorectal conditions are the cause or a contributing factor of pruritus ani.
  - Operative management that avoids further scarring or corrects fecal incontinence or leakage should be offered to pruritus patients in most cases.

Systemic Diseases

- Several systemic diseases have been associated with pruritus ani; however, the precise causative factors remain unknown.
- Diabetes mellitus (most common), liver disease, lymphoma, leukemia, pellagra, vitamin A and D deficiencies, renal failure, iron-deficiency anemia, and hyperthyroidism.

Diagnoses of Perianal Disease

- Establishing an exact diagnosis may be difficult, often resulting in dissatisfied patients who may be seen multiple times and by several doctors in different specialties.
- Consequently patients can have symptoms for many years, as well as a long list of prescribed and over-the-counter medications.
- To pinpoint the cause of dermatologic diseases of the anus, it is recommended that patients be asked about their current diet, current and previous medications, personal history of atopy, information about bowel habits, and perianal hygiene regimen, including how they routinely clean the anal area after a bowel movement.
- A review of the patient's medical history, including any history of anorectal conditions or operations.
- Other pertinent history includes previous skin infections, especially mycotic infections of the genitalia, STDs, anal seepage, and symptoms of fecal and urinary incontinence.
- A diagnostic algorithm, including a full history and physical examination, biochemical and microbiology testing, proctoscopy, and patch tests (including the patient's own products), is strongly recommended (Fig. 18.3).

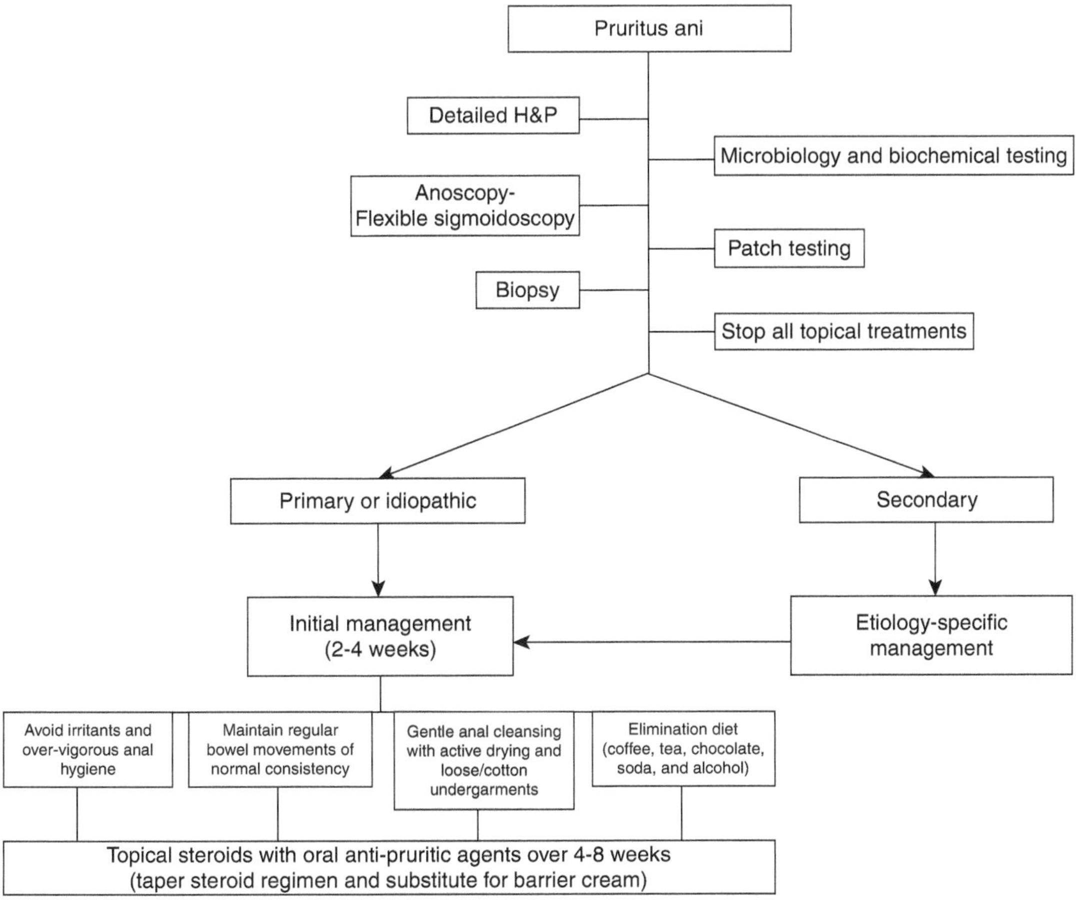

Fig. 18.3 Diagnostic and treatment algorithm for patients presenting with pruritus ani

Physical Examination

- Physical examination should also include evaluation of other related sites of skin manifestations including the groins, axillae, buttock cleft, and other intertriginous areas or skin folds.
- Response to treatment at these areas should also be documented at follow-up examinations.
- Washington Hospital classifies pruritus ani based on physical exam findings: stage 0 is normal skin, stage 1 is red and inflamed skin, stage 2 has lichenified skin, and stage 3 has lichenified skin, coarse ridges, and ulcerations.

Infectious

- In the setting of bacterial perianal dermatitis, the perianal skin typically shows a moist, bright, and erythematous eruption with distinct borders and no satellite lesions.
- Chronic infected discharge from the anus may lead to hyperpigmentation of the anorectal cleft with long-standing anorectal conditions, including pilonidal disease, anorectal fistulas, and hidradenitis suppurativa.
- Erythrasma is often associated with scaly, well-defined patches of initially reddish- and then brownish-colored lesions at other intertriginous areas (Fig. 18.4).
- When caused by *Corynebacterium minutissimum*, these lesions show a characteristic

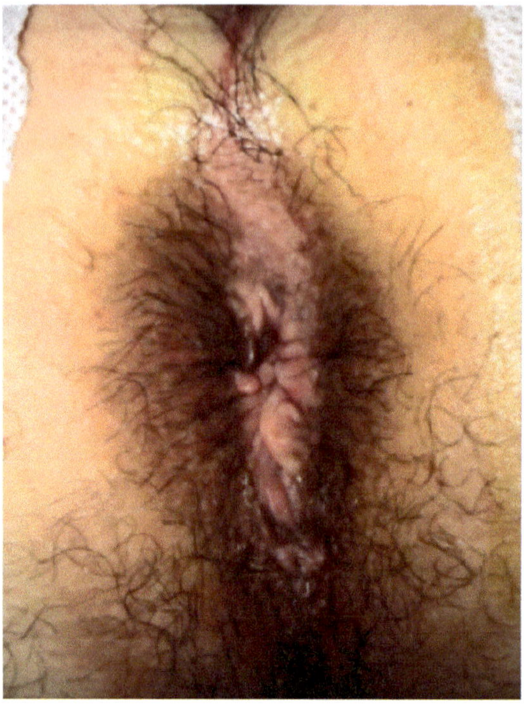

Fig. 18.4 Hyperpigmentation and perianal skin lichenification seen in a patient with erythrasma

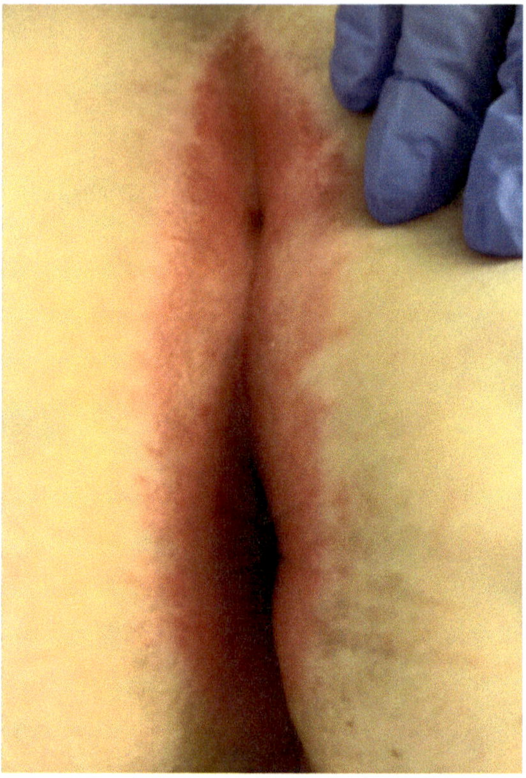

Fig. 18.5 Perianal fungal infection in a patient with anal seepage and fecal incontinence. This infection is characterized by a bright-red rash at the perianal area and intergluteal fold in a "butterfly" distribution

coral-red fluorescence when examined with a Wood's lamp.

  - *C. minutissimum* is commonly present and pathogenic at other body folds (axillae, groin, inframammary) and toe webs.
- *Molluscum contagiosum* has a distinct presentation with clusters of small, palpable, flesh-colored papules with central umbilication.
- In general, human immunodeficiency virus (HIV)-associated lesions rarely present with itching except for secondary fungal infections.
- Perianal fungal infections are characterized by a bright-red rash without the cheesy exudate sometimes seen in other parts of the body (Fig. 18.5).
  - These infections may present following treatment with systemic antibiotics and topical or systemic steroids.
  - *Candida* is commonly found in patients with pruritus secondary to common anorectal conditions (i.e., hemorrhoids, fissure) and is typically eliminated with adequate treatment of the underlying condition.
  - Infections where dermatophytes are cultured almost always present with pruritus and are considered pathogenic.
    - Topical steroids may render direct scrapings negative for hyphae but frequently facilitate dermatophyte growth.

Dermatologic

- Anal eczema or contact dermatitis is characterized by erythema, scaling, and vesicles.
- Similar findings may be located on the face, neck, and dorsum of the hands, as well as popliteal and antecubital fossas.
- Atopic dermatitis presents as nonspecific and diffuse erythema, often seen with signs of skin excoriation.
  - Associated findings include keratosis pilaris (rough sandpaper-like texture over the

posterior biceps and thighs), Morgan's folds or Morgan–Dennie lines (redundant creases beneath the eyes), "sniffer" lines (a subtle transverse crease across mid-nose), urticaria, and white dermatographism.
  - With the loss of an adequate epidermal barrier, secondary infections and irritation by contact agents are common in patients with atopic dermatitis.
- Psoriasis typically appears as well-demarcated, scaly, plaque-like lesions that are bright red in color (Fig. 18.6).
  - Typical lesions are commonly found on the scalp, elbows, knees, knuckles, and penis, but perianal psoriasis may also present as an isolated lesion.
  - In the perianal region, lesions tend to be poorly demarcated, pale, and non-scaling because of persistent maceration, hence the term inverse psoriasis.
- With seborrheic dermatitis, excessive perianal moisture is the common denominator, and special attention should be directed to the scalp, chest, ears, beard, and suprapubic areas since these regions are commonly affected, as well.
- Lichen planus presents as shiny, flat-topped papules that are darker than the surrounding skin and begin on the volar aspects of the wrists and forearms.
  - Genital and mucous membrane involvement is common.
  - Wickham striae are intersecting gray lines that can be seen if mineral oil is applied to the plaques and help to establish the diagnosis.
- Lichen sclerosus mainly involves the vulva but typically extends posteriorly toward the perianal region.
  - The first phase of this condition begins as ivory-colored, atrophic papules that break down and expose underlying erythematous raw tissue; this process is severely pruritic and painful.
  - As this heals, the area is replaced by chronic inflammation, sclerosis, and atrophy of the affected area (Fig. 18.7).
  - The classical finding is white patches around the vulva and anus.

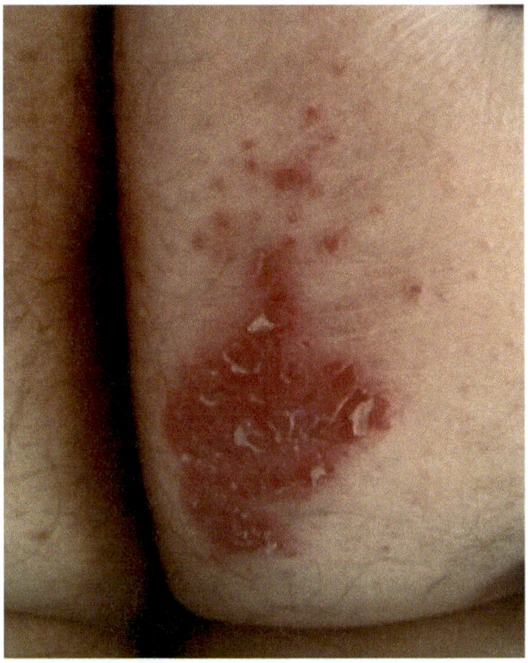

Fig. 18.6 Perianal psoriasis or psoriasis inversa showing a well-demarcated, scaly, bright-red, plaque-like lesion

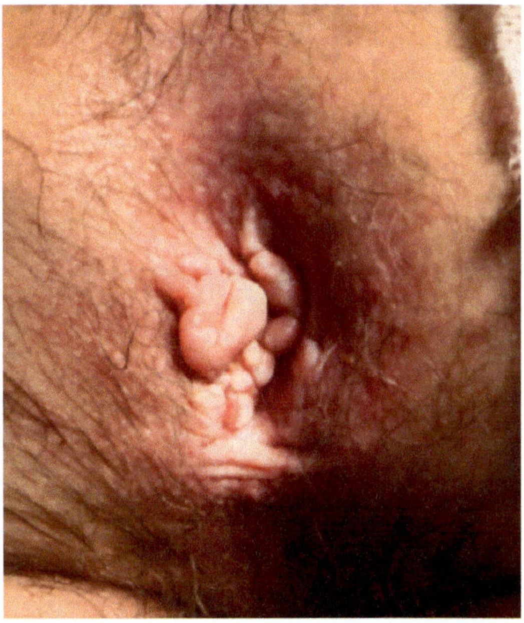

Fig. 18.7 Lichen sclerosus of the anus with chronic healing

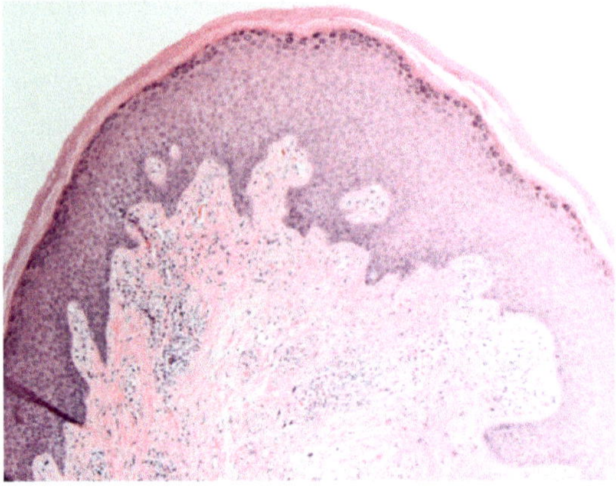

Fig. 18.8 Photomicrograph of lichen sclerosus showing signs of chronic scaring and lack of lymphocytic interface dermatitis

- Histologically, these lesions are consistent with a chronic scar, lacking a lymphocytic interface (Fig. 18.8).
- Because of a reported 4–6% risk of developing squamous cell carcinoma, all nonresponders or those with recurrent sclerosis should have a skin biopsy to rule out malignancy.
- Treatment of the disease does not appear to modify this risk.

- Lichenification is the characteristic finding seen in patients with lichen simplex chronicus or neurodermatitis.
  - The perianal skin appears thickened and is commonly described as cracking and scaling.

Neoplasms

- The presentation of dermatologic malignancies, such as Paget's and Bowen's disease, may vary from a mild rash to a florid type of eczema at times associated with indurated skin.
- The classic presentation is an erythematous and eczematoid perianal plaque (Fig. 18.9).

Biochemical Testing

- After failed topical management and if systemic disease is suspected, biochemical testing is warranted.

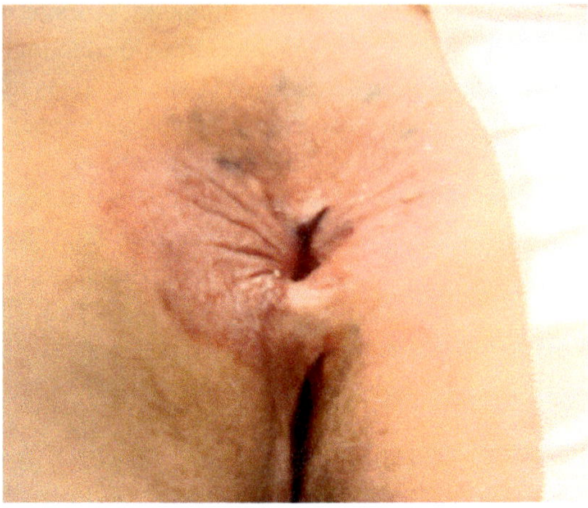

Fig. 18.9 Perianal Paget's disease presenting with anal pruritus

- Common laboratory tests to rule out systemic and infectious causes include liver and kidney function tests, blood glucose level, white blood cell count with differential, C-reactive protein, and erythrocyte sedimentation rate.

Microbiology Testing

- Cultures of perianal skin exudates and infectious material are simple and straightforward but can be misleading if not performed adequately.
- Infected material should be aspirated with a syringe and expelled into a sterile container.
- Alternatively, a swab may be used to collect a specimen, but this is less than ideal.
- Culture specimens should be placed in appropriate medias (anaerobic, bacterial, fungal, and viral) and refrigerated without delay.
- Viral cultures should be kept on ice. Fluid from vesicular lesions should be aspirated or taken with a swab from the base of an unroofed lesion and placed on a cell culture media or a microscopic slide for Tzanck smears if herpes zoster is suspected.
- Swabs should be lubricated with saline if lubricated at all because conventional water-soluble lubricant is bactericidal for some organisms including *Neisseria gonorrhoeae*.
- Skin scrapings may be submitted for fungus culture.

- Scrapings can also be examined for hyphae with KOH prep, but this test is rarely available because of the lack of trained and experienced personnel.
- It is essential to have discussed the proper arrangements with the laboratory and nursing personnel (clinic and operating room) to assure adequate specimen handling and testing well before obtaining a specimen.
- In patients with diarrhea, bacterial stool cultures as well as ova and parasites on three different stool samples can be useful.
- In patients with suspected or confirmed streptococcal or staphylococcal perianal infections, nasal or throat swabs rarely detect the offending bacteria and therefore are unnecessary.
- If pinworms are suspected, a cellophane or scotch tape test in the early morning identifies adult worms and their eggs and confirms the diagnosis.

Patch Testing

- Patients with an extensive list of allergies, both dietary and drug-related, are good candidates for patch testing.
- This usually involves a dermatologic consultation, which can be very helpful when the staff has a particular interest in perianal dermatology (Table 18.4).
- It is important to also test the patient's own products as these have been shown to be a significant etiology in pruritus ani.

Table 18.4 Patch test findings in 58 consecutive patients suspected of having allergic contact anal eczema (26)

Contact allergen	N (%)
Thimerosal	11 (19)
Patients' own products	6 (10)
Balsam of Peru (*Myroxylon pereirae*)	5 (9)
Amerchol	3 (5)
Lanolin alcohol	3 (5)
Nickel sulfate	3 (5)
Fragrances/perfumes	3 (5)
Lidocaine, benzocaine	2 (3)
Propolis	1 (2)
Neomycin	1 (2)

Anoscopy: Proctoscopy

- All patients with pruritus ani should undergo anoscopy and flexible sigmoidoscopy.
- Full colonoscopy is indicated for patients who are age-appropriate for colorectal cancer screening and those with hematochezia, iron-deficiency anemia, and positive family history of colorectal cancer.

Biopsy

- Skin lesions not responding to treatment or suspicious for malignancy require biopsy.
- This is the single most valuable test in patients with primary pruritus ani and should include an area of the lesion with adjacent normal skin.
- Specific query should be made to a pathologist with expertise in dermatologic pathology with clinically suspected diagnoses.
- Biopsy may conveniently be done with either an 11 blade or skin punch blades (Keyes dermal punches).

Evidence-Based Management

- The management of dermatologic diseases of the anus in practice is particularly challenging for several reasons.
  - These conditions are hidden on a part of the body often associated with embarrassment, and therefore patients may have advanced disease before they present to a doctor for help.
  - Additionally, there is limited class A data regarding the management of pruritus ani.

Aims of Treatment

- The aims of treatment for any form of anal dermatitis are rapid relief of symptoms, healing of dermatitis, and prevention of recurrence.

- Long-term recurrence can be prevented in many patients by avoiding contact with allergens and irritants, as well as curing the underlying anorectal disease or condition.

Primary Prutitis Ani

- Because primary or idiopathic pruritus ani is more common, a therapeutic trial of generic management is recommended.
- This will be effective in more than 90% of patients.
- This management strategy focuses on reestablishing ideal anal hygiene and providing reassurance that there is no underlying condition causing the symptoms.
  - Treatment begins with avoiding known irritants such as soaps, lotions, creams, perfumed powders, medicated baby wipes, and any product with witch hazel.
  - The patient must also know to avoid further trauma to the perianal skin, which may be caused by scratching, dry toilet paper, and vigorous scrubbing with bathing.
    - Gently blotting the skin clean with moist toilet paper, a cotton ball, or a soft, unscented, and non-medicated baby wipe is recommended.
  - An important part of the initial management of primary pruritus ani is to avoid moisture and keep the perianal area dry.
  - Patients should avoid tight-fitting, synthetic undergarments and may also use a small piece of cotton or makeup removal pad to help soak up any excess moisture.
  - The brief use of a hair dryer with cool air is an excellent way to keep the perianal skin dry after cleansing.
  - Unscented Dove® (Unilever, London, UK) is free of conventional soap and is the preferred bathing agent.
  - It is also important for patients to maintain regular bowel movements of normal consistency.
    - This is especially useful to avoid seepage and fecal contamination of the perianal skin.
    - A high-fiber diet without excessive fluid intake and the judicious use of loperamide or cholestyramine is recommended, as needed.
    - As mentioned earlier in this chapter, an elimination diet excluding "high-risk" dietary components such as coffee, tea, chocolate, soda, and alcohol for 2 weeks can be strongly considered in most patients with primary pruritus ani.
- In those patients in whom the initial management strategy is not effective after 4–6 weeks, attention is directed toward excluding the multiple potential causes of secondary pruritus ani.
  - If no secondary cause can be found, topical therapy is recommended (Table 18.5).
  - Topical steroids are an effective and safe treatment option.
    - First-line topical treatment includes preparations with a low-potency topical steroid such as 1% hydrocortisone, which should not be given for more than 8 weeks.
    - Potent or extended use of topical steroids should be avoided as they can lead to skin atrophy, infections, and worsened pruritus ani (Fig. 18.10).
  - Capsaicin has also been studied in a randomized fashion in 44 patients with primary pruritus ani.
    - This topical agent decreases levels of substance P, a neuropeptide that triggers itching and burning pain.
    - Topical capsaicin (0.006%) showed relief of symptoms in 70% of patients as compared to 2% patients who received placebo (1% menthol).
- The majority of patients with moderate symptoms and minimal skin changes will respond well to low-dose topical steroids or topical capsaicin.
- These preparations are applied at night and in the morning after bathing.
- If topical steroids are used, a tapering regimen should be set in place ending with substitution of a barrier cream such as Calmoseptine® (Calmoseptine, Inc., Huntington Beach, CA).

Table 18.5 Marketed topical products most commonly prescribed for the treatment of perianal dermatitis (66)

Active ingredients	Brand name(s)
Single active agents	
Hydrocortisone	Procto-Kit, DermoPosterisan
Tribenoside	Borraza G
Cinchocaine	Dolapostern
Glyceryl trinitrate	Rectogesic
Corticosteroids + local anesthetics	
Hydrocortisone + pramocaine or cinchocaine or lidocaine or benzocaine + amylocaine + aesculin	Pramosone, Proctofoam, Proctocreme HC, Porctosedyl, Xyloproct
Prednisolone + cinchocaine or + desonide + lidocaine + heparin + vitamins A and E	Scheriproct, Cirkan
Diflucortolone + lidocaine	Neriproct
Fluocinonide + lidocaine	Jelliproct
Fluocortolone + lidocaine or cinchocaine	Doloproct, Ultraproct
Fluocinolone + lidocaine (+ menthol + bismuth)	Synalar Rectal
Corticosteroids + antimicrobials/antiseptics	
Hydrocortisone + benzyl benzoate + Peru balsam + bismuth + zinc with or without resorcinol	Anusol HC
Corticosteroids + local anesthetics + antimicrobials/antiseptics	
Hydrocortisone + cinchocaine with neomycin + aesculin or framycetin	Proctosedyl
Local anesthetics + antimicrobials/antiseptics	
Cinchocaine + polycresulin	Faktu
Other combinations	
Trimebutine + ruscogenin	Proctolog
Peru balsam + bismuth + zinc	Anusol
Hydrocortisone + Escherichia coli suspension	Posterisan
Hydrocortisone + phenylephrine + paraffin oil + fish oil	Preparation H
Lidocaine + carraginates + zinc	Titanoreine

Products with >10,000 prescriptions in 2011 according to IMS data for Brazil, France, Germany, Japan, the UK, and the USA

- Patients with chronic perianal skin changes should be managed with a medium- or high-potency steroid (Table 18.6).
  - It is important to emphasize to patients that a high-potency steroid should be used for a limited period of time, generally 4–8 weeks.
  - Once normalization of the skin has occurred, patients are switched to a mild steroid that can be further tapered down to bi-weekly applications until total elimination.
- Nonirritating cleansers are highly recommended during the initial therapeutic trial.
  - Dilute white vinegar (one tablespoon in an 8-ounce glass of water) on a cotton ball is a cheap and effective non-soapy cleanser.
  - Tea tree oil, a volatile oil with antibacterial and antifungal properties, works well for patients with moist perianal skin and pruritus.
- Patients who come to the office with acute moderate-to-severe changes of the perianal skin may be treated with Berwick's dye (crystal violet 1% + brilliant green 1% + 95% ethanol 50% + distilled H2O q.s.ad. 100%).
  - Dried with a hair dryer and subsequently covered with benzoin tincture as a barrier and dried similarly.
  - This topical treatment will stay in place for several days if only water is used to cleanse, relieves symptoms rapidly, and allows for reepithelialization of broken-down skin.

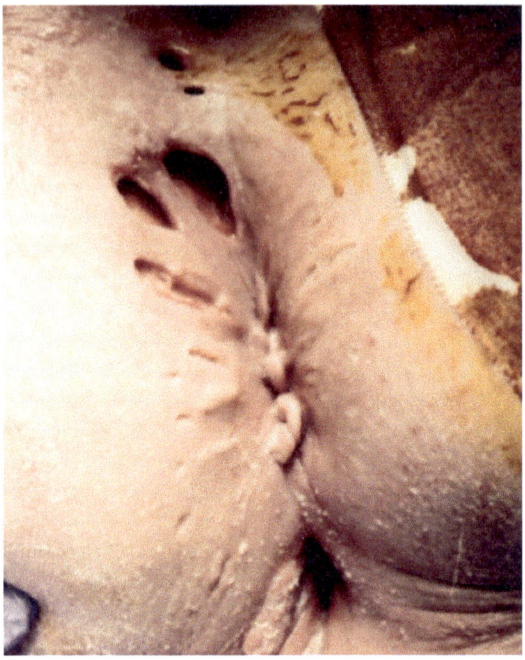

Fig. 18.10 Chronic skin changes of atrophy and ulcerations secondary to pruritus ani with associated left buttock infection in a patient who had been taking steroids for 8 years

Table 18.6 Relative potency of topical steroids

Group 1 (most potent)
Betamethasone dipropionate 0.05% (Diprolene®)
Clobetasol propionate 0.05% (Temovate®)
Group 2
Desoximetasone 0.25% (Topicort®)
Fluocinonide 0.05% (Lidex®)
Group 3
Betamethasone valerate ointment 0.1% (Valisone®)
Triamcinolone acetonide 0.5% (Aristocort®)
Group 4
Desoximetasone 0.05% (TopicortLP®)
Flurandrenolide 0.05% (Cordran®)
Group 5
Betamethasone valerate cream 0.1% (Valisone®)
Hydrocortisone butyrate 0.1% (Locoid®)
Triamcinolone acetonide 0.1% (Kenalog®)
Group 6 (least potent)
Alclometasone dipropionate 0.05% (Aclovate®)
Hydrocortisone 1%

Finne CO, Fenyk JR. Dermatology and pruritus ani. In: Fleshman JW, Wolff BG, editors. The ASCRS textbook of colon and rectal surgery. New York: Springer; 2007. p. 277–294. ©Springer

- Skin breakdown or maceration caused by scratching or over-vigorous cleansing efforts must be avoided.
- A combination of topical and systemic medications has shown the best results compared to either alone.
  - Doxepin (both topical and oral) and hydroxyzine are effective adjuncts to reduce or eliminate itching.
    - Doxepin, a tricyclic antidepressant, possesses both anti-H1 and anti-H2 activities.
    - Hydroxyzine, a potent H1 receptor inverse agonist, has shown to have equal antipruritic efficacy compared to oral doxepin but with higher sedation effects.
  - Patients may not be aware of nocturnal scratching, and this can be a serious contributing factor in many cases of primary pruritus ani.
- For intractable cases or primary pruritus ani, intradermal injection of methylene blue has been described with some efficacy (Fig. 18.11).
  - The presumed mechanism of symptomatic improvement is through the destruction of nerve endings.
  - Intracutaneous and subcutaneous injection of 30 mL of 0.25% bupivacaine with 1:200,000 epinephrine mixed with equal volumes of 0.5% lidocaine at the anoderm and perianal areas in the operating room.
  - After this, 20 to 30 mL of 0.5% methylene blue was injected at the same sites using a 25-gauge spinal needle.
  - Risk of full-thickness skin necrosis.
  - Mentes et al. used a slightly different technique.
    - Intradermal and subcutaneous injection of a mixture of 7–8 mL of 2% methylene blue with equal volumes of 0.5% lidocaine without previous local anesthesia or sedation.
    - No major complications or cases of skin necrosis were reported, likely due to a smaller injected volume.

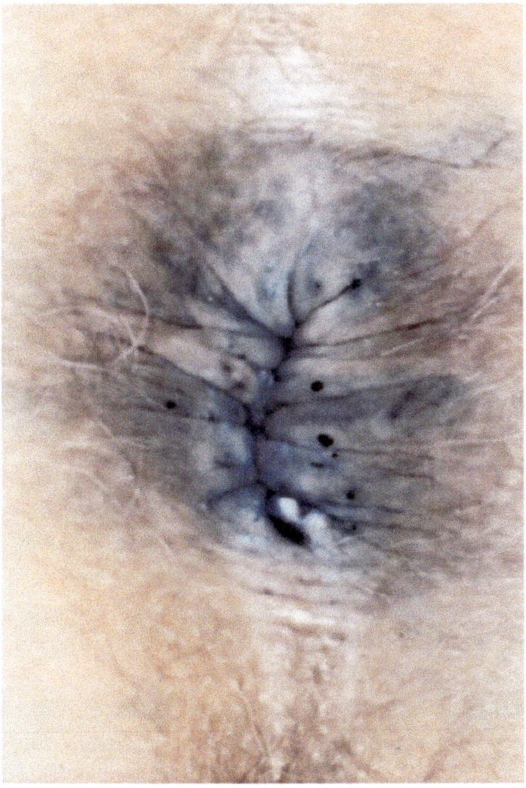

Fig. 18.11 Tattooing with methylene blue for severe refractory idiopathic pruritus ani. (Courtesy of C.O Finne, St Paul, MN)

Secondary Prutitis Ani

Infectious

- Bacterial infections of the perianal region should be treated with systemic antibiotics.
- If a specific agent has not been identified, antibiotic coverage should include Gram-positive and Gram-negative cocci.
- Parenteral antibiotics have been reported to be especially useful with *Staphylococcus aureus* infection.
- When refractory pruritus ani is associated with cultures that show growth of *Candida albicans*, antifungals should be given, especially in patients who are immunosuppressed and diabetic or who were recently treated with systemic steroids or antibiotics.
  - We have seen good results with a combination of oral fluconazole and topical luliconazole 1%, given for 2–3 weeks.
  - When dermatophytes are found in the setting of pruritus ani, this associated fungal infection should also be treated appropriately.
- The treatment of erythrasma involves systemic antibiotics, typically erythromycin 250 mg *qid* for 10 days, or tetracycline may be used as a second alternative.
- Silver sulfadiazine is an effective topical adjunct in patients with bacterial perianal dermatitis, especially in patients with ulcerations and fissuring skin as it sooths and promotes reepithelialization.

Dermatologic

- With regard to anal eczema, both the European and American Academy of Allergy, Asthma, and Immunology guidelines recommend starting treatment with basic skin care.
- Keys to success include avoiding allergens, irritants and tight constricting undergarments, liberal use of warm sitz baths for comfort, and keeping the affected area dry at all other times.
- As mentioned above, gentle but thorough cleansing of the perianal area with soap substitutes (i.e., Dove) is recommended during bathing.
- When these methods fail, mild-to-moderately potent topical corticosteroids for 2–3 weeks periods are recommended.
- Topical calcineurin inhibitors such as tacrolimus and pimecrolimus are also effective for reducing inflammation and itch in patients with anal eczema and also avoid skin atrophy.
- Although systemic gamma interferon and narrowband UVB therapy has shown promising results in patients with atopic dermatitis as well as cholestatic and uremic pruritus, no evidence in patients with pruritus ani exists.
- Treatment of atopic dermatitis begins with providing a barrier such as Vaseline® (white petrolatum USP) or Calmoseptine® (Calmoseptine, Inc., Huntington Beach, CA) and the use of anti-inflammatory agents (systemic and topical) and antipruritic agents.
- Psoriasis is not a curable condition, but symptoms can be well controlled with mild topical

steroid preparations (i.e., 1% hydrocortisone cream).

- Seborrheic dermatitis responds well to 2% sulfur with 1% hydrocortisone or miconazole lotion.
- Lichen sclerosus is initially managed with topical steroids.
  - Potent topical steroid creams, such as clobetasol 0.05%, for a short course (4–6 weeks) followed by less potent hydrocortisone cream are the mainstay of treatment.
  - Systemic steroids are given only for very severe cases.
  - Topical calcineurin inhibitors are effective alternatives in patients who have failed therapy with potent corticosteroids or who have a contraindication for the use of corticosteroids.
  - Treatment with retinoid and testosterone creams may be useful in selective cases.
- The treatment of lichen simplex chronicus or neurodermatitis
  - Begins with topical steroids to decrease the inflammation and break the itch-scratch-itch cycle.
  - Antihistamines, doxepin, or capsaicin creams are effective adjuncts to topical steroids.
  - For patients who have a poor response to topical steroids, topical acetylsalicylic acid/dichloromethane or immunomodulators, such as tacrolimus, have shown positive results.
- Treatment of perianal Paget's disease requires wide local excision.
  - Soft tissue and skin reconstruction frequently requires V-Y gluteal flaps or skin grafting, with the assistance of plastic surgery.
  - Recurrence of disease is common and may occur up to a decade after initial excision; therefore, regular and long-term follow-up is imperative.

Systemic Diseases

- Effective treatment of pruritus ani in patients with poorly controlled or exacerbated systemic disease involves appropriate management of the underlying disease.
- Appropriate skin cleansing, application of a topical barrier, and antipruritic agents are the mainstay of treatment.
- Cimetidine has been reported to eliminate itching induced by lymphoma and polycythemia vera.
- In our experience, doxepin and gabapentin are also effective antipruritic agents in patients with systemically induced pruritus ani.
- Chronic itching in these patients may also lead to lichenification and secondary infections; appropriate systemic antibiotic or antifungal therapy is warranted.

Sexually Transmitted Infections

19

Cindy J. Kin and Mark L. Welton

Key Concepts

- Nucleic acid amplification tests are superior to culture to screen for *Chlamydia trachomatis* and *Neisseria gonorrhea* infections. The best specimens are vaginal or endocervical swabs from women and first catch urine samples from men.
- Nucleic acid amplification tests for *Chlamydia trachomatis* and *Neisseria gonorrhea* can be used for rectal and oropharyngeal specimens in addition to genital sites to increase the sensitivity of testing.
- If one suspects failure of standard antibiotic treatment for gonococcal infection, then culture needs to be performed to evaluate antibiotic susceptibility.
- Infections causing rectal or genital ulcerations increase the risk for infection with HIV in both men and women, compared to patients with non-ulcerative STIs.
- Patients diagnosed with syphilis should be tested for HIV. Patients with HIV should be regularly screened for syphilis.
- Empiric treatment for proctitis in populations at high risk for STIs should be given at the time of evaluation rather than waiting for test results and should consist of treatment for gonorrhea, chlamydia/lymphogranuloma venereum, and genital herpes.
- Herpes simplex virus is a common cause of proctitis in men who have sex with men and may often present without visible external ulcerations.

C. J. Kin (✉)
Department of Surgery, Stanford University School of Medicine, Stanford, CA, USA
e-mail: cindykin@stanford.edu

M. L. Welton
Corporate Department, Fairview Health Services, Minneapolis, MN, USA

Introduction

- "Sexually transmitted diseases" (STD) and "sexually transmitted infections" (STI) are interchangeably used terms, but the latter has been increasingly adopted to emphasize that infections may not cause symptoms of disease nor may they result in development of disease.
- Clinicians must maintain a high level of suspicion for STIs to avoid delays or errors in diagnosis.
- A frank discussion of the patient's sexual history should direct STI testing and empiric therapy.
- A substantial proportion of patients with STIs are completely asymptomatic.
  - 7% of men who have sex with men (MSM) undergoing screening for STI test will be positive for at least one infection.
  - HIV-positive MSM with an STI are twice as likely to be being asymptomatic from the STI than HIV-negative MSM with an STI.

S. R. Steele et al. (eds.), *The ASCRS Manual of Colon and Rectal Surgery*,
https://doi.org/10.1007/978-3-030-01165-9_19

Screening Guidelines for Asymptomatic High-Risk Patients

- The predominant risk factor for contracting STIs is high-risk sexual behavior.
- Other risk factors include current infection with ulcerative STIs and HIV seropositivity.
- MSM, especially those who engage in unprotected receptive anal intercourse, represent the demographic group at greatest risk for STIs and should undergo regular universal testing for STIs.
- People in high-risk sexual networks such as swingers are also at very high risk for STIs and should also undergo universal testing for STIs.
- A policy of universal testing can help to stop the cycle of ongoing transmission of STIs within these networks.
- MSM and other high-risk populations including prostitutes and swingers should undergo testing for STIs (mainly, chlamydia and gonorrhea) at anorectal, oropharyngeal, and urogenital sites.
  - Isolated non-urogenital infections represented the majority of infections in both MSM and high-risk women.

Screening Guidelines for Symptomatic Patients

- Symptoms of STIs may include painful or painless perianal or genital lesions; rectal, vaginal, or urethral discharge; or proctitis.
- Table 19.1 details the suspected etiologies, recommended testing, and empiric therapy by symptom class.

Perianal or Genital Lesions

- Lesions or other symptoms involving the anus and perianal skin may be easily mistaken for other diagnoses so physical exam of the perianal skin and anal canal is crucial.
- Genital lesions in young sexually active patients are most likely to be genital herpes or syphilis.
- Less commonly, chancroid and donovanosis may also be the cause of genital ulcers.
- The genital lesions of molluscum contagiosum may cause pruritus.
- Painless lesions may be condyloma or other HPV-related dysplasia.
- Empiric treatment of the most likely pathogen should be started.

Table 19.1 Initial sexually transmitted infections (STI) testing and empiric therapy by symptom

Symptom	Suspected etiology	Testing	Empiric therapy
Genital, anal, perianal ulcers	Herpes Syphilis Chancroid Donovanosis	Syphilis serology HSV culture or PCR HIV *H. ducreyi* testing in settings where chancroid is prevalent	Treatment for HSV or syphilis depending on clinical suspicion
Proctitis	Gonorrhea Chlamydia Syphilis Herpes	Intra-anal swabs for chlamydia and gonorrhea and HSV culture or PCR	
Proctocolitis	*Campylobacter*, *Shigella*, and *Entamoeba histolytica* LGV	Stool studies NAAT for chlamydia	
Enteritis	Giardia	Stool studies	

HSV herpes simplex virus, *LGV* lymphogranuloma venerum, *PCR* polymerase chain reaction, *NAAT* nucleic acid amplification tests

Proctitis

- Proctitis is inflammation of the rectum, causing symptoms of anorectal pain, tenesmus, and discharge (Fig. 19.1).
- The suspected etiologic agents are *N. gonorrhea*, *C. trachomatis*, *T. pallidum*, and HSV.
- Patient discomfort may preclude a proctoscopic examination, but intra-anal swabs for chlamydia and gonorrhea and HSV can and should be performed.
  - Swabs should be taken before doing a rectal exam with lubricant given its bacteriostatic properties.
- Infectious proctitis is often misdiagnosed as inflammatory bowel disease so it is important to elicit a clear sexual history to help distinguish between the two.
- Anorectal pain and bleeding may also signal the presence of a malignancy such as anal or rectal cancer.
- Patients who present with both symptoms of proctitis and an anal ulceration are very likely to have HSV (83%) or gonorrhea.
- HIV-positive MSM presenting with proctitis are:
  - More likely than their HIV-negative counterparts with proctitis to be infected with HSV-1 (14% vs. 7%) or HSV-2 (22% vs. 12%), lymphogranuloma venereum (8% vs. 0.7%), or multiple STIs (18% vs. 9%)
  - Equally likely to have chlamydia or gonorrhea
- Empiric treatment for proctitis should be given at the time of evaluation rather than waiting for test results and should consist of treatment for gonorrhea (ceftriaxone 250 mg intramuscular × 1), chlamydia/LGV (doxycycline 100 mg bid × 21 days), and HSV (valacyclovir 1 g bid × 10 days).
- Symptom management with topical anesthetics and stool softeners will also be helpful.
- When test results come back, the medication regimen can be adjusted.

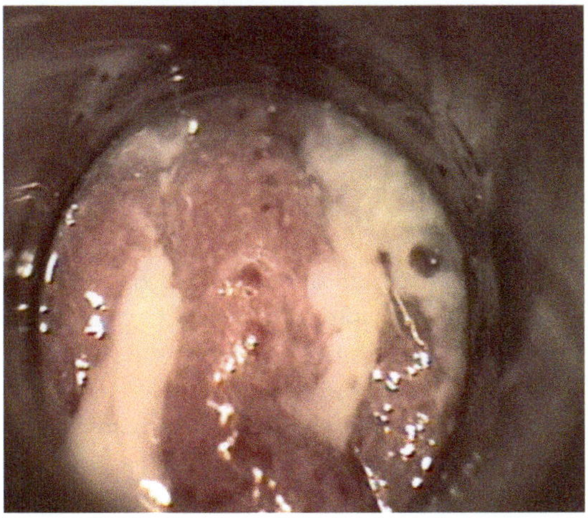

Fig. 19.1 Patients with STIs may present with proctitis, characterized by anorectal pain, tenesmus, and mucopurulent discharge. Proctoscopy may not be possible due to pain

Proctocolitis

- Proctocolitis causes symptoms of proctitis (anorectal pain, tenesmus, and discharge) along with diarrhea and abdominal cramps.
- Lower endoscopy reveals inflammation of the rectal and distal colonic mucosa.
- Stool studies may reveal fecal leukocytes.
- The suspected etiologic agents include *Campylobacter*, *Shigella*, and *Entamoeba histolytica*. LGV serovars of *C. trachomatis* may also cause proctocolitis.
- The route of transmission may be oral or oral-anal.

Enteritis

- Symptoms of enteritis include diarrhea and abdominal cramping; since the rectum is not involved, patients will not present with proctitis symptoms.
- Enteritis acquired as an STI can be attributed to oral-anal contact.
- The most common etiologic agent is *Giardia lamblia*.

Diagnosis and Management of Sexually Transmitted Bacterial Infections

Testing for Chlamydia and Gonorrhea

- Nucleic acid amplification tests (NAATs) are 86% sensitive and 97% specific for detecting gonorrhea and chlamydia.
- NAATs can be used in all circumstances to detect chlamydia and gonorrhea, except for special circumstances involving prepubescent boys and girls, and potential treatment failures in which cultures are indicated.

Gonorrhea

Epidemiology

- *Neisseria gonorrhea* is the causative agent in gonococcal infections.
  - Second most common notifiable communicable disease in the USA
  - Over 300,000 cases reported annually, likely a gross underestimation of the actual disease burden due to underdiagnosis and underreporting
- Groups suffering from particularly high rates include MSM, HIV-positive patients, African Americans, adolescents, and young adults.

Clinical Presentation

- Men
  - Urethritis manifesting as painful urination.
  - Epididymitis.
  - Proctitis, in those who engage in anal receptive intercourse.
  - Disseminated infection can also occur.
- Women
  - Tend to be asymptomatic although they can cause cervicitis, urethritis, proctitis, and, later, pelvic inflammatory disease

Screening and Testing for *N. gonorrhoeae*

- CDC recommends routine screening of oropharyngeal, anorectal, and urogenital sites for all MSM who are sexually active and at risk for STI.
  - Nucleic acid amplification tests (NAATs), with at least 86% sensitivity and 97% specificity for detecting gonorrhea and chlamydia, are the recommended testing method.
    - First catch urine and urethral swab are the recommended sample types for men.
    - In women, the recommended sample types are vaginal swabs that can be either self- or clinician-collected or endocervical swab if a pelvic examination is also indicated.
    - First catch urine in women may miss 10% of infections compared to the other sample types.
    - Rectal and oropharyngeal specimens can also be tested with NAATs.

Treatment and Management of Gonorrhea

- For uncomplicated gonococcal infections, the CDC recommends combination therapy with ceftriaxone 250 mg intramuscular injection, plus a single dose of oral azithromycin 1 g or a 7-day course of oral doxycycline 100 mg twice daily.
- Azithromycin is preferred due to the high prevalence of tetracycline resistance.
- Patients with allergies to cephalosporins can be treated with a single oral dose of azithromycin 2 g, but *N. gonorrhea* isolates have demonstrated resistance to azithromycin (Fig. 19.2).
- *N. gonorrhea* culture testing to evaluate for antibiotic susceptibility should be performed if treatment failure is clinically suspected, or NAAT positivity persists.
- Patients who have undergone treatment for gonorrhea should be referred to programs to reduce STI risk and also undergo retesting for gonorrhea at 3 months.
- Sexual partners of infected patients in the preceding 2 months should also undergo treatment with ceftriaxone and azithromycin.

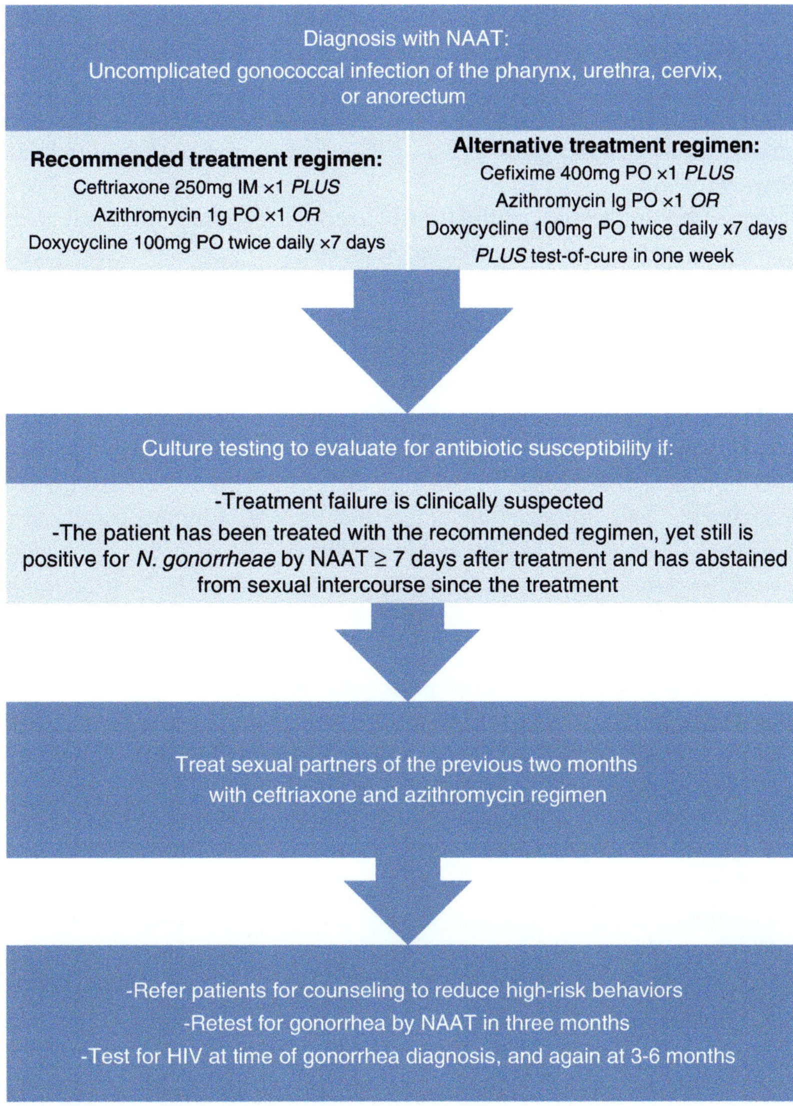

Fig. 19.2 Treatment algorithm for patients with *N. gonorrhea* infection

Emerging Antibiotic Resistance

- *N. gonorrhea* has a record of developing antibiotic resistance – to penicillins and tetracyclines in the 1980s and then to fluoroquinolones and cephalosporins in the 2000s.

Chlamydia

Epidemiology

- Infection with *Chlamydia trachomatis* is the most common notifiable disease in the USA with over 1.3 million cases reported to the CDC in 2010.

Clinical Presentation

- Most patients with chlamydia are asymptomatic or have such mild nonspecific symptoms that a visit to a physician never occurs and they never become aware that they are infected.
- Therefore, screening is crucial to controlling this disease and preventing the severe potential sequelae of pelvic inflammatory disease

that increases the risk of infertility (20%), chronic pelvic pain (18%), and ectopic pregnancy (9%).

Screening and Testing for *C. trachomatis*

- Recommended testing method for *C. trachomatis* is the NAAT, and the recommended sample type for men is a first catch urine or urethral swab and, for women, vaginal swab.
- Urine samples from women are less sensitive.
- Rectal and oropharyngeal specimens should also be used for screening to increase the sensitivity of the test.
- There is a high incidence of co-occurrence of anorectal and urogenital chlamydia in women – over 94% of women with anorectal infection also have urogenital chlamydia, and over 71% of women with urogenital infection also have anorectal infection.
- Due to its high prevalence and serious sequelae, and the potential to reduce the incidence of pelvic inflammatory disease, the CDC and the US Preventive Services Task Force recommend screening sexually active women aged 24 and younger for chlamydia, as well as older women at increased risk for infection.
- Routine universal screening for men is not recommended, as complications from chlamydia infection in men are rare.
- Screening is recommended for certain high-risk male populations including men in STI clinics, national job training programs, and juvenile detention facilities, as well as men under 30 years old who are in the military or in jail, men whose partners have been diagnosed with chlamydia, and all MSM reporting receptive anorectal intercourse.

Treatment and Repeat Testing

- A single oral dose of 1 g of azithromycin is the recommended treatment for *C. trachomatis* infection and should be given empirically for acute nongonococcal urethritis or for suspected or proven infection in women.
- A 7-day course of twice daily doxycycline 100 mg is equally effective.
- Alternative regimens include 7-day courses of erythromycin, levofloxacin, or ofloxacin (Table 19.2) (18).
- Patients should be instructed not to engage in sexual intercourse for 7 days after the single dose of azithromycin (or until they complete the full 7-day course of the other antibiotic regimens), and they should also avoid having sexual intercourse until their partners are treated as well to avoid reinfection.
- Patients should be counseled to refer anyone with whom they have had sexual contact in the 60 days prior to chlamydia diagnosis or symptoms for testing and treatment.
- Routine test-of-cure several weeks after treatment for chlamydia is not recommended by the CDC if the patient has undergone appropriate treatment and is asymptomatic with no suspicion of reinfection.

Lymphogranuloma Venereum

Epidemiology

- *C. trachomatis* serovars L1, L2, and L3 cause lymphogranuloma venereum.
  - L2b, previously undescribed, has been identified as the main causative agent of the recent epidemic.
  - LGV serovars cause severe inflammation and invasive infection.
- Hemorrhagic proctitis due to LGV has only been reported in MSM.
- Risk factors for LGV proctitis include HIV seropositivity and chlamydia with concurrent ulcerative disease, previously diagnosed STI, unprotected receptive anal intercourse with casual partners, MSM, having sex at sex parties, and having sex with HIV-positive partners.
- MSM with anorectal chlamydia should undergo LGV testing; if it is not available, then MSM with anorectal chlamydia and either proctitis, >10 white blood cells per high power field on anorectal smear, or HIV seropositivity should be treated empirically for LGV (Fig. 19.3).

Table 19.2 Centers for Disease Control recommended antibiotic regimens for bacterial sexually transmitted infections (STI)

Infection	Recommended regimens	Alternative regimens
Chlamydia trachomatis	Azithromycin 1 g oral × 1 dose or Doxycycline 100 mg orally twice daily for 7 days	Erythromycin base 500 mg orally four times daily for 7 days or Erythromycin ethylsuccinate 800 mg orally four times daily for 7 days or Levofloxacin 500 mg orally once daily for 7 days or Ofloxacin 300 mg orally twice daily for 7 days
Neisseria gonorrhea	Ceftriaxone 250 mg intramuscular injection ×1 *plus* Azithromycin 1 g orally ×1 *or* Doxycycline 100 mg orally twice daily for 7 days	Cefixime 400 mg PO ×1 *plus* Azithromycin 1 g PO ×1 *or* Doxycycline 100 mg PO twice daily ×7 days *plus* test-of-cure in 1 week
Acute proctitis in patient with recent receptive anla intercourse, with anorectal exudate or WBCs on gram-stained smear	Treat empirically with: Ceftriaxone 250 mg intramuscularly × 1 dose *plus* Doxycycline 100 mg orally twice daily for 7 days	
LGV proctitis/proctocolitis (MSM with anorectal chlamydia and proctitis or HIV)	Doxycycline 100 mg orally twice daily for 3 weeks	Erythromycin base 500 mg orally four times daily for 3 weeks
Primary, secondary, or early latent syphilis	Penicillin G benzathine 2.4 million units intramuscularly × 1 dose	Doxycycline 100 mg orally twice daily for 2 weeks or Tetracycline 500 mg four times daily for 2 weeks Pregnant women with syphilis should undergo desensitization and be treated with penicillin regimen[a]
Tertiary or late latent syphilis or syphilis of unknown duration	Penicillin G benzathine 2.4 million units intramuscularly once per week for 3 weeks	
Neurosyphilis	Aqueous crystalline penicillin G 18–24 million units per day, administered as 3–4 million units intravenously every 4 h or as a continuous infusion, for 10–14 days	
Chancroid	Ceftriaxone 250 mg intramuscularly × 1 dose or Azithromycin 1 g orally × 1 dose or Ciprofloxacin 500 mg orally twice daily for 3 days or Erythromycin base 500 mg orally three times daily for 7 days	

(continued)

Table 19.2 (continued)

Infection	Recommended regimens	Alternative regimens
Granuloma inguinale (donovanosis)	Doxycycline 100 mg orally twice daily[a]	Azithromycin 1 g orally once per week[a] or Ciprofloxacin 750 mg orally twice daily[a] or Erythromycin base 500 mg orally four times daily[a] or Trimethoprim/sulfamethoxazole 800 mg/160 mg orally twice daily[a]

WBC white blood count, *HIV* human immunodeficiency virus, *MSM* men who have sex with men, *LGV* lymphogranuloma venerum

[a]All regimens are for at least 3-week duration and should be continued until all lesions have healed

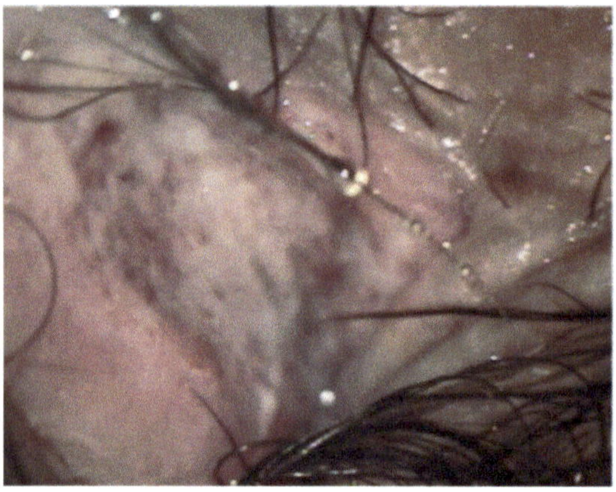

Fig. 19.3 Chlamydia infection may present with no symptoms, mild symptoms, urethritis, ulcerations, or proctitis. Pictured is an ulcer due to chlamydia infection. (Photograph courtesy of Stephen Goldstone, MD)

- A recommended algorithm for testing and treatment of chlamydia and LGV for MSM reporting anal intercourse is detailed in Fig. 19.4.

Clinical Presentation

- Depending on the site of primary inoculation (genital vs. anorectal), patients will manifest different syndromes.
- Patients with the inguinal syndrome (genital inoculation) experience unilateral painful inguinal or femoral lymphadenopathy (buboes), possibly with a genital ulcer.
- Patients with the anorectal syndrome experience ulcerative proctocolitis or proctitis characterized by mucopurulent discharge and tenesmus, along with systemic constitutional symptoms (Figs. 19.5 and 19.6).
- Untreated LGV infection can result in severe complications including colorectal fistulas and strictures, elephantiasis, infertility, and pelvic fibrosis.
- The proper diagnosis of LGV is frequently delayed because symptoms can be misleading, physicians may be unfamiliar with the disease, and there is no routine diagnostic test for LGV serovars.
- Since LGV proctocolitis presents with bleeding, pain, and tenesmus, it can be mistaken as inflammatory bowel disease.

Treatment

- The recommended treatment is twice daily doxycycline 100 mg orally for 3 weeks or for as long as anorectal symptoms persist.
- Buboes may require aspiration or incision and drainage to prevent ulcerations.
- Clinical follow-up should be continued until signs and symptoms have resolved (Table 19.2).

Syphilis

Epidemiology

- Rates of primary and secondary syphilis, after declining for many years to a nadir of 2.1 cases per 100,000 in the year 2000, have experienced a concerning resurgence to over double that rate to 5.3 per 100,000 in 2013.

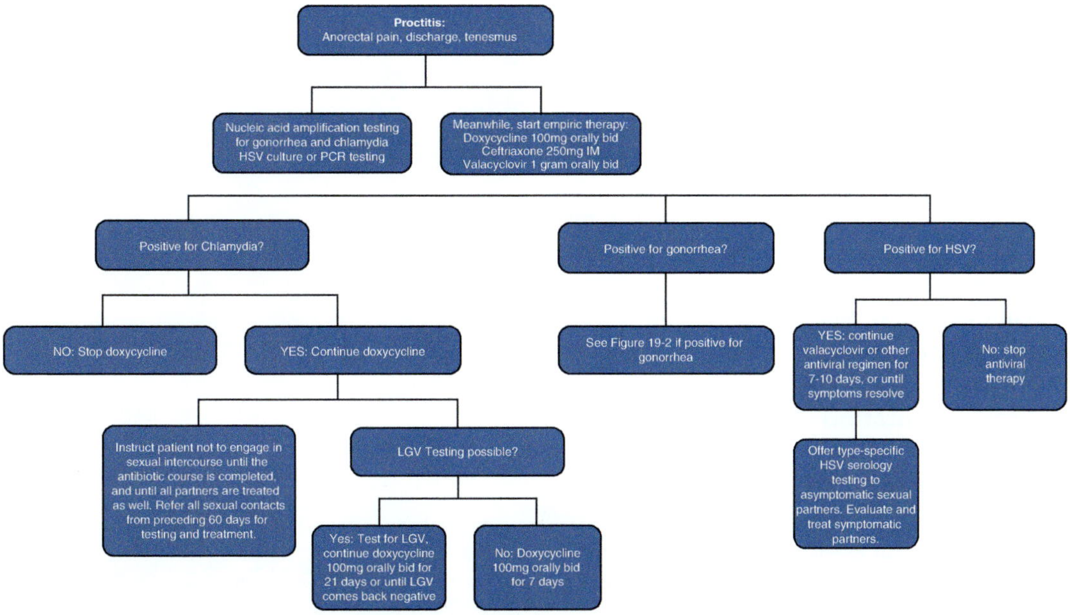

Fig. 19.4 Management algorithm for MSM with proctitis reporting receptive anal intercourse

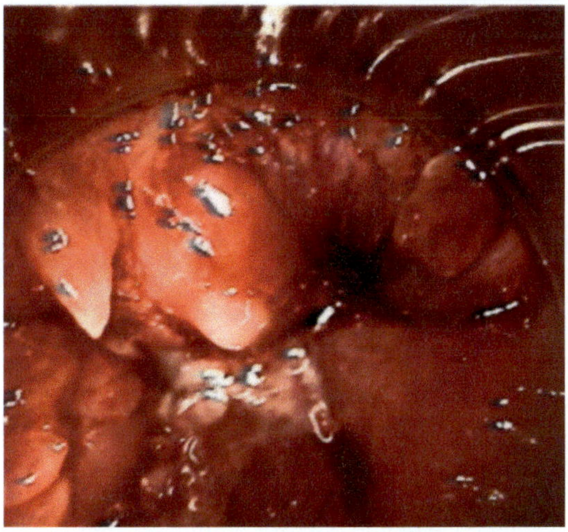

Fig. 19.5 Proctitis due to lymphogranuloma venereum, demonstrating marked inflammation 1 week after treatment started. (Photograph courtesy of Stephen Goldstone, MD)

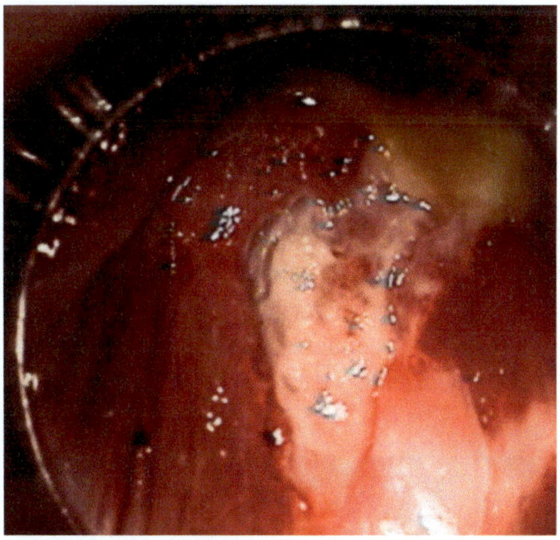

Fig. 19.6 After 2 months of treatment for lymphogranuloma venereum, proctitis has resolved and ulcerations are healing. (Photograph courtesy of Stephen Goldstone, MD)

- Over 90% of cases of primary and secondary syphilis occur in men, and the rise in syphilis rates is attributable to increases in men.
- Men in their 20s, MSM, black men, and Hispanic men have had the greatest increases.
- Similar to their male counterparts, the rate among black and Hispanic women is higher than in white women.
- Half to a third of MSM infected with syphilis are coinfected with HIV.

Clinical Presentation

- Syphilis, caused by the spirochete *Treponema pallidum,* presents classically in its primary form as a solitary nontender genital chancre, but it can also present with multiple chancres or proctitis with bleeding, pain, and tenesmus (Figs. 19.7, 19.8, and 19.9).
- Only a third of patients are diagnosed during the primary infection as the primary chancre can be quite small and unnoticeable.
- HIV-positive patients have a higher rate of asymptomatic primary syphilis, may experience more aggressive secondary infection, and are at increased risk of developing neurosyphilis.

Testing Recommendations

- Two types of serologic tests are used to make a presumptive diagnosis of syphilis.
  - The nontreponemal tests include the venereal disease research laboratory (VDRL) and RPR tests and are used for screening as they become positive within 3 weeks of the primary chancre.
    - Dark field examination to detect *T. pallidum* in lesion exudate or tissue may be successful in diagnosing early syphilis, as the nontreponemal tests may be negative in these early stages.
    - Some patients may manifest a serofast reaction, causing the nontreponemal test to be elevated for a long period of time.
  - Treponemal tests include the fluorescent treponemal antibody-absorbed tests,

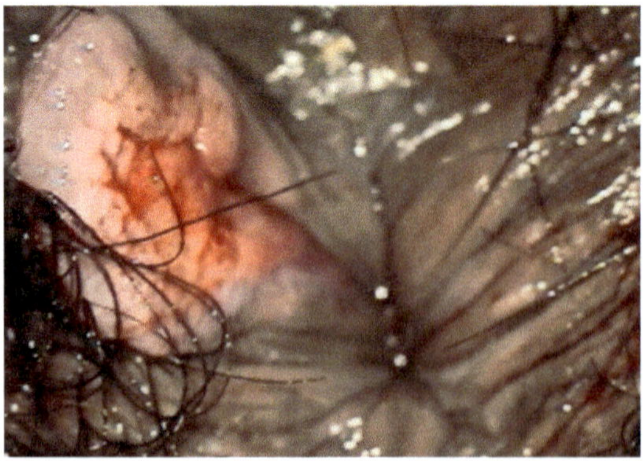

Fig. 19.7 Chancre due to primary syphilis. (Photograph courtesy of Stephen Goldstone, MD)

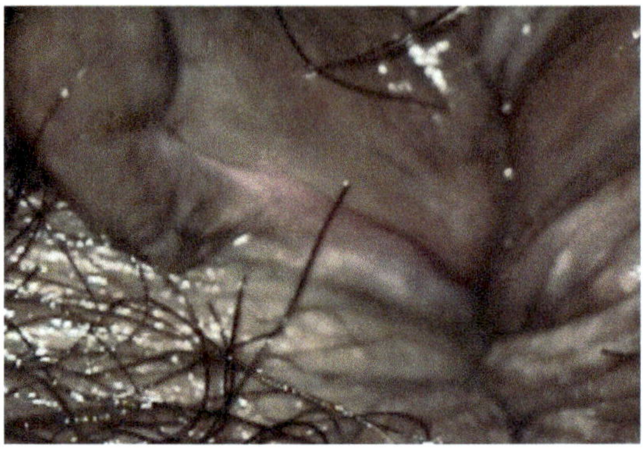

Fig. 19.8 Healed chancre after resolution of primary syphilis. (Photograph courtesy of Stephen Goldstone, MD)

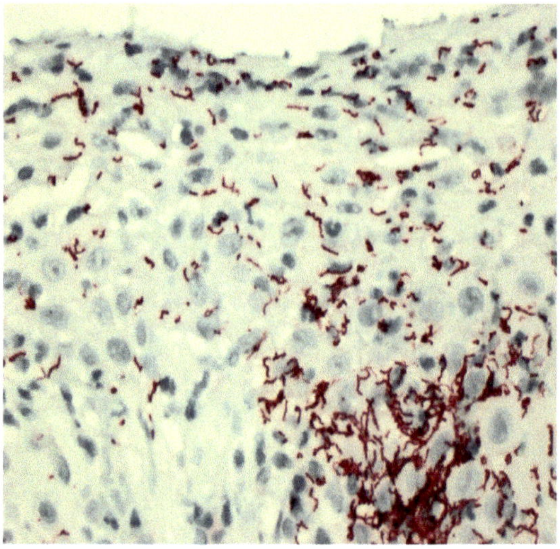

Fig. 19.9 Immunohistochemistry staining for spirochetes, indicative of syphilis infection. (Photograph courtesy of Stephen Goldstone, MD)

T. pallidum passive particle agglutination assay, and other immunoassays.
  - These tests usually remain reactive for life in patients who have had a reactive test at one point.
  - Patients with a positive nontreponemal test should undergo a confirmatory treponemal test.
- Patients with a negative VDRL or RPR but with strong clinical indicators of primary syphilis should undergo repeat nontreponemal testing 2 weeks later.
- Confirmed cases of syphilis must be reported to local and state health departments.
- Due to the rebound in syphilis rates disproportionately affecting MSM, all sexually active MSM should be screened at least annually for syphilis.
- Due to the high rate of coinfection with HIV, patients with syphilis should undergo HIV testing.

Treatment

- The CDC recommends a single intramuscular dose of 2.4 million units of penicillin G benzathine for primary, secondary, and early latent syphilis.
- Patients coinfected with HIV should be treated with the regimen recommended for the treatment of neurosyphilis and should be closely monitored due to increased rates of relapse.
- The Jarisch-Herxheimer reaction, an acute febrile reaction characterized by headache, myalgia, and fever, may develop within 24 h of treatment and occurs most commonly in patients with early syphilis.
- Patients with penicillin allergy should be treated with doxycycline, tetracycline, ceftriaxone, or azithromycin.
- Pregnant women with syphilis and a penicillin allergy should undergo desensitization and be treated with penicillin.
- Sexual contacts of patients with primary, secondary, or early latent syphilis should undergo presumptive treatment.
- Treatment of primary and secondary syphilis should result in a decline of the nontreponemal test titers over the ensuing months.
- Repeat testing with nontreponemal tests should be performed at 6 and 12 months after treatment.
- Retreatment for relapse should consist of 2.4 million units of intramuscular penicillin G benzathine weekly for 3 weeks (Table 19.2).

Chancroid

- Chancroid, caused by *Haemophilus ducreyi*, is a common cause of genital ulcer disease.
- It usually presents with multiple painful purulent genital ulcers that progress through pustular and ulcerative stages, as well as painful regional lymphadenopathy with bubo formation.
- Perianal chancroid is less common than genital chancroid but can occur in MSM.
- Diagnosis can be difficult due to its rarity.
- There are no FDA-approved tests for it in the USA.
- Thus, diagnosis of chancroid is made based on symptoms of painful genital ulceration and regional lymphadenopathy in the absence of syphilis and HSV.
- First-line treatment of chancroid includes azithromycin, erythromycin, ceftriaxone, and ciprofloxacin, detailed in Table 19.2.
- HIV-positive patients may have a higher risk of treatment failure with single-dose regimens.
- Inguinal bubo formation requires at least a 2-week course of antibiotic therapy and may also require aspiration or incision and drainage to prevent spontaneous rupture.

Granuloma Inguinale aka Donovanosis

- Granuloma inguinale is a rare tropical genitoulcerative disease caused by *Klebsiella granulomatis* (formerly *Calymmatobacterium granulomatis*), endemic in Papua New Guinea, South Africa, India, Brazil, and Australia.
- The mode of transmission is via sexual contact, fecal contamination, and autoinoculation.

- Clinical presentation includes papules or nodules that progress into a painless ulcer, usually in the genital area.
- Disseminated disease may cause cervical ulceration, pelvic lymphadenopathy, and septic arthritis and can be mistaken for cervical and ovarian cancer.
- Coinfection with HIV may worsen the course of the disease with more ulceration and tissue damage and thus the need for prolonged antibiotic therapy.
- Malignant transformation can also occur in HIV-positive patients.
- Testing is performed using tissue smears from the lesions and microscopic identification of characteristic intracytoplasmic inclusion bodies (Donovan bodies).
- PCR has recently become available as well.
- Treatment regimens include 3-week courses of doxycycline, ciprofloxacin, erythromycin base, or trimethoprim/sulfamethoxazole.

Diagnosis and Management of Sexually Transmitted Viral Infections

Herpes

Epidemiology

- Herpes simplex virus types 1 and 2 (HSV-1 and HSV-2) are common in the population with a seroprevalence of 54% and 15.7%, respectively.
- Both may cause anogenital herpes infection, while most cases are caused by HSV-2.
- Over 90% of patients with genital herpes are unaware that they have it.
- Primary prevention of genital herpes is difficult due to the high rates of unrecognized infection.
- HSV has been found to be frequently reactivated for short periods of time (less than 12 h) and then rapidly cleared without causing clinical symptoms, likely by the peripheral mucosal immune system.

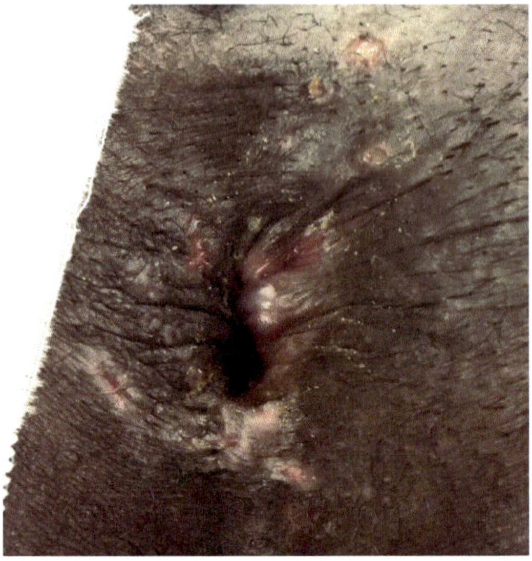

Fig. 19.10 Perianal herpes lesions that have started to resolve

- Men with HSV infection, even when asymptomatic, also have higher rates of HIV shedding which has implications for increased HIV transmission.

Clinical Presentation

- HSV infections classically presents with multiple painful vesicular ulcers, although not all infected patients have these symptoms (Fig. 19.10).
- HSV is the most common cause of proctitis among HIV-positive men, occurring in more than a third of HIV-positive MSM with proctitis.
- HSV is the cause of proctitis in 20% of HIV-negative men with proctitis.
- Only a third of patients with HSV proctitis have external ulcers as well, thus underscoring the need to test and treat for herpes in MSM with proctitis, regardless of the presence of ulcers.
- HSV-2 infection is more likely to cause recurrences than HSV-1 infection.
- Patients who also have HIV are more likely to have more severe and painful lesions and increased HSV shedding, even when they are asymptomatic.

Testing and Screening

- HSV testing can be performed with cell culture or PCR, although a negative result may be attributed to intermittent viral shedding.
- Type-specific HSV serologic assays are also available and can be used to evaluate patients with symptoms of genital herpes but with negative HSV cultures, patients who have a partner with genital herpes, patients seeking an STI evaluation, HIV-positive patients, and MSM at high risk for being infected with HIV.

Treatment

- The first clinical episode of genital herpes can cause severe ulcerations as well as systemic symptoms.
- Therefore, treatment with antiviral therapy – acyclovir, famciclovir, or valacyclovir – is recommended to shorten the course of the episode.
- Suppressive antiviral therapy can decrease the number of recurrences in patients with frequent recurrences (at least four per year).
- Suppressive therapy may also be indicated to decrease the risk for transmission to sexual partners.
- Condom use and avoidance of sexual activity during recurrences offer additional protection against transmission to HSV-negative partners.
- Recommended regimens for treatment of the first clinical episode, suppressive therapy, and episodic therapy are detailed in Table 19.3.

Table 19.3 Centers for Disease Control recommended treatment regimens for viral STIs

Infection	Recommended regimens
Genital herpes (HSV-1 or HSV-2): first clinical episode	Acyclovir 400 mg orally three times daily for 7–10 days or Acyclovir 200 mg orally five times daily for 7–10 days or Famciclovir 250 mg orally three times daily for 7–10 days or Valacyclovir 1 g orally twice daily for 7–10 days
Suppressive therapy for recurrent genital herpes (frequent recurrences)	Acyclovir 400 mg orally twice daily or Famciclovir 250 mg orally twice daily or Valacyclovir 500 mg orally once daily[a] or Valacyclovir 1 g orally once daily
Suppressive therapy for patients coinfected with HSV and HIV	Acyclovir 400–800 mg orally twice to three times per day or Famciclovir 500 mg orally twice day or Valacyclovir 500 mg orally twice daily
Episodic therapy for recurrent genital herpes	Acyclovir 400 mg orally three times daily for 5 days or Acyclovir 800 mg orally twice daily for 5 days or Acyclovir 800 mg orally three times daily for 2 days or Famciclovir 125 mg orally twice daily for 5 days or Famciclovir 1000 mg orally twice daily for 1 day or Famciclovir 500 mg once, then 250 mg orally twice daily for two more days or Valacyclovir 500 mg orally once twice daily for 3 days or Valacyclovir 1 g orally once daily for 5 days

(continued)

Table 19.3 (continued)

Infection	Recommended regimens
Episodic therapy for patients coinfected with HSV and HIV	Acyclovir 400 mg orally three times daily for 5–10 days or Famciclovir 500 mg orally twice daily for 5–10 days or Valacyclovir 1 g orally twice daily for 5–10 days
External genital warts (HPV) Patient-applied	Podofilox 0.5% solution or gel: application with cotton swab twice daily for 3 days, then 4 days without therapy; can repeat cycle up to four times (max 0.5 mL per day) or Imiquimod 5% cream: apply three times per week up to 16 weeks, washing treated area with soap and water 6–10 h afterwards or Sinecatechins 15% ointment: apply three times daily for up to 16 weeks
External genital warts (HPV) Provider-administered	Cryotherapy with liquid nitrogen or cryoprobe or Podophyllin resin 10–25% in a compound tincture of benzoin or Trichloroacetic acid (TCA) or Bichloroacetic acid (BCA) 80–90% or Surgical removal
Anal warts (HPV) Provider-administered	Cryotherapy with liquid nitrogen or Trichloroacetic acid (TCA) or bichloroacetic acid (BCA) 80–90% can be applied weekly as needed or Surgical removal

HIV human immunodeficiency virus, *HSV* herpes simplex virus, *HPV* Human papillomavirus
[a]This regimen may be less effective than the others for patients with over 10 recurrences per year

- Rarely, HSV can cause severe complicated disease requiring hospitalization and intravenous acyclovir therapy.
- For patients coinfected with HIV, suppressive herpes treatment with valacyclovir has also been shown to decrease rectal, seminal, and plasma HIV levels.
- HSV resistance to acyclovir, valacyclovir, and famciclovir may result in persistent infections, which will need to be treated with alternative regimens such as foscarnet or cidofovir.

Human Papillomavirus

Epidemiology

- Over 40 different HPV types can cause genital infection, and most infections are asymptomatic and self-limited.
- Sexually active people have at least a 50% risk of becoming infected at least once in their lifetime, if they are not vaccinated.
- Low-risk HPV types include HPV types 6 and 11, and these are the most common etiologic agents for genital warts, while the high-risk HPV types 16 and 18 are associated with cancers of the anus, cervix, penis, vulva, and vagina.
- Genital warts may also harbor more high-risk HPV types 16, 18, 31, 33, and 35 and may contain areas of high-grade dysplasia.
- These precursor lesions are common among high-risk populations such as MSM and HIV-positive patients, occurring in over half of HIV-positive MSM and over a third of HIV-negative MSM.

Clinical Presentation

- While the majority of infections with HPV are asymptomatic and self-limited, some patients may develop genital warts, dysplastic lesions, or cancer depending on the virus type.
- Genital warts, or condyloma, present as growths on the genital mucosa, anal mucosa, and perianal skin (Fig. 19.11).

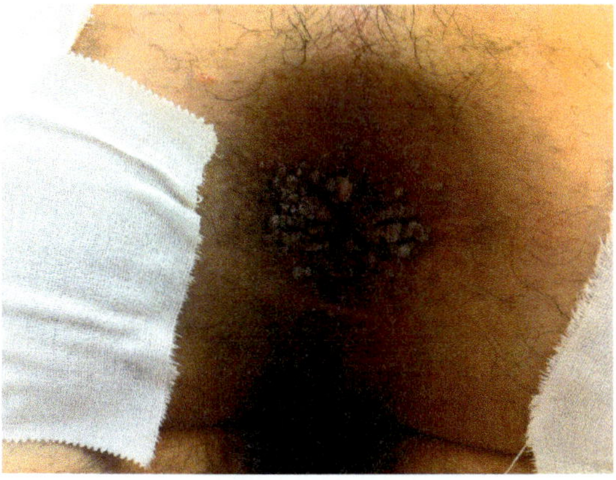

Fig. 19.11 Perianal condyloma due to HPV infection

- Patients with warts within the anal canal may have a history of receptive anal intercourse, but not necessarily.
- Symptoms may include pain, pruritus, discomfort, or bleeding, depending on the location and size of the warts.
- Patients with HIV infection or another source of immunosuppression are more likely to develop genital warts, and these warts are less likely to respond to treatment and more likely to recur.
- The high-risk HPV types can cause invasive squamous cell cancers of the anus.
  - Squamous cell carcinoma occurs more frequently in patients who are immunosuppressed, especially in patients who are coinfected with HIV.
  - Disturbances in the peripheral immune function in the anal mucosa may explain this increased risk to progress to invasive anal cancer.

Testing

- HPV testing can be used to screen women for cervical cancer, but screening for HPV is not indicated for men, sex partners of women with known HPV, adolescent women, or for other HPV-related malignancies such as anal cancer.
- As certain high-risk populations such as HIV-positive MSM have seen a rise in incidence of invasive anal squamous cell carcinoma, screening programs to detect precursor lesions have been developed to prevent progression to invasive cancer.
- Liquid-based anorectal cytology specimens are the preferred specimen type to screen for high-grade anal dysplasia.
- Self-collected samples are less sensitive than clinician-collected samples.
- Patient with positive findings should be referred to a specialist for high-resolution anoscopy or routine anoscopy and monitoring.

Treatment

- The indication to treat anogenital warts is to relieve symptoms.
- Untreated genital warts may self-resolve or worsen.
- Treatment does not affect the risk of transmission of HPV.
- External genital warts can be treated in a variety of ways (Table 19.3).
  - Patients may apply their own treatment at home using podofilox solution or gel, imiquimod cream, or sinecatechins ointment.
  - Provider-administered options include cryotherapy, podophyllin resin, or trichloroacetic or bichloroacetic acid.
  - Patients with extensive genital warts may warrant surgical management.
- Anal condyloma – including warts in the anal canal and the distal rectum – can be treated with cryotherapy, TCA or BCA, or surgical therapy.
- High-resolution anoscopy may be indicated to inspect for high-grade dysplasia as well.
- The management of high-grade anal dysplasia, the precursor to invasive squamous cell carcinoma, remains a controversial topic.
- While some clinicians view ablation or destruction of high-grade dysplasia as an important strategy to prevent progression to invasive cancer, others disagree with this approach.
- Patients with high-grade intra-anal dysplasia who undergo ablation have recurrence rates of about 50% overall (higher in HIV-positive patients) but a low risk of developing anal cancer.

Vaccine

- The two HPV vaccines available are the bivalent vaccine, which protects against high-risk oncogenic HPV types 16 and 18, and the quadrivalent vaccine which protects against HPV types 6, 11, 16, and 18 and should be given before one become sexually active.
- Both are approved for girls and boys aged 9–26 years old.
- The quadrivalent vaccine has been shown to reduce the rates of high-grade anal dysplasia among MSM and may help to reduce the risk of anal cancer.

HIV and AIDS

Epidemiology

- Over 1 million people in the USA have HIV, and over half of those infected are MSM.
- A quarter of those patients reported high-risk sexual practices such as unprotected sexual intercourse with a casual partner or sex in exchange for money or drugs, and almost half of those patients reported using noninjection drugs over the past year.

Testing

- HIV screening is recommended for all patients who present for STI testing.
- Positive screening tests for HIV antibody require confirmatory testing before a diagnosis can be made.
- If patient is suspected of having acute HIV infection, then a nucleic acid test should be performed in addition to the antibody test, and the patient should be referred immediately to an infectious disease specialist.
- The FDA has recently approved combination tests detecting both HIV antigen and antibody, as well as tests that differentiate HIV-1 from HIV-2.

Anorectal Issues

- Anorectal complaints such as pain due to fissures may be the presenting symptom of patients with HIV infection.
  - Fissures in HIV-positive patients may be a manifestation of HIV but could also represent coinfection with other STIs such as HSV or syphilis.
  - Treatment of fissures in patients with HIV should consist of the same treatment undertaken for fissures in the general population.
- Anal ulcers are another source of anal pain in patients with HIV and are located in a more proximal location within the anal canal – often above the dentate line – and are broader and more ulcerative than fissures.
- Perianal abscesses and fistulas are common in patients with HIV or AIDS.
  - Patients with well-controlled HIV and normal CD4 counts who develop abscesses and fistulas can be treated with the same surgical techniques as one would do for patients without HIV.
  - However, abscesses in patients with AIDS should be treated with smaller incisions, favoring drain placement over larger incisions.
  - Fistulas in patients with advanced or poorly controlled AIDS should be treated with placement of draining setons rather than fistulotomy to avoid the creation of a nonhealing wound.
- External thrombosed hemorrhoids and symptomatic internal hemorrhoids in patients with HIV or AIDS should be treated in the same manner as those occurring in patients without HIV.
- Hemorrhoidectomy is safe in HIV-positive patients without AIDS; patients with advanced or poorly controlled AIDS and severe hemorrhoids not amenable to banding may have wound healing problems.

Molluscum Contagiosum

- Molluscum contagiosum is a common cutaneous viral infection caused by the molluscipox virus, causing small, waxy, dome-shaped umbilicated papules (Fig. 19.12).

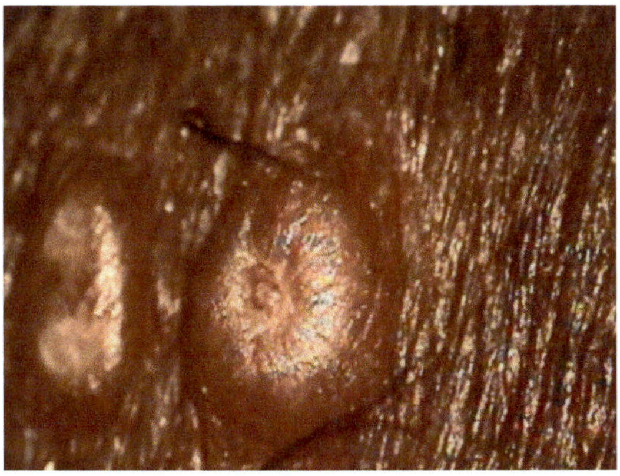

Fig. 19.12 Molluscum contagiosum lesions present as waxy dome-shaped umbilicated papules

- It is second only to genital warts as the most common non-ulcerative STI, affecting up to 5% of the population, 18% of patients with immunosuppression, and 30% of patients with advanced AIDS.
- Secondary bacterial infection may occur especially if patients tend to scratch the lesions.
- Mollusca contagiosa occur frequently in young children, but their occurrence in adults is usually considered an STI and involves the pubic area.
  - Risk factors include shaving.
  - Transmission occurs through skin-to-skin contact, and autoinoculation can also occur to spread to other sites.
  - Sexual contact can lead to transmission from the genitalia to the oral mucosa, conjunctiva, and cornea.
- Diagnosis can be made by visual inspection although if there is difficulty, then dermatoscopy revealing orifices, vessels, and specific vascular patterns can help confirm the diagnosis.
- A recent PCR test has been developed as well for the molluscum contagiosum virus.
- Immunocompetent patients will self-resolve these lesions over a period of months to years, so most patients prefer treatment.
  - Treatment consists of removal of the lesions, similar to the treatment of genital warts.
    - Curettage, excision, and cryotherapy are the most common methods of treatment.
    - These treatments should not be performed in patients with immunosuppression due to the risk of nonhealing wounds and superinfection with other bacterial, viral, or fungal organisms.
- For these patients topical treatments such as imiquimod 5% cream may be helpful without incurring the risk of open surgical wounds.

Pubic Lice: *Phthirus pubis*

- Pubic lice are obligate blood-sucking parasites, and infestation is diagnosed by finding lice on pubic hair (Fig. 19.13).
- As lice can neither jump nor fly, transmission is due to close contact.
- Therefore, the diagnosis of pubic lice should prompt testing for other STIs.

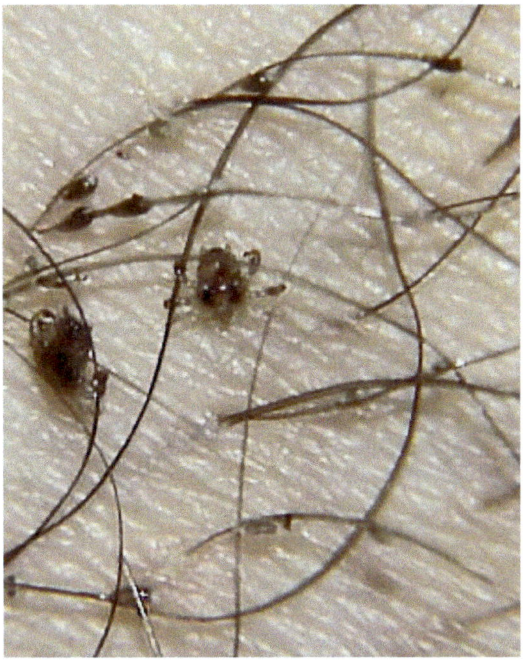

Fig. 19.13 Pubic lice infestation causes severe pruritus and can be treated with permethrin 1% cream. (Photograph courtesy of Stephen Goldstone, MD)

- The increased incidence of pubic hair removal has been associated with a lower incidence of pubic lice infections due to destruction of their natural habitat.
- The CDC recommends permethrin 1% cream or pyrethrins 0.3%/piperonyl botuxide 4% cream as first-line therapy for pubic lice.
- Alternative regimens include malathion 0.5% lotion or oral ivermectin.
- Laundering clothes and bedding in hot water should be done as well to prevent reinfection and transmission.

Scabies

- Scabies is caused by the mite *Sarcoptes scabiei* var. *hominis.*
- Scabies transmission is via skin-to-skin contact, as the mites neither jump nor fly.
- Scabies most commonly occurs in young children but can also occur in patients subject to overcrowded conditions, poor hygiene, and homelessness and via sexual contact.
- The mites burrow into the skin, creating wavy scaly lines on the skin surface, usually located on the hands and feets, typically in finger webs.
- The infestation causes an intense pruritic rash localized in a characteristic distribution in the armpits, elbow creases, wrists, and groin areas (Fig. 19.14).
- Infants, children, and immunosuppressed patients may develop a more severe vesicular and pustular rash.
- Diagnosis can be made by visual inspection and history.
- Skin scrapings of the burrows, papules, and vesicles can be performed by applying mineral oil to the skin and scraping laterally across the lesion with a scalpel and examining the scraping microscopically for mites, eggs, and fecal pellets.
- First-line treatment of scabies is with topical permethrin 5% cream, which is rather effective as there is not much resistance.
- Reapplication of the cream should be performed 1 week later to ensure eradication.
- Oral ivermectin can also be used as first-line therapy or second-line therapy if the permethrin cream does not work.
- Clothing and bedding should be washed in hot water and dried in a hot dryer to prevent re-infestation and transmission.

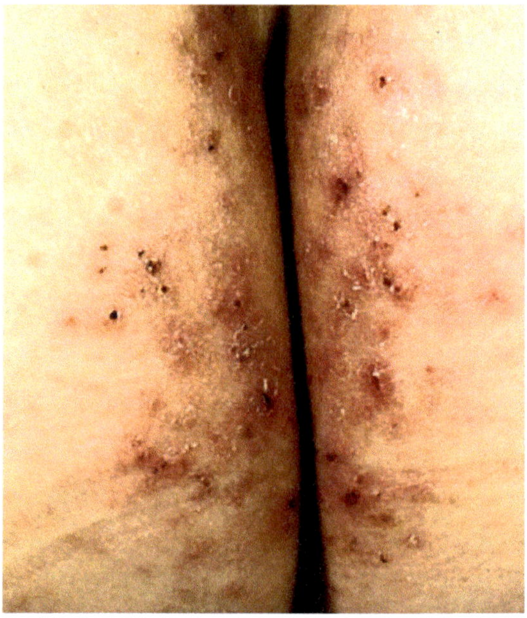

Fig. 19.14 Scabies infestation causing an intensely pruritic rash can be treated with permethrin 5% cream. (Photograph courtesy of Stephen Goldstone, MD)

20 Anal Intraepithelial Neoplasia

Rocco Ricciardi

Key Concepts

- Anal intraepithelial neoplasia is a dysplastic condition of the squamous tissue and is considered to be a premalignant stage of anal cancer.
- The histological findings and cellular abnormalities mirror cervical dysplasia.
- Anal cytology is a useful method to identify anal neoplasia in high-risk groups.
- When cytology is concerning, the evaluation of anal neoplasia can proceed with anal cytology and high-resolution microscopy, a technique similar to colposcopy.
- A targeted approach to dysplasia ablation through microscopy is more of tissue sparing than the historically practiced wide local excisions and flap advancements.
- Treatment should be tailored to the patient's degree of dysplasia, risk factors, immune status, continence, symptoms, and likelihood of progression.

Introduction

- Anal intraepithelial neoplasia is a dysplastic condition of the squamous tissue and is considered to be a premalignant stage of anal cancer.
- Anal intraepithelial neoplasia (AIN) is further stratified into three grades: AIN I, AIN II, and AIN III, defined as low-, moderate-, and high-grade dysplasia, respectively (Fig. 20.1).
- The histological findings, including the cytologic changes, mitotic activity, nuclear membrane changes, and cellular abnormalities, mirror cervical dysplasia grading.
- Terminology can be confusing as anal intraepithelial neoplasia is referred to by many names including anal dysplasia, intraepithelial carcinoma, intramucosal carcinoma, squamous cell carcinoma in situ, and Bowen's disease.
- In addition, recently the terms high-grade (HGAIN) and low-grade (LGAIN) anal intraepithelial neoplasia have been proposed that correspond to AIN III/II and AIN I, respectively.

Symptoms

- The vast majority of individuals will experience no outward manifestation of human papillomavirus (HPV) infection, and similarly most patients with AIN have no clear symptoms.
- As AIN progresses to anal cancer, symptoms become more frequently reported.
  - 50% of patients with invasive cancer describe pain and bleeding.

R. Ricciardi (✉)
Massachusetts General Hosptal,
Boston, MA, USA
e-mail: rricciardi1@mgh.harvard.edu

S. R. Steele et al. (eds.), *The ASCRS Manual of Colon and Rectal Surgery*,
https://doi.org/10.1007/978-3-030-01165-9_20

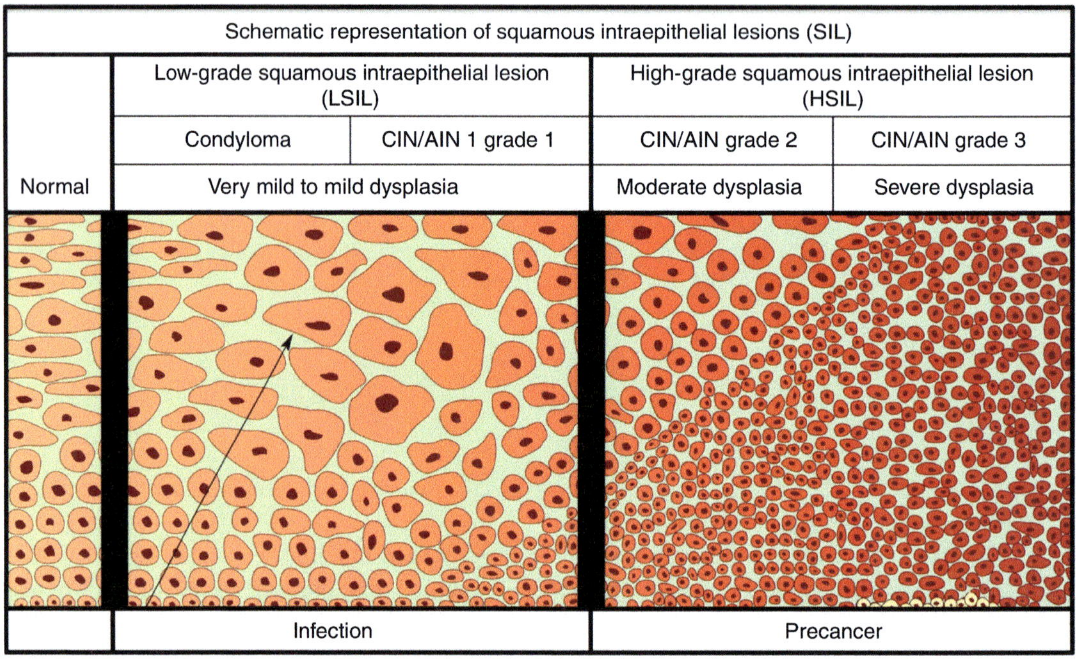

Fig. 20.1 Schematic representation of squamous intraepithelial lesions (SIL). As shown in this illustration, with increasing severity of SIL of the anus, the proportion of the epithelium replaced by immature cells with large nuclear-cytoplasmic ratios increases. Invasive cancer probably arises from one or more foci of high-grade SIL (HSIL) as depicted in the drawing by epithelial cells crossing the basement membrane below the region of HSIL. (With permission from Brickman C, Palefsky JM Human papillomavirus in the HIV-infected host: epidemiology and pathogenesis in the antiretroviral era Curr HIV/AIDS Rep 2015;12:6–15. Copyright Springer)

Epidemiology

- Anal intraepithelial neoplasia develops from HPV contact generally through direct exposure.
- It is estimated that there are more than 100 subtypes of HPV but not all have been implicated as disease causing.
- About 90% of all patients remain asymptomatic, and those that have infection resolve without any treatment within 2 years.
- A small number of patients develop persistent asymptomatic infections, while a smaller number of patients will develop condyloma.
- It is unclear why a fraction of patients develop neoplasia in the form of AIN that then may progress to squamous cell cancer.
- Explanations for why the virus causes condyloma or neoplasia in some patients but not in others are speculative.
  - It is likely related to patient's immune function, subtype of HPV, repetitive inoculation, and/or potentially concomitant infections such as other sexually transmitted infections.
  - Among HPV subtypes, types 6 and 11, cause 90% of genital warts as compared to those subtypes that are associated with cancer (i.e., types 16, 18).
- HPV, the causative exposure to AIN, is quite prevalent in both the developed and developing world.
  - Estimates indicate that at any point in time, 1 in 10 women worldwide harbors the HPV virus.
  - Prior to the introduction of the HPV vaccine, there had been a steady rise in the rate of HPV infections across the nation and the globe.
  - However, with the introduction of the HPV vaccine, prevalence of HPV types 6, 11, 16,

and 18 identified by cytology specimens decreased by over 50% among teens and young women.
  - Genital wart cases appear to have decreased since 2011, presumably because of increased vaccination (Fig. 20.2).
- Incidence data characterizing trends of HPV infection and condyloma are easily obtainable, yet it is unclear whether the rate of AIN has changed in the last several years.
  - There are no public records, and cancer surveillance data do not record incidence or treatment of dysplastic lesions.
- National cancer incidence data do reveal that the rate of anal cancer has been increasing for several years; new anal cancer cases have been rising on average 2.2% each year over the last 10 years.
  - The number of new cases of anal cancer was 1.8 per 100,000 people per year based on 2007–2011.
  - Slightly more common in women than in men.
- Much of what is known regarding the transformation of AIN to squamous cell cancer has been extracted from the cervical cancer literature.
  - Precursor high-grade squamous intraepithelial lesions.
  - Integration of the viral genome into the host occurs in order to produce genetic change.
  - Viral oncogenes are then ultimately responsible for directly coupling to oncogenic enhancers and promoters permitting continued expression through integration and immortalization.
  - Phenotypic changes of the squamous epithelium.
  - One of the most frequently reported changes in chromosomal structure is a gain in the long arm of chromosome 3q.
  - Following incorporation of the viral genome into host DNA, cellular changes and atypia of squamous tissues occur.
    - Ultimately these changes correspond to AIN I which then can progress to AIN II and AIN III and ultimately dedifferentiate into squamous cell cancer.
    - It is unclear whether the development of anal neoplasia must traverse all these steps or if squamous cell cancer can skip one or more phases, i.e., from AIN I directly to AIN III.

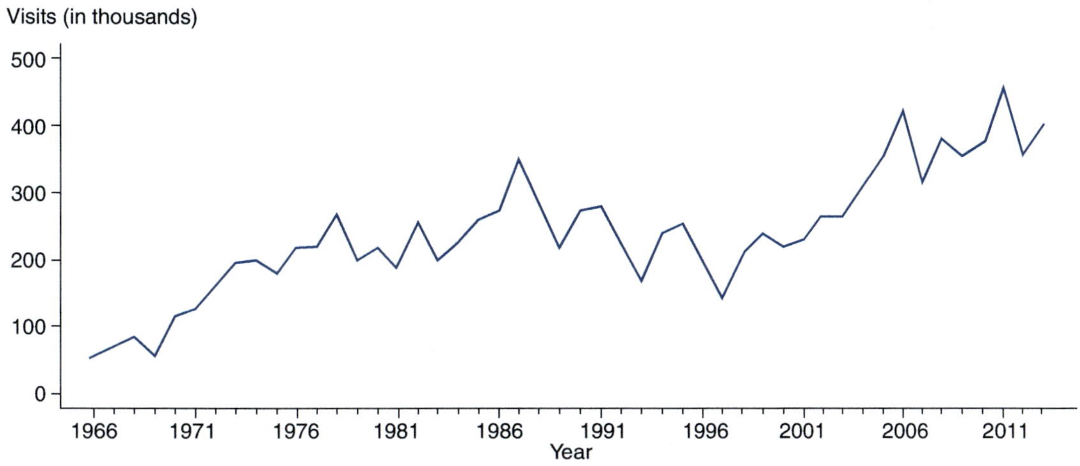

Fig. 20.2 Genital warts. Initial visits to Physicians' Offices, United States, 1966–2013, http://www.cdc.gov/std/stats13/figures/49.htm. (Source: IMS Health, Integrated Promotional Services™. IMS Health Report, 1966–2013)

Screening/Surveillance

- Most patients at risk for anal neoplasia undergo screening with digital rectal examination, anal cytology, and anoscopy.
  - Anal cytology is akin to cervical cytology, providing cellular material for review of intraepithelial lesions.
  - The cytology must be performed before any instrumentation of the anus and before lubrication is used.
  - The procedure is performed with a moist swab in the anal canal and without any preparation.
  - Following completion, a digital rectal examination and anoscopy can be performed.
- The anal cytology smear is graded by a cytologist with the same classification used in gynecologic samples.
  - Anal cytology may return as insufficient, normal, atypical squamous cells of undetermined significance, low-grade squamous intraepithelial lesion, high-grade squamous intraepithelial lesion, or anal cancer.
  - Based on these results and prior medical history, the recommendation is either continued surveillance or more detailed evaluation with high-resolution anoscopy.
    - Lesions classified as atypical squamous cells of undetermined significance or higher are generally referred for high-resolution anoscopy.
    - However, a large number of patients have abnormal cytology results leading to a considerably large population of patients to evaluate in microscopy.
    - In addition, given that the sensitivity of anal cytology ranges from 69% to 93% and specificity ranges from 32% to 59%, results can be difficult to interpret.
    - It is important to remember that anal cytology in high-risk cohorts such as men who have sex with men has false-negative rates of up to 23% in HIV-negative patient and 45% if HIV-positive.
    - Therefore, close follow-up of all high-risk patients is likely to be the best strategy (see Fig. 20.3).
- Defining the population that is high-risk and requiring evaluation is challenging because of societal and other behavioral concerns.
- Overall, the risk of anal neoplasia is highest in immunosuppressed individuals as they appear to have great difficulty in clearing the virus from their body.

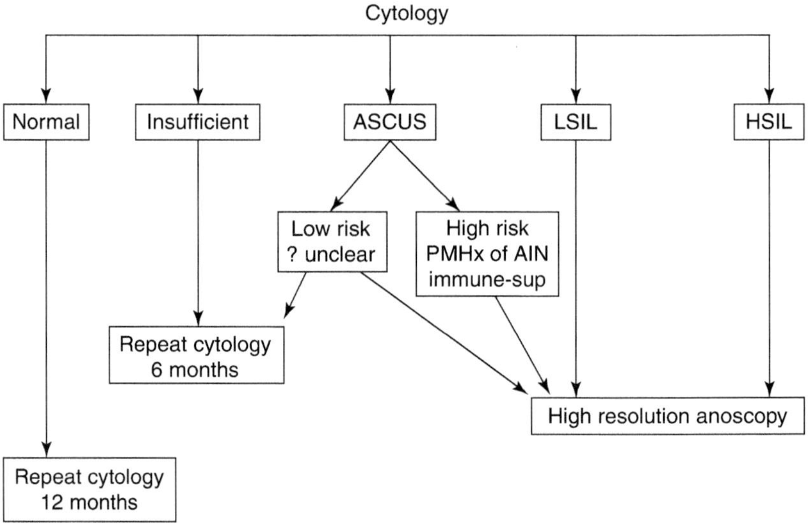

Fig. 20.3 Management algorithm for anal cytology results. General guidelines provided. Individual case management is based on many factors, which may increase or decrease the interval of evaluation

- Rates of anal dysplasia in HIV-infected patients of all sexual risk groups are substantial indicating some value for anal cancer screening in all HIV-infected patients regardless of sexual practices.
- The immunosuppressed group should also include those with organ transplants as well as other medically induced suppressive conditions.
- Men who have sex with men and a concomitant diagnosis of HIV pose the greatest risk of HPV-related illnesses and thus anal neoplasia.
- One of the highest risk groups is women with a past history of cervical, vulvar, vaginal, or perineal neoplasia.
- The proximity of the anus to the vulva may explain why patients with vulvar neoplasia were at highest risk for anal cancer, yet the increased risk with in situ neoplasia was also remarkable.
- Thus, patients with gynecologic neoplasia, and especially vulvar neoplasia, should be followed closely for potential anal cancer development.
- Individuals with a past history of sexually transmitted infections may also represent an important screening population.
  - A past history of condyloma is generally a sign of prior contact with human papillomavirus.
  - At this time, it is unclear whether those individuals who tend to develop condyloma (without any sign of dysplasia) have a tendency to develop benign warts rather than cancer.
- The value of anal cancer screening is difficult to quantify.
  - Screening HIV-positive homosexual and bisexual men for anal dysplasia with anal cytology offers quality-adjusted life expectancy benefits at a cost comparable with other accepted clinical preventive interventions.
  - Others have not come to the same conclusion indicating that many of the criteria for assessing the need for a screening program were not met for anal neoplasia screening and that cost-effectiveness remained unacceptable.
  - The lack of concordance for these models may be related to the lack of agreement with uncertainties in modeling clinical scenarios in the face of poor evidence.
  - At this time, a review of 30 regional and national guidelines for screening in HIV patients revealed that only 2 societies recommended digital and anorectal examination.
    - The "European AIDS Clinical Society Guidelines" recommends digital examination every 1–3 years for HIV-positive men who have sex with men.
    - In New York State, the Department of Health has recommended annual anal cancer screening for HIV-positive men who have sex with men, HIV-positive patients with history of condyloma, and HIV-positive women with history of gynecologic neoplasia.
    - However, the US Guidelines for the prevention and treatment of opportunistic infections in HIV-infected adults and adolescents recommended only an annual digital examination for the HIV-positive population in general.

Diagnosis

- Most patients are diagnosed with anal neoplasia through investigation with digital rectal examination, anal cytology, anoscopy, and/or endoscopy.
  - The sensitivity of digital rectal examination in identifying anal neoplasia is fairly low as many AIN lesions are not palpable.
  - Anoscopy is routinely performed by colon and rectal surgeons and can be used to identify macroscopic areas of AIN, which often appear to be benign condylomata, but may return with AIN on biopsy (Fig. 20.4).
  - In addition, endoscopic identification of AIN occurs quite commonly during endoscopy, particularly during the retroflexed view of the anus.

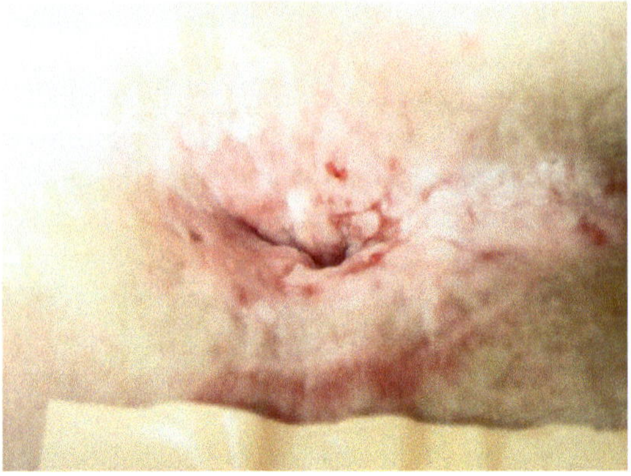

Fig. 20.4 AIN 3. (Courtesy of Richard Billingham, MD)

- Last, a large number of patients are identified with anal dysplasia on cytologic evaluation during routine screening.

- During diagnostic evaluation, it is imperative to remember that patients with AIN should have a complete and thorough history and physical examination.
- It is important to remember the link between anal dysplasia with other HPV-related diseases such as oral cancer, gynecologic neoplasia, and other genital lesions.
- Following examination of the entire body, the evaluation of AIN can proceed with anal cytology and high-resolution microscopy, a technique similar to colposcopy of gynecologic neoplasia.
  - The colposcopic appearance of variable grades of anal squamous intraepithelial lesions is similar to those described for the cervix.
  - In high-resolution anoscopy, a colposcope or other microscope is used to examine the anal verge and anal canal in close detail.
  - No bowel or anorectal preparation is necessary, and the procedure is most commonly performed without analgesia.
- After positioning, the tissues to be examined are swabbed with a 3–5% acetic acid solution for 2–5 min.
  - The acetowhitening from acetic acid with microscopic assistance is sufficient to identify dysplastic tissues.
  - The entire anal canal and anal verge should be examined, but we find that dysplastic tissues are most commonly found within the transition zone, as this area has the greatest area of susceptible and immature squamous tissues.
  - Dysplastic epithelium will absorb acetic acid and appear scaly white as compared to columnar tissues.
  - The characterization of dysplastic tissue and differentiation of AIN I, II, or III can then be performed without biopsies and in real time under high magnification.
  - Dysplastic tissues are characterized by scaly white plaques and with greater disarray of vascular patterns, the higher the grade of dysplasia.
  - We also find that high-grade dysplasia tends to be quite friable when in contact with the anoscope or a swab (Fig. 20.5).
- Some colposcopists choose to add an iodine-based Lugol's solution to further assist with the detection of dysplastic tissue.
  - The mechanism for Lugol's utility is that only healthy epithelial tissue absorbs the compound which causes normal tissue to appear wood-like.
  - Dysplastic tissues do not absorb the solution leaving these tissues with a yellowish hue.

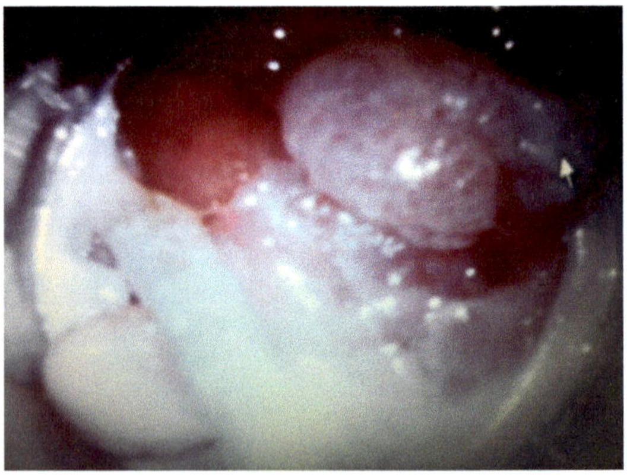

Fig. 20.5 AIN on high-resolution anoscopy. The pointer denotes area of high-grade dysplasia. (Courtesy of Rocco Ricciardi, MD)

- May interfere with proper dysplasia differentiation (i.e., AIN I versus AIN II or III).
- The equipment used for the evaluation of AIN is expensive, and the high-resolution microscopy procedure is time intensive and difficult to learn.
- Others have taken to diagnose AIN with simple anoscopy or endoscopic methods.
- At this time, data have not demonstrated that high-resolution anoscopy is superior to other methods.
  - Interestingly, a recent study from Ohio revealed no difference in anal cancer progression with simple observation versus high-resolution anoscopy.
  - Others have demonstrated a very low rate of anal cancer progression with an intense surveillance strategy involving anal cytology, digital anorectal examination, and oncogenic HPV testing in men who have sex with men.

Treatment

- It should be clear that there is no proven treatment for HPV infection.
- As stated earlier, the infection is self-limited such that treatment is directed only to the macroscopic (i.e., genital warts) or pathologic (i.e., precancerous) lesions caused by infection.
- It is thought that all subclinical HPV infections resolve without treatment, and thus, any attempt at antiviral therapies is not indicated.
- When dysplasia is present, whether in the anus, vulva, or cervix, there are a number of methods to manage or treat these neoplastic tissues ranging from no intervention to very aggressive care.
- At this time there is no clear best treatment option for all types of patients and all degrees of anal dysplasia.
- Ultimately the best method of treatment must be efficacious in preventing the progression of anal intraepithelial neoplasia to cancer while reducing the morbidity of treatment and preserving function (Table 20.1).
- Observation may be the best option for patients with low-grade dysplasia.
  - Management would consist of surveillance every 4–12 months.
  - Overall low rates of disease progression and malignant potential (especially for low-grade disease) and the increased morbidity associated with excision and repeated focal destruction.
- Topical treatments with imiquimod and 5-FU have demonstrated effectiveness for both high- and low-grade dysplasia.
  - Imiquimod is one of the most tested agents although there is a high rate of recurrence when treatment is discontinued.

Table 20.1 Common options used in the treatment of anal dysplasia

Treatment	Advantages	Disadvantages	Cure	Recurrence
Observation	Cost cheap No side effects	Low cure rate Time intensive	Poor	High
Imiquimod	Minimal pain Easy to use	Burning Moderate cost	Poor	High with DC
5-FU	Easy to use	Burning Moderate cost	Poor	High with DC
Infrared coagulation	Clinic use	Need equipment	Good	Moderate in immunosuppressed
Ablation	One application	Painful Costly	Good	Moderate in immunosuppressed
Wide local excision	Removes all tissue	Disfiguring Painful	Good	Low

    - Interestingly a recent meta-analysis failed to demonstrate any statistically significant effect of imiquimod in the management of anal intraepithelial neoplasia, but there was a trend for imiquimod to downgrade high-grade AIN to a lower risk stage.
  - 5-FU has fewer trials but is similarly effective in reducing dysplasia with complete response in 39%.
    - Unfortunately, patients treated with 5-FU similarly had high rates of recurrence (50%) and even higher rates of side effects.
- Surgery is an effective option to treat anal neoplasia.
  - Electrocautery is highly effective in inducing complete response of AIN especially in immunocompetent individuals (72%) as compared to immunosuppressed individuals (51%).
  - Ablation is generally performed in the operating room with electrocautery in conjunction with high-resolution anoscopy; yet others perform the procedure in clinic with local anesthesia.
  - The technique is highly selective with targeting of only those areas with evidence of dysplasia.
  - The operating surgeon should remember that the disease is limited to the epidermis and does not require destruction of deeper dermal tissues.
  - During ablation, the surgeon should be mindful of potential scarring, stricture formation, and the need to preserve as much healthy tissue as possible.
- In addition to ablation or excision, infrared coagulation can also be used to destroy lesions.
  - The infrared beam can be pulsed at varying intervals to prevent trauma to deeper tissues with a tissue to a depth of approximately 1 mm targeting the epithelium and destroying dysplastic tissue.
  - The technique is reportedly as effective as electrocautery and considered to be associated with less pain.
- In the past, mapping biopsies with wide local excision was recommended for patients with anal intraepithelial neoplasia.
  - Unfortunately, much healthy and uninvolved tissue was removed with the dysplastic tissues, and this treatment option was associated with high rates of recurrence between 13% and 63%.
  - In addition, because of the extensive tissue destruction, wide local excision was associated with high rates of local wound complications such as stenosis and incontinence.
- When selecting which of the above options is best for an individual patient, the physician should consider patient treatment goals, symptoms, history of immunosuppression, past history of dysplasia, and bowel function.
- An attempt at Cochrane Review failed to provide guidelines for treatment in anal intraepithelial neoplasia because of lack of high-quality randomized controlled trials.

Management Strategies

- For AIN I, a minimalist approach may be the most effective strategy (Fig. 20.6).

Progression

- Progression of anal intraepithelial neoplasia to squamous cell cancer of the anus parallels the pathway of cervical dysplasia to cervical cancer.
- Once established in the anal epithelium, dysplasia of the anus rarely regresses.
- The high rate of progression to cancer is particularly true for immunosuppressed patients as compared to immunocompetent patients.

Prevention

- As with all infectious diseases that are transmissible by sexual contact, the best method of prevention is safe sexual practices or limiting sexual contact.

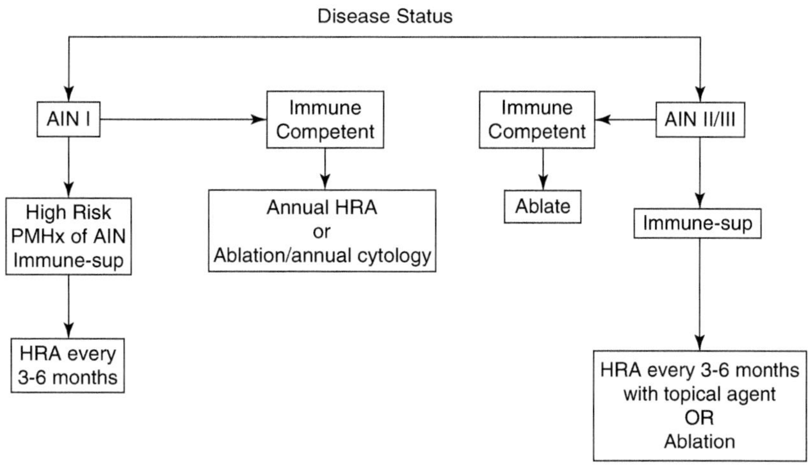

Fig. 20.6 Algorithm for the treatment of AIN based on immune status and biopsy results

- In addition to monogamy, proper and consistent use of prophylactic condoms has been shown to reduce the transmission of HPV.
- Educational interventions do have the potential to reduce the transmission of HPV and possibly reduce the incidence of squamous carcinoma.
- In addition to primary prevention techniques, vaccines have also been efficacious in reducing the incidence of HPV infection.
  - In the general screening population, HPV vaccine efficacy was almost 100% for cervical intraepithelial neoplasia, vulvar and vaginal intraepithelial neoplasia, and anogenital condyloma.
  - In men who have sex with men, use of quadrivalent HPV vaccine significantly reduced the rates of moderate and high-grade anal intraepithelial neoplasia.
  - Although the vaccinated populations were HPV naïve, there are some data indicating effectiveness of HPV vaccines in preventing reinfection or reactivation of disease.
  - Along the same reasoning, a nonconcurrent cohort study of HPV-vaccinated men who had been previously treated with high-grade anal intraepithelial neoplasia noted a reduction in anal intraepithelial neoplasia recurrence.

Part III

Malignant Disease

21 Anal Cancer

Tushar Samdani and Garrett M. Nash

Key Concepts

- Chemoradiotherapy (CRT) is the primary treatment for patient with anal squamous cell carcinoma (mitomycin + 5-FU + radiotherapy). The dosage of radiotherapy varies based on the size of the tumor and presence of lymph node involvement.
- Surgery (local excision) can be used to remove some small squamous cell carcinomas (usually measuring <1 cm or ½ in.) that do not involve the anal sphincter musculature.
- Following primary treatment with chemoradiotherapy, patients are evaluated with repeat physical examination of the anal area at approximately 8–12 weeks after completion of treatment and then at 6- to 8-week intervals until resolution of any suspicious findings. Patients with persistent but nonprogressive disease may be followed up to 6 months after chemoradiotherapy for assessment of complete remission.
- Patients with progressive disease or recurrence after chemoradiotherapy are considered for salvage abdominoperineal resection (APR).
- Dosage of radiotherapy and chemotherapy may be modified based on CD4 count and blood count in immunocompromised patients.
- Anal melanoma is very aggressive and is generally treated with local excision (LE).
- Anal adenocarcinoma is treated with APR and usually with neoadjuvant chemoradiotherapy, as in treatment for distal rectal adenocarcinoma.
- Anal cancer accounts for only 4% of all cancers of the lower alimentary tract. However, the incidence is rising – possibly due to the higher incidence of persons engaging in anal-receptive intercourse.

Anal Squamous Cell Carcinoma

- Risk factors: sexually transmitted disease; anal-receptive intercourse; more than 10 sexual partners; the presence of precancerous anal lesions such as condylomas or high-grade anal intraepithelial neoplasia and cervical, vulvar, or vaginal cancers; immunosuppression secondary to solid organ transplantation or chronic glucocorticoid therapy; HIV seropositivity, low CD4 count; and smoking.
- Anatomic Location Guides Treatment
  - Surgery alone (local excision) can be used to remove select small squamous cell

T. Samdani
Department of Colorectal Surgery, Medstar Saint Mary's Hospital, Leonardo Town, MD, USA

G. M. Nash (✉)
Department of Surgery, Memorial Sloan Kettering Cancer Center, New York, NY, USA
e-mail: nashg@mskcc.org

S. R. Steele et al. (eds.), *The ASCRS Manual of Colon and Rectal Surgery*,
https://doi.org/10.1007/978-3-030-01165-9_21

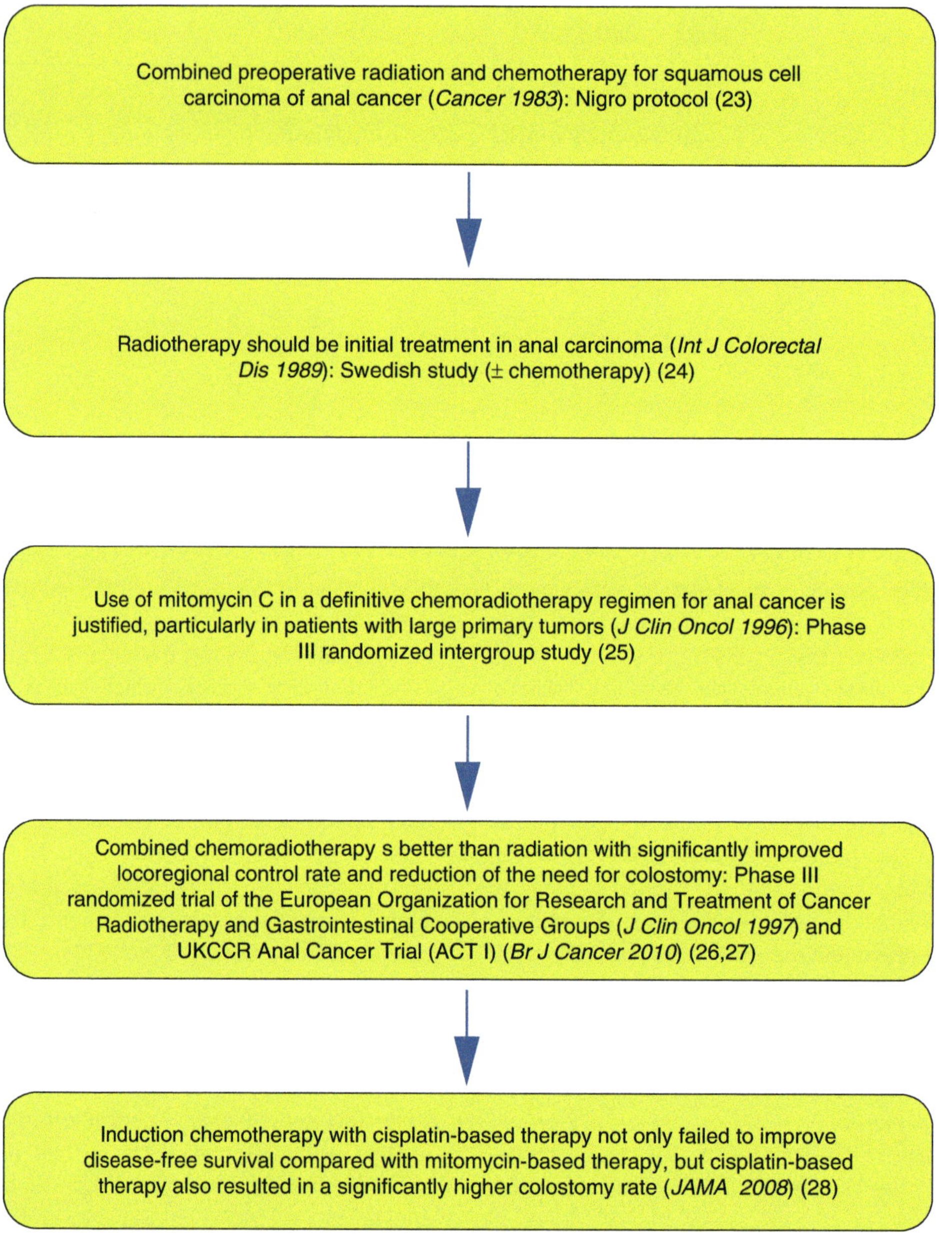

Fig. 21.1 Evolution of management of anal cancer (algorithm)

carcinomas of the perianal skin that do not involve the anal sphincter musculature and tumors of the buttock skin.

- Chemoradiotherapy (CRT, mitomycin +5-flourouracil + radiotherapy) is the primary treatment for patient with squamous cell carcinoma that involves the anal canal or anal sphincter musculature. The dosage and fields of radiotherapy vary based on the size of the tumor and presence of lymph node involvement. There has been an evolution of treatment philosophy over time (Fig. 21.1).

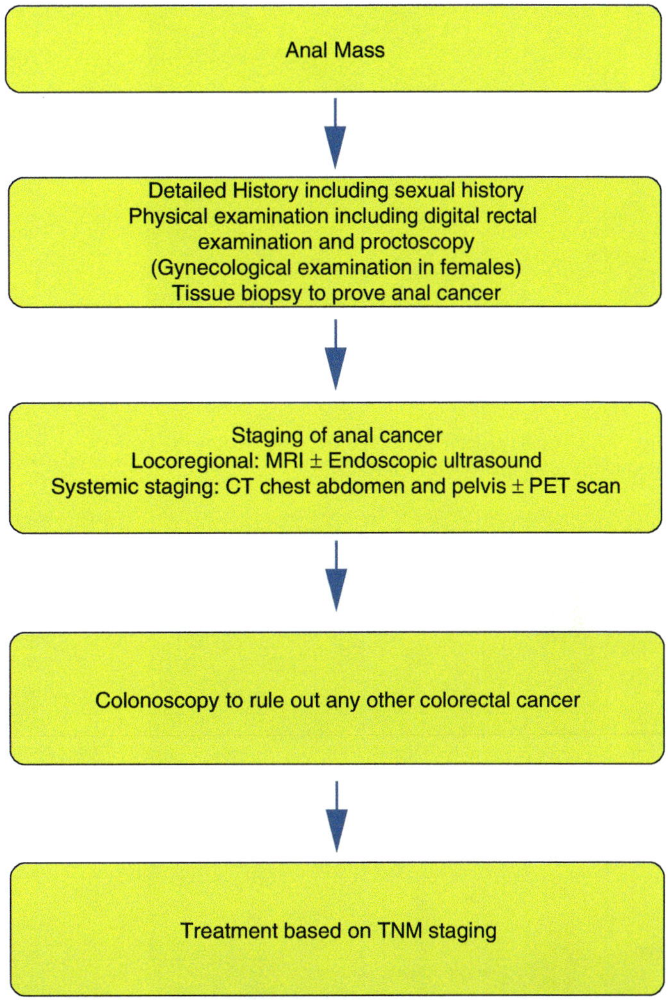

Fig. 21.2 Algorithm for anal mass evaluation and work-up

- Anal Canal Tumors: Staging/Prognosis
  - A thorough exam including assessing the primary tumor and the groins should be performed in patients with anal canal tumors (Fig. 21.2).
  - A CT of the chest, abdomen, and pelvis or whole body FDG-PET-CT should be performed to rule out distant metastasis. PET-CT is often used to assess response to therapy; thus a pretreatment PET-CT may be of value as a baseline examination (Fig. 21.3). MR of the pelvis can provide information regarding adjacent organ invasion and/or regional lymphadenopathy (Fig. 21.4). Transanal/transrectal ultrasound can occasionally be helpful with assessment of primary tumor and/or mesorectal lymph nodes.
  - Clinical/histologic staging: Unlike colorectal adenocarcinoma, anal squamous cell carcinoma T staging is based on the size of the tumor and nodal (N) staging based on the anatomic location of the nodes (Table 21.1).
  - Lymph node involvement: Studies have shown that the chance of LN involvement with a T1 primary is extremely low. However, the chance of LN involvement with a T2 primary is 24% and as high as 67% with a T3 primary.
  - The size of the primary tumor and the presence of nodal or distant metastases are the principal determinates of outcome. Patients with de novo tumors >5 cm (T3) are at increased risk of ultimately requiring APR with permanent colostomy, and such

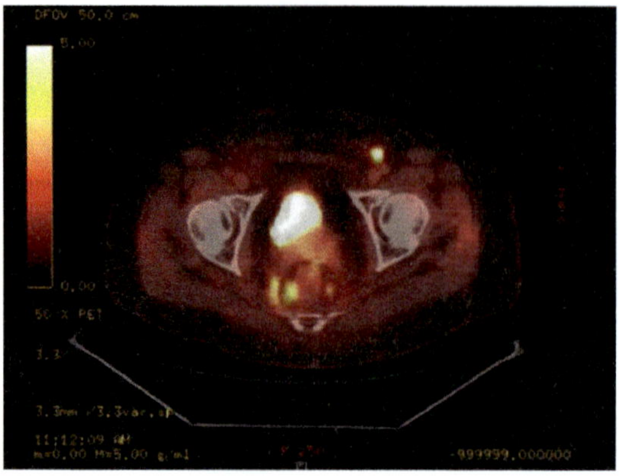

Fig. 21.3 Anal cancer: left inguinal adenopathy and mesorectal adenopathy seen on PET-CT

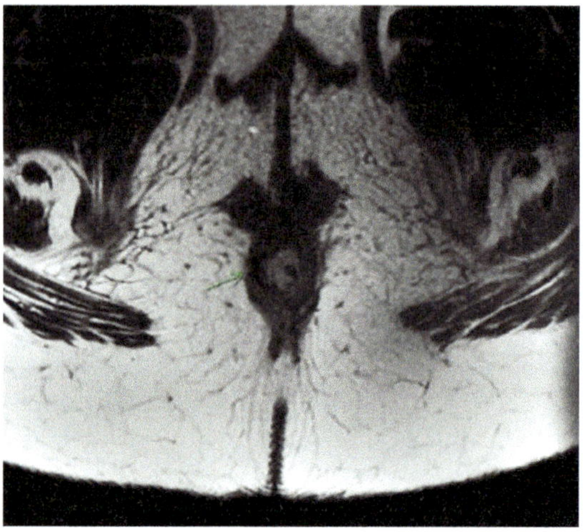

Fig. 21.4 Anal cancer: pretreatment MRI T2 oblique, suspicion for focal tumor invasion into the right lateral internal anal sphincter

tumors are associated with inferior disease-free and overall survival, compared to T1/T2 primary tumors. Male gender and HIV-positive status may portend an unfavorable long-term outcome.

- Anal Canal Tumors: Surveillance
  - Following primary treatment with chemoradiotherapy, patients are evaluated with repeat physical examination of the anal area at approximately 8–12 weeks after completion of treatment and then at 6- to 8-week intervals until resolution of any suspicious findings. Patients with persistent but nonprogressive disease may be followed for up to 6 months after chemoradiotherapy for assessment of complete remission.
  - Patients with complete remission should undergo clinical evaluation every 3–6 months for 5 years. This should include examination of the primary tumor site and the groin. CT scan of the chest, abdomen, and pelvis, or PET/CT, is performed annually for 3 years.
- Anal Canal Tumors: Persistent/Recurrent Disease
  - Approximately 10–30% of patients have persistent or recurrent disease after initial CRT. Risk factors associated with failure of initial treatment include HIV-positive status, high T and N stage at original presentation, and interruption of treatment during CRT.
  - If the patient has persistent disease at 6 months, or progressive disease develops

Table 21.1 TNM classification for anal cancer

	Primary tumor(T)
TX	Primary tumor cannot be assessed
T0	No evidence of primary tumor
Tis	Carcinoma in situ (Bowen's disease, high-grade squamous intraepithelial lesion (HISL), AIN II–III)
T1	Tumor 2 cm or less in greatest dimension
T2	Tumor more than 2 cm but not more than 5 cm in greatest dimension
T3	Tumor more than 5 cm in greatest dimension
T4	Tumor of any size invades adjacent organ(s), e.g., vagina, urethra, bladder (direct invasion of rectal wall, perirectal skin, subcutaneous tissue, or sphincter muscle is not classified as T4)
	Regional lymph node (N)
NX	Regional lymph nodes cannot be assessed
N0	No regional lymph node metastasis
N1	Metastasis in perirectal lymph nodes(s)
N2	Metastasis in unilateral internal iliac and/or unilateral inguinal lymph node(s)
N3	Metastasis in perirectal and inguinal lymph nodes and/or bilateral internal iliac and/or inguinal lymph nodes
	Distant metastases (M)
M0	No distant metastasis
M1	Distant metastasis

Source: AJCC Cancer Staging Manual plus EZTNM, 6th edition

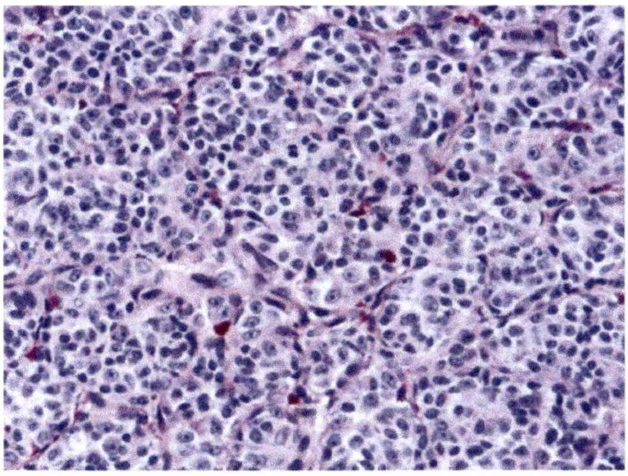

Fig. 21.5 Anal melanoma with epithelioid morphology

in the meantime, biopsy may be done to confirm cancer. Biopsy is recommended earlier when there is tumor mass progression or unsatisfactory response to treatment. However, unnecessary biopsy should be avoided to minimize the risk of soft tissue infections, tissue necrosis, or impairment of anal function.
- Patients who fail initial chemoradiotherapy, or those with local recurrence following initial response to therapy, should be restaged with PET-CT.
- Patients with isolated local disease should be considered for salvage abdominoperineal resection (APR). Salvage APR is associated with 5-year locoregional control in 30–77% of patients; overall survival at 5 years ranges from 30% to 60%. Wound complications are common, and muscle flap reconstruction of the perineum may be considered.
- Isolated recurrence in an inguinal node may be treated with RT to the groin, with or without chemotherapy, if there is no history of previous RT to the groin. If isolated recurrence develops in an inguinal node despite previous RT, inguinal node dissection may be performed without an APR. Morbidity from groin dissection may be high.
- Patients with metastatic anal cancer are treated with cisplatin-based chemotherapy with or without radiotherapy (or surgery) to control the primary tumor. Cetuximab-based treatment may be used in patients with metastatic anal cancer (KRAS wild type) after failure of cisplatin-based chemotherapy.

- Anal Canal Tumors in HIV-Positive Patients
  - Increased incidence, likely due to human papillomavirus infection and immunosuppression.
  - Dose of radiotherapy and chemoradiotherapy may need to be adjusted in patients with CD4 counts <200, due to increased toxicity.
  - Otherwise, treatment is the same as for HIV-negative patients.

Anal Melanoma

- Anal melanoma represents 1–4% of all anorectal malignancies. It is the third most common site of melanoma, after the skin and retina, accounting for less than 1% of all melanomas. These tumors arise from the transitional epithelium of the anal canal, the anoderm or the mucocutaneous junction.
- The most common symptom of anal melanoma is bleeding per rectum. Early lesions may be mistaken for hemorrhoids.
- A thorough physical exam, including assessment of the groin, should be done. Anal melanoma may be pigmented, and either polypoid or ulcerated, with raised edges. Satellite lesions may also be present. Biopsy is confirmatory.
- Histopathological Diagnosis: The features of anal melanoma resemble those of cutaneous melanomas (Fig. 21.5). The majority show a junctional component adjacent to the invasive tumor, which proves that the lesion is primary in nature. Perineural invasion is an important prognostic factor.
- Staging: Metastatic disease is common (up to 35% of patients at initial presentation). CT of the chest, abdomen, and pelvis or whole body PET-CT should be considered.
- Treatment/Prognosis. The overall prognosis of anal melanoma is dismal, with a median survival of 10–19 months after diagnosis.

Melanoma does not respond well to chemotherapy or radiotherapy; thus, surgery is the principal treatment when disease is localized. The extent of surgical resection is a matter of debate.

- Patients with tumors >1 cm are unlikely to be cured by any type of treatment. Thus, most authors advocate for local excision as the only surgical treatment which should be considered. Local excision may be curative for small tumors, which are often incidentally found in hemorrhoidectomy specimens.
- Palliative local excision can be considered for patients with local symptoms due to anal melanoma.
- APR can be considered. However, as most patients with anal melanoma die of distant metastasis, radical resection is unlikely to offer a survival advantage.

Anal Adenocarcinoma

- Primary mucinous adenocarcinoma of the anus is a rare malignancy, accounting for approximately 3% of anal cancers. Most anal adenocarcinomas originate from the colorectal zone in the upper portion of the anal canal, or from the glandular cells of the ATZ mucosa.
- Adenocarcinoma of the anal canal can be categorized based on origin:
  - Colorectal-type adenocarcinoma: Macroscopically and histologically, these lesions are indistinguishable from typical rectal adenocarcinoma. However, they carry a higher risk of nodal disease along the inguinal and femoral nodal chains.
  - Adenocarcinoma within an anorectal fistula.
  - Adenocarcinoma of the anal glands: This diagnosis is given if the tumor is primary to the anal canal and centered within the wall of the anorectal area, without a pre-existing fistula and without surface mucosa dysplasia, irrespective of the extent of mucin production.
- Anal adenocarcinomas are staged and treated as one would for a distal rectal adenocarcinoma.
- Historically, these tumors have been considered aggressive with poor prognosis. However, the rarity of the tumors and the difficulty of making the distinction between distal rectal adenocarcinoma and anal gland adenocarcinoma has made it difficult to draw firm conclusions in this regard.

Presacral Tumors

22

John Migaly and Christopher R. Mantyh

Key Concepts

- Unless contraindicated, presacral tumors should be surgically excised because of the risk of malignancy.
- MRI should be performed to characterize the lesions and to plan surgery.
- Lesions that are below sacral level S4 can be excised through a posterior/perineal approach.
- Complete, non-piecemeal excision is critical to avoiding recurrence or infection.
- Although the role of preoperative biopsy has been a source of debate, because of the fear of recurrence at or seeding of biopsy tracts, there is good single institutional data to support its selective use.
- Complete resection is critical as it drives the outcomes and prognosis for these patients.
- Lesions that are below sacral level S4 may be amenable to excision via a posterior/perineal approach.

General Considerations

- Presacral tumors are a heterogeneous group of rare tumors.
- Unless contraindicated, these tumors should be removed surgically as a third of them may be malignant and benign lesions can undergo subsequent malignant transformation.
- The diagnosis of these tumors is often delayed because of vague symptomatology, and often these lesions are advanced when found.
- MRI is essential for characterization of the tumor and surgical planning.

J. Migaly (✉)
Division of Advanced GI & Oncologic Surgery, Duke University Medical Center, Durham, NC, USA
e-mail: john.migaly@duke.edu

C. R. Mantyh
Department of Surgery, Duke University Medical Center, Durham, NC, USA

Anatomic Considerations

- The presacral or retrorectal space is a potential space posterior to the rectum, whose superior extent is the pelvic peritoneal reflection, the lateral limits are ureters and the iliac vessels; posteriorly it is defined by the sacrum, and anteriorly it is defined as the posterior wall of the rectum. The inferior border is the levator complex and the coccygeal muscles (Fig. 22.1).
- It is a unique area in that it represents a developmentally critical location where several types of embryological distinct cell lines converge for the final steps prior to completion of ontogeny. It is these changes that produce the variety of benign and malignant, solid, and cystic growths that can occur in this space.
- The retrorectal space presents a multitude of challenges to the surgeon, and this subset of

S. R. Steele et al. (eds.), *The ASCRS Manual of Colon and Rectal Surgery*,
https://doi.org/10.1007/978-3-030-01165-9_22

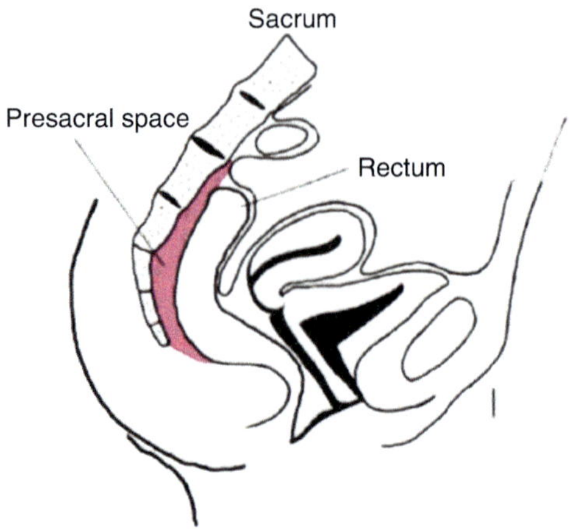

Fig. 22.1 Location of the presacral space. (Reprinted with permission from. Ghosh J, Eglinton T, Frizelle FA, Watson AJ. Presacral tumours in adults. Surgeon. 2007 Feb;5(1):31–8 © 2007, Elsevier Ltd.)

procedures is not recommended for those uninitiated in pelvic surgery. The sacral nerve rootlets are located in this retrorectal space, and thus injury to and sacrifice of these structures can have substantial implications on rectoanal and sexual function. In cases requiring the unilateral sacrifice of all of the sacral nerve rootlets, the patient will likely retain normal anorectal and sexual function. Bilateral sacrifice of the third sacral nerve rootlet will usually result in fecal incontinence.

Classification

- Congenital lesions
  - Represent two-thirds of all retrorectal lesions, which are thought to arise from various combinations of the three embryonic cell layers. These congenital lesions can be cystic or solid. In general, these lesions are more common in females than males. Can be benign or malignant.
  - *Dermoid and Epidermoid Cysts*: Line with squamous epithelial cells and may contain various skin appendages such as hair or nails (Fig. 22.2). Patients can have a post-anal dimple or sinus that can be mistaken for an abscess and errantly drained, which may account for high rate of infection of these cysts.

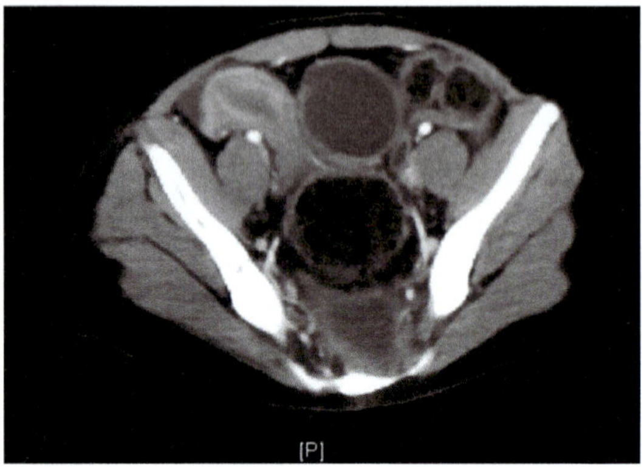

Fig. 22.2 CT image of an epidermoid cyst

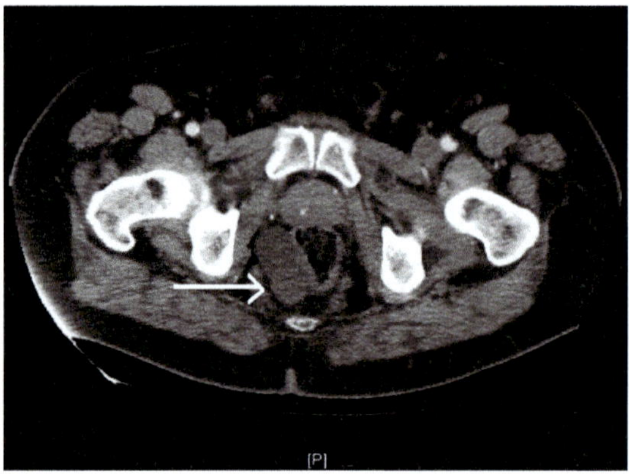

Fig. 22.3 CT image of rectal duplication cyst

  - *Enterogenous*: Unlike dermoid and epidermoid cysts, enterogenous cysts are multilocular. They arise from the endoderm of the primitive hindgut. These lesions can also undergo malignant degeneration.
  - *Tailgut Cysts* (retrorectal cystic hamartomas, rectal duplication cysts): Arise from persistence of the hindgut (Fig. 22.3). Rectal duplication cysts that contain all of the layers of the intestinal tract can undergo malignant change.
  - *Teratomas*: Contain cells from all three germ layers, can contain both solid and cystic components, and can contain tissues from almost any organ system including digestive, respiratory, or bony tissue. Up to 10% harbor malignancy cancer and thus aggressive extirpation should be pursued. Because of the diverse germ cell layers,

these lesions can become squamous cell carcinomas, rhabdomyosarcomas, or anaplastic tumors.

- *Chordomas*: The most common malignant tumor of the presacral space arises from what is believed to be the vestigial notochord tissue. Can occur almost anywhere on the spinal cord but are most commonly found in the presacral area. The 5- and 10-year survival rates are 67% and 40%, respectively, and although surgery remains a mainstay of treatment, it is associated with a high recurrence rate.
- *Anterior Sacral Meningocele*: Arise from protrusions of the dural sac through a defect in the sacrum. The classic radiologic finding of the "scimitar sign" can often be seen on plain films. Patients often have vague symptomology including headaches related to postural changes and Valsalva. Magnetic resonance imaging usually easily characterizes these lesions, and *percutaneous biopsy should be avoided* for fear of bacterial contamination of the cerebrospinal fluid and iatrogenic meningitis.

- Neurogenic tumors
  - Represent about 10% of all retrorectal tumors. They arise from peripheral nerves and include neurofibromas, schwannoma, ganglioneuroma, neuroblastomas, ganglioneuroblastoma (Fig. 22.4), and ependymoma. Ependymomas are the most common of these tumors [1, 2]. Differentiation between benign and malignant variants can be difficult, and these tumors can produce significant neuropathy as a presenting symptom.
- Osseous lesions
  - Osseous lesions include giant cell tumors, osteoblastoma, aneurysmal bone cysts, osteogenic sarcoma, Ewing's sarcoma, myeloma, and chondrosarcomas. These lesions represent 10% of all retrorectal tumors. These may be the most aggressive of all the retrorectal tumors and can be very locally destructive and have pronounced metastatic potential.

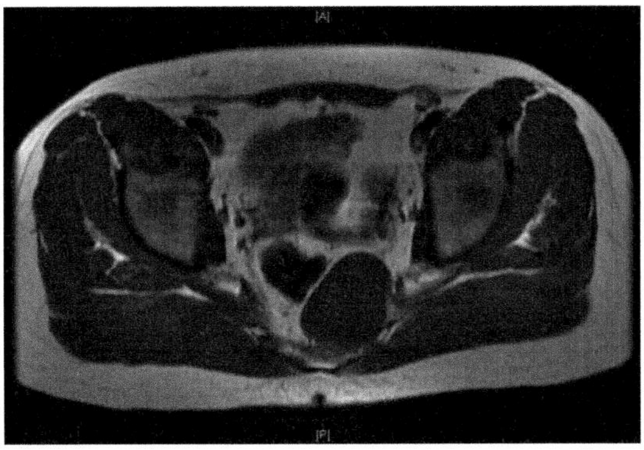

Fig. 22.4 CT image of a ganglioneuroblastoma

Diagnosis

- History and Physical
  - Symptoms are often vague. Tumors are often noted incidentally on cross-sectional imaging obtained for other indications. Occasionally presacral cystic lesions are confused with cryptoglandular abscess and fistula. Patients with advanced tumors can have constipation, sexual dysfunction, urinary incontinence, and other leg and gluteal symptoms related to local extension and mass effect.
  - Digital rectal examination can help assess the consistency and fixation of the lesion and relationship to the anal sphincter. Flexible endoscopy will often reveal subtle extrinsic mass effect on the rectosigmoid. Neurologic exam with attention to gluteal and lower extremity dysfunction allows for preoperative documentation of these defects and aids assessing the locally invasive nature of the lesion.
- Imaging Studies
  - Plain films have limited utility but can sometimes demonstrate osseous destruction of the sacrum or calcifications within the tumor itself. In patients with anterior sacral meningocele, the classic "scimitar sign" can often be seen on plain films, but usually cross-sectional imaging is required for confirmation.
  - Magnetic resonance imaging (MRI) with gadolinium is the imaging modality of

choice for retrorectal tumors. MRI is critical in the management of these tumors by facilitating accurate diagnosis, determining the anatomic extent of the lesion and selection of the optimal surgical approach.
  - Characterization of the lesion as solid or cystic is easily achievable via MRI, but subtle nodularity or septation of these lesions allows further characterization of these lesions into their various subtypes (Fig. 22.5).
  - What MRI excels at in comparison to CT scan is defining invasion of the muscular walls of the rectum, particularly in cases of sacrococcygeal chordoma.
- Preoperative Biopsy
  - In general, biopsy of cystic lesions should only be undertaken in situations where there is some question of the characterization of the lesion *after* a high-quality MRI interpreted by an experienced radiologist.
  - Biopsy of presacral lesions via the transrectal or transvaginal route is strongly discouraged, as it is possible to infect a sterile cystic lesion. In addition, biopsy via these routes necessitates either partial or complete proctectomy or vaginectomy to remove the biopsy tract in continuity with the presacral tumor in order to prevent recurrence. Biopsy of a meningocele via any route should be avoided for fear of an infection of the cerebrospinal fluid and resultant meningitis.
  - There is a role for biopsy in unresectable, sizeable, or aggressive tumors such as Ewing's sarcoma or osteogenic sarcoma where preoperative radiation or chemotherapy could be of value for systemic or local control or to improve the likelihood of resectability.
  - Many authors recommend excision of the biopsy tract and site at the time of definitive surgery.

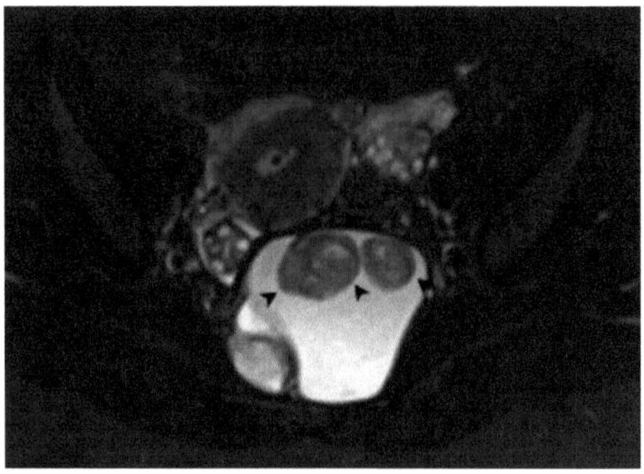

Fig. 22.5 MRI of presacral cyst. T2-weighted imaging of an epidermoid cyst shows a bilobulated cystic lesion with pools of keratin debris (arrows) inside the larger cyst. (*Reprinted Loock MT, Fornès P, Soyer P, Rousset P, Azizi L, Hoeffel C. MR imaging features of nongynaecologic cystic lesions of the pelvis. Clin Imaging 2013;37(2):211-8 © 2013 Elsevier Ltd, with Permission from Elsevier*)

Management

- Role of Preoperative Neoadjuvant Therapy
  - In cases of large locally advanced presacral tumors, where resectability is at issue, neoadjuvant radiotherapy may render some benefit in decreasing tumor size and increasing resectability.
- Surgical Treatment
  - Preoperative Planning
    - In patients that have direct invasion of the muscular wall of the rectum, proctectomy must be anticipated. In cases of bony invasion, partial sacrectomy is planned. Pelvic sidewall involvement may necessitate intraoperative radiotherapy and vascular or ureteric reconstruction. The assembly of a multispecialty team of colorectal, urologic, neurosurgical, orthopedic, vascular, and plastic surgeon is a prerequisite for many of these undertakings.
  - Choice of Surgical Approach
    - In lesions above the S4 level of the spine, a purely abdominal approach can be considered, while lesions below S4

can be approached posteriorly. Lesions spanning both above and below S4 are best approached via a combined abdominal and posterior approach.

– Posterior Approach
  - Prone jackknife position; general endotracheal anesthesia.
  - Proceed as outlined in Figs. 22.6, 22.7, and 22.8. After removal of the tumor, the operative field is submerged beneath the irrigant, and a proctoscope is used to insufflate the rectum to check for an air leak and assure that the rectum has not been violated. The soft tissue and the incision are closed in multiple layers over a closed suction drain.

– Combined Abdominal and Perineal Approach

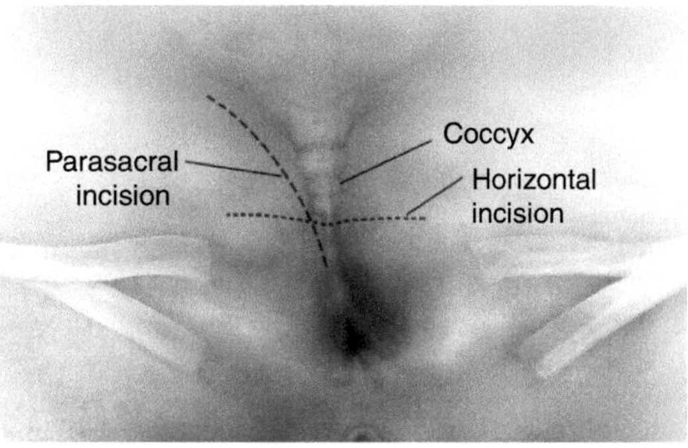

Fig. 22.6 Posterior approach to removal of a presacral tumor, placement of incision. The patient is in prone jackknife, and the incision can either be horizontal on the anococcygeal ligament or curvilinear to the left of the lower sacrum/coccyx and into the intergluteal fold. (*With permission from Ludwig KA, Kalady MF. Transacral approaches for prescral cyst: rectal tumor. Operative Techniques in General Surgery 2005;7:3–126–136* © *2005 Elsevier Ltd.*)

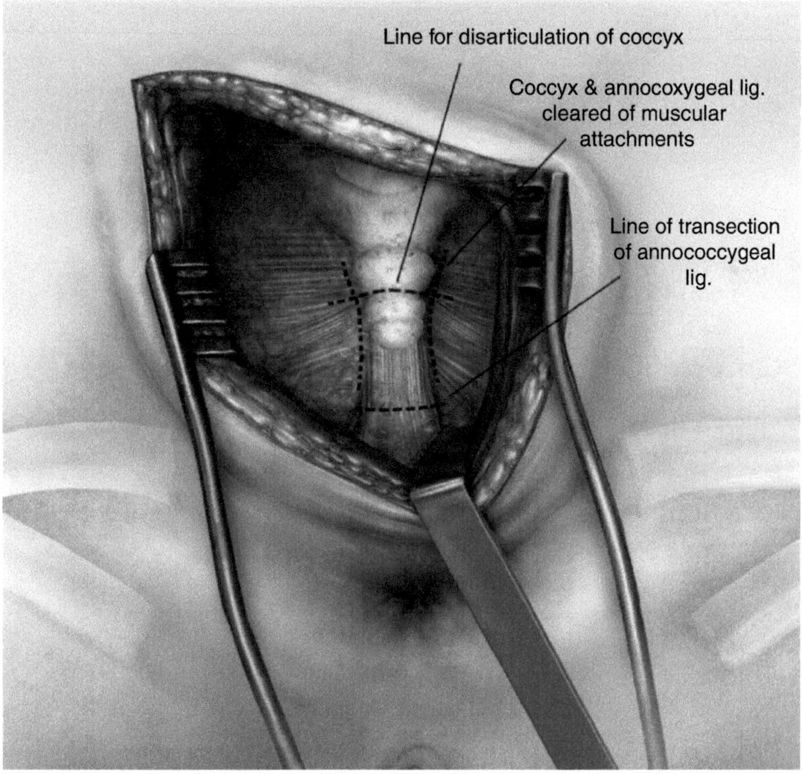

Fig. 22.7 The anococcygeal ligament is divided, and the coccyx is subsequently cleared of its lateral attachments and removed; this facilitates dissection along the sacrum. (*With permission from Ludwig KA, Kalady MF. Transacral approaches for prescral cyst: rectal tumor. Operative Techniques in General Surgery 2005;7:3–126–136* © *2005 Elsevier Ltd.*)

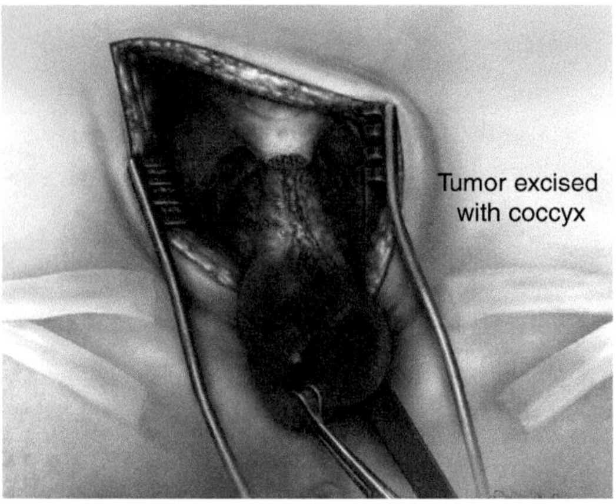

Fig. 22.8 Now with access to the presacral space, the surgeon can carefully dissect the cyst off of the sacrum and "roll" it toward himself from cephalad to caudad. (*With permission from Ludwig KA, Kalady MF. Transacral approaches for prescral cyst: rectal tumor. Operative Techniques in General Surgery 2005;7:3–126–136 © 2005 Elsevier Ltd.*)

- Lithotomy position with access to anus and perineum initially.
- Rectosigmoid mobilization.
- There is often a feeding vessel to the tumor in the midline, and ligating the middle sacral vessels can often help stem potential blood loss.
- The tumor is then dissected anteriorly off of the rectum and posteriorly off of the sacrum and laterally off of the sidewalls.
- In situations where tumor is densely adherent to the posterior rectum, a proctectomy should be performed for en bloc removal with the tumor.
- If the internal iliac artery or vein needs to be sacrificed, communication with the anesthesiologist in advance of ligation is ideal, as the sacrifice of these vessels can sometimes be associated with large volume bleeding misadventures and blood products should be on hand. If involvement of these vessels is identified preoperatively, catheter-based venous or arterial embolization can be considered in advance of surgery.
- In situations where the lower most portion of the tumor cannot be reached from the abdominal approach, there are two options: the first is to place the patient in high lithotomy and proceed via a posterior approach or the second is to close the abdomen and place the patient in prone jackknife position. The visualization and performance of the posterior approach with the patient placed in high lithotomy are challenging, and it is our preference to close the abdomen and subsequently flip the patient to the prone jackknife position.
- Transabdominal rectus abdominis or gracilis myocutaneous flaps can be transposed into the pelvis to fill large defects.

Outcomes

- The rarity of these tumors and the heterogeneous approach to them preclude rigorous assessment of outcomes. Nevertheless, patients can be cured of presacral malignancies. Lesions that are resected completely without disruption have a better prognosis than those that are not.

Molecular Basis of Colorectal Cancer and Overview of Inherited Colorectal Cancer Syndromes

23

Matthew F. Kalady and Y. Nancy You

Key Concepts

- Colorectal cancer is a genetically heterogeneous disease that arises via at least three main oncogenic pathways: chromosomal instability, microsatellite instability, and the methylator phenotype. Each pathway produces distinct but overlapping clinical phenotypes. These pathways are represented in sporadic colorectal cancer as well as in hereditary colorectal cancer syndromes.
- Identification and diagnosis of a hereditary colorectal cancer syndrome require a high level of suspicion and appropriate knowledge to evaluate the patient and at-risk family members. These syndromes have distinct genetic and clinical traits and are broadly classified into polyposis (adenomatous, hamartomatous, serrated polyps) and nonpolyposis (HNPCC and Lynch syndrome).
- Familial adenomatous polyposis is a multisystem disease that confers a near 100% colorectal cancer malignancy risk. Close endoscopic surveillance and timely prophylactic surgery are required to limit colorectal cancer formation. Desmoid disease and duodenal adenocarcinoma are other leading causes of morbidity and mortality.
- *MUTYH*-associated polyposis (MAP) is a recessively inherited syndrome that carries an approximately 75% lifetime risk of colorectal cancer. Annual colonoscopic surveillance is necessary, and surgery is indicated for uncontrolled polyp burden or the development of adenocarcinoma. Extended colectomy should be offered in healthy patients.
- The hamartomatous syndromes (Peutz-Jeghers syndrome, juvenile polyposis syndrome, and PTEN hamartoma syndrome) are rare but are associated with significant colorectal cancer and extracolonic multisystem malignancy. Early recognition and extensive screening and surveillance protocols are required.
- Serrated polyposis syndrome is characterized by numerous and/or large serrated polyps. Although no genetic etiology has been identified, it carries an approximately 25% risk of developing colorectal cancer. Annual colonoscopic surveillance is necessary, and surgery is indicated for uncontrolled polyp burden or the development of adenocarcinoma. Extended colectomy should be offered in healthy patients.
- Lynch syndrome is the most common of the hereditary syndromes and is responsible for about 3% of all colorectal cancers. Universal

M. F. Kalady (✉)
Department of Colorectal Surgery, Digestive Disease Institute, Cleveland Clinic, Cleveland, OH, USA
e-mail: kaladym@ccf.org

Y. Nancy You
Department of Surgical Oncology, University of Texas MD Anderson Cancer Center, Houston, TX, USA

S. R. Steele et al. (eds.), *The ASCRS Manual of Colon and Rectal Surgery*,
https://doi.org/10.1007/978-3-030-01165-9_23

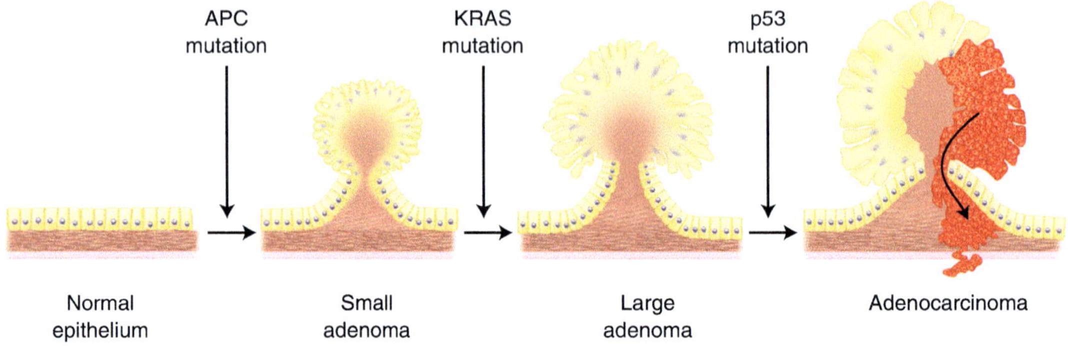

Fig. 23.1 Schematic representation of the traditional adenoma-to-carcinoma sequence resulting in chromosomal instability

screening and systematic molecular analysis of newly diagnosed colorectal cancer for DNA mismatch repair deficiency provide an effective approach to identifying patients at risk for Lynch syndrome.

- Patients with Lynch syndrome face significantly elevated risks for colorectal and extracolonic cancers in multiple organs. Lynch syndrome patients benefit from colonoscopic screening and participation in a hereditary registry.
- After development of an initial colorectal cancer, patients with Lynch syndrome have high risk for metachronous colorectal neoplasia. Extended resection (total abdominal colectomy for colon cancer and total proctocolectomy for rectal cancer) should be considered in weighing risks of future malignancy and quality of life.

Chromosomal Instability

- Chromosomal instability refers to an alteration in the chromosome copy number or structure and is the most common form of genomic instability in CRC, accounting for about 75% of all CRC. Physical loss of a chromosome segment may delete entire genes and produce loss of heterozygosity for those genes. That is, as one allele is lost, only one functional copy of the gene exists, and there is no longer redundancy for that gene. Loss of the second allele results in complete loss of that gene function. *APC* and *p53* are examples of tumor suppressor genes, whose loss via this mechanism results in chromosomal unstable CRC.
- The traditional adenoma-to-carcinoma sequence as described by Vogelstein and Fearon is characterized by the accumulation of genetic changes over time and the prototype chromosomal instability of CRC. An overview of this pathway is given in Fig. 23.1. Clinically, CRCs arising via chromosomal instability tend to be located in the left colon, have male predominance, and develop later in life. Genetically, key genes mutated in this pathway include *APC*, *KRAS*, and *p53*.

Microsatellite Instability

- Microsatellite instability results from faulty DNA mismatch repair (MMR) function. Routine DNA replication is associated with high infidelity, with specific sites along the DNA strand that are prone to errors. These sites are areas of repetitive DNA sequences, called microsatellites. Microsatellites are noncoding segments of DNA that contain repetitive sequences of one to four nucleotides. There are hundreds of thousands of microsatellites in the genome, and microsatellite patterns provide a unique DNA fingerprint. When these errors are not repaired due to MMR deficiency, the length of the microsatellite regions is altered, and the fingerprint changes; i.e., there are different lengths of the DNA fragments. Thus, the pattern of fragments detected by PCR techniques produces a different pattern of microsatellites, and thus the term microsatellite unstable or microsatellite instability-high (MSI-H).

- Functionally, loss of MMR function leads to an accumulation of unrepaired errors. Several key tumor suppressor genes have multiple short repetitive sequences that make them prone to DNA mismatch. Loss of MMR function allows accumulation of mutations in these genes that subsequently lead to adenoma and cancer formation. Cancers arising through this molecular pathway are termed the mutator phenotype as these tumors tend to be hypermutated and account for approximately 15% of CRC. Inherited mutations in one of the DNA mismatch repair genes result in Lynch syndrome.

CpG Island Methylator Phenotype (CIMP)

- Epigenetic mechanisms such as hypermethylation of DNA promoter regions can affect gene expression and protein translation without changing the inherent DNA sequence. Methylation of cytosine is a common biological phenomenon that occurs throughout the genome and controls multiple processes.
- Several key tumor suppressor genes contain cytosine-guanine (CpG) repetitive sequences, which are prone to hypermethylation in the promoter region, which silences transcription of that gene, and thus no functional protein is made. As the areas prone to hypermethylation contain regions rich in cytosine and guanine dinucleotide repeats, or CpG islands, they have been termed CpG island methylator phenotype (CIMP or CIMP-high).
- This pattern is reproducible in approximately 20% of CRCs and is associated with aberrant methylation of the mismatch repair gene, *MLH1*. Approximately 85% of MSI-H CRCs develop via loss of the expression of the MMR gene, *hMLH1*, caused by DNA hypermethylation.
- In contrast to CRC arising via chromosomal instability in which the precursor lesions are adenomatous polyps, the precursor lesions in CIMP cancers are serrated polyps.
- The most common initial mutation occurs in the *BRAF* oncogene. BRAF mutations support the transformation of normal mucosa to aberrant crypt foci or a hyperplastic polyp or sessile serrated polyp (SSP).
- Increasing methylation gives rise to CIMP and eventual methylation of *MLH1*, which in turn silences transcription. Loss of MLH1 results in MMR deficiency and thus the development of an MSI-H CRC. As CIMP CRCs develop through serrated polyp intermediates, this pathway is called the serrated pathway. An overview of this process is shown in Fig. 23.2.
- Clinically, CIMP CRC tends to develop in the right colon, at advanced age, and is more common in females.

General Approach and Classification of Suspected Hereditary Syndromes

- Awareness and suspicion are the keys to identifying hereditary CRC syndromes. Although only about 5–10% of all CRCs arise with a known hereditary syndrome, recognizing these cases and making the correct diagnosis impact care of that particular patient and their family including future generations.
- Clinical evaluation should include a personal and family history, physical examination, documentation of gastrointestinal polyps or cancers, and identification of extracolonic manifestations.
- A specific diagnosis is warranted to assign risk for cancer development and guide surveillance and prophylactic interventions. Information gained from the initial evaluation can guide the specific diagnostic tests required to make a diagnosis. Genetic counseling is a critical component to this evaluation and is recommended before genetic testing to discuss potential implications of the results. An overview of the classification of hereditary CRC syndromes is given in Table 23.1.

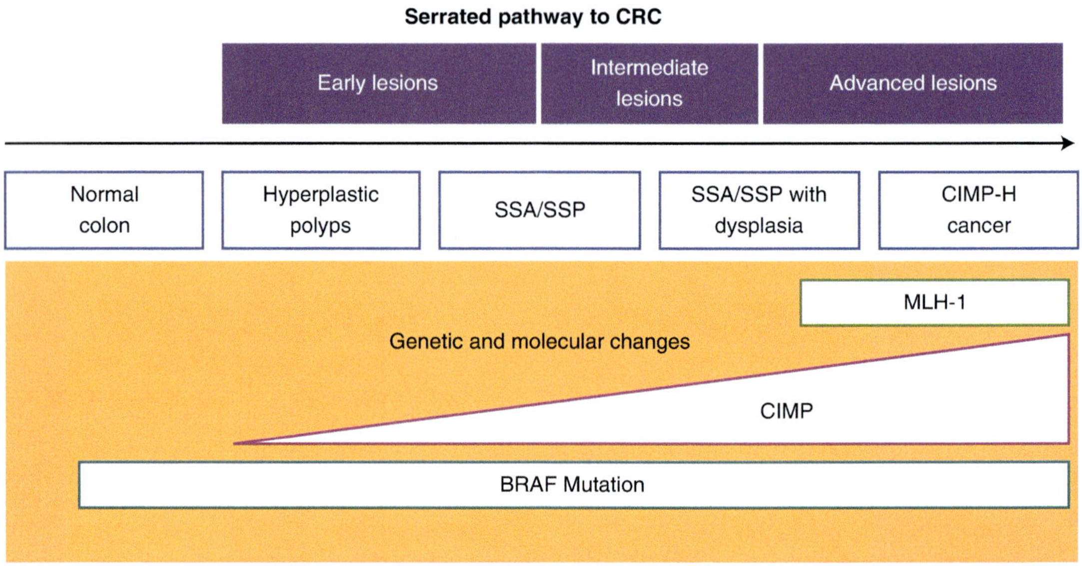

Fig. 23.2 Schematic representation of proposed serrated pathway to colorectal cancer

Table 23.1 Classification and overview of hereditary colorectal cancer syndromes

Polyposis syndromes					
Syndrome	Gene(s)	Main polyp type	Inheritance	Predominant clinical findings	Approximate CRC risk
FAP					
Classical	*APC*	Adenoma	AD	100–1000 adenomas; duodenal adenomas and carcinomas; gastric fundic gland polyps desmoid tumors, epidermoid cysts, extra teeth, osteomas	100%
Profuse	*APC*	Adenoma	AD	>1000 adenomas; duodenal adenomas and carcinomas; gastric fundic gland polyps desmoid tumors, epidermoid cysts, extra teeth, osteomas	100%
Attenuated	*APC*	Adenoma	AD	<100 adenomas; gastric fundic gland polyps desmoid tumors, epidermoid cysts, extra teeth, osteomas	80%
MAP	*MYH*	Adenoma	AR	0–1000 adenomas, CRC <50 years; gastric fundic gland polyps, duodenal adenomas and carcinomas	80%
JPS	*BMPR1A* *SMAD4*	Hamartoma	AD	≥5 juvenile polyps; Any juvenile polyp and JPS family history; HHT	40%
PJS	*STK11*	Hamartoma	AD	Peutz-Jeghers polyps; orocutaneous pigmentation; family history of PJP; cancer of small bowel, colon, stomach, pancreas, breast, ovary, testis	40%
PHTS	*PTEN*	Hamartoma	AD	Colorectal adenomas, lipomas, fibromas, ganglioneuromas, juvenile hamartomas; colorectal cancer; macrocephaly, trichilemmomas	10% (Cowden)

Table 23.1 (continued)

Polyposis syndromes					
Syndrome	Gene(s)	Main polyp type	Inheritance	Predominant clinical findings	Approximate CRC risk
SPS	Unknown	Serrated polyps	Unknown	>20 serrated polyps; Any serrated polyp and family history of SPS; >5 serrated polyps proximal to the sigmoid, 2 are >1 cm diameter	25–40%
Nonpolyposis syndromes					
Lynch syndrome	*MLH1*, *MSH2*, *MSH6*, *PMS2*, *EPCAM*	Adenoma	AD	Microsatellite-unstable CRC, advanced adenomas; gastric, duodenal, small bowel, transitional cell, gall bladder, pancreas, endometrial, and ovarian cancer	60–80%
Familial CRC type X	Unknown	Adenoma	AD	Amsterdam criteria positive, microsatellite-stable tumors	12%

With permission from Kalady MF, Heald B. Diagnostic approach to hereditary colorectal cancer syndromes. Clin Colon Rectal Surg. 2015;28(4):205–14. © Thieme

FAP familial adenomatous polyposis, *MAP MUTYH*-associated polyposis, *JPS* juvenile polyposis syndrome, *PJP* Peutz-Jeghers polyposis, *PHTS* PTEN hamartoma tumor syndromes, *SPS* serrated polyposis syndrome, *CRC* colorectal cancer, *HHT* hereditary hemorrhagic telangiectasia, *AD* autosomal dominant, *AR* autosomal recessive

Adenomatous Polyposis Syndromes

Familial Adenomatous Polyposis

Clinical Presentation

- FAP is an autosomal-dominant inherited disease that occurs in approximately 1 in 10,000 live births and affects both genders equally and all races. The hallmark feature of FAP is colorectal adenomatous polyposis, but the phenotype varies per patient, even within the same family.
- Severe FAP is characterized by thousands of colorectal adenomas. Often times there is little normal mucosa between the adenomatous polyps. Mild polyposis is described as having between 100 and 1000 colorectal adenomas. Patients with fewer than 100 adenomas are considered to have attenuated FAP. Figure 23.3 provides an example of moderate to severe polyposis.
- Nearly 100% of patients with FAP will develop CRC if left untreated.
- FAP is a multisystem disease and may present with various extracolonic lesions. Two specific subtypes of FAP are based on a specific constellation of extracolonic manifestations. Gardner's syndrome is FAP with desmoid tumors, osteomas, epidermoid cysts, or extranumery teeth. Turcot's syndrome is FAP associated with malignant tumors of the central nervous system. Both syndromes are also caused by mutations in *APC*.

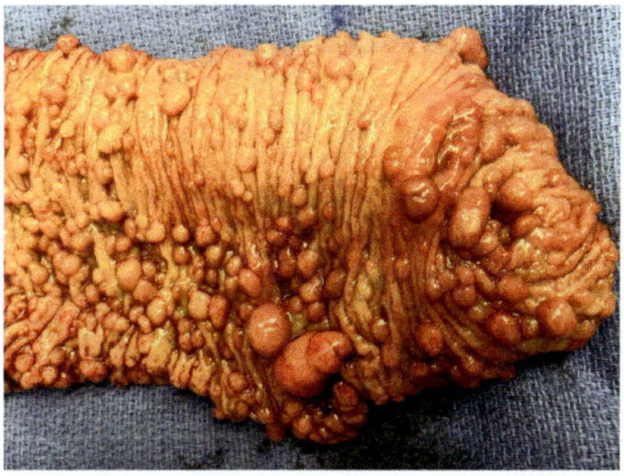

Fig. 23.3 Moderate to severe polyposis in the resected specimen of a 22-year-old woman with familial adenomatous polyposis

Underlying Genetics

- FAP is caused by an inherited mutation in the *APC* gene on chromosome 5q21. As patients

are born with only one functional copy of the "gatekeeper" gene, loss of the second allele via sporadic mechanisms leads to rapid development of hundreds to thousands of colorectal adenomas.
- More than 850 different mutations have been described, most of which produce a stop codon that ceases protein translation which yields a truncated APC protein. Depending on the location of the "stop," the truncated protein has variable functional abilities, likely accounting for some of phenotypic variation seen with different mutations. About 25% of patients with FAP have a "de novo" mutation and thus have no family history.

Diagnosis

- FAP may be diagnosed genetically or clinically. Genetic testing reveals an *APC* germline mutation in approximately 80% of cases. Indications for genetic counseling referral and testing include a family history of FAP, personal history of more than ten adenomas, personal history of adenomas, and an extracolonic manifestation of FAP.
- For at-risk individuals in families with a known mutation, genetic testing is directed for that mutation.
- Approximately 20% of patients will not have an identified germline mutation but still have the clinical phenotype.

CRC Risk

- FAP carries a near 100% CRC risk. Cancers develop at a median age of 39. The goal of surveillance and intervention is to reduce the risk of death from colorectal cancer via colectomy or proctocolectomy before cancers develop. The risk of CRC in attenuated FAP is approximately 70%, and cancers develop at a relatively later age (average 58 years) compared to classical FAP.

FAP Extracolonic Manifestations

- *Upper gastrointestinal tract*: Approximately 90% of patients with FAP develop duodenal adenomas. Despite the high incidence of adenomas, only about 5–10% of patients will develop periampullary cancer. Non-neoplastic gastric fundic gland polyps are a common finding, occurring in about 50% of patients. These have a minimal risk of malignancy. Rare gastric cancers in FAP are felt to develop from gastric adenomas that form in the gastric antrum in about 10% of FAP patients.

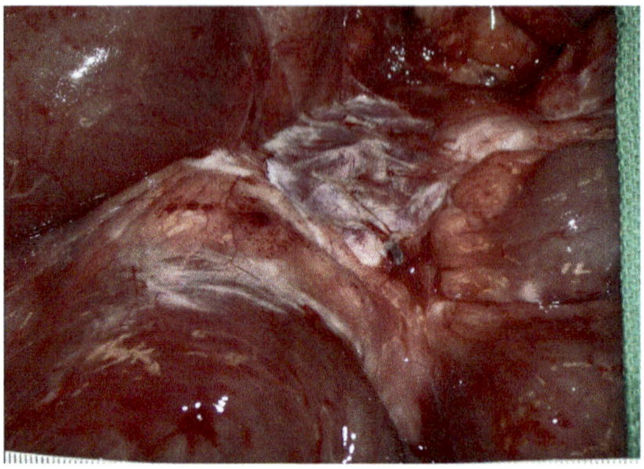

Fig. 23.4 Different manifestations of desmoid disease. (**a**) Abdominal wall desmoid occurring 1 year after total proctocolectomy for familial adenomatous polyposis. (**b**) Resected abdominal wall desmoid. (**c**) Large intra-abdominal desmoid arising from the root of the small bowel mesentery. (**d**) Sheetlike desmoid tumor arising in the mesentery with associated desmoid reaction (Photos in (**c**) and (**d**) courtesy of Dr. James Church)

- *Desmoids*: Desmoid disease affects approximately 5% of patients with FAP. About half of FAP-associated desmoid tumors arise intra-abdominally in bowel mesentery, and 40% develop in the abdominal wall. The remainder presents in the back, neck, or limbs. Desmoids can manifest as flat, fibrous, sheet-like lesions or as defined discrete masses (see Fig. 23.4).
- *Thyroid cancer*: Although the risk of thyroid cancer in FAP is only 2%, it doubles the risk of that for the general population. The incidence is 17 times higher in women than in men, and it develops at a young mean age of 27 years. The primary histology is papillary carcinoma.
- *Other malignant tumors*: There are several rare extracolonic malignant tumors associated with FAP that have a higher incidence than the general population. These include pancreatic adenocarcinomas (relative risk 4.5, lifetime risk 1.7%), hepatoblastoma in children (RR

7500–7500, absolute risk 2%), and medulloblastoma (RR 7, lifetime risk 0.025%).

- *Other benign lesions*: Several benign lesions are associated with FAP that do not necessarily require intervention but can be used to help make a diagnosis. Congenital hypertrophy of the retinal pigment epithelium (CHRPE) is characterized as well-delineated grayish-black or brown oval spots seen in 60–85% of FAP patients. Bony lesions including dental abnormalities and mandibular and skull osteomas are found in approximately 20% of patients. Multiple cutaneous and subcutaneous lesions are associated with FAP including epidermoid cysts, lipomas, and fibromas. These are benign, and intervention is not necessary unless they cause symptoms. The presence of these on the face, scalp, and extremities rather than on the back in young patients should raise suspicion for possible FAP.

Table 23.2 Scores of duodenal adenoma characteristics and management recommendations according to Spigelman criteria

Duodenal disease grading scale (points assigned)			
Assigned points	1	2	3
Number of polyps	1–4	5–20	>20
Size of polyps (mm)	1–4	5–10	>10
Histology	Tubular	Tubulovillous	Villous
Dysplasia	Mild	Moderate	Severe
Recommendations based on Spigelman score			
Total points	*Spigelman stage*	*Recommendation*	
0	0	Repeat endoscopy in 5 years	
1–4	I	Repeat endoscopy in 5 years	
5–6	II	Repeat endoscopy in 2–3 years	
7–8	III	Repeat endoscopy in 6–12 months	
9–12	IV	Surgical evaluation	

Management

Screening

- *Colorectal*: The goal of colorectal screening and surveillance in FAP is to limit CRC risk by timely intervention and surgical referral. Screening should be done on all individuals with a genetic diagnosis or in first-degree relatives of persons with a clinical diagnosis of FAP. If no genetic mutation is found in a family but they have a clinical diagnosis, all first-degree relatives should be screened. Screening begins at age 12 and can be initiated with flexible proctosigmoidoscopy. If polyps are seen, a full colonoscopy is warranted. If no polyps are identified on the initial proctosigmoidoscopy, the exam should be repeated every 1–2 years or earlier if symptoms develop. For those without a genetic diagnosis, first-degree relatives who are not found to have any polyps by age 40 can safely be transitioned to screening guidelines for the general population.
- *Duodenal and gastric*: Upper gastrointestinal endoscopic screening is a key part of FAP disease management. Screening is done with a side-viewing endoscope and should begin at age 20–25 years. Screening intervals are based on the Spigelman staging system (Table 23.2).
- *Desmoids*: There are no recommendations for routine screening for desmoid disease.
- *Thyroid*: Annual thyroid screening by ultrasound should be recommended to FAP patients.

Treatment

Colorectal

- The goals of FAP treatment are to remove or limit the CRC risk while maximizing quality of life. As CRC is near certain, surgical removal is the mainstay of treatment.

Timing of Surgery

- Patients with symptoms should be offered surgery both to treat the symptoms and to prophylactically treat potential occult cancer. For asymptomatic teenagers with FAP, surgery can be reasonably delayed until the late teen years or early twenties when they have reached physical and emotional maturity. CRC before the age of 20 is extremely rare and is usually accompanied by symptoms. Since cancer risk increases with age, patients diagnosed in their third decade or beyond should be offered surgery at the time of diagnosis.

- Delaying surgery in an asymptomatic patient with low polyp burden may be considered in specific circumstances: women who wish to have children and avoid the risk of decreased fecundity following proctectomy; morbidly obese patients who wish to lose weight to make restorative proctocolectomy with ileal pouch-anal anastomosis (IPAA) a more feasible option; and patients who have desmoids in their family, as most desmoids develop after surgery. Deferral of surgery should only be done in patients who are asymptomatic, motivated, and adherent to surveillance protocols.

Extent of Resection

- For patients *without evidence of rectal cancer*, surgical options include colectomy with ileorectal anastomosis (IRA) or total proctocolectomy (TPC) with or without restoration of gastrointestinal tract. Decisions are made based on balancing future cancer risk with quality of life associated with bowel function, as valued by both the patient and surgeon. TPC removes all or nearly all at-risk mucosa and almost completely eliminates future CRC risk. Restoration of the gastrointestinal tract via an ileal pouch-anal anastomosis (IPAA) results in more frequent bowel movements, higher incidence of incontinence, and decreased quality of life compared to colectomy and IRA. The improved function of an IRA is countered by cancer risk in the residual rectum. Patient selection is key to minimizing risk. An IRA is the preferred approach for patients who have a relatively low colorectal polyp burden. Conversely, *APC* mutations at codons 1309 and 1328 are associated with severe polyposis and are independent risk factors for proctectomy after TAC in FAP.
- For patients who develop *rectal cancer*, total proctocolectomy should be performed with restoration of the gastrointestinal tract via an IPAA when possible. In the presence of stage IV disease with limited life expectancy, a proctectomy alone may be considered if there is no cancer in the colon and the polyp burden is minimal or controlled. If the rectal cancer is locally advanced and radiotherapy is required, it should be utilized in the preoperative period or not at all, especially if a restorative proctocolectomy is planned, as postoperative radiotherapy is associated with toxicity and risk of ileal pouch loss. If an IPAA is not planned, and radiotherapy is not given preoperatively, an omental pedicle flap or pelvic inlet mesh should be considered to occlude the small bowel from the pelvis in case postoperative radiotherapy is unexpectedly required.
- In the presence of *colon cancer and metastatic disease*, decisions regarding whether to proceed with proctocolectomy instead of just colectomy should be based on the likelihood of cure and risk of metachronous cancer in the rectum if left in situ. Patients with locally advanced primary tumors (or those with possible metastatic disease) with minimal rectal polyp burden may be better served by abdominal colectomy and IRA (or proctocolectomy and ileostomy) versus restorative proctocolectomy – where complications of surgery are more common and may delay administration of adjuvant chemotherapy.
- Debate exists over the use of *mucosectomy and handsewn anastomosis versus double-stapled anastomosis during TPC and IPAA* as a means of reducing the risk of subsequent rectal cancer. Mucosectomy to the dentate line theoretically removes all colorectal mucosa at risk for neoplasia. However, this technique potentially fails if an incomplete mucosectomy results in residual mucosal cells, which are present in up to 20% of patients. This risk must be balanced against the cancer risk from a small anal transition zone that remains following a stapled IPAA. It may be preferable to have any at-risk mucosa in the lumen of the gut, where it can be observed over time, rather than implanted outside the ileal pouch at the time of mucosectomy, where it cannot be observed. In cases of rectal dysplasia or rectal cancer, many clinicians advocate mucosectomy, although definitive data regarding reduction in cancer risk are lacking.

Duodenal Adenomas

- Duodenal adenomas can progress to cancer, but this rate is relatively low, and, as such, the lesions can usually be managed endoscopically. The Spigelman staging system estimates duodenal cancer risk based on several factors as given in Table 23.2. Early-stage lesions may safely be surveyed with low risk of cancer. However, those with Spigelman stage IV disease have a 36% risk of adenocarcinoma. Adenocarcinoma, persistent or recurrent high-grade dysplasia, or Spigelman stage IV disease warrants consideration of surgery. Surgical options include pancreaticoduodenectomy or pancreas-preserving duodenectomy.

Desmoid Disease

- *Staging and medical therapy*. Desmoid disease can be clinically devastating and is the second cause of death in FAP. Clinically, presentation ranges from asymptomatic to severe pain, obstruction, or fistulization. Treatment depends on symptoms, desmoid location, size, and extent of disease. Church has proposed a staging system for abdominal desmoids (Table 23.3). The Cleveland Clinic uses this staging system to guide medical management. Stage I desmoids are either observed or treated with a nonsteroidal anti-inflammatory drug such as sulindac (150–200 mg twice daily). Stage II desmoid treatment includes sulindac and antiestrogen therapy, such as raloxifene (60 mg twice daily). Stage III desmoids are usually treated with chemotherapy agents such as methotrexate and vinorelbine or Doxil. Stage IV desmoids are difficult to control and are treated with more aggressive anti-sarcoma chemotherapy such as Doxil or Adriamycin. Although desmoid tumors are radiosensitive, the close proximity to the small bowel limits its use due to toxicity.
- Surgical therapy. Surgery for abdominal desmoids is usually reserved for treatment of disease complications such as bowel obstruction, enterocutaneous fistula, and ureteric obstruction. If possible, resection to negative margins is the goal. Intra-abdominal tumors are frequently located at the root of the small bowel mesentery and are often not resectable due to the proximity to critical small bowel blood supply. Surgery is usually the first-line treatment for symptomatic abdominal wall desmoids. Due to the location, these tumors are usually able to be safely resected with minimal complications. The defect in the abdominal wall may need to be closed with tissue flaps or mesh.

Table 23.3 Proposed intra-abdominal desmoid disease clinical staging system

Disease stage	Clinical characteristics
I	Asymptomatic disease, not growing, and < 10 cm in maximum diameter
II	Minimally symptomatic and not growing or > 10 cm in maximum diameter
III	Symptomatic disease, slowly growing, or obstructive complications
IV	Symptomatic disease and rapidly growing or severe complications (e.g., fistula)

Thyroid Neoplasia

- Thyroid disease may be detected in FAP by evaluation of symptoms or routine ultrasound screening. Since cancers tend to be multifocal, patients with thyroid cancer should be considered for total thyroidectomy and radioiodine ablation.

Evaluation of At-Risk Relatives

- As FAP is autosomal dominantly inherited, all first-degree relatives of an FAP patient have a 50% chance of also having the disease. Therefore, all first-degree relatives in an FAP family should be evaluated. Due to the implications of both positive and negative results, pretest counseling, preferably with a genetic counselor, should be done. Potentially affected family members should be evaluated at the time of diagnosis or for children, when they reach the age of 12.
- If the proband (first affected relative) has a *known APC mutation*, then germline DNA testing of at-risk relatives is appropriate.
- If the proband does *not have a detectable mutation*, then genetic testing for *APC* mutations in the family is not indicated. At-risk

relatives should undergo screening by colonoscopy. For at-risk children, flexible sigmoidoscopy should be considered at age 12 years. Subsequent testing intervals for children depend on findings at the initial proctosigmoidoscopy. If polyps are seen, a full colonoscopy is warranted. If no polyps are identified, the exam should be repeated every 1–2 years or earlier if symptoms develop. For those families without a genetic diagnosis, first-degree relatives who are not found to have any polyps by age 40 can safely be transitioned to screening guidelines for the general population.

MUTYH-Associated Polyposis

Clinical Presentation

- The syndrome is primarily characterized by multiple colorectal adenomas and an increased risk for CRC at a younger age (40s–50s), but the colorectal polyp phenotype is highly variable. Moderate polyposis (less than 100 adenomas) is the most common phenotype. Polyposis is not necessary for an MAP diagnosis and as many as 20% of patients present with colorectal cancer without a history of colorectal polyps or synchronous polyps.
- Despite the similar colorectal phenotype to FAP, patients with MAP are less likely to have the extracolonic manifestations that are commonly seen in FAP. Approximately 20% of patients with MAP will have duodenal polyposis, and gastric fundic polyps are rare. Osteomas, desmoids, and CHRPE are not associated with MAP.

Underlying Genetics

- MAP is the only hereditary CRC syndrome with an autosomal recessive inheritance pattern, and thus family history may help guide counseling and testing in patients who are suspected of having MAP. MAP is caused by inherited biallelic mutations in the *MUTYH* gene, which codes for a base excision repair protein. Approximately 1–2% of the general population carries a *MUTYH* mutation.

Diagnosis

- MAP diagnosis is confirmed by genetic testing for mutations in the *MUTYH* gene. Germline *MUTYH* testing should be offered to patients who have a recessive pattern of family history of colorectal cancer or polyposis, who have a clinical phenotype of FAP or attenuated FAP but test negative for an *APC* mutation, or who have a personal history of >10 colorectal adenomas. Nearly 30% of patients with a clinical phenotype of FAP without an identified *APC* mutation have biallelic *MUTYH* mutations.

CRC Risk

- The cumulative lifetime risk of developing colorectal cancer for patients with biallelic *MUTYH* mutations is estimated at 75% for males and 72% for females by age 70. Onset of cancer is earlier than sporadic colorectal cancer, with the mean age of diagnosis reported between 45 and 56 years old.
- The risk of CRC for monoallelic *MUTYH* carriers continues to be defined. Data from the Colon Cancer Family Registry estimate the cumulative lifetime risk of developing CRC for people with monoallelic *MUTYH* mutations at 7.2% for males and 5.6% for females by age 70.

Extracolonic Cancer Risk

- The spectrum of extracolonic neoplasia in MAP continues to be defined. An increased risk of upper gastrointestinal polyps and cancers is consistently reported. About 17% of cases have duodenal adenomas with a lifetime duodenal cancer risk of 4%. The overall incidence of malignancy outside the gastrointestinal tract is 38%, almost double that of the general population. The most common extraintestinal cancers are bladder, ovarian, and skin cancers with standard incidence ratios of 7.2, 5.7, and 2.8, respectively. Some studies report an increased risk of thyroid cancer and sebaceous gland tumors.

Management

Screening

- Most cases of MAP are diagnosed at the time of CRC detection. In the rare cases when an individual is diagnosed with biallelic *MUTYH* mutations but does not have an indication for colectomy, colonoscopy screening should begin at age 25–30 years. If no neoplasia is identified on the exam, it should be repeated every 3–5 years with consideration for decreasing the interval with advancing age. Any polyps found on colonoscopy should be removed and examined histologically. When polyps are present, the interval is shortened to 1–2 years depending on the findings. Patients with a polyp burden that cannot be controlled endoscopically should be referred for consideration of colectomy.
- Esophagoduodenoscopy with side-viewing gastroscope should be performed to evaluate for duodenal adenomatous neoplasia. This screening should start at age 30 years and repeated every 3–5 years if the exam is normal. For patients with duodenal adenomas, management is similar to the recommendations for FAP patients with duodenal adenomas. The American College of Gastroenterology also recommends annual thyroid ultrasound screening in patients with MAP.
- There is no consensus regarding screening for monoallelic carriers. Some clinicians have suggested screening these people by colonoscopy every 5 years, beginning 10 years earlier than the youngest patient afflicted with CRC in the family.

Treatment

- The phenotype dictates treatment in MAP. Indications for surgery include CRC, high-grade dysplasia in an adenoma that cannot be removed endoscopically, or a polyp burden that cannot be safely managed by colonoscopy. Surgical options include total abdominal colectomy, subtotal colectomy, or proctocolectomy. A segmental colectomy may be considered in certain circumstances such as metastatic cancer or medical comorbidities that preclude extended resection. Any remaining colorectum should be surveyed annually, with removal of subsequent polyps.
- Despite the recommendation to consider subtotal or total abdominal colectomy for patients with curable colon cancer, and proctocolectomy for patients with curable rectal cancer, there are no prospective data that show extended resection reduces the risk of death from metachronous colorectal cancers. It is unlikely that definitive studies will be performed, given the rarity of the diagnosis.

Evaluation of At-Risk Relatives

- As this syndrome is autosomal recessive, patients must have two abnormal alleles to manifest the disease. Different from other inherited colorectal cancer syndromes, it is the *siblings of patients with MAP that are at greatest risk*, rather than the parents or children. Each sibling of an affected individual has a 25% chance of also having the disease.
- Genetic counseling and testing for specific *MUTYH* mutation in the family should be offered at the age of 18 years to reduce morbidity and mortality through early diagnosis and treatment. Children of biallelic patients will be at least a monoallelic carrier. Approximately 1% of the general population is a monoallelic carrier. If the spouse of the affected patient is a carrier, then each offspring has a 50% chance of having MAP. Therefore, the partner of the affected patient should be tested to evaluate risk to the offspring.

Polymerase Proofreading-Associated Polyposis

A new syndrome has recently been reported as polymerase proofreading-associated polyposis

(PPAP). This syndrome continues to be defined and has only been characterized in a few families. It is inherited in an autosomally dominant fashion and caused by a germline mutation in proofreading regions of one of two DNA polymerases, POLE and POLD1. The clinical phenotype is one of oligo-adenomatous polyposis and early-age CRC and endometrial cancer. Guidelines are in evolution, but expert opinions support surveillance via colonoscopy every 1–2 years starting at age 20–25 and EGD every 3 years. For females with a POLD1 mutation, endometrial cancer screening by ultrasound is recommended starting at age 40 years.

Hamartomatous Polyposis Syndromes

- Hamartomas are non-neoplastic growths of an abnormal mixture of tissue that is normally found at that anatomic site. Juvenile polyps and Peutz-Jeghers polyps are hamartomatous polyps in the small bowel and colorectum. Although these lesions are generally not considered neoplastic, they can be the hallmark of inherited hamartomatous polyposis syndromes such as juvenile polyposis syndrome (JPS), Peutz-Jeghers syndrome (PJS), and the PTEN hamartoma tumor syndrome (PHTS). These syndromes are rare but clinically important as they predispose to colorectal and other cancers.

Juvenile Polyposis Syndrome

Clinical Presentation

- Juvenile polyps are usually round, smooth, cherry-red lesions that are often pedunculated on a long stalk. An abundance and overgrowth of the lamina propria with mucin-filled spaces are the characteristic histologic features. Chronic inflammatory cells are often seen which can lead to an inaccurate diagnosis of inflammatory polyp. Juvenile polyps occur throughout the gastrointestinal tract including the stomach, small bowel, colon, and rectum, starting in the first or second decade of life. The number of polyps varies from a few to hundreds. Symptoms are related to the polyps and most commonly include acute or chronic gastrointestinal bleeding, iron-deficiency anemia, prolapsed rectal polyps, abdominal pain, or diarrhea.
- JPS is also associated with extracolonic congenital malformations such as cardiac and cranial abnormalities, duplication of the renal pelvis, cleft palate, gut malrotation, and polydactyly. JPS along with a *SMAD4* mutation may present as hereditary hemorrhagic telangiectasia (HHT). HHT may manifest with skin and mucosal telangiectasias; cerebral, pulmonary, and hepatic arteriovenous malformations; and an increased risk of associated hemorrhage.

Underlying Genetics

- JPS is an autosomal dominantly inherited disease caused by germline mutations in *BMPR1A* or *SMAD4*. About 60% of JPS cases are familial, while the remaining 40% occur sporadically.

Diagnosis

- JPS diagnosis is based on clinical criteria which include the following: (1) more than five juvenile polyps of the colon or rectum, (2) juvenile polyps in the extracolonic gastrointestinal tract, or (3) any number of juvenile polyps and a positive family history. Patients who satisfy any of these criteria should be offered genetic counseling and genetic testing. A causative germline mutation is identified in approximately 50% of cases.

CRC and Extracolonic Risk

- JPS patients have an approximately 50% lifetime CRC risk, with reports of varying incidence between 17% and 68%. The mean age of CRC diagnosis is 43 years, but CRC may develop at a young age, and there is a case report of CRC in a 15-year-old patient. The stomach, duodenum, pancreas, and jejunum are at increased risk for cancer in JPS. The risk of gastric or duodenal cancer is 15–21%.

SMAD4 associations are associated with a higher risk of extracolonic cancer compared to patients with BMPR1A mutations.

Management

Screening

- Screening by colonoscopy should begin at age 12–15, or earlier if symptoms are present. The interval between colonoscopies depends on the exam findings. If there are no polyps, colonoscopy should be repeated in 2–3 years. Any polyps seen should be removed at colonoscopy and examined histologically. When polyps are present and removed, colonoscopy should be done annually until an exam is clear, after which, the interval may be extended to every 2–3 years. Upper gastrointestinal screening should begin between ages 15 and 25 or earlier if symptoms develop. Endoscopic management principles follow those as given for adenomas of the upper GI tract.

Treatment

- Surgical indications include the presence of high-grade dysplasia or cancer, or if the polyp burden cannot be effectively managed endoscopically. Prophylactic colectomy may be considered for patients with poor surveillance compliance or those with a family history of CRC. For colorectal disease, surgical options include colectomy and ileorectal anastomosis, subtotal colectomy with ileosigmoid anastomosis, or total proctocolectomy.
- Surgery for the upper gastrointestinal tract is indicated for significant symptoms, malignancy, or development of protein-losing gastropathy or enteropathy. For gastric disease, subtotal gastrectomy is usually done. For small bowel disease, treatment is segmental resection.

Evaluation of At-Risk Relatives

- If a specific mutation is identified in an individual, all at-risk family members should be counseled and tested for that mutation. Approximately 75% of patients will have an affected parent. If a parent carries the mutation, then siblings of the parent as well as siblings of the proband should be tested as they have a 50% chance of also having the mutation. Children of the proband should also be tested after counseling and testing in the early teenage years. If a mutation is not found in the family, at-risk individuals should be initially screened for gastrointestinal polyps and followed accordingly based on results.

Peutz-Jeghers Syndrome

Clinical Presentation

- Nearly 90% of PJS patients will develop hamartomatous polyps, most commonly in the small bowel, followed by the colon, stomach, and rectum in decreasing frequency. Polyps vary in size from a few millimeters to several centimeters and tend to become pedunculated as they grow larger.
- Peutz-Jeghers polyps differ histologically from juvenile polyps in that they arise due to an overgrowth of the muscularis mucosa, rather than the lamina propria. They have less inflammatory infiltrate and less mucin than juvenile polyps. Multiple branching of the muscularis mucosa gives the histologic appearance of a tree under the microscope.
- Although the polyp burden is usually low (<20), the larger size of the polyp often causes symptoms of obstruction, pain, gastrointestinal bleeding, polyp prolapse per anus, or small bowel intussusception. Symptoms usually develop by the teen years or early twenties.
- The classical extraintestinal lesion seen in PJS is benign mucocutaneous pigmentation, which is present in approximately 95% of cases. The pigmentation is usually a small, dark-brown or blue-brown macule that is obvious in infancy but may fade in adolescence.

Underlying Genetics

- PJS is autosomal dominantly inherited and caused by germline mutations in *STK11*. This gene encodes a member of the serine/threonine kinase family, which functions as a tumor suppressor.

Diagnosis

- PJS is a clinical diagnosis based on meeting any one of the following World Health Organization criteria: (1) three or more histologically confirmed Peutz-Jeghers polyps, (2) any number of Peutz-Jeghers polyps with a family history of PJS, (3) characteristic, prominent, mucocutaneous pigmentation with a family history of PJS, or (4) any number of Peutz-Jeghers polyps and characteristic prominent, mucocutaneous pigmentation. An individual meeting any of the above criteria should be offered genetic counseling and testing.

CRC and Extracolonic Risk

- Patients with PJS have an increased risk of developing colorectal and extracolonic cancers. PJS patients have more than 90% estimated lifetime risk of developing cancer of some type. The risk for developing breast, colon, pancreatic, and gastric cancer is 54%, 39%, 36%, and 29%, respectively. In addition, males are at risk for Sertoli cell testicular tumors and women for sex cord tumors with annular tubules of the ovary and adenoma malignum of the cervix.

Management

Surveillance

- Given the broad spectrum of disease in PJS, surveillance is complex and includes multiple organs. Randomized controlled trials have not been performed to evaluate the efficacy of cancer surveillance protocols, and published recommendations are based on expert opinion.
- The NCCN recommends starting screening at age 8–10 years via evaluation of the small bowel, with the interval exam based on findings. If initial exam is normal, then the repeat evaluation is recommended at age 18 years and then at 2–3 year intervals. Males should undergo annual testicular physical examination starting at age 10 years, and females should undergo annual pelvic examination and Papanicolaou stain starting at age 18–20 years. Women should have breast physical examinations every 6 months and yearly mammogram and breast MRI starting at age 25 years. Colonoscopy and upper endoscopy should be in the late teens and repeated every 2–3 years for both genders. Pancreatic cancer screening involves endoscopic ultrasound or MRCP along with serum CA19-9 every 1–2 years starting at age 25–30 years.

Polypectomy

- Endoscopic intervention plays a key role in the management of PJS. Polypectomy treats polyp-related symptoms and prophylactically prevents development of symptoms. As with the surveillance guidelines, intervention recommendations are based on expert opinion. Asymptomatic gastric or colonic polyps larger than 1 cm should be removed endoscopically. Small bowel polyps larger than 1–1.5 cm or those that have grown rapidly from prior exam should be removed to decrease future complications such as bleeding and intussusception. Some symptomatic polyps may be beyond the reach of conventional endoscopy, and intervention may require push enteroscopy or combined laparoscopy/laparotomy with endoscopy in the operating room, which allows guidance of the endoscope further distally into the small bowel.

Surgery

- Surgery is most commonly reserved for symptoms, the most common being obstruction and bleeding in the small bowel. Obstruction is often caused by intussusception. Most cases resolve spontaneously, but if the obstruction persists more than a few hours, surgery is required. The goal of surgery is to remove the affected segment, preserving as much bowel as possible. If surgery is required, a "clean sweep" at surgery is recommended to reduce the need for future operations. This technique involves evaluating the entire small bowel and removing all polyps. An endoscope may be placed through the open resection ends of the bowel or via an enterotomy.
- As in the other syndromes, the development of high-grade dysplasia, colorectal cancer, or an

uncontrolled colorectal polyp burden is an indication for colorectal surgery. Total abdominal colectomy and ileorectal anastomosis are the preferred operation unless the pathology is in the rectum.

Evaluation of At-Risk Relatives

- For individuals with a specific known mutation, at-risk family members should be tested for that mutation. Approximately 50% of individuals will have an affected parent, and parents should be evaluated for PJS traits. If one of the parents is affected, then testing should be offered to the siblings of the proband. Additionally, all children of the proband have a 50% risk of inheriting the mutation and should be tested accordingly. Genetic testing for at-risk family members may be performed at age 8 after appropriate genetic counseling and informed consent. If a specific mutation is not identified in the affected individual, at-risk family members are surveyed as if they potentially have the disease. This includes surveillance of the colon, stomach, small bowel, pancreas, breast, ovary, uterus, cervix, and testes as described above.

PTEN Hamartoma Tumor Syndrome (PHTS)

- PHTS is a spectrum of extremely rare hereditary syndromes that are characterized by hamartomatous polyps in the gastrointestinal tract and abnormalities of the skull, skeleton, and skin. The two main syndromes are Cowden syndrome and Bannayan-Riley-Ruvalcaba syndrome (BRRS).

Clinical Presentation

- About 95% of Cowden syndrome patients have colorectal polyps, ranging from few to hundreds in number and are distributed throughout the colorectum. The most common polyps are hamartomas, accounting for about 30% of all polyps. Other types of polyps include adenomas, juvenile polyps, inflammatory polyps, leiomyomas, lipomas, fibromas, neurofibromas, and ganglioneuromas. The majority of patients have multiple histologic types of polyps.
- About 30% of Cowden syndrome patients have macrocephaly. Trichilemmomas are considered to be pathognomonic. Other benign and malignant lesions of the breast, thyroid, uterus, and skin are seen in Cowden syndrome.

Underlying Genetics

- Cowden syndrome and BRRS are both autosomally dominant inherited disorders associated with a *PTEN* mutation. *PTEN* is a tumor suppressor gene that encodes a phosphatase that is involved in the PI3K/AKT signaling pathway. It plays a key role in apoptosis. Approximately 80% of patients who meet the diagnostic criteria for Cowden syndrome, and 60% of patients with BRRS, have PTEN mutations.

Diagnosis

- The International Cowden Consortium developed clinical diagnostic criteria for Cowden syndrome, including both major and minor criteria. Major criteria include breast cancer, thyroid cancer (especially follicular), macrocephaly, endometrial cancer, and Lhermitte-Duclos disease. Minor features include benign thyroid changes (such as a goiter), mental retardation, hamartomatous intestinal polyps, fibrocystic changes in the breast, lipomas, fibromas, and genitourinary tumors (such as kidney cancer or uterine fibroids) or malformations.
- Cowden syndrome is diagnosed if a patient has either macrocephaly or Lhermitte-Duclos disease and one other major feature. A diagnosis of Cowden is also made when a person has one major feature and three minor features or at least four minor features. Definitive diagnosis is based on a *PTEN* mutation.
- Specific diagnostic criteria for BRRS are not established, but patients with macrocephaly, hamartomatous colonic polyposis, lipomas, and pigmented macules of the glans penis should be considered for genetic testing.

CRC and Extracolonic Risk

- A recent study reported CRC in 13% of *PTEN* mutation carriers in Cowden syndrome with early age of onset, all before the age of 50 years. The adjusted standardized incidence ratio was 224 (95% confidence interval, 109.3–411.3; P < 0.0001). Other groups have supported a 9–16% lifetime risk for CRC cancer.
- Most of PTHS cancer risk is extracolonic. Women have a 50% lifetime risk of developing breast cancer and a 5–10% lifetime risk of developing endometrial cancer. Men and women with Cowden syndrome have a 10% lifetime risk of developing epithelial thyroid cancer.
- Approximately half of the patients with BRRS will have hamartomatous polyps in the digestive tract, particularly in the ileum and colon. These polyps can become symptomatic, but are not believed to increase the risk of colon cancer. Patients with BRRS have similar extracolonic malignancy risks as those with Cowden syndrome.

CRC Risk Management

- There is debate regarding the need for colonoscopy screening in PTHS. Given the recent findings of increased CRC risk, we recommend starting colonoscopy at age 35, with repeat examinations every 1–2 years. Colectomy should be considered if the polyp burden cannot be controlled endoscopically or if cancer develops.

Evaluation of At-Risk Relatives

- At-risk relatives should be counseled and tested for the presence of PTEN mutation. For families with PTHS but no detected gene mutation, at-risk individuals should be initially surveyed as if they have the disease. Screening includes evaluation of the colorectum, stomach, small bowel, thyroid, breast, uterine, kidney, and skin.

Serrated Polyposis Syndrome (SPS)

Clinical Presentation

- SPS is usually asymptomatic and is often detected on screening colonoscopy.
- More than 90% of SPS patients are of white European descent. It affects both men and women nearly equally with a slight female inclination. The median age at diagnosis ranges from 44 to 62 years, with extremes of age including SPS in a 10-year-old and a man in his eighties.
- SPS encompasses a variety of clinical phenotypes and is likely a heterogeneous disease that has not yet been characterized genetically.
- The primary feature of SPS is serrated polyps – a family of polyps characterized by a classic serrated or sawtooth appearance of the arrangement of glands. This includes hyperplastic polyps, sessile serrated adenomas (SSAs) which are also called sessile serrated polyps (SSPs), SSAs or SSPs with dysplasia, and serrated adenomas.
- Different phenotypes have been described based on the size and number of serrated polyps. Some patients have multiple small polyps distributed throughout the colon, while others have a few large, right-sided polyps. The cancer risk is similar for both phenotypes. In addition to serrated polyps, SPS patients often are prone to having adenomas.

Underlying Genetics

- A causative germline mutation has not been identified for SPS. There is no genetic testing for this syndrome.

Diagnosis

- SPS is diagnosed by clinical criteria as defined by the World Health Organization as follows:

(1) >20 serrated polyps of any size, distributed throughout the colon; (2) at least five serrated polyps proximal to the sigmoid colon with two or more of these being >10 mm; and (3) any number of serrated polyps proximal to the sigmoid colon in an individual who has a first-degree relative with SPS.

CRC Risk

- Although the true incidence of CRC in SPS is yet to be defined by prospective studies, it is consistently reported as increased compared to the general population. Reports are variable from multiple relatively small series, ranging from 0% to 77%, with an estimate of around 25%.
- The initial SPS diagnosis is often made at the time of cancer diagnosis, and thus the natural history progression from SPS to cancer is uncertain.

Management

Screening

- For patients with an established SPS diagnosis, colonoscopy should be performed every 1–2 years. Management guidelines are based on clinical experience and expert opinion.
- Although some studies suggest an association with extracolonic malignancies, the data are not strong enough to justify surveillance recommendations for extracolonic neoplasia.

Treatment

- Treatment is determined by the clinical phenotype and patient's wishes. The goal of treatment for SPS patients is to decrease or eliminate CRC risk by removing polyps before they become cancer.
- Expert panels recommend removing any single polyp larger than 5 mm for histologic evaluation. For clusters of small (3–4 mm) left-sided polyps, which are likely benign hyperplastic polyps, representative biopsies should be performed.
- Screening colonoscopies should be done yearly, with consideration of the number, size, and histology of the polyps to adjust the interval. If successive colonoscopies reveal no polyps, the interval to the next examination may be extended to 2–3 years, but this should be considered on a case-by-case basis.
- Endoscopic management alone is often difficult as polyps are large, flat, and right-sided. If the polyp burden cannot successfully be controlled via colonoscopy and polypectomies, surgery should be considered.
- The development of CRC or adenoma with high-grade dysplasia that cannot be adequately or safely removed endoscopically are also indications for surgery.
- As the risk of neoplasia is not limited to the specific location of the index neoplasm but rather the entire colorectal mucosa, extended surgery should be entertained. This includes a subtotal or total colectomy and ileosigmoid or ileorectal anastomosis, respectively. Decision-making for the extent of surgery should be taken for each individual and evaluated within the context of medical comorbidities and anal sphincter function. A segmental colectomy may be considered for patients with focal disease (few large right-sided polyps) and who are not medically fit for extended resection.
- Any remaining colorectum should undergo annual endoscopy to prevent and manage future neoplasia.

Evaluation of At-Risk Relatives

- Compared to the general population, first-degree relatives of patients with SPS have an approximately fivefold increased CRC incidence.
- As there is no genetic test to screen for SPS, colonoscopy serves as the screening mechanism.

- Expert panels recommend colonoscopy screening for first-degree relatives, particularly those older than 40 years. Endoscopic findings and polyp histology should guide the interval to the next colonoscopy.
- First-degree relatives do not have increased risk of extracolonic malignancy.

Lynch Syndrome

- Lynch syndrome (LS), previously used as a synonym for hereditary nonpolyposis colorectal cancer (HNPCC) syndrome, accounts for 3–5% of all CRCs and 10–19% of CRCs diagnosed before age 50.
- The underlying genetic cause is a germline mutation in a DNA mismatch repair (MMR) gene, which results in a nonfunctioning MMR protein. Lynch syndrome, as currently defined, is a genetic diagnosis.
- The syndrome follows an autosomal dominant inheritance pattern.
- Tumors are typically microsatellite unstable (MSI-H) and exhibit loss of expression of mismatch repair proteins on immunohistochemistry.
- There are several conditions that should be distinguished from LS:
  - Familial colorectal cancer type X: patients meeting Amsterdam criteria for HNPCC who have microsatellite-stable, rather than microsatellite-unstable, tumors.
    - The CRC risk is between that of the general population and patients with LS; patients develop CRC at later ages compared to LS, and do not have increased extracolonic malignancy risk. The exact genotype remains to be elucidated.
  - Constitutional mismatch repair deficiency (CMMRD) syndrome: in contrast to LS where an inherited mutation is present in one allelic copy of a MMR gene, a rare group of patients has inherited mutations of the MMR gene in both of their alleles.
    - Patients exhibit a distinct phenotype with the development of CRC at very young ages (before age 20), multiple adenomatous polyps numbering between 10 and 100, café au lait skin lesions, hematologic malignancies, and brain tumors.
  - Finally, there are patients who present with MSI-H tumors, but subsequent germline mutation testing fails to detect a pathogenic mutation in any of the major MMR genes. The terms "Lynch-like syndrome," "suspected LS," or "mutation-negative LS" have been utilized, and the molecular characterization of these patients represents areas of active research.

Underlying Genetics and Molecular Profile

- Patients with LS harbor an inherited dominant mutation in a MMR gene on one allele. This germline mutation, propagated through all somatic cells, confers susceptibility for cancer but requires a "second hit" within the specific somatic tissue for malignant transformation (Fig. 23.5). The "second hit" alters the wild-type copy of the allele, leading to loss of DNA MMR activity in the somatic cell and, further, cancer development. Thus, malignant tumor cells in patients with LS harbor DNA MMR gene mutations in both alleles (one inherited and another acquired as a "second hit").
- The four major DNA MMR genes responsible for LS are *MLH1*, *MSH2*, *MSH6*, and *PMS2*. Additionally, mutations in the gene *EPCAM* (or *TACSTD1*) upstream of *MSH2* can silence or disrupt MSH2 expression and lead to clinical features similar to LS. Based on data from 12,624 observations worldwide, it has been estimated that *MLH1* accounts for 39%, *MSH2* for 34%, *MSH6* for 20%, and *PMS2* for 8% of the entries in the International Society for Gastrointestinal Hereditary Tumours (InSiGHT) database (www.insight-group.org/mutations/), and up to 3% of the cases are due to *EPCAM* mutations.
- *Tumor phenotype*. The underlying genetic mutations and mismatch repair deficiency

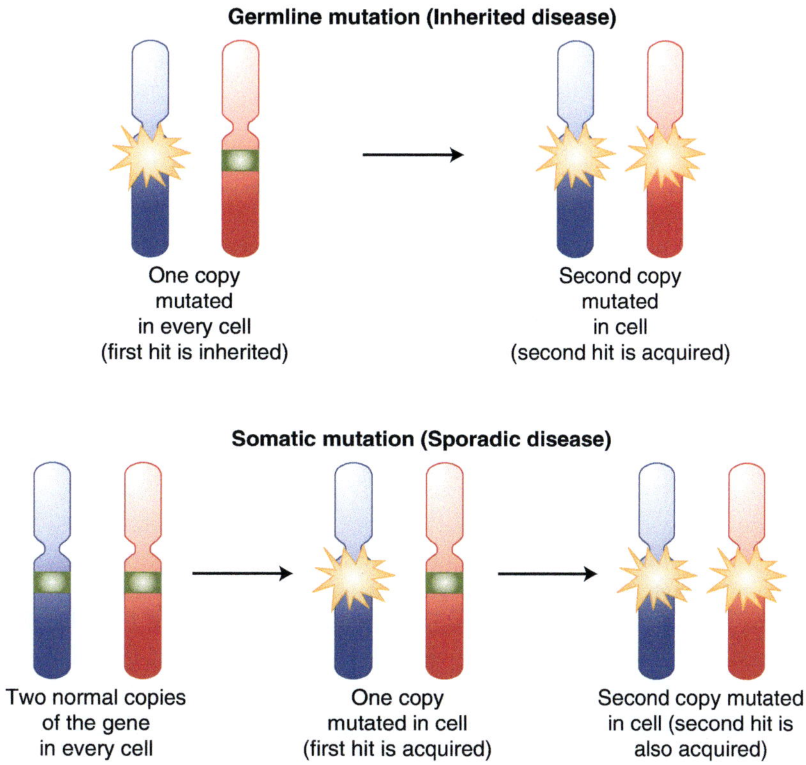

Fig. 23.5 A germline MMR gene mutation confers susceptibility for cancer but requires a "second hit" within the specific somatic tissue for it to develop into a malignancy. The "second hit" causes the wild-type copy of the allele to also become mutated, leading to loss of DNA MMR activity in the somatic cell and, further, cancer development

yield molecular changes within the tumor that can be examined as part of the screening process toward a LS diagnosis.

- *Microsatellite instability*. DNA microsatellites are tandem sequences of mono-, di-, or trinucleotide repeats that are particularly susceptible to replication errors when MMR function is impaired. These differences can be measured by the PCR-based MSI test, which assesses a standard panel of (typically five) microsatellite markers in paired tumor and normal tissue by consensus; a tumor is considered MSI-H if 30% or more of the markers tested show instability and microsatellite stable (MSS) if none of the markers are unstable. MSI-low connotation is reserved for tumors that have some markers that are unstable but fewer than 30%. MSI-low is infrequently encountered, and its clinical significance has been regarded similar to that of MSS tumors.
- *Immunohistochemistry*. Measuring expression of mismatch repair proteins using immunohistochemistry is the other means of determining mismatch repair proficiency or deficiency of a tumor. In vivo, the MMR protein products function as dimers, with MSH2 forming a complex with MSH6 and MLH1 with PMS2 protein. Thus, mutations in either *MSH2* or *EPCAM* genes typically result in loss of staining in both MSH2 and MSH6 protein products, while mutations that lead to loss of MLH1 protein result in the loss of staining for both MLH1 and PMS2 proteins. On the other hand, mutations in *MSH6* and *PMS2* genes typically result only in the loss of the respective single gene product. IHC has demonstrated 92% sensitivity for identifying defective MMR in tumors from known LS patients with a germline pathogenic mutation.

• *BRAF mutations*. As discussed above, the vast majority of MSI-H in CRC is caused by methylation of the *MLH1* gene promoter as seen in the methylator pathway. Mutations in the *BRAF* oncogene are strongly associated with the methylator pathway and are rare in

LS-related CRC. Thus, the presence of a somatic *BRAF* mutation within a CRC is often used to rule out further screening for a LS diagnosis. Patients with absence of *MLH1* expression on immunohistochemistry should have their tumor analyzed for *BRAF* mutation. If *BRAF* is mutated, then LS is unlikely. If *BRAF* is normal, LS is likely.

Distinguishing Lynch from Sporadic Epigenetic Changes: Methylation of MLH1 Gene Promoter

- Approximately 85% of mismatch repair deficiency in CRC is caused by methylation of the promoter region of *MLH1* gene. This epigenetic phenomenon silences MLH1 expression in the tumor tissue. These tumors characteristically arise in elderly female patients and in the right colon. Identifying *MLH1* promoter methylation from tumor tissue can help eliminate the diagnosis of LS. However, should *MLH1* promoter methylation be encountered in young patients with a family history suggestive of LS, the clinicians should be aware of two rare exceptions: (1) the patient may have LS with an inherited *MLH1* mutation and *MLH1* promoter methylation may have developed as the "second hit" leading to cancer development and (2) germline *MLH1* hypermethylation has been reported in rare families which exhibit characteristic cancers associated with LS.

Clinical Presentation and Spectrum of Disease

Genotype-Phenotype Correlations

- While the clinical hallmarks of LS are CRC and extracolonic malignancies, the cancer risks are highly variable within and among families with LS. Genotype-phenotype correlation studies have shown that the lifetime risks of LS-related malignancies vary by gender and the mutated gene (Table 23.4).

Muir-Torre Syndrome (MTS)

- Muir-Torre syndrome (MTS) is a clinical variant of LS, where patients are affected by skin sebaceous gland neoplasms (sebaceous

Table 23.4 Summary of reported cumulative risks of colorectal and extra-colorectal cancers by age 70 in patients with Lynch syndrome

Cancer	Mutated gene	Cumulative risk, %		Mean age at diagnosis (years)
Colorectal	*MLH1/MSH2*	Male Female	27–74 22–53	27–46
	MSH6	Male Female	18–22 10–18	54–63
	PMS2	Male Female	20 15	47–66
Endometrial	*MLH1/MSH2*		14–54	48–62
	MSH6		17–71	54–57
	PMS2		15	49
Ovary			4–20	43–45
Stomach			0.2–13	49–55
Genitourinary			0.2–25	52–60
Hepatobiliary			0.02–4	54–57
Small bowel			0.4–12	46–49
Brain/central nervous system			1–4	50
Sebaceous skin neoplasms			1–9	Unknown

Modified from Giardiello FM, Allen JI, Axilbund JE, Boland CR, Burke CA, Burt RW, et al. Guidelines on genetic evaluation and management of Lynch syndrome: a consensus statement by the US Multi-society Task Force on colorectal cancer. The American Journal of Gastroenterology. 2014;109(8):1159–79

These reported risks and mean ages of diagnosis should not be used to exclude the possibility of Lynch syndrome in a patient who has suggestive clinical feature

adenomas and carcinomas) and/or hair follicle neoplasms (keratoacanthomas).
- MTS can be associated with mutations in any of the MMR genes, but *MSH2* mutation appears most common.
- Sebaceous adenoma, especially when multiple or when arising from the trunk or extremities, is characteristic for MTS. Sebaceous tumors can occur before, with, or after the development of other cancers, and CRC and genitourinary tumors are the most common visceral malignancies associated with MTS.
- Referral for genetic counseling and for colonoscopic screening should be considered in patients with sebaceous neoplasm, especially when there is suggestive personal or family history. However, there is currently no uniform recommendation for systemic screening of sebaceous neoplasms for dMMR.

Turcot's Syndrome

- Turcot's syndrome describes patients with CRC and brain tumors. Turcot's syndrome is not considered an independent entity, and it can be associated with two main types of germline genetic defects: mutation of the *APC* gene in association with anaplastic astrocytoma, ependymoma, or medulloblastoma or mutation of an MMR gene that is usually associated with glioblastoma. Although excellent survival of more than 3 years has been reported in patients with Turcot's syndrome, whether LS patients with these tumors have more favorable prognosis remains unestablished.

Colorectal Cancer Risk

- The lifetime risk for CRC ranges from 30 to 74% among *MLH1* and *MSH2* mutation carriers, but only 15–20% among *PMS2* carriers and 10–22% among *MSH6* carriers.
- The mean age of diagnosis for LS-related CRC is 44–61 years, significantly younger than the average age of CRC onset in the United States which is 72 years.
- The LS-associated CRCs show a predilection for the right colon when compared to sporadic CRC, but left-sided colon cancers, rectal cancers, and synchronous lesions at different sites of the colon and rectum are also common presentations.
- Among LS patients who have had an initial CRC treated by less than a total colectomy, the risk for metachronous CRC is 16% at 10 years, 41% at 20 years, and 62% at 30 years.
- The adenoma-to-carcinoma progresses more rapidly in LS patients secondary to more rapid accumulation of errors due to the deficiency in MMR genes. Adenoma may progress to carcinoma within 2–3 years, compared with 4–10 years in the general population.
- Up to 70% of the mutation carriers develop at least one adenoma by age 60. The adenomas tend to be larger, flat, and are more likely to show high-grade dysplasia at the time of diagnosis.
- It has been estimated that endoscopic polypectomy can prevent one CRC for every 2.8 adenoma removed in a LS patient, compared to one CRC for every 41–119 adenomas in the general population.
- Unique histologic features have been described for MSI-H CRCs, including greater proportion of tumors showing poor differentiation, mucinous or signet ring cell histology, tumor infiltrating lymphocytes, and lymphoid (Crohn's-like pattern and/or peritumoral lymphocytes) host response.

Endometrial and Ovarian Cancer Risk

- Endometrial cancer is the most common extracolonic malignancy in patients with LS. It poses the highest risk in women with *MSH6* and *MSH2* mutations, in whom the lifetime risk can be up to 44% (Table 23.4). The lowest risk (15%) is observed among *PMS2* mutation carriers. The mean age at diagnosis ranges between 48 and 62 years. LS-associated endometrial cancers are more commonly of endometrioid histology and arise from the lower uterine segment. Synchronous endometrial and ovarian cancers have been reported in 7–21% of the women with LS.

Other LS-Associated Cancer Risk

- The spectrum of other extracolonic cancers associated with LS is wide and continues to evolve. Classically, LS is associated with increased lifetime risk of genitourinary tumors including transitional cell carcinoma of the ureter, renal pelvis, and bladder; cancers of the stomach, hepatobiliary tract, and small bowel; brain cancer (glioblastoma); and sebaceous skin neoplasms (Table 23.4).

Diagnosis

- LS is diagnosed by the identification of a germline mutation in one of the MMR genes as described above. Current commercial germline testing detects both sequence changes as well as large rearrangements in these genes. It is most commonly performed on DNA isolated from peripheral blood or buccal mucosa samples. Independent of tumor tissue, germline testing can be performed in patients who are affected or unaffected by malignancy.
- Genetic testing should be preceded by genetic counseling to ensure that the patients are fully informed of the significance, advantages, and disadvantages of genetic testing.
  - In 2008, Genetic Information Nondiscrimi nation Act (GINA) removed the finding of a pathogenic germline mutation as a pre-existing condition for health insurance or employment purposes; thus patients should not fear loss of coverage because of a genetic diagnosis of LS.

Screening and Diagnostic Strategies

CRC in a Patient Without Known LS

- This is the most frequently encountered indication for testing in clinical practice. Over the past several decades, the approach to diagnostic testing has moved from a selective approach, where patients deemed to be at elevated risk of harboring MMR mutations by clinicopathologic criteria undergo testing, to a universal approach, where CRCs are screened using MSI or immunohistochemistry.
- The selective approaches utilize clinicopathologic criteria and prediction models to select patients to undergo germline mutation testing. Although selective approaches do not depend on the availability of tumor tissue and of tumor molecular tests (i.e., IHC, MSI), they are subject to the accuracy, availability, and the recall bias of the personal and family histories obtained.
- As tumor molecular testing has become increasingly available, a universal screening approach for all CRCs for MMR deficiency has been advocated as the most sensitive strategy to identify patients at risk for LS. This two-step approach involves a screening step where all CRCs are tested for evidence of MMR deficiency independent of somatic mechanisms, followed by a confirmatory step where patients undergo germline MMR mutation testing. Tumors may be testing for MSI and/or MMR protein expression. If the tumor is MSI-H and/or if one of the MMR proteins is not expressed, further exploration is warranted.
  - Since the majority of CRC MSI is not caused by MLH1 loss secondary to hypermethylation of the *MLH1* promoter region, strategies to evaluate MSI with MLH1 IHC loss have been used before proceeding with genetic testing. CRC lacking expression of MLH1 may be further evaluated for DNA hypermethylation of the *MLH1* promoter or for *BRAF* mutations, which are highly associated with sporadic MSI-H tumors. If the tumor is methylated and/or has a BRAF mutation, the likelihood of LS is less, and testing does not need to be pursued unless there is a strong suspicion based on clinical or family history. If MSH2, MSH26, or PMS2 is lost, then it is highly likely to be caused by a germline mutation, and directed testing for that particular gene proceeds along those lines. One algorithmic approach to screening for LS in CRC is demonstrated in Fig. 23.6.

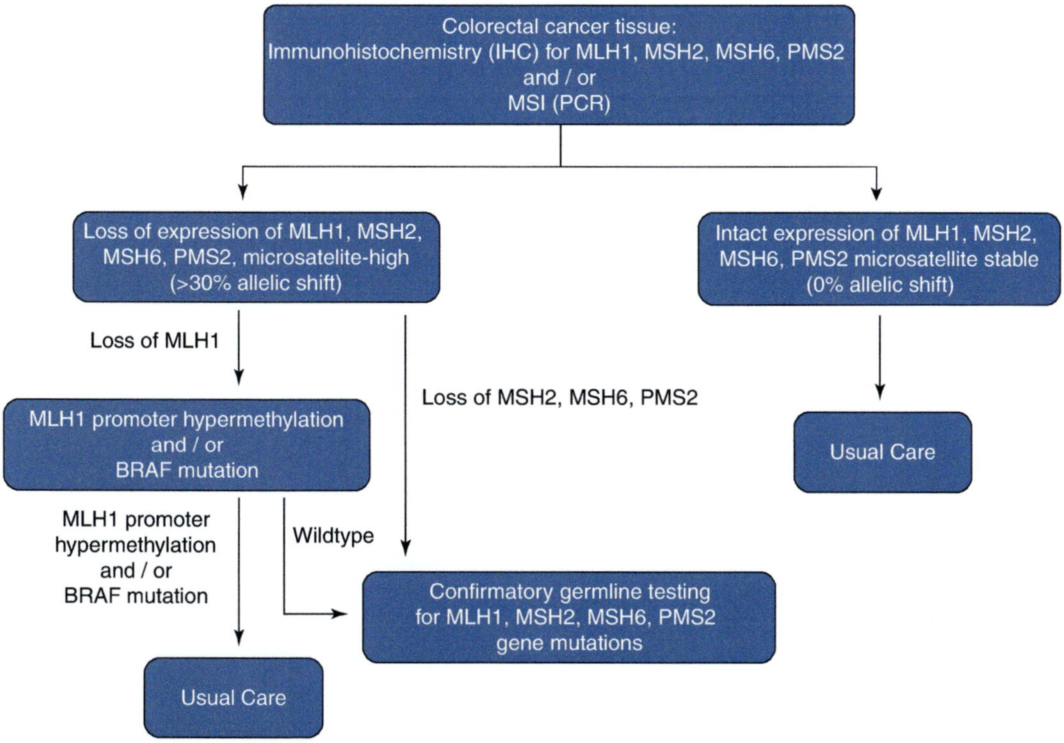

Fig. 23.6 One algorithm for testing of colorectal tumors for MMR deficiency as a first step to screen for patients with Lynch syndrome

- Whichever strategy is used, one must be able to interpret and take action on germline testing results. In general, germline testing yields one of three possible results: (1) a deleterious (pathogenic) mutation, (2) a variant of unknown significance, or (3) uninformative negative or no mutation found. Finding of a pathogenic mutation confirms the diagnosis of LS in the patient. The latter two findings should be considered inconclusive, in the setting of a dMMR tumor without evidence of *MLH1* promoter methylation and/or BRAF mutation. Patients with a MSI-H tumor and loss of MMR protein expression but without a confirmatory germline mutation are considered to have "Lynch-like syndrome." In the absence of clearly defined cancer risks for patients with Lynch-like syndrome, it remains the most prudent today to clinically manage these patients and families in the same way as LS patients. One caveat is that strategies that involve only germline testing (i.e., based on Amsterdam criteria or predictive models) without accompanying tumor MMR status testing are thus at risk for missing patients who might have "Lynch-like syndrome."

Individual with a Family Diagnosis of LS

- Once a pathogenic mutation is identified in a proband, all at-risk blood-relatives should undergo site-specific germline testing for the known family mutation.
- In these cases of site-specific testing (for affected relatives) or predictive testing (for unaffected relatives), there are two possible results: (1) true positive (when the specific mutation is identified, the individual is confirmed to have LS) and (2) true negative (this is a conclusive negative result and effectively rules out LS in the individual, who carries only general population risks for malignancies).

Table 23.5 Summary of possible surveillance regimen for Lynch syndrome patients

Cancer	Test	Frequency (years)	Age to commence (years)
Colorectal	Colonoscopy	1–2	20–25 or 2–5 years prior to earliest colon cancer before age 25
Endometrial and ovarian	Transvaginal ultrasound with endometrial sampling consideration for serum CA-125	1–2 years	30–35
Gastric/small bowel	Consideration for extended esophagoduodenoscopy	3–5	30–35
Urinary tract	Consideration for urinalysis	1	25–30
Sebaceous Neoplasms	Physical examination	1	25–30
Brain/central nervous system	Physical/neurologic examination	1	25–30

Modified from the National Comprehensive Cancer Network Guideline on Genetic/Familial High-risk Assessment: Colorectal. Version 1.2015. www.nccn.org

Individual Whose Family Meets Amsterdam Criteria but Does Not Have Any Clinical Phenotype

- It is not uncommon for a healthy individual from an Amsterdam criteria family to seek consult regarding his/her own screening recommendations. The initial evaluation should begin with a detailed personal and family cancer history. The most informative individual to evaluate would be a relative with a LS-associated cancer, particularly at a young age. If tumor is available, screening may be conducted as discussed above. If a pathogenic mutation is found, then directed germline testing can be performed for at-risk relatives. If tumor screening is not feasible, germline testing of an affected individual within the context of appropriate genetic counseling is an option. We do not recommend broad germline genetic testing for an unaffected individual as the yield is low and inconclusive results such as variant of unknown significance or uninformative negative would be clinically difficult to interpret in an unaffected individual.

Clinical Management

Screening

- For patients with LS, key elements of their lifelong care include screening for cancers in unaffected individuals and surveillance for recurrent, metachronous, or other syndromic cancers in affected individuals (Table 23.5).
- Recent guidelines have suggested varying the age to initiate colonoscopy depending on family history (at least 2–5 years younger than the earliest affected age in the family).
- LS patients are also at increased risk for developing extracolonic malignancies that can potentially benefit from screening of asymptomatic individuals. A definitive survival benefit has not been proven by prospective studies, and management is based on expert opinion and published guidelines.

Modifiers of Risk for Colorectal and Other Cancers

- High meat and high snack contents of a diet, smoking, and obesity increase the risk of developing colorectal neoplasia.
- Aspirin has been shown in some studies to be associated with reduced risk of LS-related cancers. However, currently the evidence is not sufficiently mature to recommend routine use of high-dose aspirin in LS patients.

Surgery for Colorectal Cancer

- Surgical treatment of LS-associated *colon cancer* starts with the same oncologic principles as those for sporadic colon cancer. Colectomy should be performed with adequate proximal, distal, and radial resection margin, regional lymphadenectomy, and R0 and en bloc resection of all malignant tissue.

- The extent of resection (segmental colectomy or total abdominal colectomy with ileorectal anastomosis) depends on balancing surgical morbidity, patient comorbidities and wishes, and risk of future malignancy in the remaining colorectum. Factors to consider include the presence of synchronous pathology, age of the patient, disease prognosis and life expectancy, risk of metachronous CRC, expected compliance with surveillance, morbidity of reoperation, bowel function, and patient preferences.
- The American Society of Colon and Rectal Surgeons recommends extended colectomy for patients with colon cancer and LS, based mainly on metachronous cancer risk. Multiple retrospective studies have demonstrated a higher rate of metachronous colorectal cancer following segmental colectomy compared to extended colectomy. This risk may vary depending on the compliance with endoscopic surveillance and feasibility of endoscopic removal of premalignant polyps.
- There have not been prospective studies to prove that extended colectomy improves survival in LS patients. In a Markov model, the calculated gain in life expectancy from extended compared to segmental colectomy was 2.3 years if surgery were performed at age 27 years, 1 year at age 47 years, and 0.3 years at age 67 years, and these numbers became 3.4 years at age 27 years, 1.5 years at age 47 years, and 0.4 year at age 67 years if the colon cancer were stage I. Therefore, extended colectomy may have the most benefit in young patients with early-stage disease only. Advanced CRC stage, significant medical comorbidities, and other LS-associated malignancies that pose competing risks to the patient's life expectancy should also be considered.
- Functional expectations of each operation should also be discussed with patients.
- Management of *rectal cancer* in LS involves complex decision-making. The cancer should be managed like any other rectal cancer in terms of indications for multimodality therapy and oncologic principles.
- However, just as in colon cancer in LS, the extent of the resection is determined by many factors. The surgeon and patient must decide between a proctectomy and total proctocolectomy (TPC) with or without sphincter preservation as determined by the tumor location.
- Compared to TPC with an ileal pouch reconstruction, proctectomy alone results in less frequent bowel movements and less incontinence. However, proctectomy without colectomy leaves the entire colon in situ and at risk for metachronous cancer.
- If restorative proctocolectomy with ileal pouch-anal anastomosis is contemplated, the need for, and timing of, pelvic radiotherapy should be carefully considered. Although little data exist regarding the long-term functional outcome of an IPAA performed before or after pelvic radiotherapy, there is general reluctance to radiate ileal pouch postoperatively because of the risks of radiation enteritis, pelvic fibrosis, and pouch dysfunction. Neoadjuvant radiotherapy should be better tolerated, but the risk of long-term risk of anal sphincter dysfunction due to radiotherapy, combined with functional alterations associated with the ileal pouch procedure, may sway both patient and surgeon away from a restorative proctocolectomy in this situation.

Prophylactic Surgery for Endometrial and Ovarian Cancer

- In women undergoing curative surgical treatment of CRC, concomitant prophylactic total abdominal hysterectomy and salpingo-oophorectomy should be considered.

Evaluation of At-Risk Relatives

- When LS or an MMR pathogenic mutation has been identified in an individual, genetic counseling and site-specific testing for the pathogenic mutation should be offered to all first-degree relatives (parents, siblings, and children). Due to the considerable psychoso-

cial issues associated with germline testing, it is usually not recommended for at-risk individuals younger than age 18 years.
- Screening of asymptomatic at-risk relatives for premalignant lesions or early manifestations of cancer is appropriate and has been recommended to commence 5–10 years younger than the youngest age of onset of cancer in the family or between age 20 and 25.
- A major reason to identify individuals with LS is to optimize the care of their at-risk relatives, with the goal of ultimately minimizing the morbidity and mortality of LS.
- Probands and their at-risk relatives with LS greatly benefits from enrollment in a hereditary CRC registry.

24 Colorectal Neoplasms: Screening and Surveillance After Polypectomy

Evie H. Carchman and Charles P. Heise

Key Concepts

- Screening can reduce colorectal mortality.
- Screening recommendations are based upon risk for polyp/cancer development (family history of cancer or polyps, personal history of cancer/polyps, genetic syndromes (FAP, MYH, and HNPCC), and inflammatory bowel disease).
- Surveillance after polypectomy depends on the histology of polyp and the completeness of its resection.
- The decision to perform colectomy for a polyp that contains cancer depends on the extent of invasion (Haggitt staging for pedunculated polyp and Kikuchi classification for sessile polyp).

Introduction

- Colorectal cancer is the second leading cause of cancer-related deaths in the United States in men and women combined. In 2014, the National Cancer Institute (NCI) estimated 96,000 new colon cancer and 40,000 new rectal cancer cases, and the estimated number of deaths for both colon and rectal cancer combined was 50,310.
- The fortunate news is that the death rate from colorectal cancer has been decreasing over the last 20 years. This reduction in the number of new cancer cases and cancer-related deaths is a consequence of current screening programs.
- Screening can reduce colorectal cancer-related deaths by three mechanisms: endoscopic removal of adenomatous polyps can prevent the development of cancer; early detection of asymptomatic cancers; and identification of individuals at higher risk for accelerated carcinogenesis who may benefit from more frequent screening.
- It should also be considered that if current routine screening recommendations are followed by all, there is the potential to identify large groups of patients with adenomatous polyps. Their surveillance will incur substantial cost to the healthcare system.

Recommended Screening Guidelines

- Guidelines from the American Cancer Society (ACS), the American Society of Colon and Rectal Surgeons (ASCRS), and the American Gastroenterology Association (AGA) all recommend that colorectal cancer screening begin at the age of 50 for both men and women

E. H. Carchman · C. P. Heise (✉)
Department of Surgery, University of Wisconsin – School of Medicine and Public Health, Madison, WI, USA
e-mail: heise@surgery.wisc.edu

S. R. Steele et al. (eds.), *The ASCRS Manual of Colon and Rectal Surgery*, https://doi.org/10.1007/978-3-030-01165-9_24

at average risk of colorectal cancer (i.e., no family history of colorectal cancer, no personal history of inflammatory bowel disease, and asymptomatic). These accepted guidelines are based on joint efforts set forth in 2008 by the ACS, the US Multi-Society Task Force on Colorectal Cancer, and the American College of Radiology.

- Screening regimens can be divided into two categories: fecal testing and structural examinations. While structural examinations are designed to detect both polyps and cancer, fecal testing primarily detects already established cancers or, less commonly, advanced adenomas.

Screening Options and Timing for Average-Risk Individuals

- Colonoscopy every 10 years
- CT colonography (virtual colonoscopy) every 5 years
- Flexible sigmoidoscopy every 5 years
- Double-contrast barium enema every 5 years
- Guaiac-based fecal occult blood test (gFOBT) every year
- Fecal immunochemical test (FIT) every year
- Stool DNA test (sDNA) every 3 years
- It is important to note that in order for the above to be effective, each of these screening regimens should be performed at regular intervals. In addition, if any of the non-colonoscopy screening tests listed are abnormal, a full colonoscopy is usually warranted, and the patient should be made aware of this possibility prior to initiation of screening.

Screening Guidelines for Individuals at an Increased Risk Based on Family History

- If there is a history of colorectal cancer or adenomatous polyps in a first-degree relative before age 60, or in 2 or more first-degree relatives at any age (non-hereditary syndrome), then screening should begin at age 40 or 10 years prior to the youngest case, whichever is earlier. Unless contraindicated, colonoscopy is the recommended test in this instance, with screening every 5 years.
- If there is a history of colorectal cancer or adenomatous polyps in a first-degree relative aged 60 or older, or in at least 2 or more second-degree relatives at any age, then screening should begin at age 40. Any of the screening options for average-risk individuals may be recommended along with the same screening intervals.

Screening Guidelines for Individuals Considered at High Risk Based on Genetics

- If there is positive genetic testing for familial adenomatous polyposis (FAP) or suspected FAP without testing, then screening should begin at age 10–12 years. Screening should include yearly flexible sigmoidoscopy and consideration for genetic testing if not yet performed. Consideration for colectomy is recommended when testing is positive.
- If there is a diagnosis of Lynch syndrome or an individual at increased risk for Lynch, screening should begin at age 20–25 years or 10 years prior to the youngest case. This should include colonoscopy every 1–2 years and genetic testing if not yet performed. In addition, genetic testing should be offered to all first-degree relatives if a Lynch mutation is identified.
- Individuals with inflammatory bowel disease (chronic ulcerative colitis or Crohn's disease) should begin screening 8 years after the onset of pancolitis or 12–15 years after the onset of left-sided colitis. Screening should be performed by colonoscopy every 1–2 years with biopsies assessing for dysplasia.

Screening Cessation

- The US Preventive Services Task Force recommends screening up to the age of 75.

Screening should be discontinued in individuals aged 76–85 years, if they have had routine screening. However, screening may be considered in this age group if never screened previously and according to each individual's health status and risk. Screening should not be performed in individuals after the age of 85 years.

- Age alone, however, is not an indication for screening. In average-risk persons, colorectal cancer screening should, in general, be discontinued when there are fewer than 10 years of life expectancy.

Methods of Screening

Colonoscopy

- The major advantages for colonoscopy as a screening regimen are that it allows visualization of the entire colon, along with the identification, biopsy, or removal of encountered polyps or cancer.
- Although colonoscopy is widely utilized in the United States for colorectal cancer screening, there are no prospective, randomized trials demonstrating a reduction in the incidence of, or the mortality from, colorectal cancer as a result of colonoscopy. However, as other screening modalities result in subsequent therapeutic colonoscopy after polyp detection, there is indirect evidence suggesting that colonoscopy is beneficial in reducing cancer incidence.
- Although the use of colonoscopy as a screening modality has major benefits in risk reduction, there are also associated drawbacks with this procedure. Colonoscopy is usually done with sedation and thus requires a chaperone to accompany the patient for transportation. In addition, a complete bowel preparation is required and is often the most difficult part of the process for the patient. However, it is also one of the most important components to completing the procedure successfully and is critical in terms of quality.
- Rex et al. published an update of several quality indicators set forth by the American Society for Gastrointestinal Endoscopy (ASGE) and American College of Gastroenterology (ACG) Task Force on Quality in Endoscopy. In this update, proposed quality indicators and performance targets are summarized for colonoscopy examinations in the pre-procedure, intra-procedure, and post-procedure periods (Table 24.1).
- Unfortunately, despite best efforts there are reported miss rates for both polyps and cancers with the use of colonoscopy. Miss rates for polyps $\geq$10 mm vary from 2% to 12% depending on the study and the control method, typically tandem colonoscopy or CT colonography.
- Similarly, potential miss rates for cancer are reported to be approximately 3% overall, and higher for lesions in the proximal colon (6%), based upon evaluation of patients who had undergone screening colonoscopy within 3 years prior to diagnosis.

Incomplete Colonoscopy

- Recommended rates of incomplete colonoscopy (without cecal intubation) should be <5% during screening and < 10% overall. Unfortunately, there are no apparent guidelines or consensus as to the best management strategies in cases of incomplete colonoscopy.
- When colonoscopy is incomplete, options include repeat colonoscopy, use of other endoscopic modalities (i.e., smaller endoscope, double balloon endoscopy), CT colonography, or barium enema. The decision of which modality is best suited is dependent on both the reasons for the incomplete exam and the institution-specific resources available.

Adjuncts to Colonoscopy

- In an effort to improve colonoscopy screening, more recent technical developments in colonoscopic imaging have targeted advancements in polyp detection. These advances have included (1) techniques applied to current colonoscopy methods, including

Table 24.1 Proposed quality indicators in colonoscopy

Quality indicator	Grade of recommendation	Measure type	Performance target (%)
Pre-procedure			
1. Frequency with colonoscopy is performed for an indication that is included in a published standard list of appropriate indications, and the indication is documented	IC+	Process	>80
2. Frequency with which informed consent is obtained, including specific discussion of risks associated with colonoscopy, and fully documented	IC	Process	>98
3. Frequency with which colonoscopies follow recommended post-polypectomy and post-cancer resection surveillance intervals and 10-year intervals between screening colonoscopies in average-risk patients who have negative examination results and adequate bowel cleansing (priority indicator)	IA	Process	≥90
4. Frequency with which ulcerative colitis and Crohn's colitis surveillance are recommended with proper intervals	2C	Process	≥90
Intra-procedure			
5. Frequency with which the procedure note documents the quality of preparation	3	Process	>98
6. Frequency with which bowel preparation is adequate to allow the use of recommended surveillance or screening intervals	3	Process	≥85 of outpatient exams
7. Frequency with which visualization of the cecum by notation of landmarks and photodocumentation of landmarks is documented in every procedure (priority indicator)	1C	Process	
Cecal intubation rate with photography (all examinations)			≥90
Cecal intubation rate with photography (screening)			≥95
8. Frequency with which adenomas are detected in asymptomatic average-risk individuals (screening) (priority indicator)	1C	Outcome	
Adenoma detection rate for male/female population			≥25
Adenoma detection rate for male patients			≥30
Adenoma detection rate for female patients			≥20
9a. Frequency with which withdrawal time is measured	2C	Process	>98
9b. Average withdrawal time in negative-result screening colonoscopies	2C	Process	≥6 min
10. Frequency with which biopsy specimens are obtained when colonoscopy is performed for indication of chronic diarrhea	2C	Process	>98
11. Frequency of recommended tissue sampling when colonoscopy is performed for surveillance in ulcerative colitis and Crohn's colitis	1C	Process	>98
12. Frequency with which endoscopic removal of pedunculated polyps and sessile polyps <2 cm is attempted before surgical referral	3	Outcome	>98
13. Indication of perforation by procedure type (all indications vs. colorectal cancer screening/polyp surveillance) and post-polypectomy bleeding	1C	Outcome	

Table 24.1 (continued)

Quality indicator	Grade of recommendation	Measure type	Performance target (%)
Incidence of perforation – all examinations			<1:500
Incidence of perforation – screening			<1:10,000
Incidence of post-polypectomy bleeding			<1%
14. Frequency with which post-polypectomy bleeding is managed without surgery	1C	Outcome	≥90
15. Frequency with which appropriate recommendation for timing of repeat colonoscopy is documented and provided to the patient after histologic findings are reviewed	1A	Process	≥90

With permission from Rex DK, Schoenfeld PS, Cohen J, Pike IM, Adler DG, Fennerty MB, et al. Quality indicators for colonoscopy. Am J Gastroenterol. 2015;110(1):72–90. © Nature Publishing Group
This list of potential quality indicators is meant to be a comprehensive listing of measurable end points. It is not the intention of the task force that all end points be measured in every practice setting. In most cases, validation may be required before a given end point may be adopted universally

high-definition monitors, chromoendoscopy, or cap-assisted colonoscopy (CAC), and (2) colonoscope enhancements to current imaging, such as narrow-band imaging (NBI), autofluorescence imaging (AFI), and Fujinon intelligent color enhancement (FICE).

Complications

- Complications related to colonoscopy include cardiopulmonary events, bleeding, perforation, diverticulitis, and post-polypectomy syndrome.
  - The overall 30-day risk of serious adverse events after colonoscopy is approximately 0.5% following screening colonoscopies and 0.7% after follow-up colonoscopies.
  - The overall risk readmission after colonoscopy is approximately 1%, and the risk of death varies from 0% to 0.09%.
  - The risk of unplanned cardiopulmonary events after colonoscopy is approximately 1% and is usually related to the effects of conscious sedation.
  - Perforation is rare, approximately 0.04% for screening (0.07% with polypectomy) and 0.12% after follow-up.
  - Post-polypectomy syndrome is an electrocautery full-thickness burn resulting in localized peritonitis, without definitive evidence of perforation. In a review by Ko et al., the risk of post-polypectomy syndrome ranged from 0.003% to 0.1%.
  - Most related bleeding occurs after polypectomy, with a rate of 0.27% for screening and 0.50% after polypectomy. Post-polypectomy bleeding can be immediate or delayed. Older age was associated with higher rates of perforation or bleeding.

CT Colonography (CTC) or Virtual Colonoscopy

- CT colonography or virtual colonoscopy is a minimally invasive, radiographic option for colorectal cancer screening. It utilizes computed tomography to generate two-dimensional images that allow for further three-dimensional reconstruction with the assistance of software technology. Together, evaluation of both 2D and 3D images allows for accurate neoplasia detection. Figure 24.1a–d demonstrates two-dimensional and three-dimensional imaging of a pedunculated sigmoid polyp and subsequent colonoscopic identification.
- CTC still requires adequate bowel preparation and must have gaseous distension of the colon to allow for adequate examination. This entails insertion of a rectal catheter to allow for

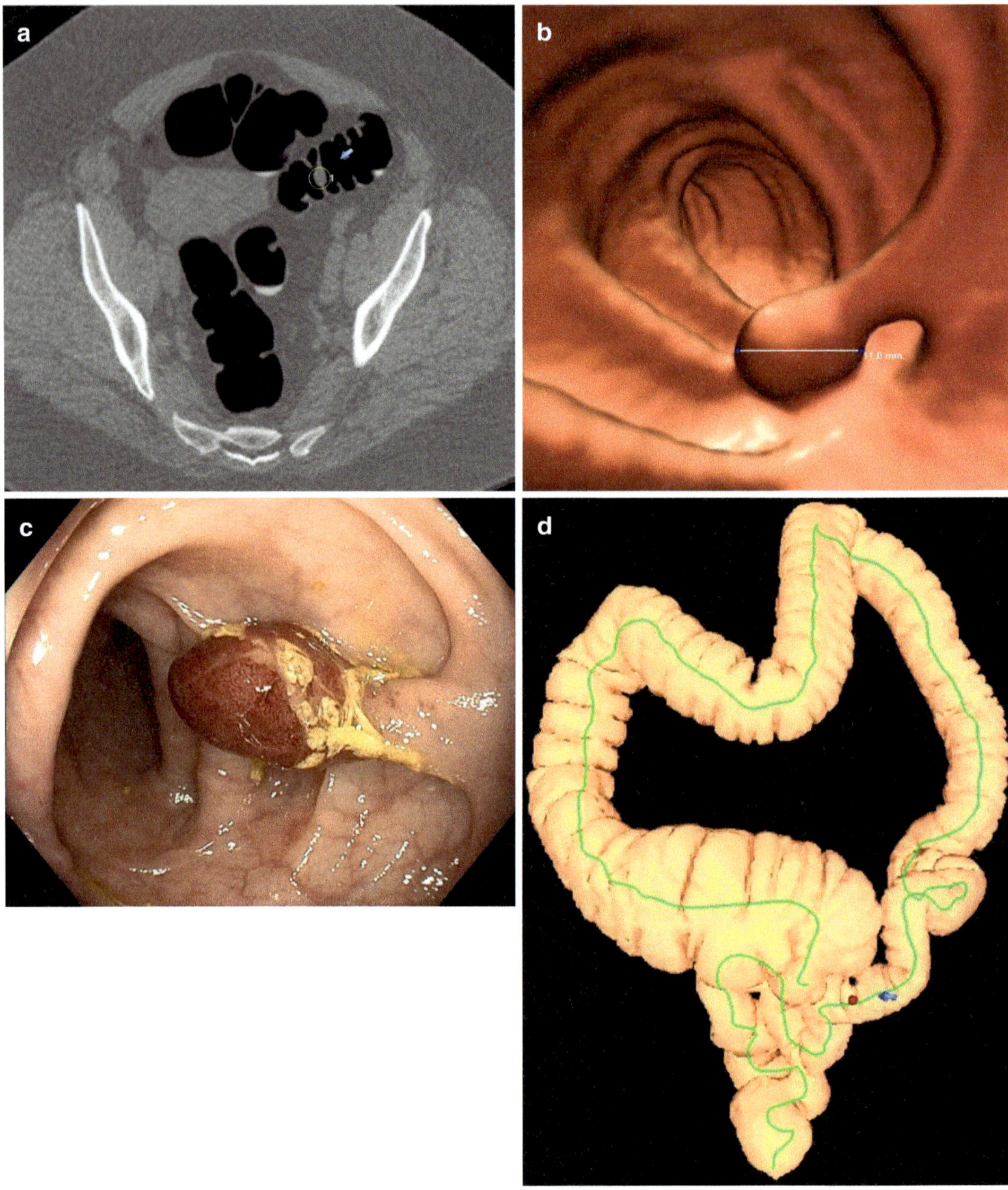

Fig. 24.1 CT colonography images demonstrate both (**a**) two-dimensional and (**b**) three-dimensional imaging of a pedunculated sigmoid polyp, and subsequent (**c**) colonoscopic identification (**d**) demonstrates the virtual location of the polyp by CT imaging

manual or automated inflation with carbon dioxide, infused continuously as images are acquired.

- Tagging of residual stool contents with an oral delivery of dilute barium (2%) and residual fluid tagging with water-soluble iodinated contrast (diatrizoate) have further increased sensitivity.
- As with optical colonoscopy, meeting appropriate quality parameters is also important in

CTC. These parameters as recommended by the American College of Radiology (ACR) should include: (1) adequate colon cleansing and distension, (2) complete anatomic coverage of the colon and rectum, (3) visualization of each colonic segment in at least one position, (4) appropriate physician training for CTC performance and interpretation, and (5) proper documentation and communication of clinical findings.

- CTC does not require sedation, and the exam can be performed rather quickly. However, in cases where polyps are detected, subsequent therapeutic colonoscopy is required for confirmation and removal. Ideally, this should be performed on the same day since bowel preparation is already complete. This requires program coordination between gastroenterology and radiology departments.
- In cases where polyps are detected, findings of one or more polyps ≥10 mm or three or more polyps ≥6 mm should be referred for subsequent colonoscopy and polypectomy. Though somewhat controversial, isolated polyps in the 6–9 mm range may also be referred for therapeutic intervention.
- Since very small polyps (≤5 mm) carry low clinical risk, reporting and referral for these isolated lesions are currently not recommended.
- A further advantage of CTC is that it allows for a limited evaluation for extracolonic findings, approximately 7% of which are clinically relevant and 2% of which patients gain clinical benefit from detection.
- Complications related to CTC are very rare. A survey of a virtual colonoscopy working group reported no perforations in more than 11,000 CTC screening examinations, and 2 perforations in more than 10,000 exams for diagnostic indications (0.02%), only one of which was symptomatic.
- Although often discussed, the radiation exposure associated with CTC is quite low, reportedly around 5 mSv for screening purposes. This is well below the 100 mSv threshold often considered when attempting to address associated health risk.
- CTC compares favorably to optical colonoscopy, with detection rates of >95% for cancer, 90–95% for adenomas ≥10 mm, and 80–90% for adenomas ≥6 mm. In parallel screening program studies utilizing both colonoscopy and CTC, similar detection rates for advanced neoplasia (polyps and cancer) are noted.

Flexible Sigmoidoscopy

- Flexible sigmoidoscopy may be useful as a component of the screening regimen for colorectal cancer.
- The standard sigmoidoscope is 60 cm in length. To be effective as a screening modality, the quality of the evaluation must be adequate. Therefore, it has been recommended that the scope be advanced to a minimum of 40 cm in order to minimize the risk of missing a distal colorectal cancer.
- If a polyp is identified, it should be biopsied in order to best determine the need for proximal colon evaluation. With adenoma detection, the risk of harboring concomitant disease more proximally is at least twofold and should prompt consideration of complete colonoscopy.
- The advantages of flexible sigmoidoscopy lie in the ability to perform the procedure without sedation (although with some potential patient discomfort), by a variety of healthcare professionals and after only minimal bowel preparation.
- The major problem with sigmoidoscopy lies in its inability to evaluate the more proximal colon. Despite this, meta-analyses have demonstrated a beneficial reduction in the incidence of colorectal cancer and long-term mortality when compared with no screening.
- Some guidelines recommend combining flexible sigmoidoscopy every 5 years with annual fecal occult blood testing (FOBT).

Complications

- The risk of complications, including perforation, with flexible sigmoidoscopy is extremely low, reported to be 0.02%.

Fecal Occult Blood Testing (FOBT)/ Fecal Immunochemical Testing (FIT)

- Fecal occult blood testing (FOBT) is aimed at detecting subtle blood loss in the gastrointestinal tract and is typically performed annually as a screening examination.
- There are two general types of FOBT based on the analyte detected: guaiac versus immunochemical. A positive test should prompt further evaluation, typically with colonoscopy.
  - A stool guaiac test (gFOBT) is done by smearing feces onto an absorbent paper that has been chemically treated. Hydrogen peroxide is then placed onto the paper, and if trace amounts of blood are present, the color will change. Optimal use depends on following strict dietary adjustments prior to collecting the stool sample. This test requires at least 2 mL of blood loss a day to become positive. There have been several randomized, controlled trials that demonstrate a benefit of FOBT in reducing mortality from CRC (about 15% reduction).
  - Fecal immunochemical testing (FIT) utilizes specific antibodies to detect globin. FIT has replaced most gFOBT tests in that it is both cheap and quantitative. There is evidence that FIT has higher sensitivity and specificity than gFOBT, and patients are not required to follow any dietary restrictions prior to testing. A recent systematic review demonstrated an overall accuracy of 95% for CRC detection with 79% sensitivity and 94% specificity. However, it does have a lower sensitivity in terms of adenoma detection (only 28%).

Stool DNA Testing

- In patients with colorectal cancer, tumor cells and their associated DNA are continuously passed into the stool. Tumor DNA constitutes a very small amount of the fecal content; therefore a large stool sample is needed for analysis. This assay tests for DNA mutations and methylations of common genes associated with colorectal cancer (i.e., KRAS mutations). This test concomitantly tests for beta-actin to allow for an estimation of total amount of human DNA present.
- These tests also assay for human hemoglobin similar to FIT.
- The results of the assay allow for a composite score that is compared to a standardized value in order to determine a positive or negative test result.
- There are no dietary restrictions with this test.
- In a recent study in asymptomatic patients, stool DNA testing detected significantly more cancers than did FIT but also had more false positives.

Double-Contrast Barium Enema (DCBE)

- With the more widespread use of the previously described screening entities, the use of contrast enema has diminished as a screening modality. However, it may still be utilized in regions where other screening modalities are not available.
- DCBE involves coating the colonic mucosal surface with barium followed by distension with air through a rectally placed catheter. Fluoroscopic and standard radiographic imaging is utilized during various positional changes to assess the entire colon. Prior bowel preparation is required to allow for removal of adherent fecal content.
- DCBE is less sensitive than colonoscopy or CT colonography for the detection of cancer and polyps. In addition, DCBE is often unattractive to both patient and radiologist, due to the nature and labor intensiveness of the exam. Therefore its current role in screening for colorectal cancer is uncertain in areas where colonoscopy and CT colonography are available.

Status of Screening in the United States

- Although there are several modalities available for colorectal cancer screening, the American Cancer Society reports that in 2012, only 59% of Americans over the age of 50 were screened according to current guidelines. Furthermore, there appears to be wide geographic variability in screening patterns.

Surveillance

Guidelines for Surveillance After Polypectomy

History

- Consensus guidelines have evolved from the recommendation for annual repeat colonoscopy following polypectomy in the 1970s to recommendations based on the number, size, location, and histologic features of the polyps removed (Table 24.2).
- Prior to making a recommendation regarding surveillance colonoscopy, the endoscopist should carefully consider the personal and family history of colorectal neoplasia, potential technical issues with colonoscopy and associated risk, and life expectancy of the patient.
- It is important to note that the current guidelines for surveillance are to be applied only after high-quality baseline colonoscopy with complete removal of all detected lesions. If either of these two criteria is not met, then repeat examination should be planned.
- Discontinuation of surveillance should be considered in patients with less than a 10-year life expectancy.
- These guidelines apply only to asymptomatic individuals; new symptoms should prompt consideration of diagnostic work-up.

Table 24.2 Recommendations for screening intervals based on consensus guidelines for patients with serrated polyps based on histology, number, location, and size

Histology	Size	Number	Location	Interval in years
HP	<10 mm	Any number+	Rectosigmoid	10+++
HP	≤5 mm	≤3	Proximal to sigmoid	10
HP	Any	≥4	Proximal to sigmoid	5
HP	> 5 mm	≥1	Proximal to sigmoid	5
SSA/P or TSA	<10 mm	<3	Any	5
SSA/P or TSA	≥10 mm	1	Any	3
SSA/P or TSA	<10 mm	≥3	Any	3
SSA/P	≥10 mm	≤2	Any	1–3+++
SSA/P/w/dysplasia	Any	Any		1–3++++

With permission from Rex DK, Ahnen DJ, Baron JA, Batts KP, Burke CA, Burt RW, et al. Serrated lesions of the colorectum: review and recommendations from an expert panel. Am J Gastroenterol. 2012;107(9):1315–29; quiz 4, 3 Reproduced with permission. © Nature Publishing Group

Note 1: Patients with both significant serrated findings and concurrent adenomas may be at a more advanced stage in the progression toward cancer. Closer follow-up may be indicated in some cases based on clinical judgment

Note 2: In general, these recommendations for surveillance are for the first follow-up. For findings with short follow-up recommendations, a longer subsequent follow-up interval may be appropriately applied when a follow-up exam shows improvement in findings, i.e., reduction in the number, size, and/or histologic severity of lesions

Note 3: Because of interobserver variation in the pathologic differentiation of HP from SSA/P, proximal colon serrated lesions >10 mm in size that are designated HP may be considered to be SSA/P by clinicians

SSA sessile serrated adenoma, *TSA* traditional serrated adenoma

+The interval recommendations presented here represent consensus opinion based on low-quality or very low-quality evidence. They are likely to change as higher-quality evidence becomes available, and alternatives may be equally reasonable

+Patients with >20HPs in the rectosigmoid meet the World Health Organization definition of serrated polyposis if there are additional serrated lesions proximal to the sigmoid

++Some panel members follow a policy of 5 years if there are multiple HPs 6–9 mm in size in the rectosigmoid

+++Patients with two or more serrated polyps ≥10 mm in the proximal colon meet the World Health Organization criteria for serrated polyps if three additional serrated lesions of any size proximal to the sigmoid are identified

++++SSA/P with cytological dysplasia is a more advanced lesion than SSA/P. Depending on the size of the lesion, the confidence in complete endoscopic resection and other associated lesions, intervals shorter than 3 years may be appropriate

Surveillance Based on Pathology of Polyp

Hyperplastic and Serrated Polyps

- Serrated lesions of the colon and rectum are classified by the World Health Organization (WHO) into three general categories based on cytological features, architectural features, and location. The categories include hyperplastic polyps, sessile serrated adenoma/polyps, and traditional serrated adenomas (Fig. 24.2a, b).
- Small hyperplastic polyps in the rectosigmoid are very common and are not believed to be associated with development of adenomatous colorectal neoplasia. If encountered, they should be biopsied to establish a diagnosis, but otherwise their presence does not alter the patient's risk stratification.
- Sessile serrated adenomas/polyps are usually located in the proximal colon, sessile or flat in morphology, pale in color, with indistinct borders, and usually have a mucus cap. Due to their indistinct appearance, there is a high rate of incomplete resection. NBI and chromoendoscopy techniques can be used to facilitate identification and delineation of borders. Given that incomplete resection rates are high for serrated adenomas greater than 1 cm, some authors have recommended routine tattooing of the polypectomy site to facilitate identification at repeat colonoscopy.
- There is increasing awareness that these lesions may be precursor lesions to cancer development in about 1/3 of colorectal cancer cases. Recent reviews on the management of serrated lesions recommended complete removal of all lesions except for ≤5 mm in sigmoid or rectum.

Adenoma

- Adenomas can be classified histologically as tubular, villous, or tubulovillous. According to the World Health Organization criteria, tubular adenomas have less than 25% villous component, tubulovillous 25–75%, and villous greater than 75%.
- Tubular adenomas are the most common type of adenoma found followed by tubulovillous and then villous. Tubular adenomas have <5% of harboring cancer, while the risk of tubulovillous is 20–25%, and villous adenomas is 35–40%.
- Screening series have reported an adenoma prevalence rate of 15–30%. With the addition of high-definition colonoscopy, this number has been quoted as high as 50%.

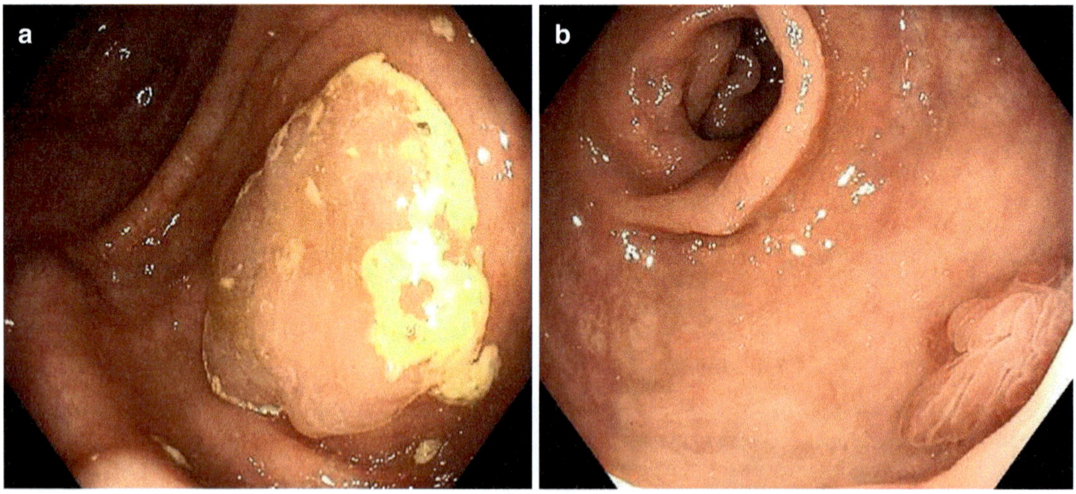

Fig. 24.2 Endoscopic views of two different types of serrated polyps. (**a**) Sessile serrated adenoma/polyp in cecum and (**b**) a traditional serrated adenoma of rectum

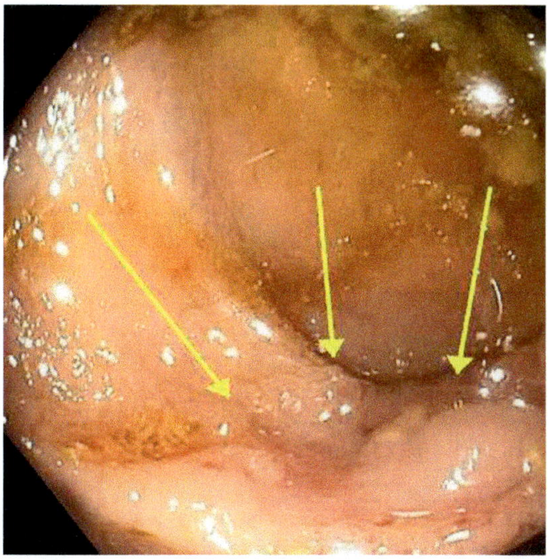

Fig. 24.3 Endoscopic view of a cecal ulceration which pathology after biopsy demonstrated colonic mucosa with adenomatous change and focal high-grade dysplasia

- The recommendations for post-polypectomy surveillance are outlined in Table 24.2.
- Those patients with sessile adenomas that were removed in piecemeal fashion should be reexamined in 2–6 months to confirm complete lack of regrowth (Fig. 24.3).
- Patients with >10 adenomas at one examination should have follow-up in less than 3 years and should be considered for referral to a genetic counselor.

Inflammatory Polyps

- Inflammatory polyps include benign lymphoid polyps and pseudopolyps (such as those seen in ulcerative colitis). Benign lymphoid polyps are composed of normal lymphoid tissue and therefore do not require any surveillance if this is seen on pathology. Pseudopolyps are discussed below in the inflammatory disease section.

Hamartomas Polyps

- Hamartomas of the colon and rectum include juvenile polyps and polyps seen in Peutz-Jeghers syndrome.
- In a patient with juvenile polyps, all polyps should be removed, and surveillance should be done yearly until no polyps are found. Thereafter, patients with juvenile polyps should undergo surveillance colonoscopy every 3 years as long as no further polyps are detected.
- Patients who meet clinical criteria for Peutz-Jeghers syndrome should undergo genetic testing for a germline mutation. In terms of surveillance, these patients should undergo a colonoscopy every 2–3 years starting in late adolescence. They should also have upper endoscopies every 2–3 years. Small bowel interrogation (CT enterography) should also occur every 2–3 years.
- Please see Chap. 23, Molecular Basis of Colorectal Cancer and Overview of Inherited Colorectal Cancer Syndromes, for a detailed description of these entities.

Inflammatory Bowel Disease

- In patients with inflammatory bowel disease (IBD), the presence of chronic inflammation puts them at an increased risk for dysplasia and cancer.
- Polyps detected in patients with IBD are referred to as a dysplasia-associated lesion or mass (DALM).
  - DALM lesions are then divided into three categories based on endoscopic appearance and location:
    1. It is a sporadic adenoma if the polyp resembles an adenoma both endoscopically and histologically and is located outside an area of histologically proven colitis. Complete polypectomy with routine surveillance is adequate with these lesions.
    2. It is an IBD-associated adenoma-like polypoid dysplasia if the lesion resembles an adenoma endoscopically and histologically and is located in an area of colitis. For these lesions, if they are not associated with flat dysplasia or carcinoma, polypectomy with surveillance at a shortened interval is recommended.
    3. Finally IBD-associated non-adenoma-like dysplasia, which is considered a true

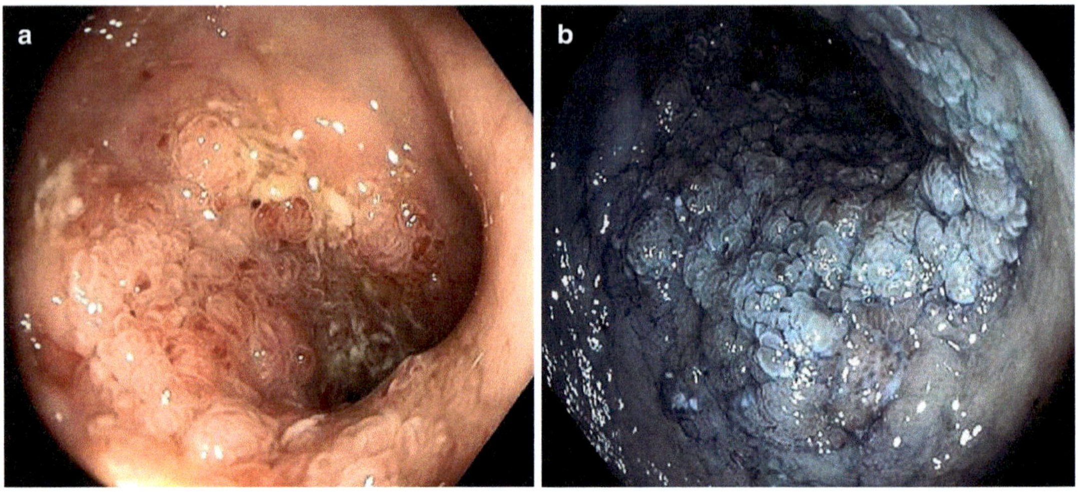

Fig. 24.4 (**a**) Endoscopic view of a polyp in the sigmoid colon of a patient with ulcerative colitis. (**b**) The use of chromoendoscopy in 4-2 allows for better visualization of the borders of the polyp compared to the images with indigo carmine in 4A

DALM, is a lesion that is irregular and broadly based and is located in an area of colitis. These lesions are at high risk for associated carcinoma and should be treated with colectomy after the diagnosis of dysplasia is confirmed by an experienced pathologist (Fig. 24.4a, b).

Surveillance with Cancer Resection

- Patients who undergo curative resection for sporadic colorectal cancer are recommended to undergo surveillance colonoscopy 1 year after resection to look for metachronous neoplasia. If the examination at 1 year is normal, then the interval should be extended to 3 years. If that subsequent colonoscopy is normal, then the interval is again increased to 5 years.
- For those patients who undergo curative resection of rectal cancer, additional digital rectal examination and proctoscopy should be performed every 3–6 months for the first 2–3 years and yearly for the next 2–3 years to look for signs of pelvic recurrence.

Early Cancer (T1) Within Polyp

- There are two classification systems that are established for the identification of cancer within a polyp. The first is Haggitt classification, which is utilized for quantifying the extent of invasion in pedunculated polyps. The second is the Kikuchi classification for sessile polyps.
- Haggitt classification for cancer in pedunculated polyps:
  - Haggitt level 0: Noninvasive.
  - Haggitt level 1: Cancer invading into the submucosa but limited to the head of the polyp.
  - Haggitt level 2: Cancer invades into the neck of the polyp.
  - Haggitt level 3: Cancer invading the stalk of the polyp.
  - Haggitt level 4: Cancer invading the submucosa of the bowel wall below the stalk.
- The risk of spread to the lymph nodes is less than 1% for levels 1–3, and if the polypectomy margin is negative, observation can be considered. For Haggitt level 4, the risk of nodal metastases ranges from 12% to 25%, and colectomy should be strongly considered.

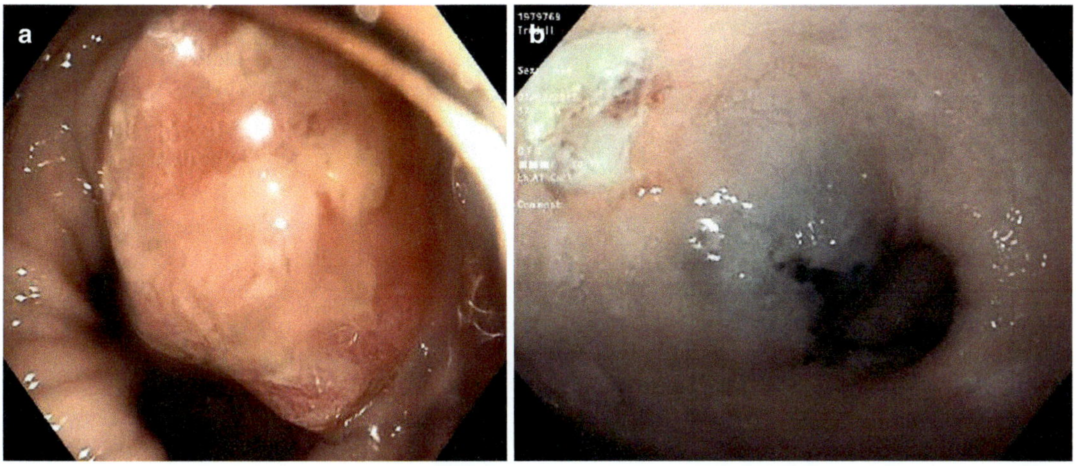

Fig. 24.5 (**a**) A 2 cm rectal polyp noted endoscopically. (**b**) Polyp was resected and tattooed based on size criteria. Final pathology demonstrated moderately differentiated invasive colonic adenocarcinoma with mucinous features arising from tubulovillous adenoma. Carcinoma present at cauterized margins

- Kikuchi classification of cancer in polyps. Invasion of the submucosa is divided into three:
  - SM1 is invasion of the upper one-third.
  - SM2 is invasion of the middle third.
  - SM3 is invasion into the lower one-third.
- Haggitt levels 1–3 are equivalent to SM1, and Haggitt level 4 can be SM1, SM2, or SM3. There have been several factors identified that increase the risk of lymph node metastases. These factors include lymphovascular invasion, poor differentiation, gender, extensive budding, and SM3 invasion.
- For low-risk cancers, Haggitt levels 1–3, Kikuchi SM1, or no evidence of poor differentiation or angioinvasion, where the lesion has been completely resected in one piece with negative margins, endoscopic or local excision is regarded as adequate treatment.
- However, patients should be made aware that although the risk of nodal metastases is very low, it is not zero and that there is no effective surveillance that will reliably detect nodal metastases prior to distant metastatic spread.
- Although surveillance colonoscopy is recommended at frequent intervals (e.g., yearly), the risk of tumor growth after resection of pedunculated polyps with a focus of cancer is in the nodes, not in the lumen, calling into question the value of frequent colonoscopy.
- Surveillance is usually continued for 5 years. There has been some debate on this matter; however, in that there are studies that demonstrate that the risk for recurrence extends past 5 years post-polypectomy.
- Formal surgical resection is indicated for high-risk cancers (Haggitt level 4, Kikuchi SM3, lymphovascular invasion, poor differentiation, or positive resection margin, cancer in sessile lesions removed in piecemeal fashion).

When to Tattoo an Area After Polypectomy

- Current guidelines strongly recommend tattooing of suspicious lesions during colonoscopy. Given that risk of cancer arising from a polyp in the National Bowel Cancer Screening Program increased significantly when the polyp was greater than 1 cm in size, most would recommend tattoo of all polyps greater than 1 cm (Fig. 24.5a, b).
- In addition, when sessile lesions are removed in piecemeal fashion, the risk of recurrence is

high. Tattoo at the site of polypectomy should be considered to help identify the area at subsequent colonoscopy.

Benefits of Surveillance

- There have been several studies that have examined the benefits of post-polypectomy surveillance in terms of cancer prevention. These studies identified the risk of colorectal cancer after adenoma resection that depended not only upon the characteristics of the adenoma (advanced or non-advanced) but also colonoscopy surveillance practices. None of these studies are randomized, controlled trials, so there is no direct evidence on the exact benefit that is obtained through surveillance.

Status of Surveillance

- Surveys demonstrated that 50% of endoscopists are not following the guidelines for post-polypectomy surveillance, often performing surveillance examinations more frequently than recommended. Some authors have suggested that failure to follow guidelines was due to uncertainty, fear of malpractice, and financial gain.

Chemoprevention

- A variety of oral agents have been evaluated as possible chemopreventive strategies for both adenoma and carcinoma formation. These agents have included nonsteroidal anti-inflammatory agents, folic acid, calcium, and various antioxidants.
- A systematic review identified several randomized, controlled trials evaluating for the potential benefits of these agents. They concluded that the use of aspirin (81–325 mg/day) in individuals with a history of adenomas or colorectal cancer (CRC) resulted in a 21% reduction in adenoma recurrence. Though not evident until after a prolonged follow-up period (23 years), a 26% reduction in CRC incidence was noted in the general population in studies evaluating a larger aspirin dose (300–1500 mg/day).
- Non-aspirin anti-inflammatory medications such as celecoxib (400 mg/day) have also demonstrated benefit in patients with a history of adenomas, revealing a 34% reduction in adenoma recurrence.
- Though the use of folic acid failed to show benefit with respect to adenoma recurrence, calcium intake (1200–2000 mg/day) was found beneficial with an 18% risk reduction after a history of prior adenomas.
- There was no significant benefit with regard to adenoma recurrence noted with antioxidant ingestion (vitamins A, C, E, beta-carotene, or selenium).

25 Colon Cancer: Preoperative Evaluation and Staging

Cary B. Aarons and Najjia N. Mahmoud

Key Concepts

- Total colonic evaluation is recommended prior to surgical intervention to exclude synchronous tumors that may alter surgical plan.
- Evaluation for metastatic disease by cross-sectional imaging is recommended prior to surgical intervention, as it may alter treatment decisions.
- Preoperative carcinoembryonic antigen (CEA) level should be obtained, as changes in CEA may herald tumor recurrence.
- Tumor location should be identified preoperatively.
- Tumor grade, lymphovascular invasion, margin status, and immunohistochemical assessment of mismatch repair proteins may have prognostic significance and should be routinely reported.

Background

- Once the diagnosis of colon cancer is made, the goal of preoperative evaluation is to establish the location of the tumor, assess for metastatic disease and adjacent organ invasion, and identify other patient and tumor factors that may affect outcome or alter the medical or surgical approach to treatment.
- The primary importance of staging in colon cancer is to rule out additional pathology and distant metastatic disease (stage IV), which can affect treatment approach. This differs from rectal cancer where estimates of locoregional tumor stage have a greater effect on treatment planning.

Clinical Presentation

- Colon cancer presents in three common ways:
  - Asymptomatic: lesion detected during routine screening examination
  - Non-specific subacute symptoms and signs that should prompt further investigation such as change in bowel habits, chronic abdominal pain, rectal bleeding, anorectal discomfort, iron-deficiency anemia, lethargy, weight loss, and fatigue
  - Emergent: perforation or obstruction
- Symptoms will often manifest differently depending on tumor location and size.
- Late findings can include palpable abdominal mass, severe weight loss, intestinal obstruction, and, in rare cases, perforation leading to peritonitis or fistulization to adjacent organs.

C. B. Aarons
Division of Colon and Rectal Surgery, Hospital of the University of Pennsylvania, Philadelphia, PA, USA

N. N. Mahmoud (✉)
Division of Colon and Rectal Surgery, Department of Surgery, University of Pennsylvania Health System, Philadelphia, PA, USA
e-mail: najjia.mahmoud@uphs.upenn.edu

S. R. Steele et al. (eds.), *The ASCRS Manual of Colon and Rectal Surgery*,
https://doi.org/10.1007/978-3-030-01165-9_25

- Approximately 20–25% of colon cancer will present with metastatic disease at the time of diagnosis; therefore, it is also critical to evaluate patients for signs and symptoms associated with metastatic disease. Widely metastatic cancers can result in constitutional symptoms such as unintentional weight loss, cachexia, weakness, and anorexia.

Preoperative Evaluation

- History: duration and severity of symptoms associated with the primary tumor such as intestinal obstructive symptoms, anemia, and abdominal pain, as well as those associated with metastatic disease such as weight loss and fatigue. History of inflammatory bowel disease.
- Family history: history of colorectal cancer or other cancers known to be associated with inherited colon cancer syndromes.
- Overall health: assess readiness for any surgical intervention.
- Physical examination: palpable mass, distant adenopathy, tenderness, or distention.

Tumor Localization

- Pitfalls
  - Colonoscopy is often inaccurate with regard to anatomic localization. Review of colon endoscopic photographs may be helpful, as anatomic landmarks (e.g., ileocecal valve) may sometimes be identified in the same image as the tumor.
  - For distal lesions, it should be remembered that estimates of distance to the anal verge are often highly inaccurate when measured with a flexible endoscope and may have little relationship to the true anatomy.
- Endoscopic localization
  - Tattoo placed adjacent to the lesion in multiple quadrants, typically just distal to the tumor, may assist in operative localization. Although visceral obesity may limit the ability to see tattoo intraoperatively, the tattoo is still valuable, as it can be identified by intraoperative colonoscopy.
  - If cancer was detected in a polyp that was removed endoscopically, and the site not tattooed at index colonoscopy, then expeditious repeat colonoscopy with tattooing of the polypectomy scar should be considered. This is usually most effective when performed by the original endoscopist.
  - Endoscopic clips may be placed at the time of polypectomy/biopsy, and plain abdominal radiographs obtained immediately post-colonoscopy. The colon will usually still be filled with gas and thus anatomic relationships appreciated. Occasionally clips will remain in situ long enough to be detected on cross-sectional imaging that is typically ordered after diagnosis is confirmed histologically.
  - For distal lesions, repeat endoscopic evaluation by the surgeon is critical. At minimum, all patients with left-sided lesions should undergo preoperative proctoscopy to ensure that the tumor is not in the rectum.
  - Intraoperative colonoscopy can localize a small tumor. This can be performed immediately prior to operation or after exploration of the abdomen. The use of carbon dioxide as an insufflation gas is preferred, in order to limit bowel dilatation. When positioning the patient at operation, access to the anus for intraoperative colonoscopy should be considered.
- Radiographic localization
  - Endoscopic clips (see above).
  - Larger tumors may be localized via cross-sectional imaging (CT, MR).

Total Colon Evaluation

- Total colon evaluation is critical to identify synchronous neoplasms that may alter the planned operation. The rate of synchronous cancers is understood to be about 5%; and the overall rate of synchronous neoplasia that would change operative approach is somewhat higher.

- If preoperative colonoscopy is not possible, CT colonography or contrast enema may be performed.
- Occasionally, high partial obstruction from the tumor will limit preoperative proximal colonic evaluation via endoscopy or contrast radiography, but the patient will be able to tolerate preoperative bowel preparation. In these cases, intraoperative colonoscopy performed via the colon proximal to the tumor may be considered.
- For cases of obstructing cancers that preclude adequate endoscopic or radiographic assessment preoperatively, intraoperative colonic lavage and colonoscopy should be considered. If this is not possible, the proximal colon should be palpated intraoperatively, and if no obvious lesions detected, a full colonoscopy should be performed when safe to do so after surgery.

Carcinoembryonic Antigen (CEA)

- CEA is a glycoprotein primarily involved in intercellular adhesion that is produced by columnar and goblet cells and can be found in normal colonic mucosa. It is found in low levels in the circulation of healthy individuals, but it is overexpressed in a variety of cancers, including colorectal cancer.
- Elevated serum levels may be identified in heavy smokers, in benign conditions such as pancreatitis and inflammatory bowel disease, as well as in malignancies outside of the gastrointestinal tract; therefore, CEA is not a sensitive or specific screening tool for colorectal cancer.
- CEA is an important tool in CRC surveillance after surgical resection since its elevation may be the first indication of locally recurrent or metastatic disease.
- Patients with preoperative serum CEA >5 ng/mL have a worse prognosis, stage for stage, than those with lower levels. Elevated preoperative CEA levels have been shown to be associated with poorer survival and increased recurrence in several studies; however, contradictory studies do exist. Therefore, there is currently insufficient evidence to support the use of elevated preoperative serum CEA levels as an absolute indication for adjuvant chemotherapy.
- Current American Society of Clinical Oncology (ASCO) guidelines recommend that serum CEA levels be obtained preoperatively in patients with demonstrated colorectal cancer for posttreatment follow-up and assessment of prognosis.
- Elevated preoperative CEA levels that do not normalize following surgical resection imply the presence of persistent disease.
- Furthermore, serial testing of CEA levels should be performed for 5 years for patients with stage II and III disease in those eligible for surgery or chemotherapy if metastatic disease is discovered. Rising CEA levels after surgical resection implies recurrent disease and should prompt consideration of radiologic and endoscopic evaluation to look for treatable disease.

Radiographic Evaluation

- Preoperative radiographic imaging is useful for initial staging of newly diagnosed or recurrent colon cancers.
- Computed tomography (CT) scans of the chest, abdomen, and pelvis with intravenous contrast provide valuable preoperative information about distant metastases, tumor localization, and possible invasion of adjacent organs.
  - CT scan has a sensitivity ranging from 75% to 90% for detecting distant metastasis; however, the ability to accurately detect nodal involvement or small peritoneal metastases is poor.
  - The routine use of CT for imaging of the chest remains controversial for initial staging of colon cancer, as compared to rectal cancers. In asymptomatic patients in whom the suspicion of lung metastasis

is low, a plain chest x-ray will suffice. Any suspicious findings on chest x-ray can be investigated with a noncontrast chest CT scan.
- Contrast-enhanced magnetic resonance imaging (MRI) is particularly valuable in evaluating smaller suspicious liver lesions (especially in the presence of fatty liver changes) with sensitivities up to 97%. In routine clinical practice, MRI should be reserved for the evaluation of suspicious liver lesions not clearly characterized on CT scan or for operative planning prior to liver metastectomy.
- Positron emission tomography–computed tomography (PET/CT) scan is useful for characterization of indeterminate possibly metastatic lesions and should be routinely employed prior to embarking on radical resection of locally recurrent or metastatic disease.
  - PET is less sensitive in the detection of mucinous tumors, given the relatively lower cell/tumor mass ratio.

Preoperative Evaluation of Coexisting Medical Conditions

- Regardless of the operative approach, colorectal procedures carry inherent risks, which can be divided into procedure-specific risks and cardiopulmonary risks. Therefore, a thorough history and physical examination encompassing the patient's comorbidities is also vital. This is immensely important because surgical morbidity and mortality can be greatly improved by a careful assessment of organ-specific risks and, if feasible, preoperative optimization.
- A detailed knowledge of the patient's prior abdominal surgery will aid in the appropriate operative planning.
- Routine preoperative testing should be obtained and should include a complete blood count (CBC), a metabolic panel, type and screen, and a 12-lead electrocardiogram in older patients with cardiac risk factors.
- Liver function tests are much less sensitive for liver metastases as compared to cross-sectional imaging and are not recommended routinely.
- Nutritional panels are not generally required unless there are significant concerns for underlying malnutrition. Complete optimization of nutritional parameters, either parenterally or enterally, typically takes weeks, which would delay surgery unnecessarily.
- Smoking cessation should be emphasized but should not delay surgery, as any substantial benefits would not be realized for several weeks. However, there may be measurable gains in improving postoperative wound healing and reducing postoperative pulmonary complications if patients can stop smoking preoperatively.
- In patients with renal insufficiency, care must be taken with choosing preoperative bowel preparation, and special attention must be paid to perioperative fluid balances. Additionally, diuretics, angiotensin-converting enzyme inhibitors, and angiotensin receptor blockers should be held the day prior to surgery to minimize the risk of profound hypotension during surgery.

Staging of Colon Cancer

- The preferred staging system for colon and rectal cancers is the TNM staging system put forth by the American Joint Committee on Cancer and the International Union Against Cancer (UICC). This system, which is summarized in Table 25.1, consists of three categories: tumor depth of invasion, nodal involvement, and distant metastasis.
- Tumor stage is the most powerful driver of prognosis and can help guide decisions regarding adjuvant therapy.
- The completeness of resection should also be noted:
- R0—complete tumor resection with negative margins
- R1—incomplete tumor resection with microscopic involvement of the margin
- R2—incomplete tumor resection with gross residual disease that was not resected

Table 25.1 TNM classification and AJCC 8th edition staging of colon cancer

Primary tumor (pT)			
TX		Primary tumor cannot be assessed	
T0		No evidence of primary tumor	
Tis		Carcinoma in situ, intramucosal carcinoma (involvement of lamina propria with no extension through muscularis mucosae)	
T1		Tumor invades submucosa (through the muscularis mucosa but not into the muscularis propria)	
T2		Tumor invades muscularis propria	
T3		Tumor invades through the muscularis propria into the pericolorectal tissues	
T4			
T4a		Tumor invades through the visceral peritoneum (including gross perforation of the bowel through tumor and continuous invasion of tumor through areas of inflammation to the surface of the visceral peritoneum)	
T4b		Tumor directly invades or adheres to other adjacent organs or structures	
Regional lymph nodes (pN)			
NX		Regional lymph nodes cannot be assessed	
N0		No regional lymph node metastasis	
N1		Metastasis in 1–3 regional lymph nodes	
N1a		Metastasis in 1 regional lymph node	
N1b		Metastasis in 2–3 regional lymph nodes	
N1c		No regional lymph nodes are positive but there are tumor deposits in the subserosa, mesentery, or nonperitonealized pericolic or perirectal/mesorectal tissues	
N2		Metastasis in 4 or more regional lymph nodes	
N2a		Metastasis in 4–6 regional lymph nodes	
N2b		Metastasis in 7 or more regional lymph nodes	
Distant metastasis (pM)			
M0		No distant metastasis by imaging; no evidence of tumor in other sites or organs (this category is *not* assigned by pathologists)	
M1		Distant metastasis	
M1a		Metastasis confined to 1 organ or site without peritoneal metastasis	
M1b		Metastasis to 2 or more sites or organs is identified without peritoneal metastasis	
M1c		Metastasis to the peritoneal surface is identified alone or with other site or organ metastases	
Stage grouping			
Stage 0	Tis	N0	M0
Stage I	T1–T2	N0	M0
Stage IIA	T3	N0	M0
Stage IIB	T4a	N0	M0
Stage IIC	T4b	N0	M0
Stage IIIA	T1–T2	N1/N1c	M0
	T1	N2a	M0
Stage IIIB	T3–T4a	N1/N1c	M0
	T2–T3	N2a	M0
	T1–T2	N2b	M0
Stage IIIC	T4a	N2a	M0
	T3–T4a	N2b	M0
	T4b	N1–N2	M0
Stage IVA	Any T	Any N	M1a
Stage IVB	Any T	Any N	M1b
Stage IVC	Any T	Any N	M1c

- Other histologic criteria that are associated with prognosis:
  - Tumor grade: low grade (well- and moderately differentiated) versus high grade (poorly differentiated and undifferentiated)
  - Tumor ("satellite") deposits
  - Lymphovascular invasion
  - Perineural invasion
  - Mucinous or signet ring cell morphology
  - Margin status (distal, proximal, and radial)
    - Non-peritonealized resection margins for all cases of neoplasia resection should be inked to allow for assessment of radial margin status. This is best performed on the fresh specimen.

Lymph Node Evaluation

- Other than radial margin status, lymph node status is the most important prognostic factor following resection of colon cancer.
- The identification of at least 12 lymph nodes has been suggested as a key quality indicator in the resection of colon cancers.
  - While there are patient-related factors that influence lymph node yield, the completeness of mesenteric resection and the interest of the pathologist in obtaining the maximal number for nodes for examination are also paramount. Numerous studies have shown that increasing the number of lymph nodes examined is associated with improved survival in stage II and stage III patients.
  - Tumor deposits that are found in the pericolonic fat that do not show any evidence of residual lymph node are not counted as lymph nodes replaced by tumor and are designated as N1c. The number of these nodules should be reported as they confer a poor prognosis.
- Lymph node ultraprocessing (microsectioning, immunohistochemical analysis, or RT-PCR) has been demonstrated to increase the number of nodes found to have tumor. However, there is no definitive evidence that treatment of patients with occult nodal metastases with chemotherapy improves survival.
- Many studies of sentinel lymph node mapping (injection of vital dye around the tumor at the time of operation as a method of identifying lymph nodes theoretically at greatest risk for metastases) have been fraught with bias. To date, sentinel node mapping for colorectal cancer has not been demonstrated to be effective.

Lynch Syndrome Phenotype

- Assessment for Lynch tumor phenotype via immunohistochemistry (IHC) looking for expression of mismatch repair (MMR) proteins (*MLH1, MSH2, MSH6, PMS2*) should be performed. Some institutions perform this selectively, based on family history, or routinely on all colon cancer specimens.
- In general, patients with absence of MMR on IHC should be considered for referral to a genetic counselor and germline mutational analysis.
- The exception to the above recommendation is when MLH1 is absent on IHC. In addition to Lynch syndrome, absence of *MLH1* on IHC can be due to mutation of *BRAF*. This is common in older female patients.
  - Prior to germline mutational analysis for Lynch, the tumor should undergo *BRAF* analysis.
  - If *BRAF* is mutated, then a sporadic mutation in MLH1 is 96% likely. Lynch is thus unlikely and, in most cases, the patient can be considered to have a sporadic cancer, and genetic testing will cease.
  - If *BRAF* is normal, then Lynch is likely, and genetic counseling and testing should be considered.
  - In some institutions, reflex *BRAF* testing is performed on any tumor specimen with absent *MLH1* on IHC.

- Microsatellite instability (MSI) in the tumor is another indicator of DNA repair defects caused by defective mismatch repair proteins.
  - It is typically assessed by PCR amplification of repeated single-nucleotide units of DNA, or microsatellites, in tumor tissue.
  - Tumors are characterized as MSI-high (MSI-H) or MSI-low (MSI-L) based on the number of microsatellite sequences that appear.
    - If the tumor has two or more mutated sequences, it is termed MSI-H, while if only one sequence is mutated, it is classified as MSI-L. Finally, if no mutation is present, then the tumor is microsatellite stable (MSS).
- Patients with MSI-H tumors should be considered for genetic counseling and germline mutational analysis to look for Lynch syndrome.
- IHC for MMR has replaced MSI testing in most institutions because of the reduced cost and the fact that it is a direct measurement of protein product.

The Surgical Management of Colon Cancer

26

Matthew G. Mutch

Key Concepts

- Complete clinical staging for colon cancer includes a total colon exam, computed tomography of the chest, abdomen, and pelvis, and measurement of serum CEA level.
- The principles of an oncologic resection include a total mesocolic resection, ligation of the primary vessel at its origin, a wide mesenteric resection with >12 lymph nodes examined, and at least a 5 cm resection margin.
- There is no difference in cancer-related outcomes for open and laparoscopic resections.
- Anastomotic assessment for left-sided anastomosis is associated with a decreased leak rate.
- Surgical resection is the most effective therapy for patients who present with obstruction colon cancers.
- Endoscopic stenting of an obstructing colon cancer is an effective bridge to surgery within 72 h.
- Perforated cancers should be treated with an oncologic resection.
- First-line therapy for patients with metastatic colon cancer and an asymptomatic primary tumor is chemotherapy.

M. G. Mutch (✉)
Section of Colon and Rectal Surgery, Department of Surgery, Washington University School of Medicine, St. Louis, MO, USA
e-mail: mutchm@wudosis.wustl.edu

Preoperative Preparation

Physiologic Assessment

- A variety of scoring systems are available for stratifying a patient's risk of perioperative morbidity and mortality after undergoing major digestive system surgery. Each scoring system differs in the included parameters and the outcomes that they measure.
  - The most widely utilized scoring system is the American Society of Anesthesiologists (ASA) Score, but it only provides assessment of an anesthesia complication for a given patient's physiologic status.
  - In contrast, the POSSUM and modified Portsmouth-POSSUM scoring systems provide an assessment of the risk of postoperative mortality and morbidity.
    - In an effort to improve the performance prediction of patients undergoing colorectal resections, a colorectal-specific POSSUM (CR-POSSUM) score was developed.
  - The American College of Surgeons developed a surgical risk calculator using data from NSQIP to provide patient-specific postoperative risks of various complications. The NSQIP risk calculator has been shown to underestimate the risk of complications for colorectal resections, and more

S. R. Steele et al. (eds.), *The ASCRS Manual of Colon and Rectal Surgery*,
https://doi.org/10.1007/978-3-030-01165-9_26

surgeon- and patient-specific data are needed. However, it remains a useful tool to preoperatively assess morbidity and mortality risk. The risk calculator is available at http://riskcalculator.facs.org.

Tumor Localization

- Accurate tumor localization is a critical component of the preoperative assessment of the patient and operative planning. Intraoperative tumor localization can be challenging from several standpoints such as small or early tumor, obese patient, adhesions, laparoscopy, or inadequate tattooing.
  - The utilization of intraluminal anatomic markings for tumor localization is inaccurate 10–15% of the time and may be higher if cecal and rectal tumors are excluded. In other words, the colonoscopy will not accurately locate the tumor one out of seven times.
  - Localization with endoscopic tattooing provides the most accurate method for localization. The tattoo should be placed distal to the lesion and in three separate areas around the circumference of the lumen (Fig. 26.1). A single injection into the mesenteric border or sprayed into the peritoneal cavity may be difficult to identify.
  - Alternatively, endoscopic placement of metal clips at the site of the tumor with immediate plain radiograph (or CT) will localize the tumor with a high degree of accuracy.
  - The ultimate fallback to identify a lesion is intraoperative colonoscopy, ideally using carbon dioxide as the insufflation gas to limit bowel dilatation.
  - Patients who present with endoscopically obstructing lesions can be effectively evaluated with CT colonography to complete their total colon exam prior to surgery. CT colonography has replaced contrast enema studies in many situations because of improved accuracy in detecting synchronous lesions and often provides better tumor localization.

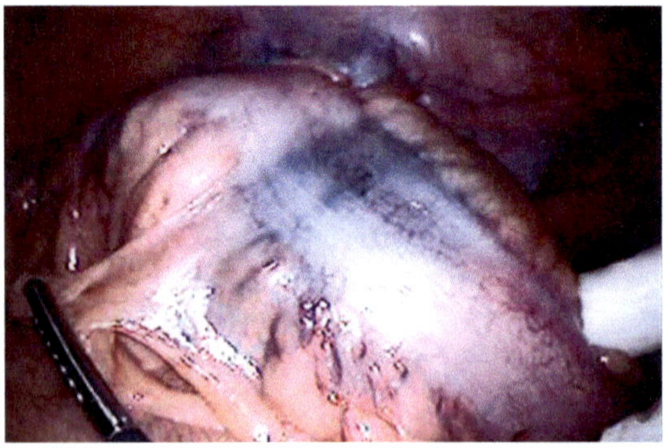

Fig. 26.1 Tattoo localization of a sigmoid colon cancer

Surgical Technique

Extent of Resection

- The National Comprehensive Cancer Network provides the recommended principles of surgical resection for colon cancer, which include obtaining an adequate proximal margin, distal margin, and lymphadenectomy.
- Colon cancers tend to grow circumferentially around the lumen of the colon and extend out radially and, to a lesser degree, longitudinally along the bowel. Therefore, a 5 cm proximal or distal margin has always been recommended. This is important to remove all tumor-bearing mucosa but also to resect all lymph nodes with potential to drain tumor cells.
- In order to obtain an adequate lymphadenectomy, the named feeding vessel to the resected segment of the colon should be taken at its origin. The goal is to clear all regional lymph nodes and provide a minimum of 12 lymph nodes for pathologic evaluation.

Mesocolic Resection

- Just as the mesorectum is enveloped in a fascia, the mesocolon also has a visceral fascial plane that separates it for the retroperitoneum (parietal fascia). A serosal surface on the bowel and mesentery excludes the anterior aspect of the mesentery from the perineal cavity.

- Complete mesocolic excision (CME), as popularized by Hohenberger et al., is the sharp dissection of the visceral fascia from the parietal fascia of the retroperitoneum and central ligation of the primary vasculature.

Right Colectomy

- Tumors located anywhere from the cecum to the proximal transverse colon can safely be treated with a right colectomy. The basic tenets of resection of a right-sided tumor include full abdominal exploration, full mobilization of the right colon, and hepatic flexure with a mesenteric resection including ligation of the ileocolic and right branch of the middle colic vessels at their origin. The resection can be performed safely and effectively via either an open or laparoscopic approach. Data regarding laparoscopy and colorectal cancer is presented in detail below.
- The initial approach to mobilization can vary based on the anatomy of the tumor and the preference of the surgeon. It is often helpful to completely mobilize the colon and mesentery away from the site of the tumor before embarking on dissection in the area of the tumor, especially when the cancer is locally advanced and invasive into the retroperitoneum.
- All of the surgical approaches contain the same steps. They are typically named according to the initial approach to mobilization.

Open Approach

- The peritoneal cavity can be accessed with a midline or right-sided transverse or oblique incision.
- Once the abdomen is opened and explored and the tumor is located, the wound should be protected with a wound protector.
- The colon and its mesentery are separated from the retroperitoneum, returning the colon to its embryologic position in the midline. Care is taken to preserve retroperitoneal structures such as the duodenum, pancreas, and ureter. The hepatic flexure is mobilized. The omentum is divided in the midline and the right side of the omentum resected en bloc with the colon. With the colon completely mobilized, the vascular pedicles can be ligated.
- The "approaches" are named for their initial maneuvers. However, regardless of the named technique, the steps are the same, and only their order is different.

Lateral-to-Medial Approach

- The surgeon stands on the patient's left side and the first assistant on the patient's right side.
- The right colon is grasped, and the peritoneum is incised just anterior to the white line of Toldt from the cecum to the hepatic flexure. This allows access to the avascular plane between the visceral and parietal planes of the colon and retroperitoneum. It is important not to violate the mesenteric side of this plane in order to ensure a total mesocolic resection.
- Under tension, the right colon is separated sharply from the retroperitoneum. The duodenum should be identified and reflected into the retroperitoneum. The cecum is then mobilized off the retroperitoneum, and the posterior attachments of the small bowel mesentery are divided all the way up to the duodenum. This provides the mobility of the small bowel for the anastomosis.
- With the duodenum safely reflected posteriorly, the hepatic flexure can be mobilized. The surgeon's left hand is placed under the colon and its mesentery and brought out laterally to expose the superior attachments along the inferior edge of the liver.
- Eventually, the lesser sac is entered and the lesser omentum is divided. Care must be taken so the plane between the omentum and the transverse colon mesentery is separated, and dissection into the transverse colon is avoided. These two planes are typically fused up to the midline, and beyond this point, the proper lesser sac is entered.

- After the right colon and hepatic flexure are completely mobilized, the cecum is put on stretch, and the ileocolic pedicle can easily be identified. Since the right colon and its mesentery have been mobilized, there should be bare areas on the cephalad and caudad aspects of the ileocolic pedicle. The peritoneum is incised along the lines of resection for both bare areas allowing isolation of the pedicle so it can be ligated at its origin on the superior mesenteric vessels.
- The terminal ileal mesentery is divided so that an adequate amount of ileal mesentery is included with the specimen, depending on the location of the tumor.
- The right branch of the middle colic vessels is identified by elevating the transverse colon mesentery. The pedicle should become evident either by bowstringing it under tension or there should be another bare area where the omentum has been dissected free during the exposure of the lesser sac. The peritoneum should be incised from the distal site of transection of the colon to the base of the pedicle and across the pedicle to the cut edge of the right colon mesentery. The pedicle can then be ligated at its origin.

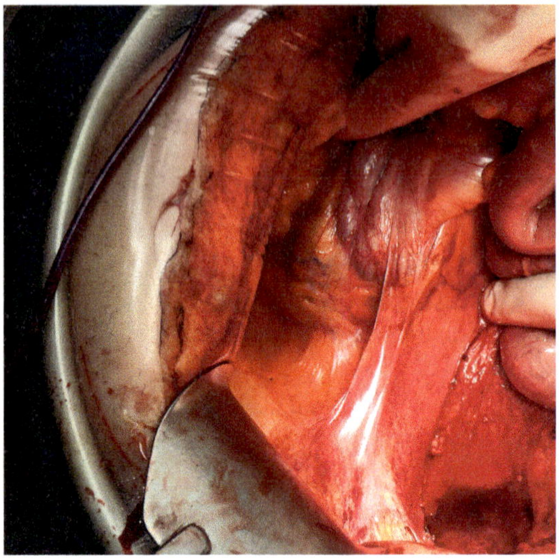

Fig. 26.2 Exposure of the posterior aspect of the small bowel mesentery for the posterior approach to the right colon

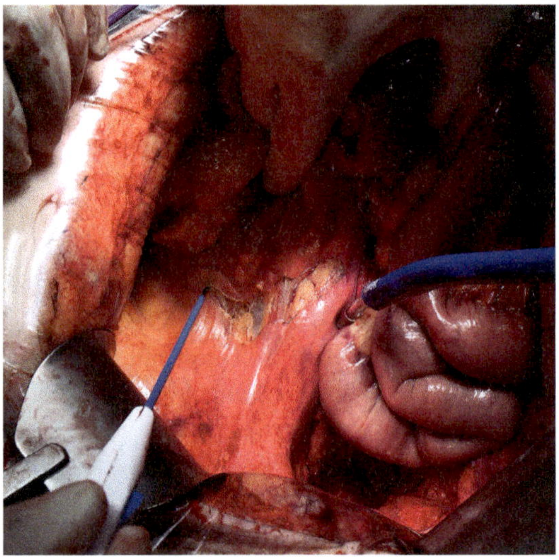

Fig. 26.3 Entry into the retroperitoneum from the posterior approach to a right colectomy

Posterior (Inferior-to-Superior) Approach

- The principal difference between this approach and the lateral-to-medial approach is that the initial step in the operation is to mobilize the root of the ileal mesentery first to the level of the duodenum.
- The small bowel is eviscerated and reflected toward the right upper quadrant to expose the posterior aspect of the small bowel mesentery from the ligament of Treitz to the cecum (Fig. 26.2).
- The peritoneum is incised along the root of the ileal mesentery to the midline, and the plane between the mesentery and the retroperitoneum is entered (Fig. 26.3). The duodenum is readily identified and reflected into the retroperitoneum.
- The right colon mesentery is elevated off the retroperitoneum out beyond the ascending colon laterally and the transverse colon superiorly.
- The further this dissection can be performed from a medial-to-lateral direction beyond the transverse colon, hepatic flexure, and ascending colon, the easier the lateral dissection becomes as all that remains are the lateral peritoneal and lesser omental attachments. At

this point, starting at the level of the cecum, the surgeon, while standing on the patient's left side, places their left hand under the right colon mesentery and lateral to the colon to expose the lateral peritoneal attachments. These are then divided heading up toward the hepatic flexure.

- If the dissection is continuing easily, the lesser omentum is separated from the transverse colon mesentery in order to enter the lesser sac. If this plane is difficult to develop, the distal site of transection is identified, and the lesser sac can be entered at this point. This begins by dividing the greater omentum to the level of the colon, and the lesser omentum is bluntly separated from the colon and its mesentery to enter the lesser sac. Once the lesser sac is entered, this plane is developed toward the hepatic flexure. Eventually, the posterior retroperitoneal dissection plane is entered. With the duodenum free, the remaining attachments along the inferior liver can be safely divided. The right colon and hepatic flexure are completely mobilized so the vascular pedicles can be ligated, and the mesentery can be resected as described above.

Superior to Inferior Approach

- The principal difference between this approach and the lateral-to-medial and inferior-to-superior approaches is that the initial step in the operation is to divide the omentum over the transverse mesocolon and mobilize hepatic flexure first.
- The superior approach is useful for locally advanced tumors of the cecum and proximal ascending colon with possible retroperitoneal invasion because it allows for complete mobilization of the colon and mesentery before addressing the site of the tumor.
- The dissection begins at the distal site of transection of the transverse colon. This is accomplished by elevating the transverse colon to expose its inferior aspect of the mesentery so the right branch of the middle colon vessels can be identified. It is the first pedicle medial to the bare area of the duodenum and should bowstring under the tension of the elevating the transverse colon. The greater omentum is divided up to the transverse colon, and the lesser omentum is separated from the colon and mesentery to enter the lesser sac.
- As this plane is developed toward the hepatic flexure, the lesser omentum is divided. The stomach superiorly and duodenum posteriorly should be identified and separated from the colon mesentery.
- Once the lesser omentum or hepatic attachments to the colon are divided beyond the hepatic flexure, the hepatic flexure can be elevated under tension to develop the retroperitoneal plane, identify and free the duodenum, and divide the lateral peritoneal attachments of the right colon.
- With the peritoneal attachments divided, the remaining colon is mobilized in the same manner as described in the lateral approach.

Medial-to-Lateral Approach

- This approach is helpful when the tumor is invasive into the retroperitoneum over the kidney and/or duodenum or there is question of ureteral involvement.
- The dissection begins at the root of the ileocolic mesentery from the medial aspect. The ileocolic vessels are isolated and divided and the right colon mesentery dissected away from the duodenum and pancreas, if they are not involved with tumor.
- The mobilization continues inferiorly lifting the ileal mesentery away from the retroperitoneum, taking care to preserve the ureter and gonadal vessels.
- The ileal mesentery and terminal ileum can be divided at this point.
- The omentum is divided over the transverse mesocolon, allowing control of the mesocolon from both superior and inferior aspects.
- The right branch of the middle colic vessels is divided. The remainder of the transverse mesocolon is divided. The transverse colon is divided.
- This leaves the lateral attachments of the colon. The surgeon can then assess the degree of invasion of the tumor into the retroperitoneum and make a decision whether en bloc

resection of any adjacent organs is required. The ureter should be free from a medial aspect, so if retroperitoneal en bloc excision is required, there should be little risk of ureteral injury.

Anastomosis

- Ileocolic anastomosis can be accomplished via handsewn or stapled techniques.
- Handsewn anastomosis may be performed in end-to-end or side-to-side fashion and can be created using a single or double layer of sutures. However, an end-to-end anastomosis is often difficult given the significant size discrepancies between the lumens of the small bowel and colon.
- Stapled anastomoses are most commonly performed in a side to side fashion but can also be performed in a side to end configuration as well. The traditional side to side, stapled anastomosis is created by individually dividing the proximal (Fig. 26.4) and distal limbs (Fig. 26.5) of the bowel with a stapler.
- The anti-mesenteric corner of each staple line is then excised, and the forks of the stapler are placed into the lumen of each limb of the intestine. The stapler is reassembled and fired with the bowel in an antiperistaltic and antimesenteric fashion (Fig. 26.6).
- The resulting common enterotomy is reapproximated so the longitudinal staple lines are offset, which prevents the intersection of more than two staple lines (Fig. 26.7).
- The common enterotomy can be closed with suture or staples (Figs. 26.8 and 26.9).
- An alternative method for creating the side to side anastomosis is not to divide the proximal and distal bowel. Enterotomies are made on the anti-mesenteric side at the chosen site of transection proximally and distally. The forks of the staple are then passed through each enterotomy where they are reassembled and fired in an anti-mesenteric position, as above. The common enterotomy is closed by firing the linear cutting stapler again, across the

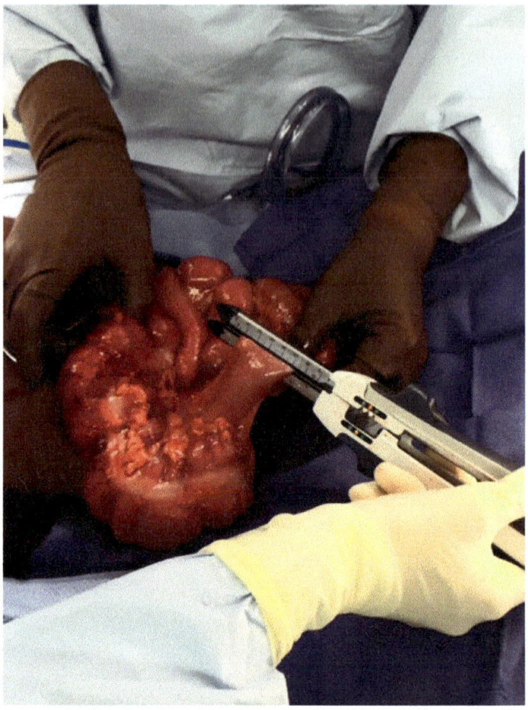

Fig. 26.4 Division of the terminal ileum. (Courtesy of Howard Ross, MD)

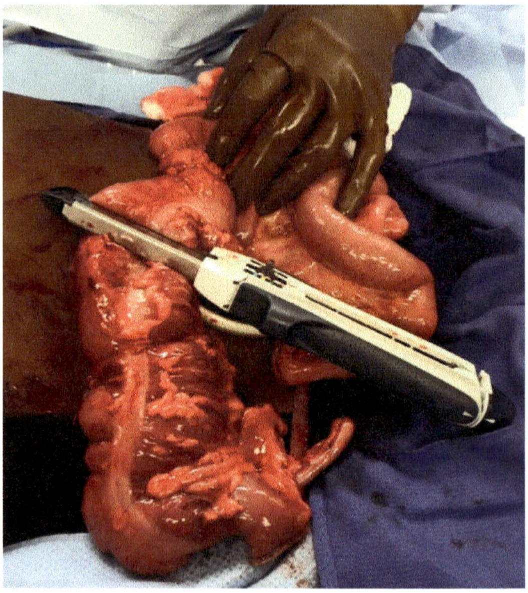

Fig. 26.5 Division of the transverse colon. (Courtesy of Howard Ross, MD)

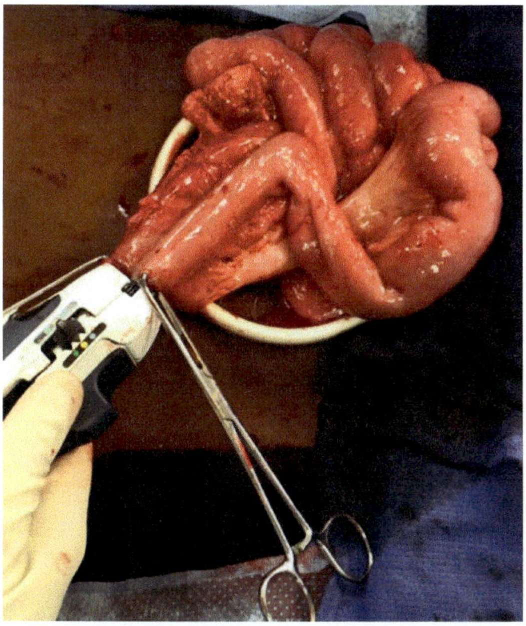

Fig. 26.6 Firing of the linear stapler for a side to side stapled anastomosis. (Courtesy of Howard Ross, MD)

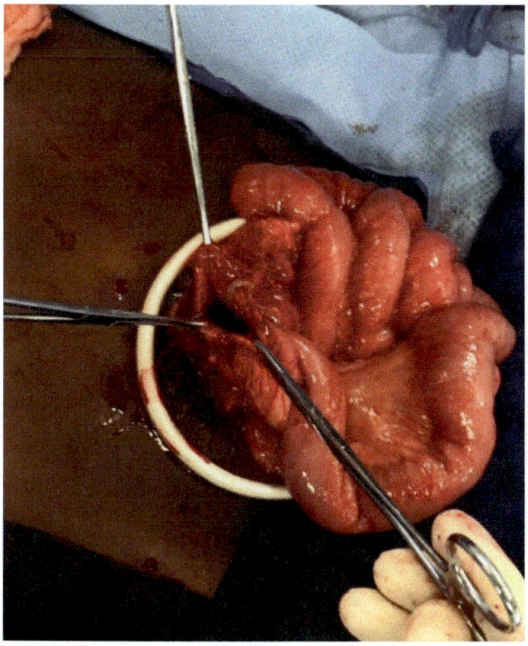

Fig. 26.7 Closing the common enterotomy by offsetting the longitudinal staple line. (Courtesy of Howard Ross, MD)

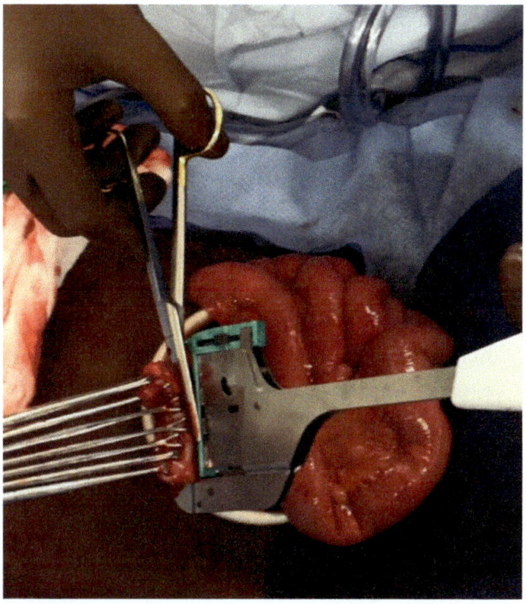

Fig. 26.8 Closing the common enterotomy for a side to side anastomosis. (Courtesy of Howard Ross, MD)

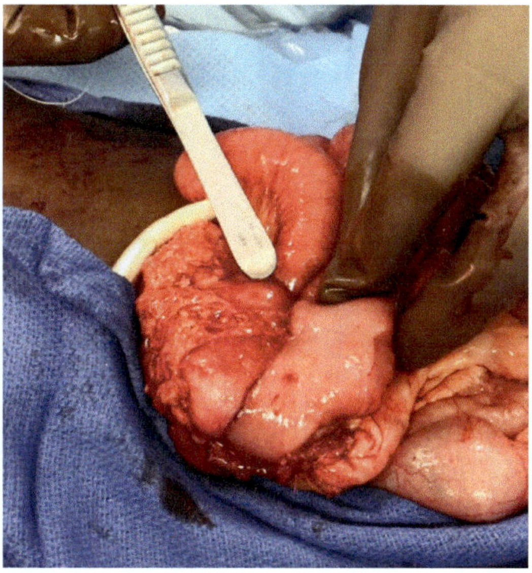

Fig. 26.9 Complete side to side ileocolic anastomosis. (Courtesy of Howard Ross, MD)

proximal and distal limbs that incorporate the proximal and distal limbs of the bowel. This technique saves the use of two stapler loads but does involve passing the blade of the stapler through two rows of staples, when the intestine is divided.

- A stapled anastomosis can also be created in a side-to-end fashion, using an end-to-end anastomotic (EEA) stapler to create an anastomosis between the end of the ileum and the side of the transverse colon and the end of the open end of the transverse colon. The spike should be positioned proximal enough so the distal aspect of the circular staple line is at least 4 cm proximal to the cut edge of the bowel. This is important to ensure that distal strip of the bowel remains viable once the enterotomy is closed. The transverse colon is then closed with suture or a linear stapler. This creates the appearance of normal anatomy, although offers no obvious advantage over the techniques described above.

Laparoscopic Approach

- Proper room setup and instrumentation are critical for success. A mechanical bed is essential so the patient can be placed in extremes of positions to maximize the use of gravity for retraction and exposure. The patient needs to be safely secured to the bed, and there are a myriad of techniques to accomplish this such as beanbags, nonskid pads, or shoulder braces. Placing the patient in supine split-leg position or lithotomy may sometimes be helpful, as it has the advantage of allowing the assistant or surgeon to stand between the legs.
- Instrumentation is up to surgeon's preference, but the use of atraumatic graspers is recommended. There are several energy devices available such as monopolar cautery, bipolar vessel sealers, and ultrasonic sealers that can be used for dissection and ligation of appropriate vessels.
- With regard to port placement, there are no hard set rules, and they should be based on the surgical approach and surgeon's preference (Fig. 26.10a, b). Laparoscopic colectomy is a multi-quadrant procedure so placement of the camera port as to maximize visualization is important. The most optimal place for the camera port is at the apex of the pneumoperitoneum. This is typically in the midline and at the midpoint between the xiphoid process and the pubic symphysis, which can either be above or below the umbilicus.

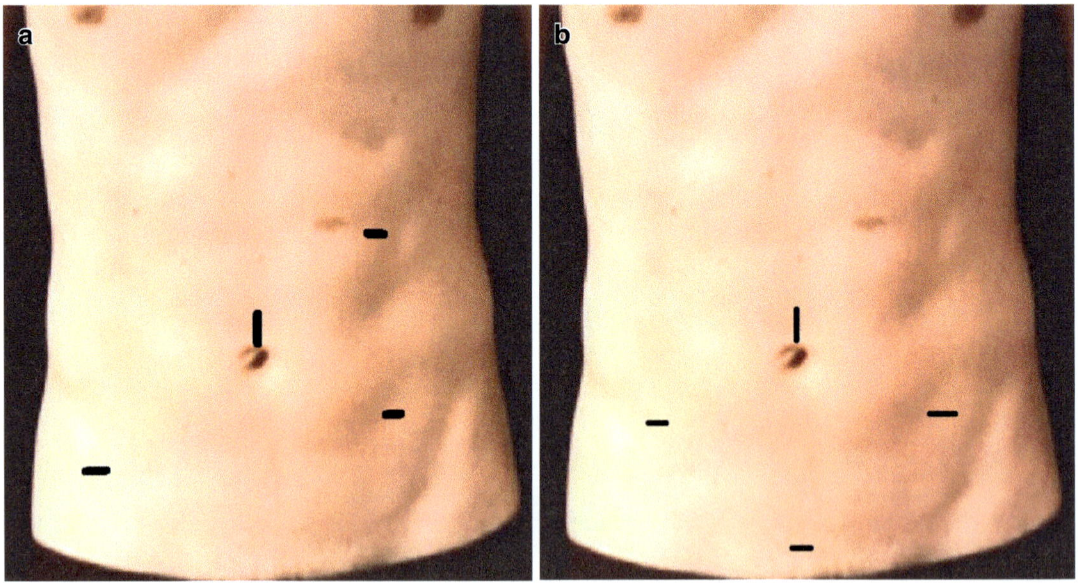

Fig. 26.10 (**a**) Port placement for a laparoscopic right colectomy; (**b**) port placement for a laparoscopic right colectomy

- Once pneumoperitoneum is established and the abdomen is adequately explored, the dissection can be carried out in a medial-to-lateral, lateral-to-medial, inferior-to-superior, or superior-to-inferior approach. The medial-to-lateral approach is favored by many surgeons, as the operation is conducted in-line with the camera view. This approach and the inferior-to-superior approach will be described below.

Medial-to-Lateral Approach

- The patient is tilted with the right side up in very slight Trendelenburg position. The omentum is placed in the upper abdomen to expose the transverse colon and the hepatic flexure. The small bowel is moved to the left side of the abdomen with the terminal ileum in the pelvis to fully expose the right colon mesentery.
- The first step of the dissection is to grab the mesentery at the junction of the terminal ileum and cecum and pull it to the right lower quadrant. This puts the ileocolic pedicle on tension and can be identified as it creates a bowstring in the mesentery. The peritoneum on the caudad aspect is incised parallel to the arc of the ileocolic vessels connecting with the ileal arcades. A wider incision in the peritoneum provides better exposure.
- Blunt dissection is used to enter into the plane between the retroperitoneum and the mesentery. The goal is to identify the duodenum and to dissect anterior to the duodenum and pancreas. If this is difficult from an approach inferior to the root of the ileocolic vessels, the peritoneum just inferior to the sweep of the duodenum should be opened and the mesentery dissected free from the retroperitoneum working in this avascular space. The two dissection planes can then be connected safely.
- The dissection is carried cephalad and lateral as far as possible to safely separate the duodenum from the right colon mesentery, which allows the ileocolic pedicle to be isolated and ligated at its origin from the superior mesenteric vessels. The pedicle can be ligated with clips, staples, looped suture, or bipolar vessel-sealing devices.
- Other steps in the operation proceed at the discretion of the surgeon. It is often helpful to divide the omentum over the transverse colon and mobilize the hepatic flexure in retrograde fashion, connecting the planes of dissection anterior to the duodenum prior to dividing the right branch of the middle colic vessels. The lateral attachments of the colon are divided to the pelvic brim. The root of the ileal mesentery is then mobilized to the midline with the patient in steeper Trendelenburg position. The right colon should now be returned to its embryologic midline position.
- In cases of visceral obesity, it may be helpful to divide the remaining transverse mesocolon and ileal mesentery and omentum prior to extracting the specimen. The colon can be extracted via the surgeon's site of choice. For cancer cases, the use of a wound protector for extraction is recommended to minimize the risk of a wound contamination. Once the colon is extracted, it is resected, and the anastomosis can be created using one of the techniques described earlier.

Posterior (Inferior-to-Superior) Approach

- The patient is placed in steep Trendelenburg, and the omentum is reflected over the transverse colon to expose the hepatic flexure. The small bowel is placed in the right upper quadrant to expose the posterior aspect of the small bowel mesentery. The patient remains in neutral right to left position so the small bowel will stay in the right upper quadrant.
- To obtain the exposure, the terminal ileum is identified and reflected toward the right colon. This will expose the fold of where the small bowel mesentery joins the retroperitoneum. Moving the small bowel to the right upper quadrant and following this fold in a cephalad direction will expose the forth portion of the duodenum (Fig. 26.11).
- An instrument in the surgeon's right hand elevates the proximal aspect of the small bowel

mesentery under tension, and the first assistant via a right lower quadrant port elevates the distal aspect of the small bowel mesentery, which provides exposure of the duodenum and posterior peritoneum of the small bowel mesentery. With the use of an energy source, the peritoneum is incised from the duodenum to the cecum allowing access to the retroperitoneum, and the right colon mesentery can be elevated off the retroperitoneum.

- The duodenum is reflected posteriorly, and mesentery is elevated from the mid-transverse colon, out to the hepatic flexure, and down the ascending colon to the cecum (Fig. 26.12). The further this dissection is carried beyond the colon laterally and superiorly, the easier the lateral and hepatic flexure mobilization will be.
- Now the patient is airplaned right side up, and the small bowel and omentum are pulled to the left side of the abdomen to expose the lateral aspect of the right colon. The lateral attachments are divided by grabbing the cecum and retracting it medial and cephalad toward the spleen (Fig. 26.13). The attachments are divided toward the hepatic flexure as far as possible.
- Just like described in the medial-to-lateral approach, if the lesser sac can be easily developed and entered, the dissection can proceed in this direction. If this approach is too difficult, place the colon back in its anatomic position, and identify the distal site where the colon will be divided. This is accomplished by elevating the transverse colon mesentery and putting the right branch of the middle colic vessels on stretch (Fig. 26.14). The vessel is

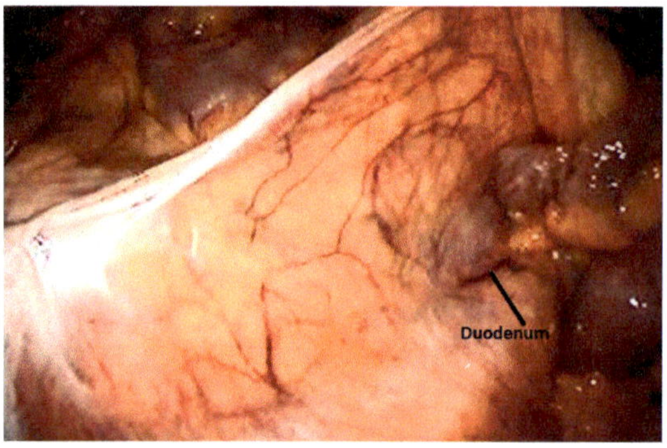

Fig. 26.11 Exposure of posterior aspect of the small bowel mesentery for a laparoscopic posterior approach

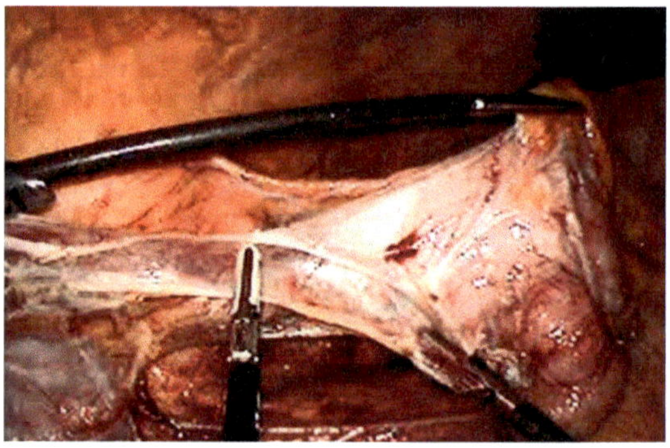

Fig. 26.13 Exposure of the lateral attachments after the posterior dissection

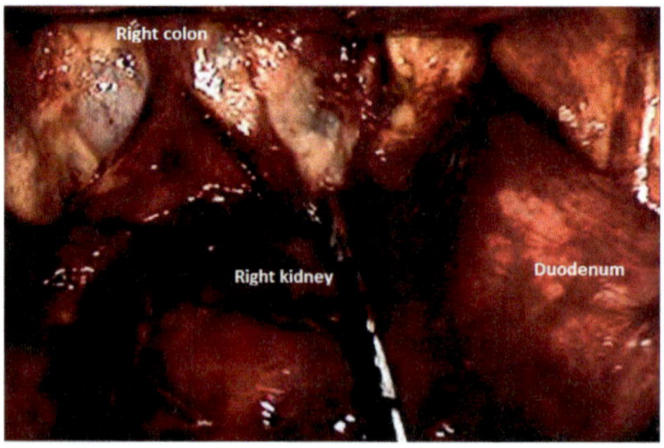

Fig. 26.12 Posterior mobilization of the right colon mesentery off the retroperitoneum

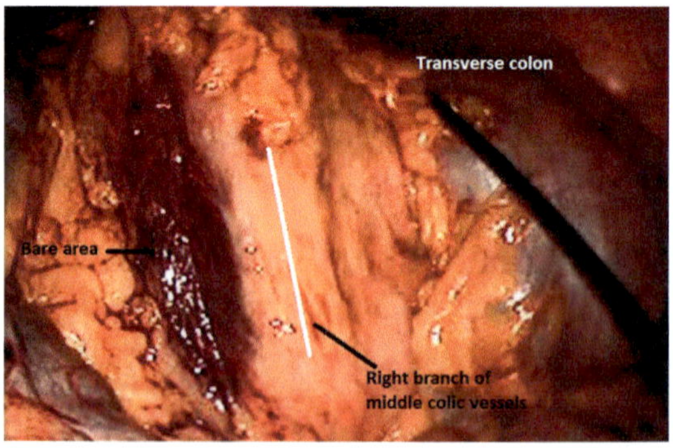

Fig. 26.14 Exposure of the right branch of the middle colic vessels

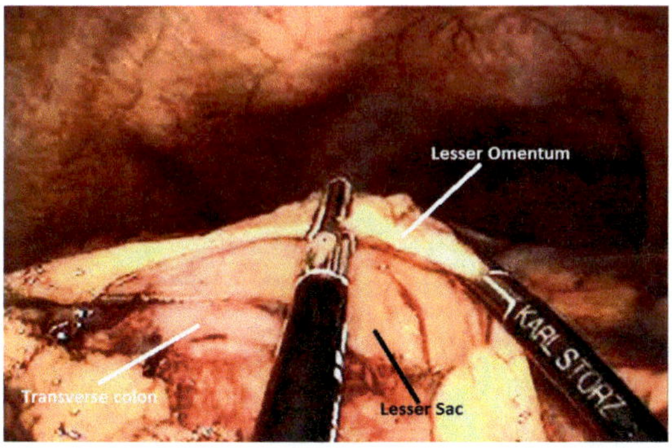

Fig. 26.15 Entering the lesser sac by separating the lesser omentum from the transverse colon at the distal site of transection

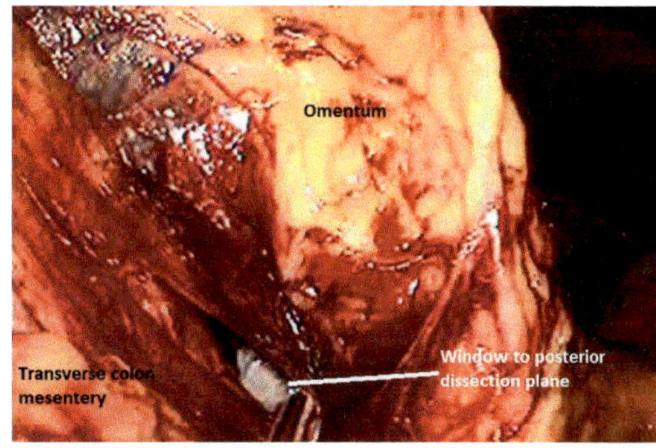

Fig. 26.16 Exposure of posterior dissection plane from the superior approach

medial to the bare area of the right colon mesentery.

- The greater omentum is then divided at this point, and the lesser sac is entered by separating the lesser omentum from the transverse colon and its mesentery (Fig. 26.15). This is an avascular plane so it can be separated bluntly under tension. Once this plan has been developed, the dissection progresses toward the hepatic flexure by dividing the lesser omentum.
- As the dissection progresses beyond the pylorus, the retroperitoneal dissection plane can be identified by the purplish tissue planes indicative of the previous posterior dissection. This plane can be safely entered, and the remaining attachments along the liver can be safely divided because the duodenum has been dissected free of the right colon mesentery (Fig. 26.16). At this point, the right colon and hepatic flexure have been completely mobilized.
- The next step is to isolate and ligate the vasculature. The ileocolic pedicles are identified by grasping the mesentery on the inside of the ileocecal valve and pulling to the right lower quadrant. The pedicle will bowstring, and because it has been mobilized off the retroperitoneum, bare areas can be seen on the caudad and cephalad (bare area over the duodenum) aspects (Fig. 26.17). The peritoneum on the caudad aspect is scored parallel to the pedicle, and blunt dissection through the mesentery will allow entry into the retroperitoneum. The duodenum can be visualized to ensure it is completely free of the pedicle.

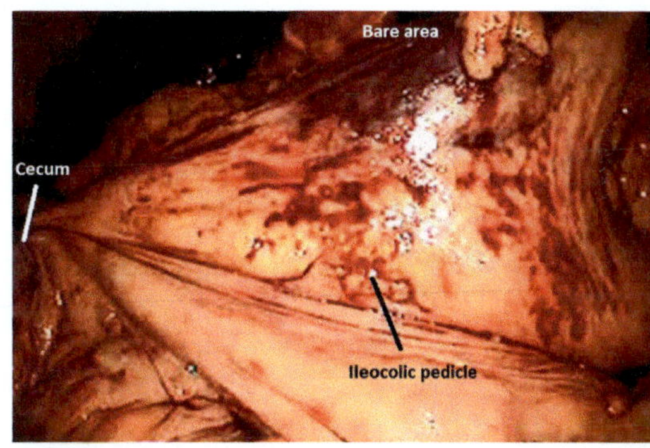

Fig. 26.17 Identification of the ileocolic pedicle

- The peritoneum is then scored over the base of the pedicle toward the cephalad bare area, and the pedicle is safely isolated and ligated.
- The medial cut edge of the mesentery near the right branch of the middle colic vessels is grasped and reflected to the video right, allowing any remaining attachments to the duodenum, stomach, or omentum which can be seen and gently swept free. The transverse colon mesentery is then elevated under tension, which allows for the right branch to bowstring, and ideally, a bare area is seen medial to the vessel (Fig. 26.18). The peritoneum is then scored from the colon down to the base of the vessel and then across it to connect with the cut edge of the mesentery. Blunt dissection of the bare area will allow access into the

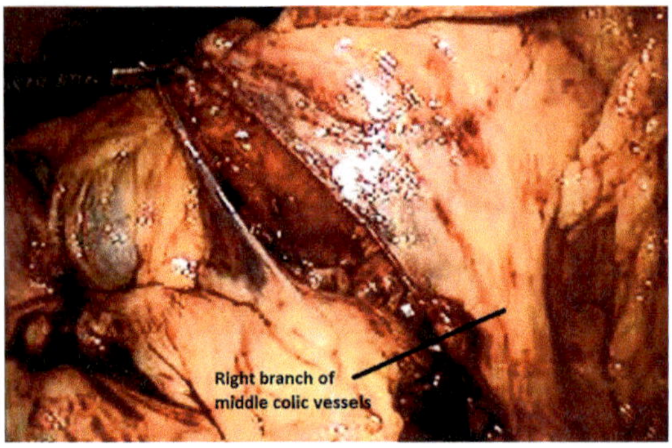

Fig. 26.18 Identification of the right branch of the middle colic vessels

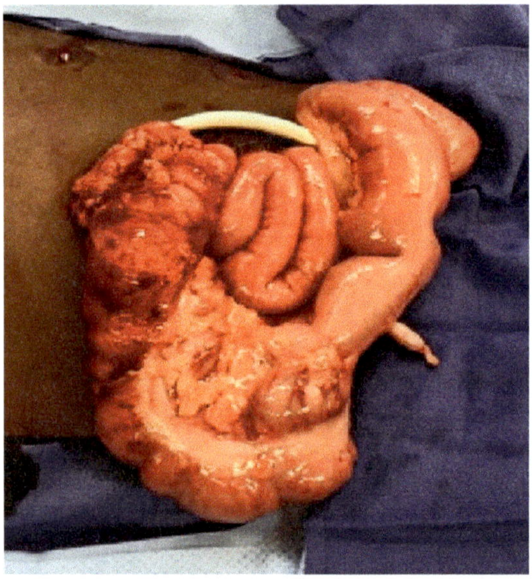

Fig. 26.19 Extraction of the right colon

lesser sac and for safe ligation of the pedicle. Because the omentum has been previously dissected free from entering the lesser sac, the vessel can be safely ligated without the risk of injury to surrounding structures.

- The colon can now be extracted and resected and the anastomosis created as described in the medial-to-lateral section (Fig. 26.19).

Left Colectomy

Open

- The patient is placed in the supine split-leg or lithotomy position to have access to the anus

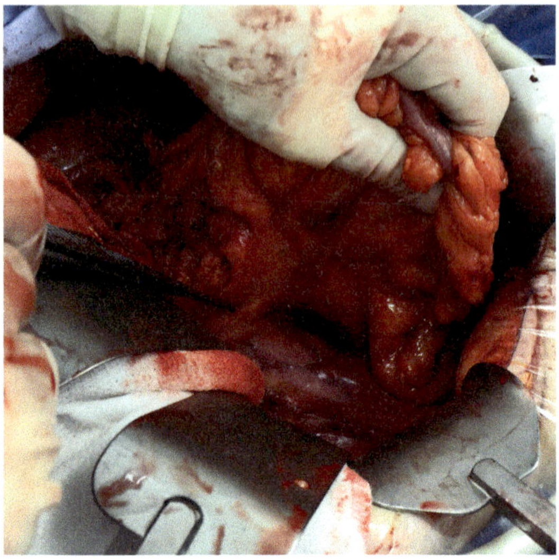

Fig. 26.20 Medial exposure of the IMA

for the anastomosis and anastomotic assessment. One or both of the patient's arms can be tucked to their side, and the Mayo stand for the scrub nurse can be placed over the patient's head, or the scrub nurse can stand off one of the patient's hips. The peritoneum is entered via a midline incision that allows for complete exploration and mobilization of the splenic flexure. With the abdomen open, a wound protector can be inserted, and a self-retaining retractor can be utilized.

- Initial exposure of the left colon anatomy is accomplished by packing the small bowel in the right upper quadrant to the base of left colon mesentery, which includes exposing the inferior mesenteric artery (IMA) at its origin (Fig. 26.20) and the inferior mesenteric vein (IMV) as it courses near the ligament of Treitz and inferior border of the pancreas (Fig. 26.21). The cecum and terminal ileum are also packed away to provide complete exposure into the pelvis and the sacral promontory.
- The dissection begins with division of the lateral attachments of the sigmoid colon to allow for visualization of the white line of Toldt from the upper rectum to the proximal descending colon. The sigmoid colon and descending colon are elevated and retracted medially, and a long incision is made in the peritoneum to enter the retroperitoneal plane. With adequate

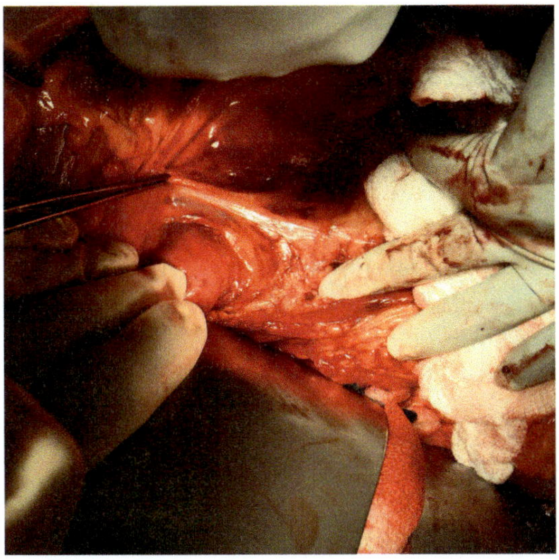

Fig. 26.21 Medial exposure of the IMV

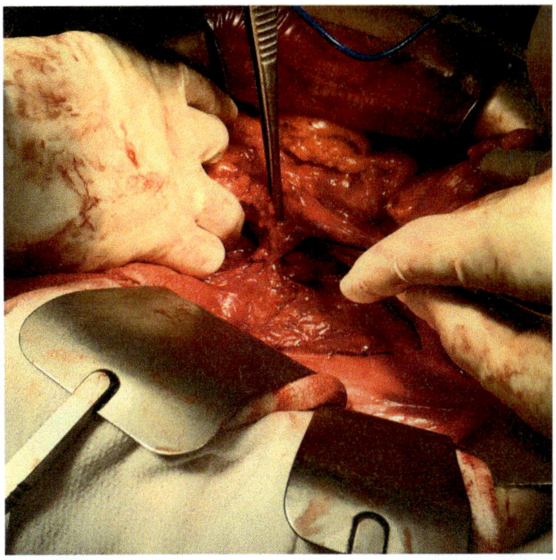

Fig. 26.22 Isolation of the IMA

tension on the colon and its mesentery, the areolar plane of dissection along the retroperitoneal plane is easily identified.

- The sigmoid colon and its mesentery should be completely medialized to the midline to expose and identify the left ureter. The dissection is then carried toward the splenic flexure. Mobilization of the splenic flexure can be facilitated by dissecting the posterior aspect of the mesentery up to the inferior border of the pancreas. The anatomy of the splenic flexure can be obscured by attachments of the omentum to the descending colon or medial aspect of the transverse colon. Separating these attachments restores normal anatomy, which can make the splenic flexure mobilization much easier.
- The next goal is to enter the lesser sac, and this is accomplished by separating the omentum from the transverse colon. By incising the peritoneal layer along the length of transverse colon, the lesser sac is eventually entered, and the posterior attachments of the omentum to the colon mesentery can be exposed and divided. This will allow the lesser sac to be completely exposed from the flexure to beyond midline. This will also expose the remaining lateral attachments of the flexure which can be divided by either retracting the colon medially or placing a hand into the retroperitoneum and rolling the colon medially over the hand.
- With the lesser sac completely open and the flexure mobilized, the posterior attachments along the inferior border of the pancreas can be divided. With the posterior mesenteric dissection carried all the way up to the inferior border of the pancreas, the surgeon's right hand is passed into the retroperitoneum in the lateral-to-medial direction. The fold of the splenic flexure mesentery can be palpated and separated from the inferior aspect of the pancreas, and the overlying peritoneum is divided to the midline. Care should be taken not to injure the inferior mesenteric vein as the dissection is carried medially.
- With the left colon and splenic flexure completely mobilized, the vascular pedicles can be isolated and ligated. The sigmoid colon is elevated and retracted laterally to expose the base of the mesentery at the level of the sacral promontory.
- The peritoneum is incised from just below the promontory toward the attachments of the proximal jejunum and ligament of Treitz. This will allow for the superior rectal artery to be elevated off the retroperitoneum and expose the lateral plane of dissection.
- The surgeon can then pass their right hand under the superior rectal artery and divide the cephalad attachments so the IMA can be isolated at its origin from the aorta (Fig. 26.22).

The artery is isolated by creating a window on its cephalad side and medial to the IMV. It can then be ligated once the left ureter is clearly out of harm's way.

- The IMV is now elevated off the retroperitoneum and isolated at the inferior border of the pancreas, and its ligation will ensure adequate mobilization for a tension-free anastomosis (Fig. 26.23). This allows for complete exposure of the retroperitoneum (Fig. 26.24).

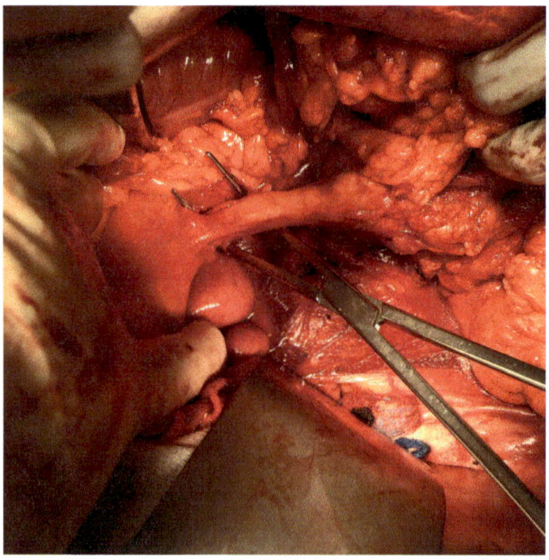

Fig. 26.23 Isolation of the IMV

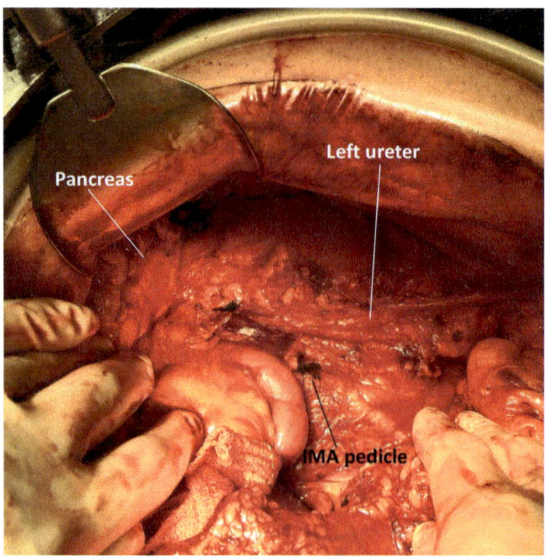

Fig. 26.24 Left retroperitoneum

- The proximal site of bowel transection is dependent up on the location of the tumor and should ensure a minimum of a 5 cm margin. The distal site of transection should be at the proximal rectum to ensure an adequate distal margin and avoid having distal sigmoid colon included in the anastomosis. The rectum is stapled and divided with a linear stapler for future double-stapled anastomosis or left attached for future double purse-string anastomosis (see Chap. 9).

Anastomotic Assessment

- Anastomotic assessment with either an air leak test alone or combined with endoscopic visualization is critical to ensuring a safe anastomosis. Anastomotic assessment has been shown to be associated with a decreased incidence of anastomotic leak from left-sided anastomosis. Endoluminal visualization may help to ensure that there is adequate mucosal blood flow and assess for arterial hemorrhage at the anastomosis, which can usually be controlled with endoscopic clips. Carbon dioxide insufflation gas is helpful to avoid distention of the bowel.

Straight Laparoscopic Medial-to-Lateral Approach

- The patient is positioned and secured to the operating table in the same manner as described above for the laparoscopic right colectomy. Typically, both arms are tucked to the patient's sides, and the legs are in the lithotomy or supine split-leg position. The abdomen is accessed via an open or closed technique in the supraumbilical position.
- There are various options for port placement, and the choice is dependent upon surgeon's preference (Fig. 26.25). Typically there are three or four working ports – two for the surgeon and one or two for the assistant.
- Once the abdomen has been thoroughly explored and the lesion located, the patient is placed in steep Trendelenburg and airplaned so the left side is up. This allows gravity to retract the small bowel to the right upper quadrant and expose the left colon mesentery.

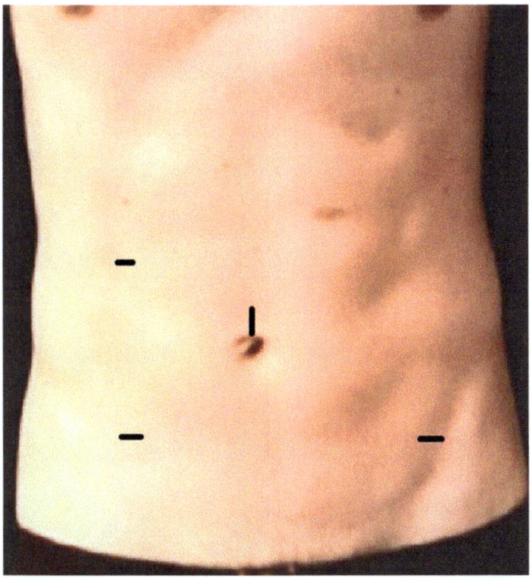

Fig. 26.25 Port placement for laparoscopic left colectomy

The omentum is reflected cephalad to the transverse colon to expose it and the splenic flexure.

- The inferior mesenteric vein and the superior rectal artery are the vascular landmarks to be identified. At the level of the sacral promontory, the superior rectal artery is grasped and elevated with the surgeon's right hand. This will allow for the course of the artery to be seen and traced to its origin. With the energy source of choice in the left hand, the peritoneum is incised from below the sacral promontory to the IMA origin on the aorta. The wider the incision, the wider the window to the retroperitoneum will be, and this will maximize visualization of the retroperitoneum.
- The retroperitoneum is swept posteriorly until the left ureter is identified. If the left ureter is difficult to identify, an alternative approach should be taken, and it will be described below. Once the left ureter is safely swept into the retroperitoneum, the superior rectal artery is dissected free to the origin of the IMA at the aorta.
- The peritoneum is then scored across the base of the IMA and medial to the IMV. The vein is then grasped and elevated off the retroperitoneum by scoring the peritoneum up to the ligament of Treitz. This will allow access into the retroperitoneum once again, and the plane is developed in a caudad direction to join with the original retroperitoneal dissection plane.
- The IMA is safely isolated, and the left ureter can be traced from the pelvic brim up to near the kidney. The IMA can be ligated with any energy source of choice. Next the IMV can be isolated by separating the mesentery from the retroperitoneum to the inferior border of the pancreas. Once isolated, it can be safely ligated.
- Now there is a large window into the space between the mesentery and the retroperitoneum, and left colon mesentery is mobilized out beyond the colon laterally. This dissection should extend from the sigmoid colon up to the splenic flexure so all that remains are the lateral attachments. Beginning near the pelvic brim, the lateral peritoneum is incised by retracting the sigmoid colon medially and cephalad.
- As the splenic flexure is neared, there needs to be a transition from dividing the lateral peritoneal attachments to separating the omentum from the colon, and this is dependent upon the adhesions between the two structures. Mobilization of the splenic flexure usually requires a third working instrument. The omentum just above its attachment to the colon is retracted anteriorly, and the colon is retracted posteriorly, which puts the plane to be incised in a vertical position. This superficial peritoneal plane is incised toward the midline, and the lesser sac is eventually entered.
- Once the lesser sac is entered, the deeper attachments of the omentum and transverse colon can be divided. These deeper attachments are identified by pulling the colon down to the lower abdomen and watching for where the omentum moves or is attached. The omentum and colon are grabbed at this point, and by making the plane vertical, they are divided.
- The lesser sac is completely opened in this fashion so that all that remains are the peritoneal attachments to the inferior border of the

pancreas. These attachments are divided by retracting the splenic flexure medially and caudad while elevating it off the retroperitoneum. This will allow for visualization along the retroperitoneal and lesser sac sides of this attachment. Division of this attachment to the midline will allow for adequate mobilization for extraction, resection, and a tension-free anastomosis.

- The rectum can be divided either intra-corporally or in an open fashion through a suprapubic extraction site. If the rectum is divided intra-corporally, the colon can be extracted through either a left lower quadrant or suprapubic site. With either method of rectal division, the colon is extracted and resected, and the anvil is placed in the same method as described for an end-to-end anastomosis.
- The proximal colon is then returned to the abdomen, and the extraction port can be closed temporarily or definitively. Under laparoscopic visualization, the stapler is passed transanally up to the top of the rectal stump, and the anvil is reassembled making sure there is no twist in the left colon and its mesentery. An air leak test or endoscopic assessment is performed under laparoscopic visualization.
- Typically, only 10–12 mm port sites need to have the fascial defect closed, and this can be accomplished open via the skin incision or laparoscopically using a transfascial suture passer.

Hand-Assisted Medial-to-Lateral Approach

- Patient preparation and position are the same as for the straight laparoscopic approach. The hand port can be placed in the suprapubic, periumbilical, or left lower quadrant based on surgeon's preference (Fig. 26.26). A suprapubic hand port has the advantage of having direct access to the pelvis to aid the pelvic dissection, divide the rectum, perform the anastomosis, and manage anastomotic complications. The port can be placed through a vertical midline or Pfannenstiel incision.
- For a suprapubic hand port, the camera port is placed in the supraumbilical position to avoid interfering with the hand port. A working port is placed on the right side, half the distance between the hand and camera ports and lateral to the rectum muscle. A second working port is placed in the left lower quadrant to help with the lateral and splenic flexure mobilization. This port is placed lateral to the rectus muscle and as low as possible to minimize the time working against the camera.

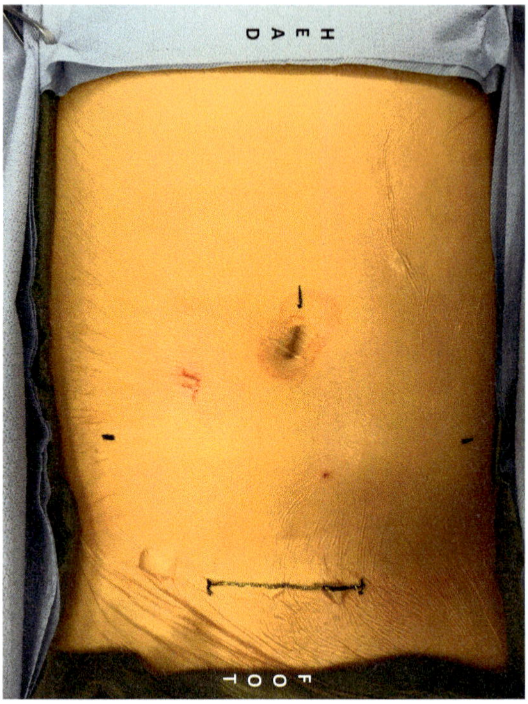

Fig. 26.26 Port placement for HALS left colectomy

- With the patient placed in steep Trendelenburg and left side up, the small bowel is put in the right upper quadrant, and the omentum is reflected to the upper abdomen. This exposes the left colon mesentery and splenic flexure as previously described. The surgeon stands on the patient's right side and places their right hand in the abdomen.
- The superior rectal artery at the level of the sacral promontory is grasped and elevated (Fig. 26.27), and the peritoneum is incised as described above (Fig. 26.28). The hand acting as a retractor elevates the vessel to expose the retroperitoneum. The identification of the left ureter and its reflection into the retroperitoneum is the same as described above (Fig. 26.29).

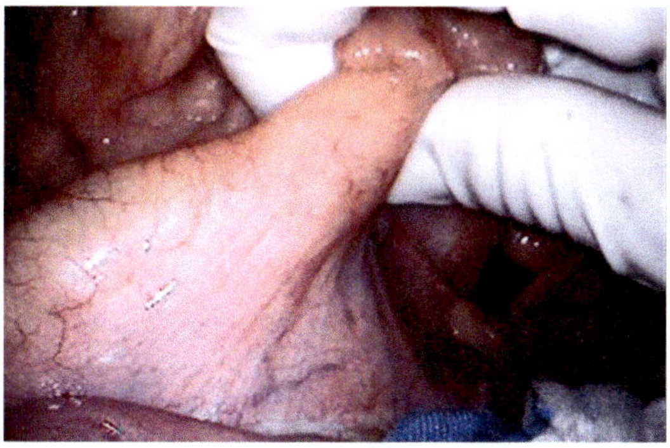

Fig. 26.27 Isolation of the superior rectal artery at the level of the sacral promontory

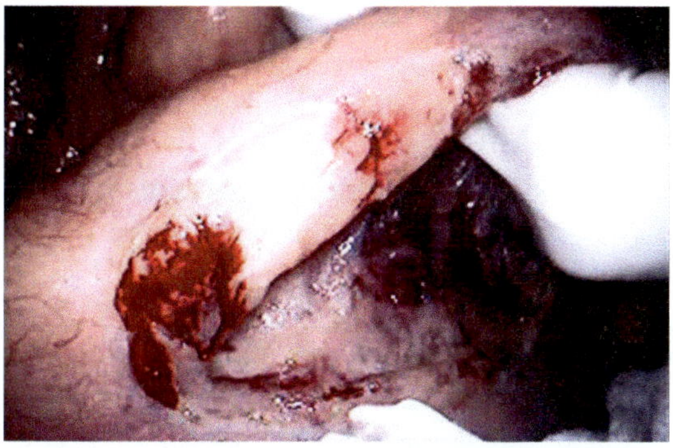

Fig. 26.28 Accessing the retroperitoneum at the level of the sacral promontory

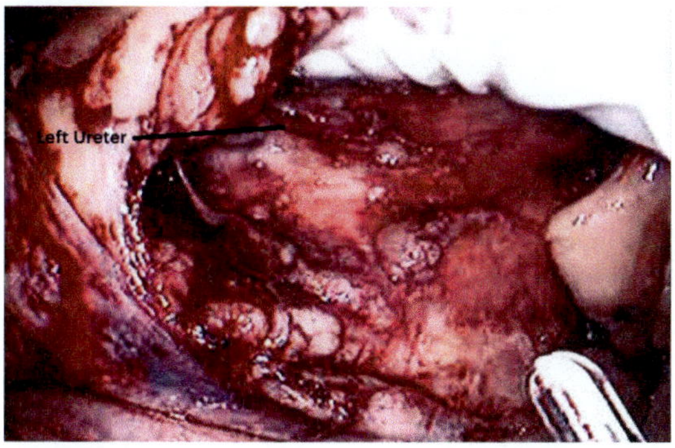

Fig. 26.29 Identification of the left ureter from a medial-to-lateral approach

- Once the left ureter is identified and separated from the mesentery, the index finger is used to elevate the superior rectal artery under tension. The middle finger can then bluntly sweep down the retroperitoneum working toward the origin of the IMA (Fig. 26.30).

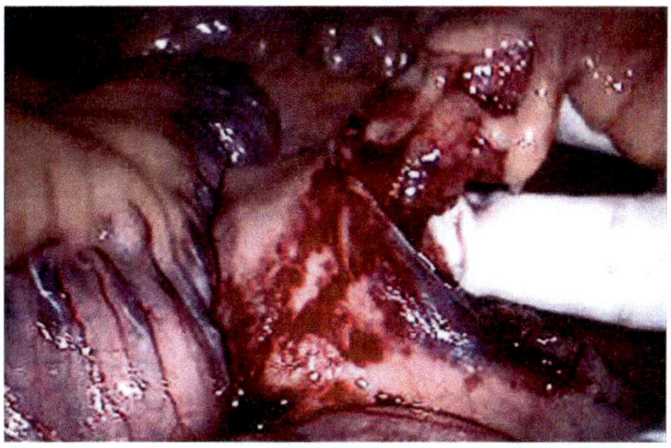

Fig. 26.30 Isolating the IMA at its origin

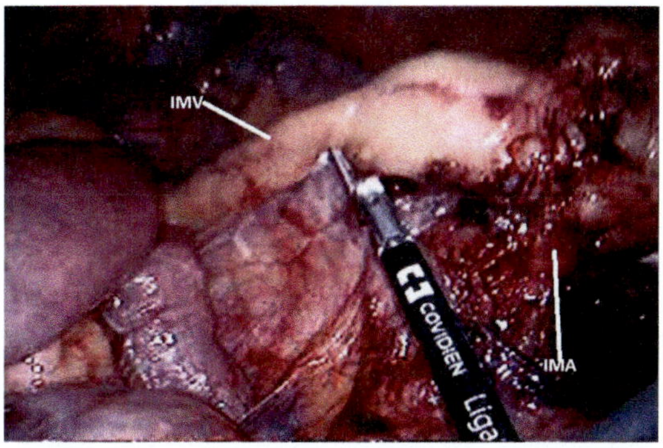

Fig. 26.31 Accessing the retroperitoneum medial to the IMV

- Care should be used to sweep the retroperitoneal tissue and associated sympathetic nerves posteriorly to avoid injury during the ligation of the vessel. This dissection is carried cephalad to the vessel to expose and elevate the window medial to the IMV. The peritoneum is incised across the IMA origin, and the retroperitoneum can be entered medial to the IMV.
- The hand now elevates the IMV, and the peritoneum is incised up to the ligament of Treitz (Fig. 26.31). The retroperitoneum is swept down, and the thumb elevates the IMV and mesentery to keep it on tension. Once the retroperitoneal plane is adequately developed, the index finger elevates the IMV, and the middle finger sweeps the retroperitoneum down as the IVM is elevated to isolate it at the inferior border of the pancreas (Fig. 26.32).
- Now that both vascular structures are safely isolated and the left ureter is safely in the

retroperitoneum, both vessels can be ligated (Fig. 26.33). For ligating both the artery and vein, the index and middle fingers are placed in the retroperitoneum behind the vessel to create space, the fourth and fifth fingers lay in front of the vessel to protect the small bowel, and the thumb can help elevate any mesentery or fat obscuring the view (Fig. 26.34).

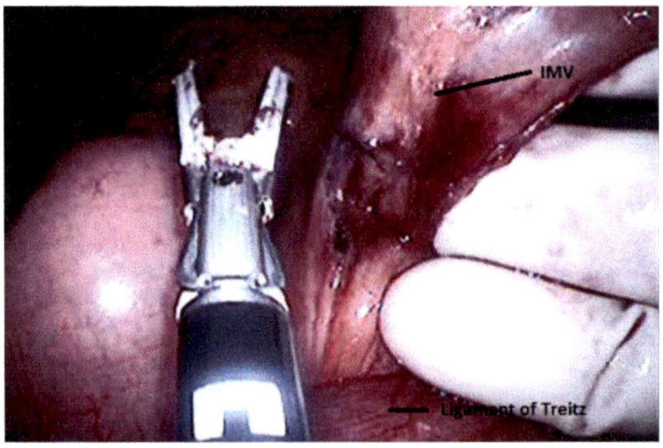

Fig. 26.32 Isolating the IMV near the ligament of Treitz and the inferior border of the pancreas

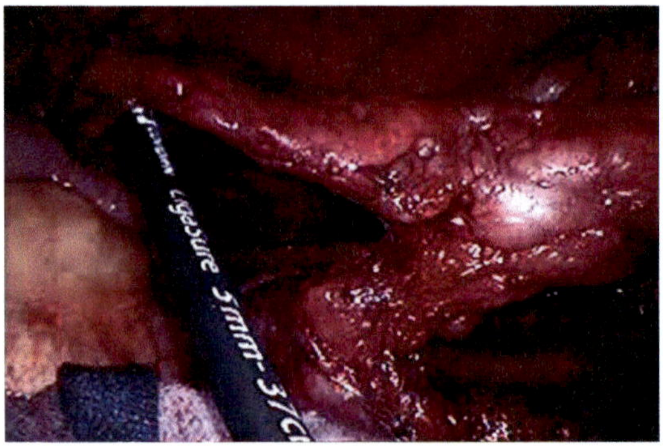

Fig. 26.33 Safe isolation of the IMA

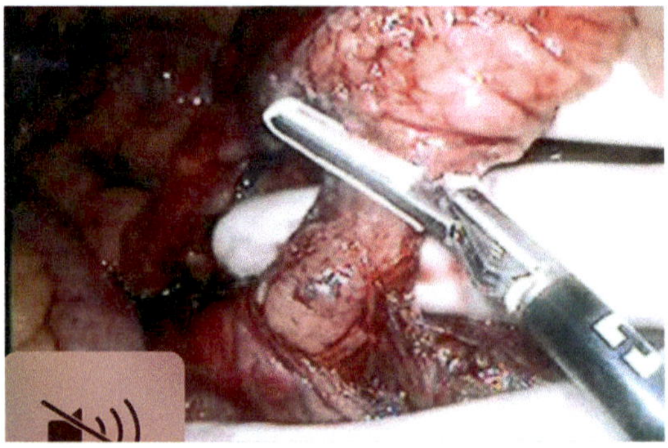

Fig. 26.34 Hand position for ligating the IMA and IMV

- With both pedicles ligated, the hand is placed palm down under the mesentery. It elevates the mesentery under tension so the retroperitoneal dissection can be carried out laterally beyond the colon (Fig. 26.35). The extent of the dissection should be from the sigmoid colon caudad up to the splenic flexure cephalad and along the inferior border of the pancreas medially.
- The lateral dissection begins by mobilizing the sigmoid colon. Often the hand gets in the way for this dissection so solutions include depressing the sigmoid colon with the fingers and passing the energy device between the fingers to get the proper angle or removing the hand and placing an instrument through the hand port to begin the dissection straight laparoscopically.
- Once the retroperitoneal dissection plane is entered (Fig. 26.36), the hand can be passed

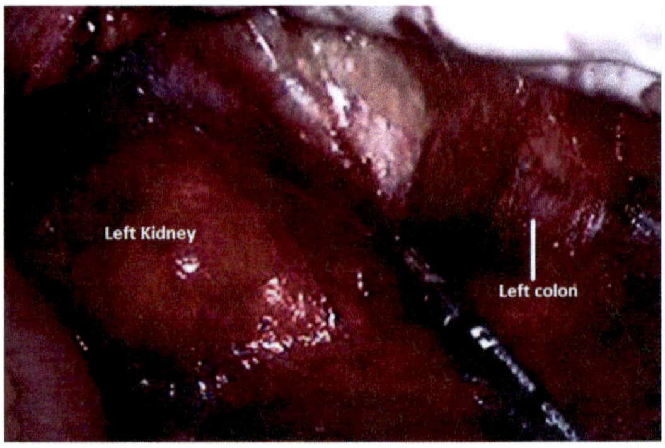

Fig. 26.35 Medial-to-lateral mobilization of the left colon mesentery off the retroperitoneum

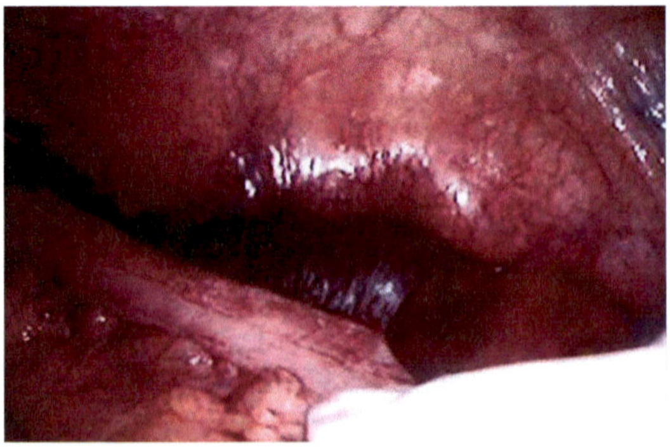

Fig. 26.36 Incision of the lateral attachments and entry into the retroperitoneal plane

into the retroperitoneum, and the lateral attachments can be exposed on the hand just like an open case (Fig. 26.37). The assistant stands between the legs and uses the left lower quadrant port to divide the tissue.

- The dissection continues toward the splenic flexure until the need to transition to the omentum. At the omental attachments, the omentum is elevated and pulled to the video right with the grasper, and the colon is retracted down with the hand (Fig. 26.38). Pulling with the grasper to the right helps to keep it out of the way from energy device during this dissection. The peritoneum is incised along the transverse colon, and the lesser sac is eventually entered.
- With the hand and instrument, the colon is pulled to the lower abdomen, and the next level of omental attachments is identified. At this point, the omentum is elevated, and the colon is depressed allowing for the attachments to be divided. This is continued until the lesser sac is wide open from the splenic flexure to the midline (Fig. 26.39). The only remaining attachments are along the inferior border of the pancreas. With the colon pulled to the lower abdomen, the lateral cut edge of the mobilization is seen. The hand is passed into the retroperitoneum along the inferior border of the pancreas. Much like the open approach, the fold of the mesentery can be palpated and separated from the pancreas allowing for safe division to the midline (Fig. 26.40).
- The colon is completely mobilized at this point and can be extracted for resection and anastomosis. Typically, the proximal colon is divided, the stapling anvil is placed, and the rectum is divided. This procedure has been previously described. However, this can be

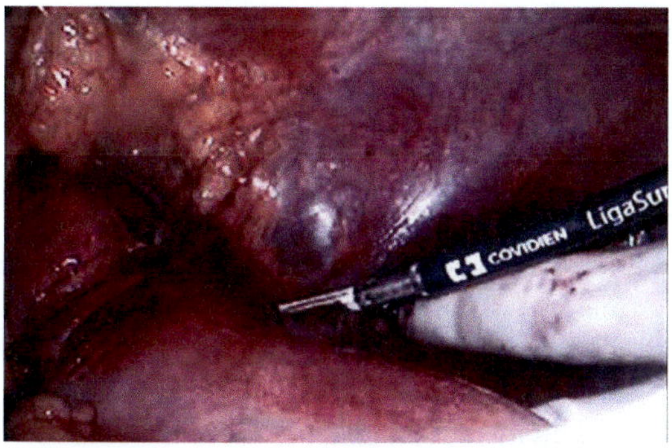

Fig. 26.37 Lateral mobilization of the left colon

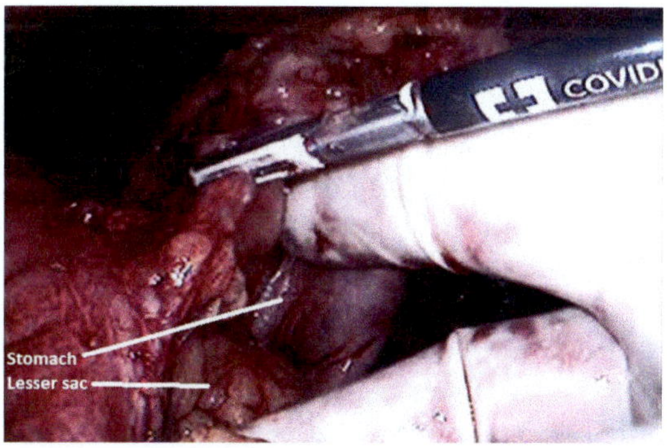

Fig. 26.39 Completing the opening of the lesser sac

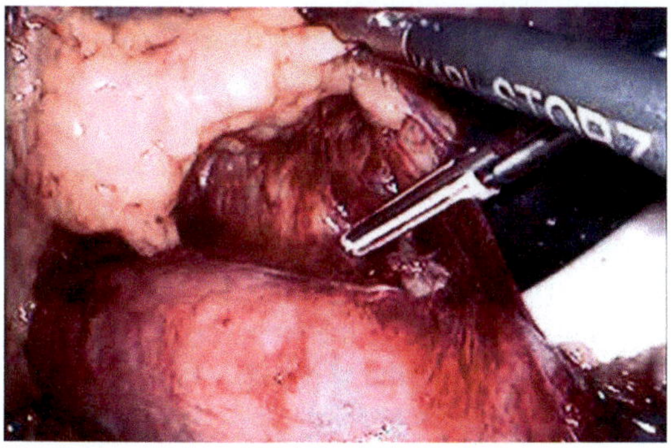

Fig. 26.38 Entering the lesser sac by separating the omentum from the transverse colon

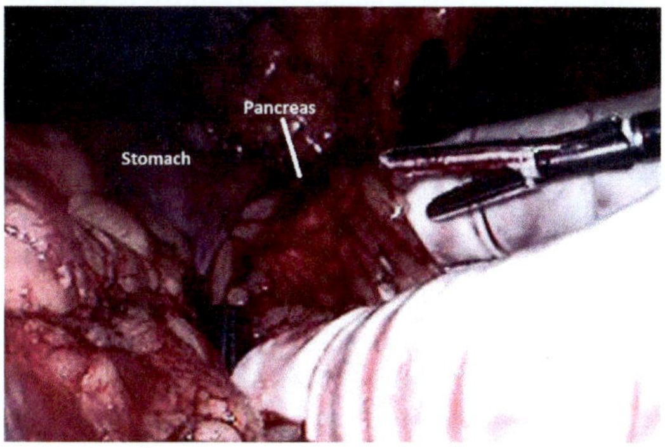

Fig. 26.40 Division of the peritoneal attachments between the transverse colon mesentery and the inferior border of the pancreas

difficult in patients with a fat or bulky mesentery. This can be managed by dividing the rectum and the mesorectum first allowing for easier extraction of the proximal colon. The anastomosis and anastomotic assessment can be performed under direct vision via the hand port or laparoscopically.

Laparoscopic Identification of the Left Ureter

- The IMA or IMV should not be ligated until the left ureter is clearly identified and safely dissected free of the left colon mesentery. There is a simple three-step algorithm that can help facilitate safe identification of the left ureter. The first approach is at the level of the superior rectal artery as the retroperitoneum is accessed at the level of the sacral promontory as described above. If the ureter is not easily identified, the approach should change to the IMV.
- The IMV is grasped and elevated, and medial aspect of the peritoneum is incised. The retroperitoneum is accessed and the plane developed. This part of the retroperitoneum is flat so identification of the proper plane is much easier. Once in the proper plane, the dissection can be directed in a caudad direction to see if the original plane started at the level of the sacral promontory can be entered to identify the ureter.
- If the left ureter can still not be identified, the colon can be mobilized in a lateral-to-medial direction. If unable to identify the ureter at this point, consider conversion to an open procedure or, if using a hand port, remove the top of the port, and identify it in an open fashion through the hand port. Ureteral stent should be employed at the discretion of the surgeon.

Subtotal Colectomy

- Tumors of the transverse colon often increase the complexity of the required resection because of the need to divide most or all of the branches of the middle colic vessels. An extended right colectomy can adequately treat a tumor from the hepatic flexure to mid-transverse colon. With complete mobilization of the small bowel mesentery and widely opening the lesser sac toward the splenic flexure, there should be adequate mobilization to create an ileocolic anastomosis with proper bowel orientation and without tension from either an open or laparoscopic approach.
- However, distal transverse colon tumors tend be more difficult to manage. Some surgeons advocate a transverse colectomy, but challenges associated with this type of resection include obtaining an adequate mesenteric resection and mobilization of the right and left colon to create a safe, tension-free anastomosis. For patients with a redundant and mobile transverse colon, it may be feasible to perform an extended left colectomy. If the transverse colon cannot be mobilized enough to reach the top of the rectum, it may be more appropriate to perform a subtotal colectomy. This entails resection of the right and transverse colon and creation of an ileo-descending colon anastomosis.

Open Approach

- The right colon mobilization begins as describe above, and as the hepatic flexure is mobilized, the lesser sac is entered by separating the omentum from the transverse colon mesentery. The plane to the right of the midline tends to be fused, but it is an avascular plane so it can be developed bluntly. With careful dissection under tension, the plane can be developed, and the proper lesser sac is entered. The lesser omentum is divided toward the splenic flexure as far as possible.
- With the right colon and hepatic flexure mobilized and the lesser sac completely open, the mesentery can be ligated. This begins with isolation and ligation of the ileocolic pedicle and division of the terminal ileum and its mesentery as described in the open right colectomy section. The middle colic vessels are isolated by pulling the transverse colon caudad and having the surgeon, who is standing on the patient's left side, pass their left hand through the ileocolic mesenteric defect from the retroperitoneal to peritoneal side. The index finger is elevated against the junction of

the SMA and the origins of the middle colic vessels, which allows for a safe high ligation of these vessels.

- Now the left colon needs to be mobilized, and the surgeon switches to the patient's right side packing the small bowel into the right upper quadrant. The sigmoid colon, left colon, and splenic flexure are mobilized as described in the open left colectomy section. The IMV is isolated by grasping and elevating it so the peritoneum medial to it can be incised. This allows access into the retroperitoneal dissection plane, and the IMV can be isolated and ligated at the inferior border of the pancreas.
- The IMA is not isolated or ligated to preserve the blood supply to the distal colon. The distal bowel and mesentery are divided to provide an adequate distal margin. For the creation of a side to side ileocolic anastomosis, the orientation of the small bowel is very important. If the stapled end of the terminal ileum is brought over the top of the small bowel to perform a side to side anastomosis on the left side, this will create the potential for the small bowel to volvulize through the mesenteric defect. To avoid this complication, the small bowel needs to be rotated counterclockwise 180 degrees so the cut edge of the mesentery is brought underneath the remaining small bowel. This allows for the cut edge of the small bowel mesentery to pass under the small bowel and face the patients left side in a straight line. Also, the entire small bowel from the ligament of Treitz to the anastomosis is on top of the mesenteric defect so there is no risk of a small bowel volvulus. This will allow for a side to side stapled anastomosis to be performed. Some surgeons will suture close the mesenteric defect with the intent to minimize risk of volvulus of the small bowel.

Laparoscopic Approach

- This extended resection can occur either straight laparoscopically or hand-assisted. For the straight laparoscopic approach, the right colon is mobilized in the same fashion as described for right colectomy. Once the lesser sac is entered, the lesser omentum is divided as far as possible toward the splenic flexure. This exposes the lesser sac as much as possible and facilitates ligation of the middle colic vessels by clearing any posterior mesenteric attachments.
- With the ileocolic vessel ligated, the middle colic vessels are exposed. This is accomplished with the first assistant via one or two right-sided ports elevating the transverse colon. The peritoneum near the ligament of Treitz is scored across the base of the vessels to the cut edge of the mesentery on the right. This allows the individual branches of the middle colic vessels to be isolated and safely ligated.
- With the right colon and transverse colon mobilized and mesentery ligated, attention is turned to the left colon. The patient is positioned as described for a laparoscopic left colon.
- The IMV is identified and elevated so the peritoneum can be incised allowing access to the retroperitoneum. The IMV is mobilized, isolated, and ligated at the inferior border of the pancreas. The mesenteric side of the IMV and the cut edge of the transverse colon mesentery are elevated, and the intervening mesentery is divided. Ideally, there should not be any remaining vessels in this remaining bit of mesentery.
- With the mesentery of the colon to be resected completely divided, the left colon mesentery is mobilized out laterally beyond the colon. To ensure adequate mobilization for extraction and the anastomosis, the sigmoid colon should be mobilized. The lateral attachments starting at the sigmoid colon are incised and divided toward the splenic flexure. The splenic flexure is mobilized as described in the left colectomy section.
- Once the colon is completely mobilized and before it can be extracted, the IMV needs to be divided again along the line of the distal resection margin. If it is not divided before extraction, the specimen will be tethered by this vessel preventing adequate exposure. Some surgeons will divide the entire specimen intracorporeally.

- Prior to performing the anastomosis, the small bowel and its mesentery must be oriented as described above. The specimen can then be extracted via a midline incision.
- For a hand-assisted approach, one option is to use the same port placement as described for left colectomy. If the patient has favorable anatomy, some of the sigmoid and ileocecal mobilization can be performed directly through the hand-assisted incision prior to starting the dissection. Occasionally, in patients with a redundant transverse colon, the transverse colon can be brought to the lower abdomen, out through the incision, and a portion of the omentum mobilized off of the colon.
- The dissection begins either with the right or left colon. The posterior (inferior-to-superior) approach to the right colon as initial maneuver will be described here. The small bowel is placed in the right upper quadrant exposing the posterior attachments of the small bowel mesentery to the retroperitoneum. The mesentery is grasped and elevated with the middle finger and thumb of the left hand. The index finger pointing toward the head swings over the pedicle to further expose the duodenum (Fig. 26.41). The peritoneum is incised from the duodenum to the cecum. With the hand palm down, the fingers elevate this peritoneal incision, and the retroperitoneum is entered.
- The hand continues to elevate the right colon mesentery, and duodenum is exposed and reflected posteriorly (Fig. 26.42). This dissection is continued superiorly and laterally beyond the transverse colon, hepatic flexure, and ascending colon.
- The patient is then tilted right side up to move the small bowel to the left side of the abdomen and expose the lateral planes. The lateral dissection begins at the level of the cecum by placing the hand in the retroperitoneal plane and lateral to the cecum and right colon to expose the lateral attachments (Fig. 26.43). They are divided heading toward the hepatic flexure, which is mobilized by entering the lesser sac. The lesser sac is entered by separating the lesser omentum from the transverse colon mesentery (Fig. 26.44).
- Once the plane is developed, the cut edge of the lesser omentum is grasped with a grasper and elevated so the hand can control the colon and develop the plane into the lesser sac. The lesser omentum is divided out toward the

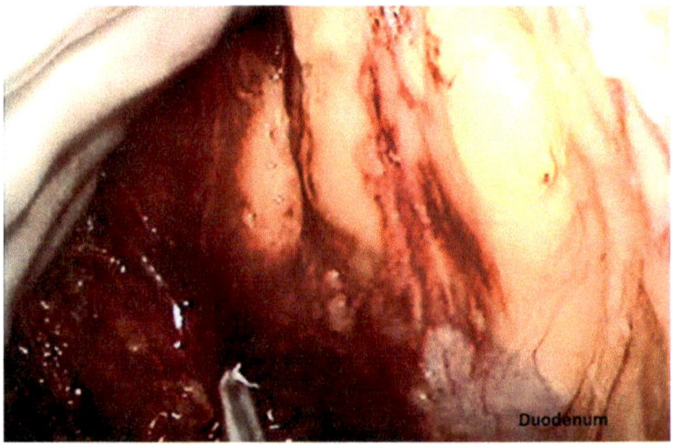

Fig. 26.42 Accessing the retroperitoneal plan: elevating the right colon mesentery and dissection the duodenum posteriorly

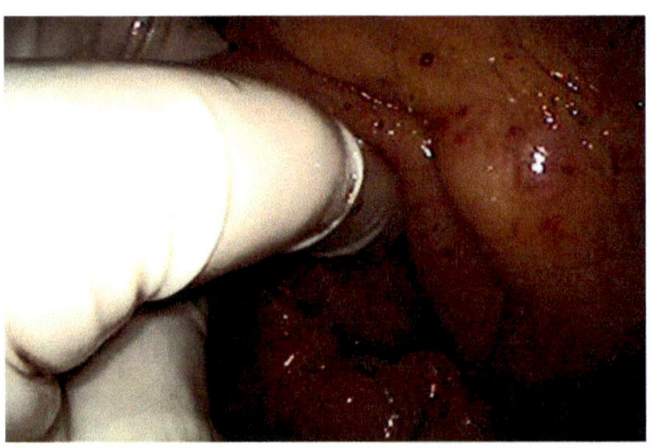

Fig. 26.41 HALS exposure of the posterior aspect of the small bowel mesentery for the right colon dissection

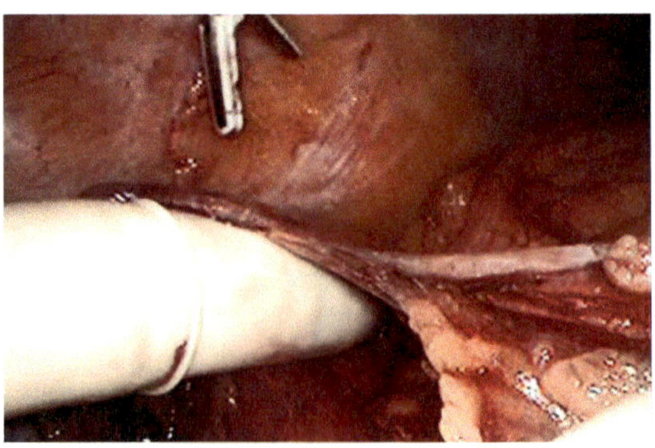

Fig. 26.43 Division of the lateral attachments of the right colon

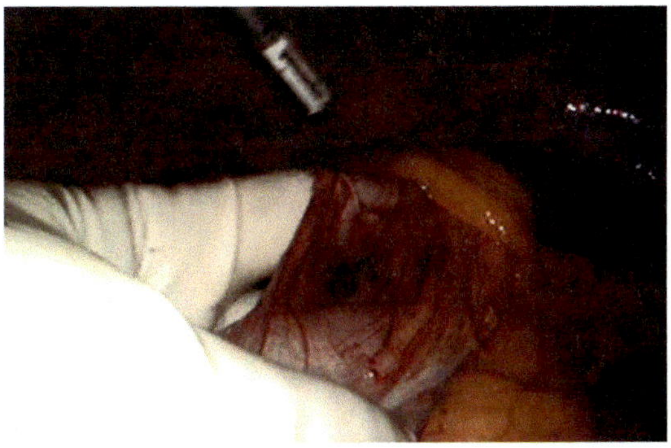

Fig. 26.44 Mobilization of the hepatic flexure by entering the lesser sac

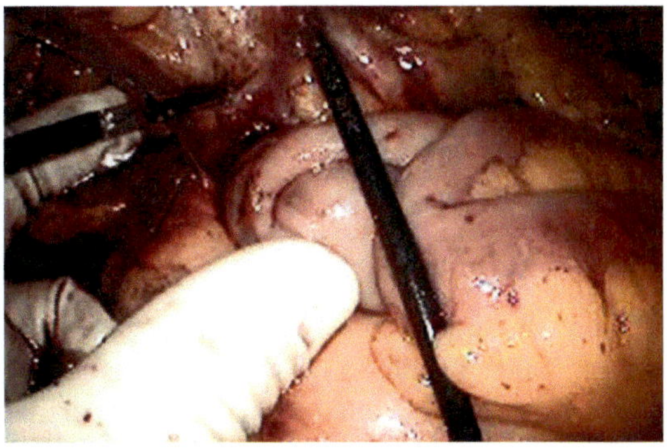

Fig. 26.46 Exposure of the middle colic vessels

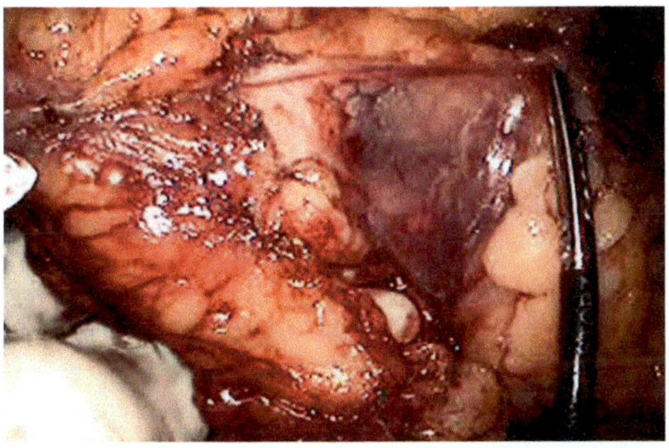

Fig. 26.45 Isolation of the ileocolic pedicle by passing the hand through the mesenteric defect on the ileal side of the pedicle

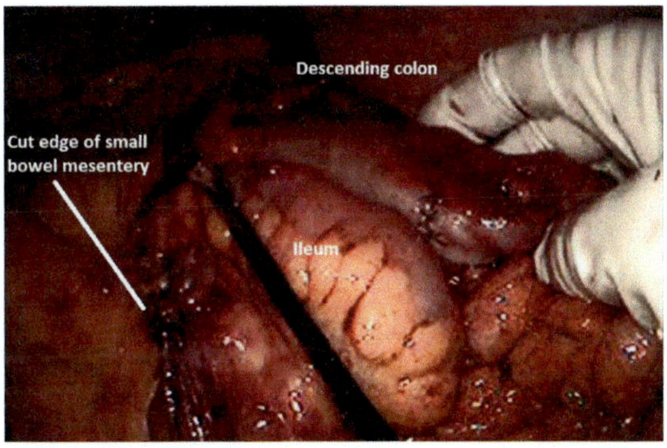

Fig. 26.47 Orientation of the small bowel mesentery for an ileo-descending colon anastomosis

splenic flexure as far as possible. Now the right colon and transverse colon mesentery can be ligated.

- The ileocolic pedicle is isolated by pulling to the right lower quadrant. The peritoneum on the caudad aspect is incised, and the mesentery is dissected to expose the retroperitoneum. The index and middle fingers are passed through the mesenteric defect to expose the vessels and the bare area on their cephalad aspect (Fig. 26.45). The bare area is incised along the lines of resection to isolate and ligate the ileocolic pedicles.
- To isolate the middle colic vessels, the left hand is passed through the mesenteric defect into the retroperitoneum and lesser sac. The transverse colon mesentery is exposed by elevating the hand, and the first assistant via right lower quadrant port elevates the distal transverse colon (Fig. 26.46). The peritoneum is incised from the ligament of Treitz to the cut edge of the right colon mesentery. The hand is able to palpate each middle colic vessel to facilitate its isolation and ligation.
- With the right and transverse colon mesentery divided, attention is turned to the left colon, and the left colon is mobilized as described in the paragraph above but using the hand-assisted technique for the left colon.
- The IMA is preserved to maintain blood supply to the sigmoid and descending colon. The IMV is then again divided at the distal resection margin, and the colon is then extracted through the hand port for resection.
- Just as described for the open approach, the small bowel and its mesentery are rotated 180 degrees counterclockwise to allow the cut edge of the mesentery to face the patient's left side (Fig. 26.47). After the small bowel is

properly oriented, a side to side anastomosis can be performed via the hand port.

Total Abdominal Colectomy with Ileorectal Anastomosis

- Total abdominal colectomy may be indicated for patients with synchronous tumors or hereditary cancer syndromes such as hereditary nonpolyposis colorectal cancer or familial adenomatous polyposis. The entire abdominal colon is resected, and an ileorectal anastomosis can be performed in either an end-to-end, end-to-side, or isoperistaltic side-to-side fashion. Postoperative cancer surveillance can often be performed in the office, without sedation using either a rigid or flexible endoscopy.
- The operation is virtually identical to subtotal colectomy, with the exception that the majority of the sigmoid is resected and anastomosis performed between the terminal ileum and rectosigmoid junction.

Special Circumstances

Laparoscopy

- The introduction of laparoscopy for the treatment of colorectal adenocarcinoma provoked considerable controversy regarding its oncologic appropriateness. Prospective multicenter randomized trials were initiated to compare laparoscopic with open techniques. Over two decades later, there appears to be abundant evidence indicating that laparoscopic surgery is at least as safe and oncologically sound for the treatment of intraperitoneal colon cancer compared to open techniques, when performed by experienced surgeons. At least five prospective, randomized clinical trials have demonstrated modest short-term benefits for the laparoscopic approach with no differences in long-term overall survival, disease-free survival, and recurrence rates as compared to open colectomy. The phenomenon of port-site recurrence following resection of early stage cancer appears to be related more to suboptimal operative technique than to a change in the local environment due to carbon dioxide pneumoperitoneum that would potentially enhance tumor deposition and growth. Therefore, it is safe and effective to employ the laparoscopic approach for the surgical management of colon cancer if the principles of oncologic resection are observed.

Obstructing Colon Cancers

- The management of obstructing colon cancers presents unique challenges in that the treatment of the acute or subacute obstructive process often dictates the oncologic management of the cancer.
- The overall outcome in terms of survival and recurrence is worse for patients whose initial presentation is with obstruction or obstructive symptoms.
- By the time a tumor grows to the point of luminal obstruction, it is frequently a T3 or T4 lesion, and these tumors have a higher incidence of lymph node, peritoneal, or distant metastasis.
- The management options for obstructing colon cancers are many, and there are no well-established guidelines.
- Proximal diversion alleviates the obstruction but does not address the cancer, and resection of the primary tumor addresses both issues but carries significant morbidity and a high stoma rate.
- The introduction of self-expanding stents as a means for a bridge to therapy (surgery vs chemotherapy) or as palliation in the setting of unresectable tumors is an additional option. The morbidity associated with urgent resection with ostomy creation or primary anastomosis can be as high as 60% with wound complications, deep organ space infections, respiratory complications, and intensive care unit admissions being some of the most common. Therefore, the concept of endoscopically alleviating the obstruction, which would

allow for complete colonic evaluation and elective, one-step resection, has significant appeal.

- Initial single institution reports demonstrated significant benefit of endoscopic stenting as a bridge to surgery compared to emergent surgery. These studies have reported a high incidence of technical and clinical success of greater than 90% of cases and are associated with a stoma-free rate of 60–90%. The major complications associated with endoscopic stents are perforation, migration, and bleeding, which have been reported as being relatively low.
- It must be kept in mind that retrospective, single institution studies suffer from many potential sources of bias such as patient selection, small numbers, and missing data.
- A multicenter, prospective, randomized trial of colonic stenting versus emergent surgery for acute left-sided malignant colon obstruction was undertaken in the Netherlands. The study was scheduled to enroll 60 patients in each arm with the primary outcome being mean global quality of life and secondary outcomes morbidity and mortality. The study was stopped after the enrollment of 47 patients in the stenting arm and 51 in the surgery arm due to 6 procedures related to perforations in the stent arm. The technical success rate of 70% was felt to be too low compared to the previous published literature, and the study was stopped. Interestingly, there was no statistical difference between the two arms with regard to global quality of life, morbidity/mortality profiles, and stoma rates.
- Endoscopic stenting clearly has a role in the management of obstructing colon cancers, but proper patient selection is of paramount importance to its success. Completely obstructing cancers, particularly when confirmed by contrast enema, have a low rate of technical success and increased likelihood of a stent-related complication. Stenting should also be avoided in patients with peritonitis, hemodynamic instability, or concern for impending perforation.

- Surgical intervention remains the mainstay of managing obstructed colon cancers as it provides alleviation of the obstruction and resection of the tumor in one setting. The extent of the operative procedure is highly dependent upon the condition of the patient and the extent of the obstruction.
  - Proximal diversion alone should be performed only in selected situations such as complete obstruction with dilated small bowel that makes resection too difficult or in a setting where neoadjuvant therapy would be beneficial. The extent of resection and restoration of intestinal continuity remain to be debated and are dependent upon the physiology of the patient and the intraoperative findings.
  - If there is evidence of impending perforation or ischemia of the proximal colon, resection of the entire colon proximal to the obstruction is recommended, and performing a primary anastomosis should be avoided. However, if the proximal colon is dilated but healthy, a segmental versus extended colectomy can be performed based on the clinical situation.
  - The decision to perform a primary anastomosis is dependent upon the condition of the patient and quality of the proximal bowel.

Perforated Colon Cancers

- Perforated colon cancers present the challenge of adequately addressing the sepsis associated with a perforated colon while attempting to maintain the oncologic principles of resection for the malignant disease.
- The acute septic injury has the greatest impact on short-term outcomes, which in turn impacts the long-term outcome of the cancer. These patients typically present with a contained perforation much like diverticulitis or with a free perforation requiring an emergent operation. Either scenario results in a poorer outcome compared to non-perforated cancers.
- Patients who present with perforated tumors should undergo an oncologically based resection

if their physiologic state will allow as this will provide them with the best cancer-related outcome.
- If the patient has diffuse peritonitis or is in septic shock, emergent operation is indicated. If possible, oncologic resection of the primary tumor should be considered at the time. Postoperative adjuvant chemotherapy should be considered.
- If the patient has a contained perforation and is not in shock, then medical management initially can be considered. Neoadjuvant chemotherapy can also be considered given that there is likely spread of tumor cells in the peritoneal cavity due to the perforation.

Management of Primary Colon Cancer in the Setting of Distant Metastasis

- Advances in chemotherapy have greatly impacted our management strategies of patients who present with metastatic colon cancer. Current recommendations are for patients with symptomatic (bleeding or obstructing) primary tumors to undergo resection of their primary tumor before initiating systemic therapy for their metastatic disease.
- If the tumor is asymptomatic and the patient has a good performance status, the first-line treatment should be systemic chemotherapy. The rationale being that most patients will succumb to their metastatic disease before the primary tumor causes complications.
  - Non-randomized retrospective studies which have demonstrated a purported survival benefit with colectomy in this setting are plagued by selection bias, and should not be utilized for decision-making.

Outcomes for Colon Cancer

Short-Term Outcomes

- Short-term outcomes for colectomy for cancer include morbidity, mortality, length of hospital stay, and intraoperative parameters such as conversion from laparoscopy.
- Recent prospective randomized trials comparing laparoscopic versus open colectomy for cancer provide some of the best data regarding short-term outcomes. Overall complication rates range from 20% to 30%, equal between laparoscopic and open operations. Overall mortality rate is 1–4%.
  - It must be kept in mind that there were ASA and BMI exclusions for these studies, which would be expected to bias the results toward reduced morbidity and mortality as compared with the general population.
  - As mentioned in the beginning of the chapter, the ACS-NSQIP risk calculator can provide a reasonable assessment of operative and perioperative complication risk.

Long-Term Outcomes

- The 5-year survival and recurrence rates for colon cancer are dependent upon the stage of disease at the time of surgery.
  - Based on the data published from 2012 by the Surveillance, Epidemiology, and End Results (SEERS) Program , the 5-year overall relative survival for stage I is 90%, stage IIA is 87%, stage IIB is 63%, stage IIIA is 89%, stage IIIB is 69%, stage IIIC is 53%, and stage IV is 13%.
  - Survival has improved every 5 years since 1975, which reflects improvements in detection, surgical technique, and adjuvant therapy.
- Surgeons play a critical role in the referral of cancer patients to medical oncologist so a comprehensive knowledge of the indications for adjuvant chemotherapy is essential.
  - Administration of adjuvant FOLFOX chemotherapy to patients with node-positive colon cancer improves 5-year disease-free survival.
  - Patients with stage IIB (T4,N0,M0) colon cancer behave similarly to patients with

stage IIIB (T3-T4a,N1,M0; T2-T3,N2a,M0; or T1-T2,N2b,M0).

- Therefore, it is imperative for the surgeon to understand and recognize that patients with stage IIB and III cancers should be appropriately referred for adjuvant therapy in a timely fashion.

- The other notable observation is that patients with stage IIIA (T1-T2,N1,M0 or T1,N2a,M0) do as well as those with stage IIA (T3,N0,M0). This highlights the importance of surgical technique and the importance of resecting all potentially metastatic lymph nodes.

27 Rectal Cancer: Preoperative Evaluation and Staging

Jorge Marcet

Key Concepts

- Accurate preoperative staging of patients with rectal cancer helps identify patients at risk for local or distant metastasis and guides treatment decisions.
- Endorectal ultrasound (ERUS) is effective for staging the depth of invasion (T stage), especially for early-stage rectal tumors (uT0, uT1) that may be considered for local excision.
- Magnetic resonance (MR) has the ability to delineate the extent of locally advanced tumors and estimate involvement of the mesorectal fascia.
- ERUS and MR use surrogate markers to estimate nodal involvement—size, node morphology—and are not particularly accurate in predicting nodal metastatic spread unless there are multiple large nodes in the mesorectum.
- The potential for understaging and overstaging of patients should be realized and taken into account when making treatment decisions.
- High-resolution computed tomography (CT) can detect distant metastatic lesions greater than 1 cm in diameter.
- Positron emission tomography (PET) scan is the most accurate assessment of total body tumor burden, especially when combined with CT (PET-CT).
- PET-CT is indicated when there are equivocal findings on CT, and finding distant metastatic disease would alter therapeutic decisions.

Introduction

- Preoperative staging is performed according to the TNM classification of malignant tumors, estimating the depth of invasion into the rectal wall (cT), the presence or absence of lymph node metastasis (cN), and presence of distant metastasis (cM). Also of importance is the determination of invasion of the anal sphincter and pelvic floor musculature, adjacent pelvic organs, or pelvic sidewall, all with significant consequences of planning and treatment to the patient.
- The prefix "c" is used to indicate clinical staging, which is the estimate of stage based on physical examination and radiographic studies. Unfortunately, there is often confusion regarding this distinction, with some authors describing treatment recommendations for "T3N0" tumors as determined by pretreatment staging, when instead they should describe the tumor as "cT3N0." The difference at first glance appears trivial but can have significant consequences if

J. Marcet (✉)
Department of Surgery, Tampa General Hospital, Tampa, FL, USA
e-mail: jmarcet@health.usf.edu

S. R. Steele et al. (eds.), *The ASCRS Manual of Colon and Rectal Surgery*,
https://doi.org/10.1007/978-3-030-01165-9_27

the clinician fails to understand that estimates of tumor stage are just that, estimates, and that treatment planning must take into account the potential inaccuracy of these estimates. For example, understaging of the cancer preoperatively may result in the omission of preoperative radiotherapy/chemoradiotherapy and lead to an increased risk of local recurrence. Conversely, overstaging may lead to overtreatment, increasing the overall morbidity and cost of treatment.

- Pretreatment evaluation begins with physical examination and colonoscopic evaluation. Radiographic studies may include computed tomography (CT), endorectal ultrasound (ERUS), magnetic resonance imaging (MRI), and positron emission tomography (PET). These tests are complimentary, each with their own advantages and disadvantages, and may be used in combination. Laboratory evaluation includes determination of the carcinoembryologic antigen (CEA) level.

History and Physical Examination

- When evaluating a patient diagnosed with rectal cancer, the patient's history is recorded, and an inquiry is made as to the duration of symptoms, changes in weight, bowel habits, bowel control, and presence of pain.
- If restorative proctectomy or local excision is to be contemplated, a detailed assessment of anal sphincter function and prior trauma (e.g., obstetrical history, prior anal operations) should be obtained.
- A general physical examination is performed with special attention for signs of muscle wasting, abdominal distension, hepatomegaly, and lymphadenopathy.
- A careful digital rectal examination is performed, noting the distance of the tumor from the anal verge and its proximity to the anal sphincter and pelvic floor. Tumors located in the anterior portion of the rectum have the risk of invasion into the genital structures, and special attention should be made to the potential for fixation to adjacent structures (i.e., prostate, vagina, sacrum, puborectalis). In a woman with an anterior rectal cancer, a pelvic examination should be done to ensure there is no invasion of the vaginal wall that may affect treatment. When the tumor is located in the posterior or lateral rectal wall, pelvic sidewall invasion should be considered.
- If restorative proctectomy is being considered, assessment of anal sphincter bulk and tone is important as it may help predict postoperative function.
- The texture of the tumor also gives a clue as to the stage. Benign adenomas are soft, and the tumor may occasionally be difficult to detect on digital rectal examination. When a tumor invades the rectal wall, a desmoplastic reaction occurs, and the resulting fibrosis will be felt as firm tissue.
- Evaluating the mobility of the tumor can also give information on how deep the tumor invades. A tumor tethered to the rectal wall, but that is otherwise mobile, is likely to invade into but not through the wall. Tumors that are fixed within the pelvis and are not mobile are locally advanced, deeply invading the full thickness of the rectal wall and possibly invading surrounding pelvic structures.
- The digital rectal examination may occasionally also detect peritumoral lymphadenopathy, though this is often difficult. It should be noted that digital rectal examination has limitations in that only tumors of the distal rectal rectum can be adequately assessed. Furthermore, accuracy in staging depth of invasion is better for advanced tumors than for early tumors and improves with the surgeon's experience.

Endoscopic Evaluation of the Rectum

- Flexible sigmoidoscopy or proctoscopy should be performed to help localize the tumor anatomically and assess its appearance.
- The endoscopic appearance of a tumor also gives a clue as to the relative degree of invasion, with benign tumors soft to manipulation with the endoscope or endoscopic forceps and

malignant tumors being firm. Ulceration of the tumor implies invasion into the rectal wall, while deep ulceration may be a sign of transmural invasion.

- Distance to the anal verge is best assessed by rigid proctoscopy, although this measurement is of limited utility as it can vary greatly based on differences in body habitus. It is more important to assess the distance of the distal margin of the tumor from the anorectal muscular ring as this will often guide the decision between restorative and non-restorative proctectomy. Another assessment which is helpful is the relationship of the tumor to the folds of Houston.
- As noted in other chapters, the surgeon should always examine the rectum of any patient referred with a lesion in the left colon prior to operation, as flexible endoscopic measurements of distance by non-surgeons are notoriously inaccurate. Many lesions described as being proximal to "15 cm" are actually in the true rectum. This discovery may fundamentally alter treatment planning.

Total Colon Evaluation

- Evaluation of the proximal colon, preferably by complete colonoscopy, should be performed in all patients with rectal cancer to exclude synchronous lesions and to confirm the histopathology of the tumor via biopsy.
- Other radiological testing may occasionally be used (i.e., CT colonography, air-contrast enema) for patients who cannot undergo complete colonoscopy, though each has inherent limitations that providers should be aware of such as the need for an adequate preparation or failure to identify small lesions.
- Patients that are unable to be cleared prior to surgery due to an obstructing lesion should undergo proximal colon evaluation within 6 months after their operation.
- In select cases of an apparent benign lesion, pretreatment evaluation may be limited to digital rectal examination, colonoscopy, and CEA prior to surgery.
- For patients with known or suspected rectal invasive adenocarcinoma, additional pretreatment staging is appropriate.

Locoregional Imaging

Computed Tomography

- Although computed tomography (CT) is routinely performed to exclude distant metastatic disease, it has limited ability to define the mesorectal fascial layers and layers of the rectal wall. Although CT can suggest tumor invasion into surrounding structures, tumor involvement of an adjacent organ or the pelvic sidewall is not entirely accurate and is only inferred by the loss of the fat plane between the tumor and the adjacent organ or structure.

Endorectal Ultrasound

- On endorectal ultrasound (ERUS), the bowel wall is defined by five distinct sonographic layers of alternating hyper- and hypoechoic qualities. Extending from the lumen outward, these layers correspond to (1) the interface between the ultrasound probe and the mucosa, (2) the interface between the mucosa and muscularis mucosa, (3) the submucosa, (4) the muscularis propria, and (5) the serosa or pericolic fat. The prefix "u" is used to describe ERUS, T, and N staging of rectal cancer (Figs. 27.1, 27.2, 27.3, 27.4 and 27.5).
- The advantage of ERUS is that it can be performed in the surgeon's office as part of the initial evaluation of the patient, and it is inexpensive compared to CT or MR. The patient is given an enema to evacuate the rectum prior to the procedure. The procedure is often combined with a flexible or rigid proctosigmoidoscopy. The probe can be passed through a rigid proctoscope to assess proximal tumors.
- The ultrasound probe needs to pass proximal to the tumor in order to evaluate the entire extent of the tumor, thus making it difficult or impossible with obstructing lesions.

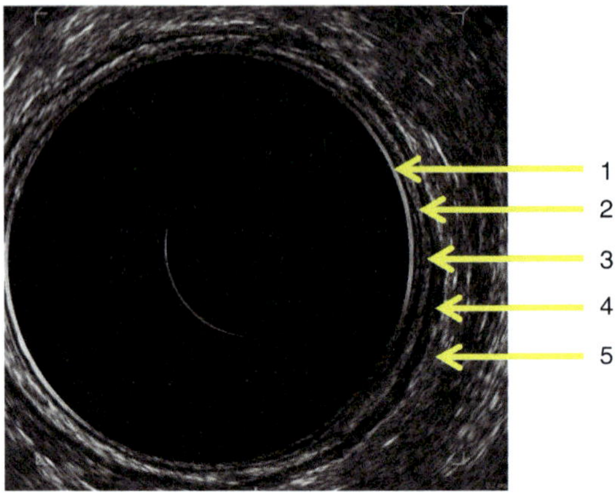

Fig. 27.1 Endosonographic layers of the rectal wall. (1) Interphase of endoscopic balloon with mucosa. (2) Interphase of mucosa/submucosa. (3) Submucosa. (4) Muscularis propria. (5) Serosa and pericolic fat

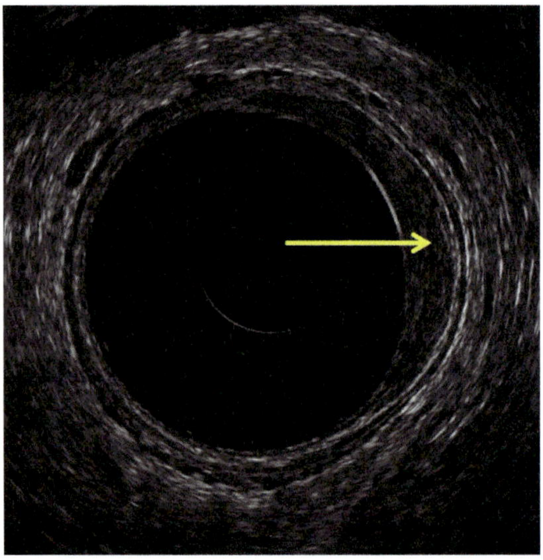

Fig. 27.2 ERUS of uT0 tumor. Hypoechoic tumor (arrow) does not invade into the first hyperechoic layer. Notice the submucosa (white layer) remains intact

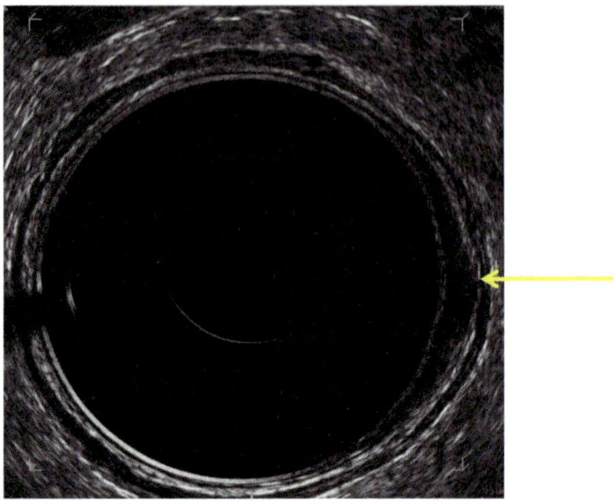

Fig. 27.3 ERUS of uT1 tumor. Hypoechoic tumor invades into the middle hyperechoic layer (arrow) but does not invade the outer hypoechoic layer

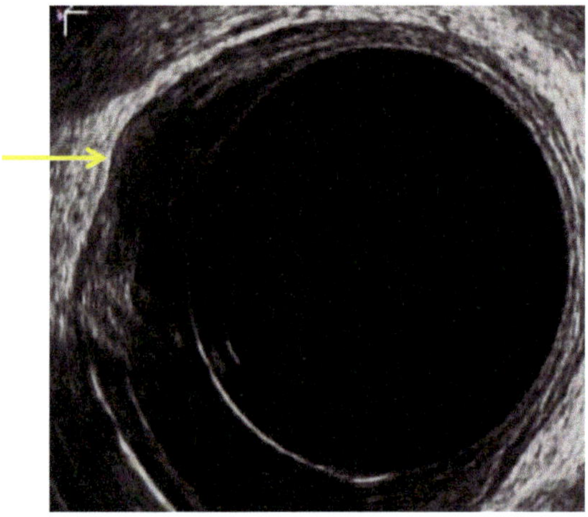

Fig. 27.4 ERUS of uT2 tumor. Hypoechoic tumor invades through the middle hyperechoic layer and into the outer hypoechoic layer

- 3-D ultrasonography records the image in real time and allows for subsequent manipulation of the image for axial, coronal, and sagittal evaluation.
- Malignant lymph nodes appear as hypoechoic and rounded peritumoral structures, whereas benign lymph nodes are less likely to be detected as they are isoechoic with the perirectal fat.
- Limitations to ERUS for staging rectal cancer include incomplete exams due to tumors that are bulky or stenotic and inadequate contact of the ultrasound probe with the tumor due to air or stool in the rectum or angulation of the tumor. Operator experience has also been shown to play a role in the accuracy of ERUS staging. Some patients require sedation to allay discomfort or anxiety.

T Staging

- The reported accuracy of ERUS in accessing the T stage of rectal cancer ranges from 63% to 96% (Table 27.1).

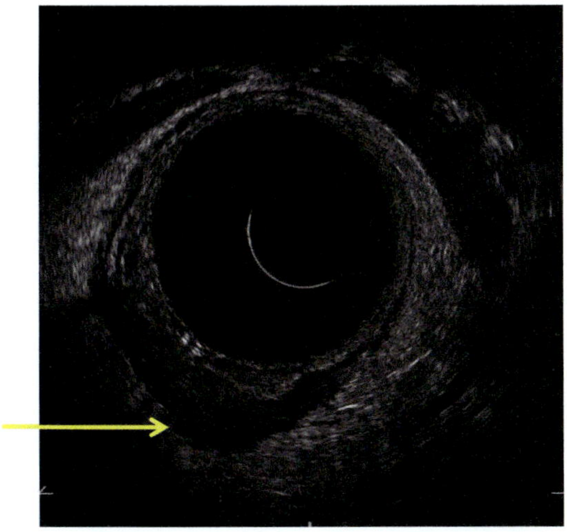

Fig. 27.5 ERUS of uT3 tumor. Tumor extends through the second hypoechoic layer and into the outer hyperechoic layer (arrow)

Table 27.1 ERUS accuracy compared to histological stage

T Stage	Pooled sensitivity	Pooled specificity
T1	87.8% (95% CI 85.3–90.0%)	98.3% (95% CI 97.8–98.7%)
T2	80.5% (95% CI 77.9–82.9%)	95.6% (95% CI 94.9–96.3%)
T3	96.4% (95% CI 95.4–97.2%)	90.6% (95% CI 89.5–91.7%)
T4	95.4% (95% CI 92.4–97.5%)	98.3% (95% CI 97.8–98.7%)

Meta-analysis of 42 studies, $N = 5039$ patients
Adapted from Puli S, et al. How good is endoscopic ultrasound in differentiating various t stages of rectal cancer? Meta-analysis and systematic review. Ann Surg Oncol. 2009; 16:254–65

- As with many interpretive studies, operator experience plays a significant role in staging accuracy.
- Several investigators have demonstrated a lower accuracy of ERUS in detecting T2 tumors compared to T1, T3, or T4.
- However, other investigators have demonstrated the utility of ERUS in the selection of patients with early-stage rectal cancer (T0, T1) who may benefit from transanal excision instead of traditional transabdominal rectal resection.

Table 27.2 Meta-analysis of magnetic resonance accuracy in T stage, N stage, and circumferential resection margin (CRM)

	Specificity
T stage 19 studies ($N = 1986$)	75% (95% CI 68–80)
N stage 12 studies ($N = 1249$)	71% (95% CI 59–81)
CRM 10 studies ($N = 986$)	94% (95% CI 88–97)

Adapted from Al-Sukhni E, et al. Diagnostic accuracy of MRI for assessment of T category, lymph node metastases, and circumferential resection margin involvement in patients with rectal cancer: a systematic review and meta-analysis. Ann Surge Oncol. 2012; 19:2212–23

N Staging

- Accuracy for detecting metastatic lymph nodes by endorectal ultrasound is less precise than for T staging, with a variable accuracy in reported studies of 63%–85%.
- Further complicating the analysis is that different investigators have used different size and morphology criteria for nodal involvement with tumor.
- Staging accuracy for lymph node metastasis improves when the findings are associated with the T stage, with a higher risk of metastasis correlating with higher T stage.

Magnetic Resonance

- High-resolution magnetic resonance (MR) with phased array pelvic coils is being increasingly used in the preoperative assessment of rectal cancer given its improved ability to evaluate the at-risk surgical circumferential resection margin (Table 27.2).
- The pelvic coil is a wraparound surface coil placed around the pelvis. Patients are prepared with an enema on the morning of the examination. Thin-section (3-mm) T2-weighted fast spin-echo sequences are obtained in a plane orthogonal to the tumor. Higher-resolution MRI allows improved definition of bowel and tumor infiltration.
- MR with endorectal coil is no longer recommended. Although endorectal MRI can show five layers of the rectal wall, the field of view is limited, and the mesorectal fascia is not

always visible. Additionally, the endorectal coil is more uncomfortable to the patient than the external coil and cannot be inserted in stenosing tumors. Endorectal coil also has the potential to distort the tissues.

- Three layers of the rectal are visible on a phased array external MR. The innermost mucosa is thin and hypointense, the middle submucosa is hyperintense, and the outer muscularis propria is darkly hypointense.
- Below the peritoneal reflection, the rectum is surrounded by the mesorectal fat (MRF) which is limited by the thin mesorectal fascia, which fuses with the retroprostatic or retrovaginal fascia anteriorly and the presacral fascia posteriorly. The MRF surrounds the rectum completely only in the lower third and is best seen laterally as a thin hypointense line on T2W sequences. Inferiorly, the MRF thins out as it reaches the levator ani, which forms the roof of the ischiorectal fossa.
- MR is the best imaging modality to identify this avascular plane surrounding the mesorectum, which includes the mesorectum in its fascial envelope—the circumferential radial margin (CRM) (Fig. 27.6) and invasion of the anal sphincter musculature (Fig. 27.7).
- As with other radiographic techniques, prediction of N stage is less accurate than for T stage. However, MR appears to be the most

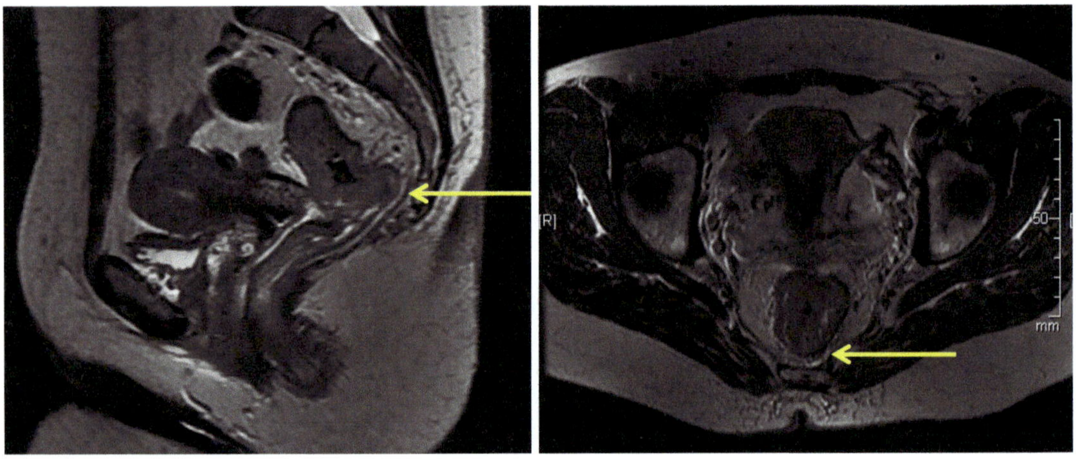

Fig. 27.6 MR of cT3 tumor. Circumferential resection margin is preserved (arrows)

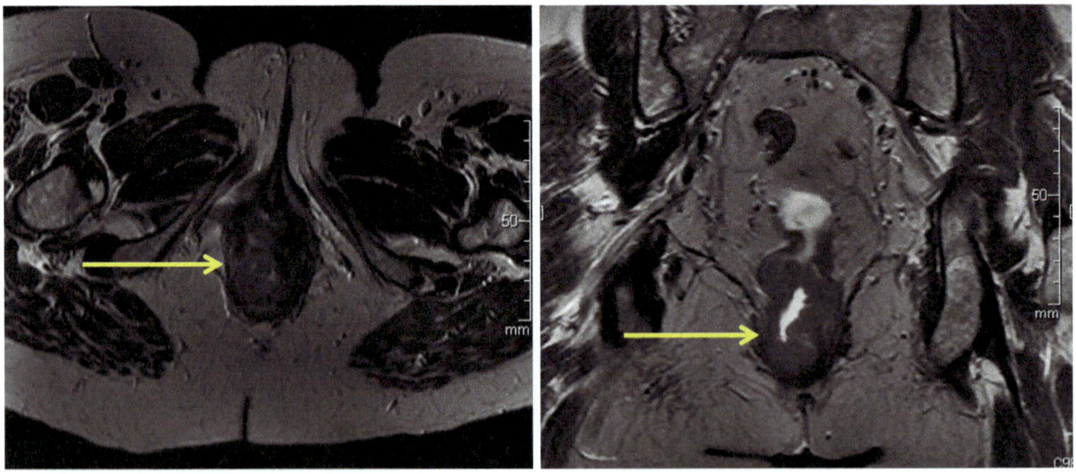

Fig. 27.7 MR of cT4 tumor. Tumor invades the anal sphincter and levator ani (arrows)

accurate of the imaging modalities currently employed. A variety of advanced techniques are being employed by various investigators in an attempt to improve nodal staging accuracy with MR.

- MR limitations include foreign bodies in patients that are MR incompatible. Foreign bodies that are compatible, such as surgical clips, may also obscure images. Movement-related artifacts may preclude accurate visualization of the rectal wall. MR is not portable to the operating room and is more expensive than ERUS.
- Many referral centers with an expertise in rectal cancer treatment are now utilizing MR as the preferred locoregional staging evaluation, especially for locally advanced tumors. ERUS is utilized for evaluation of early-stage lesions or used in combination with MR for select patients.

Whole-Body Imaging

Computed Tomography

- CT of the chest, abdomen, and pelvis is indicated in patients with rectal cancer to evaluate for distant metastasis, primarily of the liver and lung (Fig. 27.8). The overall sensitivity of CT for liver metastases ranges from 77% to 94%. Most lesions measuring over 1 cm in size can be reliably differentiated from benign liver lesions (such as cysts or hemangiomas). However, for lesions under 1 cm in size, sensitivities drop to as low as 40%. The finding of small nonspecific hypodensities measuring <1 cm (also known as "too small to characterize" hypodensities) is very common, perhaps present in as many as 17% of all patients. In the majority of cases, even in those patients with a known underlying malignancy, these small hypodensities in the liver are likely to be benign (~90%) and can be further evaluated with liver MR or simply followed over time.
- Evaluation of lung metastases is also an important component of CT staging.

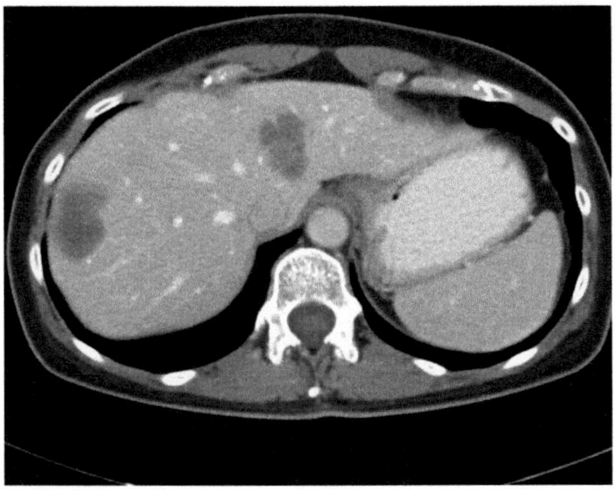

Fig. 27.8 CT of the abdomen demonstrating two liver metastases

Positron Emission Tomography (PET)

- PET is a whole-body nuclear medicine imaging examination utilizing 2-[18F] fluoro-2-deoxy-D-glucose (FDG) that exploits the increased rate of glycolysis in tumor cells to detect tumor. FDG is a glucose analog that is taken up by cellular glucose transport mechanisms and is phosphorylated by hexokinase. Most malignant cells have an increased metabolism of glucose and thus take up the FDG at a greater rate than surrounding tissues. FDG-6-phosphate then becomes metabolically "trapped" intracellularly, because of the relative lack of glucose-6-phosphatase activity in tumor cells. PET detects the increased FDG uptake.
- FDG uptake can be assessed both qualitatively (via visual examination of the degree of uptake of a tumor relative to other tissues) and quantitatively (via a SUV value). While PET was traditionally performed as a stand-alone examination, these studies are now typically performed in conjunction with CT to allow for more precise correlation of FDG activity with anatomy.
- Although PET has been demonstrated to be more accurate in the assessment of whole-body tumor burden than a combination of conventional imaging, it does have limitations.

There is a limit to the resolution of the scan, and lesions less than 1–2 cm may be missed. This makes accurate assessment of nodal metastases difficult. In addition, the activity of the primary tumor may interfere with detection of mesorectal lymph nodes due to the proximity of the primary rectal tumor. Lastly, mucinous adenocarcinomas may not be detected, given that the FDG uptake per unit volume of tissue is reduced as compared to non-mucinous tumor.

- The role of PET in the management of patients with primary rectal adenocarcinoma is to investigate equivocal findings on CT, when the detection of metastatic disease would change treatment strategy. In addition, PET should also be performed prior to consideration of resection of distant metastatic disease or local pelvic recurrence, to exclude incurable occult disease that would make operation palliative rather than curative. PET is extremely useful in the differentiation of pelvic scar from recurrent tumor in those patients who have undergone proctectomy for rectal adenocarcinoma.
- PET has been evaluated as a potential technique to determine histologic response to neoadjuvant chemoradiotherapy and better identify patients for local excision or nonoperative therapy, but, like CT, MR and ERUS, has not been found to be accurate in the assessment of residual tumor in the pelvis. At present, PET is not recommended in the routine evaluation of patients presenting with primary rectal adenocarcinoma but is utilized to evaluate equivocal findings on CT when finding distant metastatic disease would alter management.

Rectal Cancer: Neoadjuvant Therapy

28

Andrea Cercek and Julio Garcia-Aguilar

Key Concepts

- Neoadjuvant radiotherapy is associated with an improvement in local pelvic control following proctectomy for rectal cancer as compared to surgery alone.
- Neoadjuvant chemoradiotherapy is associated with an improvement in local pelvic control and has lower toxicity as compared to postoperative chemoradiotherapy.
- Short-course neoadjuvant radiotherapy has been demonstrated to have similar outcomes in terms of overall survival, disease-free survival, and local pelvic control when compared to long-course neoadjuvant chemoradiotherapy and is associated with lower cost and shorter time to multidrug systemic cytotoxic chemotherapy.
- Current research is focused on limiting the morbidity of therapy, by omitting either proctectomy or radiotherapy in select patients.

A. Cercek
Department of Medicine, Memorial Sloan Kettering Cancer Center, New York, NY, USA

J. Garcia-Aguilar (✉)
Department of Surgery, Memorial Sloan Kettering Cancer Center, New York, NY, USA
e-mail: garciaaj@mskcc.org

S. R. Steele et al. (eds.), *The ASCRS Manual of Colon and Rectal Surgery*,
https://doi.org/10.1007/978-3-030-01165-9_28

Introduction

- Neoadjuvant therapy is a critical component of the multidisciplinary treatment of patients with rectal cancer. The objective of neoadjuvant therapy, either radiotherapy, combined chemoradiotherapy, or chemotherapy alone, is to reduce the risk of local recurrence in patients with locally advanced rectal cancer undergoing surgical resection.
- Neoadjuvant therapy provides other potential advantages to rectal cancer patients. It allows early assessment of tumor responsiveness to therapy, which is closely correlated with long-term oncologic outcomes.
- Neoadjuvant therapy could potentially enable the consideration of organ preservation by allowing for more effective local excision and nonoperative management strategies.
- Delivering systemic chemotherapy before surgery in patients at risk for distant metastasis has the potential to improve survival by addressing micrometastatic disease earlier and improving treatment compliance.
- In this chapter, we will focus primarily on neoadjuvant therapy for locally advanced rectal cancer (LARC), widely accepted to be clinical stage II (cT3–T4, cN0) or stage III (any cT, cN1–N2) invasive adenocarcinomas of the rectum.

Historical Context

- The story of neoadjuvant radiotherapy and chemoradiotherapy for patients suffering from rectal cancer is long and convoluted, and although much has been published on the topic, there is no universally agreed upon treatment strategy. It is important for the reader to understand how we arrived at our current state of affairs so that the data from published trials can be put in the proper context.
- The concept of neoadjuvant therapy for rectal cancer was first introduced by Janeway and Quick in c. 1917, who noted significant tumor response when gold-filtered radon emanation seeds were implanted directly into rectal cancers. In the era when the surgical mortality and morbidity for a rectal cancer operation were prohibitive, contact radiation with emanation seeds containing radium salts or radon was explored as a curative treatment. Surgery was considered a salvage procedure for patients with tumors resistant to radiation.
- As surgery became safer and the limitations of contact radiation as the only treatment modality became apparent, radiation lost its role as a primary treatment and became an adjuvant to surgical resection. In fact, for many years, proctectomy alone became the standard treatment for rectal cancer.
- It was eventually realized that the outcomes of surgery alone were often suboptimal, with 5-year local recurrence rates in published trials of 25–30%. It was demonstrated that adjuvant chemoradiotherapy improved oncologic outcomes, and in 1990 the National Institutes of Health advocated adjuvant external beam radiotherapy and chemotherapy for patients with stage II and stage III tumors. In the United States, except for a few select referral centers, upfront proctectomy followed by selective postoperative chemoradiotherapy was the regimen utilized for most patients.
- However, postoperative radiotherapy is associated with relatively high toxicity and is poorly tolerated by many patients. Investigators in Europe and select US centers explored utilizing neoadjuvant radiotherapy and chemoradiotherapy, and eventually the benefits of administering radiotherapy in the preoperative period were demonstrated.
- In response to these data, many US clinicians simply moved the chemoradiotherapy package from the postoperative to the preoperative period.
- It is puzzling that, although much of the data demonstrating the benefits of neoadjuvant radiotherapy came from trials of short-course radiotherapy, and neoadjuvant short-course radiotherapy has been demonstrated to have similar oncologic outcomes as neoadjuvant long-course chemoradiotherapy in two prospective randomized trials, the use of short-course radiotherapy has been limited in the United States.
- At the same time that neoadjuvant radiotherapy was demonstrated to be more effective and less toxic than postoperative radiotherapy, there was a realization that oncologic outcomes following proctectomy for rectal cancer were highly technique dependent. Wide variability in outcomes was seen, depending on who did the operation and how it was performed.
- So once again the wheel of opinion turned full circle, with some surgeons arguing that radiotherapy primarily compensated for "sloppy" surgery and that there was no need for the patient with non-fixed tumors to undergo radiotherapy if proctectomy was performed properly. Data from the Dutch rectal cancer trial and others, however, suggested that the oncologic benefits of neoadjuvant radiotherapy and good surgical technique were additive, not compensatory, with regard to pelvic control.
- Clinicians understand that our therapies for rectal cancer are morbid, unfortunately with the most effective treatment (i.e., proctectomy) associated with the greatest chance of lasting morbidity. We continue to search for treatment regimens in which morbidity can be lessened while preserving the chance for cure, especially in patients with non-fixed tumors. Definitive chemoradiotherapy, or local

excision +/– adjuvant chemoradiotherapy, would avoid proctectomy.

- Chemotherapy regimens are now more effective, and there is interest in upfront proctectomy in patients with mesorectal margins that are not threatened based on preoperative imaging followed by selective use of postoperative chemotherapy. In addition, there is interest in the use of neoadjuvant chemotherapy alone. Both of these strategies would avoid the toxicity of radiotherapy.
- Another approach that has been utilized extensively in Europe and in select US centers is to administer neoadjuvant short-course radiotherapy, followed by proctectomy and selective use of postoperative chemotherapy.
- The three aforementioned strategies allow the patient to receive effective systemic chemotherapy faster than the regimen commonly employed in the United States – long-course chemoradiotherapy (in which the patient receives only a radiosensitizing chemotherapeutic agent) followed by delayed proctectomy. This concept has intrinsic appeal given that most patients with rectal cancer who ultimately fail treatment succumb to distant metastatic disease, not local pelvic recurrence, and that the benefit of neoadjuvant radiotherapy has primarily been to improve pelvic control without improvement in overall survival.
- One of the difficulties in constructing guidelines for treatment of patients with rectal cancer is that treatment decisions must take into account multiple variables: tumor fixation, circumferential position in the rectum, relation to the pelvic floor musculature, pelvic morphology, clinical T and N stage, presence of symptoms, presence of metastases, continence status, planned operation, etc. It is virtually impossible to publish straightforward guidelines that account for all of these variables.
- At present, the clinician caring for the patient with rectal cancer must have a firm grasp of the rationale for, and the data supporting, any proposed treatment algorithm and be facile enough to tailor recommendations for therapy based on the characteristics of the patient and the tumor.

Postoperative Radiotherapy

- Although currently out of favor, one of the advantages of the strategy of upfront proctectomy followed by selective chemoradiotherapy is that the exact stage of the tumor is known prior to initiation of radiotherapy, and radiation can be avoided in patients with early-stage tumors who may not derive benefit.
- A number of studies demonstrated that surgery followed by radiation, delivered in 180–200 cGy a day for a total dose of 45–50 Gy, was more effective than surgery alone in achieving a local control in patients with stage II or III rectal cancer.
- However, postoperative chemoradiotherapy has been clearly demonstrated to be less effective and more toxic than neoadjuvant chemoradiotherapy and should thus be reserved for unusual circumstances.

Preoperative Radiotherapy

- Neoadjuvant radiotherapy has been demonstrated to improve local pelvic control versus surgery alone. Most of these trials were performed using short-course radiotherapy.
  - The Swedish Rectal Cancer Trial demonstrated that short-course preoperative radiation (25 Gy of radiation delivered in five equal doses in five consecutive days) not only improved local recurrence but also overall survival.
  - However, this study was later criticized because surgery was not standardized and the rate of local recurrence in the control arm was considered high for those years' standards.
  - The Dutch Rectal Cancer Trial (CKVO 95-04) was the first to prove that preoperative radiation also reduced the risk of local recurrence rate in patients having optimal surgery according to the principles of total mesorectal excision. While no benefit in overall survival was observed for the entire group, the 12-year updated results

demonstrated that preoperative short-term radiotherapy significantly improved 10-year survival in patients with stage III disease and negative circumferential margins, and the benefit in terms of local control persisted.

Radiosensitizing Agents

- Further improvements in local tumor control have been achieved by adding systemic chemotherapy to radiotherapy. Numerous chemotherapeutic agents including fluoropyrimidines (5-FU) and capecitabine; irinotecan, oxaliplatin, and anti-epidermal growth factor agents; and cetuximab and panitumumab have been tested in the neoadjuvant setting with radiotherapy. With the exception of fluoropyrimidines, however, none have been effectively validated in prospective trials.

Preoperative Versus Postoperative Radiation

- Although there was once great debate on this subject, the preponderance of the evidence supports the use of neoadjuvant radiotherapy versus postoperative adjuvant radiotherapy.
- The rationale for this approach is logical: neoadjuvant radiotherapy requires less of a dose to achieve the same biologic effect, most likely due to the absence of postoperative scarring and tissue hypoxia in the pelvis.
- The toxicity, both short term and long term, of neoadjuvant therapy is markedly reduced compared to postoperative radiotherapy, especially when the patient undergoes neorectal reconstruction.
- The proportion of patients who can complete that therapy is markedly improved when radiotherapy is administered in the preoperative period.
- A commonly employed treatment paradigm for locally advanced rectal cancer is preoperative 5-FU-based chemoradiotherapy, followed by proctectomy and additional 5-FU-based adjuvant chemotherapy. Specifically, patients receive combined radiation (180 cGy/day/5 days a week for 5 weeks followed by a 540 cGy boost) and chemotherapy (either continuous infusion 5-FU or capecitabine), followed by proctectomy 6–8 weeks later, and postoperative systemic adjuvant chemotherapy, usually mFOLFOX6 (Fig. 28.1).

Short- Versus Long-Course Preoperative Radiotherapy

- To compare different dose-fractionation schedules, radiation therapists have introduced the concept of biologically equivalent doses. The most common dose-fractionation schedules used in rectal cancer, 1.8–2 Gy per day, 5 days per week for 5 weeks (usually in combination with a fluoropyrimidine), and 5 Gy per day for 5 consecutive days, are considered biologically equivalent.
- The advantages and disadvantages of each one of these regimens have been the subject of a heated debate. Proponents of long-course chemoradiotherapy point to a greater tumor response, although this may be an artifact of the greater time delay prior to proctectomy typically utilized after long-course chemoradiotherapy (typically 6–8 weeks) as compared to after short-course radiotherapy (typically 1 week). Those in favor of short-course radiation argue that improved patient convenience, lower cost, reduced toxicity in the neoadjuvant treatment period, and faster time to effective systemic chemotherapy are important advantages. Two trials have compared these two approaches directly.
- Three prospective randomized trials have demonstrated no obvious oncologic differences between neoadjuvant long-course chemoradiotherapy and neoadjuvant short-course radiotherapy for patients with cT3 and cT4 disease.
- The short-course/long-course divide has remained somewhat static across national boundaries, with a Western preference for long-course chemoradiotherapy and a majority of

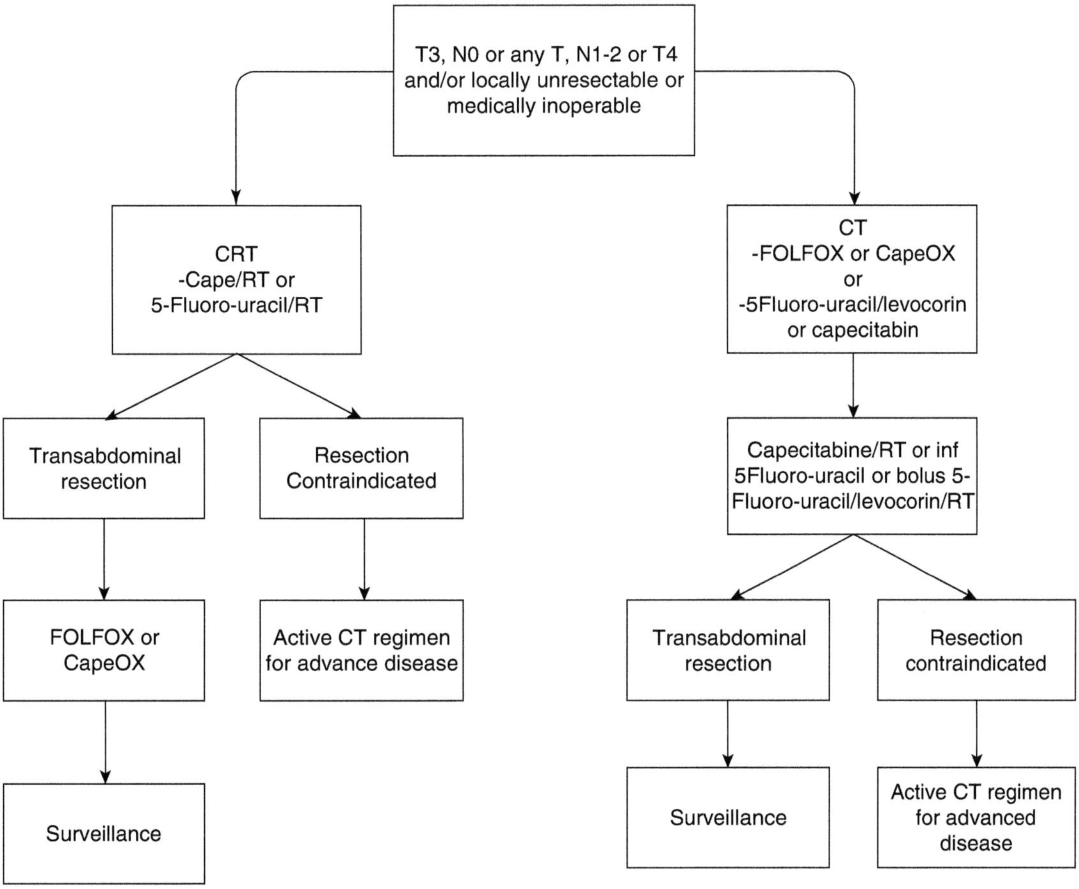

Fig. 28.1 National Comprehensive Cancer Network guidelines for locally advanced rectal cancer. Permission from JCO/NCCN (Cape, capecitabine; CapeOx, capecitabine plus oxaliplatin; CRT chemoradiation, CT chemotherapy, FLOX fluorouracil, leucovorin, and oxaliplatin, FOLFOX infusional fluorouracil, leucovorin, and oxaliplatin, FU fluorouracil, inf. infusional, LR local recurrence, LV leucovorin, MRF mesorectal fascia, RT radiotherapy, TME total mesorectal excision). (With permission from Neoadjuvant chemoradiation therapy and pathological complete response in rectal cancer. Gastroenterology Report. Gastroenterol Rep 2015. https://doi.org/10.1093/gastro/gov039, http://gastro.oxfordjournals.org/content/early/2015/08/19/gastro.gov039.full. Copyright ©2015 Oxford University Press and Digestive Science Publishing Co. Limited)

European countries favoring short-course radiotherapy. It is puzzling that, except for a few expert centers, short-course radiotherapy has not been embraced by US physicians. One could argue that it is the best-studied neoadjuvant radiotherapy regimen, with demonstrated efficacy in prospective randomized trials of neoadjuvant radiotherapy versus surgery alone, and shortens the time to administration of full-dose adjuvant cytotoxic chemotherapy, which is of critical importance given that most patients treated by experienced surgeons who die of their disease suffer from distant metastases rather than local failure.

- Because of a current trend exploring the incorporation of therapies traditionally reserved for the adjuvant period into the neoadjuvant regimen, combinations of either short-course radiotherapy or long-course chemoradiotherapy with systemic therapies are being explored and gaining greater traction. Therefore it may never be clearly determined whether short-course or long-course RT is more effective as independent modalities.

- Future treatment of patients with rectal cancer may involve "total neoadjuvant therapy," in which a complete course of chemotherapy is administered, with neoadjuvant short- or long-course radiotherapy administered prior to proctectomy or, if a complete clinical response is appreciated, enrollment in a nonoperative observation protocol.

Impact of Pelvic Radiotherapy on Quality of Life

- Another quoted advantage of preoperative radiotherapy is the potential ability to downstage tumors and to increase the potential for sphincter-sparing surgery, which can improve long-term quality of life for patients with low-lying rectal cancers. The issue of sphincter salvage, however, is complicated. As one might imagine, the assessment of whether a restorative proctectomy could possibly be performed based on initial evaluation of a patient is somewhat subjective. In addition, given that radiotherapy does not kill tumor in a wavefront, and that multiple studies have demonstrated residual tumor scattered throughout the bed of the initial volume of tissue involved with the tumor, many surgeons would argue that changing the operation based on the clinically observed effect of radiotherapy is potentially dangerous.
- Unfortunately, pelvic radiotherapy remains associated with significant short- and long-term side effects. Overall short-term toxicity has been reported in as many as 50% of patients. Long-term side effects of pelvic radiotherapy include fibrosis and autonomic nerve injury, which can lead to bowel and bladder dysfunction, sexual dysfunction, and infertility due to hormonal effects and uterine incompetence. Moreover, because the pelvis is an active site of bone marrow function, patients who undergo pelvic irradiation can suffer from diminished hematopoiesis.
- The fact that prospective randomized trials have demonstrated improvements in local pelvic control without improvements in overall survival raises the issue of an adverse effect of radiotherapy that is, to date, not well characterized. Otherwise, one would logically assume that improvement in pelvic control should produce an equal improvement in survival.

Adjuvant Systemic Chemotherapy in Patients Treated with Chemoradiotherapy and Proctectomy

- Although prevention of local recurrences is important for patients' quality of life, most patients with rectal cancer succumb to metastatic disease. Consequently, similar to patients with stage III colon cancer, patients with locally advanced rectal cancer treated with neoadjuvant chemoradiotherapy and proctectomy are considered for postoperative adjuvant chemotherapy independent of the histologic tumor stage in the proctectomy specimen.
- Patients with clinical stage II and III rectal cancer treated with preoperative chemoradiotherapy and proctectomy usually receive 5-FU or capecitabine plus oxaliplatin-based adjuvant chemotherapy.
- While the use of postoperative adjuvant chemotherapy in rectal cancer is not supported unequivocally by a prospective randomized trial, a recent meta-analysis of 21 randomized controlled trials concluded that postoperative 5-FU-based chemotherapy is effective in patients with locally advanced rectal cancer.
- Due to the low rate of completion of planned postoperative adjuvant therapy, splitting adjuvant chemotherapy and delivering a limited number of cycles pre-chemoradiotherapy and then delivering the remaining cycles post-surgery have been proposed to increase tumor response in locally advanced rectal cancer patients. A number of randomized phase II trials have reported mixed results, without clear survival advantage for the split neoadjuvant or the postoperative regimen.
- Another potential approach is to deliver all chemotherapies upfront. This neoadjuvant

chemotherapy has several potential advantages compared to the standard adjuvant chemotherapy; it theoretically treats occult micrometastasis several months earlier and increases treatment compliance, potentially enhancing the efficacy of chemotherapy and ultimately improving survival. Other benefits of neoadjuvant chemotherapy include increased response of the primary tumor, early identification of nonresponders, and earlier takedown of the loop ileostomy if patients have had a restorative proctectomy. Induction chemotherapy before chemoradiation and proctectomy is now considered as a valid alternative to the more widely accepted neoadjuvant chemoradiation, proctectomy, and postoperative systemic chemotherapy (Fig. 28.1).

- Chemotherapy can also be delivered as consolidation (after chemoradiotherapy completion and before surgery). Although solid data from large prospective studies are still lacking, in the most recent edition of the NCCN guidelines, neoadjuvant chemotherapy is contemplated as an option for the treatment of locally advanced rectal cancer patients.

Choosing Optimal Treatment Regimens

- Chemoradiotherapy has proved itself useful at improving local tumor control in patients with locally advanced rectal cancer. We find that the weight of evidence is also demonstrating that systemic chemotherapy – when applied in the neoadjuvant setting – is able to similarly control tumor progression, possibly acting on micrometastatic disease to improve distant control. But while the benefits of these intensive neoadjuvant regimens are alluring, they have also sparked a heated debate about whether all patients require such intensive treatment. The oncologic success in treating locally advanced rectal cancer has been achieved at the cost of significant morbidity and compromised quality of life. The task before us is to develop treatment approaches that maximize oncological outcome while preserving quality of life by minimizing morbidity associated with this intense multimodality approach. Do all patients with locally advanced rectal cancer really require chemoradiotherapy, chemotherapy, and proctectomy? The necessity of this intense multimodality approach is called into question.

The European Approach

- In a number of European countries, treatment decisions are driven by MRI-based measures of tumor aggressiveness. A risk stratification system that covers all rectal cancers and that incorporates the proximity of the primary rectal cancer to the mesorectal fascia, the depth of tumor invasion, the presence of metastatic lymph nodes, and the presence of venous invasion is used to classify locally advanced rectal cancer into "the good," "the bad," and "the ugly." For the low-risk, "good" tumors, proctectomy alone is recommended; for intermediate-risk "bad" tumors, the recommendation is short-course radiotherapy followed by proctectomy; and for high-risk "ugly" tumors, it is chemoradiotherapy followed by proctectomy (Table 28.1). These MRI-based risk stratification schemas have been incorporated into clinical practice guidelines and clinical trial design (e.g., Expert-C and RAPIDO). However, the treatment approach guided by MRI risk categorization is based on prospective observational studies conducted in institutions with significant expertise in rectal cancer and has not been tested in prospective randomized trials. In addition, given that prospective, randomized trials have demonstrated that neoadjuvant short-course radiotherapy produces similar or better oncologic outcomes when combined with cytotoxic chemotherapy, it begs the question as to the choices for "bad" and "ugly" tumors.

Table 28.1 European/Scandinavian model of stratification for patients with locally advanced rectal cancer based on magnetic resonance imaging and subsequent treatment decisions

Risk	Treatment
Low risk T1–T3 (<5 mm) mid-/upper rectum T1–T3 (superficial) lower rectum N0 Extramural vascular invasion: no mesorectal fascia clear Risk of local recurrence <10%	Total mesorectal excision (TME)
Intermediate risk T3 (<5 mm) T4 (posterior vaginal wall only), or N1/2, or Extramural vascular invasion: yes Mesorectal fascia clear (<1 mm) Risk of local recurrence: 10–20%	Preoperative short-course radiation Total mesorectal excision Adjuvant chemotherapy
High risk T4 (other than posterior vaginal wall N01/2 Mesorectal fascia involved Risk of local recurrence >20%	Preoperative chemoradiation Total mesorectal excision Adjuvant chemotherapy

Modified from Smith JJ, Garcia-Aguilar J. Advances and challenges in treatment of locally advanced rectal cancer. J Clin Oncol 2005

Selected Adjuvant Systemic Chemotherapy

- Many locally advanced rectal cancer patients experience variable degrees of response to chemoradiotherapy, and tumor response is now one of the most important prognosticators in locally advanced rectal cancer patients.
- The need for adjuvant chemotherapy in patients with a complete or near-complete response after chemoradiotherapy has been questioned. Data from recent trials suggest that patients with ypN+ disease derive more benefit from postoperative adjuvant chemotherapy than patients with ypN0 disease.
- Identification of those patients most likely to derive benefit from adjuvant treatment will be better informed by carefully conducted correlative studies that more accurately delineate molecular, pathologic, and clinical markers of resistance.

Chemotherapy Only to Improve Local Tumor Control

- The risk of local pelvic failure in locally advanced rectal cancer depends on tumor stage, but also on the distance of the tumor from the anal verge, and the proximity of the tumor from the mesorectal fascia. Upper rectal tumors away from the mesorectal fascia have a low risk of local recurrence when treated with proctectomy. The added benefit of radiotherapy in these patients has been questioned.
- A growing body of evidence suggests that radiotherapy could be safely avoided in patients with intermediate-risk rectal cancer (e.g., rectal cancers located between 5 and 12 cm from the anal verge that do not threaten the mesorectal fascia) on MRI.
- In the ongoing CALGB PROSPECT Study (*P*reoperative *R*adiation *O*r *S*elective *P*reoperative *E*valuation of *C*hemotherapy and *T*ME), patients with mid-proximal rectal cancer are randomized to either the standard arm (chemoradiotherapy, surgery, and adjuvant FOLFOX chemotherapy) or the selective arm with FOLFOX × 6 cycles, evaluation of response followed by surgery or standard therapy with chemoradiotherapy if the reduction in the primary tumor is <20% (Fig. 28.2).

Selective Nonoperative Management

- Proctectomy is the cornerstone of the treatment algorithm for locally advanced rectal cancer patients. However, up to 33% of locally advanced rectal cancer patients treated with neoadjuvant chemoradiotherapy exhibit a pathologic complete response (pCR) at the time of surgical resection.
- Patients with a pCR have improved oncologic outcomes with local recurrence rates of less than 1% and a 5-year survival rate of over 90%, leading us to question the added benefit of proctectomy for these patients. The potential gains of avoiding proctectomy – reduced morbidity, improvement in quality of life, and

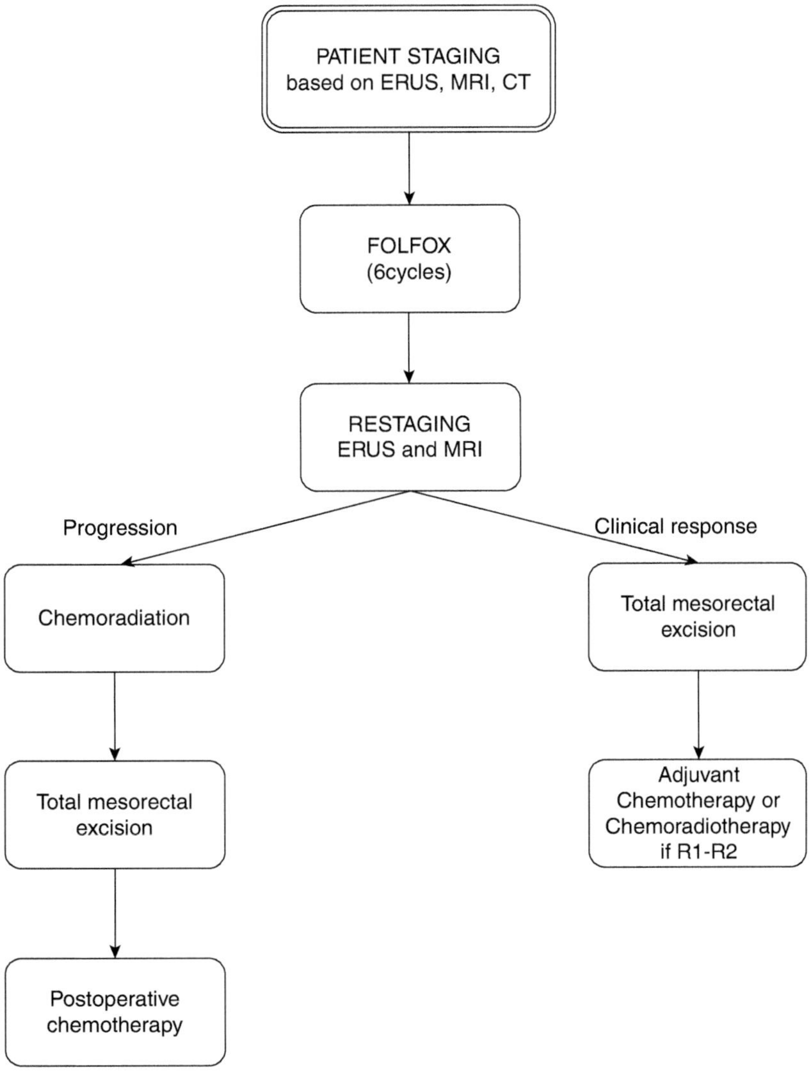

Fig. 28.2 PROSPECT (chemotherapy alone or chemotherapy plus radiation therapy in treating patients with locally advanced cancer undergoing surgery) trial schema. A phase II/III randomized study designed to evaluate the impact of the selective use of radiotherapy compared with nonselective use of chemoradiation for patients with locally advanced rectal cancer. (*FOLFOX* infusional fluorouracil, leucovorin, and oxaliplatin, LAR low anterior resection, FUCMT fluorouracil or capecitabine plus radiotherapy, TME total mesorectal excision). (With permission from Neoadjuvant chemoradiation therapy and pathological complete response in rectal cancer. Gastroenterology Report. Gastroenterol Rep 2015. https://doi.org/10.1093/gastro/gov039, http://gastro.oxfordjournals.org/content/early/2015/08/19/gastro.gov039.full. Copyright ©2015 Oxford University Press and Digestive Science Publishing Co. Limited)

potential reduction of healthcare expenses – could be significant.

- The current challenge lies in accurately identifying which patients have achieved a pCR and could safely avoid proctectomy. Although cCR does not always correlate with pCR, and current imaging modalities cannot distinguish with certainty tumor remnants from tissue fibrosis, a number of institutions have reported their experience with the selective use of an organ-preserving or nonoperative management approach in patients with a complete clinical response after chemoradiotherapy, with mixed results (Table 28.2).

Table 28.2 Summary of the most representative series, nonoperative vs. operative management of LARC after CRT

					OS				DFS			
					NOM		Operative arm		NOM		Operative arm	
Series	# cCRs	%	Mean interval to LR	# of patients	Survival	%	Survival	%	Survival	%	Survival	%
Habr-Gama et al.	71	27	60	2	5 years	100	5 years	88	5 years	92	5 years	83
Habr-Gama et al.	90	49	17	28	5 years	91	NA		5 years	68	NA	
Mass et al.	21	11	22	1	2 years	100	2 years	91	2 years	89	2 years	93
Smith et al.	32	NA	11	6	2 years	97	2 years	88	2 years	100	2 years	88
Dalton	12	24	24[a]	6	26 months	100	26 months	100	26 months	100	26 months	100[b]

cCR clinical complete response, *CRT* chemoradiotherapy, *DFS* disease-free survival, *LARC* locally advanced rectal cancer, *LR* local recurrence, *NA* not available, *NOM* nonoperative management, *OS* overall survival, *RT* radiotherapy, *pCR* pathological complete response

[a]mean time to surgery

[b]all 6 with pCR

- Although there are clearly some patients who can be cured without proctectomy, problems with methodology in the reported trials have limited our ability to understand the exact outcomes. In some reports, results were heavily biased in favor of the nonoperative management group.
- The safety and efficacy of the nonoperative management approach outside of centers specializing in the treatment of rectal cancer are controversial. It is now clear that even with strict complete clinical response definitions, some patients will later develop local recurrence, emphasizing the importance of close surveillance, because the success of this approach relies on the early diagnosis of recurrences and timely salvage therapy. In addition, the risk of distant metastases in patients with an apparent complete clinical response that develop local tumor regrowth and subsequent outcomes is unknown.
- The design of large, prospective randomized trials investigating the efficacy of the nonoperative management approach is challenging, given the relatively small proportion of patients with a complete clinical response to standard neoadjuvant chemoradiotherapy and the disparity of the treatment arms – observation versus proctectomy. However a number of prospective observational studies and phase II trials are underway to test the feasibility of incorporating a nonoperative management approach to the multimodality treatment of rectal cancer in a multi-institutional setting.

29 Local Excision of Rectal Neoplasia

Mark H. Whiteford

Key Concepts

1. When anatomically appropriate, local excision is preferred over proctectomy for benign rectal polyps due to high success rates and lower morbidity.
2. If local excision is to be utilized as definitive surgical therapy for rectal cancer, the depth of dissection should be full thickness of the rectal wall.
3. Histologic predictors of lymph node metastasis in early rectal cancers include tumor depth, lymphatic and vascular invasion, poor differentiation, and tumor budding.
4. Five-year disease-free survival after local excision of rectal cancer is lower than after proctectomy, although it is unclear whether overall survival is different.
5. Survival and local recurrence rates for T2 rectal cancers treated with neoadjuvant chemoradiation and local excision appear to be similar to those of T1 cancers treated with local excision alone.
6. Transanal endoscopic surgery may be associated with improved outcomes as compared to conventional transanal excision, although the quality of comparative studies is suboptimal.

M. H. Whiteford (✉)
Providence Portland Medical Center, Providence Cancer Center, Portland, OR, USA

The Oregon Clinic, Gastrointestinal and Minimally Invasive Surgery, Portland, OR, USA

Oregon Health & Science University, Portland, OR, USA
e-mail: mwhiteford@orclinic.com

Transanal Surgery: A Historical Perspective

- The initial report of transanal excision of a rectal tumor is attributed to Dr. Jacques Lisfranc in the early 1800s whereby a protruding and painful rectal tumor was excised via a prolapsing and incising technique. There was no mention of anesthesia, no defect closure was attempted, and hemostasis was eventually maintained with serial intrarectal packing.
- Sir Alan Parks popularized the era of modern transanal excision in the 1960s. This more familiar technique employed anesthesia, a self-retaining rectal retractor, epinephrine injection, a submucosal resection plane, use of stay sutures, and primary closure of the defect.
- In the early 1980s, Prof. Gerhard Buess, inspired by the poor visibility and limited reach of conventional transanal excision, ushered in the era of transanal endoscopic surgery (TES) when he invented a new technique and series of instruments for removal of rectal tumors. His technique and instruments were termed transanal endoscopic microsurgery (TEM, Richard Wolf, GmbH, Knittlingen,

S. R. Steele et al. (eds.), *The ASCRS Manual of Colon and Rectal Surgery*,
https://doi.org/10.1007/978-3-030-01165-9_29

Germany). TEM involves a 4 × 12 (or 20) cm cylindrical metal reusable operating rectoscope mounted to the operating table. The rectoscope has a sealed faceplate with multiple access ports that permit simultaneous pneumodistention of the rectum along with passage of a stereoscopic camera and modified laparoscopic instruments into the rectum. Stable pneumorectum is maintained with a dedicated TEM suction-CO_2 insufflation pump. TEM instruments could now remove larger lesions as well as lesions up to the rectosigmoid junction (~17 cm from the anal verge). A similar reusable rigid proctoscopic transanal endoscopic operation (TEO®) system is also commercially available (Karl Storz, GmbH, Tuttlingen, Germany).

- In 2010, Atallah first described the use of a commercially available single-port laparoscopic platform placed transanally in conjunction with standard laparoscopic instruments and insufflators to perform transanal surgery. This technique has been coined transanal minimally invasive surgery (TAMIS). Due to the similarities of the techniques and clinical results, TEM, TEO, and TAMIS are collectively termed transanal endoscopic surgery (TES).

Techniques

Technique for Conventional Transanal Excision

- Preoperative examination should include digital rectal examination with proctoscopy to determine and document the longitudinal and circumferential location, extent of the lesion, and its proximity to the sphincter. Repeat or deeper biopsy can also be performed if colonoscopic biopsy was nondiagnostic. When concern for malignancy exists, then additional imaging studies such as endoscopic ultrasound, MRI, and CT scan may be considered.
- The patient usually receives a full mechanical bowel prep and perioperative antibiotics. General anesthesia is the most common mode of anesthesia, but spinal anesthesia is an acceptable option.
- Patient positioning is chosen such that the target pathology is placed dependently: lithotomy position for posterior lesions and prone jackknife for anterior and lateral lesions.
- Exposure is obtained via the surgeon's preferred method of self-retaining anal retractor, lighted anoscope, operating proctoscope, and Lone Star® retractor (Cooper Surgical, Inc., Trumbull, CT). A headlight provides ideal illumination in the tightly confined operating field.
- Electrocautery is then utilized to demarcate a 5–10 mm margin around the lesion. Stay sutures may be placed on the normal rectal wall away from the tumor for retraction and improved visibility. Dissection progresses distally, laterally, and then proximally with sharp or electrocautery dissection.
- Depth of dissection is in the submucosal plane for benign-appearing lesions or to avoid sphincter injury and full-thickness dissection for biopsy-proven malignant lesions or lesions with gross features of malignancy.
- Most authors advocate for primary transverse closure as longitudinal closure is thought to predispose to stricture. At times, there may be too much tension to close the defect. These can then either be partially closed or left open to heal by secondary intention if the defect is extraperitoneal (Fig. 29.1).

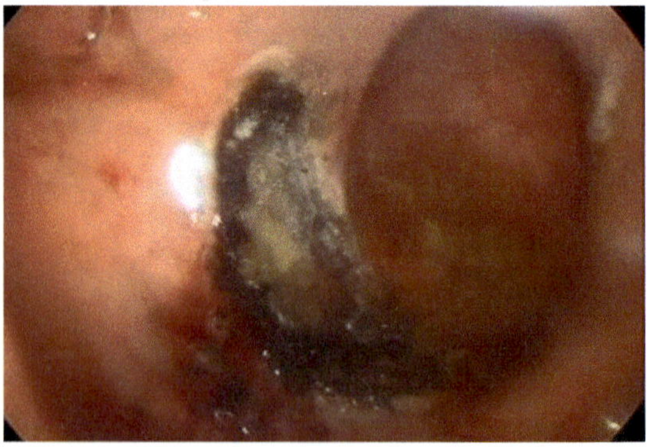

Fig. 29.1 Open wound following local excision

Technique for TEM and TEO

- Bowel preparation, anesthetic choice, and positioning are the same as transanal excision.
- Gentle digital dilation is performed to accommodate the 4-cm-diameter proctoscope, which is then inserted and attached to the table mount. Both 12 and 20 cm lengths are available. The faceplate is attached and tubing connected to the suction insufflator unit. Pneumorectum is established and the proctoscope adjusted to view the target lesion through the stereoscopic microscope or the laparoscopic video monitor.
- Three 5–9 mm instrument ports are available for use of the modified angled TEM laparoscopic instruments. Needle tip electrocautery is utilized to demarcate a 5–10 mm margin around the lesion.
- Submucosal or full-thickness dissection is then initiated. This is most easily started in the distal right corner of the lesion with progression toward the proximal left corner. Partial en bloc resection of the mesorectum has also been described for deeper malignant lesions.
- Continuous suction functions to clear the cautery smoke during the procedure. The integrated suction-insufflation unit prevents loss of pneumorectum from the suctioning.
- Following specimen removal, the defect is closed transversely using a running absorbable suture. A metal clip is locked at each end of the suture in lieu of intracorporeal knot tying. With the increased proximal reach of TEM, intraperitoneal entry occasionally occurs and, in experienced hands, can safely be closed via the TEM instrumentation.
- TEM does suffer from technical limitations of the rigid proctoscope causing significant instrument conflict and has a longer learning curve for both technique and instrument troubleshooting than compared to other transanal techniques (Figs. 29.2, 29.3, and 29.4).

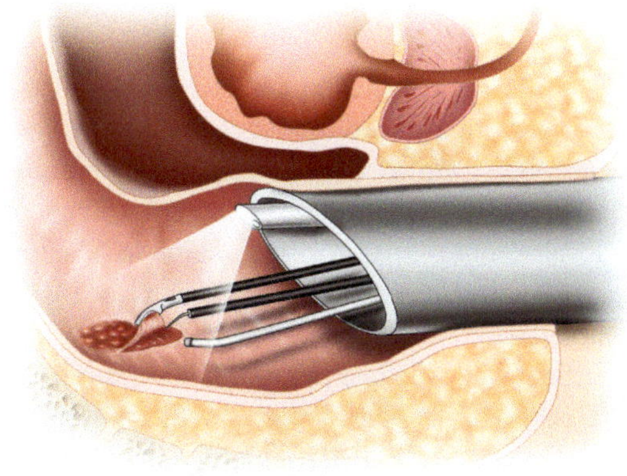

Fig. 29.2 Transanal endoscopic microsurgery

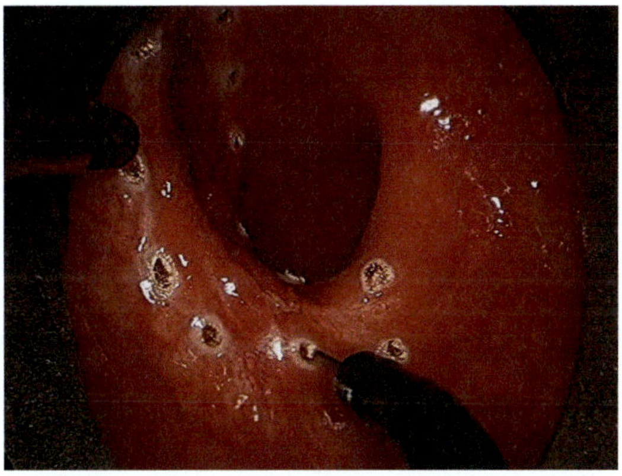

Fig. 29.3 Margin around sessile polyp demarcated with monopolar cautery during TEM. (Courtesy Mark Whiteford, MD)

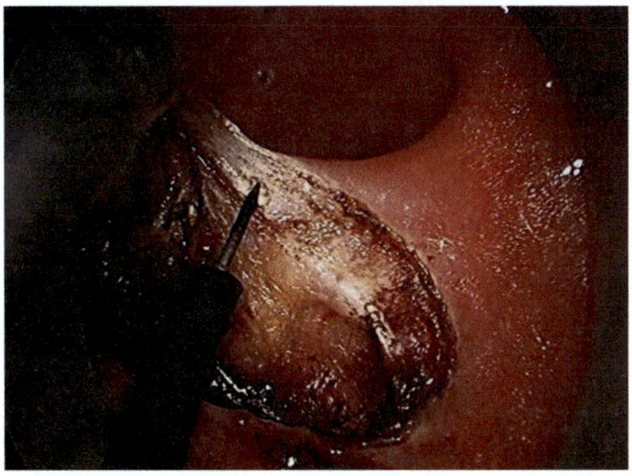

Fig. 29.4 Full-thickness depth of excision during TEM. (Courtesy Mark Whiteford, MD)

Technique for TAMIS

- TAMIS is a modification of TEM whereby the reusable rigid 4-cm-diameter operating proctoscope is replaced by a flexible, disposable single-port laparoscopic platform. Standard laparoscopic insufflators, camera, instruments, and vessel-sealing devices are also utilized.
- Patient selection and preparation are similar to TAE and TEM. The shorter length and flexible platform of the TAMIS technique more easily permit operating on the nondependent (downward) wall of the rectum. For this reason, the majority of cases can be done in the lithotomy position.
- Dissection is performed in a similar fashion as with TEM.
- Laparoscopic suctioning must be done judiciously as not to lose pneumorectum and exposure. A more liberal use of laparoscopic vessel-sealing devices provides improved hemostasis over that of monopolar cautery, thereby reducing the need for suctioning.
- Defect closure techniques vary among authors and include the use of different laparoscopic suturing devices or barbed sutures.
- Intraperitoneal entry during TAMIS is more likely to require laparoscopic assistance for defect closure due to loss of the rectum and visualization of the defect via the transanal device.
- Since the TAMIS devices rely on radial fixation to the top of the sphincter complex, low-lying rectal polyps become partially obscured by the transanal device and require a hybrid TAMIS and TAE resection technique. This involves dissection of the proximal portion of the lesion utilizing the TAMIS technique and then removal of the TAMIS device followed by the conventional TAE technique to complete the distal dissection and defect closure.
- All forms of transanal excision techniques have limitations such as the potential for incomplete resection or the requirement for conversion to an alternate technique, such as staged transanal procedures or need for an abdominal approach to complete the resection or defect closure. These events are more likely when the tumor is too bulky to permit adequate working space, the proximal extent of tumor cannot be visualized around a fold or sigmoid bend, uncontrolled bleeding is encountered, or there is an inadequate bowel preparation.
- Transcoccygeal (Kraske) and transsphincteric (York-Mason) approaches to locally excise rectal neoplasia have largely been supplanted by these purely transanal techniques.

Transanal Excision of Benign Rectal Polyps

- The ideal indication for transanal excision is for the complete removal of benign lesions in the rectum. Radical surgery, in the form of proctectomy, which includes a complete regional lymphadenectomy, provides no clinical benefit over transanal excision in the setting of benign disease yet subjects the patient to considerable perioperative morbidity and significant long-term risk of urinary, sexual, and defecatory dysfunction.
- Local excision also has the advantage of acting as a "total biopsy" to assess for completeness of resection and presence of otherwise occult cancer.
- Most rectal polyps are detected on screening colonoscopy in asymptomatic patients. While most small polyps are readily removed using colonoscopic polypectomy, larger polyps that would generally require piecemeal snare polypectomy are better served with transanal excision which provides a higher chance of complete polyp removal and a resultant lower chance of polyp recurrence. Endoscopists should thus be encouraged to avoid piecemeal endoscopic resection of large rectal polyps and instead refer them for consideration of en bloc transanal excision.
- Larger rectal polyps, particularly villous adenomas, have a higher incidence of harboring an occult cancer despite benign appearance and biopsies. For this reason preoperative assessment with endoscopic ultrasound is

reasonable to further assess tumor and nodal staging.

- Benign polyps can be removed using either a partial-thickness (submucosal plane) or full-thickness technique (deep to muscularis propria). Partial-thickness dissection is facilitated through the use of submucosal injection of saline with or without epinephrine to help raise the polyp and mucosa off the muscularis propria. A non-lifting sign is worrisome for invasive cancer and is an indication for consideration of conversion to full-thickness excision for complete histologic assessment. A true submucosal dissection does not require defect closure provided there is no concern for full-thickness intraperitoneal entry. Alternatively, the mucosa is usually fairly mobile, and most defects can be closed primarily.
- It should be noted that the submucosal plane is much more likely to be scarred or obliterated if the patient has undergone prior piecemeal hot snare polypectomy or multiple attempts at endoscopic excision. Full-thickness excision may be required in this situation if the layers of the rectal wall are fused by scar. This is just another reason why piecemeal endoscopic resection should be avoided for large rectal polyps.

Results

- Local excision with TAE, TEM, and TAMIS is typically performed in the outpatient setting. The goal of transanal excision is complete en bloc removal of the target pathology with minimal morbidity and mortality. Numerous case series and several comparison trials demonstrate a low perioperative complication rate (10–17%) and a less than 1% mortality rate following TAE and TEM.
- There are some nonrandomized studies that suggest that the quality of TEM excision, however, is better than TAE with the incidence of specimen fragmentation, positive margins, and local recurrence favoring TEM.
- However, the quality of the studies of outcomes following local excision is distressingly suboptimal. Heterogeneous study populations (mixing benign and malignant pathology of various T stages), lack of appropriate time-to-event analysis, retrospective study design, and selection bias plague much of the published literature on the topic. It should also be remembered that, as of this writing, there have been no prospective, randomized comparisons of local excision techniques. It remains unclear whether any surgical technique is truly superior to any other, especially for lesions in the distal rectum.
- While there are no guidelines that mandate a recommended follow-up strategy following TES for benign rectal polyps, many surgeons performed endoscopy every 6–12 months for 2–3 years. Routine endoscopic ultrasound and imaging are not recommended for benign disease.
- Some newer advanced colonoscopic techniques, endoscopic mucosal resection (EMR) and endoscopic submucosal dissection (ESD), are being utilized for excision of benign colorectal polyps. EMR is usually a piecemeal resection, whereas ESD attempts a single en bloc resection. These techniques are primarily utilized in Asia with limited North American and European experience.

TES for Rectal Cancer

- Curative surgery for rectal cancer aims to maximize the oncologic clearance of the primary tumor as well as the mesorectal lymph nodes. Proctectomy is the accepted gold standard surgical procedure for rectal cancer with 5-year local recurrence rates in the 5–10% range. The procedure, however, comes with significant risk of perioperative complications; long-term defecatory, urinary, and sexual dysfunction; and frequent need for temporary or permanent ostomies.
- Local excision has long been an appealing option for rectal cancer because of its low risk of morbidity and mortality, relative paucity of long-term functional sequelae, and the

potential for curative treatment of disease limited to the bowel wall. The ideal candidate for local excision is a patient who has no lymph node metastasis and has a primary tumor which can be excised with negative margins. In such a situation, local excision should be curative. The great controversy, however, is that our ability to predict lymph node metastases is disappointingly poor and local recurrence following transanal excision remains much higher than with radical surgery.

- Local excision can be utilized as a tool to gain additional information regarding tumor biology and risk of lymph node metastasis. This may help guide clinical judgment in deciding whether or not a patient can be spared radical surgery. It is wise to clarify this concept with the patient preoperatively. The local excision will be utilized as a "total biopsy" to help guide treatment recommendations.
- If this total biopsy reveals high-risk histologic features, then a recommendation for subsequent radical surgery will be made. However, if no high-risk features are identified and the priorities and values of a patient are such that they accept a potentially higher risk of local recurrence than with proctectomy, local excision may be considered acceptable treatment. Local excision remains most appealing in patients who are unfit or unwilling to undergo radical surgery.
- Lymph node status dramatically effects patient prognosis as well as our treatment decisions and recommendations. Current efforts to predict lymph node status consist of identifying high-risk histopathologic features from biopsy specimens. This is complemented with selected imaging modalities. When considering patients for local excision, it is imperative to choose those with the lowest risk of harboring locoregional metastatic disease.

Predicting Risk of Lymph Node Metastasis

- Prediction of lymph node metastasis for rectal cancer is an imprecise science. No single histologic feature can solely predict risk of lymph node metastasis nor is there any currently available genetic or molecular marker that is predictive.
- Through a combination of histopathologic characteristics and imaging modalities, the surgeon and the patient try to roughly generate a risk-benefit calculation to guide clinical strategies related to local excision versus radical surgery.
- Colonoscopic biopsies alone sample but a small portion of the tumor, whereas an excisional full-thickness biopsy allows the fullest examination of the tumor histology, death of invasion, and margin status. Unfavorable histologic features are not only independently predictive of lymph node metastasis, but multiple unfavorable features also have an additive risk.

Depth of Invasion

- Depth of tumor invasion into the wall of the bowel has traditionally been one of the best predictors of lymph node metastasis and is an assessable variable in nearly all complete excisions.
  - T1 tumors, which are limited to the submucosa, are associated with a 10–15% incidence of occult lymph node metastases detected at the time of radical surgery.
  - T2 tumors, which invade into but not through the muscularis propria, are associated with a 20–26% risk of lymph node metastasis.
- Kikuchi further identified the importance of depth of submucosal invasion on lymph node metastases and local recurrence among T1 cancers. They analyzed a large series of patients subdivided by the cancer depth of invasion into the upper, middle, and lower thirds of the submucosa (SM1, SM2, SM3) and demonstrated an incremental increase in risk of lymph node metastasis or local recurrences with deeper depth of invasion. Tumors invading to the SM3 level were shown to have a similar risk of lymph node metastasis and local recurrence as T2 cancers.

Table 29.1 Local recurrence rates (percentage) at 36 months following TEM excision of rectal cancer

		Maximum tumor diameter (cm)					
Depth of invasion	Lymphatic invasion	≤1	1.1–2	2.1–3	3.1–4	4.1–5	≥5.1
pT1 sm1	No	3.0	3.6	4.4	5.4	6.6	8.1
	Yes	5.2	6.4	7.7	9.4	11.4	13.7
pT1 sm2–3	No	10.5	12.7	15.3	18.5	22.1	26.4
	Yes	17.8	21.4	25.5	30.3	35.7	41.8
pT2	No	9.8	11.9	14.3	17.3	20.7	24.7
	Yes	16.7	20.0	23.9	28.5	33.7	39.5
pT3	No	19.7	23.6	28.0	33.2	39.0	45.4
	Yes	32.2	37.9	44.1	51.0	58.3	65.7

With permission from Bach SP, Hill J, Monson JR, Simson JN, Lane L, Merrie A, Warren B, Mortensen NJ. Transanal Endoscopic Microsurgery (TEM) Collaboration. A predictive model for local recurrence after transanal endoscopic microsurgery for rectal cancer. Br J Surg. 2009;96(3):280–90. Copyright © 2009 John Wiley & Sons, *Inc*

pT pathological tumor stage, *sm*1 and *sm*2–3 Kikuchi submucosal stage

Lymphovascular Invasion

- Lymphovascular invasion is found in 12–32 percent of T1 rectal cancers and is a strong predictor of lymph node metastasis with an odds ratio between 3.0 and 11.5 reported on multivariate analysis.
- The predicted incidence of local recurrence at 36 months following TEM, based on depth of invasion, lymphatic invasion, and tumor diameter, is shown in Table 29.1.

Poor Differentiation

- Poorly differentiated histology also predicts for lymph node metastases in rectal cancer; however this trait is seen infrequently, present in only 2–4% of early rectal cancers. Odds ratio for probably poorly differentiated tumors having lymph node metastasis is 4.8–6.1.

Tumor Budding

- Tumor budding, defined as small nests of five or more, usually poorly differentiated, cancer cells along the invasive front, is a histologic trait not routinely mentioned on biopsy reports in North America but has been extensively reported in the Asian gastroenterology literature as a strong predictor of lymph node metastasis in colon and rectal cancer. Tumor budding is present in 16–25% of T1 cancers, and multivariate analysis has demonstrated an odds ratio of 5.1–5.8 in predicting lymph node metastasis.

Location and Mucinous Histology

- Location of the cancer within the rectum may also be a risk factor for lymph node metastasis. Distal rectal cancers may have up to a threefold increased risk of mesorectal lymph node metastasis as compared to mid and proximal rectal cancers. Mucinous histology and gender have not consistently been associated with increased risk of lymph node metastasis. Molecular markers are not yet able to reliably predict nodal status. (Fig. 29.5)

Imaging for Early Rectal Cancer Staging

- Imaging is a standard recommendation for the staging of rectal cancer. At present, rectal endoscopic ultrasound (EUS) is the imaging modality of choice to distinguish between T1 and T2 rectal cancers. CT scan and MRI do not have adequate resolution to differentiate between layers of the bowel wall in T1 and T2 rectal cancers, but they are better than EUS at determining deeper T3 and T4 tumors.

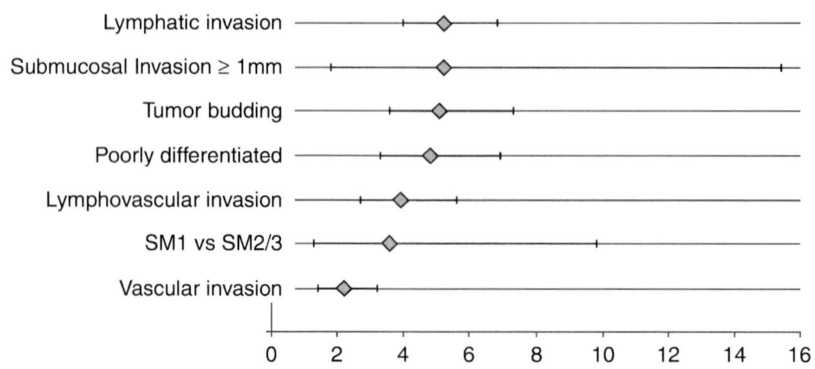

Fig. 29.5 Relative risk (95% confidence intervals) of lymph node metastases in pT1 rectal cancers. SM1, invasion into superficial third of submucosa. SM2/3, invasion into middle and deep third of submucosa. (With permission from Bosch SL, Teerenstra S, de Wilt JH, Cunningham C, Nagtegaal ID. Predicting lymph node metastasis in pT1 colorectal cancer: a systematic review of risk factors providing rationale for therapy decisions. Endoscopy. 2013 Oct;45(10):827–34)

- Despite innumerable technological advances in medicine, however, imaging remains an unreliable and inadequate measure of lymph node metastasis for rectal cancer. Imaging features that are suspicious for malignant lymph nodes include the presence of a round shape, internal heterogeneity, and irregular border and, to a lesser extent, size.
- Lymph node size alone is not a reliable indicator of node positivity, but nodes greater than 8 mm are considered highly suspicious on EUS, CT, and MRI.
- MRI and EUS are the more reliable modalities for assessing lymph node metastasis in early rectal cancer. CT and MRI are more accurate than EUS in the setting of locally advanced and metastatic disease.

Oncologic Results Following Local Excision of Rectal Cancer

- As noted above, the methodology of many reported series of local excision for rectal neoplasia is suspect. In addition to the problems noted above, trials of local excision for rectal cancer suffer from additional issues.
  - One problem is inclusion of patients who have cancer in a polyp that is completely or mostly removed by endoscopic polypectomy, and local excision is performed for unclear margins. Many of these patients will have no residual tumor in the local excision specimen and have an extremely low risk of local pelvic failure, biasing the results of the series in favor of local excision.
  - Another problem is retrospective subgroup analysis, in which patients are only included in the analysis after review of the histology. This allows for exclusion of patients who have positive margins of resection, greater than T1 stage, or other unfavorable histologic features. This obviously biases the analysis in favor of local excision but fails to replicate the true clinical situation in which margins and T stage cannot be known with certainty preoperatively.
  - Nonrandomized comparative trials of local excision versus proctectomy suffer from lack of information regarding mesorectal nodal status in the local excision group, which would most likely favor proctectomy. Although this bias can be mitigated by inclusion of patients in each group based on T stage alone, it cannot be completely eliminated as there may be hidden selection bias.

- It is thus difficult to make firm conclusions regarding the optimal place for local excision in our armamentarium of therapies for patients suffering from rectal cancer.

Local Excision for T1 Cancer

- Local excision of T1 rectal cancer is a widely available and technically feasible procedure with low risk of short-term morbidity and mortality. Approximately 15% of all rectal cancers present at stage 1 with no metastatic lymph nodes and tumor confined to the bowel wall. In theory, these patients will gain no clinical benefit from the lymphadenectomy associated with a low anterior or abdomino-perineal resection.
- The reported rate of local recurrence following transanal excision varies considerably in the literature but is universally higher than for proctectomy. For these reasons, proctectomy remains the oncologic gold standard for rectal cancer surgery.
- However, despite the oncologic advantages of proctectomy as compared to local excision, it remains unclear as to whether the oncologic benefit translates into a survival benefit for select patients with small, apparently low-risk tumors. Data regarding this topic have been of moderate to low quality and conflicting.

Local Excision for T2NX Cancer

- The deeper T2 rectal cancers invade into the muscularis propria permitting them greater access to the lymphatics. As a consequence, the incidence of lymph node metastasis and local recurrence is double that of T1 cancers. Proctectomy is the oncologic procedure of choice.
- However, as with T1 cancers, organ-sparing options have been explored in conjunction with the use of neoadjuvant or adjuvant chemoradiotherapy.
  - Preoperative chemoradiotherapy
    - Advantage: better prediction of nodal metastasis rate based on response to neoadjuvant therapy (i.e., ypT0–1 tumors have very low rates of ypN+ status)
    - Disadvantage: problems with healing of TAE site
  - Postoperative chemoradiotherapy
    - Advantage: better assessment of presenting T stage and histologic features and better wound healing
    - Disadvantage: unknown response to chemoradiotherapy and less accurate prediction of nodal status
- At present, transanal excision and chemoradiotherapy for cT2 or pT2 tumors should be reserved for patients unfit or unwilling to undergo proctectomy.

Surveillance and Salvage Following Local Excision of Rectal Cancer

- Surveillance following local excision is recommended to assess for early identification of local recurrence. It should be understood that if the margins of resection were negative, then the recurrence will begin in the mesorectum and only be apparent luminally at a late stage.
- No formal guidelines are in place, but a summary of several retrospective series suggests a follow-up strategy of proctoscopy or flexible sigmoidoscopy with high-resolution rectal MRI or endorectal ultrasound every 3–6 months for 3 years; then q 6–12 months through year 5; colonoscopy at years 1, 4, and 9; and CT of the abdomen and chest annually.
- Median time to recurrence diagnosis ranges from 13 to 47 months with most discovered between 12 and 24 months. The addition of radiation therapy often delays identification of local recurrence an additional 1–2 years.
- Despite close follow-up, recurrences have a relatively poor prognosis. Patients with local only recurrences who were candidates for resection had an R0 resection in 79–96% of

cases resulting in a 53–58% disease-free survival.

- These poor results of salvage therapy should provide a sobering reminder that the best chance of curing a patient suffering from rectal cancer is with initial treatment. Trying to "mop up" after local pelvic or distant failure has occurred is often futile. In addition, it should be remembered that patients undergoing local excision are typically those with the smallest, early-stage lesions and those most easily cured by proctectomy.

Complications of TAE

- Complications following local excision of rectal polyps and cancers occur in 5–25% with mortality rates in the 0.3–0.6% range.
  - Bleeding
  - Peritoneal entry
  - Urinary retention
  - Transient fecal incontinence

Rectal Cancer: Watch and Wait

30

George J. Chang

Key Concepts

- Pathologic complete treatment response following neoadjuvant chemoradiation therapy and surgery for rectal cancer is associated with favorable prognosis.
- Pathologic complete treatment response is observed in approximately 10–20% of rectal cancer patients following chemoradiation therapy.
- Clinical and radiographic assessment of neoadjuvant therapy treatment response is suboptimal and remains a primary challenge for safe implementation of watch and wait strategies.
- Approximately one in three patients exhibiting clinical complete response will develop tumor regrowth.
- At present, watch and wait should be offered to patients only in the context of a clinical trial.
- Local excision following neoadjuvant chemoradiation therapy may help predict mesorectal nodal status but is associated with significant risk for pain and poor wound healing.

Introduction

- Despite advances in rectal cancer treatment, multimodal therapy for rectal cancer is associated with a significant impact on long-term functional and quality-of-life outcomes including risks for bowel, bladder, and sexual dysfunction, pain, and potential need for permanent colostomy. Therefore there is great interest in strategies to decrease the toxicity of treatment, including strategies that employ the selective use of radiation, chemotherapy, or even surgery.
- The modern concept of selective use of surgery following chemoradiation therapy for patients with rectal cancer is based on the fact that pathologic complete response (pCR) is observed in approximately 10–20% of patients following long-course chemoradiation therapy.
- While definitive surgical resection remains the standard of care for all patients with nonmetastatic rectal cancer, a growing number of studies are providing supportive evidence for a watch and wait, organ-preserving approach in highly selected patients with rectal cancer who have a complete clinical response to chemoradiotherapy.

G. J. Chang (✉)
Department of Surgical Oncology, The University of MD Anderson Cancer Center, Houston, TX, USA
e-mail: gchang@mdanderson.org

S. R. Steele et al. (eds.), *The ASCRS Manual of Colon and Rectal Surgery*,
https://doi.org/10.1007/978-3-030-01165-9_30

Neoadjuvant Chemoradiotherapy

- Preoperative chemoradiotherapy has typically been administered in a "long-course" fashion, with radiotherapy and a radiosensitizing chemotherapeutic agent administered over a 5–6-week period with a 6–10-week treatment break prior to proctectomy. This extended period of time allows for tumor regression, if the tumor is sensitive to the therapy.
- It is now widely recognized that tumor regression in response to neoadjuvant treatment is an important prognostic indicator of long-term outcome. It can be associated with tumor volume reduction, downstaging, and nodal sterilization, and a number of pathologic grading systems now exist to describe the extent of response (Table 30.1).
- Following completion of CRT, up to 50% of patients will experience a clinical complete response (cCR) as defined by replacement of the tumor bed by scar or normal appearing mucosa on clinical and endoscopic examination.
- Pathologic complete response (pCR—specimen without evidence of residual tumor cells) or pathologic near-complete response (specimen with only single or small groups of tumor cells) can be observed in 10–40% of patients following neoadjuvant chemoradiation therapy (nCRT).
- Complete clinical response, however, is not necessarily predictive of pathologic response.
- With improved surgical techniques, distant, rather than local, disease recurrence has emerged as the primary cause of tumor-related death.

The Watch and Wait Approach

- In 2004 Habr-Gama and her group first reported outcomes for selective surgery with a nonoperative (aka "watch and wait" or "wait and see") strategy in select patients who achieved a clinical complete response following chemoradiation therapy.
- Following Habr-Gama's original report, other investigators initially reported a wide range of success with an initially nonoperative approach, including a locoregional treatment failure rate of up to 50–60%, much higher than the 3% failure rate initially reported by Habr-Gama. While not fully explained, the reasons for this discrepancy may have included differences in initial tumor burden, selection

Table 30.1 Tumor regression grading systems

TRG	Mandard (1)	Dworak (2)	Rödel (3)	Ryan (4)	CAP (5)
0		No regression	No regression		No residual tumor cells
1	No residual cancer cells	Dominant tumor mass with obvious fibrosis and/or vasculopathy	Fibrosis <25% of tumor mass	No residual cancer cells or single cells	Single or small groups of cancer cells
2	Rare residual cancer cells	Dominantly fibrotic changes with few tumor cells or groups	Fibrosis 25–50% of tumor mass	Residual cancer outgrown by fibrosis	Residual cancer outgrown by fibrosis
3	Fibrosis greater than residual cancer	Very few (difficult to find microscopically) tumor cells in fibrotic tissue with or without mucous substance	Fibrosis >50% of tumor mass	Significant cancer outgrown by cancer or no fibrosis with extensive residual cancer	Minimal evidence of fibrosis
4	Residual cancer greater than fibrosis	Complete regression	Complete regression		
5	No regression				

of patients for a watch and wait approach following neoadjuvant therapy, method and timing of assessment, or the neoadjuvant treatment regimen.

- In addition, the method of selection of patients for inclusion in the nonoperative therapy arm in Habr-Gama's initial report may have played a major role. Specifically, patients were not included in the study (observation) group until they had been followed for 12 months following chemoradiotherapy. Put another way, patients initially selected for nonoperative therapy who then failed in the first 12 months were excluded from analysis. This has the potential to bias the results heavily in favor of the observation group.
- Recent data, including from an updated report by Habr-Gama, indicates that the true risk for locoregional treatment failure is approximately 30%. This suggests that a number of patients initially thought to have a pCR based on clinical assessment of complete response actually had undetected viable tumor, highlighting one of the major challenges and pitfalls of the watch and wait approach.
- One potential solution to the challenge of clinically identifying patients with a pCR is to ensure a close follow-up strategy. This will only be effective, however, if salvage treatment is proven to be effective.
- Although no specific follow-up regimen has been compared prospectively to any other, it is reasonable to consider frequent digital rectal and endoluminal examination combined with carcinoembryonic antigen level determination (some investigators recommend a 3–4-month interval) and relatively frequent pelvic magnetic resonance imaging (MR) with rectal cancer protocol (some investigators recommend a 3–6-month interval) with biopsy of any suspicious lesions.
- The majority of tumor regrowth is usually detected within the first 12–24 months, in which case patients may be eligible for curative resection.
- There is concern that a longer delay to surgery will result in making the salvage resection more difficult. Although it has been reported that salvage surgical resection after nonoperative management is feasible, longer delays in identification of regrowth have been associated with more than a 50% decrease in the ability to perform sphincter-preserving salvage surgery.
  - Tumor regrowth occurring deep to the mucosa may be difficult to identify before more extensive sphincter involvement, and the addition of radiation-induced posttreatment fibrosis along the pelvic floor or anal sphincter complex may also preclude subsequent sphincter-preserving resection.
- Before a nonoperative strategy can be broadly applied, it is important to ensure that oncologic outcomes are not being compromised, particularly for this group of patients who are expected to have excellent outcomes, with an extremely low risk for either local or distant disease recurrence, with proctectomy.
- Finally, what remains to be settled is if leaving the rectum containing residual viable tumor in patients with cCR but not pCR increases the risk for distant failure.
- Despite these concerns, the evidence in support of a watch and wait approach is growing. A limited number of prospective series have been reported on nCRT followed by observation (Table 30.2). A review of the wait and see approach published in 2012 identified 30 publications from 9 series including 650 patients. While demonstrating proof of principle, significant heterogeneity of the studies in staging, inclusion criteria, study design, and follow-up rigor limit our ability to draw firm conclusions.

Clinical Assessment of Treatment Response

- The clinical assessment of treatment response is difficult and is perhaps the greatest challenge and limiting factor for safe implementation of the watch and wait approach.
- A number of different strategies have been considered including clinical assessment, full-thickness local excision, metabolic imaging, and high-resolution pelvic MRI imaging.

Table 30.2 Comparison of selected modern studies

Series	Number of patients observed	Number of patients operated	Median follow-up (months)	cCR	Local regrowth	Outcome
Mass 2011	21	20	15 (observed) 35 (operated)	100%	1 patient	2-year OS 100% 2-year DFS 89%
Dalton 2012	12	37	25.5 (mean)	24%	50%	Disease free at follow-up
Habr-Gama 2014	93	90	60	49%	31%	5-year OS 91% 5-year LRFS 69% 5-year DFS 68%
Smith 2015	73	72			26%	4-year OS 91% (obs) vs. 95% (surg) 4-year DSS 91% (obs) vs. 96% (surg)
Smith 2015	18	30	68.4 (mean)		1 patient	Alive with pelvic disease at 54 months

- The concordance between clinical and pathologic evaluation has traditionally been poor both in terms of sensitivity (~25%) for detecting pCR and specificity (~60–90%) for excluding residual disease.
- There has not existed a standard method for the clinical evaluation of complete response. Investigators have advocated for a combination of digital rectal examination and endoluminal visualization to identify residual mass, ulceration, nodularity, or stenosis, all of which may suggest persistent tumor. Findings in support of a complete response include regular and smooth mucosa and changes such as whitening or presence of telangiectasias.
- Given the challenges for clinical assessment of residual disease within the bowel wall, a number of investigators have considered local excision of the tumor bed as both a diagnostic test to assess pathologic treatment response and a therapeutic maneuver to excise any residual tumor cells residing within the bowel wall.
  - Endoscopic biopsy alone has the obvious limitation of being able to provide only a superficial sampling of the tumor bed that can miss residual disease that may be present more deeply within the bowel wall or away from the site of biopsy.
  - Full-thickness excision of the entire tumor bed may be performed through a variety of approaches including transanal excision, transanal endoscopic microsurgery (TEM), or transanal minimally invasive surgery (TAMIS).
    - Complete pathologic assessment of the bowel wall can be performed, and ypT stage has prognostic implications regarding ypN stage, but it is not a perfect correlation.
    - An additional major limitation of full-thickness excision following nCRT is that it is associated with significant treatment-associated toxicity including poor healing and pain.
    - Finally, the watch and wait strategy may perhaps have the greatest appeal for patients whose tumors involve the anal sphincter for whom sphincter preservation would be impossible. Full-thickness excision in this circumstance would necessitate at least partial resection of the internal sphincter. Thus the role for full-thickness excision in a watch and wait approach remains limited.
- Two primary approaches to radiologic imaging for the assessment of treatment response have been investigated:
  - ^{18}Fluorodeoxyglucose positron emission computed tomography (PET-CT): Despite its utility in signaling response to systemic

Table 30.3 MRI tumor regression grade (mrTRG)

mrTRG	Description
1	Tumor bed with low signal intensity signaling fibrosis with no residual intermediate tumor signal
2	Tumor bed with predominance of fibrosis with minimal residual intermediate tumor signal
3	Substantial intermediate intensity tumor signal present, but does not predominate over low-intensity fibrosis
4	Minimal fibrosis
5	No change from baseline

therapy for a variety of malignant diseases, metabolic imaging with PET has not been shown to be reliable for the identification of complete responders.

- MR: This is currently the most useful imaging modality in watch and wait strategies.
  - Areas of treatment response and fibrosis are characterized by low signal intensity on T2-weighted imaging. The presence of uniform low signal intensity with the absence of areas of intermediate signal intensity within it is suggestive of a pCR.
  - Based on these findings and a comparison to pretreatment MRI, a tumor regression grade has been proposed by the MERCURY study investigators (Table 30.3).
    - The so-called mrTRG of 1–3 correlated with better survival outcomes when compared to mrTRG 4–5, comparable to the difference in survival observed when comparing ypT0-3a vs. ypT3b or greater.
    - There is currently great interest in the potential for the addition of diffusion weighting or functional dynamic contrast-enhanced MRI to improve the detection of response, and other technologies may still be on the horizon.

Increasing the Rate of Complete Response

- Based on the presumption that patients with pCR are eligible for an organ-preserving watch and wait approach, a number of investigators have tried to improve the rate of PCR with neoadjuvant therapy using one or more of the following techniques:
  - Radiotherapy dose intensification including contact radiation
  - Utilization of more active chemotherapeutic regimens
  - Utilization of induction or consolidation chemotherapy
  - Increasing the time interval from chemoradiotherapy to surgery
- However, it is critical to understand that increasing the pCR rate by simply increasing the time interval from neoadjuvant therapy to surgery alone may have no impact on prognosis.
  - Tumor cell death is initiated immediately (during neoadjuvant therapy), but the pCR rate can be manipulated by changing the duration of delay prior to proctectomy. Therefore, one cannot assume that one neoadjuvant therapy regimen is superior to another based on pCR rate if proctectomy occurs at different intervals following neoadjuvant therapy.

31 Proctectomy

Emmanouil P. Pappou and Martin R. Weiser

Key Concepts

- A proper proctectomy with sharp dissection along the visceral and parietal layers of the endovascular fascia facilitates margin-negative resection, reduces local recurrence, and limits nerve injury associated with sexual dysfunction.
- Precise understanding of pelvic anatomy including fascial planes, autonomic nerves, and pelvic floor musculature is critical in performing a proper proctectomy.
- The quality of mesorectal excision and the distance of the circumferential radial margin are associated with local pelvic control.
- Proctectomy can be performed using open, laparoscopic, and robot-assisted techniques.

Background and General Concepts

- At the beginning of the twentieth century, the majority of patients diagnosed with rectal cancer in Europe and the United States underwent perineal proctectomy which was highly morbid, with poor oncologic results.
- In 1908, William Ernest Miles of St. Mark's Hospital in London advocated the abdominal perineal excision (APE) or, as it came to be called, abdominoperineal resection (APR) to more completely remove the lymphovascular supply of the rectum.
  - APR soon became the surgical procedure of choice for treatment of carcinoma of the rectum. Compared with perineal proctectomy, long-term outcomes following this new operation improved considerably.
- Miles' emphasis on the necessity of removing the mesorectum in its entirety would become the guiding principle of what is now known as total mesorectal excision (TME). Today, TME remains the gold standard in rectal cancer surgery.
- TME entails sharp—rather than blunt—dissection of the visceral and parietal layers of the endopelvic fascia, resulting in intact removal of the rectum and mesorectum. In Miles' time, however, most surgeons continued to perform traditional blunt dissection, limiting the benefits of APR and resulting in a 25% rate of positive resection margins, with high rates of recurrence and mortality.
- The absolute necessity of sharp dissection in every rectal cancer operation—i.e., meticulous removal of the entire mesorectum along the areolar plane outside of the rectal fascia

E. P. Pappou
Department of Colorectal Surgery, Columbia University, New York, NY, USA

M. R. Weiser (✉)
Department of Surgery, Memorial Sloan Kettering Cancer Center, New York, NY, USA
e-mail: weiser1@mskcc.org

S. R. Steele et al. (eds.), *The ASCRS Manual of Colon and Rectal Surgery*,
https://doi.org/10.1007/978-3-030-01165-9_31

propria—was reemphasized in 1982 by Bill Heald.

- The aims of TME are to excise the rectum and surrounding mesorectum, including its blood vessels and pararectal lymph nodes, within an intact visceral fascial "envelope"; to complete en bloc resection of the lymph nodes along the superior rectal and inferior mesenteric arteries; and to achieve clear resection margins.
- Advocates of "total mesorectal excision" have focused attention on two critical components of oncologic proctectomy: the lateral (radial) margin and the distal margin of mesorectal excision.
  - Sharp dissection in the avascular plane surrounding the mesorectum, so as to remove the mesorectum in its fascial envelope and achieve a wide circumferential radial margin (CRM), has been demonstrated to be essential in avoiding local recurrence of tumor in the pelvis.
  - The second component of total mesorectal excision, as advocated initially by Heald et al., is the removal of the entire mesorectum distal to the tumor. However, the necessity of removing mesorectum more than 4–5 cm distal to a proximal rectal tumor is not supported by pathologic studies of lymph node involvement in the mesorectum.
    - At present, many advocates of "total mesorectal excision" limit mesorectal resection to 4–5 cm distal to proximal rectal tumors, although some authors still refer to this technique as "total" mesorectal excision, which has caused confusion. Other groups have termed the concept of tailoring the mesorectal excision to the position of the tumor "tumor-specific mesorectal excision," which may be more accurate.
- In summary, for all patients with rectal cancer, it is critical that the primary tumor is removed in its entirety. In addition, mesenteric tissue at greatest risk for nodal metastases should also be resected.
  - For patients with mid and distal rectal cancers, appropriate proctectomy technique will involve removing the entire mesorectum.
  - For patients with proximal rectal cancers, it is important to remove the mesorectum for a distance of approximately 4–5 cm distal to the tumor, although resecting the mesorectum distal to that point does not appear to confer benefit.

Anatomy of the Mesorectum/Rectal Fascia

- The rectum is surrounded by a recognizable annular envelope: the rectal fascia (or mesorectum, as it is better known to surgeons). The mesorectum contains the lymphovascular supply of the rectum and upper anal canal. It encloses the branches of the superior rectal artery and the perirectal lymph nodes, which drain in a caudal direction toward the inferior mesenteric artery. Around the rectum is an avascular plane, surgically recognizable as a cobweb of areolar tissue.
- The mesorectum is asymmetrically distributed. The bulk of it sits posterior to the rectum, identified by two protruding bulges (the "mesorectal cheeks"); anteriorly and laterally, the perirectal tissue is thinner. Similarly, the mesorectal fascia is most developed on the posterior aspect. Anteriorly the mesorectum is thinner and bordered by the recto-genital septum known as Denonvilliers' fascia.
- In men, Denonvilliers' fascia separates the rectum and mesorectum from the prostate and seminal vesicles. In women, the thinner rectovaginal fascia separates the rectum from the vagina. Ligaments below and lateral to the peritoneal reflection connect to the parietal fascia on the pelvic sidewall.
- The sympathetic autonomous system is responsible for urinary continence and ejaculation, whereas the parasympathetic system controls micturition, as well as genital erection and lubrication.
  - The sympathetic autonomic plexus arises from lumbar sympathetic nerves originating in the T12-L2 spinal junction, which

pass anterior to the aorta and form a network in close proximity to the origin of the inferior mesenteric artery. This is known as the superior hypogastric plexus. The superior hypogastric plexus enters the pelvic cavity anterior to the sacral promontory and splits into fairly well-defined left and right hypogastric nerves (Fig. 31.1). Damage to this sympathetic plexus during ligation of the inferior mesenteric artery, or damage to the hypogastric nerve trunks during mesorectal mobilization, can lead to urinary incontinence and retrograde ejaculation.

 - The hypogastric nerves course posterolateral to the mesorectum and ultimately join parasympathetic nerves—also known as the pelvic plexus, pelvic splanchnic nerves, or nervi erigentes—to form the inferior hypogastric plexus.
 - The parasympathetic nerves that join the sympathetic system originate from the S2–S4 sacral spinal nerve roots, lying posterolaterally along the mesorectal fascia. Preservation of the pelvic splanchnic nerves and the inferior hypogastric plexus, and careful separation of these from the rectum, is one of the most challenging aspects of proctectomy. The inferior hypogastric plexus forms an extensive network of interlocking fibers of the sympathetic left and right hypogastric nerves and parasympathetic pelvic splanchnic nerves are situated on the pelvic sidewall.

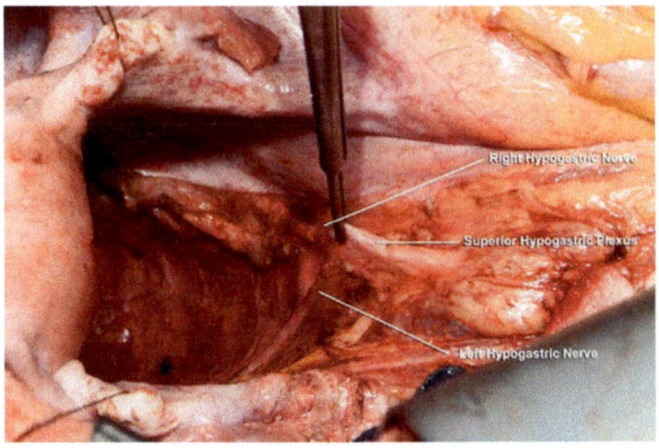

Fig. 31.1 The superior hypogastric plexus splits into the right and left hypogastric nerves as it enters the pelvic cavity. Parasympathetic pelvic splanchnic nerves, also known as nervi erigentes, arise from sacral spinal nerves S2-S4 and pierce the presacral fascia on the left and right side to join the hypogastric nerves, forming the inferior hypogastric plexus (not shown). (With permission from Lee-Kong et al. Autonomic nerve preservation during rectal cancer resection. J Gastrointest Surg. 2010;14:416–22. © Springer)

 - Various nerves leave the inferior hypogastric plexus to enter the rectal wall, while the remaining neurovascular bundles extend anterolaterally to the seminal vesicles, distal ureters, vasa deferentia, urinary bladder, and prostate and cavernous bodies in men and in the similar anatomic area in women, for whom the lower portion of the inferior hypogastric plexus runs along the lower lateral wall of the vagina.

- Laterally the mesorectum is sometimes not completely covered by a layer of fascia and is penetrated by the middle rectal vessels (coming from the internal iliac vessels, present in about 10–20% of patients) and autonomic nerves from the inferior hypogastric plexus.
- Posterior to the mesorectum is the presacral fascia, which follows the concavity of the sacrum. The presacral fascia is a thickened parietal fascia that covers the presacral veins and fat, extending laterally to join Denonvilliers' fascia anteriorly. Inferiorly, between the levels of the third and fourth sacral vertebra, the mesorectum and the presacral fascia fuse. The thick connective tissue bridging these two separate fascias is also known as the rectosacral fascia or Waldeyer's fascia.
   - Waldeyer's fascia is an important surgical landmark during posterior rectal mobilization, because of its close relationship to the sympathetic hypogastric nerves and the inferior hypogastric plexus. Inaccurate dissection at this level can lead anteriorly to breach of the mesorectum and posteriorly to tearing of the fascia, resulting in considerable bleeding from the presacral veins.
- At the most distal part of the rectum, the mesorectum thins out as a recognizable structure so that it is virtually absent over the final 1 cm of the rectum. Distal rectal can-

cers are thus at greater risk of invading surrounding structures than proximal rectal cancers, particularly the pelvic floor/external anal sphincter, vagina, or prostate, because of the relative paucity of mesorectum at this level.

Surgical Principles of Proctectomy for Rectal Cancer

The basic principles of proctectomy are as follows:

1. Sharp dissection circumferentially around the mesorectum in an avascular areolar plane between the visceral and parietal layers of the endopelvic fascia (Figure 31.2a).
2. Identification and preservation of the autonomic nerve plexus that controls bladder and sexual function (Figure 31.2b).
3. Achievement of a circumferential margin that is macroscopically and microscopically clear of tumor.
4. Preservation of the anal sphincter complex and pelvic floor, with restoration of gastrointestinal continuity when appropriate.

Pathological Assessment

- Pathological analysis of the excised proctectomy specimen provides important prognostic information on the stage and biology of the tumor.
- In addition to assessment of proximal, distal, and circumferential radial margins, pathologists should grade the quality of the mesorectal specimen. This has been demonstrated to have prognostic significance.
- Pathologic analysis is also a means of assessing the quality of surgery, because margin status and quality of mesorectal excision can be used as surrogates for oncologic outcome assessment.
- The College of American Pathologists (CAP) has implemented standardized assessment of rectal cancer specimens.
  - The surgeon or pathologist should ink the non-peritonealized radial margin of the fresh resection specimen to help guide this analysis.
  - A standardized synoptic report should include a subjective assessment of mesorectal grade and quantitative measurement of CRM in millimeters.

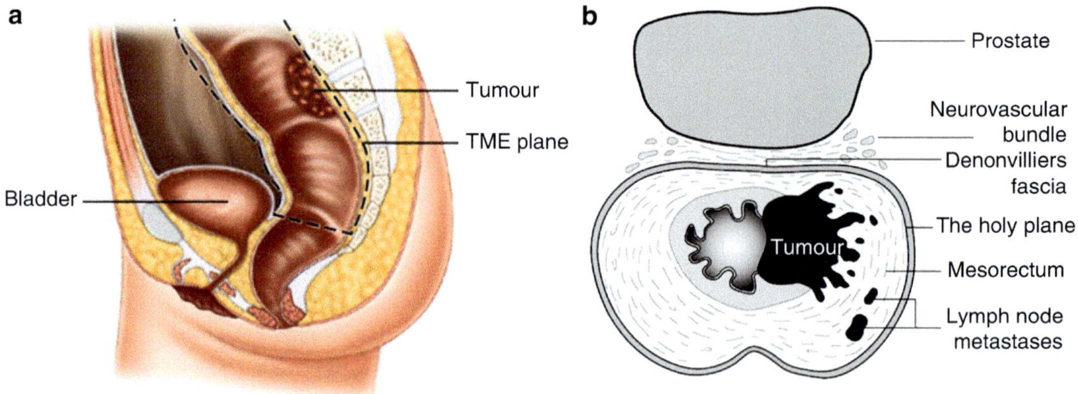

Fig. 31.2 Total mesorectal excision. (**a**) Dissection follows the dotted line. Tumor deposits are often present within the lymphovascular tissue surrounding the rectum (mesorectum). Incomplete resection leaves residual deposits which are most likely the origin of local treatment failure. (With permission from Janjua AZ, Moran B, Heald RJ. Open surgical management of rectal cancer. Patel HRH, Mould T, Joseph JV, Delaney CP, editors. Pelvic cancer surgery: modern breakthroughs and future advances. New York: Springer; 2015. p. 531. © Springer 2015). (**b**). The plane of total mesorectal excision allows complete removal of regional lymph nodes while sparing the neurovascular bundles. (With permission from Heald RJ, et al. Embryology and anatomy of the rectum. Semin Surg Oncol. 1998 Sep;15(2):66–71. © John Wiley and Sons)

- A margin is considered positive if the primary tumor or involved lymph node extends to within 1 mm of the resection margin.

Preoperative Preparation

- Oral mechanical bowel preparation with oral antibiotics
  - In addition to the impact of bowel preparation on wound infection, cathartic bowel preparation will:
    - Clear the rectosigmoid of stool, in order to accurately assess the position of the tumor intraoperatively.
    - Facilitate division of the colon and rectum.
    - Clear the intervening colon free of stool, which is important in the case of anastomotic leak following restorative.
- Preoperative broad-spectrum intravenous antibiotics
- Thromboembolic prophylaxis with unfractionated heparin or low molecular weight heparin combined with intermittent pneumatic compression devices
- Discussion of potential impact on fertility with all individuals of childbearing potential
- Discussion of potential function consequences of restorative and non-restorative proctectomy
- Preoperative stoma site marking and stoma teaching, preferably by an enterostomal therapist.

Operative Approaches

Abdominal Exploration and Decision-Making

- The abdominal cavity is explored thoroughly, especially the liver and the peritoneum, to identify signs of distant metastatic disease. If unresectable distant metastatic disease is encountered, then the surgeon should carefully consider whether low pelvic anastomosis is warranted.
  - Patients with unresectable distant metastatic spread often undergo prolonged treatment with chemotherapy; and the presence of a temporary diverting ileostomy may increase the severity of chemotherapy-induced enteritis.
  - The added risk of colorectal or coloanal anastomotic leak may not be warranted because if leak occurs, systemic chemotherapy may be delayed. In addition, chemotherapy must be stopped temporarily to close the ileostomy; if complications ensue from this second procedure, systemic chemotherapy may again be delayed. Lastly, the functional derangements associated with low pelvic anastomosis will only be exacerbated if the patient receives cytotoxic chemotherapy, which may produce enteritis.
- It may be preferable to simply perform a Hartmann's resection for mid and distal rectal adenocarcinoma that does not invade the pelvic floor or anal sphincter, in patients with unresectable distant metastatic disease.
- For patients with proximal rectal cancer who may not require temporary fecal diversion and are at low risk for anastomotic complications, it is reasonable to perform anterior resection with primary anastomosis, even in the setting of unresectable distant metastatic disease (if this was the original plan).
- If the primary tumor is felt to be unresectable, then fecal diversion alone should be considered. Except in rare circumstances, there is little value in debulking rectal cancer.

Open Low Anterior Resection (LAR)

- The patient is placed in a modified lithotomy or supine split-leg position.
- A variety of incisions can be utilized; however, it is important to keep the incision line away from the area of potential stoma and stoma appliance, so as to not interfere with management of the stoma postoperatively.
- Our preferences regarding the technical aspects of restorative proctectomy are described as follows:
  - The small bowel is carefully packed and retracted to the right, providing access to the pelvis.

- The sigmoid and descending colon are mobilized to the midline.
- The space deep to the superior rectal (hemorrhoidal) vessels is mobilized taking care to avoid damage to the sympathetic plexus/hypogastric nerves.
- The superior rectal artery (just distal to the left colic artery) or inferior mesenteric artery, at its origin 1–2 cm from the aorta, is ligated and divided to preserve the sympathetic plexus. High ligation of the IMA may be useful when bulky adenopathy is present at the base of the vessel or when a coloanal anastomosis is necessary and maximal length of the left colon is required.
  - When the inferior mesenteric artery is ligated, care must be taken to preserve the marginal artery, which provides the blood supply from the middle colic vessels to the left colon and anastomosis.
- The inferior mesenteric vein is ligated at the paraduodenal (ligament of Treitz) location just inferior to the pancreas and again adjacent to the ligation site of the inferior mesenteric artery.
  - Dividing the vein at the ligament of Treitz is critical in order to accommodate full mobilization of the splenic flexure, which is then allowed to rotate into the pelvis for maximal length.
- Splenic flexure mobilization is performed. Colonic attachments to the pancreas are then taken down, and care is taken to avoid aggressive retraction on the colon, which can tear the splenic capsule. Omental attachments are then taken down from the distal transverse colon to complete the mobilization.

- The distal descending/proximal sigmoid mesentery is divided to the bowel wall.
- The colon is divided with a purse-string instrument and staple anvil inserted (for restorative proctectomy with stapled anastomosis) or linear cutting stapler (for APR or coloanal anastomosis).
- The left colon is packed superiorly, facilitating visualization of the pelvis.
- The distal segment is retracted anteriorly, which opens the perimesorectal planes. A sharp dissection is carried out under direct vision, circumferentially around the mesorectum.
- The presence of the superior hypogastric plexus posteriorly must be kept in mind throughout the dissection (Figure 31.3a). Starting the dissection in the posterior and then the lateral plane, in a stepwise manner,

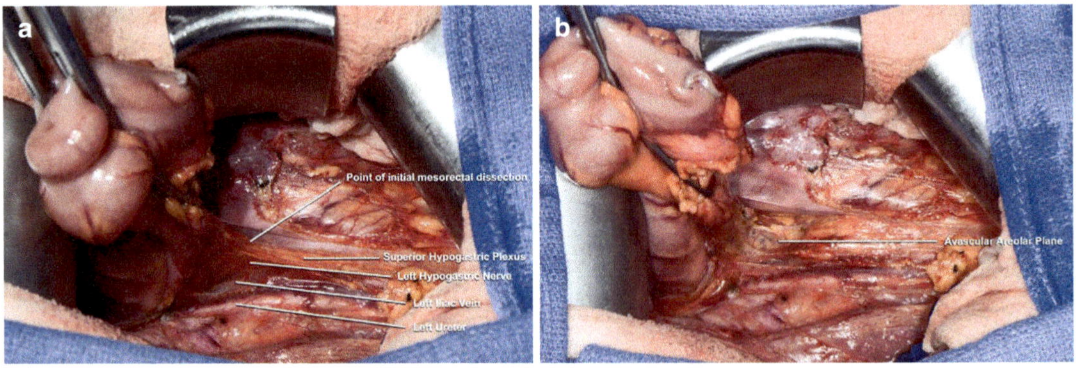

Fig. 31.3 (**a**) The distal sigmoid/proximal rectum is elevated anteriorly, exposing the aortic bifurcation and sacral promontory, with identification of the left ureter, left iliac vein, and superior hypogastric plexus. The hypogastric nerves may appear as an obvious discrete band of tissue or as multiple smaller bands. (**b**) Careful dissection of the sigmoid mesentery distally results in an avascular, areolar plane separating the mesorectal fascia propria from the presacral fascia. (With permission from Lee-Kong et al. Autonomic nerve preservation during rectal cancer resection. J Gastrointest Surg. 2010;14:416–22. © Springer)

facilitates identification of the correct mesorectal plane (Figure 31.3b).

- The lateral dissection is carried out by extending the posterior plane of dissection anteriorly and around the sidewalls of the pelvis. At this point in the dissection, the inferior hypogastric plexuses curve around the surface of the mesorectum and are vulnerable to inadvertent injury.
  - While retracting the divided rectosigmoid forward, the tangentially running hypogastric and pelvic parasympathetic nerves are carefully identified and dissected away from the mesorectal surface on each side (Figure 31.4a).
- As the lateral dissection moves deeper into the pelvis, one or two middle rectal arteries may be encountered. Middle rectal arteries are present in fewer than 20% of patients and, if encountered, can be easily divided with cautery or bipolar vessel energy sealing devices.
- Dissection anteriorly progresses along Denonvilliers' fascia down to the pelvic floor (Figure 31.4b). Forward retraction with the help of the retractor facilitates the development of the space anteriorly.
  - Anterior tumors require resection of Denonvilliers' fascia, which puts the parasympathetic nerves at risk, as they extend anteriorly toward the prostate.
  - For posterior tumors, dissection can proceed below Denonvilliers' fascia.
- Adequacy of the dissection distal to the lower edge of the tumor is examined by palpation and/or endoscopy to ensure a proper distal margin.
- When mesorectal mobilization down to the pelvic floor is considered complete on both anterior and posterior sides, the rectum is elevated above the pelvic floor and cross-clamped. At this point, washout of the anorectal stump can be performed with saline solution or water.
- The rectum is typically transected with a stapler and the specimen is removed. The anastomosis between the colon conduit and the rectal stump is constructed with a circular stapler (Figure 31.5a).
  - The serosa and mucosa are visually evaluated for adequate vascular supply.
  - Intraoperative anastomotic air testing of the colorectal anastomosis is performed by filling the pelvis with saline solution and insufflating the rectum with air through a sigmoidoscope.
- A handsewn coloanal anastomosis is shown in Figure 31.5b and is discussed separately below.

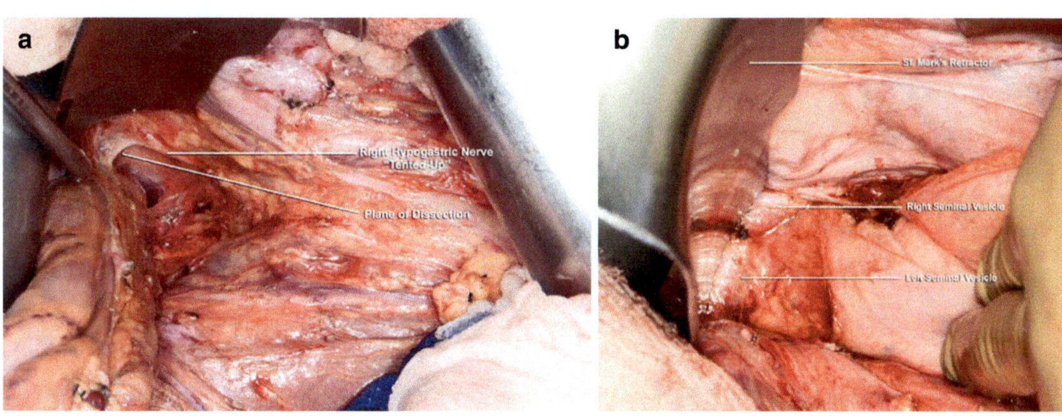

Fig. 31.4 (**a**) Caudal dissection in the posterior midline while lifting the rectum "toward the ceiling" may cause the hypogastric nerves to "tent up," as they often adhere to the mesorectal fascia. (**b**) Anterior dissection during TME. (With permission from Lee-Kong et al. Autonomic nerve preservation during rectal cancer resection. J Gastrointest Surg. 2010;14:416–22. © Springer)

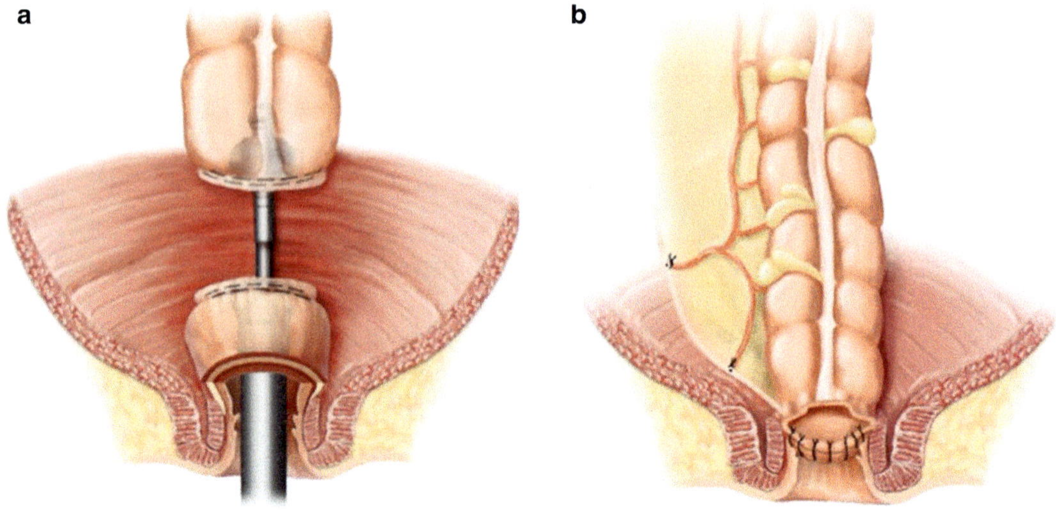

Fig. 31.5 (**a**) Stapled end-to-end colorectal anastomosis. (**b**) Handsewn end-to-end coloanal anastomosis. (With permission from Wexner SD, Fleshman JW, editors. Colon and rectal surgery: abdominal operations, master techniques in surgery. Philadelphia: Lippincott Williams & Wilkins; 2012)

Laparoscopic Low Anterior Resection

- Our preferred approach is described below.
- The patient is placed in a modified lithotomy position. A five-trocar technique is generally utilized, with an umbilical camera port, two left-sided and two right-sided working (Fig. 31.6).
- The dissection is performed in a medial-to-lateral fashion, first dissecting the vessels, followed by takedown of the splenic flexure and then the lateral colonic attachments before entering the pelvis for rectal resection.
- For pelvic dissection, it may be necessary to position the patient in a more head-down position, often with less rotation to the right. The rectum is mobilized circumferentially, applying standard open TME surgical principles. Dissection can be performed with cautery, ultrasonic dissector, or vessel sealing devices.
- After TME dissection is completed, the level of rectal transection is confirmed with digital rectal and endoscopic examinations. The rectum is irrigated and then stapled and divided with endoscopic staplers. The specimen is extracted via a wound protector at the umbilical camera port or the future diverting ileostomy site.
- The proximal sigmoid/left colon is divided, and the anvil secured for laparoscopic circular anastomosis. An air leak test confirms the integrity of the anastomosis, and a diverting ileostomy is fashioned selectively.
- In patients with a narrow pelvis or elevated body mass index, pelvic dissection can be challenging. In such cases, a lower midline or Pfannenstiel incision may be utilized to allow open pelvic dissection, rectal division, and restoration of intestinal continuity. A combination of laparoscopic and open surgery in this manner is often referred to as a "hybrid" approach.

Robotic Low Anterior Resection

- Some surgeons find the robot a useful technology in pelvic dissection, which may have advantages with respect to manual dexterity versus standard laparoscopy.
- A single-docking technique using the da Vinci® Si™ robot is first described. This entails single docking of the robot for the entire procedure, from colon mobilization to pelvic dissection.

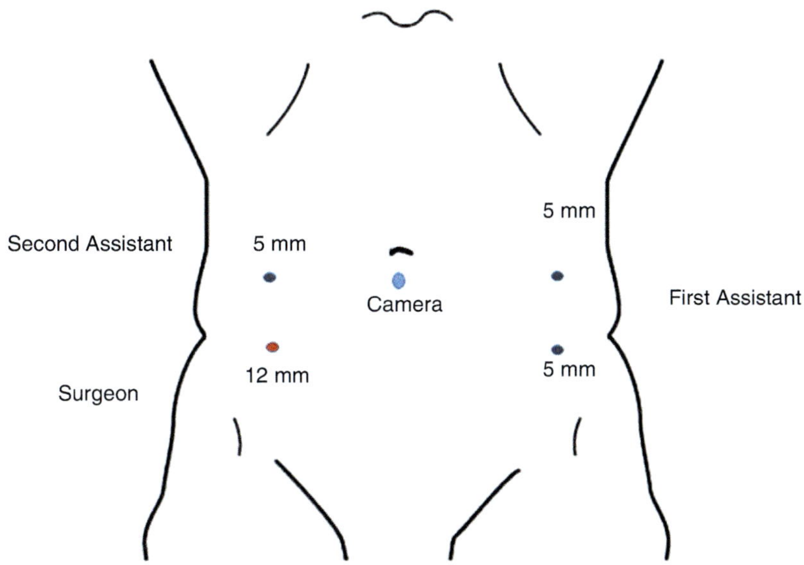

Fig. 31.6 Preferred port placement for laparoscopic LAR with TME

- The patient is placed in a modified lithotomy position. Pneumoperitoneum is established with a Hasson technique through a supraumbilical incision. The abdominal cavity is examined using the robotic camera. Four additional robotic ports are inserted, along with an assistant port, as shown in Figure 31.7a.
- The greater omentum and the small bowel are retracted out of the pelvis. The patient is placed in Trendelenburg position, with right-side down.
- The robotic cart is brought to the left lower quadrant. The robotic arms are first docked, with robot arm 1 in the right lower quadrant using monopolar curved scissors or vessel sealer; robot arm 2 in the right upper abdomen using a fenestrated bipolar forceps; and robot arm 3 in the left mid-abdomen using a ProGrasp™ or Cadiere forceps for retraction. Arm 3 begins on the left side of the robot, on the same side as arm 1.
- Dissection proceeds in a medial-to-lateral fashion, as in standard laparoscopic dissection. Following division of the IMA and IMV, splenic flexure mobilization, and division of the left colic mesentery, robot arm 3 is repositioned (Figure 31.7b). The robot does not need to be moved, and patient position can be maintained.
- On occasion, a slightly more accentuated head-down and minimal tilt are utilized for the pelvic dissection, in order to keep the small bowel out of the pelvis. This configuration ensures that all instruments can reach the pelvic floor without conflict.
- Proctectomy proceeds, as described above for standard laparoscopy, but with a few exceptions. Care is taken to maintain dissection along the mesorectal plane laterally and avoid dissection into the pelvic sidewall. This is facilitated by early anterior dissection, which is easily visualized with the camera setup, as described, and use of articulating instruments.
- We often use a tie around the rectum (such as thin vaginal packing) to facilitate rectal retraction. During pelvic dissection, the bedside assistant utilizes the lateral assistant port and the right upper quadrant robotic port (which was used for pedicle ligation and flexure takedown).
- Intraoperative endoscopy, with picture-in-picture technology, allows the operating surgeon to visualize the rectal tumor at the robotic console and optimize the distal resection margin. We use the robotic sta-

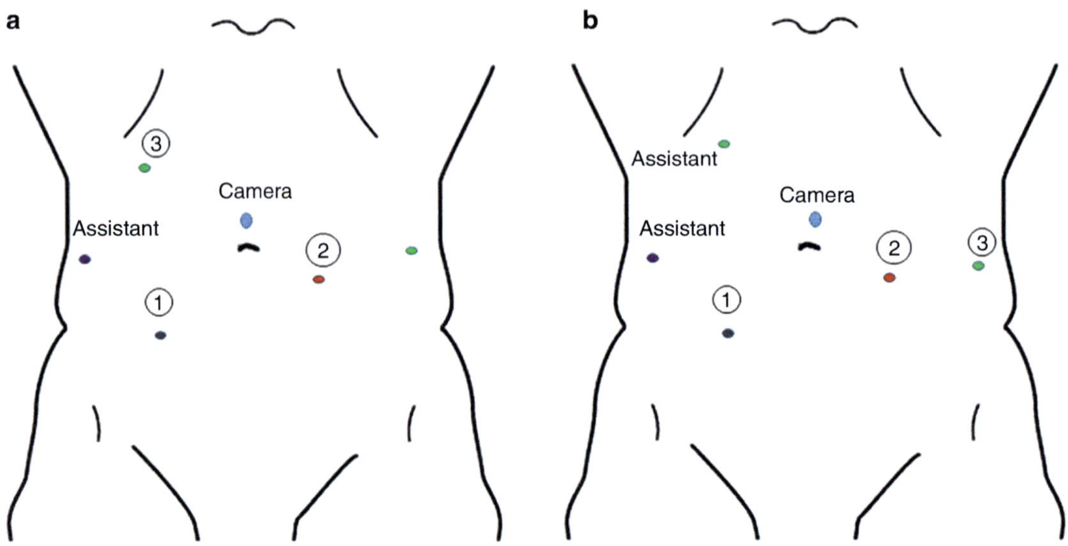

Fig. 31.7 Trocar placement for robotic LAR using the da Vinci® Si™ robot with the two separate phases of the operation: (**a**) pedicle ligation and splenic flexure mobilization and (**b**) pelvic dissection

pler (EndoWrist® Stapler 45) to achieve low pelvic stapling.
- When the distal rectum has been divided, the robot is undocked and the rectum extracted via a wound protector at the umbilical port or future stoma site. The descending colon is divided, the anvil secured, and laparoscopic anastomosis performed.

- A similar setup is utilized with the da Vinci® Xi™ robot.
  - This system has more flexibility, as the camera is 8 mm and can be used in any port. This is referred to as "port hopping" and is useful if dissection becomes difficult and a new vantage point is needed.
  - The da Vinci® Xi™ robot instruments are longer, eliminating problems related to reaching the splenic flexure and the deep pelvis. Port setup is shown in Fig. 31.8 a and b.

Abdominoperineal Resection (APR)

- APR is appropriate for distal rectal cancers that invade the external sphincter or the levator muscles.
  - Relative indications include patients with poor preoperative baseline bowel function who are not candidates for a Hartmann resection.
  - Furthermore, care should be taken when planning surgery in patients with bulky low tumors that show minimal response or progression on neoadjuvant chemoradiation. This portends aggressive tumor biology with extension along lymphovascular and perineural spaces, making complete margin-negative resection more challenging. Wide resection, including APR, should be considered in such cases.
- During APR, left colon/splenic flexure mobilization is not required.
- Dissection is generally taken down to the pelvic floor, and then the perineal phase is begun.
- Perineal dissection can be performed in lithotomy or prone position. Some assert that the prone dissection is more comfortable for the surgeon and facilitates anterior dissection but requires abdominal closure and stoma maturation prior to repositioning the patient facedown.
- When beginning the perineal phase, additional skin preparation is utilized, and the anus is sutured to reduce contamination.

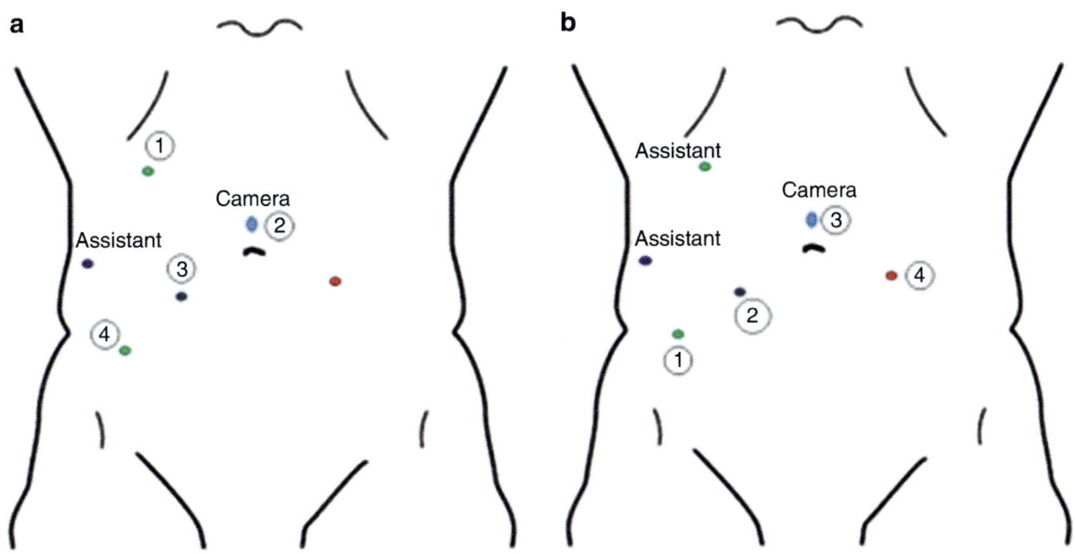

Fig. 31.8 Trocar placement for a robotic LAR using the da Vinci® Xi™ robot. (**a**) Configuration used for pedicle ligation and splenic flexure mobilization. (**b**) Configuration used for pelvic dissection

- A wide elliptical incision is created to encompass the sphincter complex, and dissection proceeds into the ischiorectal space.
- The dissection proceeds just anterior to the coccyx, where the pelvic floor is divided and the perineal dissection meets the anterior dissection.
- The lateral pelvic floor musculature is divided widely, and the anterior dissection is then performed, carefully avoiding injury to the vagina or membranous portion of the urethra.
- Following specimen removal and pelvic irrigation, what remains of the levators are re-approximated, and the perineum is closed in multiple layers to eliminate the dead space. Pelvic drains are used to reduce fluid buildup in the pelvis.

Extralevator or "Cylindrical" APR

- Patients undergoing APR have higher rates of local recurrence and poorer survival as compared to patients undergoing restorative proctectomy. The difference in oncologic outcomes may be explained to a substantial degree by the increased risk of tumor-involved margins (CRM) and inadvertent bowel perforations associated with APR, as both of these factors are significantly related to local control and survival.
- It is important to keep in mind that the distal rectum is devoid of surrounding mesorectum; therefore, tumor extension beyond the muscularis propria can invade surrounding tissues, resulting in positive CRM with standard resection techniques.
- An approach to reduce CRM involvement and specimen perforation, proposed by the Karolinska Institute in Stockholm and termed extralevator or "cylindrical" APR, involves wide resection of the levator muscles en bloc with the sphincter muscles, anal canal, and mesorectum (Figure 31.9a–d).
- The abdominal component of the procedure terminates higher in the pelvis, and the levator ani muscle is divided along its attachments to the sidewall to avoid a "waist" in the specimen (Figure 31.10a, b).
- The perineal phase widely resects the ischiorectal space and completes the dissection.
- In a report comparing cylindrical to conventional APR specimens, Holm and colleagues demonstrated a marked reduction in CRM

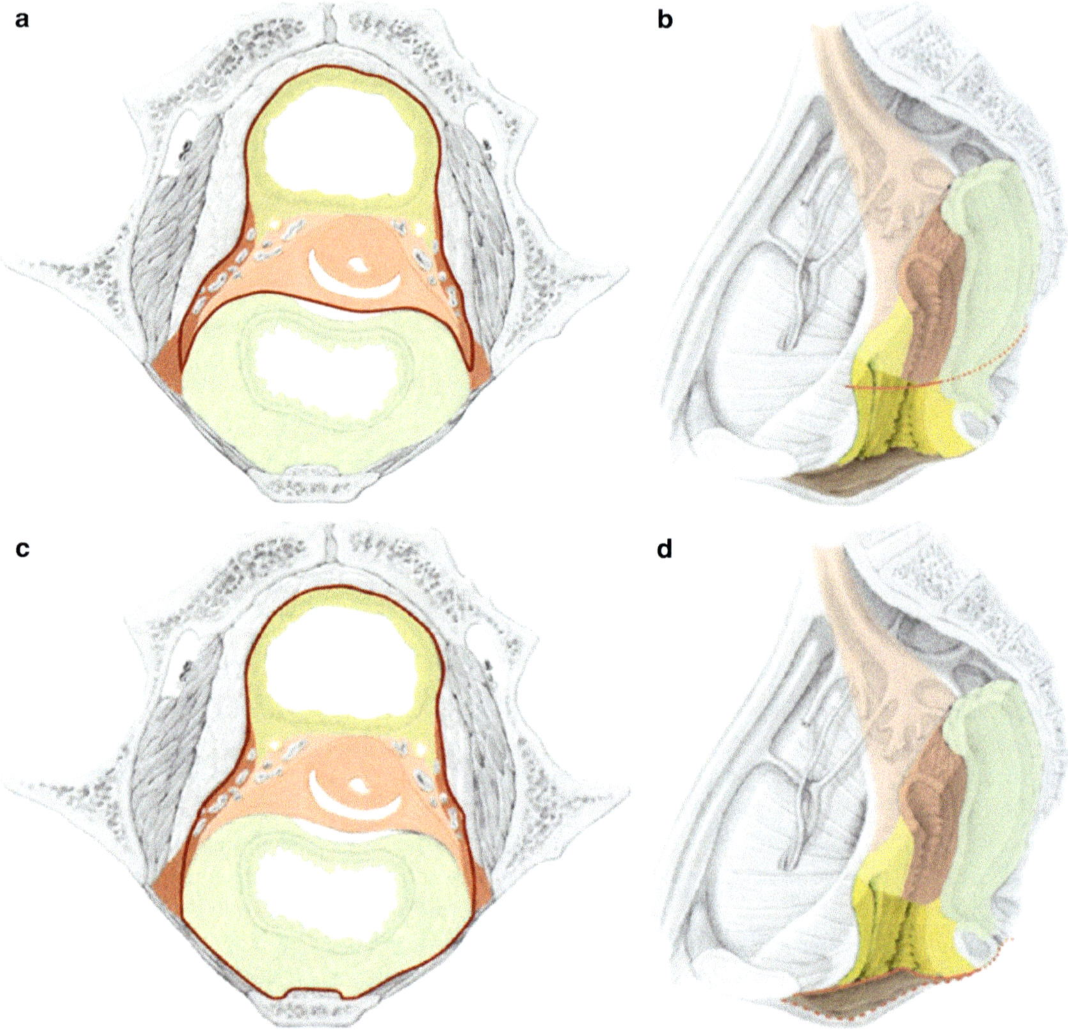

Fig. 31.9 Schematic representation of the major types of extended endopelvic resection. (**a**) Anterior endopelvic resection (transverse place, circumferential resection line highlighted). (**b**) Abdominal pelvic resection (sagittal plane, caudal resection line highlighted). (**c**) Total endopelvic resection (transverse plane, circumferential resection line highlighted). (**d**) Abdominoperineal endopelvic resection (sagittal plane, caudal resection line highlighted). (With permission from Hockel M. Laterally extended endopelvic resection for the treatment of locally advanced and recurrent cervical cancer. In: Patel HRH, Mould T, Joseph JV, Delaney CP, editors. Pelvic cancer surgery: modern breakthroughs and future advances. New York: Springer; 2005. © Springer 2005)

involvement and perforation with cylindrical APR; however, flap closure is usually required, and perineal wound complications and chronic pain were significantly increased in the extralevator group.

- Many advocate "selective extralevator dissection" in areas of tumor, stressing the need for accurate preoperative imaging and examination.

Special Considerations

Distal Margin

- The distal resection margin is an important consideration in rectal cancer surgery. Although lymphatic drainage of the rectum generally occurs in a cephalad direction toward the major lymph node stations, pathological studies have

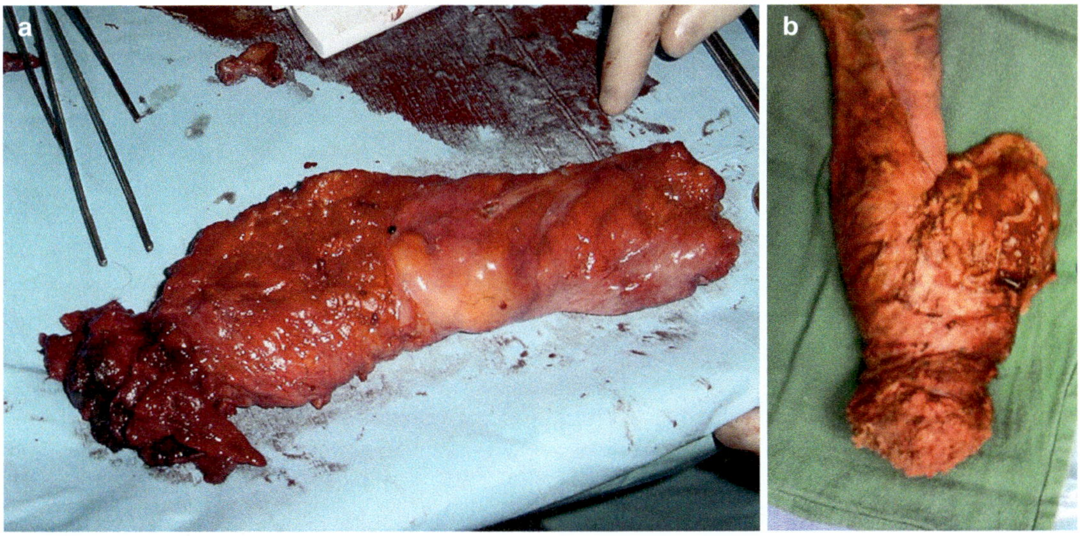

Fig. 31.10 Abdominoperineal resection specimens. Dissections from above and below meet above the anal canal. (**a**) APR specimen with a waist. Courtesy of Eric K Johnson, MD. (**b**) Specimen with a cylindrical resection and no waist (intact mesorectum). Courtesy of Conor Delaney, MD

shown distal mesorectal spread as far as 2–3 cm below the lower palpable edge of the tumor.

- Thus, for upper rectal cancers, mesorectal resection should include mesorectum at least 4–5 cm distal to the lower edge of the tumor and the mesorectum divided perpendicular to the longitudinal access of the rectum for a tumor-specific mesorectal excision. It is critical not to "cone in" and leave mesorectum behind when performing this maneuver.
- For mid to low rectal cancers, dissection 4–5 cm below the tumor generally ends at the pelvic floor. Thus, as long as the entire mesorectum can be removed and negative margins of resection obtained for the primary tumor, it is reasonable to consider restorative proctectomy with coloanal anastomosis for patients with distal cancers.
- The exact distance that constitutes an adequate distal mural margin in this situation is the subject of debate, but an attempt to achieve 1–2 cm seems reasonable.

Coloanal Anastomosis

- In carefully selected cases in the setting of an ultralow rectal cancer, continued dissection along the intersphincteric plane (which is an extension of the muscularis propria of the rectum) may facilitate sphincter preservation.
- A handsewn anastomosis is commonly performed, with good oncologic outcomes, especially in patients with a significant response to preoperative chemoradiotherapy.
- Patient selection and counseling are critical, as patients with coloanal anastomosis have worse bowel function and potentially poorer quality of life than those with a standard stapled colorectal anastomosis.

Options for Reconstruction of the Gastrointestinal Tract

- Following rectal resection, patients often describe frequent bowel movements, incomplete evacuation, clustering, urgency, and, at times, incontinence.
- In order to mitigate these symptoms, which are collectively known as low anterior resection syndrome, various techniques have been attempted to recreate the reservoir function of the resected rectum. These are known as colonic neorectal reservoirs and include the colonic J-pouch and the end-to-side (or "Baker-type") anastomosis.

- A colonic J-pouch is constructed in similar fashion to an ileal J-pouch; however, the colonic J-pouch is much smaller, about 6–8 cm in length. Randomized trials, a meta-analysis, and Cochrane review have all concluded that a colonic J-pouch results in improvement of symptoms (decreased frequency, urgency, and nocturnal bowel movements) and a better quality of life for at least 1 year after surgery, compared to an end-to-end anastomosis.
- Coloplasty, longitudinal colotomy closed transversely, was proposed for patients with a narrow pelvis for whom J-pouch was not technically feasible; however, this has not been shown to be an improvement over straight anastomosis. The additional suture line has a risk of leak that can be difficult to treat, and generally coloplasty has fallen out of favor.
- It is difficult to interpret the results of some trials, given the variation in surgical technique: specifically, the use of either sigmoid colon or descending colon for construction of the neorectum.
  - Use of the sigmoid colon for construction of the neorectum in patients with significant muscular hypertrophy or diverticular disease may negatively impact postoperative function.
- An end-to-side or Baker anastomosis, first described in 1950, has recently been revisited as another option for improving postoperative bowel function. This side-to-end anastomosis appears to confer many of the functional advantages of the colonic J-pouch. Compared to a straight anastomosis, it is associated with significantly fewer anastomotic leaks, and overall it is safe and easier and faster to create than the colonic J-pouch.
- Ensuring sufficient length of the bowel to adequately sacralize in the pelvis is crucial to healing and function. Some experts prefer to avoid the multiple staple lines associated with reservoirs, and the risk of anastomotic leaks, which are difficult to remedy.

Fecal Diversion

- Anastomotic leakage following proctectomy occurs in up to one-quarter of patients.
- Creation of a defunctioning stoma following restorative proctectomy decreases the rate of clinically apparent leak and minimizes the sequelae of anastomotic leak.
- However, diversion requires a second operation to restore intestinal continuity, may result in dehydration if an ileostomy is constructed, entails an increased risk of bowel obstruction, and is not popular with patients. Therefore, most centers divert selectively, based on anastomotic height, patient-related factors such as diabetes and previous pelvic radiation, and the results of intraoperative leak test.

Extended Resection

- Up to 10% of patients with rectal cancer present with tumor invading adjacent structures, necessitating en bloc resection of the affected organ(s). En bloc resection of adjacent pelvic organs has been associated with good oncologic outcomes when pathologically negative microscopic (R0) margins can be achieved.
- Involvement of the uterus and vagina in women is best treated with en bloc resection of the rectum with the uterus and the posterior vaginal wall, in order to achieve R0 resection. Closure can be done easily after partial vaginectomy by flap reconstruction or primary closure, preserving sexual function.
- Involvement of the seminal vesicles on one or both sides in men can be managed by dissection anterior to the vesicles, removing them en bloc with the rectum.
  - The neurovascular bundles arising from the inferior hypogastric plexus, which control urinary and sexual function, are at risk during this dissection—as are the distal ureters, which should be identified and preserved.
- Involvement of the prostate by rectal cancer requires urologic consultation and is usually treated either with a partial prostatectomy or a

pelvic exenteration, depending on the extent of tumor invasion.
  - It should be noted that en bloc resection of the seminal vesicles only, with preservation of the bladder and prostate, is a challenging operation, often much more difficult than pelvic exenteration.
- Involvement of the distal ureters by a locally advanced rectal tumor is rare. However, if encountered, it is best managed with en bloc resection of the ureter, with primary ureteric anastomosis over a stent or a psoas hitch, depending on the length of the ureteric defect. Rectal cancers that adhere to the urinary bladder require partial or total cystectomy, especially when the trigone is involved.
- Lateral pelvic sidewall lymph node involvement has been reported in up to 20% of T3/T4 rectal cancer cases. In general, pelvic sidewall lymph node involvement is associated with low-lying tumors and worse prognosis.
  - In Japanese studies, selective use of lateral pelvic lymphadenectomy has reportedly led to good outcomes. A meta-analysis of 20 studies demonstrated no improvement in survival or local recurrence when an extended lymphadenectomy was performed compared to standard proctectomy.
  - In selected cases where lymphatic spread is suspected clinically or radiographically, an extended lymphadenectomy may be warranted.

Intraoperative Radiation Therapy

- Intraoperative radiation therapy (IORT) has been used in patients with locally advanced primary rectal cancer and an involved or threatened CRM following surgical resection.
- The goal of IORT is to sterilize any microscopic foci of tumor, thus decreasing the risk of local recurrence.
- During IORT the radiosensitive bladder and bowel can be excluded from the radiation field, allowing a higher dose to be delivered to the tumor bed.
- In the United States, IORT is most commonly administered by two different techniques: intraoperative electron beam radiation therapy (IOERT) or high-dose-rate (HDR) brachytherapy.
  - IOERT is delivered by means of a linear accelerator over the course of a few minutes; it can be used in any operating room because electrons do not penetrate the tissue as deeply as conventional radiation. The radiation is delivered through a cone, usually toward the tumor bed.
  - HDR treatment, however, can be administered only in adequately shielded rooms. It is delivered through parallel catheters in a flexible plastic flap, which can be cut to fit the region at risk and packed onto the curving pelvic surface. HDR brachytherapy may take up to an hour.
- IORT has been used in locally advanced rectal cancer for more than 30 years, yet there is no convincing evidence that it decreases local recurrence or improves survival.
  - The only multicenter randomized trial to date included 142 patients with locally advanced rectal cancer, who had received preoperative chemoradiation and were randomly assigned to either surgical resection alone or surgery plus IORT. After a 5-year follow-up, the trial did not demonstrate any significant improvement in local recurrence or disease-free survival.
- In the setting of locally advanced primary rectal cancers, we recommend having IORT available for patients if a close or threatened CRM is highly suspected, based on preoperative imaging.
- IORT is more commonly utilized in resection of recurrent rectal cancer if tissue planes have been previously disrupted and discontinued foci of tumor may be present.

Flap Closure Following Abdominoperineal Resection

- Special attention to perineal closure is required after APR. The bony confines of the pelvis prevent tissue collapse, leading to significant dead space. Pelvic infection requiring opening of the perineum, prolonged wound healing, and chronic perineal sinuses are not uncommon. Multilayered closure to reduce dead space and liberal use of drains are common.
- However, in some cases, rotating a well-vascularized omentum or a myocutaneous flap [39] into the pelvis should be considered, in order to reduce dead space and facilitate perineal healing after APR, especially in patients who have received pelvic radiation.
- A properly designed omental pedicle graft can be easily devised by dividing the gastrocolic omental attachments, detaching the left omentum from the spleen, and ligating the left gastroepiploic pedicle and the short gastric vessels. Care is taken to avoid injury to the right gastroepiploic, which allows the bulk of well-vascularized left omentum to rotate into and fill the pelvis. Rotation of the right omentum, based on the left gastroepiploic, is also feasible.
- In cases of exenteration, sacrectomy, extensive perineal skin loss, or requirement of vaginal reconstruction, a myocutaneous (vertical rectus abdominus myocutaneous, gracilis, or gluteal) flap is utilized.

Functional Outcomes

- High rates of postoperative sexual and urinary dysfunction were a well-known phenomenon in the early years of rectal cancer surgery.
- Improved surgical technique has resulted in less frequent rates of sexual dysfunction; however it is still a major issue for patients undergoing proctectomy.
- Type of surgery (APR compared to LAR) and age greater than 60 years are associated with male sexual dysfunction postoperatively.
- Serious urinary dysfunction, such as neurogenic bladder, is now rare.
- In patients with extensive pelvic disease, autonomic nerve preservation may not be feasible or oncologically sound. Involvement of the autonomic nerves by tumor, or lymphadenopathy in the pelvic sidewall, generally requires a resection that will affect nerve function permanently.
- In patients who undergo LAR, poor bowel function has been associated with the level of the anastomosis and the administration of pelvic radiotherapy. Low anastomoses (<3 cm) and coloanal anastomoses are associated with more incontinence of gas and solid stools compared to higher anastomoses.
- Despite suffering defecation problems, quality of life has consistently been shown to be better following an LAR compared an APR. This has been confirmed by comparative studies and in a meta-analysis of several studies. Body image is consistently higher in patients undergoing an LAR versus APR, which may contribute to the inferior sexual function associated with APR.
- Neoadjuvant radiation therapy causes fibrosis, leading to reduced compliance of the remaining rectum and damage to the myenteric (Auerbach's) plexus, and has been associated with higher rates of urgency, frequency, and fecal incontinence.

Oncologic Outcomes

- Attention to detail during proctectomy, especially with regard to appropriate mesorectal excision, has been associated with improved local control and survival rates. Local pelvic failure rates following proctectomy at centers of excellence are now in the single digits. This is a substantial improvement compared to the local pelvic failure rates following proctectomy in the past, which were 3 to 5 times higher.
- The impact of training in proper proctectomy technique has been well documented. Surgical TME educational programs in Sweden,

Norway, and the Netherlands have been shown to markedly reduce local recurrence, improve survival, and reduce the rate of permanent stomas.

- In Sweden, implementation of specialized proctectomy training, utilization of neoadjuvant short-course radiotherapy, and referral of patients with rectal cancer to specialists have led to a fall in local recurrence rates.
- During the same period, the proportion of APR procedures performed in Sweden decreased by more than 50%.
- Another factor associated with oncologic outcome is the training and experience of the operating surgeon. Studies have shown that subspecialty training, surgeon experience, volume of cases, and treatment in high-volume tertiary care centers influence and enhance patient outcomes with respect to postoperative morbidity and mortality, local recurrence, and long-term survival.

Multidisciplinary Rectal Cancer Care

- There is increasing evidence that multidisciplinary team management is associated with improved clinical decision-making, superior outcomes, and better patient experience in several types of cancer, including rectal cancer.
- Cancer centers of excellence have been successfully established in several European countries over the past decade to address variability and disparity in the quality of rectal cancer care.
- Similar efforts in optimizing care to improve outcome have now gained traction in the United States. These efforts are appropriate, given the wide variability in oncologic outcomes, permanent stoma rates, and use of neoadjuvant radiotherapy and chemotherapy demonstrated in multiple studies.

32 Rectal Cancer Decision-Making

W. Donald Buie and Anthony R. MacLean

Key Concepts

- Sound decision-making requires a full assessment of the primary lesion, the presence of metastatic disease, the patients' surgical risk, and goals of care.
- A submucosal excision may be used as a radical biopsy to assess a polyp for adverse features without compromising future radical excision.
- Following endoscopic excision of a malignant polyp, the pathology should be re-reviewed and strict criteria adhered to regarding the need for radical surgery.
- While cT2 (clinical stage T2) lesions can be treated with radical excision alone, neoadjuvant treatment can be selectively given to patients with cT3 lesions, based on preoperative staging by MRI and multidisciplinary discussion.
- Pre-treatment staging can be inaccurate, especially with regard to mesorectal nodal status. Treatment planning should include a discussion of what will be recommended if stage changes based on histologic analysis. This is especially true if patients are assumed to be node negative, undergo up-front proctectomy, and are found to be node positive or if patients undergo local excision and are found to have higher T stage than anticipated.
- Most operative decisions should be made prior to entering the operating room. The patient and the surgeon must be prepared for all eventualities. In some situations the ultimate surgical decision may depend on intraoperative findings.
- Patients with potentially curable stage IV disease require multidisciplinary discussion with early involvement of hepatobiliary surgeons and medical oncologists to determine the optimal sequence of treatment.

Assessment

- When first encountering a patient with a rectal neoplasm, our first step is to gather information.
  - Lesion size, location (distance from anal verge, distance from the superior aspect of the anorectal muscular ring and circumferential position—anterior/posterior/lateral), morphology, fixation (fixed, tethered, mobile), and general appearance.
  - Anatomy and function of the anal sphincters.
  - Presence of metastatic disease.
  - Assess the patient for surgical risk including anesthetic risk, procedural risk, and patient risk.

W. D. Buie (✉) · A. R. MacLean
Department of Surgery, Foothills Medical Centre, University of Calgary, Calgary, AB, Canada
e-mail: wdbuie@ucalgary.ca

S. R. Steele et al. (eds.), *The ASCRS Manual of Colon and Rectal Surgery*, https://doi.org/10.1007/978-3-030-01165-9_32

- As the surgeon you are responsible for ensuring that each patient is fully evaluated and optimized for the required treatment, the right procedure at the right time as safely as possible.
- An important part of assessment includes goals of care. Oncologic surgery is a balance of cure versus morbidity, mortality, and quality of life.
  - Patients with significant comorbidity or those who are elderly may place greater emphasis on quality rather than quantity of life and make decisions accordingly.
  - The risk-benefit profile of each potential treatment should be outlined and discussed thoroughly.
- The final part of assessment is a firm understanding of your own strengths, skills, and limitations.
  - Utilizing senior colleagues for a second opinion or as an intraoperative assist is a sign of good judgment.
  - The management of rectal cancer is multidisciplinary, and you must cultivate strong relationships with your colleagues in the associated disciplines of diagnostic radiology, radiation oncology, medical oncology, pathology, and hepatobiliary surgery to provide optimal patient care.
  - Ideally rectal cancer patients should be discussed at regular multidisciplinary conferences which have been shown to enhance care and outcomes.

Early Rectal Neoplasms

Local Excision

- For rectal lesions that appear to be benign or cT1 cancer, we would typically arrange for local staging, most commonly with endorectal ultrasound to examine the depth of invasion.
- Pelvic MRI can also be considered for staging regional nodes and to document the baseline appearance of the pelvis going forward.
- If the lesion has a malignant appearance or is a proven cancer on biopsy, we also arrange systemic staging with a CT scan of the chest, abdomen, and pelvis.
- CEA should be obtained preoperatively for all neoplasms.
- As long as there are no features on biopsy or imaging that are high risk for nodal disease, we would offer transanal excision using any of a variety of techniques as a "radical biopsy."
- While the prevailing opinion described in most textbooks advocates for full-thickness excision in all cases, we tend to be more selective in our approach.
- For lesions that appear benign on biopsy and imaging or at worst T1, we try to gauge the patient's thoughts on what their wishes would be in response to the biopsy results.
  - If the patient decides that he or she would want a radical excision for anything other than the most early, most favorable cancer, we feel that a partial-thickness excision is a very reasonable option, as it provides definitive histology and allows assessment of high-risk features, including differentiation, lymphovascular invasion, tumor budding, and depth of invasion in microns (Table 32.1).
    - For lesions invading to <1000 microns with no adverse pathologic features, particularly with no evidence of high-grade budding, local excision alone is felt to be acceptable treatment, with close follow-up.
- Additional reasons to consider a partial-thickness excision also include less perioperative risk and no significant change in the perirectal fat that can affect the difficulty of (and complications from) subsequent radical excision in cases with unfavorable histologic features.
- Most importantly, if the lesion is proven to be benign, then excision in the submucosal plane should be curative and will avoid the added morbidity of full-thickness excision.
- On the other hand, if the patient is more strongly in favor of avoiding radical surgery and would tolerate a slightly higher risk of local recurrence, we feel that a full-thickness excision is warranted for lesions

Table 32.1 Risk of nodal involvement

	# tumors	Nodal involvement (%)	Odds ratio	P value
Tumor grade				
Favorable	176	5.7		
Unfavorable	75	29.2	2.9	0.023
Vascular invasion				
Absent	176	5.7		
Present	75	30.7	2.7	0.039
Cribriform pattern				
Absent	192	7.3		
Present	59	32.2	3.9	0.002
Tumor budding				
Negative	213	8.0		
Positive	38	42.1	3.7	0.008

With permission from Ueno H, Mochizuki H, Hasiguchi Y, et al. Risk factors for an adverse outcome in early invasive colorectal carcinoma. Gastroenterology 2004; 127:385–94 © Elsevier 2004

that are proven on biopsy to be adenocarcinoma preoperatively or have gross features of malignancy, which again allows for histologic evaluation but also provides a wider deep margin for more significant lesions.

- Once the histologic information is available (for which we also typically request a second opinion from an experienced GI pathologist), we have a thorough discussion with the patient about the results and define their risk of lymph node disease.
  - For patients with T1 adenocarcinoma with high-risk features and/or depth of invasion greater than 1000 microns (or Kikuchi level SM2), we recommend radical excision.
  - However, in situations where the patient understands the risks, and prefers to avoid radical excision, close follow-up is an acceptable alternative.
- For patients who are frail or have significant comorbidity that would preclude a radical excision, we consider extending our indications for local excision to more significant lesions.
- Our follow-up depends somewhat on the characteristics of the lesion excised and the patient's age and comorbidity but, in general, would include:
  - Digital rectal and sigmoidoscopic examination at 3–4-month intervals for the first 2 years when the risk of recurrence appears to be highest and then at 6-month intervals for an additional 2 years with colonoscopic evaluation as indicated for surveillance at year 1 and year 4,
  - Pelvic MRI scans at 6-month intervals for the first 2 years to look for nodal recurrence,
  - Yearly CT scans of the chest, abdomen, and pelvis for the first 3 years to look for metastatic disease.

Endoscopically Excised Malignant Polyps

- Occasionally we will be referred to a patient who has had endoscopic excision of a malignant rectal polyp. In these situations, we obtain a pathologic review and then try to determine the risk of intraluminal recurrence as well as the risk of nodal disease and systemic recurrence.
- We examine the polypectomy site with sigmoidoscopy and, if not already done, mark it with a tattoo especially if completely excised.
- The patient is staged as in the early rectal cancer section above.
  - However, it is important to remember that imaging can be affected by the thermal injury to the bowel wall from a large polypectomy. Occasionally lymphadenopathy

related to local inflammation will be seen that can be confused for nodal metastases.

- The risk of intraluminal recurrence is dependent on the margin of excision—while many textbooks advocate a 2 mm minimal margin, current evidence suggests that in the absence of other high-risk histologic features, a 1 mm margin is adequate.
- In terms of the risk of nodal disease, important factors include differentiation, lymphovascular invasion, tumor budding, and depth of invasion (see Table 32.1).
- When all histologic features are favorable and the margin is greater than 1 mm, close follow-up is recommended.
- When all histologic features are favorable, but the margin is <1 mm, we discuss re-excision transanally versus radical excision.
- When high-risk features for nodal metastases are present, we typically recommend radical excision assuming the patient is a suitable candidate. In high-risk patients where radical excision is not an option, we extend our indications for observation.

Operable and Locally Advanced Lesions

- For lesions that are not amenable to local excision, our approach is to again assess the lesion as described above but to usually forgo ultrasound and instead proceed directly to pelvic MR with rectal cancer protocol for local staging and systemic staging with a CT of the chest abdomen and pelvis. We do not routinely advocate the use of PET scan in the preoperative staging of rectal cancer, except to help resolve an indeterminate lesion identified on CT or MRI.
- For lesions that are cT2 on imaging, we typically advocate a radical excision. We do not currently feel that there is sufficient evidence to recommend local excision in association with neoadjuvant or adjuvant chemoradiation, though there is ongoing interest in this approach and further evidence could possibly change that opinion in the future.
- The current "standard of care" for all clinical stage II and III rectal cancers is to receive neoadjuvant therapy followed by radical surgery and to receive postoperative chemoradiotherapy when final pathology unexpectedly demonstrates stage II or III disease.
- However, it has become clear that many of these patients derive very little benefit from chemoradiotherapy, as this treatment primarily impacts local control, not overall survival. For patients treated at centers of excellence with optimal surgical technique, their primarily risk of death from rectal cancer is from distant disease, not local pelvic failure.
- In addition, patients who receive postoperative radiotherapy often suffer long-term complications, including fibrosis/stricture of the anorectum and other issues with bowel, bladder, and sexual function. It is also clear that receiving postoperative radiotherapy is less effective than neoadjuvant radiotherapy.
- Thus identifying those patients who are likely to derive the most benefit from radiotherapy is important.
- Current staging modalities are fairly accurate at determining T stage, and distance to the expected mesorectal margin, but are much less accurate in determining mesorectal nodal status.
  - All the techniques suffer from the inherent limitation that they do not detect tumor but rather the size and morphology of the node.
  - Tumor deposits in lymph nodes do not reliably produce lymphadenopathy greater than 1 cm; in fact more than 50% of all positive nodes will be less than 5 mm in size.
  - In addition, the inflammatory reaction from previous biopsies, or from the tumor itself, can result in nodal enlargement without tumor involvement, resulting in false positives.
  - Metabolic imaging with 18-fluorodeoxy glucose positron emission tomography (FDG-PET) may not be effective in detecting mesorectal nodal status because emission from the primary tumor may obscure adjacent nodal signal or because of the

small size of some of the nodal metastases.

- Locally advanced lesions require a considerable amount of careful thought when deciding on the most appropriate course of treatment.
- We generally use the MERCURY study group criteria to help decide which patients should be referred for neoadjuvant therapy.
  - cT3a tumors with less than 5 mm of intrusion into the perirectal fat and predicted negative resection margins generally behave more as T2 lesions and thus can be spared the negative consequences of radiation therapy (Fig. 32.1).
  - For cT3 lesions with a close but predicted negative (>2 mm) margin based on staging MRI, we believe that neoadjuvant therapy is warranted.
  - In this situation, both short course radiation and long-course chemoradiation can be considered. For cT3 lesions with a predicted positive margin, and for cT4 lesions, long-course neoadjuvant chemoradiation is typically used to shrink the tumor to make pelvic surgery less challenging.
- However, preoperative staging alone should not drive all treatment algorithms with regard to neoadjuvant therapy. Pelvic morphology and tumor position may have a significant effect on decision-making.
  - For example, a proctectomy in an obese man with a narrow pelvis and an anteriorly based tumor of the mid or distal rectum can be very challenging. Such a patient should be considered for neoadjuvant therapy and should be discussed in a multidisciplinary setting, ideally with radiologic review.
  - Alternatively, proctectomy in a thin woman with a wide pelvis and a posteriorly based tumor should be relatively straightforward

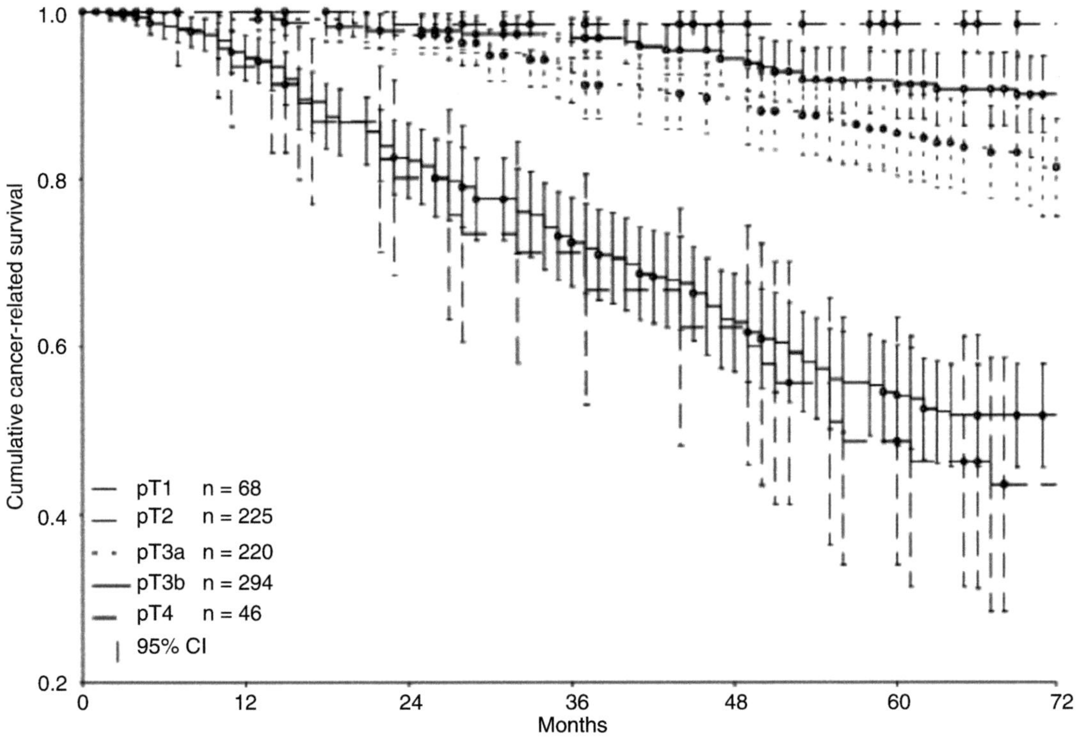

Fig. 32.1 Cancer-related survival in relation to extended pT classification based on depth of invasion: *pT1* submucosa, *pT2* muscularis propria, *pT3a* < 5 mm extramural disease, *pT3b* > 5 mm extramural disease; *pT4* other organs. (With permission from Merkel S Mansmann U, Siassi M, Papadopoulos T, et al. The prognostic inhomogeneity in pT3 rectal carcinomas. Int J Colorectal Dis. 2001;16:298–304 © Springer 2001)

with little chance of positive margin if the tumor does not extend beyond the mesorectal fascia on preoperative imaging.

- At present, we do not possess a reliable method to predict nodal status prior to embarking on a treatment course. This is of particular concern for patients who undergo proctectomy as a first step in treatment. Some of these patients who are staged preoperatively as cN0 are upstaged to pN1+ following histologic review of the proctectomy specimen.
- Prior to simply recommending postoperative radiotherapy because of N + status, it should be remembered that postoperative radiotherapy is not as effective as preoperative radiotherapy, must be administered at a higher dose with concurrent chemotherapy to achieve similar oncologic benefit, and has the downside of higher toxicity.
- One strategy to avoid the issue of radiating patients postoperatively who are found unexpectedly to have node-positive disease at proctectomy is to radiate all patients regardless of pre-treatment imaging results.
  - Short course radiotherapy is probably the best regimen for patients with non-fixed tumors if this strategy is adopted, as the oncologic results are equivalent to long-course chemoradiotherapy. In addition, short-course radiotherapy can be administered more quickly (shortening the time to full-dose cytotoxic chemotherapy in appropriate patients), is less costly, and is associated with less toxicity in the neoadjuvant period.
  - The main downside of this approach is the large number of patients who would be treated and exposed to the long-term consequences of radiotherapy without deriving any significant benefit.
- Another approach is to agree at the initial multidisciplinary conference that patients recommended for up-front proctectomy will not be considered for postoperative radiotherapy unless margins of resection are positive and will be treated with chemotherapy alone if they are found to be node positive and resection margin negative.
  - This strategy will also shorten the time to full-dose cytotoxic chemotherapy and avoid the toxicity of postoperative radiotherapy, which can be substantial.
  - The argument that this is not "standard of care" is based on recommendations from decades past, when trials were conducted without surgery or pathology quality control, radial margins were not assessed, and chemotherapeutic agents were less effective.
  - This is our current treatment approach for patients who are upstaged on pathologic review following proctectomy.
- Lastly, there is continued interest in a "watch and wait" approach following neoadjuvant therapy with complete clinical response. The issue remains that complete clinical response does not always equate with complete pathologic response. Except in situations of compromise due to patient frailty or comorbidity, we feel that this approach should be relegated to participation in a clinical trial. This opinion may change as additional information becomes available.
- As one may see from the above discussion, decision-making for patients with rectal cancer is complex and nuanced. Unfortunately, this complexity cannot be easily transformed into simple treatment guidelines.

Surgical Considerations

Intraoperative Decisions

- Most operative decisions should be made prior to entering the operating room. There is no substitute for advance preparation having thought through the potential problems and solutions away from the OR when planning and reflection can occur without distraction and emotion. The accuracy of current cross-sectional imaging modalities should make major unexpected findings at abdominal exploration (other than small volume peritoneal disease) a thing of the past.

- However, there are occasions where the final decision can only be made at the time of surgery. The surgeon must be flexible and have very precisely articulated goals of care; know why you are there and what you are trying to accomplish. In exceptional cases, this may include backing out if the situation requires more than what has been planned for. It is better to return on another day when the patient and surgeon are emotionally and physically prepared for the operation that is required.

Midrectal Cancers

- As mesorectal spread can extend up to 3 to 4 cm distal to the gross tumor margin, a 5 cm mesorectal margin is required to ensure complete removal of at-risk nodal tissue. We advocate a tumor-specific mesorectal excision for tumors in the upper third of the rectum, preserving rectal length and function without compromising cure. When the tumor is located in the distal third of the rectum, 5 cm or less from the end of the mesorectum, we advocate a total mesorectal excision (TME) to remove all nodal tissue.
- For tumors in the middle third especially in obese patients, it may be very difficult to perform a tumor-specific mesorectal excision and save 2–3 cm of viable rectum above the pelvic floor. We feel it is often technically easier and safer for the patient to extend the resection for an additional 2 or 3 cm to complete a TME. The decision is based primarily on the technical feasibility of dissecting through the distal mesorectum at that level while preserving the viability of the rectal stump.

Low Rectal Cancers

- Surgical decision-making in low rectal cancer is often complex, balancing cure with function.
- In most situations, the decision to proceed with a sphincter-preserving procedure rather than an abdominoperineal resection is made preoperatively based on history, physical examination, imaging studies, response to chemoradiation, and the ability to obtain clear surgical margins.
  - Patient factors including age, comorbidities, body habitus, continence, and patient's wishes must be considered.
  - Good quality MRI with careful interpretation is important to identify any absolute indications for APR including involvement of the levators or external sphincter.
- On rare occasions due to body habitus, tumor size, or pelvic shape, it may be difficult to predict preoperatively whether a tumor can be successfully resected with sphincter-preserving techniques.
  - In this situation the patient must be fully informed and all options discussed in detail including the reasoning behind the decision, the expected outcomes, and potential complications.
  - We consent the patient for "a low anterior resection possible abdominoperineal resection" and emphasize that we are operating for local control and will proceed with sphincter preservation provided that cure is not compromised.
  - The patient should be counseled and marked for both a colostomy and a loop ileostomy.
- Preoperatively, all approaches that enhance distal dissection should be considered including a stapled coloanal anastomosis and a hand-sewn coloanal anastomosis with or without intersphincteric resection.
- Although a stapled anastomosis results in better function and less morbidity, an intersphincteric dissection provides additional distal margin length.
  - We restrict this technique to very low tumors that are contained within the rectal wall, which do not invade the pelvic floor or anal sphincters, in patients who can tolerate and accept the functional compromise.
  - The functional results depend on preoperative sphincter function, the effect of neoadjuvant radiation, and the variable amount

of residual internal sphincter left below the dentate line.

- Generally speaking for distal rectal cancer, given that the entire mesorectum will be removed as a matter of course, the distal margin (and circumferential margin) should simply be negative for tumor.
  - Every effort should be made prior to rectal division to ascertain if the margin will be adequate.
  - If neoadjuvant therapy was administered, all tissue that was once involved with tumor should be resected. Put another way, resection should be based on initial staging.
    - Because radiotherapy does not kill in a wave front, to change the margin of resection based on response to radiotherapy is subjecting the patient to risk of leaving viable cancer cells *in situ*.
  - Once the rectum is divided and the specimen has been removed, it should be examined off table and if possible in concert with the pathologist. If the distal mural margin is inadequate, we would proceed directly with a completion proctectomy after repositioning in prone jackknife position.
- In the obese male with a bulky tumor and relatively small pelvis, distal mesorectal dissection under direct vision and thus sphincter preservation may be impossible using standard open or laparoscopic techniques such that an APR may be required to obtain clear margins.
- Transanal TME (taTME) with either TEM or TAMIS is a new wrinkle on the old technique of approaching the perineal portion of the dissection first in cases where there is likely to be a technically difficult distal dissection.
  - The distal margin and lower mesorectum are dissected transanally under direct vision and extended proximally using minimally invasive techniques. The plane of dissection is then met from the superior approach using standard laparoscopic or open proctectomy techniques.
  - While the initial case series are promising, this technique is not ready for universal adoption as the oncologic results are not mature, indications and contraindications remain to be refined, and the learning curve is yet to be established.
- A clear circumferential margin is also critical to local control. Every effort should be made preoperatively in conjunction with your radiologist to identify potentially difficult areas of dissection where the margin may be compromised with steps taken to extend resection to an uninvolved plane as necessary.
- If the decision is to proceed with an APR is made intraoperatively, it should be made as soon as possible to maximize the circumferential tumor margin with a cylindrical dissection.
  - It should be remembered that the mesorectal plane will lead the surgeon through the levator hiatus onto the bare area of the rectum with potential compromise to the circumferential margin in an ultralow tumor.
  - All options need to be considered prior to entering this area of dissection.
  - Intraoperatively, as we proceed distally, we frequently don an extra glove and bimanually palpate the tumor changing gloves prior to reentry into the operative field.
  - If we feel that sphincter preservation will compromise the circumferential margin, we stop and proceed with a proctectomy in prone jackknife position.

Low Hartmann Resection Versus APR

- Patients with poor preoperative anal sphincter function who would normally have a low anterior resection with a coloanal anastomosis may also be treated with a low Hartmann resection.
- While this obviates the need for a perineal wound with its attendant risks of non-healing and chronically draining sinus tract, a low Hartmann resection is occasionally complicated by blowout of the stump and chronic pelvic sepsis.

Special Situations

Obstructing Rectal Cancer

- Patient with incurable disease
  - Endoluminal stenting is a reasonable option in patients with limited life expectancy provided that the bottom of the stent will lie clearly above the anorectal ring, to avoid causing pain and tenesmus.
    - It should be remembered that stents will often ultimately erode through the wall of the rectum and are thus not appropriate as long-term solutions.
  - In patients with partial obstructive symptoms and without evidence of proximal colonic dilatation, administration of chemoradiotherapy will usually relieve the obstructive symptoms if instituted without delay.
  - Alternatively, construction of proximal fecal diversion, preferably colostomy, can palliate near complete or complete obstruction.
    - The surgeon should vent the distal segment via loop colostomy or divided end-loop colostomy to avoid distal stump blowout.
    - Laparoscopic or trephine techniques are preferred, if possible, to shorten recovery and allow administration of chemotherapy expeditiously.
- Patients with curable disease
  - In general, endoluminal stents should be avoided.
    - For distal tumors the stent will impinge upon the anal sphincter or protrude from the anus.
    - For more proximal tumors, the stent will impinge upon and potentially damage normal rectum that may ultimately be utilized for anastomosis.
    - In cases of obstructing proximal rectal/rectosigmoid cancer, endoluminal stenting may be followed by semi-urgent radical resection.
  - In cases requiring fecal diversion where an abdominoperineal resection will ultimately be required, we recommend using a loop or divided end-loop colostomy for fecal diversion.
    - At the time of the APR, the distal limb of the stoma can be divided, leaving the colostomy in situ if it is functioning well, or it can be revised to an end colostomy if needed.
  - In cases requiring fecal diversion where an eventual reconstructive surgery is anticipated, decision-making can be more complex.
    - In patients with partial obstructive symptoms and without evidence of proximal colonic dilatation, administration of chemoradiotherapy will usually relieve the obstructive symptoms if instituted without delay.
    - In the "near-obstructing" but not clinically obstructed situation, a diverting loop ileostomy is preferred. This can be left in situ following low anterior resection and ultimately closed after completion of adjuvant therapy.
    - If the lesion is completely obstructing and there is concern for impending colon ischemia, then we would generally construct a diverting loop sigmoid or distal transverse colostomy, the choice dictated by patient anatomy.
      - This prevents the possibility of a "closed loop" developing between the tumor and a competent ileocecal valve should the lesion swell and obstruct during neoadjuvant therapy.
      - It also allows us to perform a colonoscopy preoperatively through the stoma to clear the rest of the colon.
      - If a loop sigmoid colostomy was constructed, it can be taken down and the distal limb included with the resected specimen and loop ileostomy brought through the previous left-sided loop colostomy site.
      - If a distal transverse loop colostomy is constructed, it may be left in situ after definitive resection, depending on colon anatomy.

Perforated Rectal Cancer

- Free intraperitoneal perforation.
  - Urgent surgery is generally required.
  - The operation ideally should include an oncologic resection of the primary tumor.
  - The decision on whether to perform a primary anastomosis (with or without and proximal diverting stoma) or a Hartmann procedure depends on several factors, including the overall health of the patient, their perioperative stability, the duration and extent of fecal contamination, and the anticipated intraoperative technical difficulties.
  - Rarely should one simply divert these patients, as they risk having ongoing intraperitoneal tumor dissemination.
- Contained intraperitoneal perforation.
  - Percutaneous drainage and medical management.
  - Once the patient is stable and the perforation controlled, complete staging.
  - Treatment decisions must take into account the fact that tumor cells are likely spread outside the rectum and mesorectum.
    - Typically neoadjuvant chemotherapy or chemoradiotherapy is administered.
    - The benefit of neoadjuvant therapy should be balanced against the risk of sepsis in an immunocompromised patient. However, many patients will tolerate neoadjuvant radiotherapy or chemoradiotherapy in this situation.
- Contained extraperitoneal perforation.
  - We typically advocate proximal fecal diversion, drainage of sepsis, neoadjuvant chemoradiation, followed by radical excision, to include all tissues felt to have been contaminated by the perforation. This can require an exenterative procedure and/or an extrafascial dissection.
- In the situation where a rectal cancer presents with perianal sepsis and fistulas, we generally ensure that the sepsis is well controlled, strongly consider fecal diversion with a laparoscopic loop sigmoid colostomy, and then arrange for neoadjuvant chemoradiotherapy. This is then followed by an APR with wide pelvic and perineal excision. These patients typically have large perineal wounds, and many benefit from a rectus abdominis myocutaneous flap for perineal reconstruction.

Synchronous Hepatic Metastases

- Advancements in liver surgery, nonsurgical treatment of hepatic metastases, and systemic chemotherapy have made it possible to consider a myriad of approaches for patients suffering from stage IV rectal cancer with synchronous hepatic metastases (Table 32.2).
- Assuming that the patient is a surgical candidate, there are three overriding questions that need to be answered:
  - Is the primary tumor resectable?
  - Is the metastatic liver disease resectable?
  - Is there extrahepatic metastatic disease?
- Both the primary and hepatic metastases are resectable, and there is no extrahepatic disease.
  - Multiple options are available, with their inherent advantages and disadvantages.
  - Neoadjuvant therapy.
    - Cytotoxic chemotherapy will treat both the tumor and the metastatic disease. Tumor response in the liver can be assessed prior to embarking upon resection.

Table 32.2 Ideal criteria for liver-first protocol

1	Local-regional control does not require downstaging with neoadjuvant therapy
2	Liver metastases are very clearly resectable for cure with adequate residual liver
3	Good overall operative risk patient with normal physiologic status and no known risk factors for perioperative infectious complications and major morbidity
4	Surgery can be performed in a high-volume liver unit with low operative mortality and acceptable morbidity
5	Delays due to unexpected postoperative complications will not jeopardize local control or cure

- Long-course pelvic radiotherapy will treat only the primary and delay definitive treatment of metastatic disease.
  - It should be remembered that the typical chemotherapy utilized for long-course chemoradiotherapy treatment of rectal cancer is inadequate treatment of distant metastases.
- Short course pelvic radiotherapy is an attractive option as it is administered in a single week and has been proven to be equally effective as long-course chemoradiotherapy, even with locally advanced primary tumors. It can be administered after chemotherapy, just prior to surgery.

– Surgical resection.
  - Synchronous resection of the liver disease and primary tumor can be contemplated if the patient is healthy and the lesions are amenable to relatively straightforward operation by experienced teams.
    - The patient should be brought to the operating room with the understanding that if there is any concern regarding physiologic response to the initial resection, the secondary resection will be postponed.
  - Philosophy of staged resections.
    - If the primary tumor is asymptomatic, it may be preferable to embark upon the liver resection first, as clearance of the liver disease may drive decisions regarding proctectomy.
    - If the primary tumor is symptomatic or bulky with threatened resection margins, strong consideration should be given to resecting the rectal tumor first.

- Extrahepatic disease.
  - Generally believed to be a contraindication to hepatic resection for cure in stage IV disease.
  - However, in select situations, in a good risk, highly motivated patient, we will consider a lung resection following curative resection of the primary and all liver lesions.
  - Surgery should be done sequentially at a reasonable time interval after recovery from the previous resections to ensure that the disease remains localized and the patient is fully optimized.

Colorectal Cancer: Postoperative Adjuvant Therapy

33

Stephen M. Sentovich and Marwan Fakih

Key Concepts

- Patients with stage III colon cancer should be considered for adjuvant chemotherapy.
- Oxaliplatin-based adjuvant chemotherapy regimens improve survival of stage III colon cancer patients by an absolute 20–25% at 5 years versus no chemotherapy.
- Adjuvant chemotherapy has not been demonstrated to have significant impact on survival for stage II colon cancer patients, but it can be considered for patients whose tumors have high-risk features.
- In colon cancer patients, radiotherapy should be considered when tumors penetrate other fixed structures (T4) and can be guided by placing surgical clips at the time of operation.
- Patients with clinical stage II and III rectal cancers who undergo neoadjuvant chemoradiotherapy should be considered for postoperative adjuvant chemotherapy, regardless of the final pathologic staging, although the efficacy of adjuvant chemotherapy in this setting has not been firmly established.

S. M. Sentovich (✉)
Department of Surgical Oncology, City of Hope, Duarte, CA, USA
e-mail: ssentovich@coh.org

M. Fakih
Department of Medical Oncology and Therapeutic Diagnostics, City of Hope Medical Center, Duarte, CA, USA

Colon Cancer

Stage III Colon Cancer

- Adjuvant chemotherapy is recommended for all stage III colon cancer patients because it decreases recurrence and increases survival when compared to surgery alone.
  - After surgery alone for stage III colon cancer, overall 5-year survival is 40–60%. Current chemotherapeutic regimens improve overall survival to 70–80%. Thus, 5-year overall survival of stage III colon cancer patients improves by an absolute 20–25% with adjuvant chemotherapy.
  - Table 33.1 summarizes the results of key clinical trials establishing the efficacy of adjuvant chemotherapy for nonmetastatic colon cancer. If all patients with stage III colon cancer receive adjuvant chemotherapy, roughly 1/3 to 1/2 of disease recurrences would be prevented.
- The National Quality Forum has endorsed two metrics regarding the treatment of stage III colon cancer patients.
  - The first metric (measure 0385) determines the percentage of patients ≥18 years old who are either referred for adjuvant

S. R. Steele et al. (eds.), *The ASCRS Manual of Colon and Rectal Surgery*,
https://doi.org/10.1007/978-3-030-01165-9_33

Table 33.1 Key clinical trials establishing the efficacy of adjuvant chemotherapy for colon cancer

Trial	Tumor stage	Comparison	Results	Conclusion
INT 0035 1990	Stage III	Surgery alone vs. 5-FU/levamisole	3-year survival 5-FU/levamisole 71% Surgery alone 55%	Post-op adjuvant chemo improves survival for stage III colon cancer
IMPACT 1995	Stage III	Surgery alone vs. 5-FU/leucovorin	3-year survival 5-FU/leucovorin 71% Surgery alone 62%	Post-op adjuvant chemo improves survival for stage III colon cancer
QUASAR 2000	Stage III	5-FU/levamisole vs. 5-FU/folinic acid vs. 5-FU/placebo	Decreased survival and increased recurrence with levamisole compared with placebo	Post-op adjuvant chemo with levamisole inferior to placebo
IMPACT 1999	Stage II	Surgery alone vs. 5-FU/leucovorin	5-year survival = no difference 5-FU/leucovorin 82% Surgery alone 80%	Post-op adjuvant chemo does not improve survival for stage II colon cancer
NSABP (CO-1, CO-2, CO-3, and CO-4) 1999	Stage II	Surgery alone vs. 5-FU +	5-year survival improved with adjuvant treatment 30% mortality reduction with adjuvant treatment	Post-op adjuvant chemo improves survival for stage II colon cancer
MOSAIC 2009	Stage II and III	FOLFOX vs. 5-FU/leucovorin	6-year survival in stage III only FOLFOX 73% 5-FU/leucovorin 68%	FOLFOX superior to 5-FU/LV for stage III colon cancer
XELOXA 2011	Stage III	XELOX vs. 5-FU/leucovorin	3-year disease-free survival: XELOX 71% 5-FU/leucovorin 67%	Capecitabine plus oxaliplatin superior to 5-FU/leucovorin

Table 33.2 Current recommended adjuvant chemotherapy regimens for stage III colon cancer

Regimen	Agents and dosage	Frequency
mFOLFOX6	Oxaliplatin 85 mg/m^2 IV over 2 h, day 1 Leucovorin 400 mg/m^2 IV over 2 h, day 1 5-FU 400 mg/m^2 IV bolus on day 1 and then 1200 mg/m^2/day x 2 days IV continuous infusion	Every 2 weeks
CapeOx	Oxaliplatin 130 mg/m^2 IV over 2 h, day 1 Capecitabine 850–1000 mg/m^2 PO twice daily for 14 days	Every 3 weeks

chemotherapy, prescribed adjuvant chemotherapy, or have previously received adjuvant chemotherapy in the last 12 months.

  – The other metric (measure 0223) determines the percentage of patients under the age of 80 for whom adjuvant chemotherapy is considered or administered within 4 months of the *diagnosis*.

- For patients with stage III colon cancer, the National Comprehensive Cancer Network (NCCN) guidelines recommend adjuvant treatment with FOLFOX or CapeOx for 6 months (Table 33.2).
- While used frequently in patients with metastatic disease, biologic therapy with antibodies directed at VEGF-A (bevacizumab) and EGFR antibody (panitumumab, cetuximab) is not recommended for adjuvant therapy of stage III disease.

Stage II Colon Cancer

- Unlike stage III disease, the role of adjuvant chemotherapy in stage II disease remains controversial, with some studies showing a benefit and others showing no benefit.
- Following surgery for stage II colon cancer, the current NCCN guidelines (February 2015) recommend observation (surgery alone), enrollment in a clinical trial, or adjuvant che-

motherapy. To sort out these options, a detailed discussion with the patient is recommended to highlight the potential benefits and risks of chemotherapy.

- Any high-risk features should be identified and discussed (Table 33.3).
    - Patients with or without high-risk features should consider observation, clinical trial, or chemotherapy with capecitabine or 5-FU/leucovorin.
    - In general, only those patients with high-risk features should be considered candidates for FOLFOX or CapeOx regimens.

- Decision-making regarding the use of adjuvant chemotherapy for stage II disease may be aided by performing genetic testing of the tumor after surgical resection.
  - High microsatellite instability (MSI-H) or defective mismatch repair (dMMR) status has been shown to be associated with a lower recurrence rate (11% vs. 26%) after surgical resection alone.
  - In addition, MSI-H tumors do not benefit from 5-FU adjuvant therapy. Thus, MSI/MMR testing is recommended in all patients with stage II disease in order to avoid giving adjuvant chemotherapy in patients who will derive no benefit from it.
  - In addition to MSI/MMR testing, multigene colon cancer assays such as Oncotype Dx, ColoPrint, and ColDx are now available that can also predict prognosis and risk of recurrence. All three of these multigene assays predict recurrence independent from other factors such as TNM stage, MMR status, tumor grade, and nodes. While these assays provide additional information regarding prognosis and recurrence risk, they are not predictive of the potential benefit of chemotherapy and consequently are, to date, of limited clinical value.

Table 33.3 High-risk factors for recurrence

Poorly differentiated histology (exclusive of those that are MSI-H)
Lymphatic/vascular invasion
Perineural invasion
Close, indeterminate, or positive margins
Bowel obstruction
Localized perforation
Less than 12 lymph nodes examined

Radiotherapy for Colon Cancer

- Radiotherapy plays a limited role in patients with colon cancer.
- A few retrospective, single institution studies have shown that adjuvant radiotherapy improves local control for colon cancer patients at high risk of recurrence after surgery. Unfortunately, the single randomized prospective trial comparing chemotherapy alone with combined chemotherapy and radiotherapy lacks sufficient power to draw valid conclusions.
- Current NCCN guidelines recommend that radiotherapy for colon cancer be considered in patients with T4 tumors with penetration to a fixed structure. The radiation field should include the tumor bed as defined by preoperative imaging and the placement of surgical clips at the time of operation.
  - Thus, the colorectal surgeon should always be ready to place clips in and around the tumor bed during operations involving the resection of a fixed T4 colon tumor in order to help direct postoperative radiotherapy.
- Neoadjuvant chemoradiotherapy can be considered for select patients with bulky tumors invading other structures.

Rectal Cancer

- Decisions regarding postoperative adjuvant treatment for rectal cancer are based primarily on tumor location, clinical stage, histologic stage, and history of neoadjuvant therapy.
- Proximal rectal/rectosigmoid tumors are located at least 12 cm proximal to the anal verge and are above the peritoneal reflection. Although somewhat controversial, non-advanced proximal rectal/rectosigmoid

tumors are treated in the same fashion as tumors elsewhere in the colon, with surgical resection followed by postoperative chemotherapy for stage III and select stage II tumors.

- Tumors of the middle/lower rectum are located from 0–12 cm from the anal verge as measured by rigid proctoscopy. They typically have a worse prognosis, stage for stage, when compared to more proximal tumors, and thus treatment recommendations are slightly different.

Patients Who Did Not Undergo Neoadjuvant Therapy

- Like stage I colon cancer, 5-year survival after surgery alone for stage I rectal cancer exceeds 90%. Thus, no adjuvant treatment is recommended for patients undergoing proctectomy alone who are found to have T1-2N0M0 disease, assuming that margins of resection are negative for tumor.
- For those found to have stage II or III disease after proctectomy, decision-making is more complex. Postoperative chemotherapy is indicated for patients with stage III disease, but the benefit for stage II disease is less certain.
- Postoperative radiotherapy should be considered for patients with stage II and III disease, but this recommendation is highly controversial, as it is primarily based on data from the past, when there was little emphasis on surgical quality or assessment of circumferential radial margins.
  - Postoperative radiotherapy is also associated with substantial long-term toxicity, most notable in patients undergoing restorative proctectomy.
  - The recommendation for routine postoperative radiotherapy for patients with T3 N0 disease with negative circumferential margins has thus been questioned, including in the most recent iteration of the ASCRS Practice Parameters for the Management of Rectal Cancer.
  - Even for patients with N+ disease, it is unclear whether the small benefit of postoperative radiotherapy in terms of local control is worth the risk of toxicity, which can be substantial.
- If patients are to be treated with postoperative chemoradiotherapy, it is usually administered using a sandwich technique. This involves giving chemotherapy (FOLFOX or CapeOx) followed by chemoradiotherapy (capecitabine + radiation or infusional 5FU + radiation) followed by more chemotherapy (FOLFOX or CapeOx).
- In stage II and III rectal cancer patients, postoperative chemotherapy should be administered as soon as the patient has recovered from surgery as each 4-week delay in chemotherapy results in a 14% decrease in overall survival.

Patients Who Underwent Neoadjuvant Radiotherapy/Chemoradiotherapy

- Overall, there is a paucity of data on which to rely when making decisions regarding postoperative chemotherapy for patients with rectal cancer because neoadjuvant therapy regimens, surgical quality control, and pathologic processing have evolved so rapidly in the past 30 years.
- Traditionally, patients with ypT3 or ypN+ disease have been recommended to undergo postoperative chemotherapy. However, a recent meta-analysis of published data found that adjuvant fluorouracil-based chemotherapy did not improve overall survival, disease-free survival, or distant recur-

Table 33.4 Neoadjuvant and adjuvant treatment of stage II and III rectal cancer

	Step 1		Step 2		Step 3
Option I	Capecitabine + Radiotherapy OR Infusional 5-FU + Radiotherapy	➡	Surgery	➡	FOLFOX OR Capecitabine + Oxalplatin
Option II	FOLFOX OR Capecitabine + Oxaliplatin	➡	Capecitabine + Radiotherapy OR Infusional 5-FU + Radiotherapy	➡	Surgery

rences, calling these recommendations into question.

- If chemotherapy is utilized, it is also controversial as to which regimen to utilize. Two randomized clinical trials have reported a disease-free survival advantage to FOLFOX vs. fluoropyrimidine monotherapy in patients previously treated with neoadjuvant chemoradiotherapy followed by rectal surgery.
- Clinicians should be aware that current NCCN guidelines for clinical stage II and III rectal cancer recommend either (1) preoperative chemoradiotherapy, surgery, and then postoperative chemotherapy or (2) preoperative chemotherapy followed by preoperative chemoradiotherapy and then surgery (see Table 33.4). The total duration of perioperative therapy (preoperative chemoradiotherapy and chemotherapy) should not exceed 6 months. However, as noted above, these recommendations are based on incomplete and sometimes conflicting data.
- A summary of several key clinical trials regarding chemoradiotherapy for rectal cancer is shown in Table 33.4.

Patients Undergoing Local Excision

- Due to the oncologically inferior results of local excision as compared to proctectomy, even in highly select patients, many authors have recommended treatment with adjuvant chemoradiotherapy, either in the preoperative or postoperative period.
  - The advantage of utilizing chemoradiotherapy in the postoperative period is that T stage can be known with certainty, and one can ensure healing of the wound prior to institution of radiotherapy.
  - The advantage of utilizing neoadjuvant chemoradiotherapy is that ypT stage correlates more closely with ypN stage than T stage correlates with N stage and there may be downsizing of the tumor prior to excision. The major downside of neoadjuvant therapy combined with local excision is that wound healing may be impaired, and patients may suffer substantial morbidity as a result.
- Table 33.5 lists key clinical trials establishing the efficacy of chemoradiotherapy for rectal cancer.

Table 33.5 Key clinical trials establishing the efficacy of chemoradiotherapy for rectal cancer

Trial	Tumor stage	Comparison	Results	Conclusion
Swedish Rectal Cancer Trial 1993	Stage II and III	Surgery alone vs. preop short course XRT	Local recurrence: 27% vs. 12% 5-yr survival: 48% vs. 58%	Preop XRT decreases local recurrence, improves survival (?)
Dutch TME Rectal Cancer Trial 2001	Stage II and III	TME alone vs. preop XRT + TME	Local recurrence: 11.4% vs. 5.6% Survival: no difference	Preop XRT improves local recurrence even with TME Preop XRT no effect on survival
German CAO/ARO/AIO-94 2003/2004	Stage II and III	Preop chemoXRT vs. postop chemo XRT	Local recurrence: 13% vs. 6% Toxicity: 40% vs. 27% Survival: no difference	Decreased toxicity and local recurrence with preop chemoXRT Pre vs. post: no effect on survival
EORTC 22921 2006	Stage II and III	XRT vs. chemoXRT	Survival benefit for ypT0–2 responders	Chemo in addition to XRT can improve survival in the subgroup of responders
Cochran Review: Postop Chemo 2012	Stage II and III	No postop chemo vs. postop chemo after neoadjuvant	Recurrence reduced 25% Deaths reduced 17%	Postop chemo reduces recurrence and death rate after neoadjuvant
ADORE 2014	Stage II and III	FOLFOX vs. 5-FU/leucovorin after neoadjuvant	3-yr disease-free survival: 72% vs. 62%	Postop FOLFOX superior to 5-FU after neoadjuvant
German CAO/ARO/AIO-04 2012/2014	Stage II and III	Neoadjuvant and adjuvant FOLFOX vs. 5-FU/leucovorin	Complete pathologic response: 17% vs. 13% 3-yr survival: 76% vs. 71%	Preop and postop addition of oxaliplatin improves survival and pathologic response

XRT radiation therapy, *TME* total mesorectal excision, *preop* preoperative, *postop* postoperative, *yr.* year, *chemoxrt* combined chemoradiation therapy

34 Colorectal Cancer: Surveillance After Curative-Intent Therapy

Scott E. Regenbogen and Karin M. Hardiman

Key Concepts

- Liver metastases and locoregional recurrence are more likely to be amenable to curative-intent salvage resection when detected in asymptomatic patients. Therefore, active surveillance is indicated for patients who are candidates for liver and/or intestinal resection.
- Use of carcinoembryonic antigen testing and computed tomography (CT) scans is associated with increased detection of asymptomatic recurrence after curative resection for colorectal cancer. There is no evidence to support the use of any other laboratory testing or positron emission tomography (PET) scans in routine surveillance.
- Patients with advanced age and comorbidity, who would not be fit to undergo therapy for recurrence should not be subjected to active surveillance. They should, however, receive evaluation and treatment for symptoms suggestive of recurrence.
- Patients with resected rectal cancers are at greater risk for locoregional recurrence. This risk is increased by omission of chemoradiotherapy for locally advanced tumors, close or positive margins, T4 and N2 histology. Consideration should therefore be given to local pelvic surveillance both endoluminally and extraluminally in these patients at highest risk.
- Surveillance after resection of Stage I colorectal cancer remains controversial. While the recurrence rates are low, in general, there are markers of relatively greater risk, including margin positivity, unknown lymph node status (e.g., local excision), inadequate lymph node sampling, lymphovascular invasion, poorly differentiated histology, and/or T2 disease. Active surveillance may be considered for patients with one or more of these risk factors.

Introduction

- With improvements in screening, diagnosis, surgical technique, and adjuvant therapy for colon and rectal cancers, nearly two thirds of patients who undergo surgical resection survive 5 years or more.
- As a result, there is a rapidly growing population of colorectal cancer survivors, exceeding 1.2 million in the United States alone.
- These individuals face varying risk for subsequent colorectal cancer throughout their lifetime, yet there is little consensus on optimal

S. E. Regenbogen (✉) · K. M. Hardiman
Division of Colorectal Surgery, University of Michigan, Ann Arbor, MI, USA
e-mail: sregenbo@med.umich.edu

S. R. Steele et al. (eds.), *The ASCRS Manual of Colon and Rectal Surgery*,
https://doi.org/10.1007/978-3-030-01165-9_34

regimens for surveillance and survivorship care.

- At face value, the primary goal of colorectal cancer surveillance is to detect treatable recurrent, metastatic, or metachronous colorectal malignancy and optimize the opportunities for potentially curative intervention.
- Ultimately, however, the success of colorectal cancer surveillance should be measured by improvements in overall survival, cancer-specific survival, disability, or quality of life.
- Some studies have evaluated proxy measures, such as the rate of curative-intent metastasectomy or resection of colorectal neoplasia, but it is not clear to what degree these additional interventions benefit colorectal cancer survivors more broadly.
- Interpretation and synthesis of findings of published studies are complicated by the heterogeneity of the interventions and comparisons – the surveillance intervention in one trial may be no more intensive than the control group regimen of another – and the challenges of obtaining adequate power to detect meaningful differences in survival and other objective oncologic outcomes in such studies.
- It is also important to consider the appropriateness of surveillance for patients who might not be eligible for, or willing to undergo, treatment for recurrence. Recognizing that older adults account for the majority of colorectal cancer patients, patient preferences, age, comorbidities, and functional status must all contribute to the decision to pursue active surveillance.
  - There is little need, for example, to conduct surveillance for asymptomatic liver metastases for a patient unwilling or unable to undergo hepatic resection and/or chemotherapy. For such patients, symptom-driven evaluations may suffice.
- At the same time, the landscape around both the detection and treatment of recurrence continues to evolve. It remains unclear whether increased detection and aggressive treatment of local or distant recurrence results in true benefit to patients or whether stage migration and lead time bias produces apparent gains.

Timing and Choice of Surveillance Modalities

Intensity of Surveillance

- There are various clinical, laboratory, radiographic, and endoscopic methods available for surveillance after treatment of colorectal cancer. Recommendations regarding their application and frequency of use vary between agencies involved in scripting guidelines for colorectal cancer care and are summarized in Table 34.1.
- Most guidelines include more intensive early surveillance, with diminishing frequency after 2–5 years, due to the recognition that 80% of recurrences are detected within 3 years after initial curative-intent surgical therapy, and at least 95% are evident within 5 years.
- After 3 years without evidence of disease, cancer-specific mortality declines significantly, and conditional survival thereafter is very high.
- There have been at least eight prospective randomized trials addressing outcomes of surveillance after curative resection.
  - Overall, there is a lack of high-level evidence to support specific choices among surveillance regimens, but their interpretation is complicated by the heterogeneity of the surveillance regimens, changes in the diagnostic and therapeutic technologies available at the times they were conducted, and limitations of sample size and duration of follow-up.
  - Nevertheless, we can likely conclude that more frequent testing and the use of advanced imaging will result in more potentially curative surgery for recurrence and a measurable, but small, improvement in survival.

Table 34.1 Summary of surveillance guidelines

Modality	American Society of Colon and Rectal Surgeons	National Comprehensive Cancer Network	American Cancer Society, US Multisociety Task Force on Colorectal Cancer	American Society of Clinical Oncology	Cancer Care Ontario	European Society of Medical Oncology	British Society of Gastroenterology, Association of Coloproctology for Great Britain and Ireland
History and physical exam	Every 3–6 months for 2 years, then every 6 months to 5 years	Every 3–6 months for 2 years, then every 6 months to 5 years	Not addressed	Every 3–6 months for 5 years	Every 6 months for 5 years	Every 3–6 months for 3 years, then every 6 months to 5 years.	Not addressed
CEA	Every 3–6 months for 2 years, then every 6 months to 5 years	Every 3–6 months for 2 years, then every 6 months to 5 years	Not addressed	Every 3–6 months for 5 years	Every 6 months for 5 years	Every 3–6 months for 3 years, then every 6 months to 5 years	"Role of CEA is uncertain"
Other laboratory testing	Not recommended	Not recommended	Not addressed	Not recommended	Not recommended	Not recommended	Not recommended
Abdominal Imaging	CT scan annually for 5 years. Consider more frequent for highest risk[a]	CT scan annually for 5 years	Not addressed	CT scan annually for 3 years. Consider 6–12 months for high risk	CT scan annually for 3 years. US every 6–12 months may be substituted	CT scan or contrast-enhanced ultrasound every 6–12 months for 3 years for patients at higher risk of recurrence	"Reasonable to offer" CT of the liver within 2 years of resection
Pelvic imaging	CT scan annually for 5 years. Consider more frequent for highest risk[b]	CT scan annually for 5 years	Not addressed	CT scans every 6–12 months for 2–3 years, then annually up to 5 years	CT scan annually for 3 years for rectal cancers only	Not specifically recommended	Not specifically recommended

(continued)

Table 34.1 (continued)

Chest Imaging	CT scan annually for 5 years. Consider more frequent for highest risk[b]	CT scan annually for 5 years	Not addressed	CT scan annually for 3 years. Consider 6–12 months for high risk	CT scan annually for 3 years. CXR every 6–12 months may be substituted	CT scan every 6–12 months for 3 years for patients at higher risk of recurrence	Not specifically recommended
PET Scan	Not recommended for routine surveillance	Not recommended for routine surveillance	Not addressed	Not recommended for routine surveillance	Not recommended for routine surveillance	Not recommended for routine surveillance	Not recommended
Colonoscopy	1 year after resection (or within 6 months if previously incomplete). If normal, repeat in 3 years. If adenomas, repeat in 1 year. Annual colonoscopy for patients with suspected familial syndromes who have not undergone proctocolectomy	1 year after resection (or within 6 months if previously incomplete). If normal, repeat in 3 years, then 5 years. If advanced adenoma, repeat in 1 year. Annual colonoscopy for patients with suspected familial syndromes who have not undergone proctocolectomy	1 year after resection (or 1 year after colonoscopy that cleared synchronous disease before primary treatment). If normal, repeat in 3 years, then 5 years. More frequent if high-risk adenoma(s) or suspicion for Lynch syndrome	1 year after resection or upon completion of adjuvant therapy if previously incomplete. If normal, repeat in 5 years. Otherwise, according to endoscopic findings	1 year after resection (or within 6 months if previously incomplete). If normal, repeat in 5 years	1 year after resection, then every 3–5 years thereafter	Every 5 years after resection, until benefits outweighed by comorbidity

Stage-specific recommendations	Stage 1: high risk only[c] Stage 2: all Stage 3: all Stage 4: when metastases are resected for cure	Stage 1: colonoscopic surveillance only Stage 2: all Stage 3: all Stage 4: when metastases are resected for cure, CT scan every 3–6 months for 2 years, then every 6–12 months to 5 years	Not addressed	Recommendations apply to Stage II and III disease only. Insufficient data to make recommendations for Stage I	Recommendations apply to Stage II and III disease only	Not addressed	Not addressed
Rectal surveillance	Proctoscopy every 6–12 months for patients with anastomosis, every 6 months after local excision, for 3–5 years. Endorectal ultrasound for high risk[d]	No additional testing specifically recommended	Proctoscopy, flexible sigmoidoscopy, or endorectal ultrasound every 3–6 months for patients with anastomosis	Proctosigmoidoscopy every 6 months for 2–5 years for patients who did not receive radiotherapy, those with T4 or N2 tumors. Pelvic imaging for rectal tumors only	Proctosigmoidoscopy every 6 months for 2–5 years for patients who did not receive radiotherapy. Pelvic imaging for rectal tumors only	No additional testing specifically recommended	Not addressed

CEA carcinoembryonic antigen, *CT* computed tomography, *PET* positron emission tomography

[a]High risk of recurrence in Stage I disease is to be defined by provider(s) according to features such as margin positivity, unknown lymph node status (e.g. local excision), inadequate lymph node sampling, lymphovascular invasion, poorly differentiated histology, and/or T2 disease

[b]Highest risk for systemic recurrence includes patients with N2 disease or after curative-intent metastasectomy

[c]High risk of recurrence in Stage I disease is to be defined by provider(s) according to features such as margin positivity, unknown lymph node status (e.g., local excision), inadequate lymph node sampling, lymphovascular invasion, poorly differentiated histology, and/or T2 disease

[d]High risk for local recurrence includes local excisions with poor histology (T2+, poorly differentiated), positive margins, T4 or N2 disease

Physical Examination

- Most of the major societies' guidelines include periodic clinical examination, including assessment of symptoms and physical examination.
  - Findings suggestive of disease recurrence may include weight loss, fatigue, anemia, cough, abdominal pain, rectal bleeding, or changes in bowel habits.
    - Symptomatic recurrences, however, are far less likely to be amenable to curative-intent therapy.
  - Physical examination should focus on the abdomen, including evaluation for wound implants, lymph nodes, and rectal exam (or perineal wound exam after abdominoperineal resection).
- In addition to their role in colorectal cancer surveillance, these visits also serve an important survivorship role in overall health maintenance and management of physical and psychosocial function after colorectal resections.
- The American Society of Colon and Rectal Surgeons (ASCRS) recommends visits every 3–6 months for 2 years, followed by every 6 months until 5 years.

Laboratory Testing

- None of the major guidelines currently endorse the routine evaluation of complete blood count, liver function tests, fecal occult blood testing, or blood chemistries.
- It is recommended to check levels of carcinoembryonic antigen (CEA), an oncofetal antigen that may be elevated in patients with recurrent colorectal cancer.
  - CEA detects about 30–60% of recurrences, the positive predictive value of CEA is about 65%, and more than 15% of patients in surveillance have falsely elevated CEA in the absence of recurrence.
  - Yet, elevations in CEA may precede symptomatic presentation of metastasis, and the trials showing greatest benefit to intensive surveillance have included regular CEA evaluations.
  - CEA elevations identify disease in the absence of abnormal imaging in up to 23% of patients with recurrent colorectal cancer but may be more commonly elevated with metachronous liver metastases than with pulmonary metastases and luminal or locoregional recurrences.
  - About a third of colorectal cancers do not produce CEA, but the significance of CEA elevation during surveillance seems to be independent of the preoperative CEA level.
- Recommendations for management of asymptomatic CEA elevation are outlined in guidelines from both NCCN and ASCRS.
  - After confirmation of serial elevation in CEA level, a complete physical examination, endoscopy, and CT imaging of the chest, abdomen, and pelvis are performed.
  - If these are all negative, consideration is given to PET-CT and/or repeat imaging every 3 months until levels decline or recurrence is detected.

Abdominal Imaging

- The most common site of metachronous metastatic colorectal cancer is the liver.
- A Cochrane collaborative meta-analysis concluded that there was a survival benefit associated with liver imaging, with an odds ratio for mortality of 0.64 (95% confidence interval 0.49–0.85).
  - This conclusion was derived from the results of five randomized trials, which used varying combinations of liver ultrasonography, abdominal CT, or both.
- The current ASCRS practice parameter and recommendations from other US-based agencies recommend CT imaging, due to increased sensitivity for identifying early liver lesions, and the opportunity to evaluate the remainder of the abdomen and pelvis for other sites of metastasis (such as retroperitoneal lymph

nodes and ovaries) and to identify local recurrence in the resection bed.

- There is currently no organization that endorses routine use of PET-CT scans or liver MRI.

Chest Imaging

- Whereas plain radiography was the mainstay of surveillance for pulmonary metastasis in the past, most of the major guidelines now recommend the use of cross-sectional imaging at least annually.
- This change has come with the recognition that pulmonary metastasis may present as a solitary site of disease recurrence and may even represent the most common site of distant metastasis for distal rectal cancers.
- However, it should be noted that cross-sectional chest imaging is recommended in spite of a lack of high-level evidence to support its effectiveness in practice.

Colonoscopy

- Surveillance endoscopy after colorectal cancer resection can serve three purposes:
  - Clearance of remaining colon when preoperative colonoscopy was incomplete
  - Anastomotic surveillance for detection of local luminal recurrence, which should be a rare event
  - Most importantly, detection of metachronous neoplasia.
    - The BSG/ACPGBI guidelines suggest waiting until 5 years after resection, whereas all of the other guidelines include a complete colonoscopy at 1 year, though the rate of clinically significant findings may be low.
    - The ASCRS guideline recommends that the subsequent colonoscopy schedule be tailored to the findings at the 1-year examination and to other patient-specific risk factors and circumstances.
    - Patients with high-risk adenomas (high-grade dysplasia, size greater than 1 cm or more than three adenomas) and those with a diagnosed or suspected hereditary colorectal cancer syndrome may require annual colonoscopy for more intensive surveillance.
    - On the other hand, the very elderly and patients with limited life expectancy are unlikely to benefit from the detection of an asymptomatic cancer and may be selected for less frequent, or no, endoscopic surveillance.

Stage 1 Disease

- Most of the major guidelines for and studies of colorectal cancer surveillance pertain primarily to Stage II–III disease and to Stage IV tumors that have been resected with curative intent.
- Stage I patients have been largely excluded from many of the randomized trials of surveillance.
- As a result, there remains controversy regarding approaches to the surveillance of resected Stage I colon cancers (see Table 34.1).
- Against routine imaging surveillance for Stage I disease
  - Several of the guidelines specifically recommend against routine imaging.
    - For example, NCCN and ASCO recommend only endoscopic surveillance for anastomotic recurrence or metachronous cancers.
  - There is presumed to be a low incidence of systemic recurrence, as 5-year colon cancer survival rates exceed 90%, and very few operations for metachronous metastatic recurrence occur in patients who initially presented with a Stage I tumor.
  - There is concern that surveillance will identify more incidental findings than treatable recurrences. It is estimated that it would take nearly 200 patients with Stage I disease in surveillance to detect each cur-

able metastasis, and many authors caution against over-testing in this setting.

- For routine imaging surveillance for Stage I disease
  - Some authors have found equivalent rates of salvage and better survival for recurrences after resection of early-stage disease and have thus recommended active survival for patients with early-stage disease, though they do not distinguish between Stage I (T1–2, N0) and Stage 2a (T3 N0) in their studies.
  - The most recent ASCRS Practice Guideline recommends consideration of active surveillance for Stage I patients but limits the recommendation to those designated at higher risk – for example, close or positive margins, unknown lymph node status (e.g., local or endoscopic excision), inadequate lymph node sampling, lymphovascular invasion, poorly differentiated histology, and/or T2 disease.

Local Surveillance for Rectal Cancer

- Additional surveillance recommendations for rectal cancer are predicated on the greater risk of locoregional recurrence, compared with colon cancers, due to both anatomic and biologic differences between the tumors.
- Locoregional recurrence of rectal cancer can occur either intraluminally, typically at the site of anastomosis, or extraluminally, likely associated with residual lymphatic disease, close radial margins, or tumor shed during resection.
- Although the use of total mesorectal excision (TME) and chemoradiotherapy for locally advanced rectal cancers have substantially reduced local failure after primary resection, between 4% and 22% of patients still experience local recurrence.
- The resulting downstaging that may occur with the use of preoperative therapy for rectal cancer also may create confusion about how to classify future risk of recurrence.
  - In the ASCRS practice guidelines, it is recommended that pre-treatment clinical staging be used to guide surveillance intensity.
- Early identification of local recurrence may offer the opportunity for curative-intent salvage resection. Therefore, surveillance of colorectal anastomosis and pelvic imaging are recommended beyond what is performed for colon cancer surveillance.
- Physical assessment
  - Pelvic and groin examinations should be performed every 6 months. For patients with a low anastomosis or distal tumor with local excision or non-operative management, digital exam of the anastomosis or tumor site should be included.
  - For patients who have undergone abdominoperineal resection (APR), careful palpation of the perineum and, in women, the posterior wall of the vagina is recommended.
  - Special attention should be paid to areas of nodularity or changes over time.
  - Any suspicious lesions should undergo biopsy as local recurrences after APR are frequently perineal or presacral.
- Proctosigmoidoscopy
  - Endoluminal evaluation of the rectum is recommended in the most recent ASCRS practice parameters every 6–12 months for 3–5 years for those who have undergone a low anterior resection with anastomosis and more frequently for those considered to be at higher risk of local recurrence.
- Imaging
  - Endorectal ultrasonography (ERUS).
    - The most recent ASCRS and ACS/MSTF guidelines also suggest consideration of ERUS for patients considered high-risk for local recurrence. Although controversial, there are a handful of studies that suggest that ERUS can identify asymptomatic rectal cancer recurrence that was otherwise undetected by digital exam, endoscopy, CT, or CEA.
  - Cross-sectional imaging
    - ASCO and CCO both recommend pelvic CT imaging for rectal cancers only,

as a means of detection of local recurrence. MRI of the pelvis can also be used and is highly accurate for the diagnosis of pelvic recurrence, but its use in routine surveillance did not improve the detection of resectable recurrence in a single trial, and its cost-effectiveness has not been evaluated.

- Rectal cancer initially treated by local excision
  - Particular attention must be paid to both endoluminal and mesorectal surveillance due to the relatively high risk of local pelvic failure
    - At least semiannual digital rectal examination and rectal endoscopic surveillance after local excision are highly recommended, and consideration may be given to the use of ERUS for these patients.
- Rectal cancer initially treated by definitive chemoradiotherapy
  - Because non-operative treatment is primarily limited to clinical trials, none of the guidelines include formal recommendations for such patients.
  - However, the non-operative trials reported to date have employed remarkably intensive surveillance, including very frequent physical examination, endoscopy, and imaging, often with pelvic MRI.

Compliance with Guidelines

- Despite published recommendations for surveillance after resection for colorectal cancer, compliance with surveillance remains challenging both for patients and their physicians.
- There is evidence that patients who adhere to recommended surveillance have a greater likelihood of curative-intent reoperation for recurrence and improved overall and disease-specific 5-year survival.
- Yet anywhere from 25% to 42% of patients have poor completion of recommended surveillance, and 11–21% have no surveillance at all.
- There is also little consensus regarding who should manage cancer surveillance – the operating surgeon, medical oncologist, gastroenterologist, or primary care doctor.
  - This ambiguity may contribute to nonadherence in many patients, as responsibility for ordering and managing testing can be undefined.

Quality of Life

- Apart from the cancer-specific outcomes of surveillance, an essential question is the effect of intensive surveillance on psychological health and quality of life. While reassuring surveillance examinations may allay fears of cancer recurrence for some patients, there could be others for whom the conduct of surveillance examinations subjects them to additional unwarranted worry and investigations for false positive or incidental findings.
- Most patients in surveillance report, however, that these anxieties and inconveniences are outweighed by the reassurance and optimism imparted by negative results.

Cost

- As recommendations for surveillance imaging have expanded in recent guidelines, another important consideration will be the costs of surveillance.
- Total costs of the surveillance regimens in published studies vary 28-fold, without a clear correlation between cost and efficacy.
- Between 1999 and 2006, the use of CT and MRI scans in the follow-up of patients with colorectal cancer increased at an annual rate of more than 5%, and the use of PET scans more than tripled.
- We can conclude from limited data that the cost-effectiveness of colorectal cancer surveillance is likely to be within the range of other interventions considered acceptably costly. Caution must be taken, however, if an increase in the cost, complexity, and frequency of recommended testing is contemplated.

Colorectal Cancer: Management of Local Recurrence

35

Eric J. Dozois and Dorin T. Colibaseanu

Key Concepts

- Patients with colorectal cancer at the highest risk for local recurrence are those who present with obstruction or perforation, higher-stage disease, and adverse pathologic features or undergo an operation that does not adhere to standard oncologic principles.
- The most significant predictor of survival following surgery for local recurrence is the ability to achieve a negative-margin (R0) resection.
- The probability of achieving an R0 resection is much greater in patients with recurrences involving an anastomosis or urogynecologic structures compared with those involving the para-aortic tissue, sacrum, or lateral pelvic sidewall.
- A dedicated multidisciplinary team at an institution experienced in the management of patients with local colorectal cancer recurrence can facilitate complex surgical decision-making and greatly enhance patient outcomes.
- A multimodality approach that includes chemotherapy and radiotherapy improves local control and improves 5-year survival in patients with local recurrence.

E. J. Dozois (✉) · D. T. Colibaseanu
Department of Surgery, Mayo Clinic, Rochester, MN, USA
e-mail: Dozois.Eric@mayo.edu

Introduction

- In the United States, despite improvements in surgical technique and advances in adjuvant treatment paradigms, local failure (recurrence) remains a problem.
  - Colon cancer: 8%–12%
  - Rectal cancer: 5%–30%
- Patients with colorectal cancer at the highest risk for local recurrence are those that have higher-stage disease, high-grade tumors, lymphovascular involvement, and positive resection margins or present with obstruction, perforation, or a locally advanced tumor at the time of presentation.
- Operations done by noncolorectal-trained surgeons, or by surgeons who perform less than 20 rectal cancer resections per year, have been reported to have higher local recurrence rates.
- All efforts to reduce the risk of local recurrence should be made when managing primary colorectal cancer, and the best results are achieved when patients are managed by experienced teams.
- When patients with colorectal cancer develop local recurrence, surgery offers the best opportunity for cure.

S. R. Steele et al. (eds.), *The ASCRS Manual of Colon and Rectal Surgery*,
https://doi.org/10.1007/978-3-030-01165-9_35

- Due to the complexity of medical and surgical decision-making, in addition to the surgical expertise required to perform these technically challenging operations, the treatment of patients with local recurrence should preferentially occur at centers that have dedicated and experienced multidisciplinary team.

Diagnosis of Local Recurrence

- The majority of colorectal cancer relapses following surgery occur within 3 years of resection.
- Most, but not all, patients with local failure will have symptoms from recurrent disease, and these will include pain, malaise, bleeding, and symptoms of partial obstruction.
- In some patients, carcinoembryonic antigen (CEA) levels will be elevated, and this finding in the asymptomatic patient should trigger a workup for recurrence.
- In patients with suspected local recurrence, every attempt should be made to obtain tissue for confirmation.
  - Most patients with recurrent colon cancer will have obvious findings on imaging to confidently diagnose them with recurrence, and a transabdominal biopsy should be avoided.
  - In contrast, every attempt should be made to obtain tissue confirmation in patients with suspected pelvic recurrence. One should be hesitant to undertake a major pelvic resection without tissue confirmation of recurrence.
    - In our experience, computed tomography (CT)-guided percutaneous biopsy has been very useful to confirm or refute the presence of recurrence.
    - In the absence of a tissue diagnosis, a rising CEA, with a notable change in the size of the lesion on serial imaging, and lesions that are positron emission tomography (PET)-avid can be considered consistent with recurrent disease.

Preoperative Evaluation and Patient Selection

- History and physical examination
  - All records of previous treatments (surgical and chemoradiotherapy) should be reviewed.
  - Pain and neurologic dysfunction may be a sign of advanced pelvic disease.
  - Bilateral lower extremity edema is an indicator of venous or lymphatic obstruction.
  - If the rectum is intact, a digital rectal exam can assess the relationship of the recurrent cancer to the sphincter complex, prostate, or posterior vaginal wall.
  - Overall assessment of ability to withstand long complex surgery.
- Colonoscopy
  - A full colonoscopy should be done to rule out any synchronous lesions.
- Carcinoembryonic antigen (CEA)
  - A significantly elevated CEA should raise concern for occult metastatic disease.
- Imaging
  - PET-CT to assess for distant metastatic disease.
  - Pelvic magnetic resonance imaging (MRI) for recurrent rectal cancers to assess for local invasion of surrounding structures.
- Enterostomal therapy marking and teaching
- Determining appropriateness for surgical resection
  - If palliation is the goal, surgery must have a high probability of symptomatic relief and not be significantly morbid.
  - If oncologic cure is the goal, the ability to confidently achieve a margin-negative (R0) resection must be highly probable.
    - Based on multiple studies in patients with recurrent colorectal cancer, the number one determinant of oncologic benefit is the ability to achieve an R0 resection.
    - Multiple points of tumor fixation may limit the surgeon's ability to achieve an R0 resection, and this finding on evaluation has been associated with poor outcomes.

    - Patients operated for central recurrences that extend anteriorly (urogenital, gynecologic organs) have the best opportunity for an R0 resection and, therefore, good outcomes following surgery.
    - When a recurrence in the pelvis extends posteriorly to the sacrum, or lateral to the pelvic sidewall, the ability to achieve an R0 resection becomes much less certain.
    - In cases where there is significant lateral extension of the tumor, specifically through the sciatic notch, a positive margin is almost certain unless an extended resection such as a hemipelvectomy is done.
- Relative contraindications to surgery will vary from institution to institution and from surgeon to surgeon.
    - Local recurrences that involve major vascular structures, the high sacrum, or extensive pelvic sidewall disease were frequently listed in publications as contraindications to surgery in the past.
    - In the modern era, several well-recognized and respected centers have expanded their indications in light of increasing data demonstrating meaningful survival in patients undergoing extended resections.
    - In the author's view, contraindications to surgery should be based primarily on the inability to completely clear the tumor with the understanding that limited survival benefit is achieved if gross residual tumor remains.

Classification of Local Recurrence

- Locoregional recurrence in patients with colon cancer:
  - Peri-anastomotic (mural disease).
  - Mesenteric (regional nodal disease).
  - Retroperitoneal or pelvic (drop metastases, distant nodal disease, or residual disease transmural disease).
  - Peritoneal metastases.
  - Some cases of recurrence can be directly attributed to inadequate mesenteric resections at the time of original surgery. However, most nodal-based relapses are found at nodal sites (iliac, para-aortic) not typically removed during standard oncologic resection.
- Pelvic recurrence of rectal cancer (Fig. 35.1):

a

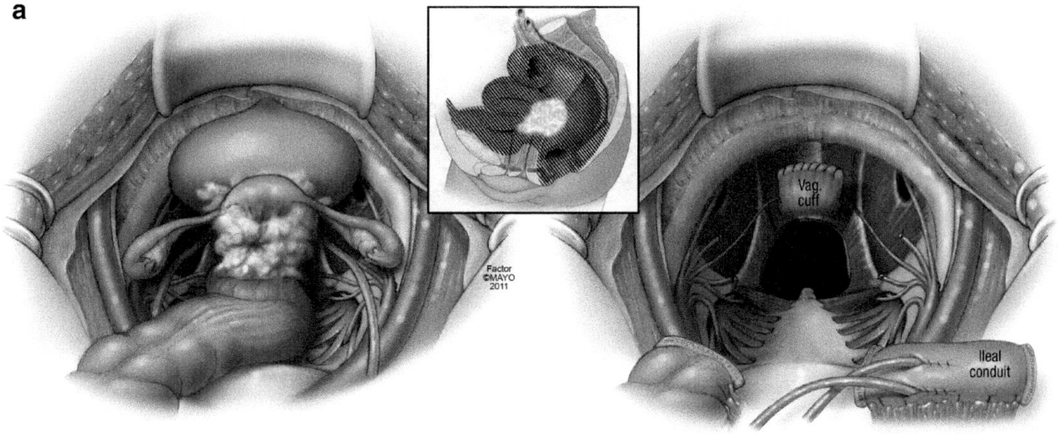

Fig. 35.1 Classification of recurrence. (**a**) Anterior: involves structures anterior to the neorectum. (**b**) Posterior: involves structures posterior to the neorectum. (**c**) Lateral: involves pelvic sidewall and associated structures. (**d**) Combined anterior-posterior: tumor includes anterior and posterior structures. (©By permission of Mayo Clinic Foundation for Medical Education and Research. All rights reserved)

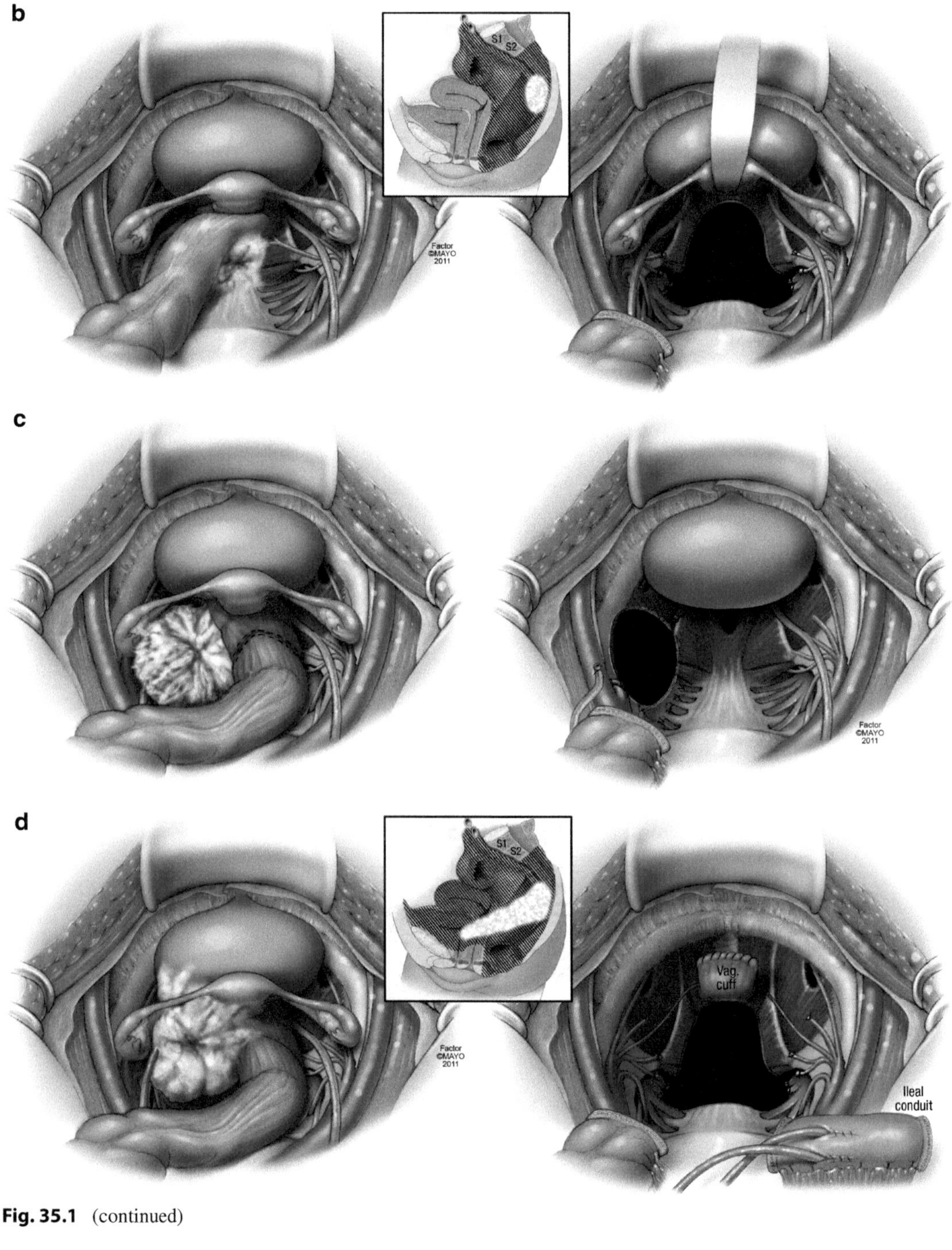

Fig. 35.1 (continued)

- Anterior: resection of the rectum and urogynecologic structures.
- Posterior: resection of the rectum and a portion of the sacrum.
- Lateral: resection of the rectum and iliac vessels and or components of the lumbosacral plexus.
- "Combined resection" or "composite resection" includes any combination of anterior, posterior, or lateral structures.

Determining Resectability

- For recurrent colon cancer, CT imaging is our study of choice to make decisions regarding resectability.
- For recurrent rectal cancer, magnetic resonance imaging of the pelvis is our study of choice to assess neuromuscular and bony involvement and for surgical planning (Fig. 35.2).
  - We use a musculoskeletal protocol that is done with and without gadolinium and includes sagittal, axial, and coronal oblique views.
  - For tumors with posterior and lateral extension, MRI can determine proximal sacral extent, involvement of lumbosacral nerves, and whether or not a margin can be obtained on the lateral pelvic sidewall.

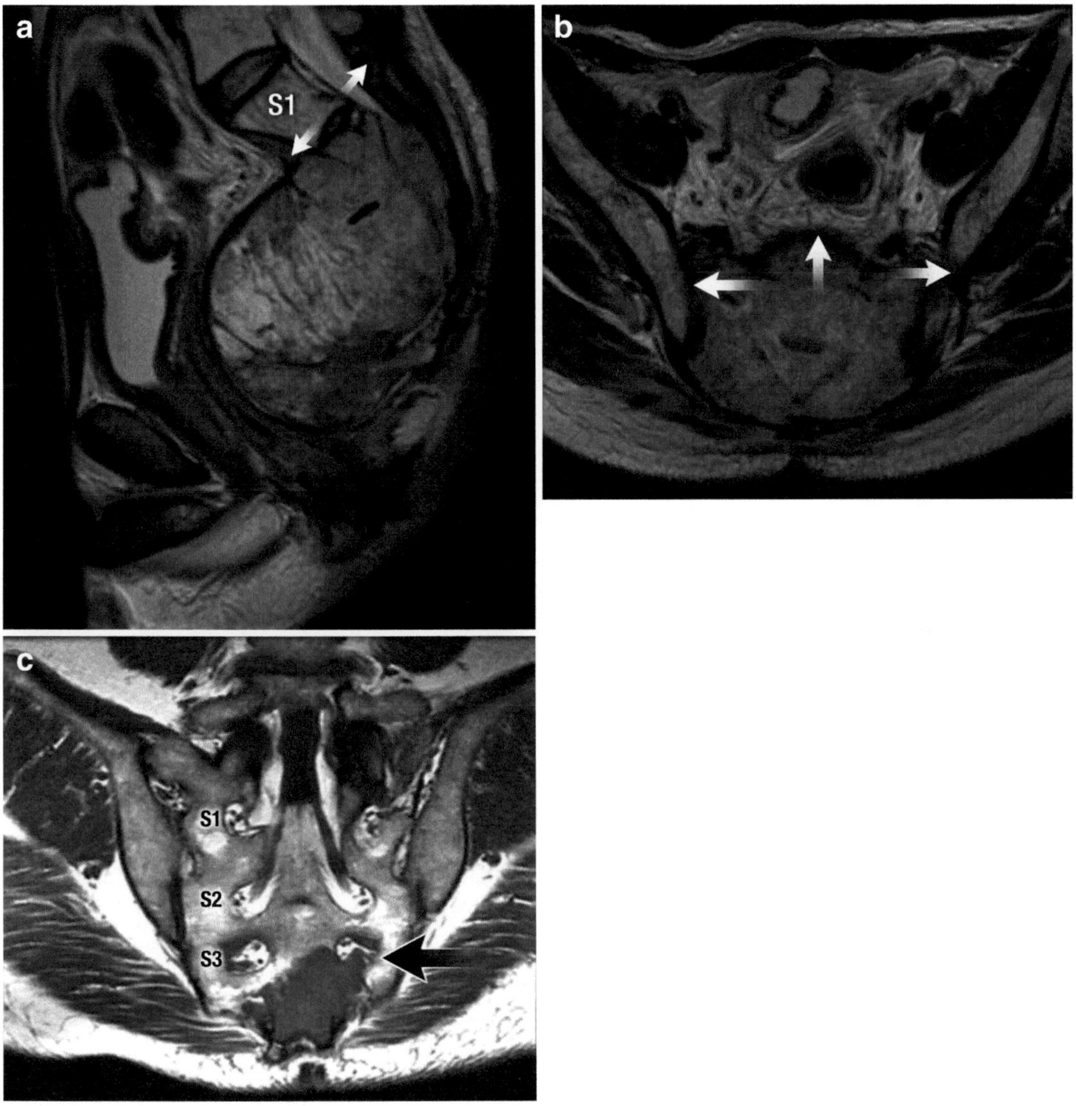

Fig. 35.2 MRI imaging assessing neuromuscular and bony involvement for surgical planning in recurrent rectal cancer. (**a**) Sagittal section showing cephalad and posterior extension of the recurrence to the first sacral body (S1). White arrows demonstrating lines of resection necessary for R0 resection. (**b**) Coronal section demonstrating soft tissue extension anteriorly and laterally, with viscera and bilateral iliac involvement (white arrows). (**c**) Coronal/oblique view showing left nerve root involvement (black arrow)

  - Computerized tomography or MR angiogram or venogram may add additional information regarding vascular involvement and indicate the need for a vascular surgeon to be a member of the multidisciplinary surgical team.
- A major challenge from a surgical planning perspective in many cases of local recurrence is the fact that the borders of recurrences can be indiscrete and ill-defined on imaging.
  - Recurrences may be infiltrative and sheet-like and sometimes have islands of intervening normal tissue. This makes it difficult to preoperatively determine where the "true margins" are.
  - Because of this, one must be prepared to alter the surgical plan intraoperatively as findings may differ significantly from what the preoperative imaging suggested. Intraoperative frozen section pathologic analysis can be very useful to ensure that further resection can be done if there is a persistent microscopic margin discovered at the time of surgery.
- Another challenge in the management of local recurrence is differentiating both postoperative and radiation-induced fibrosis from actual tumor.
  - MR imaging with T2-weighted imaging can assist because fibrosis and tumor demonstrate different signal intensities. Gadolinium-enhanced MRI is reported to have an 88% and 95% sensitivity and specificity, for the detection of pelvic recurrences in the setting of previous surgery and radiation.
  - PET is also helpful in distinguishing between scar and tumor, although fine anatomic detail is lacking compared to MR.

Multimodal Therapy Including Intraoperative Radiation

- Multimodal therapy in the management of locally recurrent colorectal cancer refers to a treatment approach that includes pre- and postoperative systemic chemotherapy, preoperative external beam radiotherapy (EBRT), and, in some protocols, intraoperative radiation therapy (IORT).
  - The authors have used this approach very selectively in patients with recurrent colon cancer and in almost all cases of recurrent rectal cancer.
  - Our protocol includes neoadjuvant chemotherapy and EBRT, IORT, and postoperative chemotherapy.
    - Patients who are radiation naïve receive 50.4 Gy of EBRT with concurrent 5-FU-based chemotherapy over 5 weeks followed by a 6–8-week recovery period before surgery.
    - In patients who have received previous irradiation, we give 20–30 Gy with concurrent 5-FU-based chemotherapy, over a 3-week period followed by surgery within 7 days of the last dose of radiation.
    - The amount of radiation given intraoperatively to the tumor resection bed depends on the margin status at the time of resection.
- Though there is a paucity of randomized data, many authors agree that a multimodality approach can significantly decrease local relapse and improve 5-year survival in colorectal cancer patients with local recurrence.
- Several centers have shown good results with the use of IORT in patients with recurrent colorectal cancer and 5-year survival rates range from 29% to 60% in patients undergoing R0 resection (Table 35.1).
- Five-year survival rates after IORT in patients having R1 or R2 resection can be as high as 16% and 27%, respectively (Table 35.2).
  - In most series where IORT is not included in the management of patients whom had an R2 resection, no long-term survival in seen.
- Radiation-induced toxicity is a significant concern in patients receiving multimodality therapy that includes IORT.
  - In many cases it may be hard to separate IORT-related complications from surgical ones.

Table 35.1 Survival and local recurrence after intraoperative radiation therapy in patients undergoing R0 resection

Study	Patients (no.)	IORT dose (Gy)	EBRT dose (Gy[a])	5-year survival rate (%[b])	5-year local control rate (%[b])
Vermaas et al. (2005)	17	10	50	45 (3-year)	35 (3-year)
Alektiar et al. (2000)	53	10–18	45–50.4	36	43
Abuchaibe et al. (1993)	8	15	40–50	29	50
Dresen et al. (2008)	84	10–15	50.4 or 30.6[c]	59 (3-year)	75 (3-year)
Lindel et al. (2001)	25	10–20	50.4	40	56
Eble et al. (1998)	14	12	41.4	71 (4-year)	79 (4-year)
Wiig et al. (2002)	18	15	46–50	60	70
Valentini et al. (1999)	11	10–15	45–47	41	80
Haddock et al. (2011)	226	12.5 (median)	30.6–50.4[c]	46	72

EBRT external beam radiation therapy, *IORT* intraoperative radiation therapy. EBRT generally was delivered only to patients not previously treated with radiation, except for patients in Dresen et al. (2008) (39) and the current series.
[a]Five-year rates are shown unless otherwise indicated
[b]Lower doses were administered in previously irradiated patients
[c]Individualized per patient
With permission from Haddock MG, Gunderson LL, Nelson H, Cha SS, Devine RM, Dozois RR, et al. Intraoperative irradiation for locally recurrent colorectal cancer in previously irradiated patients. *International Journal of Radiation Oncology, Biology, Physics*. 2001;49(5):1267–74. (21) ©Elsevier 2001

Table 35.2 Survival and local control after intraoperative radiation therapy in patients undergoing R1 and R2 resection

Study	Patients (no.)	Surgical margins	IORT dose(Gy)	5-year survival rate (%[a])	5-year local control rate (%)
Vermaas et al. (2005)	10	R1–R2	10	21 (3-year)	21 (3-year)
Alektiar et al. (2000)	21	R1	10–18	11	26
Abuchaibe et al. (1993)	19	R1–R2	15	7	16
Dresen et al. (2008)	34	R1	12.5	27 (3-year)	29 (3-year)
	29	R2	15–17.5	24 (3-year)	29 (3-year)
Lindel et al. (2001)	9	R1	10–15	11	33
	15	R2	15–20	13	12
Eble et al. (1998)	9	R1	10–20	33 (4-year RFS)	67
	8	R2	10–20	25 (4-year RFS)	63
Martinez-Mong et al. (1999)	39	R1	10–15	6	26
	41	R2	15–20	7	29
Wiig et al. (2002)	29	R1	15	20	50
	12	R2	17.5–20	0	–
Haddock et al. (2011)	224	R1	15 (median)	27	68
	156	R2	20 (median)	16	68

IORT intraoperative radiation therapy, *RFS* relapse-free survival
[a]Five-year rates are shown unless otherwise indicated
With permission from Haddock MG, Gunderson LL, Nelson H, Cha SS, Devine RM, Dozois RR, et al. Intraoperative irradiation for locally recurrent colorectal cancer in previously irradiated patients. *International Journal of Radiation Oncology, Biology, Physics*. 2001;49(5):1267–74. (21) © Elsevier 2001

Technical Aspects of Surgical Resection

General Considerations

- We use ureteral stents for all operations in patients with local recurrence in the pelvis.
- The Lloyd-Davies position is used to allow access to the perineum.
- Care is taken to protect the extremities from nerve injury with adequate padding of both the tucked arms and lateral lower extremities in the stirrups.
- An exploratory laparotomy is carried out through a midline incision to confirm absence of extra-pelvic disease and determine local resectability. Any lesions suspicious for metastatic disease are biopsied and sent for frozen section analysis.

- The presence of metastatic disease typically precludes resection for cure, and proceeding on to resection of the local recurrence has to be weighed carefully.
- All adherent tissue to the recurrent tumor should be resected en bloc.
- In general, the technical approach to local recurrence in the abdomen or in the pelvis is carried out by widely mobilizing normal surrounding tissues and organs in preserved embryologic planes when feasible and working toward the distorted anatomy and malignant pathology.
  - Vascular pedicles and collateral vasculature should be well delineated prior to ultimate mobilization of the recurrence and surrounding adherent tissue or organs, so that when significant bleeding is encountered, proximal and distal vascular control can be achieved safely.
- Most cases for recurrence at our institution are done in a dedicated IORT operating room. This suite houses our linear accelerator and mobile anesthesia equipment that allows the patient to move into the optimal position for IORT (Fig. 35.3).
  - The radiation dose and field are selected based on tumor margin status.
  - At our institution, Lucite cones are used to focus the beam of radiation delivered by the linear accelerator and protect the small bowel and other organs from radiation injury (Fig. 35.4). The radiation oncologist and surgeon position the cone together for optimal radiation delivery.

Recurrent Colon Cancer

- Luminal and locoregional nodal recurrences are generally straightforward technically, and surgery involves resection of additional colon and adjacent mesentery.
  - During operations in patients with retained mesentery from incomplete previous surgery, it is the author's experience that isolation and ligation of the vascular pedicles of the original tumor (that should have been removed during the index operation) are a good initial step to allow safe mobilization of the recurrence that lies within the retained mesentery.
- In cases where para-aortic or para-iliac nodes are involved, major vascular reconstruction may be necessary in addition to en bloc resection of surrounding structures (Fig. 35.5).

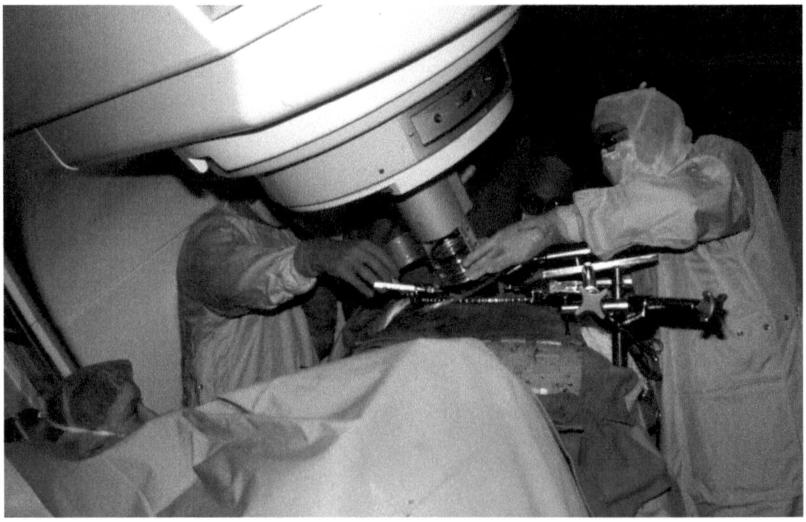

Fig. 35.3 The IORT suite; the operating table is positioned under the linear accelerator by the radiation oncologist, and the appropriate Lucite cone is affixed to direct the beam

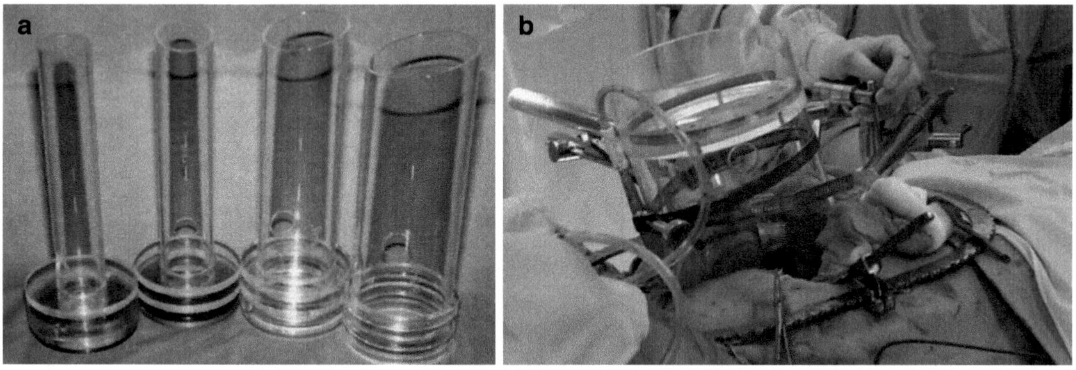

Fig. 35.4 (a) Assortment of Lucite cones of different sizes used to direct the IORT field. (b) In situ placement of the Lucite tube

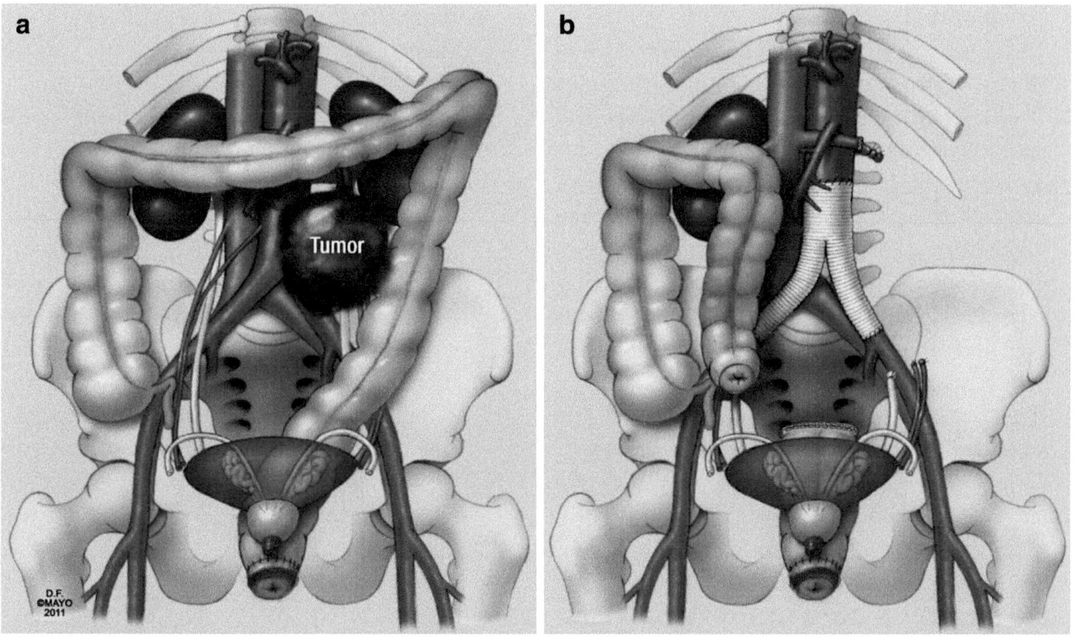

Fig. 35.5 (a) Illustration of a local recurrence involving the aortic bifurcation, colon, kidney, and ureter. (b) En bloc resection with aortoiliac reconstruction

- In cases where recurrence occurs in the previous resection bed, locoregional structures associated with the course of the colon are often involved (kidney, ureters, psoas muscle, stomach, spleen, duodenum, and pancreas).
- The most complex resections done for local recurrence after right colon resection are those that involve the duodenum and the head of the pancreas. When a Whipple operation is required, we involve a hepatobiliary surgeon to assist with resection and reconstruction.
- In cases where IORT will be used, radiation is delivered to the at-risk tumor bed just prior to closure.

Recurrent Rectal Cancer

Recurrences that Extend Anteriorly

- After ruling out metastatic disease, the left colon is fully mobilized and transected at the appropriate level for subsequent end-colostomy (in patients who have intestinal continuity).
- The entrance to the pelvis is cleared of loops of small bowel for optimal pelvic exposure.
- Dissection begins in the lower abdomen before entering the presacral space along the lower aorta and continues distally over the iliac vessels and ureters.
- Vasiloops are used to retract the ureters and vascular structures.
- In the re-operative pelvis, dense fibrosis and distorted anatomy require careful, meticulous dissection to avoid inadvertent injuries and major bleeding complications.
- In the author's experience, the most at-risk region for significant bleeding occurs during mobilization of the left common iliac vein, and this dissection should proceed with caution. Posterior lumbar branches, if not identified and injured, can lead to significant blood loss if avulsed.
- The anterior and lateral lines of resection (decided upon during preoperative review of imaging) are delineated and confirmed, and the involved structures and organs are mobilized widely for subsequent en bloc resection.
- The presacral space is further developed, and the dissection is carried down along the anterior sacrum being careful to stay anterior to Waldeyer's fascia to avoid the presacral venous plexus.
- The dissection is then carried laterally along the pelvic sidewall on each side with careful protection of the lumbosacral plexus and internal iliac vessels.
- The deepest part of the pelvic dissection will be the pelvic floor musculature, which can be incised during the abdominal portion of the procedure.
- When the transabdominal portion reaches this point, a combined transperineal approach facilitates final tumor removal.
  - The transperineal portion begins with purse-string closure of the anus (if present), and then a wide, elliptical incision is made to include the sphincter complex and as much pelvic floor musculature as possible.
  - With a surgeon working above, the two dissection planes can be joined safely and with careful attention to the tumor margins.
- In women, anterior involvement may require resection of the posterior wall of vagina, and this portion of the operation is approached transvaginally and transabdominally simultaneously.
- In men, anterior fixation often requires cysto-prostatectomy due to invasion of the trigone and prostate.
  - Partial cystectomy may be sufficient in rare cases. When a urinary conduit is necessary, the ureters are mobilized as close to the bladder as possible to provide adequate length to reach the conduit.
  - To mobilize the bladder, the space of Retzius is entered to fully mobilize the anterior portion of the bladder. The blood supply to the bladder (superior and inferior pedicles) is taken serially along the pelvic sidewall off the internal iliac vessels.
  - The wings of peritoneum to the bladder are then taken down until the bilateral vasa are identified and clipped.
  - The endopelvic fascia is opened bilaterally.
  - The dorsal venous complex is subsequently ligated.
  - The urethra is then delivered into the wound and transected.
- Once the tumor is out, the surgeon orients the specimen for the pathologist, and frozen section margins are assessed.
  - If margins are not clear, further resection is undertaken when safe to achieve an R0 resection.
- At this point IORT is given to the at-risk resection bed.
- Creation of end-colostomy and urinary conduit completes the procedure.

- In women in whom a large portion of the posterior vaginal wall is removal, a vertical rectus abdominis myocutaneous (VRAM) flap is used for vaginal reconstruction.

Resection that Includes Sacrectomy

Stage I: Anterior Component

- This dissection begins as outlined above for anterior recurrences.
- Vascular exposure often requires mobilization of the lower aorta and vena cava, in addition to the iliac arteries and veins.
  - If vascular structures need to be resected en bloc with the tumor, the decision to do so is made here.
  - If the resection does not require aortoiliac reconstruction, circumferential mobilization of the common and external iliac arteries will facilitate exposure of the veins.
  - The internal iliac artery branches are ligated and divided first, distal to the takeoff of the posterior division superior gluteal artery branch, to preserve blood flow to the gluteal muscles and soft tissue of the perineum.
  - Multiple internal iliac vein branches are then ligated after control of the main trunk(s) of the internal iliac vein has been achieved.
    - The branches are ligated and divided before ligation of the main trunk to avoid venous distention of the branches, which can lead to troublesome bleeding (Fig. 35.6).
    - Lateral and middle sacral vein branches, which drain into the posterior aspect of the left common iliac vein and caval confluence, are ligated and divided.
    - Suture ligature is preferable for short, broad-based internal iliac vein branches.
    - The vascular dissection is carried along both sides of the sacrum onto the pelvic floor.
    - In general, the internal iliac vessels are taken at their confluence as part of any sacrectomy above the third sacral body. For sacrectomy at or below the third sacral body, we generally preserve the internal iliac vessels.
- Once the most proximal lumbosacral level of transection is determined, unicortical anterior osteotomies are performed at the bony level of resection (Fig. 35.7).
  - Prior to closing the abdomen, a thick silastic mesh is placed anterior to the sacrum and posterior to the ureters, aorta, iliac vessels, and soft tissue structures to protect against injury when blind osteotomies are performed during the second stage of the procedure, at which point the patient is in prone position.
  - A titanium screw is also placed at the level of the osteotomy site to facilitate performing the posterior osteotomies by using intraoperative fluoroscopy (Fig. 35.8).
- During the anterior stage of the operation, IORT may be delivered prior to final tumor resection if orientation of the Lucite cone in the prone position will not be feasible to radiate the at-risk tumor bed.
- A colostomy and ileal or colonic urinary conduit are fashioned as needed, and a VRAM flap is then elevated for subsequent perineal reconstruction.

Stage II: Posterior Component

- The second stage of the procedure is typically carried out 2 days after the anterior portion.
- With the patient in the prone position, a posterior midline incision is made along the midportion of the sacrum, and the gluteus maximus muscles are dissected away from the sacral attachments.
- The sacrospinous and sacrotuberous ligaments are divided to access the pelvic cavity posteriorly.
- The pyriformis muscles are divided while protecting the sciatic and pudendal nerves.
- Laminectomy, dural sac ligation, and posterior sacral osteotomies are then carried out (Fig. 35.9).
- Final osteotomies are performed based on the preoperative MRI studies and intraoperative

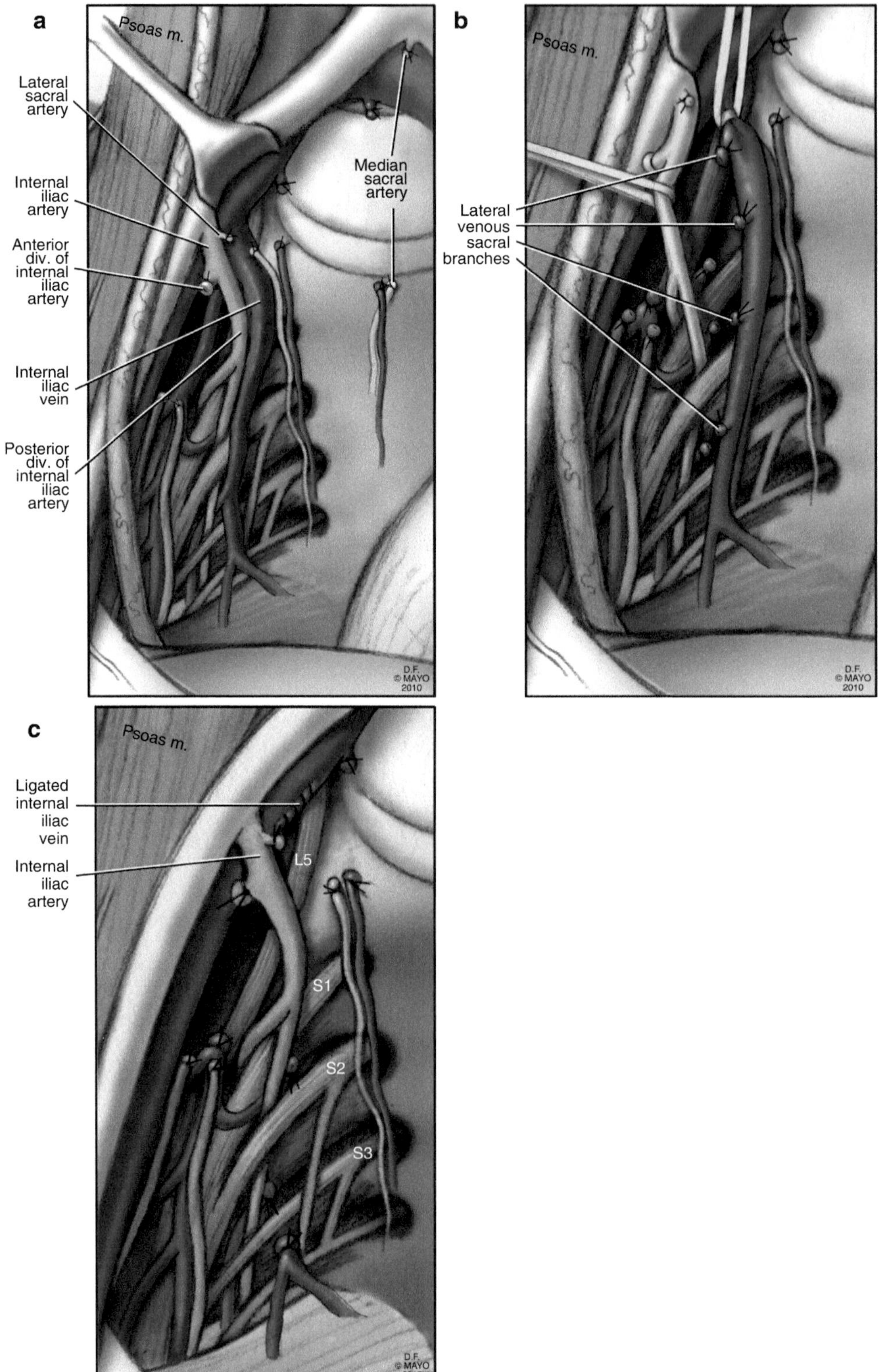

Fig. 35.6 (**a**) Pelvic vascular anatomy. Ligation of anterior division of internal iliac artery, lateral sacral arteries and veins, and sacral artery and vein. (**b**) Ligation of lateral venous sacral branches. (**c**) Ligation of internal iliac vein

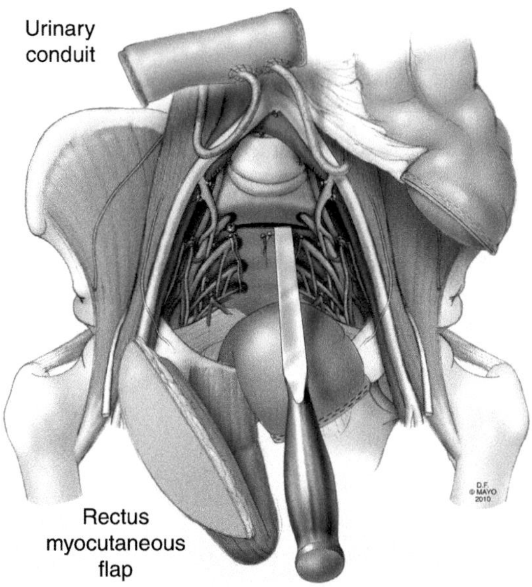

Fig. 35.7 Unicortical anterior transverse osteotomy

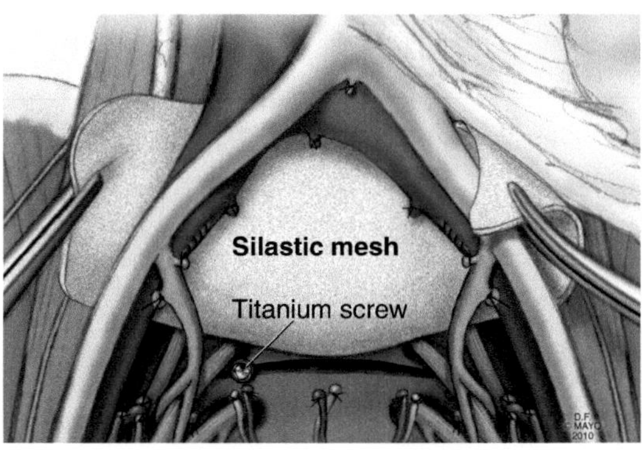

Fig. 35.8 Placement of silastic mesh to protect pelvic vasculature during the posterior osteotomies. Titanium screw marks the level of the anterior osteotomy to guide fluoroscopic identification of anterior osteotomy level when performing posterior osteotomy

fluoroscopy to identify the anterior positioned titanium screw.

- After resection, the surgical team meets with the pathologist to accurately orient the specimen, and together they assess the completeness of resection.
  - If frozen section analysis demonstrates an R1 or R2 margin, wider resection is undertaken as it can be done safely.

Before soft tissue wound reconstruction is done, IORT is given (if not given during Stage I), and the dose is based on tumor margin status, as discussed above.

Stage III: Spinal Reconstructive Component

- In cases where the lumbosacral line is transected, spinopelvic stability is compromised, and patients will require instrumented reconstruction.
  - For resections above the level of the S1 neuroforamen but below the lumbosacral junction, clinical experience and biomechanical studies have shown that in situ spinopelvic stabilization is beneficial to avoid collapse of the residual sacrum.
  - In these cases, an instrumented posterior spinopelvic fusion is made from the lower lumbar spine to the remaining pelvis.
- Resections done through the lumbosacral junction, or higher, disrupt spinopelvic continuity. These patients undergo reconstruction using a combination of dual fibula grafts and instrumented stabilization from the lower lumbar spine to the remaining pelvis (Fig. 35.10). The decision to use fibula allo- or autografts is individualized.
- A concurrent hemipelvectomy is considered if the local extent of disease leads to sacrifice of both the femoral nerve and the lumbosacral plexus/sciatic nerve or the hip joint and the femoral or sciatic nerves.
  - Resections of this magnitude would otherwise leave a nonfunctional limb. In addition, patients will have such a large soft tissue defect that a pedicled quadriceps apron flap is necessary for closure.
  - In these cases, the fibula from the amputated limb can be preserved on a pedicle at the end of the quadriceps flap for reconstruction. This is then used to restore spinopelvic continuity.

Soft Tissue Reconstruction

- Nonhealing perineal wounds following an abdominal-perineal approach to complex pelvic tumors are reported to occur in 7%–66% of patients.

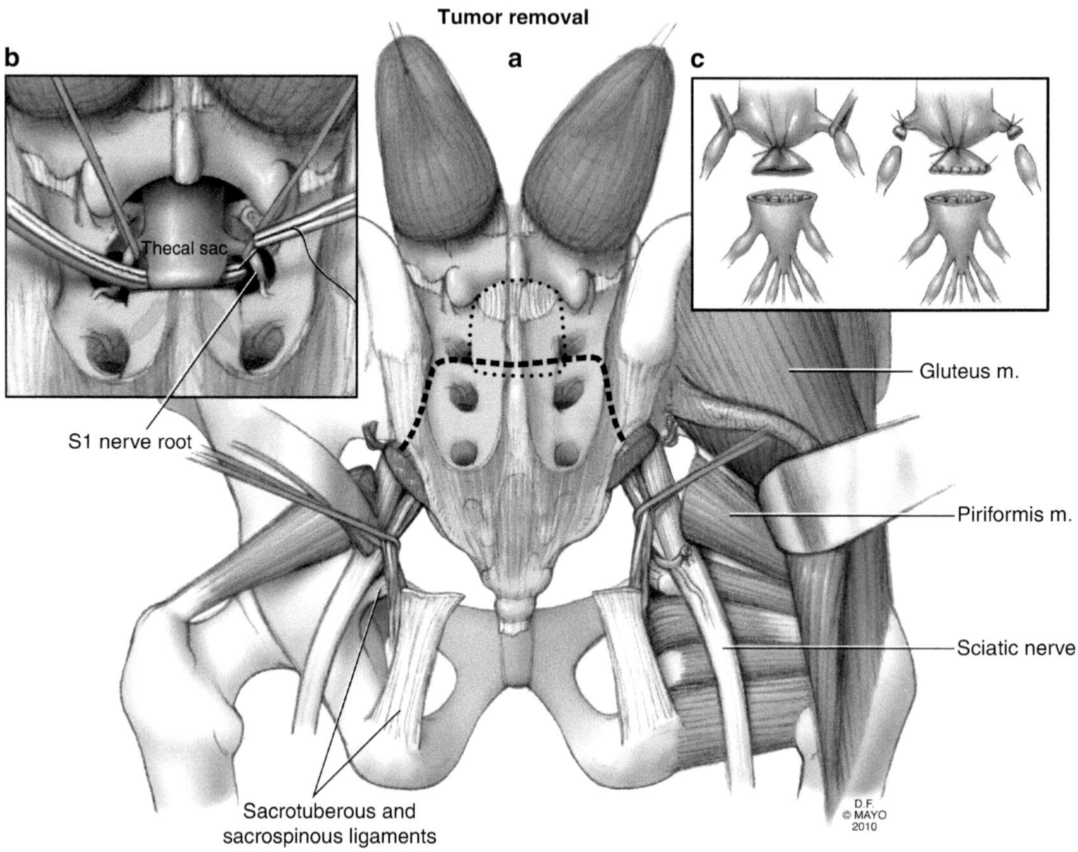

Fig. 35.9 (**a**) Posterior transverse osteotomy (thick dotted black line). Sacrospinous and sacrotuberous ligament transection. Gluteus maximus muscle is reflected laterally to expose obturator vessels and sciatic nerve. (**b**) Laminectomy to identify thecal sac. (**c**) Dural sac and sacral root ligation

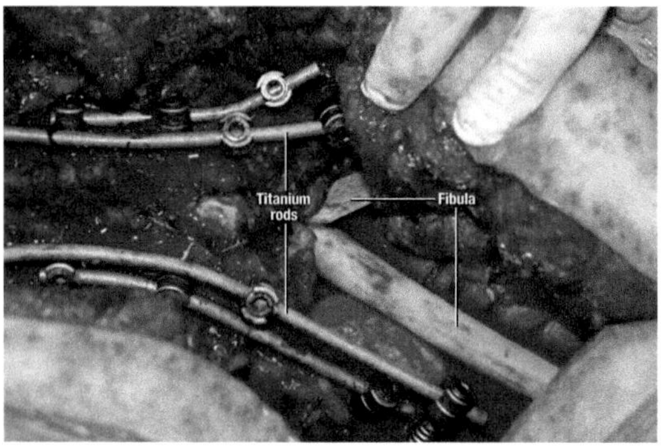

Fig. 35.10 Intraoperative photograph of fibula grafts and instrumented spinopelvic reconstruction following total sacrectomy

- We, as well as others, have found that the use of a VRAM flap is associated with fewer perineal wound complications.
  – The VRAM provides a well-vascularized, bulky tissue paddle that not only fills dead space but also can be used to reconstruct the perineal skin defect.
  – In cases where the rectus in not available, a pedicled omental flap can be a good second choice if it is robust. It can fill the pelvic dead space providing vascularized tissue and has been shown to decrease risk of pelvic sepsis following surgery.
  – Moreover, the omentum can line the raw surfaces of the pelvis, preventing the small bowel from getting trapped in the deep pelvis, which is a common cause of small bowel obstruction following exenteration.

- Thigh fillet flaps are used after hindquarter amputation and are based on the superior and inferior gluteal vessels.
- Long anterior hemipelvectomy flaps are based on the vascular muscle distribution supplied by the superficial femoral artery.

Results of Surgery

Recurrent Colon Cancer

- Limited data exist on surgical and oncologic outcomes in patients with locally advanced recurrent colon cancer.
- Few centers have published their experience, and patient groups are small and heterogeneous, making definitive conclusions regarding management difficult.
- The best oncologic outcomes are achieved in patients undergoing R0 resection.

Margin status and location of recurrence appear to be the most important predictors of outcome in patients with recurrent colon cancer.

Recurrent Rectal Cancer

- Published series of surgery for locally recurrent rectal cancer have been limited by small numbers and heterogeneous patient groups.
- However, it is clear that for select patients, R0 resection is possible and overall 5-year survival can be as high as 40%.
- In series published where IORT is a component of multimodality therapy, meaningful survival can also be achieved in patients who have R1 or R2 resections.
- Aggressive surgery that includes more lateral pelvic resections (pelvic sidewall tumors) and higher sacral resection (above the third sacral body) is increasingly reported by experienced centers with good results.
- The importance of an R0 resection in patients undergoing surgery for recurrent rectal cancer cannot be overstated.
  - Patients undergoing an R0 resection survive on average 2 years than those undergoing R1 resection and 4 years longer than those undergoing R2 resection.

Surgery for Re-recurrent Disease

- In the author's view, a second colorectal cancer recurrence is not a contraindication to curative resection as long as the principles of determining resectability for primary recurrence are followed.

Resection that Includes the Aortoiliac Axis

- Small series have demonstrated that despite the complexity of the technique, the surgery can be performed safely when done by expert multidisciplinary teams, and overall DFS is comparable to outcomes seen with locally advanced disease to nonvascular structures.

Sacropelvic Resections

- Owing to the complex anatomical relationships of the pelvic structures, some local recurrences involve multiple fixation points and will require both multivisceral and neuromusculoskeletal resection to achieve a negative-margin resection.
- Operations for recurrences involving the lateral pelvic sidewall or high lumbosacral skeletal components are among the most technically challenging to perform.
- In the past, limited data existed regarding both the safety and the oncologic benefits of surgery in these patients. Once thought to be a common contraindication to surgery for recurrent colorectal cancer, high sacral and other complex sacropelvic resections are being done by several centers around the world.
- In series from specialized centers, authors have shown that surgery in these complex patients can be done safely and with meaningful oncologic outcomes.

Postoperative Complications and Quality of Life

- Despite the complex nature and magnitude of surgery for local recurrence, several recent series have demonstrated that these cases can be done with an operative mortality rate that ranges from 0% to 3%.
- When it does occur, 30-day mortality is usually a result of uncontrolled sepsis.
- This is a dramatic improvement compared to series published 20 years ago, where operative mortality could be as high as 8.5%.
- Several factors are responsible for the significant decrease in operative mortality: better patient selection, improved surgical technique by experienced specialists, better anesthesia, and better postoperative ICU management.
- Early and late complications following surgery for local recurrence remain a significant challenge.
  - Most series report intra-abdominal /pelvic sepsis and wound-related complications as the most significant cause of morbidity.
  - Other common complications are postoperative bleeding requiring transfusion, voiding dysfunction, prolonged ileus, delayed small bowel perforation, and late fistulas.
- Universally, higher complication rates are associated with extended resections such a sacrectomy and exenteration.
- Urologic complications both early (ureteral obstruction, leak) and late (ureteral stricture) are reported in many series.
- Little information exists about the impact of major surgical intervention on quality of life in patients with recurrent colorectal cancer.
- While oncologic outcomes remain the most important outcome measure for patients and physicians deciding on an aggressive surgical approach, quality of life after surgery must be considered and discussed with patients so that they are well informed.

Palliative Approach

- Patients with an asymptomatic recurrence which is unresectable, either due to presence of concurrent metastases or because of local factors, do not warrant surgical intervention.
- In symptomatic patients, external beam radiotherapy can sometimes relieve obstruction, decrease bleeding, and reduce pain.
- Endoscopic stenting is especially helpful with malignant obstructions and can in some cases be used to palliate malignant fistulas that are inoperable.
- Patients not candidates for stents may need a colostomy for symptomatic relief.
- Chemotherapy has been shown to prolong survival and palliate symptoms in patients with primary metastatic colorectal cancer, and the treatment of unresectable recurrent colorectal cancer is based on extrapolations from this data.
- Patients in whom a palliative approach is taken will benefit greatly by meeting with a palliative medicine team to discuss treatment goals and assist with end-of-life decisions. In addition, a cancer pain specialist can assist in reducing suffering through optimal pain management, and this should be the goal in patients undergoing a palliative approach.

Colorectal Cancer: Management of Stage IV Disease

36

Glenn T. Ault and Kyle G. Cologne

Key Concepts

- Multidisciplinary evaluation is of paramount importance in the treatment of metastatic colorectal cancer.
- Positron emission tomography (PET) scan should be used in the evaluation of metastatic disease prior to potentially curative surgical therapy or in cases of equivocal disease, but not for routine detection of metastatic disease.
- Patients with incurable metastatic disease and asymptomatic primary tumors should be considered for initial treatment with chemotherapy.
- For metastatic colorectal liver lesions, synchronous resection and liver-first or colon-first strategies are all acceptable means of surgical treatment.
- Resection, ablation, or a combination of ablative and resection techniques can be used to minimize parenchymal liver resection and preserve function when treating metastatic colorectal metastases.
- Cytoreduction and hepatic artery infusion of chemotherapy (HIPEC) may be considered in appropriately selected patients treated at specialized centers with expertise in this technique, although it has not been demonstrated to be superior to modern systemic chemotherapy.
- Metastases to organs other than the liver, lung, ovary, or peritoneum are uncommon and commonly occur in conjunction with widely metastatic disease. Thus, resection rarely has an impact on overall survival and should only be undertaken in select circumstances after multidisciplinary evaluation.
- Treatment of metastatic disease in the elderly requires consideration of the performance status, frailty, and impact of various treatments on quality of life.

G. T. Ault
Division of Colorectal Surgery, Department of Surgery, University of Southern California, Los Angeles, CA, USA

K. G. Cologne (✉)
Department of Surgery, Division of Colorectal, University of Southern California Keck School of Medicine, Los Angeles, CA, USA
e-mail: Kyle.Cologne@med.usc.edu

Introduction

- Despite screening protocols, approximately 20% of colorectal cancer patients present with established distant metastasis.
- While there has been considerable progress in the treatment of advanced colorectal cancer, the vast majority of stage IV patients are

S. R. Steele et al. (eds.), *The ASCRS Manual of Colon and Rectal Surgery*,
https://doi.org/10.1007/978-3-030-01165-9_36

unfortunately not curable by current treatment protocols.
- Computed tomography (CT) scan or magnetic resonance imaging (MRI) generally detects metastases at the time of the initial staging of the cancer.
- Once the diagnosis of stage IV disease is made, a multidisciplinary team should plan appropriate curative or palliative therapy.
- Treatment approaches must be individualized based on the extent of resectability of local and distant disease, the presence or absence of symptoms, performance status, and comorbidities.
- For patients with good performance status and minimal symptoms from the primary site of the cancer, standard treatment is systemic chemotherapy, which has been proven to prolong survival and quality of life.
  – Surgical resection of the primary tumor is indicated if symptoms cannot be controlled with chemotherapy.
- Select patients can be considered for resection of the primary tumor and metastatic lesions, which may be curative.
- First-line therapy with either FOLFOX or FOLFIRI now has been shown to yield major responses in up to 50% of previously untreated patients and achieves minor responses or stable disease in an additional 20% of patients.
- Over the past 15 years, the median survival for patients with metastatic disease who are treated with chemotherapy has improved from 9 to 12months and is currently greater than 24 months and may be as long as 36 months.

Diagnostic Strategies

- Part of the evaluation of newly diagnosed colorectal cancer includes systemic staging with cross-sectional imaging of the chest, abdomen, and pelvis.
- 20–30% of patients will present with evidence of metastatic disease on this staging workup.
- Increased suspicion should be given to the presence of metastatic disease when the CEA level is greater than 20 ng/mL.
- No imaging modality is infallible, and in cases of uncertainty, multiple imaging modalities or tissue biopsy may be required to confirm the diagnosis, as it dramatically changes the prognosis and perhaps the treatment strategy as well.

Computed Tomography

- Computed tomography has been the mainstay of distant staging workup for colorectal cancer.
- Triple-phase scans allow improved delineation of hepatic metastases (Fig. 36.1).
- Though enhancement characteristics differ, most metastatic lesions are hypoattenuating on portal venous phases of an abdominal CT.
- Up to 25% of hepatic liver metastases may be missed on high-quality CT, due mostly either to size or confusion with other disease processes.

Positron Emission Tomography (PET)

- PET and combined PET-CT scans are a modality used both for initial staging and for

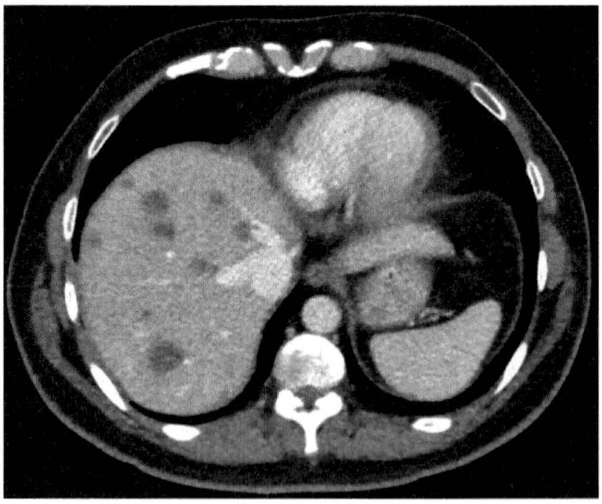

Fig. 36.1 CT of the abdomen demonstrating liver metastases involving multiple segments of the liver. Treatment of these requires advanced planning and input in a multidisciplinary setting involving hepatobiliary, interventional radiology, oncology, and other specialties to determine planned interventions and timing

follow-up imaging. The technology has dramatically improved recently and can now provide very clear pictures of tumor deposits in distant locations (Fig. 36.2).

- Sensitivity of PET-CT for detecting metastatic lesions ranges from 87% to 100%, which compares favorably with regular CT where sensitivities range from 52 to 69%).
- Specificity of PET-CT is also good and ranges from 94% to 100% (compared with 80–94% for regular CT).
- Limitations include a size resolution of about 1 cm and limited ability to detect mucinous tumors due to low tumor cell/volume ratio.
- National Comprehensive Cancer Network (NCCN) guidelines do not recommend routine use of PET-CT to evaluate metastatic lesions except in equivocal findings or in cases where patients are allergic to IV contrast which would otherwise limit the usefulness of regular CT.
- In cases where patients are being considered for potentially curative resection of recurrent/metastatic tumor, PET-CT will change management in up to 20% of cases, primarily by detecting occult metastases, which would render the planned resection palliative.

Magnetic Resonance Imaging

- MRI is particularly helpful in characterizing equivocal lesions of the liver, especially those that fall below the resolution of PET.
- Sensitivity of MRI at detecting response of liver lesions to neoadjuvant treatments may be better than PET.

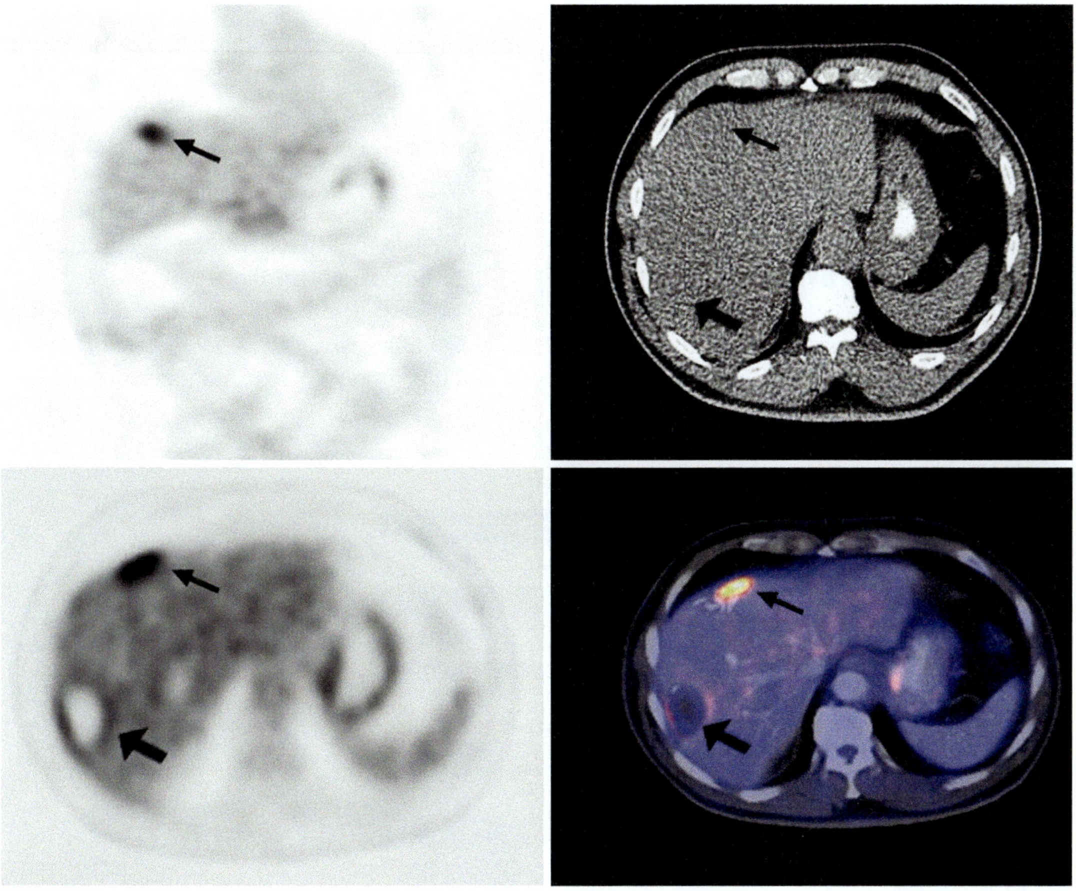

Fig. 36.2 PET-CT scan and various phases. Lesions may not always show up or appear active on all phases of imaging

- MRI cannot routinely be used in patients with pacemakers, implantable cardiac defibrillators, cochlear implants, and other orbital foreign bodies.

Contrast-Enhanced Ultrasound

- Contrast-enhanced ultrasound (CEUS) is a relatively new imaging modality to assess the liver.
- It is highly operator dependent but in experienced hands may be highly accurate.
- A potential limitation is that chemotherapy-induced fatty infiltration of the liver may limit diagnostic accuracy.

Biopsy

- In equivocal cases where imaging characteristics are not suspicious of colorectal metastases, tissue biopsy confirmation remains an option. A small percentage of patients will have a histologic process other than the primary malignancy.

Multidisciplinary Evaluation

- Multidisciplinary evaluation is of critical importance to caring for patients with metastatic disease.
- As there is often no one agreed-upon absolute treatment strategy, it is important to have consensus from treating oncologists, radiation oncologists, and various surgical disciplines such as colorectal, hepatobiliary, thoracic, and gynecology.
- It is estimated that only 20–30% of patients with identified metastatic disease will have potentially resectable disease.
- Goals of multidisciplinary evaluation should include relief of symptoms, quality of life improvement, and determining the best means of prolonging life expectancy. A typical algorithm can be found in Fig. 36.3.

Surgical Emergency

- Tumors at the primary site may cause a surgical emergency, even in the setting of metastatic disease.
- In these cases, surgical intervention should be undertaken to relieve the immediate, life-threatening issue, such as perforation with peritonitis, lower GI bleeding, or large bowel obstruction.
- If possible, and if it can be performed with limited morbidity, an oncologic surgical resection should be performed.
- A primary anastomosis can be performed in select, low-risk patients but carries the potential that it may delay chemotherapy and other

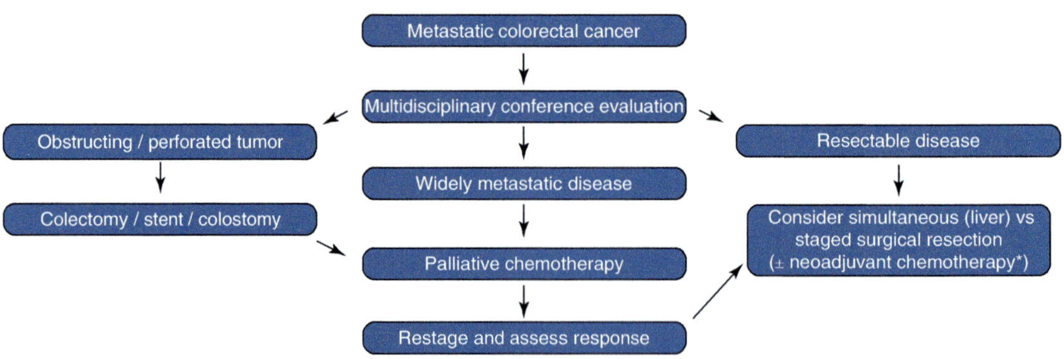

Fig. 36.3 Treatment algorithm for metastatic colorectal cancer

life-sustaining treatments if an anastomotic leak should occur.

Palliative Management of Primary Cancer: Laser, Fulguration, and Stents

Incidence and Presentation

- Approximately 8–29% of patients with colorectal cancer initially present with symptoms of partial or complete bowel obstruction.
- The majority of patients with obstructing colorectal carcinomas have either stage III or stage IV disease.
- Acute malignant colon or rectal obstruction is an indication for emergent surgical intervention.
  - However, these emergency operations are associated with a mortality rate of 15–34% and a morbidity rate of 32–64% despite advances in perioperative care.
  - Therefore, alternative palliative endoluminal strategies aimed at relieving obstruction have gained increasing popularity over the past decades.
- If the patient has minimal symptoms and there is no radiographic evidence of high-grade obstruction, many patients with partially obstructing colon and rectal cancers will respond to aggressive chemotherapy.
- In those patients with partially obstructing rectal cancers, the addition of radiation therapy is also well tolerated and can be highly effective.
- Patients must be instructed to monitor their symptoms closely and to report any signs of worsening obstruction immediately.
- For patients with advanced obstruction, nonsurgical palliative options include laser therapy, fulguration, and colonic self-expanding metal stents.
- If less invasive endoluminal strategies are not successful in patients with unresectable malignant obstruction of the colon and rectum, surgical creation of palliative proximal diverting stoma or intestinal bypass should be performed.

Laser Therapy and Fulguration

- Laser therapy has been utilized for palliation of obstructing rectal cancers.
- Although it can be effective in palliating obstruction, multiple sessions are often required in order to achieve lasting relief of symptom.
- Serious complications like bleeding, perforation, and severe pain have been reported in 5–15% of patients, especially those undergoing multiple treatment sessions.
- Surgical fulguration of rectal cancers is another method of opening the rectal lumen and relieving obstruction.
- Fulguration, in combination with endoluminal debulking, can remove a large volume of tumor.
- However, unlike laser therapy, fulguration and debulking require hospital admission and regional or general anesthesia.
- In general, both fulguration and laser therapy have given way to stenting.

Self-Expanding Intraluminal Metal Stents

- Since their introduction in 1991, colonic stents have become an effective method of palliation for obstruction in colorectal cancer patients, especially those with unresectable metastatic disease or used in an effort to decompress an obstructed patient preoperatively.
- Especially in nonoperative stage IV patients or those that have significant comorbidities, these self-expanding metallic stents can potentially dilate the lumen, providing quick relief of symptoms.
- Stents can be placed in patients using moderate sedation in the endoscopy suite with the aid of fluoroscopy.
- It should be noted emergency surgery is recommended over stent placement in those

patients with evidence of colonic obstruction and systemic toxicity. Presence of systemic toxicity may indicate the presence of ischemia and/or perforation, which requires immediate evaluation and the potential for emergency surgery.

- Stenting can achieve long-term palliation in patients who are not operative candidates.
  - More than 75% of patients can achieve adequate palliation with stenting, although tumor ingrowth, stent migration, and perforation, especially those receiving bevacizumab, may occur.
  - If these stent-related complications occur, it may necessitate reintervention either with an additional stent or with other palliative measures such as laser or argon plasma coagulation therapy or surgery.
- There are limited data evaluating stent placement proximal to the splenic flexure.
- Complications reported in the literature for colonic and rectal stents include stent malpositioning, perforation, stent migration, tumor ingrowth (through the stent interstices), tumor overgrowth (beyond the ends of a stent), stool impaction, bleeding, tenesmus, and post-procedure pain (Fig. 36.4). Perforation and stent migration occur with the highest frequency.
- Stenting of cancers in the mid to low rectum may result in urgency, pain, and incontinence.

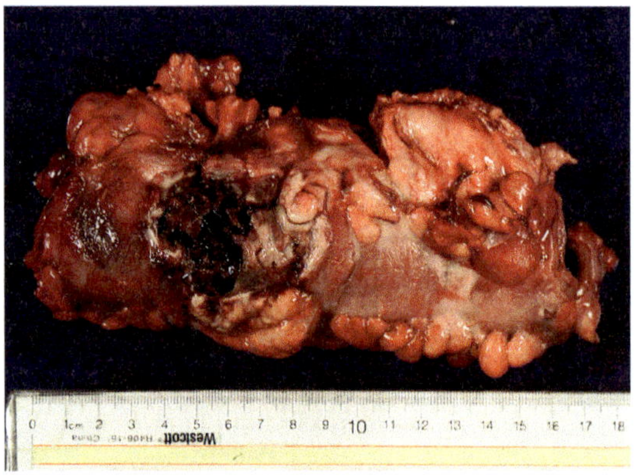

Fig. 36.4 Perforation of the bowel in a colonic stent. (Courtesy of Philip Y. Pearson, MD)

- Stents left in situ for long periods (many months or years) may erode through the bowel wall and cause significant morbidity to adjacent organ involvement, subacute perforation, fistulas, etc.
- While the complications associated with stents and other less invasive endoluminal strategies should not be taken lightly, one must keep in mind that emergency operations for malignant colon and rectal obstruction have a significant mortality rate of 15–34% and a high morbidity rate of 32–64%.

The Challenge of Primary Tumor Management in Asymptomatic Stage IV Colorectal Cancer: To Resect or Not to Resect?

- Optimal first-line therapy for patients who present initially with unresectable stage IV disease remains controversial. Some advocate initial resection of the primary, while others recommend initial chemotherapy if the primary tumor is asymptomatic.
- In the era of modern chemotherapy, patients can experience increased length and quality of life with 5-FU-based multi-agent chemotherapy.
- Prophylactic resection of the primary tumor can provide long-term local control.
  - This must be weighed against the risk of surgical complications resulting in delay in chemotherapy and other palliative treatments.
  - Particularly in rectal cancer, complications arising from surgery have been shown to delay initiation of chemotherapy beyond 8 weeks postoperatively.
- There is a paucity of prospective randomized, controlled trials addressing the question of whether patients with asymptomatic or minimally symptomatic primary tumors and stage IV disease should have the primary resected as a first step.
  - Virtually all studies have been retrospective, and selection bias has been inherent to the study design, making firm conclusions impossible.

- Currently, routine surgery for the asymptomatic primary tumor in the setting of unresectable metastatic disease is not recommended.

Surgical Therapy of Liver Metastases

- Liver metastases are a common occurrence, and surgical resection represents the best opportunity for long-term cure.
- Approximately 20–30% of patients have potentially resectable lesions at the time of diagnosis.
- With appropriate selection, 5-year survival has been reported around 30% (range 15–67%).
- Even with modern chemotherapy for colorectal cancer, surgery for metastatic cancer (if possible) has consistently been shown to improve 5-year survival and quality of life and should be considered when possible.
- Newer liver strategies may allow a staged resection, portal vein embolization, or a combination of resection, embolization, and other strategies to ablate or otherwise treat or downsize liver lesions, which may allow a greater percentage of patients to undergo some form of treatment.
  - This underscores the importance of multidisciplinary evaluation of these patients.
- The main reason for failure in treated patients is intrahepatic recurrence of the tumor, which occurs in 60–70% of patients, one third of whom die within 2 years of surgery for hepatic metastases.
- Evidence to support each of these strategies below is very limited and largely based on small, single-institution series. Survival analyses across multiple studies suggest there is little difference between simultaneous, colon-first and liver-first strategies. As such, the agreed-upon treatment strategy should depend on the local expertise at an individual institution.

Combination Liver and Colon Resection

- There is evidence to suggest that this approach results in a similar long-term outcome when compared to those undergoing staged therapy.
- Similarly, simultaneous resection does not increase overall morbidity, though there is an inherent selection bias in trials examining this issue.
- This approach is typically done for relatively minor resections, which can include lobectomy.

Liver-First Strategy

- In patients with liver metastases from colorectal cancer, it is the metastatic disease in the liver (particularly if >3 cm in size) that is the primary determinant of overall survival.
  - This is a potential reason for addressing the liver disease first, particularly in the setting of larger metastatic lesions where the primary lesion is asymptomatic.
  - As there is some evidence to suggest the primary lesion has a low chance of becoming symptomatic during follow-up, it is reasonable to proceed with treatment of the metastatic disease first.
- This also may avoid unnecessary colorectal surgery (and its associated morbidity) in patients who go on to develop incurable metastatic disease.
- There is evidence to suggest that a "liver-first" strategy may still allow patients with potentially curable disease to undergo both liver and colon resection over time.
- The liver-first approach can be combined with neoadjuvant chemotherapy for borderline resectable lesions or to allow tumor biology to dictate those lesions that are likely to progress rapidly prior to surgery.
  - While this has been recommended as standard of care by some, others have disputed this and still recommend surgical resection followed by adjuvant chemotherapy due to the effect of chemotherapy-associated steatosis that can increase surgical morbidity.
- The liver-first strategy has a particular advantage in the setting or rectal cancer, where the

process of neoadjuvant chemoradiotherapy can potentially take up to 3 months.
  - This may allow surgery on the metastatic disease while treatment for the primary lesion is still ongoing.
  - Alternatively, radiotherapy on rectal lesions can be reserved for overall disease that responds favorably to initial treatments – particularly the short-course variety.
- The data for the liver-first approach are limited, and largely based on non-randomized data, but seem to remain a viable method with reasonable long-term results.

Colon-First Strategy

- Proponents of the colon-first strategy hypothesize that the colon or rectum acts as an ongoing source of seeding metastatic disease.
- Additionally, the primary tumor represents a potential source of bowel-related morbidity in the form of bleeding, obstruction, or perforation.
- Some authors suggest the rates of this can be as high as 20%, but others suggest it is much lower than this.
- Additionally, the risk of morbidity associated with a colorectal anastomosis may be increased by addition of a liver procedure, where anesthesia and surgical techniques may include a low-flow state or temporary alteration in portal blood circulation (e.g., a Pringle maneuver), which may affect blood flow to the bowel.
- Resection of the colon first may allow detection of new or occult liver metastases which can then be removed with definitive surgery.

Margin Status

- Excision to negative margins in hepatic resection results in improved disease-free and overall survival.
- A consensus statement from the Society of Surgical Oncology concluded that while wide margins of >1 cm are desirable, a close margin should not preclude resection. Another study suggested that a margin <5 mm is a risk factor for local recurrence.

Ablation of Liver Metastases

- There are a variety of techniques for ablation of liver metastases that do not require tissue resection: percutaneous ethanol ablation, radiofrequency ablation, microwave ablation, cryoablation, and irreversible electroporation (or nanoknife).
- Radiofrequency ablation is the most commonly employed technique, though all can be used successfully and also used in conjunction with other forms of therapy (e.g., surgical resection).
- Several different treatments may be used simultaneously or in a staged approach.

Other Liver Metastasis Strategies: Hepatic Intra-arterial Chemotherapy/Chemoembolization

- Regional chemotherapy through the hepatic artery is a therapeutic option for patients with isolated liver metastasis that are not amenable to surgical resection or local ablation.
- This method can also be combined with other forms of treatment.
- This mode of therapy is based upon the fact that liver macrometastases derive more than 80% of their blood supply from the hepatic arterial circulation, while normal hepatocytes are supplied primarily by the portal circulation. This allows selective delivery of drug to the tumor with relative sparing of the normal hepatocytes.
- There is also a marked increase in the local concentration of the chemotherapy that is achieved by injection into the hepatic artery. Regional administration of agents that are rapidly metabolized in the liver by a first-pass effect leads to higher levels of drug exposure and minimizes side effects.

Pulmonary Metastasis

- Approximately 10% of patients with colorectal cancer develop pulmonary metastasis.
- The vast majority of patients with metastatic colorectal cancer to the lungs have advanced

disease and are therefore treated with systemic chemotherapy or best supportive care.

- Due to differences in blood supply, pulmonary metastases may be more common after rectal (vs. colon) cancer due to the dual blood supply of the rectum (portal and systemic).
- Due to the retrospective nature of the reported information in the literature, clinical outcome data after metastasectomy for colorectal lung metastases must be interpreted with caution.
- Improved clinical outcome and survival data is more likely due to ideal patient selection and tumor biology rather than the surgical intervention in and of itself. In addition, there are no adequate control groups in these reports; therefore, survival statistics are difficult to interpret.
- However, there are patients who undergo pulmonary metastasectomy with no evidence of disease after long-term follow-up. In addition, long-term survival without complete resection is very rare, suggesting that select patients do occasionally benefit from pulmonary metastasectomy. Input on the resectability of lung lesions by a thoracic surgeon at multidisciplinary evaluation is essential.
- Modern series of lung resection for metastatic colorectal cancer report operative mortalities of less than 2% (Table 36.1).
- Radiation therapy for colorectal cancer pulmonary metastasis has been of limited utility in the past due to radiation-induced pneumonitis, rib and spinal fractures, and skin toxicities. However, these toxicities can be minimized with the advent of robotic-assisted Gamma Knife radiotherapy or "Cyberknife."
- While it appears that certain colorectal cancer patients would benefit from pulmonary metastasectomy even in the presence of liver metastases, no randomized controlled trials have been conducted and reported, and the effectiveness of pulmonary metastasectomy has been suggested mostly by results of retrospective analyses.

Peritoneal Metastasis

- The peritoneal surface is involved in approximately 10–15% of colorectal cancer patients at time of initial presentation (synchronous metastases) and in 20–50% of patients who develop recurrence (metachronous metastases).
- As a site of colorectal cancer metastasis, the peritoneal surface ranks second only to the liver.
- It is characterized by intraperitoneal spread of metastatic nodules.
- The most frequent signs/symptoms are ascites and bowel obstruction.

Table 36.1 Outcome of patients undergoing pulmonary metastasectomy for colorectal cancer

Study	*n*	Operative mortality (%)	5-yr survival (%)	Significant risk factors
Mori et al.	35	–	38	None found
McCormack et al.	144	0	44	Margin
McAfee et al.	139	1	31	Number of lesions, CEA
Yano et al.	27	–	41	Number of lesions
Saclarides et al.	23	–	16	Number of lesions
van Halteren et al.	38	–	43	DFI
Shirouzu et al.	22	–	37	Number of lesions, size
Girard et al.	86	1	24	CEA, margin
Okumura et al.	159	2	41	Number of lesions, LN status
Zanella et al.	22	0	62	None found
Zink	110	0	33	Size, CEA
Dahabre et al.	52	–	33	None found

n number of patients, *yr* year, *LN* lymph nodes, *DFI* disease-free interval
Adapted from Rizk NP, Downey RJ. Resection of pulmonary metastases from colorectal cancer. Semin Thorac Cardiovasc Surg. 2002;14(1):29–34

- Peritoneal metastasis occurs by direct implantation of cancer cells via one of four mechanisms: (1) spontaneous intraperitoneal seeding from a T4 colorectal cancer that has penetrated the serosal surface of the colon, (2) extravasation of tumor cells at the time of colon perforation from an obstructing cancer, (3) iatrogenic tumor perforation through an area of serosal injury or enterotomy at the time of colon resection, and (4) leakage of tumor cells from transected lymphatics or veins at the time of colon resection.
- The risk of peritoneal metastasis is therefore highest in the setting of locally advanced cancers, and until recently, most oncologists viewed peritoneal carcinomatosis as a terminal condition, to be palliated only with systemic chemotherapy.
- However, in a small set of cases, the peritoneal cavity is determined to be the only site of metastatic disease after a detailed workup of the lungs and liver. This has led some to hypothesize that in some cases, peritoneal carcinomatosis may represent a first site of dissemination, and therefore, not necessarily indicative of generalized disease.
- Preoperative detection of peritoneal metastases is not reliable. Noninvasive imaging frequently misses small peritoneal lesions, even when these are widely disseminated.
- The extent of carcinomatosis is a major prognostic factor and is best assessed by either laparoscopic or open exploration.
  - Two different peritoneal carcinomatosis staging systems (Gilly's classification and Peritoneal Cancer Index of Sugarbaker) can be used to assess the extent of carcinomatosis. These staging systems have both shown utility in determining the prognosis and treatment of patients with peritoneal carcinomatosis.
- Standard management of patients known to have peritoneal metastases at initial presentation (if known preoperatively) is systemic chemotherapy.
- Colon resection plays an important role for patients with obstructing primary cancers and also for patients with occult metastases that are first detected in the operating room.
- Historically, the median survival for patients with unresected peritoneal metastasis treated with 5-fluorouracil-based systemic chemotherapy was very poor (6–8 months).
  - However, patient survival is highly variable, depending on the extent of metastatic disease and response to chemotherapy.
  - Contemporary combination chemotherapy regimens have significantly greater efficacy and can produce long periods of disease control in certain patients.
- Despite the grim prognosis for patients with peritoneal carcinomatosis from colorectal cancer, a subset of patients once thought unsalvageable are now being considered for surgery with curative intent.
  - Pioneered by Sugarbaker, the goal of cytoreductive surgery and intraperitoneal (IP) chemotherapy is to remove all macroscopic disease with peritonectomy procedures and visceral resections followed by perioperative IP chemotherapy to destroy residual microscopic disease.
  - IP delivery offers pharmacokinetic advantage over standard intravenous delivery by producing high regional concentrations of drug while simultaneously minimizing systemic toxicities.
  - For patients with isolated peritoneal carcinomatosis from colorectal cancer, radical surgery to achieve an R0 resection (if it can be accomplished) remains the mainstay of treatment.
- Benefit from cytoreductive surgery with heated intraperitoneal chemotherapy has been suggested in several retrospective case series, a multi-institutional registry review, two randomized trials, and a systematic review.
  - These randomized trials must be interpreted with caution as neither used modern combination chemotherapy as the control arm.
  - While patients who undergo complete cytoreduction followed by HIPEC may seem to have a more favorable prognosis than can be achieved with systemic chemo-

therapy alone, there remains insufficient evidence to conclude whether the survival advantage is due to treatment or to biologic features that allow these patients to undergo complete cytoreductive surgery (selection bias).

- In published series, the overall treatment-related morbidity rates range from 23% to 44% and mortality rates from 0% to 12%.
- Many important unanswered questions remain, including which patients with colorectal cancer peritoneal carcinomatosis have a higher or considerably lower likelihood of long-term survival after cytoreductive surgery and HIPEC (Fig. 36.5) and whether results in any population are better than could be achieved using modern oxaliplatin and/or irinotecan-based systemic chemotherapy with or without biologic agents.
  - In addition, the quality of the cytoreductive surgery is dependent upon the skills and level of experience of the surgeon. The favorable results (particularly with regard to treatment-related toxicity achieved by international experts in the field) may not be replicated in routine clinical practice.
- Because of all of these issues, the National Comprehensive Cancer Network [NCCN] believes this approach should not be considered standard at present and only pursued in centers with demonstrated expertise, preferably in the context of a clinical trial.

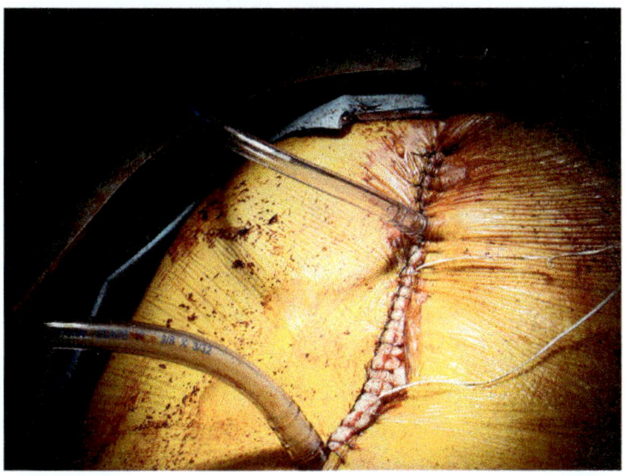

Fig. 36.5 Hyperthermic intraperitoneal chemotherapy (HIPEC). (Courtesy of Eric K. Johnson, MD)

Ovarian Metastases

- Approximately 4–30% of ovarian neoplasms are metastatic cancers with the most common being colorectal and breast cancer.
- A recent autopsy study demonstrated that of all women dying with colorectal cancer, between 6% and 14% were found to have ovarian metastasis at the time of death.
- For those women with stage IV disease, the risk of developing ovarian metastases is substantially higher and approaches 90% for those with established peritoneal metastasis.
- Therefore in a woman with a recent diagnosis of advanced colorectal cancer, any ovarian mass should be considered a metastasis from colorectal cancer until proven otherwise.
- The removal of macroscopically normal ovaries (prophylactic oophorectomy) in women with colorectal cancer is controversial and remains the subject of much debate.
  - Proponents of removal argue that resection improves the cure rate by removing potential microscopic "undetectable" synchronous disease, eliminates the risk of ovarian cancer, and removes the risk of future metachronous ovarian metastatic disease.
  - Others argue that the low incidence of ovarian metastasis, the small amount of supportive data, and few clinical correlations with predictive value make the additional resection of the ovaries unnecessary.
- Clinical studies attempting to document the benefit of ovarian metastasectomy in patients with colorectal cancer are small and retrospective.
  - The majority of studies to date, however, fail to show any survival benefit for prophylactic oophorectomy, and most studies demonstrate that when ovarian metastasis is present, it is a very poor prognostic sign.
- Based on available information, it is reasonable to offer prophylactic oophorectomy to all postmenopausal patients, in particular to those women who have undergone pelvic radiation as part of their treatment for rectal cancer.
- For premenopausal patients, only those with established peritoneal metastases, those that

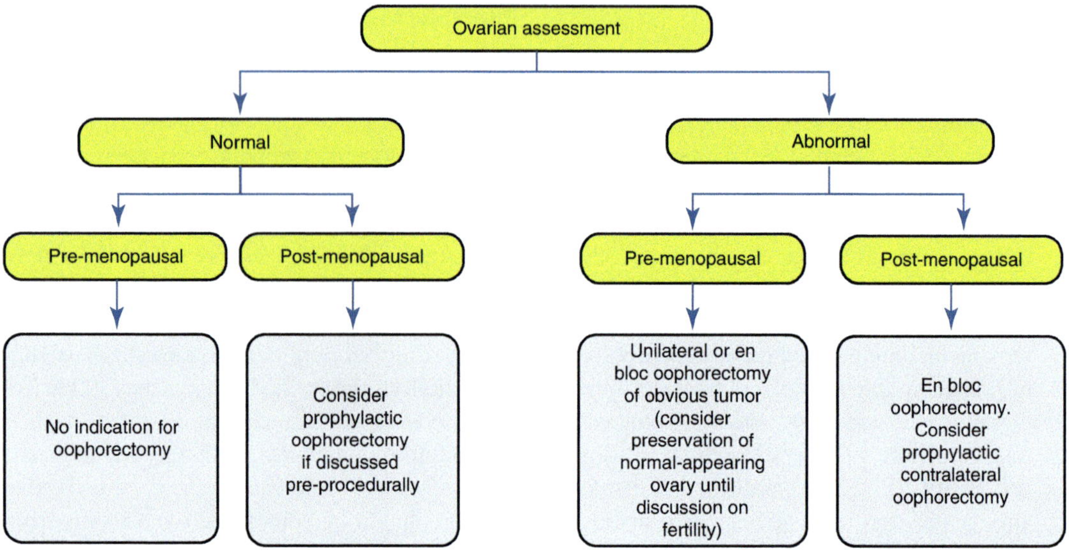

Fig. 36.6 Treatment algorithm for ovarian metastases

are proven to have an increased risk of developing ovarian carcinoma (strong family history, known carriers of breast cancer (BRCA), or those with a HNPCC mutation), or those who have already completed their families should be considered for prophylactic oophorectomy.

- See Fig. 36.6 for an algorithm outlining the treatment of ovarian metastases.

Other Sites of Metastasis

Bone

- Before the introduction of modern chemotherapy and targeted treatment options, bone metastases were reported in as high as 24% of cases. With modern therapies, bone metastases from colorectal cancer reportedly occur now in 7–9% of cases and most often present in the context of widespread metastatic disease.
- Routine diagnostic bone imaging is not indicated in colorectal cancer patients, unless there are specific bone-related symptoms.
- When bone metastasis occurs, it most commonly occurs in the spine (65%), followed by the hip/pelvis (34%) and long bones (17%).
- There are no curative modalities, but palliation of pain, fractures, and spinal cord involvement are important issues for these patients.
  - Symptomatic relief from bony metastases can usually be accomplished with radiation, chemotherapy, as well as bisphosphonate therapy with zoledronic acid.
  - Pathologic fractures are best treated by operative internal fixation.
  - The systemic issues related to bone metastases are serious and include debilitation, immobility, hypercalcemia, and thromboembolic disease.

Brain

- Cerebral metastases from colorectal cancer are uncommon, occurring in 1–4% of colorectal cancer cases.
- Colorectal tumors account for approximately 3% of all metastatic brain tumors.
- These are generally found in the context of widespread metastases to multiple organ sites but on rare occasion can present as an isolated brain metastasis.
- There is no role for routine brain imaging at primary presentation or at presentation with

metastases elsewhere, unless there are specific neurologic symptoms.
- Once brain metastases occur, symptoms are common; palliative therapies include steroids to decrease swelling and anticonvulsants to control seizures.
- Definitive therapy of colorectal brain metastases usually involves surgery, radiation, or a combination of the two.
- For isolated, single brain metastases, resection can result in survival beyond 1–2 years; however because brain metastases are infrequently the sole site of metastatic disease, and because survival is dismal regardless of therapy chosen, craniotomy is rarely indicated.

Pancreas

- The pancreas is an uncommon location for solitary metastases from other primary cancers.
- While the prevalence of pancreatic metastases has been described as high as 6% to 11%, reports of solitary resectable pancreatic metastases from colorectal cancer are extremely rare.
- Although long-term survival is rare, surgical resection can be performed safely in patients with isolated pancreatic metastases from colorectal cancer and in selected patients with extrapancreatic disease.
- As with other sites of multiorgan metastases, a multimodality approach is strongly recommended, and consideration for surgical resection should be taken in context with an overall treatment plan and chances for improving survival while maintaining quality of life.

Adrenal

- Adrenal metastases are uncommon with 14% found in one autopsy series.
- Isolated adrenal metastases are even rarer.
- Aggressive surgical resection for isolated adrenal metastases is described in only a few case reports or small series.
- In contrast to the situation with isolated adrenal metastases, the development of adrenal metastases after liver resection for colorectal cancer is associated with a poor prognosis, and adrenalectomy is not warranted.

Retroperitoneal Lymph Nodes

- Isolated retroperitoneal nodal recurrence occurs in less than 2% of patients following a colorectal cancer resection with curative intent.
- Salvage surgery has been previously avoided due to the poor prognosis; however this concept is being challenged, and surgical resection can be entertained in select cases.

Metastatic Disease in the Elderly

- Colorectal cancer remains one of the most commonly diagnosed cancers in the world with 60% of patients being over 70 years old and 43% over 75.
- Therefore multidisciplinary teams will increasingly see older patients with colorectal cancer, and management of this distinct group deserves special mention.
- When considering surgery – comorbidity, functional dependency, and older age are associated with early postoperative mortality in patients with gastrointestinal malignancies, with 30-day postoperative mortality rates underestimating postoperative mortality in older patients.
- In regard to chemotherapy, the data available indicates that older patients derive the same benefit and have the same degree of toxicity as younger patients. The clinical trial data however may not be reflective of the average elderly patient seen in practice that is often suffering from more comorbidities and has greater functional impairment.
  - For these reasons, the International Society of Geriatric Oncology (SIOG) previously recommended that colorectal cancer patients >65 years of age requiring surgery

should undergo a preoperative whole patient evaluation of the most common physiological side effects of aging, physical and mental ability, and social support.
  - Further for those patients assessed as having physical or psychological comorbidities, it was recommended that a geriatrician was involved in the patient management.
- Since those original recommendations, there have been multiple frailty indices proposed to detect vulnerability in elderly patients with cancer so that treatment can be adjusted accordingly.
  - The process of these assessments, however, can be time-consuming, and prescreening is often used to identify fit patients who are able to receive standard treatment versus those in whom a full comprehensive geriatric assessment should be done.
  - The four most common indices utilized appear to be the abbreviated *Comprehensive Geriatric Assessment* (aCGA), the Vulnerable Elders Survey-13 (VES-13), the Groningen Frailty Indicator (GFI), and the Geriatric 8 (G8).
  - Unfortunately at present, there is no universal screening tool that adequately identifies frailty in at-risk older patients, and sensitivity and specificity for these indices ranged from 67% to 87% and 59% to 73%, respectively, which questions the value they may offer to the clinician.
  - The American College of Surgeons NSQIP Risk Calculator (http://riskcalculator.facs.org) also uses degree of independence and other comorbidity variables that can be used to assess surgical risk in the elderly. In particular, it also gives an assessment of the risk of discharge to a long-term care facility in addition to the risk of common complications.

Appendiceal Neoplasms

37

Constantine P. Spanos and Andreas M. Kaiser

Abbreviations

AJCC	American Joint Committee on Cancer
DPAM	Disseminated peritoneal adenomucinosis
ENETS	European Neuroendocrine Tumor Society
HIPEC	Hyperthermic (or heated) intraperitoneal chemotherapy
LAMNs	Low-grade appendiceal mucinous neoplasms
PCI	Peritoneal carcinomatosis index
PMAC	Peritoneal mucinous adenocarcinomatosis
PMCA	Peritoneal mucinous carcinomatosis
PMP	Pseudomyxoma peritonei

C. P. Spanos
Department of Colorectal Surgery, Keck School of Medicine, University of Southern California, Los Angeles, CA, USA

Department of Surgery, Aristotelian University of Thessaloniki, Panorama-Thessaloniki, Greece

A. M. Kaiser (✉)
Keck Medical Center of the University of Southern California, Los Angeles, CA, USA
e-mail: akaiser@usc.edu

Key Concepts

- Although appendectomy for appendicitis is the most commonly performed emergency operation performed by general surgeons, primary neoplasms of the vermiform appendix are rare, and each individual general surgeon will have limited experience in the management of such lesions.
- Most primary neoplasms of the appendix are not associated with specific signs or symptoms and are incidentally diagnosed after pathological analysis of the appendectomy specimen or detected incidentally on computed tomography (CT) for other indications.
- Primary neoplasms of the appendix can generally be divided into epithelial, non-epithelial, and mixed lesions. Epithelial lesions include adenoma and adenocarcinoma. Non-epithelial tumors include neuroendocrine tumors (carcinoids), lymphoma, leiomyoma, leiomyosarcoma, and other even rarer rarities. Goblet cell carcinoids are mixed lesions with features of carcinoid as well as mucinous adenocarcinoma.
- Epithelial tumors, and specifically mucinous adenocarcinomas, are the most common primary appendiceal neoplasms.
- Pseudomyxoma peritonei is the result of a perforation and peritoneal dissemination of a mucin-producing epithelial neoplasm, most commonly originating from the appendix or the ovaries. In select patients, cytoreductive surgery with HIPEC should be considered.

S. R. Steele et al. (eds.), *The ASCRS Manual of Colon and Rectal Surgery*,
https://doi.org/10.1007/978-3-030-01165-9_37

- A mucocele is a morphologic cystic manifestation of an epithelial appendiceal neoplasm. Perforation leads to pseudomyxoma peritonei. Therefore, intact removal en bloc is of utmost importance.
- Appendiceal carcinoids are rarely associated with carcinoid syndrome or multicentricity.
- The newest tumor staging guidelines distinguish appendiceal tumors from colon cancer and separate between epithelial and non-epithelial lesions.
- The extent of surgical resection depends on the cell type, the preoperative staging, the ability to achieve negative resection margins, and the probability of nodal disease.
- Surgery is the primary treatment for localized disease, whereas its role in metastatic disease needs to be individually analyzed and weighed against systemic chemotherapy.

Introduction

- Appendectomy is the most frequent emergency operation performed by general surgeons with close to 300,000 performed in the United States annually.
- On comparably rare occasion, the pathology of the appendectomy specimen incidentally reveals an appendiceal neoplasm ("incidentaloma"), which sometimes is recognized even before or at least during surgery, but more often only after the patient has already been discharged from the hospital.
- Paradoxically and despite the fact that abdominal surgeons at all levels are very frequently involved in treating appendiceal pathology, appendiceal neoplasms are quite infrequent but may cause rather complex intellectual, management, and technical challenges in subsequent surgical interventions (Table 37.1).

Epidemiology

- Primary neoplasms of the appendix have an incidence of 0.12 cases per 1,000,000 person-years and are found in 0.9–1.4% of appendectomy specimens.
- They can be asymptomatic, be associated with appendicitis, or cause noninflammatory symptoms.
- Preoperative diagnosis based on symptoms, imaging, and laboratory results is extremely rare.
- Even intraoperatively, less than 50% appendiceal neoplasms are recognized as such.
- A retrospective cohort analysis of the Surveillance, Epidemiology, and End Results database suggested that the incidence of appendiceal neoplasms has increased significantly in the past few decades from 0.63 to 0.97 per 100,000 population.
  - It is unclear though whether this is a true increase or a simple reflection of higher awareness and reclassification as a separate entity. The increase appears to have affected all histological subtypes in an equal fashion (Table 37.2).
- Historically, carcinoid tumors were considered the most frequent neoplasms originating within the appendix, although more recent publications demonstrate that epithelial neoplasms are more frequent and represent 58% of malignant appendiceal tumors.
- At the time of diagnosis, a total of 74% of appendiceal cancer cases have already spread and developed regional or distant metastases in 39% and 35%, respectively.

Anatomical Pathology and Staging

- The literature unfortunately has for a long time shown little consistency and used a variety of nomenclatures, classification systems, and descriptive terms when referring to appendiceal neoplasms. Many synonyms for lesions of such rarity undoubtedly have led to confounding terminology.
- From an anatomical point of view, the appendix in essence has a smaller diameter but otherwise a similar layered wall structure as the rest of the large intestine; however there is a higher representation of immunological tissue components (GALT, gut-associated lymphoid tissue).

Table 37.1 Clinical scenarios depending on the type and timing of diagnosis of appendiceal neoplasms

Scenario	Acute symptoms	Presumptive preoperative diagnosis	Surgery	Pre-/intraop evidence of perforation (P) or dissemination (D)	Timing of tumor recognition	Impact/action in decision-making
1. Acute	Y	Appendicitis	N	–	N	Rely on indirect signs/risk factors for identification of affected individuals Re-imaging?
2. Acute	Y	Appendicitis	Y	P– D–	(a) Intraoperative (b) Only on final pathology (c) Not recognized at all (missed opportunity)	Primary or secondary evaluation for more extensive/oncological surgery/treatment
3. Acute	Y	Appendicitis	Y	P+ D–	(a) Intraoperative (b) Only on final pathology (c) Not recognized at all (missed opportunity)	Appropriate treatment for perforation with primary or secondary evaluation for more extensive/oncological surgery/treatment
4. Acute	Y	Appendicitis	Y	P+ D+	Intraoperative	Primary appropriate treatment for perforation Secondary assessment for more extensive surgery/treatment
5. Acute	Y	Appendicitis	Y	P– D–	Intraoperative: evidence of localized mucocele or tumor involving the appendix/cecum	Intraoperative determination of appropriate extent of resection Possible frozen section
6. Elective	Y/N	Localized mucocele/tumor involving appendix/cecum – no signs of PMP	Y	P– D+	Preoperative	Oncological resection Preparedness for HIPEC
7. Elective	Y/N	Localized mucocele/tumor of appendix/cecum and signs of PMP	TBD	P– D+	Preoperative	PCI Systemic treatment and evaluation for CRS/HIPEC
8. Elective	Y/N	PMP, but no obvious cecal pathology	TBD	P– D+	Preoperative	Evaluation for other potential primary tumor locations PCI Systemic treatment and evaluation for CRS/HIPEC
9. Elective	Y/N	PMP + distant metastases	N	P– D+	Pre-treatment	Systemic treatment

Table 37.2 Reported incidence over time of appendiceal neoplasms in SEER database

Subtype	1973–2001 (N = 2514)	2000–2009 (N = 4765)
Mucinous adenocarcinoma	38%	38%
Non-mucinous adenocarcinoma	26%	27%
Carcinoid tumors Goblet cell carcinoids	17% 15%	28%
Signet ring cell tumors	4%	7%

- The appendix does not participate in processing of intestinal contents but produces 2–3 mL of mucin per day and may participate in immunological functions.
- The arterial blood supply originates from the appendicular artery which branches off the ileocolic artery; the venous drainage is via the superior mesenteric vein to the portal vein system; the lymphatic drainage follows the vascular structures and due to variability may parallel the ileocolic, right colic, and right branch of the middle colic artery.
- Appendiceal neoplasms should be categorized according to the tissue of origin as well as the pattern of growth, expansion, and spreading (Table 37.3).

Epithelial Neoplasms

- Epithelial neoplasms are divided into mucinous and non-mucinous neoplasms.
- Mucinous neoplasms of the appendix are classified according to the grade and aggressiveness of the tumor.
  - Descriptively, these lesions characteristically can form mucoceles of the appendix, a morphologic term describing the dilation of the appendix with intraluminal accumulation of mucoid material (Fig. 37.1).
  - The obstruction can either be caused by the epithelial neoplasm itself, an independent tumor, or a benign process (retention cysts, mucosal hyperplasia).
  - Rupture of a mucocele results in peritoneal spillage and spread of mucin and – depending on the malignant potential of the lesion – of cellular elements, which are the basis for mucinosis, pseudomyxoma peritonei, and carcinomatosis.
- Low-grade appendiceal mucinous neoplasms (LAMNs) are well-differentiated neoplasms that morphologically resemble adenomas.
- LAMN has become the neutral term for a number of entities such as appendiceal villous or serrated adenoma, cystadenoma, borderline tumor of the appendix, and mucinous tumors of uncertain malignant potential.
- These lesions which tend to grow slowly and grossly are characterized by a well-defined structure, cystic dilation, and mucinous content.
- The appendiceal wall is fibrotic and – as a sign of chronicity – may sometimes contain calcifications.
- Gross rupture (spontaneously or as a result of surgical manipulation) may be evident as mucin extruding onto the serosal surface or seeding of more distant peritoneal surfaces as evidenced by the presence of mucin lakes.
- Prognosis of LAMN depends on the presence or absence of epithelial cells outside the appendix.
  - Tumors confined to the appendix generally have an excellent prognosis.
  - However, LAMN may proliferate outside the appendix in a malignant fashion, producing pseudomyxoma peritonei and/or distant metastases.
- Pseudomyxoma peritonei (PMP) derived from perforation of a LAMN is characterized by abundant extracellular mucin, hyalinized fibrotic stroma, and harboring scant strips of low-grade mucinous epithelium.
  - The term is not strictly limited to appendiceal neoplasms, but the condition can result from other tumor origins such as ovaries, gallbladder, and others.
- The prognosis of a ruptured LAMN is dependent on the amount and cellularity of mucin deposits, and recurrence rates increase when epithelial cells are present in the mucin.

Table 37.3 Tumor classifications and manifestations

	Localized[a]	Disseminated	Pattern of dissemination[b]
Epithelial	Adenoma (B)		L, H, P
	Adenocarcinoma (M)	Adenocarcinoma	L, H, P
	Mucocele (B)	PMP: mucinosis peritonei	P
	Mucinous cystadenoma (IM, LAMN)	PMP: disseminated peritoneal adenomucinosis (DPAM)	P
	Mucinous (cyst) adenocarcinoma (M)	PMP: peritoneal mucinous adenocarcinomatosis (PMAC)	P, L, H
		PMP: peritoneal mucinous carcinomatosis (PMCA)	P, L, H
	Signet ring cell carcinoma (M)	Advanced/metastatic signet ring cell carcinoma	DI, P, L, H
Mixed	Goblet cell carcinoid (adenocarcinoid)	Metastatic goblet cell adenocarcinoid	P, L, H
Non-epithelial	Carcinoid <1 cm (B) 1–2 cm (IM) >2 cm (M)	Metastatic carcinoid	L, H
	Lymphoma (M)	Lymphoma	Systemic
	Leiomyoma (B)		
	Leiomyosarcoma (M)	Metastatic leiomyosarcoma	H, L
	Kaposi sarcoma (M)	Disseminated Kaposi sarcoma	Systemic

LAMN low-grade mucinous neoplasia, *PMP* pseudomyxoma peritonei
[a]*B* benign, *IM* intermediate malignant potential, *M* malignant
[b]*P* peritoneal, *L* lymphatic, *H* hematogenous, *DI* diffuse infiltrative

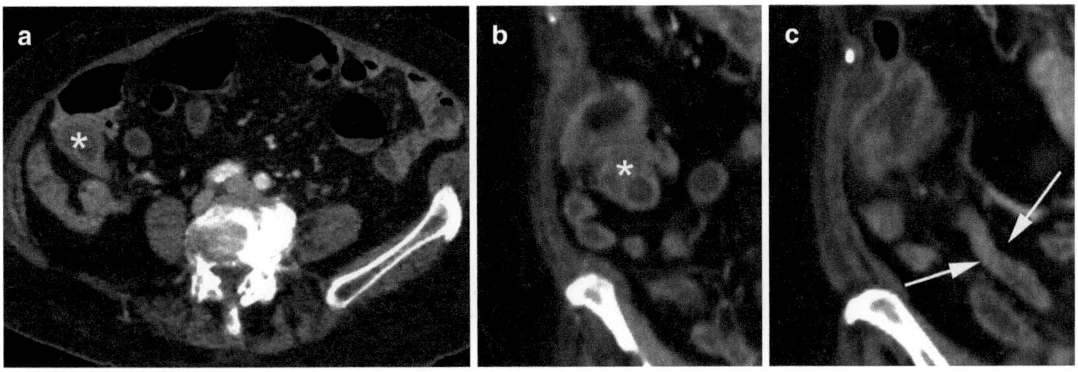

Fig. 37.1 Appendiceal mucocele: the computed tomography shows the cystic enlargement at the base of the appendix (asterisk, panels **A** and **B**), as well as the moderately enlarged appendix (in-between arrows, panel **C**)

- Most instances of PMP resulting from LAMN remain confined to the right lower quadrant. Even if the spread of PMP goes beyond the immediate vicinity, the lesion may pursue an indolent but progressive course.
- The superordinate term "PMP" has been categorized into disseminated peritoneal adenomucinosis (DPAM) and peritoneal mucinous (adeno)carcinomatosis (PMAC or PMCA).
  - The former reflects a low-grade pseudomyxoma arising from LAMNs, whereas the latter indicates peritoneal carcinomatosis.
  - DPAM lesions contain scarce strips of low-grade mucinous epithelium with mild

atypia and no significant mitotic activity; these low-grade lesions usually cover but do not infiltrate the surface of the organs to which they adhere.

- Appendiceal adenocarcinoma is also divided into mucinous and non-mucinous types.
- Mucinous adenocarcinoma of the appendix is characterized by a destructive growth pattern with tumor invasion of the appendiceal wall beyond the muscularis mucosae; infiltrating pools of mucin harbor cytologically malignant glandular epithelium arranged in strips, clusters, and complex proliferations.
- Mucinous adenocarcinoma due to the increasing pressure of accumulating mucin is prone to rupture, spreading and seeding into the peritoneal cavity, leading to formation of pseudomyxoma peritonei.
- Mucinous tumors spread along peritoneal surfaces, even in the absence of lymph node metastases. Peritoneal mucinous (adeno)carcinomatosis (PMAC/PMCA) results from secondary peritoneal proliferation of appendiceal or intestinal mucinous adenocarcinoma nests that lead to invasion of parenchymal and visceral organs and the omentum and potentially trigger secondary lymph node metastases at those sites.
- Non-mucinous adenocarcinomas behave similarly to colonic adenocarcinomas, infiltrating the appendiceal wall and metastasizing to regional lymph nodes and the liver.
- Non-mucinous adenocarcinomas show a spectrum of morphological features of the invasive component.
  - In some cases the tumor is identical to colonic adenocarcinoma with malignant (pseudo-)glandular formations, increased stratification, and disorganization (compared to the regular columnar epithelium).
  - In other cases, the malignant glands are tubular in shape, lined by cuboidal epithelium, associated with modest amount of extracellular mucin.
- Signet ring cell carcinoma is a rare but aggressive subentity of mucinous adenocarcinoma, characterized by dissolute growth and infiltration of mucin-containing cancer cells (signet rings); it almost never remains confined and may display an infiltrative growth below intact appearing mucosal surfaces as well as a rapid dissemination within the peritoneal cavity.
- Signet ring cell carcinoma is typically associated with a poor prognosis.
- Prognosis of appendiceal adenocarcinomas – similar to colon cancer – is primarily determined by the stage, but within stage IV also depends on the histological subtype and grading as well as the route of dissemination.
- Within each stage and histological subtype, poor differentiation is associated with unfavorable outcomes.
- Mucinous adenocarcinomas have a markedly worse outcome (reduced cancer-specific survival) than non-mucinous adenocarcinomas of the appendix (Table 37.4).
- This observation, which was based on published data analysis of the National Cancer Database (NCDB), was recently implemented into the current staging guidelines by the American Joint Committee on Cancer (AJCC).
  - Appendiceal carcinomas for the first time are classified separately from colonic adenocarcinoma, and distinction is made between mucinous and non-mucinous types; histologic grading for mucinous tumors is considered of particular importance for metastatic tumors (Table 37.5).

Table 37.4 Cancer-specific survival for appendiceal adenocarcinoma stratified by stage and grade

Subtype	Stages I–III (%)	Stage IV (%)
Mucinous adenocarcinoma (N = 1375)		
Well differentiated	82	71
Moderately differentiated	64	51
Poorly differentiated	50	0
Non-mucinous adenocarcinoma (N = 860)		
Well differentiated	69	48
Moderately differentiated	73	9
Poorly differentiated	55	5

Table 37.5 TNM staging by AJCC for appendiceal adenocarcinoma

Stage	T	N	M
X	Primary tumor not determined or any T	Regional lymph nodes not determined or any N	Metastatic disease not determined or any M
0	No evidence of primary tumor	No regional lymph node metastasis	No distant metastasis
Is	Carcinoma in situ: intraepithelial or invasion of lamina propria	–	–
1	Tumor invades submucosa	Metastasis in 1 to 3 regional lymph nodes	1a: intraperitoneal metastasis beyond the right lower quadrant, including pseudomyxoma peritonei 1b: non-peritoneal metastases
2	Tumor invades muscularis propria	Metastasis in 4 or more regional lymph nodes	
3	Tumor invades through muscularis propria into subserosa or into mesoappendix		
4	4a: tumor penetrates visceral peritoneum, including mucinous peritoneal tumor within the right lower quadrant 4b: tumor directly invades other organs or structures		

Stage I, T1–T2 N0 M0; stage II, T3–T4 N0 M0; stage III, Tx N1–N2 M0; stage IV, Tx Nx M1

Neuroendocrine Appendiceal Lesions/Carcinoid Tumors

- The WHO classification utilizes the terms "neuroendocrine tumor" (NET), "neuroendocrine carcinoma" (NEC), and "mixed adeno-neuroendocrine carcinomas" (MANEC).
  - Synonyms for NET include carcinoid tumors and well-differentiated endocrine tumors/carcinoma.
  - Synonyms for NEC are poorly differentiated endocrine carcinoma and small cell/large cell endocrine carcinoma.
  - Goblet cell carcinoids (now called carcinomas) are MANEC.
- Carcinoids or carcinoid tumors represent neuroendocrine tumors grade 1 and are derived from a variety of dispersed neuroendocrine cells (formerly labeled as amine precursor uptake and decarboxylation cells, APUD cells). These cells and the resulting tumors are not only found in the appendix but in the entire gastrointestinal tract and other organs and are therefore addressed more comprehensively in the next chapter.
- Nonetheless, appendiceal carcinoids are only extremely rarely associated with multicentricity, and there is no known association with multiple endocrine neoplasia (MEN syndrome).
- On gross examination, carcinoid tumors of the appendix are yellow-tan firm nodules. 75% are located at the tip, 15% in the mid-appendix, and 10% at the base of the organ.
- At the time of diagnosis, the majority (80%) are less than 1 cm, 14% measure between 1 and 2 cm, and 6% are greater than 2 cm in size.
- Histologically, carcinoids are characterized by submucosal uniform cell conglomerates with a nested or insular pattern. The cytoplasm has a modestly eosinophilic, fine granularity, and the nuclei show the classic endocrine "salt-and-pepper" chromatin pattern.
- Ki67 is used to determine the proliferative capacity of the tumor for grading according to the current WHO classification.
- AJCC staging for carcinoids is based on tumor size as it correlates with the incidence of metastases and represents the most important prognostic parameter, whereas the depth of

invasion, lymphatic, perineural, or serosal invasion, lacks prognostic power (Table 37.6).
  - Lymph node metastases are rare for lesions of less than 10 mm diameter but occur in 20–30% of patients with carcinoids greater than 2 cm in size (Table 37.7); distant metastases are comparably rare in appendiceal carcinoids.
- Five-year survival rates for patients with local, regional, and distant metastatic disease are 95%, 81%, and 31%, respectively.

Goblet Cell Carcinoids

- This term may add confusion to the classification of appendiceal lesions. It is considered a hybrid between epithelial and neuroendocrine tumors and is also referred to as mucinous adeno-neuroendocrine carcinoma.
- These tumors have a mean age of presentation in the fifth decade and behave more like adenocarcinoma than carcinoid.
- Clinically, goblet cell carcinoids in the middle third of the appendix may in fact cause appendicitis.
- At surgical exploration, 10% or more of the tumors are found to have already widespread metastatic disease; two-thirds of goblet cell carcinoids are incidental findings on appendectomy and ileocecectomy specimens.
- Five-year survival rates are worse than for regular carcinoids and for stages I, II, III, and IV were 100%, 76%, 22%, and 14%, respectively, i.e., range from 50% to 80% for locoregional disease to less than 20% for patients with distant metastases.

Clinical Features

- Appendiceal epithelial neoplasms are notorious for the absence of any specific signs or symptoms, especially at early stages.
- The complicating factor is that they escape detection by routine screening efforts such as colonoscopy.

Table 37.6 TNM staging (by AJCC and ENETS) for neuroendocrine appendiceal tumors

Stage	T (AJCC)	T (ENETS)	N (AJCC/ ENETS)	M (AJCC/ ENETS)
X	Primary tumor not determined or any T	Primary tumor not determined or any T	Lymph nodes not determined or any N	Metastatic disease not determined or any M
0	No evidence of primary tumor	No evidence of primary tumor	No lymph node metastasis	No distant metastasis
1	1a: tumor ≤1 cm 1b: tumor 1–2 cm	T1 tumor ≤1 cm invading submucosa and muscularis propria	Lymph node metastasis	Distant metastasis
2	Tumor 2–4 cm or with extension to the cecum	Tumor ≤2 cm with invasion of submucosa or muscularis propria and/ or minimal invasion (up to 3 mm) of subserosa/mesoappendix		
3	Tumor >4 cm or with extension to the ileum	Tumor >2 cm and/or extensive invasion (>3 mm) of subserosa/ mesoappendix		
4	Tumor directly invades other adjacent organs or structures, e.g., abdominal wall and skeletal muscle[a]	Tumor invades peritoneum/other organs		

Stage I, T1 N0 M0; stage II, T2–T3 N0 M0; stage III, T4 N0 M0 or Tx N1 M0; stage IV, Tx Nx M1
[a]Tumor adherent to other organs or structures grossly classified as cT4 but if microscopically negative adhesion as pT1-3 depending on depth of wall invasion

Table 37.7 Impact of appendiceal carcinoid size on lymph node metastasis and survival

Carcinoid size	LN metastases (%)	5-/10-year survival rates (%)
< 1 cm	<1.0–15.0	92–100
1–2 cm	3.0–47.0	81
> 2 cm	20–86	31

- If a tumor is concentric and causes obstruction of the lumen, clinical symptomatology of appendicitis may ensue.
  - Red flags in patients with signs of "appendicitis" should include any age above 50, family history of colorectal cancer or inflammatory bowel disease, prolonged history, or anemia.
- At later stages, epithelial appendiceal neoplasms may present as a localized abdominal or pelvic mass, bowel obstruction, or progressive, painless, abdominal distention when large volumes of mucin accumulate in the peritoneal cavity (pseudomyxoma peritonei).
- Even hormone-active tumors such as carcinoids remain silent and are only incidentally detected.
  - Since they are frequently located at the tip of the appendix, they may not even trigger appendicitis.
  - Carcinoid syndrome is extremely rare (less than 5%) and requires the presence of significant metastatic disease to allow these substances to escape the hepatic first-pass effect and be released into the systemic circulation.
- Given the incredible variability of clinical circumstances under which an appendiceal neoplasm may be diagnosed, clinicians will have to develop concepts and algorithms to optimize and standardize their management (Table 37.1).

Diagnostic Procedures

- Clinical examination is expectedly unreliable in detecting, confirming, or ruling out an appendiceal neoplasm.
- Tumor markers are limited and include nonspecific carcinoembryonic antigen (CEA) for epithelial lesions or 5-HIAA metabolites in the urine for carcinoids. Neither marker is suited for screening or as a negative predictive test.
- Cross-sectional imaging (CT, MRI) is of greatest value in evaluating a suspected appendiceal neoplasm.
- Tumors of sufficient size can be demonstrated as a moderately enhancing soft tissue mass or a cystic dilatation of the appendix beyond 15 mm, which should raise suspicion if noted as an incidental finding.
- Bowel displacement is an indirect sign of a pathological extraluminal process and is best visualized by adequate opacification of the terminal ileum and cecum by means of intraluminal contrast and differs from an abscess by the lack of inflammatory signs.
- Features of a mucocele include well-encapsulated and smooth lesions in the right lower quadrant with regular wall and low attenuation that depends on the amount of mucin in the tissue and the center of the lesion.
- The presence of punctate, curvilinear calcifications in a right lower quadrant cystic lesion is highly suggestive of a mucocele: they develop as a dystrophic response to a chronic inflammatory process.
- Pseudomyxoma peritonei is characterized by low-attenuation ascites and serosal implants which when not obvious are best seen as scalloping of the liver contour, at peritoneal reflections, or the pouch of Douglas (Fig. 37.2).
- For treatment strategy and prognosis, it is important to quantify areas affected by PMP. The peritoneal carcinomatosis index (PCI) is a summary score with a maximum of 39 points from nine abdominal squares and four small bowel segments, whereby each area is scored between 0 and 3 when deposits are >5 cm.
- Positron emission tomography (PET) scan may have a role for detection or monitoring of systemic metastatic disease but is notoriously ineffective in assessing pseudomyxoma peritonei.

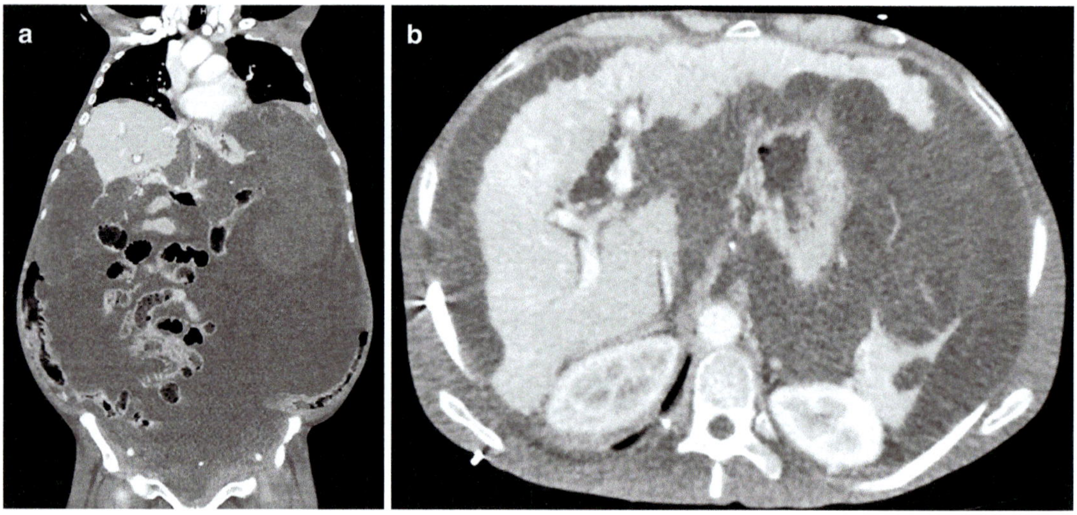

Fig. 37.2 Pseudomyxoma peritonei: the computed tomography in a coronal view (panel **A**) and axial view (panel **B**) of a patient with massive deposits of low-attenuation mucin throughout the entire abdomen with scalloping of the liver contour and widening of the spaces between the compressed bowel loops

- Since most carcinoids are surgical/pathological incidentalomas, most diagnostic investigations are performed after the initial operation.
- For the majority of incidentally diagnosed, well-differentiated appendiceal neuroendocrine tumors of <10 mm, no postoperative diagnostic procedure is necessary.
- After complete resection of 10–20 mm lesions, a single CT or MRI to rule out lymph node and distant metastases is recommended, but without level I evidence.
- For lesions >20 mm, CT and/or MRI of the abdomen is recommended; in addition a PET scan or a somatostatin receptor scan in combination with SPECT/CT (or somatostatin receptor PET with three-phase CT scan) may be considered to detect or rule out distant tumor spread.
- Appendiceal neoplasms typically evade detection by colonoscopy. Occasionally, a protrusion of the appendiceal orifice or release of mucoid material may be recognized (Fig. 37.3).
  - However, colonic evaluation (colonoscopy, CT colonography) is recommended prior to any elective intervention for a suspected or proven appendiceal neoplasm, because both epithelial and neuroendocrine tumors may be multicentric and/or be associated with synchronous lesions in up to 10–20%.

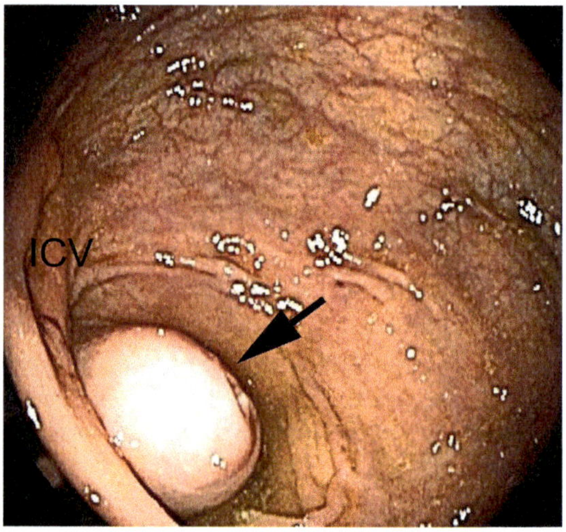

Fig. 37.3 Colonoscopic appearance: even though appendiceal neoplasms frequently escape endoscopic detection, they occasionally lead to an extramucosal protrusion (asterisk) of the appendiceal orifice into the cecal lumen. ICV ileocecal valve

Medical Management

- Management of localized appendiceal neoplasms is primarily surgical.
- Nonsurgical modalities come into play for locally advanced or metastatic lesions as well as for primarily systemic neoplasms such as leukemia or lymphoma.
- Adjuvant and palliative systemic chemotherapy are still largely based on 5-fluorouracil and typically combined with other conventional agents (oxaliplatin and others) or biological drugs such as bevacizumab.
- Somatostatin is being used for metastatic and particularly symptomatic carcinoid tumors.
- Radiation treatment is not part of routine management of any appendiceal tumor and is reserved for special circumstances on an individualized basis.

Surgical Treatment of Appendiceal Lesions

- Surgery is the primary treatment for localized disease with the goal to achieve a curative R0 resection; in metastatic disease, the role of surgery needs to be individually analyzed and weighed against systemic chemotherapy or best palliative care.
- Surgical decision-making should therefore take five questions into consideration as also alluded to in the previously listed clinical scenarios:
  1. Has the primary tumor already been removed?
  2. Was the clinical situation associated with possible tumor spillage?
  3. For a given tumor, what entails an adequate margin?
  4. What is the probability of nodal involvement?
  5. In case of locally advanced or metastatic disease, is aggressive surgical intervention superior to conservative management?
- Depending on the answers, there are four possible surgical responses (Table 37.8): (a) appendectomy only, (b) hemicolectomy or completion hemicolectomy, (c) cytoreductive surgery and peritonectomy with or without HIPEC, or (d) conservative management.

Table 37.8 Operations performed for appendiceal neoplasms

Appendectomy	Right hemicolectomy	Cytoreduction+HIPEC	Nonsurgical
Intact mucocele Adenocarcinoma Tis	Invasive adenocarcinoma	PMP with PCI ≤ 16 (−20):[a] Diffuse mucinous adenomucinosis peritonei Peritoneal mucinous (adeno)carcinomatosis Perforated appendiceal neoplasm without visible PMP?	PMP with PCI > (16-)20?[a] Adenocarcinoma with diffuse systemic metastases Adenocarcinoma with peritoneal disease and systemic metastases
Appendiceal carcinoid <1 cm, R0	Appendiceal carcinoid 1–2 cm, R0? Appendiceal carcinoid >2 cm Any carcinoid with insufficient margin (R1, questionable R), multifocality, invasion of mesoappendix >3 mm Any carcinoid with nodal involvement Any carcinoid with systemic metastases to the liver only		Carcinoid with diffuse systemic metastases beyond 1 organ
	Goblet cell carcinoid	PMP from goblet cell carcinoid	

[a]*PMP* pseudomyxoma peritonei, *PCI* peritoneal carcinomatosis index

Appendectomy

- Appendectomy alone should be reserved for premalignant lesions, carcinoma in situ (Tis), or carcinoids of less than 1 cm diameter provided that a sufficient margin can be obtained.
- Carcinoids of 1–2 cm represent a gray zone but may be associated with a higher than previously reported incidence of nodal disease, suggesting that appendectomy may not suffice.
- An appendiceal mucocele requires careful dissection to avoid perforation of the lesion.
  - If the case is approached laparoscopically, placement of the whole appendix/cecum into a specimen bag prior to starting the dissection may be a strategy to avoid rupture and spillage or conversion to a laparotomy.

Right Hemicolectomy

- For non-perforated appendiceal adenocarcinoma, carcinoids larger than 2 cm, and any of the previously mentioned lesions with unfavorable features or whose margins are insufficient with an appendectomy alone, an oncological right hemicolectomy with a mesocolic lymph node dissection is indicated.
  - Oncological resection for adenocarcinoma achieves better 5-year survival rates than appendectomy alone.
- The incidence of lymph node metastases in appendiceal carcinoid tumors increases with size of the tumor (Table 37.7).
- There is a controversy regarding the surgical management of patients in which perforation of a mucinous appendiceal neoplasm has occurred resulting in pseudomyxoma peritonei.
- Some argue that a right hemicolectomy is not necessary in this situation as the outcome is determined by the peritoneal disease rather than the lymph nodes.

Cytoreductive Surgery and HIPEC

- In cases of advanced peritoneal dissemination, cytoreductive surgery with HIPEC is performed in selected cases.
- If pseudomyxoma peritonei is unexpectedly encountered during an operative exploration, the patient would be best served by careful retrieval and cytological analysis of any mucinous fluid present and referral to a specialized center with expertise in cytoreductive surgery and HIPEC. Minimization of surgical manipulation and mobilization of intra-abdominal viscera will facilitate the subsequent cytoreductive surgery performed later.
- The mainstay of surgical treatment for disseminated peritoneal disease is the arduous operative task of cytoreductive surgery and heated intraperitoneal chemotherapy (HIPEC) (Fig. 37.4).
- In retrospective series, this surgical modality has demonstrated favorable results in carefully selected patients but at the same time was associated with a substantial morbidity and mortality; in addition, most series note that incomplete cytoreduction was unable to achieve a relevant benefit as the recurrence rates were very high.
- It seems rather obvious that the outcomes depend on the extent of the initial disease whereby a number of authors recommended

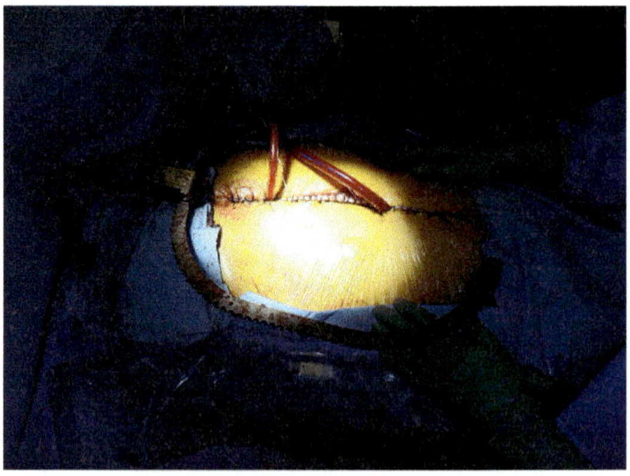

Fig. 37.4 Hyperthermic intraperitoneal chemotherapy (HIPEC). (Courtesy of Eric K. Johnson, MD)

to limit cytoreductive surgery and HIPEC to patients with a PCI of less than (16-)20.

- In reviewing the evidence supporting the use of cytoreduction and HIPEC, it should be noted that the literature on the technique and outcomes continues to have significant limitations.
  - Most series are retrospective and inconsistent in regard to inclusion criteria, extent of disease, concomitant treatment, protocols, and follow-up. Selection bias is inherent to their study designs.
  - Favorable results of prior trials have been challenged by availability of more aggressive systemic chemotherapy regimens, the latter of which parenthetically has been found to increase the risk of complications after HIPEC.
  - Most importantly, however, there is a lack of prospective randomized data on direct comparison of HIPEC and cytoreductive surgery with modern systemic chemotherapy alone.
  - A heated debate continues as to whether HIPEC should be considered the standard of care or still an experimental approach.
- In preparation for cytoreductive surgery and HIPEC, adequate staging and quantitative assessment using the PCI, colonic clearance, aggressive hydration, and bowel cleansing are essential.
  - Considerations include provisions for stomas, timely prophylactic vaccination for splenectomy (against pneumococcus, meningococcus, and *H. influenzae*), and placement of a gastrostomy tube and feeding jejunostomy tube.
- Cytoreductive surgery aims at removing or reducing all visible tumor implants to less than 2 mm in size as only complete cytoreduction allows for adequate drug penetration into residual tumor deposits.
  - It typically includes omentectomy and stripping of all parietal peritoneal surfaces, including the subdiaphragmatic spaces and the paracolic recesses (peritonectomy).
  - However, it may also involve aggressive multi-organ resection including tumor-involved bowel (colon, small bowel) or other organs (gallbladder, spleen, uterus/ovaries, and others), or the posterior rectus sheath may be removed.
  - For the HIPEC phase of the procedure, a number of open or closed techniques have been reported.
    - We have typically used the closed technique to minimize heat dissipation, spillage of perfusate, and safety hazard to health personnel.
    - The incision is temporarily closed to the size of a gel port through which large-bore afferent and efferent cannulas are placed to the peritoneal cavity.
    - The heated chemotherapeutic drugs are circulated throughout the abdominal cavity via pumps and heat exchangers (heart-lung machine).
    - The most frequently used drug is mitomycin-c, which is administered for a duration of 60–120 min at a temperature of 41–43° C.
    - Reconstructions and anastomoses are to be performed after the hyperthermic perfusion phase.
- Cytoreductive surgery and HIPEC are associated with formidable morbidity that may exceed 50% (Table 37.9).
  - Apart from myelosuppression and nephrotoxicity with intensified diuresis, complications include sepsis, respiratory failure, ileus, anastomotic leak, abscess, enterocutaneous fistula, acute renal failure, thromboembolic events, and in the long run formation of hostile adhesions.
  - The mortality rates in initial reports were approximately 10% but could be reduced significantly in more recent series (Table 37.9).
- In the majority of reports, PCI score, PMCA tumor type, and completeness of cytoreduction were significant prognostic factors. Perioperative or neoadjuvant chemotherapy is currently a matter of debate and is not routinely used.

Table 37.9 Selected series on cytoreductive surgery and HIPEC for appendiceal neoplasms

Institution	Year	N	Appendiceal origin (%)	Complete CR[a] (%)	M/M[b]	RR[c]	SV[d]
Washington Cancer Institute	1999	200	75	n/a	27/2	n/a	n/a
University of Cincinnati College of Medicine	2004	33	67	67	27/0	>33	(49)e (3 yr)
Wake Forest University, NC	2006	110	100	28	38/4	n/a	53.4 (5y)
Istituto dei Tumori, Milan, Italy	2008	96	100	67	27/1	61	71.9 (5 yr)
Washington Cancer Institute	2008	472	85	100	n/a	26	n/a
Mercy Medical Center, Baltimore, MD	2012	77	100	65	27/0	n/a	40 (3y)
International Multicenter	2012	2298	100	51	24/2	n/a	63 (10y)
National Cancer Centre Singapore	2013	100	20	90	55/0	74	50.9 (5y)
Mount Sinai Medical Ctr, NY	2014	170	29	37	52/4	40–79	30.6 (3y)
Basingstoke/North Hampshire Hospital, UK	2015	752	100	68	46/2	50	64.5 (5 yr)
Wake Forest University, NC	2015	430	100	44	28/3	n/a	53.4 (5y)

[a]*CR* cytoreduction
[b]*M/M* 30-day morbidity and mortality
[c]*RR* recurrence rate
[d]*SV* survival
[e]Number calculated from graph by weighted average

Carcinoids, GISTs, and Lymphomas of the Colon and Rectum

38

David J. Maron

Key Concepts

- Treatment of colonic carcinoids is segmental resection including mesenteric lymph nodes.
- Somatostatin analogues control the symptoms of carcinoid syndrome and help limit progression of disease.
- Rectal carcinoids less than 1 cm may be treated by local excision, while tumors greater than 2 cm require radical resection.
- Imatinib blocks activation of the KIT oncoprotein in gastrointestinal stromal tumors.
- Patients with colonic lymphomas that produce symptoms are best treated with surgical resection prior to chemotherapy.

Electronic Supplementary Material The online version of this chapter (https://doi.org/10.1007/978-3-030-01165-9_38) contains supplementary material, which is available to authorized users.

D. J. Maron (✉)
Department of Colorectal Surgery, Cleveland Clinic Florida, Weston, FL, USA
e-mail: marond@ccf.org

Carcinoid Tumors

Histology

- Carcinoids are slow-growing tumors of the neuroectodermal origin and belong to the amine precursor uptake and decarboxylation (APUD) system.
- They originate from Kulchitsky or basogranular enterochromaffin cells located in the crypts of Lieberkuhn.
- Microscopically, these tumors are composed of monotonous sheets of small round cells with uniform nuclei and cytoplasm.
- The cells contain very dense neurosecretory granules that contain various secretory peptides; these granules are similar to synaptic vesicles found in neurons.
- The cytoplasmic features are typically benign-appearing, and mitotic figures are infrequent.
- Five histologic patterns of carcinoid tumors include insular, trabecular, glandular, undifferentiated, and mixed. Insular and trabecular patterns are typically associated with a more favorable prognosis.
- Distinguishing between benign and malignant carcinoids can be difficult; however increased cellular atypia, high mitotic activity, and necrosis are often associated with more aggressive tumors.

S. R. Steele et al. (eds.), *The ASCRS Manual of Colon and Rectal Surgery*,
https://doi.org/10.1007/978-3-030-01165-9_38

- Carcinoid tumors have specific staining patterns related to the amines and peptides they produce as well as cytoplasmic proteins they contain.
  - Serotonin is capable of reducing silver salts to metallic silver, and therefore carcinoid tumors that produce serotonin and stain positive with silver stains are described as "argentaffin positive."
  - Some tumors are capable of silver uptake but not reduction, and these may be demonstrated by the addition of an external reducing agent; these tumors are referred to as "argyrophilic."
    - Carcinoid tumors of the midgut are typically argentaffin positive, while those in the hindgut are often mixed (6–70% argyrophilic and 8–16% argentaffin positive).
  - Silver staining has been abandoned in favor of immunohistochemical staining for cytoplasmic proteins, including chromogranin-, synaptophysin-, and neuron-specific enolase.
- Carcinoid tumors have been shown to produce at least 30 bioactive compounds.
  - These compounds include amines such as serotonin and histamine, proteins (including various hormones and kinins), and prostaglandins.
  - Metabolism of serotonin occurs first in the liver (monoamine oxidase) and then in the kidney (aldehyde dehydrogenase) to produce 5-hydroxyindoleacetic acid (5-HIAA), which is excreted in the urine.

Incidence and Distribution

- Carcinoid tumors may originate in the foregut, midgut, or hindgut.
  - Foregut tumors arise in the thymus, respiratory tract, stomach, duodenum, and pancreas.
  - Midgut carcinoids originate in the jejunum, ileum, appendix, and proximal colon.
  - Hindgut tumors arise in the distal colon and rectum.
- Carcinoid tumors are associated with an increased risk of synchronous colorectal and small bowel tumors, as well as metachronous lung, prostate, and urinary tract neoplasms.

Clinical Presentation

- Approximately half of all gastrointestinal carcinoids are diagnosed following appendectomy for suspected appendicitis. Carcinoids of the appendix are discussed in detail in Chap. 37.
- Colonic carcinoids most commonly occur in the seventh or eighth decade of life and are more common in women than in men.
  - They may present as a polyp or as a mass that is indistinguishable from a colon carcinoma, both grossly and on radiographic visualization.
  - Many patients with colonic carcinoids are asymptomatic or have symptoms from another condition that prompt an investigation that leads to the diagnosis.
  - Those tumors that are symptomatic produce symptoms similar to colonic carcinomas (bleeding, abdominal pain, change in bowel habits).
- Symptoms of rectal carcinoids, when present, are typically rectal bleeding or change in bowel habits. Most rectal carcinoids, however, are asymptomatic and are found at the time of colorectal cancer screening.
- The incidence of rectal carcinoids in all patients undergoing sigmoidoscopy is estimated at 0.05%.
- These tumors typically appear as a solitary 1–1.5 cm mobile submucosal nodule with an intact overlying normal mucosa.
- Malignancy is frequently associated with carcinoids larger than 2 cm and/or invasion through the muscularis propria.
  - These tumors often will appear ulcerated and present with rectal bleeding.
  - Metastatic disease tends to occur less frequently in carcinoid tumors of the hindgut (rectum 18%) when compared with midgut

carcinoids (small bowel 34%, colon 60%) and foregut tumors (stomach 23%, bronchopulmonary 21%).

Carcinoid Syndrome

- Systemic symptoms produced by carcinoid tumors are referred to as the carcinoid syndrome.
- Although classically described as the hallmark of carcinoid tumors, carcinoid syndrome occurs in only 10–18% of patients with carcinoids and in only 50% of patients with advanced disease.
- The symptoms include flushing of the skin, non-bloody diarrhea, and abdominal pain.
  - The symptoms are often episodic and may be precipitated by stress or the ingestion of certain foods, caffeine, or alcohol.
  - The flushing may involve the face or the entire body and may occur for a few minutes or last for several hours.
  - Flushing may also be associated with excessive tearing, salivation, and bronchopulmonary spasm leading to wheezing.
  - Patients with carcinoid syndrome may also develop right-sided heart failure.
- Treatment of symptoms of diarrhea includes loperamide, diphenoxylate/atropine, and other antidiarrheal medications.
- Antihistamines or H2 receptor antagonists may be helpful in reducing flushing symptoms.
- The liver is capable of metabolizing and inactivating most of the peptide hormones secreted by carcinoid tumors. It is for this reason that the carcinoid syndrome typically develops only after the tumor has developed metastases in the liver.
- Carcinoid syndrome occurs most frequently in patients with metastatic disease from a midgut carcinoid tumor. In contrast, foregut tumors typically lack the enzyme required to convert 5-hydroxytryptophan into serotonin, and hindgut carcinoids rarely produce serotonin. Therefore rectal carcinoids, even in the presence of metastatic disease in the liver, almost never result in the carcinoid syndrome.

Diagnostic Tests

- The majority of carcinoid tumors of the colon and rectum are found during colonoscopy or are discovered during abdominal exploration for another condition.
- Full endoscopic evaluation of the colon and rectum should be performed to evaluate for synchronous malignancies.
- Endoscopic ultrasonography has been used in the evaluation of rectal carcinoids and has been shown to have a 75% accuracy rate in determining the depth of invasion and presence of lymph node metastases.
- This may be helpful in determining whether the carcinoid is amenable to endoscopic resection.
- When endoscopic biopsy is not feasible, biochemical tests may help to make the diagnosis of carcinoid.
  - Although carcinoid tumors may produce a variety of hormones, the most widely used tests are related to serotonin.
  - The most useful biochemical test for diagnosing carcinoid in the symptomatic patient is the 24-h urine 5-HIAA assay.
- In addition to a CT scan of the chest, abdomen, and pelvis to evaluate for metastatic disease, somatostatin receptor scintigraphy (SRS) may be helpful in identifying occult metastases and to determine if the patient is likely to respond to treatment with octreotide.
- Whole-body positron emission tomography (PET) using ^{18}F-DOPA may also be useful in detecting carcinoid tumors.
- The TNM staging of carcinoid tumors is similar to that of adenocarcinomas of the colon (Table 38.1).

Treatment

- The treatment of carcinoid tumors is surgical resection.
- The type of surgery depends on a variety of factors, including whether the tumor is amenable to local or endoscopic resection and whether surgical debulking of tumor may help

Table 38.1 TNM staging of carcinoid tumors

Stage	Characteristics
Tumor	
T1	Tumor invades submucosa
T2	Tumor invades muscularis propria
T3	Tumor invades through muscularis propria into subserosa or nonperitonealized pericolic or perirectal tissues
T4	Tumor directly invades other organs or structures and/or perforates visceral peritoneum
Regional nodal metastases	
NX	Regional lymph nodes cannot be assessed
N0	No nodal metastasis
N1	Metastasis in one to three pericolic or perirectal nodes
N2	Metastasis in four to more pericolic or perirectal nodes
N3	Metastasis in any node along the course of a named vascular trunk and/or metastasis to apical node
Distant metastasis	
MX	Presence of distant metastasis cannot be assessed
M0	No distant metastasis
M1	Distant metastasis

Adapted from the *AJCC Cancer Staging Manuel, 7ed.* (Eds. Edge, Byrd, Compton, Fritz, Green, Trotti) Publ. Springer. NY, NY. 2010

to reduce the symptoms of the carcinoid syndrome.

- The choice of the appropriate procedure is based on the location of the tumor, the likelihood of residual primary disease, and the presence of lymph node or metastatic disease. Guidelines for resection are summarized in Table 38.2.
- Carcinoids of the small bowel are frequently multicentric and have a propensity for developing obstruction secondary to intussusception, mesenteric fibrosis, and kinking of the bowel (Fig. 38.1a, b).
- Metastasis to regional lymph nodes approaches 50%, and tumors less than 1 cm in diameter are associated with a 20–30% incidence of lymph node involvement.
- Size of the tumor is a poor predictor of distant metastasis, as tumors less than 0.5 cm have been shown to metastasize to the liver.
- Surgical management should therefore include a formal small bowel resection with wide mesenteric excision of the associated lymph nodes.

Table 38.2 Guidelines for resection

Primary tumor	Factor	Extent of resection
Small bowel	Locally limited disease	Resection of primary and metastatic tumors
	Extensive disease	Resection or bypass of primary tumor
		Debulking of metastasis
Colon		Colectomy
Rectum	<1 cm	Local excision
	1–1.9 cm	Local excision or proctectomy
	>2 cm	Proctectomy

  - This should be performed even in the presence of metastatic disease to reduce the incidence of small bowel obstruction due to tumor or fibrosis of the mesentery.
- As one-third of carcinoids of the small bowel may be multicentric, it is important to examine the entire small intestine to evaluate for synchronous lesions.
- Carcinoids arising in the colon are often asymptomatic until they develop into large tumors with lymph node metastases.
  - Colonic resection similar to that performed for adenocarcinoma is therefore recommended, with the extent determined by the location of the disease.
  - Outcomes following colectomy for colonic carcinoids are varied.
  - Location of the primary tumor may affect outcomes, as in one series cecal tumors were found to have an incidence of 71% metastases, while tumors elsewhere in the colon had only a 33% incidence.
  - Small tumors confined to the mucosa may be appropriately treated by endoscopic resection.
- As carcinoid tumors of the rectum may be amenable to local excision, less invasive treatment may be an option in some patients.
  - It is important to balance the benefits of a less morbid intervention with the risks of local recurrence and nodal involvement (and hence the risk of metastatic disease).
  - Transanal or endoscopic excision is adequate for most tumors less than 1 cm in diameter.

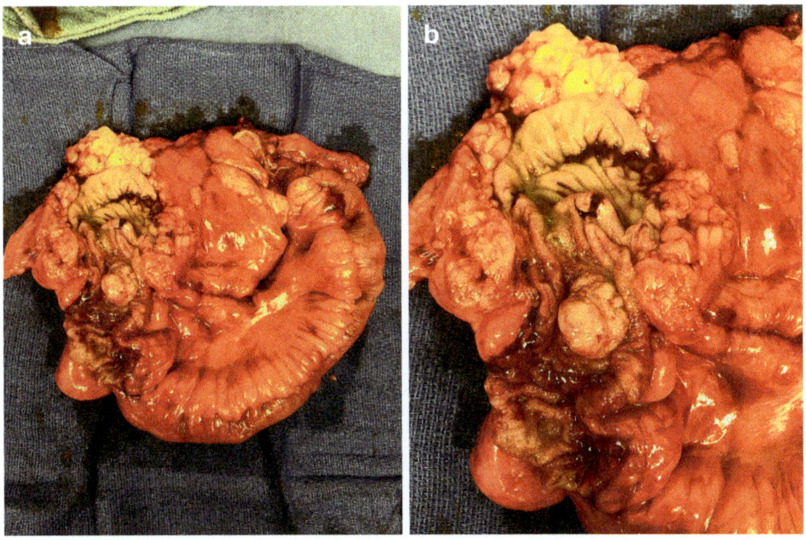

Fig. 38.1 (**a**) Surgical specimen demonstrating a terminal ileal carcinoid. Note the desmoplastic response of the mesentery. (**b**) Close-up view of the lesion

  - Formal transanal excision of the full thickness of the rectal wall allows for a precise assessment of the depth of penetration and is more likely to result in negative margins of resection.
    - However, this may not be necessary for many patients, as recurrence is rare even when there is an involved margin following endoscopic excision of tumors less than 1 cm in diameter.
- Invasion of the muscularis propria (T2) has been associated with lymph node metastases in up to 47% of patients, and therefore oncologic proctectomy should be considered.
- In addition to muscularis propria invasion, rectal carcinoids whose size is greater than 2 cm in diameter are also at significant risk of lymph node metastases.
  - Patients should therefore be considered for proctectomy with excision of the mesorectum to allow for assessment and clearance of the nodal basin.
- The treatment of rectal carcinoids measuring between 1 cm and 1.9 cm remains uncertain and must be individualized based on tumor features and the overall health of the patient.
- Carcinoid tumors are typically slow-growing, and patients often exhibit favorable 5- and 10-year survival rates despite the presence of extensive metastatic disease.
- Surgical treatment of metastatic carcinoid in the liver may be of benefit in improving survival and may help to provide long-term palliation of hormone-related symptoms in patients who are unable to tolerate or do not respond to medical treatment with somatostatin analogues.
  - Various techniques have been employed, including hepatic resection, radiofrequency ablation, cryosurgery, and chemoembolization.
  - Wedge resection or lobectomy of hepatic metastases not only improves symptoms associated with the carcinoid syndrome but also has been shown to prolong survival.
  - As metastatic carcinoid tumors derive the majority of their blood supply from the hepatic artery (while hepatocytes receive blood supply primarily from the portal venous system), chemoembolization may play an important role in patients who are unable to tolerate hepatic resection.
  - Liver transplantation has also been employed in patients with metastatic carcinoid, with outcome similar to those seen in patients who undergo transplantation for hepatocellular carcinoma.
- The efficacy of systemic chemotherapy in the treatment of metastatic carcinoid is limited.

  - Various agents have been used, including 5-FU, streptozotocin, cisplatin, doxorubicin, etoposide, and dacarbazine, either as monotherapy or in combination.
- More than 80% of carcinoid tumors express surface receptors for somatostatin (especially receptor subtype 2), and therapeutic strategies have therefore focused on the development of agents that target these receptors.
  - Activation of these receptors results in reduced hormone synthesis and secretion, thereby leading to complete or partial relief of symptoms associated with the carcinoid syndrome in up to 90% of patients.
  - Somatostatin analogues that have been used in the treatment of carcinoid include octreotide and lanreotide.
  - Octreotide may be given as a subcutaneous, intramuscular, or long-acting depot injection.
  - Lanreotide has a longer half-life than octreotide; however its use is not currently approved for use in the United States.
  - In addition to the ability to control symptoms, somatostatin analogues may also help to limit the progression of disease.

GISTs

- Gastrointestinal stromal tumors (GISTs) are the most common mesenchymal neoplasm of the gastrointestinal tract and account for approximately 0.1–3% of all intestinal cancers.
- GISTs were first described by Mazur and Clark, who used electron microscopy to differentiate these tumors from other soft tissue sarcomas.
  - Most tumors arising from mesenchymal elements of the gastrointestinal tract were considered leiomyomas, leiomyosarcomas, and leiomyoblastomas; however it was discovered that GISTs lack features associated with smooth muscle cells.
  - Instead, it is believed that GISTs arise from the interstitial cells of Cajal or other pluripotential mesenchymal stem cells.

Histology

- Histologically, gastrointestinal stromal tumors typically have a spindle cell appearance and stain positive for the CD117 antigen, a marker for the KIT tyrosine kinase oncoprotein.
- In addition, 60–70% of GISTs will stain positive for CD34, a hematopoietic progenitor cell antigen.
- These features help to differentiate GISTs from other sarcomas; leiomyomas stain negative for KIT and CD34 but positive for desmin, smooth muscle actin, and S100.

Incidence and Distribution

- GISTs typically occur in the sixth to seventh decade of life and affect men and women equally.
- Most tumors are sporadic; however several hereditary syndromes are associated with GISTs.
  - Carney's triad consists of (1) synchronous or metachronous GISTs, (2) extra-adrenal paraganglionomas, and (3) pulmonary chondromas.
  - This is usually seen in women before age 30 and is not associated with a KIT mutation.
  - Patients with neurofibromatosis type I are also more commonly affected with GISTs. Tumors in these patients are more likely to occur at a younger age and often present with multiple small intestinal GISTs.
- Gastrointestinal stromal tumors are most commonly found in the stomach (approximately two-thirds of cases), followed by the small intestine (about one-quarter of cases).
- Tumors located in the colon and rectum account for only 10–20% of GISTs, and of those, the majority arise in the rectum.

Clinical Presentation

- GISTs are usually slow-growing lesions and are often discovered incidentally during

endoscopy or in the treatment of other conditions.
- The most common clinical symptoms are rectal bleeding and abdominal or rectal pain.
- Advanced lesions may present with a palpable mass, obstruction, or perforation (Fig. 38.2).
- Metastatic disease most frequently occurs in the liver and peritoneum; metastatic disease in the lymph nodes is uncommon.

Diagnostic Tests

- Evaluation of a patient with a suspected GIST includes colonoscopy as well as endoscopic ultrasound, if feasible.
- Lesions are usually submucosal; however, biopsy may be aided with the use of endoscopic ultrasound-guided fine needle aspiration.
  - Care must be taken as these tumors are frequently associated with neovascularization and biopsy may result in significant hemorrhage.
  - Percutaneous biopsy with fine or core needle aspiration is an option for tumors that cannot be reached endoscopically; however, concern over tumor rupture and spread has been reported.
- CT and MRI may aid in staging and determining whether surgical resection is feasible. GISTs typically involve the muscularis propria and radiographically have a characteristic appearance of a well-circumscribed intramural mass. Larger lesions may have evidence of central necrosis.
- PET scanning is not helpful in diagnosis and, however, may be of benefit in evaluating the response to treatment.

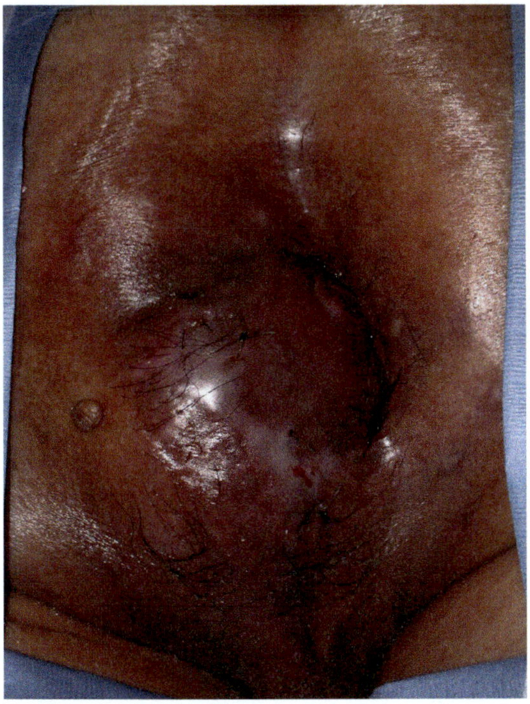

Fig. 38.2 GIST of the rectum presenting as a perianal mass

Treatment

- Surgical resection of GISTs offers the best chance for cure and is therefore the treatment of choice.
- It is recommended that resection include the tumor en bloc with any associated contiguous tissues with margins of at least 1 cm.
- As GISTs rarely metastasize to the lymphatic system, lymphadenectomy is not necessary.
- Although many gastrointestinal stromal tumors may have a pseudocapsule, enucleation of the tumor without resection of the pseudocapsule should be avoided, as this has been associated with increased risk of tumor recurrence.
- Resection of rectal GISTs may be accomplished by radical resection (low anterior resection or abdominoperineal resection) or local excision (transanal excision or transanal endoscopic microsurgery), provided that the tumor and pseudocapsule can be removed with adequate margins (Video 38.1).
- The development of imatinib has significantly impacted the treatment of gastrointestinal stromal tumors. Imatinib is a selective tyrosine kinase inhibitor which blocks activation of the KIT oncoprotein.

- When used in adjuvant therapy, imatinib has been shown to significantly decrease the risk of recurrence.
- Imatinib has also been used in patients where the tumor was felt to be too large to resect. In this situation, the use of imatinib has been shown to result in tumor shrinkage in more than 50% of patients, thereby allowing surgical resection in selected patients.
- Neoadjuvant imatinib therapy for rectal gastrointestinal stromal tumors has also been reported.
- The reported incidence of local recurrence and metastatic disease following complete surgical resection of GISTs varies but approaches 50% in some series.
- In patients whose tumors develop resistance to imatinib, sunitinib has been used as a second-line treatment with some success. Patients with unresectable hepatic metastases may also be candidates for radiofrequency ablation or hepatic artery embolization.

Lymphomas

- The gastrointestinal tract is the most common site of extranodal lymphoma.
- While the majority of these lymphomas arise in the stomach (74.6%), small bowel and colonic lymphoma are less common, accounting for 8.6% and 7%, respectively.

Histology

- Most lymphomas of the gastrointestinal tract are non-Hodgkin's lymphoma.
- Diffuse large B-cell lymphoma is the most common histologic type seen in the colon.
- Other pathologic types in the colon include MALT-associated low-grade B-cell lymphoma, mantle cell lymphoma, and T-cell lymphoma.
- Correct determination of the subtype is important for optimal treatment and prognosis.
- Differentiating between primary gastrointestinal lymphoma and secondary involvement of the intestinal tract by systemic lymphoma is important to guide treatment.
  – The diagnosis of primary lymphoma can be made: (1) in the absence of enlarged superficial lymph nodes, (2) absence of enlarged mediastinal lymph nodes, (3) normal total and differential and white cell count, (4) at laparotomy, only regional lymph nodes have metastatic disease, and (5) the liver and spleen are unaffected.

Incidence and Distribution

- Most colonic lymphomas arise in the cecum or ascending colon, likely due to the increased lymphoid tissue in this segment of the colon.
- Patients are typically between the ages of 50 and 70; sex predominance varies among different reports.
- Prolonged steroid use, inflammatory bowel disease, HIV, and EBV have been postulated as possible risk factors for the development of colonic lymphoma.
- Both a modified Ann Arbor staging system and the TNM system have been used to stage gastrointestinal lymphomas.

Clinical Presentation and Diagnostic Tests

- The most common presenting symptom of lymphomas of the colon is abdominal pain.
- Other symptoms mimic those of adenocarcinoma and include weight loss, rectal bleeding, change in bowel habits, anemia, weakness, and possibly fever.
- Tender abdominal masses may be present in up to 80% of patients at the time of presentation.
- Growth of the lesions leads to obstruction in 20–25% of cases; however perforation is uncommon (Fig. 38.3).
- Colonoscopy with biopsy should be performed; however in some cases, superficial biopsies may not be sufficient to confirm the diagnosis.

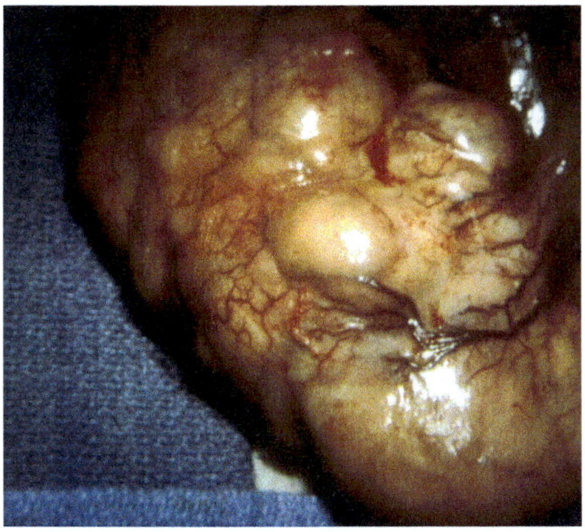

Fig. 38.3 Lymphoma of the sigmoid colon invading the ileum. (Courtesy of the ASCRS Image Library, Bruce Orkin, MD)

- CT scan of the chest, abdomen, and pelvis should be obtained to extraintestinal disease.

Treatment

- In patients with lymphoma that is confined to the bowel, treatment is surgical excision or systemic chemotherapy.
- Historically, given that a sizeable fraction of patients presented with symptomatic disease that required semi-urgent operation or underwent operation to establish a diagnosis, surgical resection was most often employed as therapy.
  - In patients with localized disease where the diagnosis can be made preoperatively, the rationale for surgical treatment is to remove tumor that has the potential to obstruct, perforate, bleed, and cure the patient if the tumor has not yet spread.
  - Adjuvant chemotherapy, typically vincristine, cyclophosphamide, bleomycin, and doxorubicin, has been used to improve survival.
  - Radiation therapy has also been advocated following resection of rectal lymphomas.
- An alternative strategy is to treat with systemic chemotherapy and potentially avoid operation.
  - One of the potential risks is perforation of the bowel if chemotherapy causes tumor necrosis.
  - Given the low incidence of the disease, there are no randomized controlled trials to rely upon when making treatment decisions.

39 Diverticular Disease

Jason Hall

Key Concepts

- The optimal diagnostic test to allow for optimal assessment of severity of diverticulitis is CT imaging.
- The majority of patients with acute diverticulitis will respond to antibiotic therapy alone.
- CT drainage of localized abscesses in diverticulitis will often avoid the need for emergency operations, even in patients who may not initially respond to medical therapy alone.
- Hartmann's resection can often be avoided in most patients requiring surgery for an acute attack. Resection with primary anastomosis, with or without proximal diversion (loop ileostomy), can be performed safely in the absence of physiologic instability.
- The indications for elective resection after an acute attack of diverticulitis are evolving but should be considered in patients who remain symptomatic or develop a definite complication (stricture, fistula, etc.).

J. Hall (✉)
Division of Colon and Rectal Surgery, Boston University Medical Center, Boston, MA, USA

Tufts University School of Medicine, Boston, MA, USA
e-mail: Jason.Hall@bmc.org

Introduction

- Most patients with diverticulosis are asymptomatic.
- Symptomatic diverticular disease represents a whole range of conditions ranging from mild abdominal pain and bloating to free perforation with peritonitis and sepsis.
- These presentations are stratified into complicated or uncomplicated diverticulitis.
- Complicated presentations are defined as episodes of free perforation, obstruction, stricture, fistula, or hemorrhage.
- Diverticular hemorrhage is associated with diverticulosis and not diverticulitis.

Incidence

- In the twentieth century, there has been a rising prevalence of diverticular disease in industrialized nations.
- The incidence of this colonic finding rises with age such that over 40% of patients develop diverticula by the age of 60 years. Over 60% of patients over 80 years have diverticular disease identified.
- In Asian countries, however, diverticulosis occurs more commonly on the right side.
- Administrative data sources suggest that the incidence of diverticulitis is increasing.

S. R. Steele et al. (eds.), *The ASCRS Manual of Colon and Rectal Surgery*,
https://doi.org/10.1007/978-3-030-01165-9_39

- There also appeared to be conflicting data regarding the incidence of complicated diverticular disease. The proportion of diverticular abscess discharges increased from 5.9% in 1991 to 9.6% in 2005 ($p < 0.0001$). The proportion of free diverticular perforations, however, has remained unchanged (1.5%) (see Fig. 39.1a, b).
- Rates of hospitalization for diverticular bleeding per 100,000 patients have declined from 32.5 to 27.1 from 2000 to 2010.

Pathophysiology, Etiology, and Epidemiology

- Most colonic diverticula are pulsion or false diverticula and contain only the mucosal and muscularis mucosal layers.
- Diverticula penetrate the colonic wall where vasa recta penetrate the circular muscle layer (Fig. 39.2).
- The pathogenesis of progression from diverticulosis to diverticulitis is unknown.

Histology and Pathology

- Microscopic features of diverticulitis include thickening of the lamina propria, mucin depletion, and Paneth cell hyperplasia.
- Hinchey developed pathologic criteria to classify the severity of diverticular disease. This classification has been used and is divided into Stages I–IV.
  - Stage I are patients with diverticulitis and a pericolic abscess.

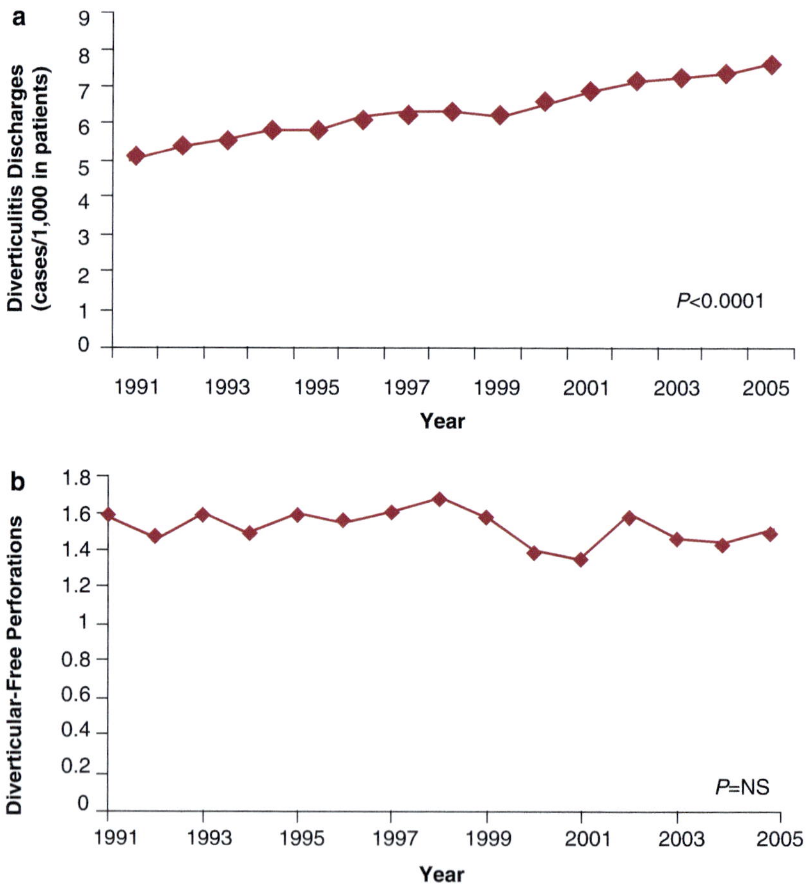

Fig. 39.1 (**a**) Diverticulitis discharges (uncomplicated and complicated) in Nationwide Inpatient Sample from 1991 to 2005. (**b**) Proportion of patient discharges for free diverticular perforation among all patients with diverticulitis in Nationwide Inpatient Sample from 1991 to 2005. (With permission from Ricciardi et al. Dis Colon Rectum. 2009 Sep;52(9):1558–63 ©Wolters Kluwer 2009)

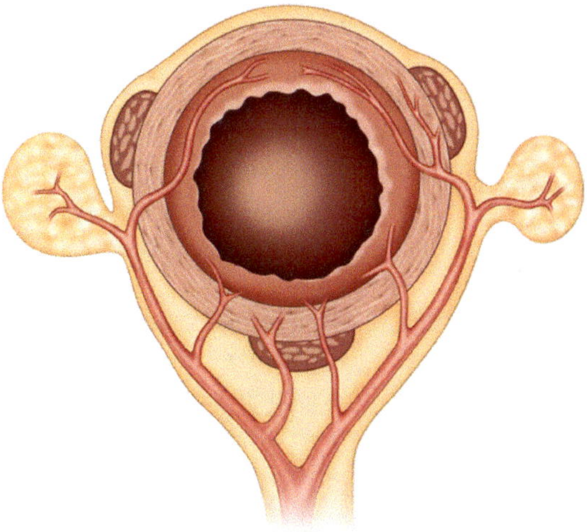

Fig. 39.2 Vasa recta penetrate the colonic wall at taenia libera, omentalis, and mesocolica. This allows herniation of mucosa and submucosa at these sites

- Stage II represents patients with distant abscesses such as a pelvic or retroperitoneal abscess.
  - Stage III and IV are patients with purulent and feculent peritonitis, respectively (Table 39.1).

Role of Fiber

- Studies demonstrate an inverse association between diverticular disease incidence and fiber intake.
- Fiber found in fruits and vegetables confers the most protective effect (compared with fiber from cereal).
- Popcorn, nut, and seed consumptions are inversely correlated with diverticulosis or diverticular complications, refuting the adage that "nuts, corn, seeds, and popcorn" cause diverticulitis.

Alternative Pathophysiology Pathways and Taenia-Specific Elastosis

- Histologic studies have determined that colonic walls are thickened secondary to elastin deposition and not muscular hypertrophy or hyperplasia.
- It is likely that a number of processes including impaired motility, low-fiber intake, inflammation, and elastin deposition contribute to the pathogenesis of diverticular disease.

Table 39.1 Hinchey classification system

Stage1	Pericolic or mesenteric abscess
Stage II	Pelvic or retroperitoneal abscess
Stage III	Purulent peritonitis
Stage IV	Feculent peritonitis

Additional Risk Factors

Age

- Diverticular disease incidence rises from 5% at age 40 to 80% by age 80.
- Acute diverticulitis has a striking male predominance in younger patients.

Geographic Factors

- Diverticulitis in Asian populations involves the right-sided colon in up to 70% of cases.
- There is a direct relationship between increasing industrialization and incidence of diverticular disease.

Obesity

- A number of retrospective case series have noted a striking preponderance of obese patients with diverticulitis, particularly patients under the age of 40.

Clinical Manifestations and Physical Findings

- There are three main clinical presentations of diverticular disease (Table 39.2).

Table 39.2 Typical presentation patterns of diverticulitis

Acute diverticulitis
Typical, relapsing (chronic)
Subacute
Complicated diverticulitis
Obstruction
Mass/abscess
Fistula
Hemorrhage
Perforation
Chronic diverticulitis
Atypical
Atypical site (transverse, ascending)

- The most common clinical presentation of diverticulitis is uncomplicated diverticulitis.
  - Presentation is characterized by left-sided abdominal pain with or without an associated mass, fever, and leukocytosis.
  - Most patients can be treated as outpatients.
- Another manifestation is smoldering diverticulitis.
  - Patients only partially improve on antibiotics and medical therapy.
  - Such patients have recurrent symptoms which can manifest with ongoing low-grade fever and left-sided abdominal pain.
  - CT scans on such patients generally will demonstrate a persistent phlegmon, and these patients often require resection to treat ongoing symptoms.
- Finally, a small group of patients have chronic left lower-quadrant pain.
  - They lack objective evidence of diverticulitis such as leukocytosis, fever, or objective findings on CT scan.
  - Many patients with atypical presentations of "diverticulitis" may have irritable bowel syndrome. Surgeons therefore must be facile with the difference between both conditions.

Symptoms

- Patients with acute diverticulitis typically present with left-sided abdominal pain, fever, and leukocytosis.
- Physical findings consist of left lower-quadrant pain and tenderness on examination.
- Patients with free perforation will typically present with diffuse peritonitis and signs of systemic toxicity.
- If present, rectal bleeding is more suggestive of ischemic colitis or inflammatory bowel disease.
- In complicated presentations, an inflammatory phlegmon can be associated with a small or large bowel obstruction.
- Patients who develop colovesical fistulas may present with pneumaturia, pyuria, or fecaluria.
- Patients with colovaginal fistulas may present with vaginal discharge, vaginal air, or stool per vagina.

Diagnostic Evaluation

- Many patients with acute diverticulitis present with leukocytosis.
- Patients with a colovesical fistula may have an abnormal urinalysis and/or a culture with enteric organisms.
- Flat and upright plain films of the abdomen are commonly obtained in the evaluation of the patient with acute abdominal pain to exclude obstruction or free intraperitoneal air.
- Computed tomography has emerged as the study of choice.
  - CT findings include the presence of diverticula, pericolic fat stranding, colonic wall thickening more than 4 mm, and abscess formation.
  - CT has the ability to stage the severity of disease and may enable percutaneous drainage of an associated abscess.
  - CT has the added advantage of detecting other intraperitoneal findings including hepatic abscesses, pyelophlebitis, small bowel obstruction, colonic strictures/obstruction, and colovesical fistulas.
  - CT findings consistent with mild diverticulitis include localized wall thickening (> 5 mm) and inflammation of the pericolic fat.

- CT findings with severe diverticulitis are the combination of localized wall thickening and inflammation of the pericolic fat with abscess, extraluminal air, or extraluminal contrast (Table 39.3).
- Patients with severe CT findings undergo operative intervention more frequently than those patients with mild findings.
- Patients with findings of severe diverticulitis on CT scan are more likely to have recurrent attacks.
- CT findings may be classified based on the modified Hinchey classification system (Table 39.4).
- In grade 0 there is colonic wall thickening but not pericolonic fat stranding.
- Grade 1a consists of wall thickening and pericolonic fat stranding, while grade 1b includes a pericolonic or mesocolic abscess.
- Patients with grade 2 disease have distant intra-abdominal or pelvic abscesses.
- Patients with grade 3 and grade 4 disease have purulent and fecal peritonitis, respectively. CT is somewhat limited in distinguishing between patients with grade 3 and grade 4 disease (Figs. 39.3, 39.4, and 39.5a–d).

Table 39.3 Ambrosetti CT criteria for diverticulitis severity

Mild diverticulitis	Wall thickening (> 5 mm) Pericolic fat stranding
Severe diverticulitis	Wall thickening (> 5 mm) Pericolic fat stranding with Abscess Extraluminal air Extraluminal contrast

Table 39.4 Modified Hinchey classification system

Stage 0	Mild clinical diverticulitis
Stage Ia	Confined pericolic inflammation-phlegmon
Stage Ib	Confined pericolic abscess (within sigmoid mesocolon)
Stage II	Pelvic, distant intra-abdominal or intraperitoneal abscess
Stage III	Generalized purulent peritonitis
Stage IV	Fecal peritonitis

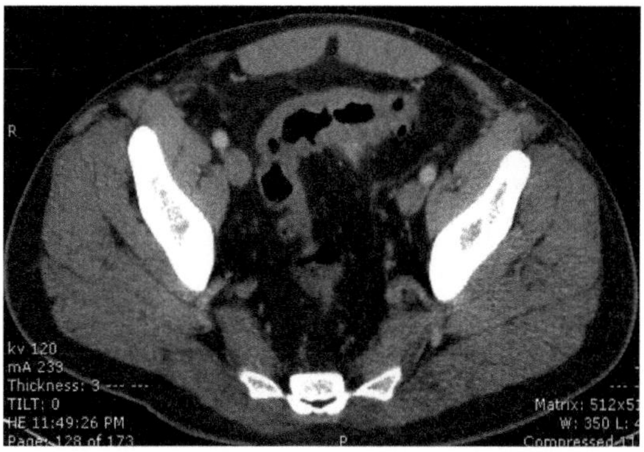

Fig. 39.3 Modified Hinchey Stage Ia diverticulitis – arrow points to pericolic inflammation and phlegmon

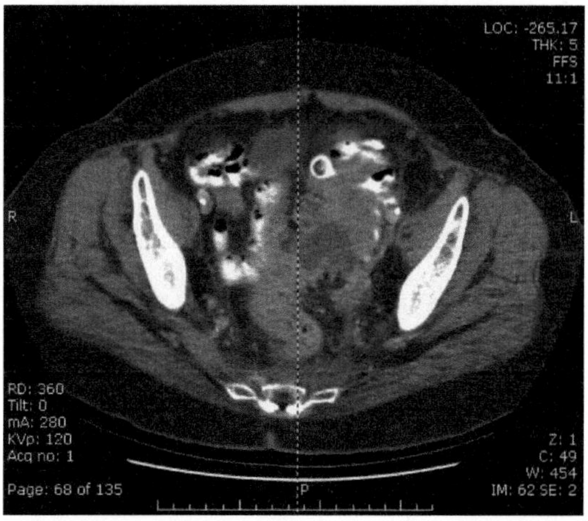

Fig. 39.4 Modified Hinchey Stage II diverticulitis – arrow points to pelvic abscess

Endoscopic Evaluation

- Endoscopic evaluation of the colon is generally advocated following an acute episode of diverticulitis to exclude the presence of a malignancy or an alternative diagnosis such as ischemic colitis, cancer, or inflammatory bowel disease.
- In actual practice, finding a malignancy is rare.

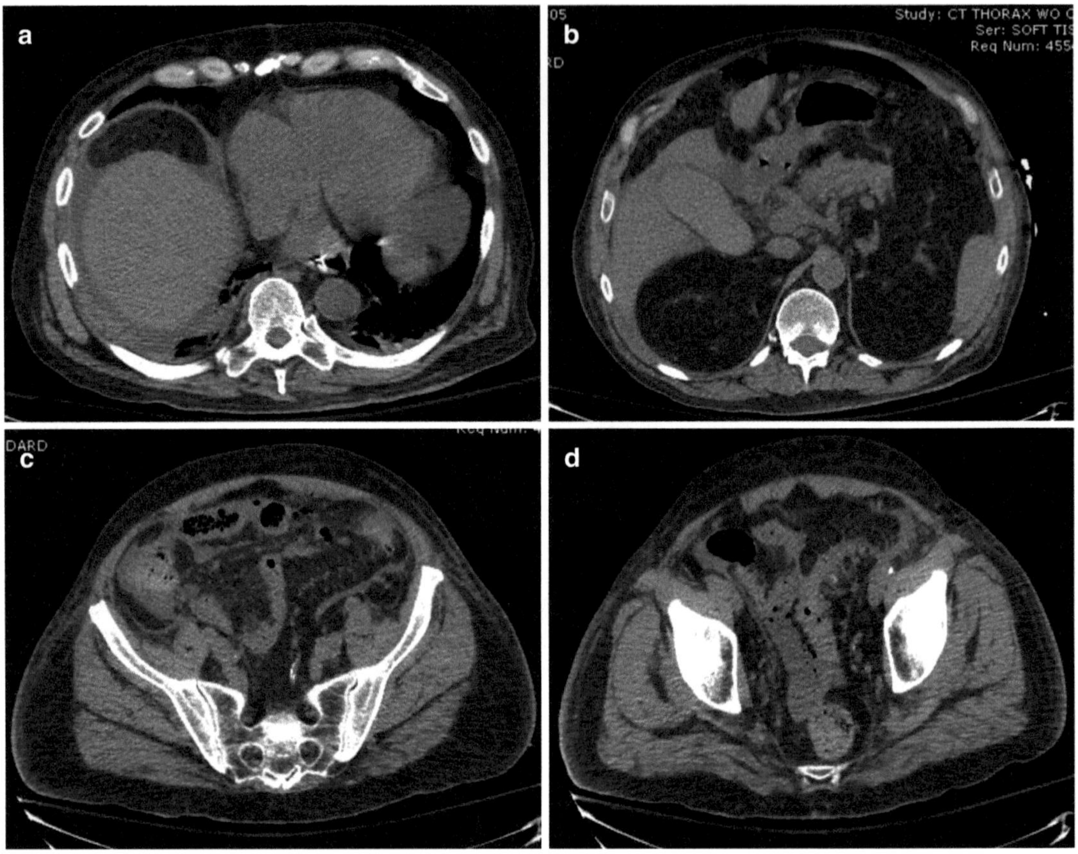

Fig. 39.5 (**a**) Modified Hinchey Stage III diverticulitis – arrow points to free fluid. (**b**) Modified Hinchey Stage III diverticulitis – arrow points to free air. (**c**) Modified Hinchey Stage III diverticulitis – demonstrates intra-abdominal free fluid. (**d**) Modified Hinchey Stage III diverticulitis – arrow points to pelvic fluid

- Flexible sigmoidoscopy or colonoscopy is generally not advocated during an acute episode of diverticulitis. A delay of 6 weeks following resolution of symptoms is recommended.

Differential Diagnosis

- Modern cross-sectional imaging is often helpful in differentiating other clinical entities such as appendicitis, bowel obstruction, colorectal cancer, ischemic colitis, pyelonephritis, gynecologic disease, inflammatory bowel disease, and irritable bowel syndrome.

Treatment of Acute Diverticulitis

Treatment of Uncomplicated Diverticulitis

Antibiotics

- In practice, antibiotic therapy remains the cornerstone of management in patients with acute uncomplicated diverticulitis.
  - However, high-quality studies show no difference between antibiotic administration and no antibiotic administration.
- Antibiotic therapy should be selected to provide adequate coverage of the most common colonic organisms. Single and combination regimens are equally effective.
- Approximately one-third of patients will have a recurrence.

- Patients with minimal symptoms and mild signs of peritoneal irritation can typically be treated as outpatients.
- Patients who present with fever, systemic symptoms, or inability to tolerate oral intake are usually hospitalized.
  - Parenteral antibiotics are typically administered until the acute symptoms resolve. Once there is clinical improvement, the antibiotic route is changed to oral administration.

Elective Surgical Management of Recurrent Uncomplicated Diverticulitis

- The recommendation for elective surgery should be individualized based on the age and medical condition of the patient, the severity and frequency of the attacks, and by the presence of ongoing symptoms.
- The number of attacks of uncomplicated diverticulitis is not necessarily an overriding factor in defining the appropriateness of surgery.
- Most patients who present with complicated diverticulitis will have complicated disease on the first attack.
- Resection after recovery from uncomplicated diverticulitis does not prevent the development of complicated diverticulitis. Therefore, recommending elective surgery to avoid future stoma formation is not generally justified.

Young Patients

- Given the current level of evidence, there is no clear mandate to treat patients with young patients with diverticulitis differently than other age groups.

Complicated Diverticular Disease

- Complicated diverticulitis is defined as diverticulitis associated with perforation, fistula, abscess, stricture, or obstruction.

Diverticular Abscess

- The initial approach to patients with diverticular abscess includes bowel rest, antibiotics, and close observation.
- Abscesses less than 4 cm in size often resolve with intravenous antibiotics alone without the need for further procedures.
- For those patients with diverticular abscess who do not improve on initial antibiotic therapy and continue to have signs of sepsis, percutaneous drainage is preferred.
  - The preferred approach for percutaneous drainage is usually by a transabdominal route (Fig. 39.6).

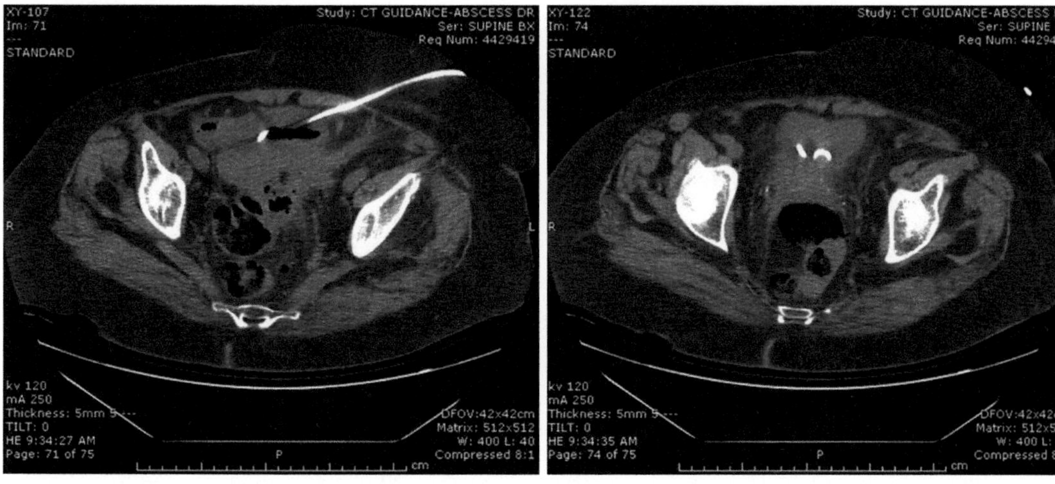

Fig. 39.6 Pigtail catheter in a complex diverticular pelvic abscess

  - If the abscess is not accessible by this route, a transgluteal, transperineal, or transrectal routes may be employed.
- The decision for surgery following successful drainage of a diverticular abscess should be approached on a case-by-case basis.
- Sigmoid resection is recommended for selected patients, particularly those with more complex or larger abscesses and those with recurrent or persistent symptoms such as colocutaneous fistula.

Perforated Diverticulitis

- Approximately 1% of patients with diverticulitis develop free perforation which may include purulent or fecal peritonitis (Fig. 39.1b).
- Free perforation almost exclusively develops on the first attack of diverticulitis.
- Patients with perforated diverticulitis manifested by purulent peritonitis or feculent peritonitis require operative intervention.
- The mainstay of treatment for perforated diverticulitis over the last several decades has been the Hartmann procedure.
  - A disadvantage of the procedure is the requirement for a second major surgical procedure to reverse the colostomy and the attendant morbidity and potential mortality of the procedure; at least one-third of patients never undergo reversal.
- Resection and primary anastomosis are superior to Hartmann resection in selected patients with Hinchey III and Hinchey IV diverticulitis.
- In clinical practice, the decision to perform a primary anastomosis should be done on a case-by-case basis.
  - Hemodynamic instability, ischemia, or significant edema of the bowel at an intended site of anastomosis and anemia, malnutrition, and immunocompromised state are general contraindications to a primary anastomosis.
- Selected patients with purulent peritonitis from diverticulitis may be successfully treated with laparoscopic lavage without resection of the affected segment of the colon. The appropriateness and role of this procedure remain uncertain.

Fistulas

- Fistulas occur in 2% of patients with diverticular disease.
- Colovesical fistulas are mostly common (65%), followed by other types of fistulas including colovaginal, coloenteric, colouterine, and colocutaneous fistulas.

Colovesical Fistulas

- Colovesical fistulas are more common in men than in women.
- Women affected with a colovesical fistula have usually undergone a prior hysterectomy.
- Patients often present with prominent urinary symptoms including polymicrobial urinary tract infections, pneumaturia, and fecaluria.
- CT scanning reveals air and/or contrast in the bladder in the absence of prior instrumentation (Fig. 39.7a–c).
- Colovesical fistulas may also be associated with locally advanced bladder or primary colon cancer. Cystoscopy and colonoscopy may be appropriate to exclude a malignancy under the appropriate clinical circumstances.
- The surgical principles for treatment of colovesical fistulas due to diverticular disease include resection of the affected segment; primary anastomosis can usually be performed safely.
- The fistula is generally small and may be simply pinched off with or without suture repair of the bladder.
- Omentum is used to interpose between the anastomosis and the bladder.

Colovaginal Fistulas

- Colovaginal fistulas occur almost exclusively in women who have undergone a prior hysterectomy (Fig. 39.8).
- Signs and symptoms include vaginal discharge and passage of air per vagina.

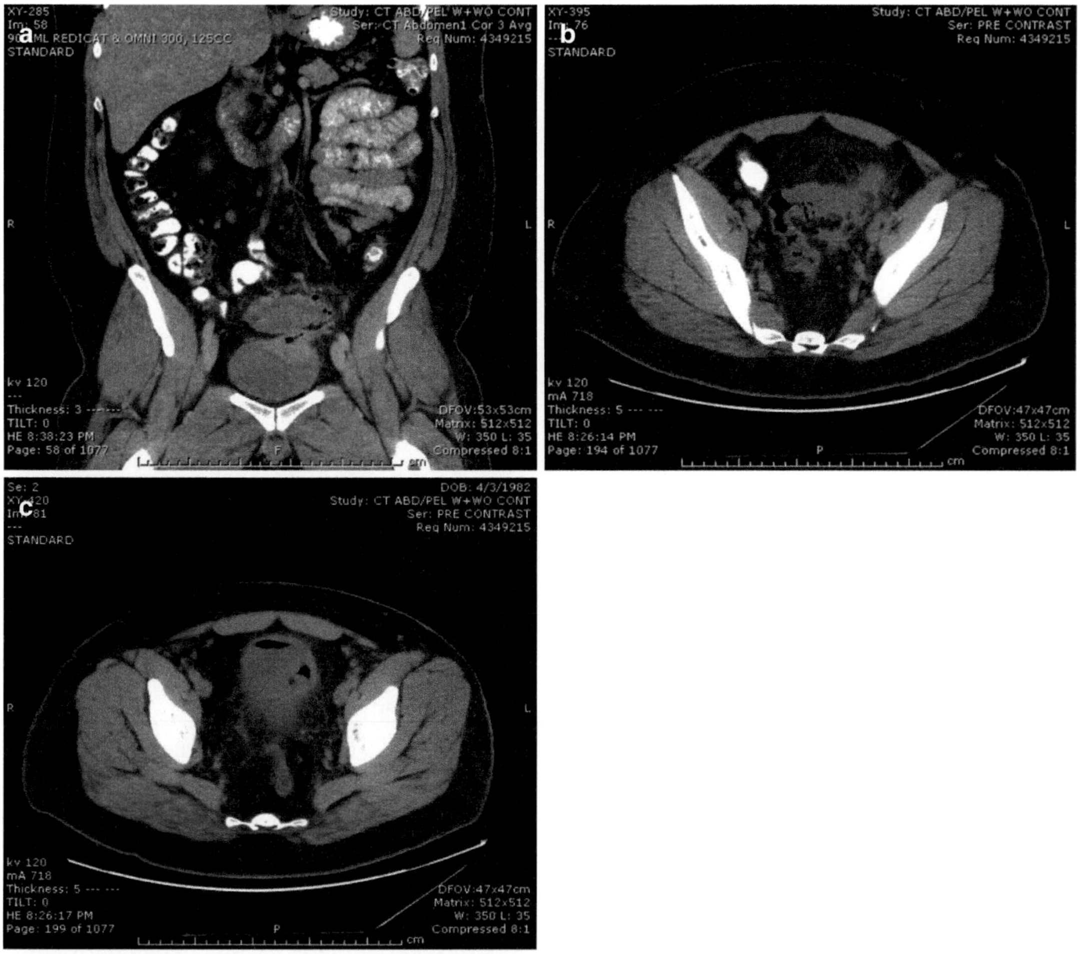

Fig. 39.7 (**a**) Arrow points to colovesical fistula. (**b**) Inflamed sigmoid colon adjacent to fistula. (**c**) Air in non-catheterized bladder consistent with colovesical fistula

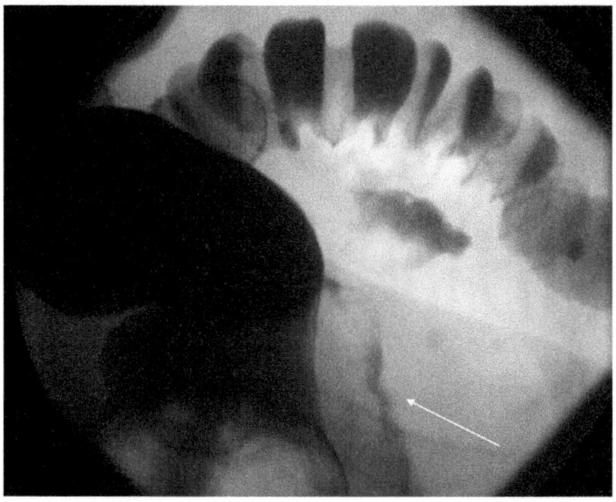

Fig. 39.8 Colovaginal fistula. Arrow demonstrates vaginal filling with contrast from pericolonic abscess

- A single-stage sigmoid resection can generally be performed, pinching off the site of the fistula and interposing omentum.

Colocutaneous Fistula

- Colocutaneous fistulas rarely occur de novo and are generally seen in patients who have undergone prior colectomy or percutaneous drainage.

Diverticular Stricture/Obstruction

- Repeated attacks of diverticulitis may be associated with the development of a sigmoid stricture (Fig. 39.9).

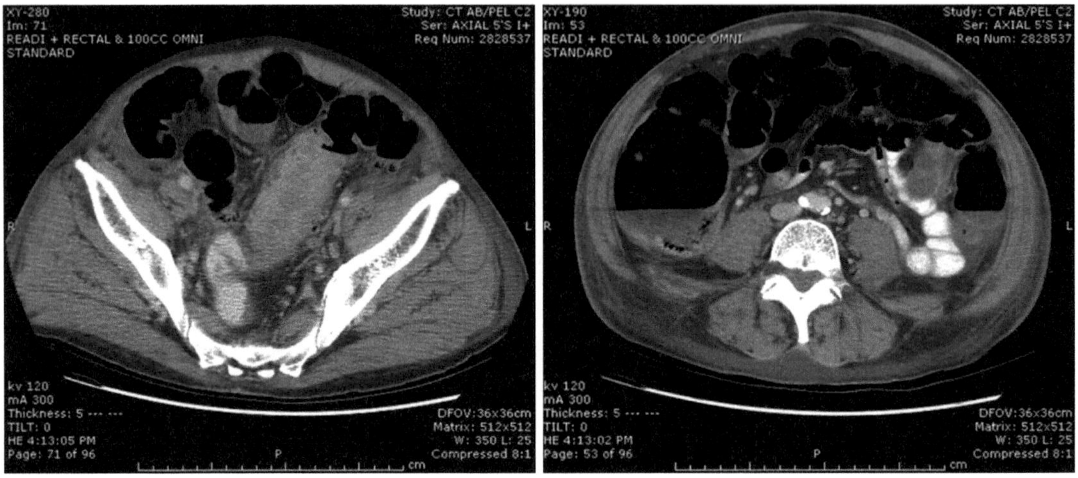

Fig. 39.9 Large sigmoid phlegmon causing a large bowel obstruction. Arrow shows a retrograde injection of contrast within the rectum which is unable to pass the obstruction

- The major differential diagnosis is with obstructing colon cancer.
- Small bowel can also become adherent to a focus of inflamed colonic tissue leading to associated small bowel obstruction.
- Patients with a partial obstruction that resolves with bowel rest, intravenous hydration, and antibiotics may be able to undergo elective resection.
- For patients with complete obstruction, the mainstay of surgical treatment is the Hartmann procedure because of concern about the increased risk of anastomotic leakage in patients who have dilated, edematous, and unprepared bowel.
- Other options include sigmoid resection with primary anastomosis and diverting proximal stoma (usually a loop ileostomy), on table lavage and primary anastomosis, or colonic stenting placement followed by semi-elective sigmoid resection.

Operative Therapy

Elective Management

- The proximal resection margin should be in soft pliable bowel; it is not necessary to resect all proximal diverticula.
- The distal resection margin is the proximal rectum, as anastomosis to the distal sigmoid is associated with a higher risk of recurrent diverticulitis.
- Ureteral stents are generally not necessary but may be used in selected cases.

Minimally Invasive Surgery

- Conventional laparoscopic techniques allow the surgeon to perform all the major portions of the case, including the anastomosis, through small 5 or 12 mm trocars (Fig. 39.9). "Hand-assisted" technique may also be useful.
- The dissection can be carried out using a medial to lateral or lateral to medial approach.
- It may be necessary to mobilize the splenic flexure to perform a tension-free anastomosis.
- The anastomosis can be performed in an intracorporeal fashion. Alternatively, the anastomosis can be fashioned through the specimen extraction site. Use of the extraction site in cases of fistulas or abscesses often allows the laparoscopic completion of colectomies in patients with severe disease without conversion. There are a wide range of published conversion rates.

- Minimally invasive colectomy has a number of benefits including shorter ileus and length of stay; decreased postoperative pain, wound infection rates, and operative blood loss; less transfusions; and a faster return to preoperative activity levels.

Urgent and Emergent Procedures

- The Hartmann procedure resects the diseased segment of the bowel, eliminates the septic focus, and allows for restoration of bowel continuity on an elective basis.
- All diseased and thickened bowel should be resected, and the resection margin should ideally be the proximal rectum. Alternatively, distal sigmoid, if not inflamed, can be left in place for later resection at the intended Hartmann reversal.
- The colostomy is generally left in place for at least 3 months, allowing the patient to sufficiently heal and facilitate identification of the Hartmann stump.
- Selection of patients who may safely undergo resection and primary anastomosis in the acute setting requires considerable judgment and must consider patient-related and disease-related factors.

Minimally Invasive Colectomy for Complicated Disease

- Patients with complicated disease undergo conversion to open procedures more frequently.

"Special Situations"

Recurrent Diverticulitis

- Recurrent diverticulitis following resection is uncommon. In the patient presenting with abdominal pain following resection for diverticulitis, a systematic evaluation should be performed to exclude other causes of pain.
- The most established risk factor for recurrent diverticulitis following resection is the level of anastomosis; the entire sigmoid should be resected and anastomosis performed to the proximal rectum.

Giant Colonic Diverticulum

- Two theories have been put forth for development of giant diverticulum; one proposed theory is that the diverticulum becomes massive because of a ball-valve mechanism allowing air into but not out of the diverticulum. Another theory suggests that air is trapped into the diverticulum because of gas-forming microorganisms without obstruction at the neck of the diverticulum.
  - Treatment consists of sigmoid resection with anastomosis.

Diverticulitis: Other Sites

Right Colonic Diverticulitis

- Right-sided diverticulitis is rare in Western countries and more common in the Far East.
- Cecal diverticula are of two types, both true and false.
  - True diverticula contain all layers of the bowel wall and are usually congenital and tend to be solitary.
  - Acquired diverticula of the cecum are false, containing mucosa and muscularis mucosa, tend to be multiple, and tend to be associated with diverticula elsewhere in the colon.
- Patients with cecal diverticulitis present at a younger age than the average patient with sigmoid diverticulitis.
- The main differential diagnosis is that of acute appendicitis, and it may be difficult in the patient with right-sided abdominal pain, fever, and leukocytosis to distinguish cecal diverticulitis from acute appendicitis.

Table 39.5 Cecal diverticulitis classification system

Grade 1	Easily recognizable projecting inflamed cecal diverticulum
Grade II	Inflamed cecal mass
Grade III	Localized abscess or fistula
Grade IV	Free perforation or ruptured abscess with diffuse peritonitis

- Laparoscopy is sometimes helpful to distinguish between cecal diverticulitis and appendicitis.
- In the absence of peritoneal signs, patients may be treated with antibiotics.
- For those patients with repeated attacks or complications including perforation or abscess, resection is indicated.
- A grading system has been suggested to aid with management of cecal diverticulitis (Table 39.5).

Rectal Diverticulitis

- Rectal diverticula are rare, are typically solitary, and are true diverticula including all layers of the bowel wall.

Transverse Colonic Diverticulitis

- Diverticulitis involving the transverse colon is rare; the prevalence of transverse colon diverticulitis has been found to be 2.6%.

Immunocompromised Patients

- Immunocompromised patients include patients on systemic steroids, patients with diabetes mellitus or renal failure, transplant patients who are immunosuppressed, patients with cirrhosis, patients with underlying malignancy, and patients being treated with chemotherapy.
- Patients who are immunosuppressed are more likely to present with free perforation and are therefore more likely to require emergency surgery with resultant increased postoperative morbidity and mortality.
- Immunocompromised patients who present with acute diverticulitis and require emergent laparotomy should typically undergo resection with colostomy and should not undergo primary anastomosis.

40 Large Bowel Obstruction

Karim Alavi and Charles M. Friel

Key Concepts

- Initial management of large bowel obstruction should include early correction of fluid and electrolyte abnormalities and surgical or endoscopic decompression.
- The current indications of endoluminal colonic stents include palliation in cancer and in patients who are medically unfit.
- After correction of fluid and electrolyte abnormalities in patients with acute colonic pseudo-obstruction, intravenous neostigmine should be attempted as the next step in management.
- Following successful endoscopic decompression of a sigmoid volvulus, given the high recurrence rates, the next step in management should be a segmental resection during the same hospitalization.
- CT scan is the imaging modality of choice for the diagnosis and subsequent management of large bowel obstruction.

Introduction

- Large bowel obstruction (LBO) is a common surgical emergency.
- While most causes are mechanical, a nonmechanical etiology (pseudo-obstruction) may be responsible.

Etiology

- Most LBOs are due to progressive narrowing of the bowel lumen caused by intrinsic lesions of the bowel wall (Table 40.1).
- The most common example of an intrinsic lesion is colorectal cancer, which accounts for nearly 50% of all LBOs.
- Approximately 10% of all colorectal cancer will present with evidence of a LBO.
- Diverticular disease also causes intrinsic compression of the lumen and is generally considered the second most common cause of LBO (~10–20%).
- Other less common examples of intrinsic narrowing include Crohn's disease, ischemia, endometriosis, and radiation, all of which can be difficult to distinguish from colorectal cancer.

K. Alavi (✉)
Department of Surgery, University of Massachusetts Medical School, Worcester, MA, USA
e-mail: karim.alavi@umassmemorial.org

C. M. Friel
Department of Surgery, University of Virginia Medical Center, Charlottesville, VA, USA

S. R. Steele et al. (eds.), *The ASCRS Manual of Colon and Rectal Surgery*,
https://doi.org/10.1007/978-3-030-01165-9_40

Table 40.1 Etiology of large bowel obstruction (LBO)

1. Intrinsic lesions
Colon cancer[a]
Diverticular disease[b]
Crohn's disease[c]
Endometriosis[c]
Radiation[c]
Ischemia[c]
2. Extrinsic lesions[c]
Non-colorectal malignancy (e.g., ovarian cancer)
Hernia
Adhesions
3. Volvulus[b]
4. Other[c]
Foreign body
Impaction
Acute colonic pseudo-obstruction (ACPO)

[a]Most common cause of LBO
[b]Common causes of LBO
[c]Uncommon causes of LBO

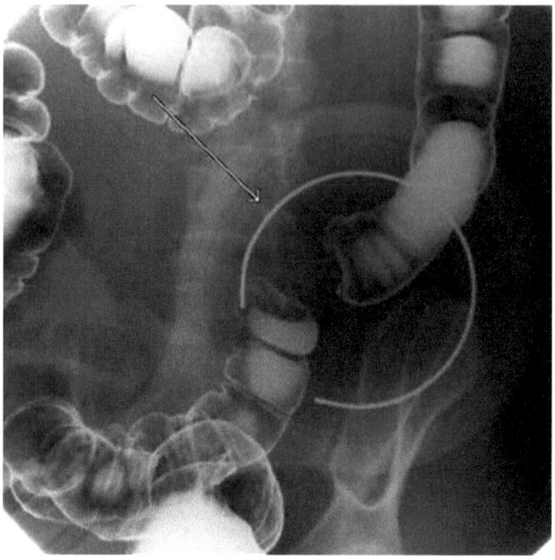

Fig. 40.1 Air contrast enema demonstrating apple-core lesion of the sigmoid colon

- The most common extrinsic compression is caused by a non-colorectal malignancy, such as ovarian cancer.
- Because both intrinsic and extrinsic compressions are slowly progressive, the clinical presentation of LBO is often insidious.
- Clinical presentation can be quite varied, and management strategies will have to be adjusted accordingly.
- Mild obstruction, or bowel stenosis, may cause symptoms such as pain, cramps, and constipation.
  - At colonoscopy, the endoscope may not pass through the stricture, and on barium enema the patient may have a classic "apple-core" lesion (Fig. 40.1).
  - Surgery can be planned on a semi-elective basis.
- Moderate obstruction will present with proximal bowel dilation and accumulation of feces and fluid upstream. These patients will be very distended on exam but may only have mild tenderness (Fig. 40.2).
- Severe obstruction will present similarly except signs of systemic toxicity are now present. These patients need immediate resuscitation and often require emergent surgery.

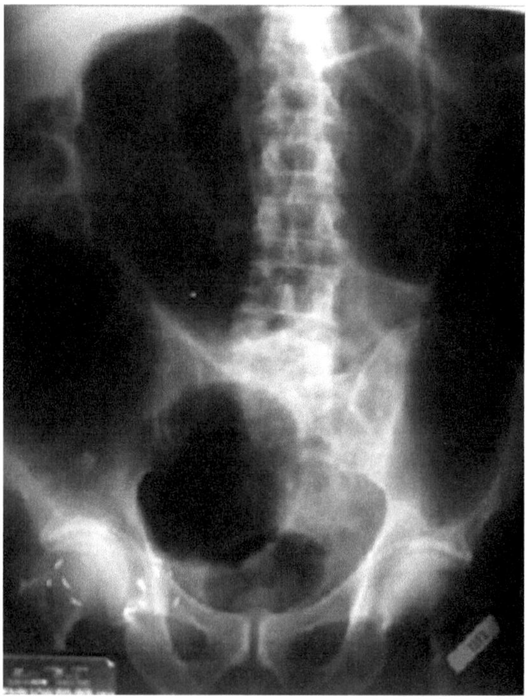

Fig. 40.2 Plain radiograph demonstrating a diffusely dilated colon

- The last major category of LBO is volvulus, a twisting of the redundant colon about the colonic mesentery (Fig. 40.3).

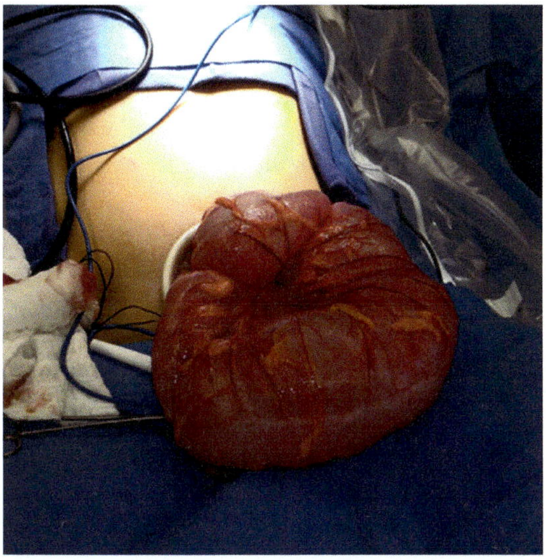

Fig. 40.3 Surgical findings of sigmoid volvulus

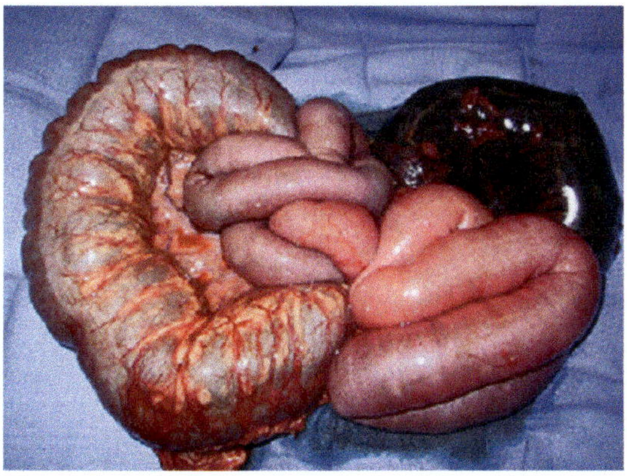

Fig. 40.4 Necrotic sigmoid colon in the setting of sigmoid volvulus and distended proximal colon

- Colonic volvulus accounts for approximately 10–15% of all LBOs reported in Western countries.
- Worldwide, however, colonic volvulus accounts for a significantly higher proportion of LBO.
- Sigmoid and cecal are by far the most common.
- Cecal volvulus tends to be in younger patients and has a slight female predilection.
- Lack of fixation of the cecum and ascending colon to the retroperitoneum seems to be a predisposing factor.
- Sigmoid volvulus seems associated with chronic constipation and elongation of the colon, indicative of an acquired pathology.
- Unlike other causes of LBO, a volvulus often presents acutely with rapid onset of distension and pain; the risk of strangulation and ischemia is significantly higher (Fig. 40.4).

Pathophysiology

- LBO, in the setting of a competent ileocecal valve and a distal obstruction or colonic volvulus, results in a closed-loop obstruction.
- As intraluminal pressure rises, intramucosal and intramural hypoperfusion leads to venous occlusion, followed by arterial occlusion, thrombosis, and eventual necrosis.
- The risk of progression to ischemia and subsequent necrosis is lessened to some degree by the presence of an incompetent ileocecal valve.
- According to Laplace's law (pressure = tension/radius), the tensile force on the wall of the colon is equal to the intraluminal pressure multiplied by the diameter of the segment in question; as such, the cecum is at the greatest risk for ischemia/perforation.
  - The cutoff for cecal diameter on plain abdominal film has long been cited to be 12 cm, above which the risk of ischemia and perforation increases.

Presentation

- Patients with LBO present with abdominal distension, crampy abdominal pain, and obstipation.
- On physical examination, patients present with a distended and tympanic abdomen.
- In the setting of ischemia, localized peritonitis along with signs of systemic sepsis may be present demanding urgent surgical exploration.

- There may be signs of intravascular volume depletion as the obstructed colonic segment becomes distended with fluid and gas.
- A digital rectal examination should be performed on all patients to evaluate for a distal neoplasm or fecal impaction.

Initial Resuscitation (Fig. 40.5)

- A flat and upright abdominal film can rapidly establish the diagnosis and exclude ischemia and/or associated perforation.
- Given the significant derangement in fluid and electrolytes, patients are usually in need of aggressive fluid resuscitation and correction of electrolyte abnormalities.
- The adequacy of resuscitation should typically be monitored with insertion of a urinary catheter.

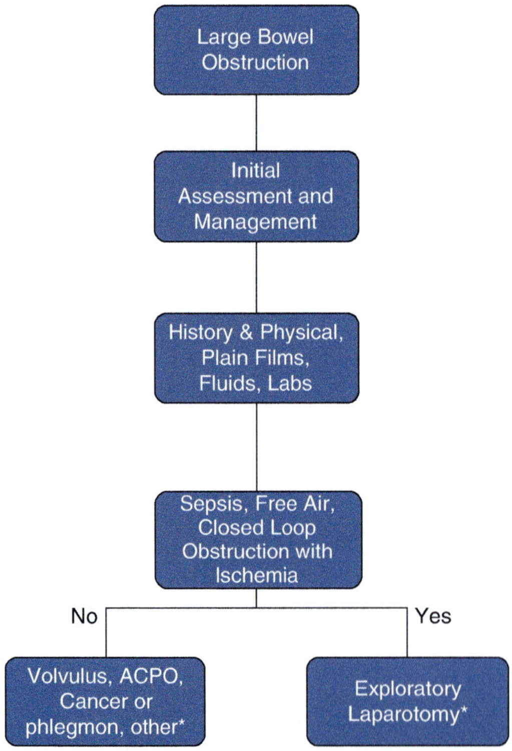

Fig. 40.5 Proposed algorithm for initial presentation and management of LBO. ACPO, acute colonic pseudo-obstruction; *see Algorithms 40.9, 40.10, 40.18, and 40.21

- Stable patients, without signs of localized or systemic sepsis, can be studied further with radiologic imaging.
- Diffuse peritonitis, however, mandates emergent surgical exploration.

Diagnostic Imaging

Abdominal Plain Film

- Plain abdominal films are usually the first diagnostic imaging performed as they are quick and inexpensive and provide immediate feedback.
  - They provide an estimation of colonic diameter, with a cecal diameter of 9–12 cm often considered concerning for impending perforation; however, the absolute cecal diameter associated with impending perforation is debatable.
  - Other variables such as the duration of distension appear to be important.
  - In some cases, such as foreign body or volvulus, a plain film may be all that is necessary.
  - Plain films may confirm the diagnosis of sigmoid volvulus by the classic presence of a "bent inner tube" or an "omega loop" pointing to the right upper quadrant (Fig. 40.6). However, these findings are present in only 50–70% of cases.
  - Conversely, cecal volvulus presents with a "coffee bean" deformity pointing to the left upper quadrant (Fig. 40.7).
- If the patient's condition permits, additional studies may be necessary to establish the diagnosis.

Contrast Enema (CE)

- CE may establish the diagnosis and localize the site of obstruction.
- Water-soluble contrast is preferred as the mortality of peritonitis secondary to barium is high if perforation is encountered.

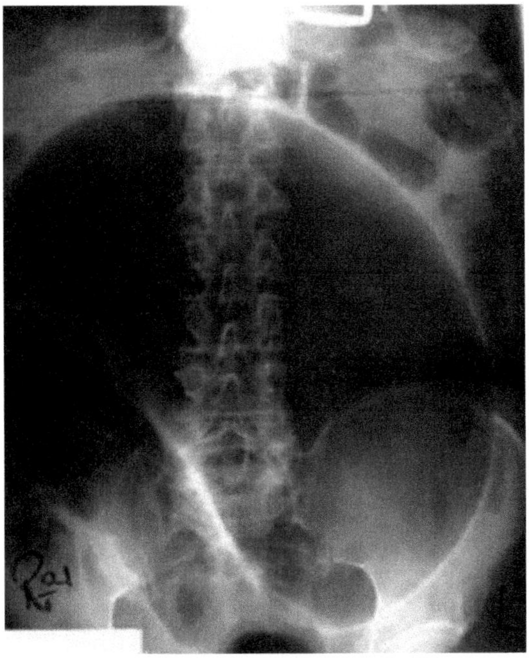

Fig. 40.6 Plain radiograph demonstrating "bent inner tube" sign of sigmoid volvulus with apex pointing to the right

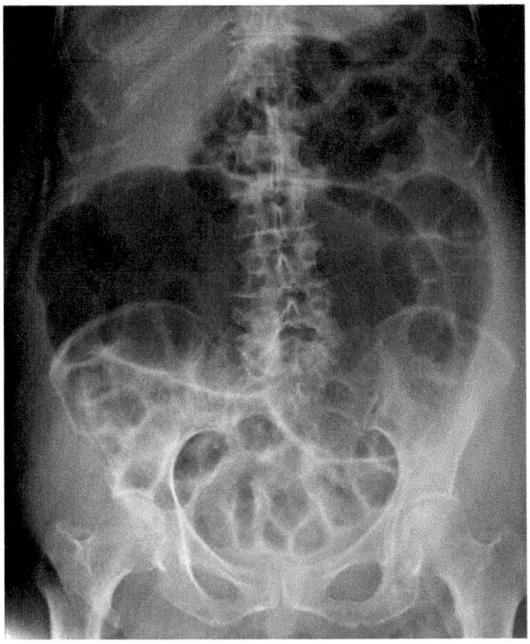

Fig. 40.7 Plain radiograph demonstrating "coffee bean "sign of cecal volvulus with apex pointing to the left

- CE classically shows a "bird's beak" deformity at the site of the torsion or obstruction.

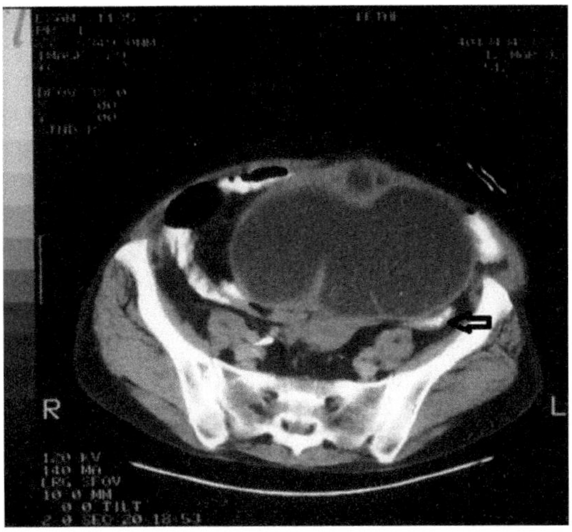

Fig. 40.8 Pelvic extra-colonic lesion causing LBO due to extrinsic compression. Arrow points to compressed descending colon

- CE in colonic pseudo-obstruction will show free flow of contrast proximally with no obstruction or transition point.
- CE may demonstrate a wisp of contrast through a narrowed channel and provide insight into the role of endoluminal stenting.

Computed Tomography

- Computed tomography (CT) is often the imaging modality of choice and provides valuable diagnostic information, such as the presence of proximal lesions, extrinsic disease, closed-loop obstruction, or distant metastasis, helping guide management (Fig. 40.8).
- Generally, CT is easier to obtain and has largely supplanted CE as the diagnostic modality of choice for the diagnosis of LBO.

Management

- Management of LBO is complex and can challenge even the most experienced surgeon.
- The rapidity with which decompression is achieved depends on the severity of the stenosis, acuity of the presentation, baseline clinical status of the patient, and the presence of overt sepsis.

- The treatment algorithm is often guided by provider expertise, availability of resources, and resectability/location of the obstructing lesion.

Emergent Setting (Fig. 40.5)

- Regardless of the etiology, patients presenting with LBO and signs of peritonitis, perforation, or closed-loop obstruction with evidence of ischemia or gangrene require emergent surgery following initial resuscitative efforts. If the patient's condition permits, the stoma site should be marked preoperatively.
- Broad-spectrum antibiotics should be administered with good aerobic and anaerobic coverage.
- Entry of the abdomen is usually best achieved through a midline incision as the distended colon often precludes laparoscopic exploration.
- The proximal dilated colon can be decompressed by passage of a 12-gauge needle obliquely through the taenia coli of the transverse colon and attaching it to suction. This allows for immediate decompression and enhances handling.

Unresectable Lesion (Fig. 40.9)

- Proximal diversion without resection of the primary obstructing lesion may be required in the setting of diffuse carcinomatosis, hemodynamic instability, or an unresectable mass.
- Proximal diversion, such as loop colostomy, is also appropriate in the setting of an obstructing

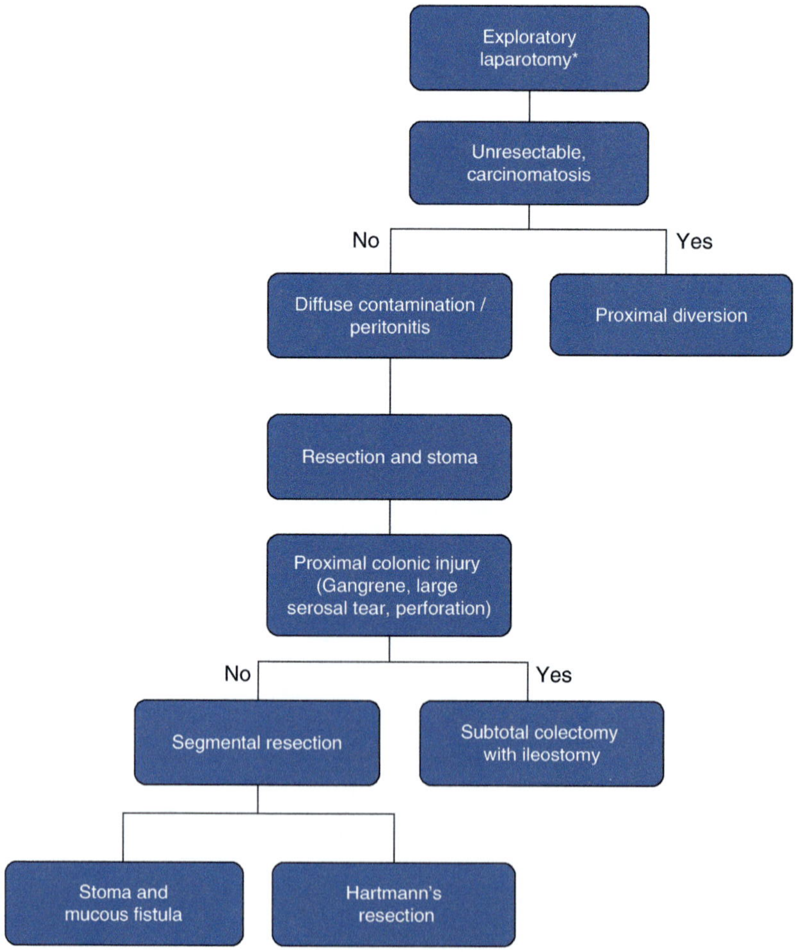

Fig. 40.9 Proposed algorithm for patients presenting with LBO and associated closed-loop obstruction with ischemia, free air, or sepsis

rectal cancer; this allows time for treatment with neoadjuvant chemoradiation, improving resectability of the primary lesion when indicated.

Resectable Lesion (Fig. 40.10)

- Following resection of the obstructing lesion, the decision to restore intestinal continuity is dependent of the intraoperative findings and the general condition of the patient.
- If anastomosis is deemed unwise, the distal colon conduit should be exteriorized as a mucous fistula or buried in the subcutaneous tissue in the inferior pole of the midline incision or at the stoma site when possible. This allows for ease of access and early identification during reversal surgery.
- In the presence of proximal ischemia, perforation, coexisting lesion, or large serosal injury of the cecum, a subtotal colectomy may be indicated (Fig. 40.11).
- Given the difficulty in identifying the underlying etiology in an emergent setting, efforts should be made to perform an en bloc resection following oncologic principles where appropriate.

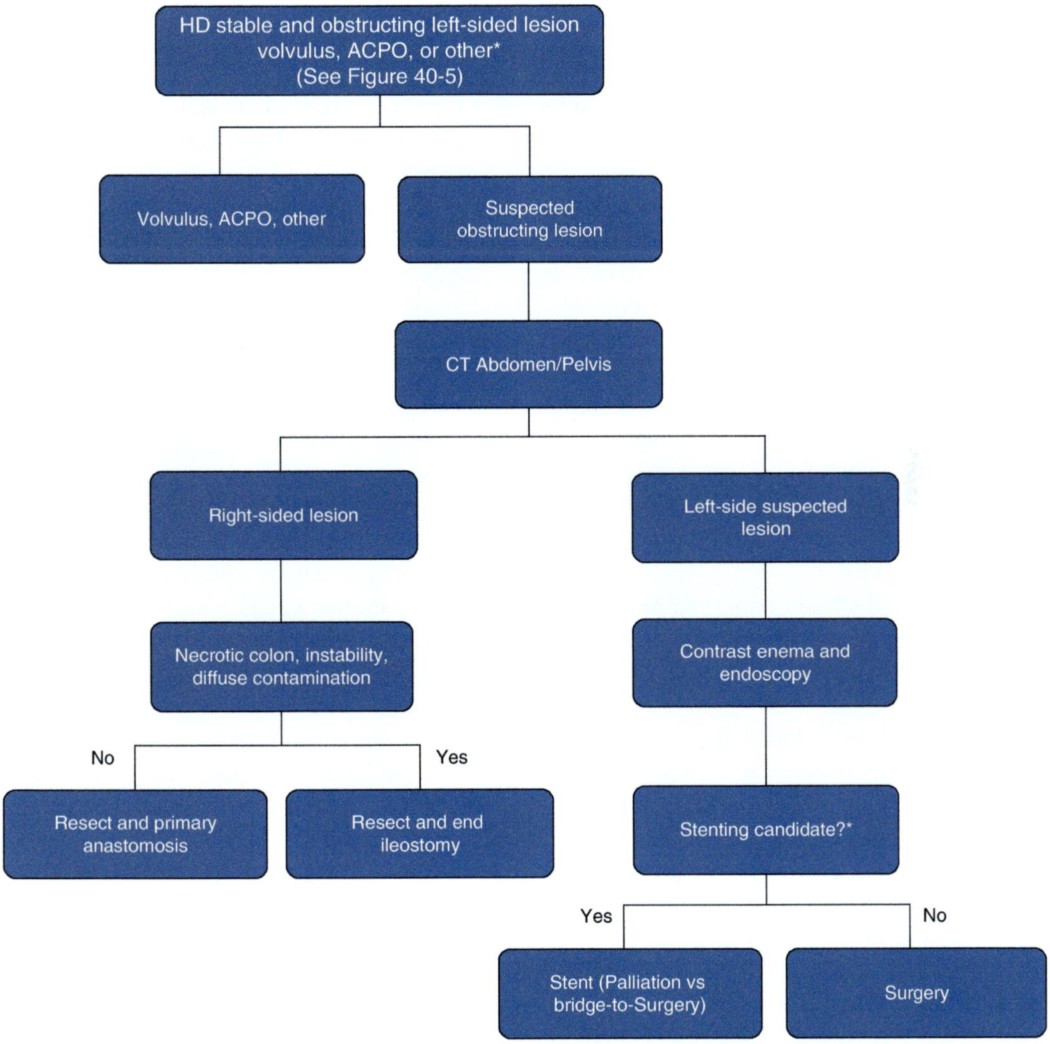

Fig. 40.10 Proposed algorithm for LBO in a stable patient secondary to a left-sided lesion (diverticular or Crohn's phlegmon, cancer, or unclear etiology)

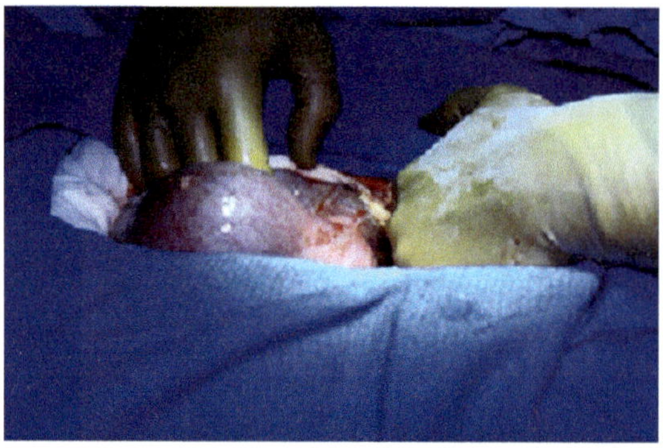

Fig. 40.11 Distended and tense cecum with large serosal tear along the antimesenteric wall

Non-emergent Setting (Fig. 40.10)

- LBO proximal to the splenic flexure should be managed by primary resection and anastomosis in a hemodynamically stable patient with no overt signs of sepsis, free air, or generalized peritonitis.
- The management of LBO secondary to lesions distal to the splenic flexure is more complex, challenging, and controversial. Endoluminal stenting, resection/primary anastomosis with or without proximal fecal diversion, staged resection with end stoma, on-table colonic lavage, and subtotal colectomy may all be applicable options.

Endoscopy and CE

- Endoscopy and CE are important tools in the initial management of LBO and should be considered early, both as part of diagnosis and management.
- Endoscopy aids in the initial diagnosis. The risk of perforation and worsening obstruction can be obviated by the use of CO2 insufflation.
- If a colonic stent is contemplated, a CE is often obtained first to define the presence and anatomy of the channel and its suitability for stent deployment.

Self-Expanding Metallic Stents

- Over the last several decades, enteral stenting has emerged as an alternative to surgery for many obstructions of the GI tract.
- Colonic stenting is an alternative to relieve colonic obstruction, potentially obviating the need for emergency surgery and the associated morbidity.
- SEMS are used either for palliation or as a "bridge to surgery."
- Patients who present with incurable disease and who have limited life expectancy may be able to avoid major surgery and the need for a colostomy with the successful placement of a colonic stent.
- Obstructed patients with curable disease may be stented and then prepared for an elective procedure, allowing the opportunity to medically optimize patients, to complete a full colonoscopy, and to decompress a distended colon. Patients may then be candidates for a minimally invasive approach and a primary anastomosis.
- Complications of stents include technical failure, stent migration, re-obstruction, and perforation.
- A wide range of perforation rates have been reported in the literature (0–83%) with a median of 4.5%. Perforations can either be immediate, often from the guidewire, or delayed.
- Perforation is also more likely with the use of balloon dilation, which causes a rapid expansion of the strictured area, and should be avoided.
- Delayed perforations are more common with stents that are placed for palliation as these stents are present for a prolonged period.
- Several studies suggest a high rate of stent perforations in patients who are receiving bevacizumab for treatment of metastatic disease.
- In the setting of potentially curable cancer, these perforations could negatively impact oncologic outcomes and remain a major concern with the use of colonic stents.

Technique

- The majority of the literature on colonic stenting focuses on obstruction secondary to left-sided colon cancer.
- When even a small amount of contrast passes through the lesion, the likelihood of passing a wire should also increase, which is the first important step in successful deployment of a stent (Fig. 40.12).

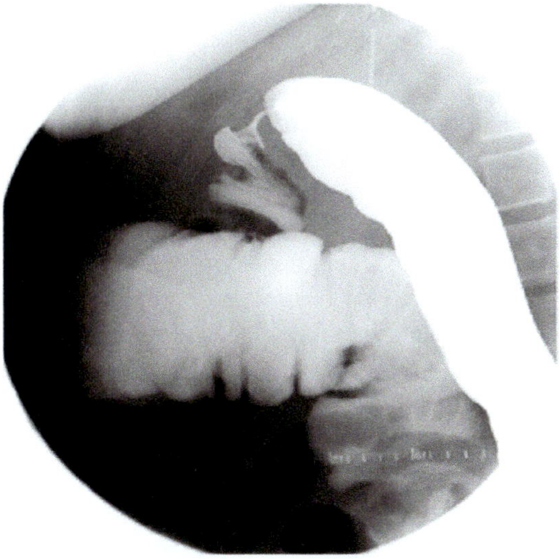

Fig. 40.12 Water-soluble contrast enema in a patient with LBO demonstrating narrow channel and apple-core lesion with proximal colon dilatation

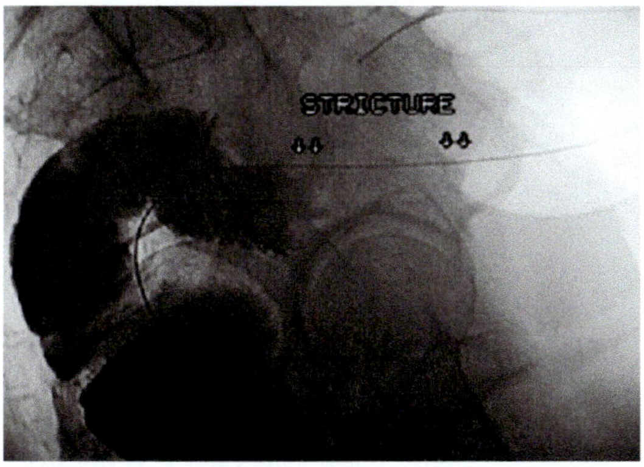

Fig. 40.13 Fluoroscopy demonstrating successful passage of guidewire across stricture

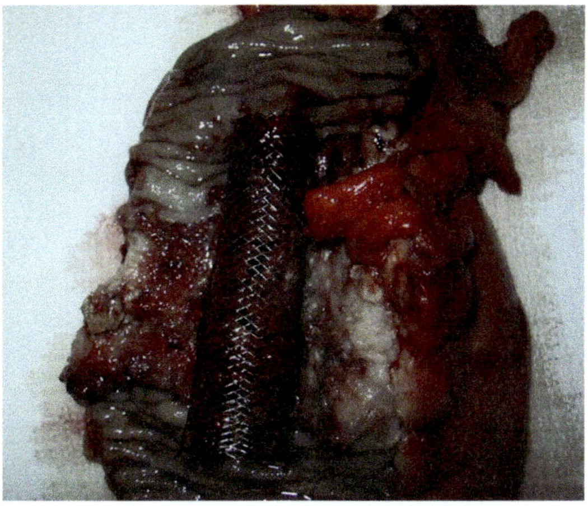

Fig. 40.14 Gross picture of stent across tumor with appropriate overlap above and below tumor

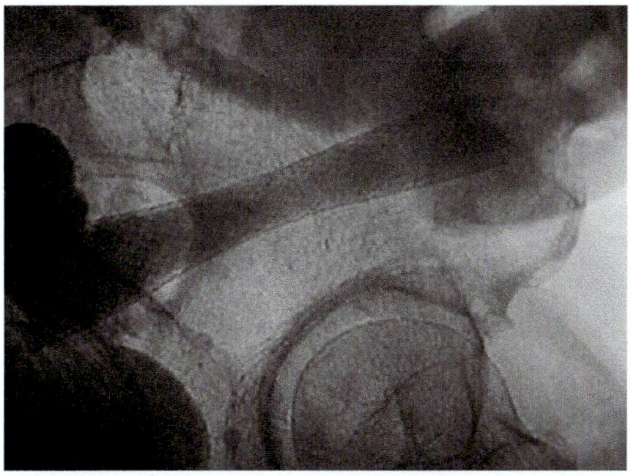

Fig. 40.15 Radiograph demonstrating excellent positioning of the stent across stricture with the characteristic waisting at mid-stent

- SEMS have been placed using fluoroscopic guidance alone or with a combination of endoscopy and fluoroscopy.
- The colonoscope can be passed to the lesion and the area inspected. Contrast can then be injected to outline the extent of the lesion and to estimate its length and contour.
- A guidewire is then passed through the strictured area and the location confirmed using fluoroscopy (Fig. 40.13).
- Once the guidewire is in place, two colonic stent systems have been described. The "through-the-scope" (TTS) system will allow the stent to be placed through the therapeutic channel of the colonoscope and then over the wire. Alternatively, if the stent will not fit through the channel, the stent can be placed entirely over the wire using the "over-the-wire" (OTW) technique.
- Ideally the stent should be deployed with at least 2 cm of overlap above and below the stricture (Fig. 40.14).
- Upon completion, plain films can be obtained to confirm stent location, demonstrating appropriate waisting at mid-stent, and to ensure colonic decompression (Fig. 40.15).
- Once successfully deployed, the obstruction should resolve over the next few days allowing patient evaluation to be completed. For patients with resectable tumors, definitive surgery is best done within 7–14 days of stent placement.

Results

"Bridge to Surgery"

- Technical success rate is approximately 90%.
- Multicenter, prospective, randomized trials looking at immediate emergency surgery compared with stenting followed by surgery have reported technical successes in only 53% and 70% of patients. Furthermore, stoma rates did not differ between the surgery and stenting arms. Of particular concern were the rates of perforation, reported at 19% in one study:
  - There were a number of "silent" perforations that were not clinically identified but were discovered at the time of surgery and pathological evaluation.
  - These studies were prematurely closed due to safety concerns with colonic stents. The major criticism of these studies is the low success rate of stent placement and the complication rates observed.

Palliation

- Colonic stenting may be appropriate for patients presenting with inoperable cancer. This is particularly true of patients with short life expectancy due to advanced disease. Many of these patients can be successfully palliated without the need for a stoma or a major abdominal procedure.
- Stents are more likely to re-obstruct over time than with surgery, but can often be treated with additional procedures, including a second stent.
- Stent complications accumulate over time, and at 6 months nearly 40% of the patients have had some complication related to the stent. Despite these problems, however, only a small number require a colostomy for palliation.

Benign Disease and Right-Sided Lesions

- The role of stenting for benign diseases, such as diverticular disease and Crohn's disease, remains unclear:
  - These strictures tend to be long and tortuous, making for a challenging stenting procedure. Complication rates seem to be higher.
  - Long-term uses of stents under these conditions are often associated with perforations, fistula, and pain and should be avoided.
- While there are reports of stenting right-sided obstructions, the rationale for this approach is less clear since obstructions proximal to the splenic flexure can be managed with a primary anastomosis.

Resection

- A traditional three-stage operation is rarely performed but may be necessary in the setting of diffuse carcinomatosis, non-resectable inflammatory phlegmon, cancer with dense adherence to critical pelvic or retroperitoneal structures, or inexperience of the surgical team.
- A two-stage operation, with either resection of the obstructed segment or primary anastomosis with proximal diversion (Hartmann's procedure), is more commonly performed.
- The advantages of the Hartmann's procedure include avoidance of an anastomosis and shorter operative times. However, 35–55% of colostomies are not reversed, either due to patient wishes or existing comorbidities. Further, reversal of the Hartmann's procedure is associated with substantial morbidity, including anastomotic leak rates ranging from 4% to 16%.
- Primary anastomosis, when feasible and advisable, should be the procedure of choice for LBO. Variables influencing the decision to perform a primary anastomosis include the degree of proximal colon dilatation, clinical condition of the patient, and operative findings, such as diffuse fecal contamination, peritonitis, cecal perforation, and synchronous neoplasm.
- Subtotal colectomy with a primary anastomosis is a viable option in select patients presenting with a left-sided LBO. Accepted indications for subtotal colectomy include cecal perforation, synchronous proximal lesion, ischemia of the proximal colon, or serosal injury of the

cecum. In general, the decision to perform a subtotal colectomy depends on the overall condition of the patient, operative findings, continence status, and comorbidities.

On-Table Colonic Lavage

- When patients are clinically stable, an on-table colonic lavage may successfully relieve the colonic distension and fecal loading, enabling primary anastomosis.

Technique

- On-table colonic lavage is best accomplished once the obstructing lesion has been resected.
- Mobilizations of both flexures are done to facilitate the procedure.
- An appendectomy is performed and a large-bore catheter inserted into the cecum, secured with a purse string. Alternatively, if the cecum is distended and thin-walled, the catheter can be inserted in the terminal ileum with a purse string.
- Sterile corrugating tubing is then secured to the descending colon using an umbilical tape. The tubing is draped over the bed into a waste container (Fig. 40.16).
- Saline can then be used to irrigate the colon until it is clear which usually requires approximately 3–6 liters. Initially flow can be slow due to the solid stool, and the surgeon may need to milk some of these contents through the tubing. However, once the stool becomes more liquid, the cleansing process flows smoothly.

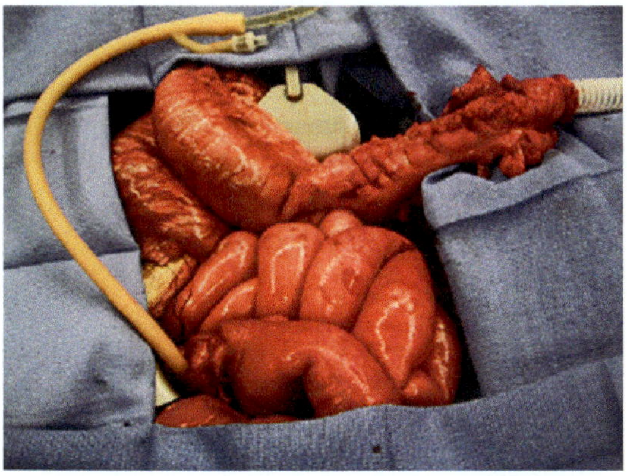

Fig. 40.16 Technique for on-table lavage prior to creation of the anastomosis following a left colectomy for LBO. Sterile corrugated tubing is secured to the descending colon using umbilical tape. Both the hepatic and splenic flexures have been mobilized to aid in the evacuation

- Upon completion of this procedure, the colon is often significantly decompressed, and an anastomosis can be performed.
- Alternatively, a Y connector and a long colonic tube may be placed through the descending colon just proximal to the obstructing lesion and passed into the cecum. The warmed saline can then be administered through the tubing, and fluid is evacuated out the other side of the Y connector (Fig. 40.17).

Results

- Major disadvantages include the additional time to perform, which can be as much as 60 min, and the additional dissection it often requires.
- Anastomotic leak rates appear acceptable.

Special Circumstances

Volvulus

Sigmoid Volvulus

Presentation and Diagnosis

- If peritonitis is present, then ischemia and/or gangrene of the colon must be assumed, and further diagnostic testing is unnecessary. Emergent exploration and resection, with or without a stoma, is recommended.
- In the non-emergent setting, an abdominal radiograph is usually the first diagnostic test obtained. Plain radiographs are diagnostic for a sigmoid volvulus in 57–90% of patients. However, the classic "coffee bean" or "bent inner tube" sign is present in <60% of cases (Fig. 40.6).
- CT scan or CE may confirm the presence of a sigmoid volvulus by a bird's beak deformity on the left side compared to a right upper quadrant location for a cecal volvulus.
- Sigmoid volvulus is the most common cause of intestinal obstruction in pregnancy worldwide.

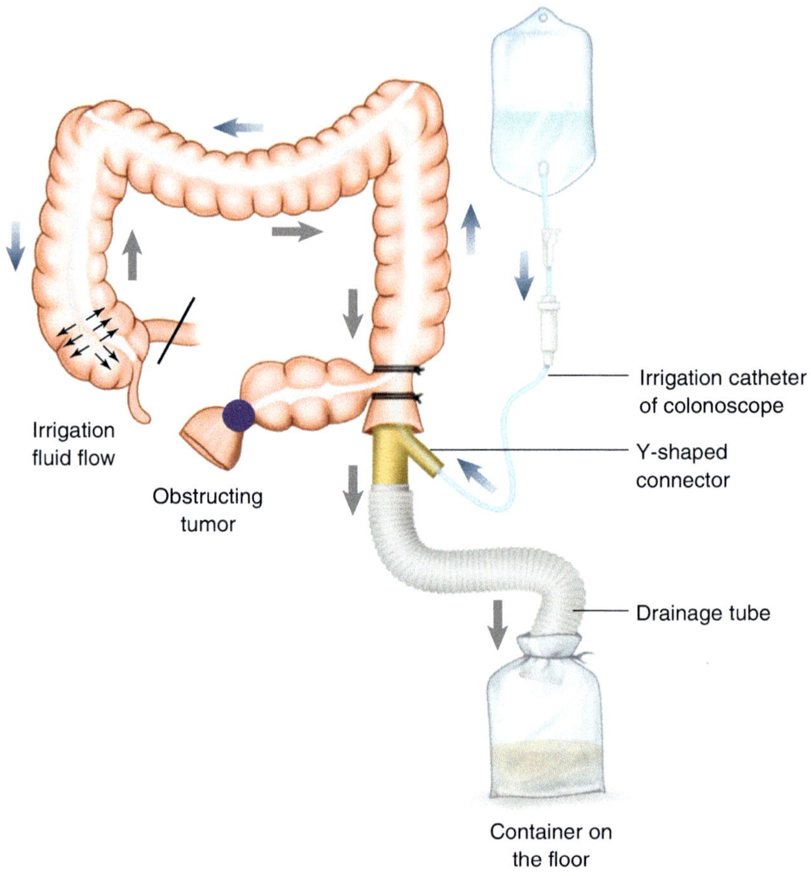

Fig. 40.17 The new device for intraoperative colonic lavage, with an irrigation catheter or colonoscope entering the proximal colon through the Y-shaped connector up to the cecum. Flow of prewarmed saline solution irrigation (clear arrow). Flow-back of feces (black arrow)

Treatment

- Endoscopic reduction and decompression are the initial treatments of choice in uncomplicated sigmoid volvulus.
- Flexible endoscopy is preferred due to its overall safety and ability to inspect the mucosa of the involved segment for ischemia. The characteristic finding on endoscopy includes a "pinwheel" configuration of the mucosa (Fig. 40.18). Detorsion and decompression are successful in 60–80% of cases.
- A long flexible tube, such as a small caliber chest tube or nasogastric tube, may be left in place to allow for continued decompression and to prevent retorsion.
- Elective resection, preferably during the same hospital setting, following successful reduction is strongly recommended as endoscopic decompression alone has recurrence rates ranging from 20% to 90%.
- The standard procedure includes a sigmoid resection and primary anastomosis accomplished using either open or minimally invasive techniques. Due to the redundancy of the colon and elongated and narrowed mesentery of the sigmoid colon, an open approach utilizing a mini-laparotomy incision is usually all that is required.
- If endoscopic decompression is unsuccessful or if there is concern for gangrene of the colon, emergent exploratory laparotomy and sigmoid resection are indicated.
- Emergent surgery for sigmoid volvulus is associated with significant morbidity and mortality and should be avoided if possible.

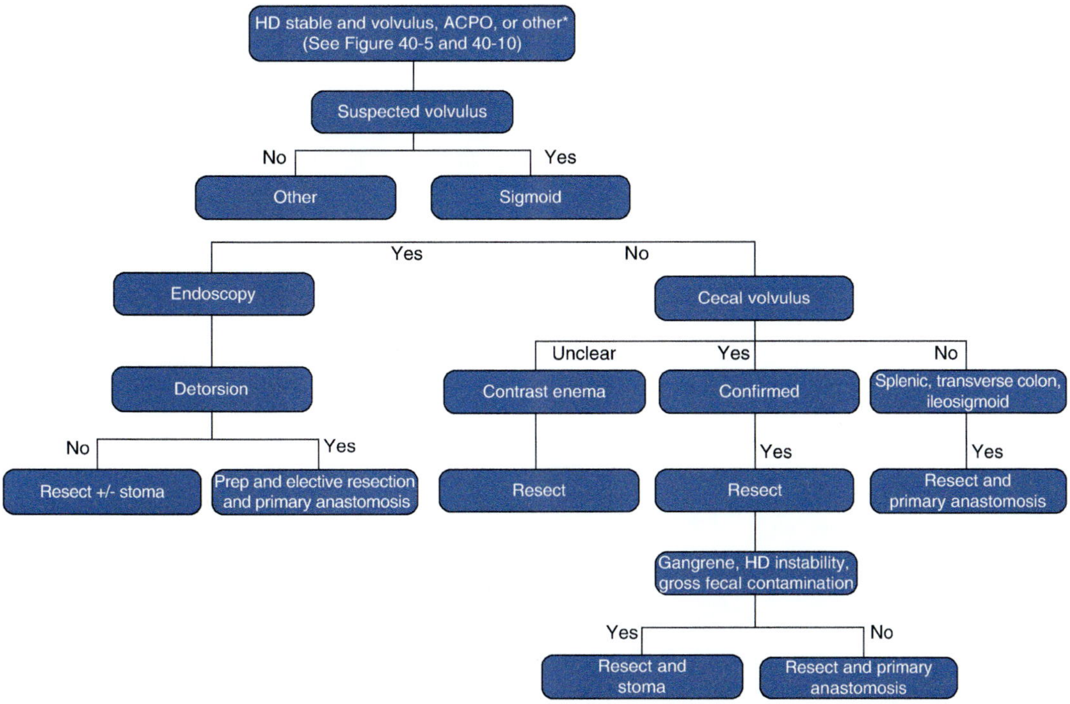

Fig. 40.18 Proposed algorithm for LBO secondary to a volvulus in a stable patient

Cecal Volvulus

Presentation and Diagnosis

- Cecal volvulus involves the axial clockwise rotation of the colon around its mesentery. Findings such as abdominal distension, pain, nausea, vomiting, and obstipation can mimic signs and symptoms of small bowel obstruction.
- Diagnosis is suspected by the classic appearance of a dilated colon in the shape of a "coffee bean" with the apex pointing to the left upper quadrant (Fig. 40.7).
- This classic radiographic finding, however, is present in less than 20% of cases. If the diagnosis is in question, a CE can provide clarity by demonstrating the characteristic column of contrast ending in a "bird's beak," with the site of the torsion in the right upper quadrant. If CE is unavailable or the diagnosis remains in question, a CT scan may be helpful in establishing the diagnosis.
- In cecal bascule, there is no axial twist but an anterior-superior folding of the cecum over the proximal ascending colon, without rotation (Fig. 40.19). The cecum is often located in the right upper quadrant on imaging.

Treatment

- Endoscopic attempts at decompression of a cecal volvulus are typically unsuccessful and should not be attempted.
- Exploratory laparotomy is the treatment of choice.
- In the setting of a gangrenous colon, attempts should not be made to untwist the colon prior to resection due to the risk of the release of toxins and ensuing shock. The extent of hemodynamic instability, contamination, malnutrition, and comorbidities will determine the safety of a primary anastomosis following resection.
- Non-resection techniques such as cecopexy have also been described, but their role, if any, is unclear.

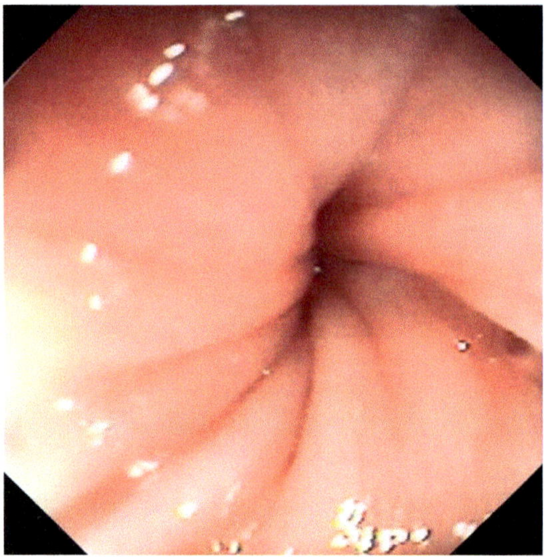

Fig. 40.19 Classic endoscopic "pinwheel" appearance of a sigmoid volvulus

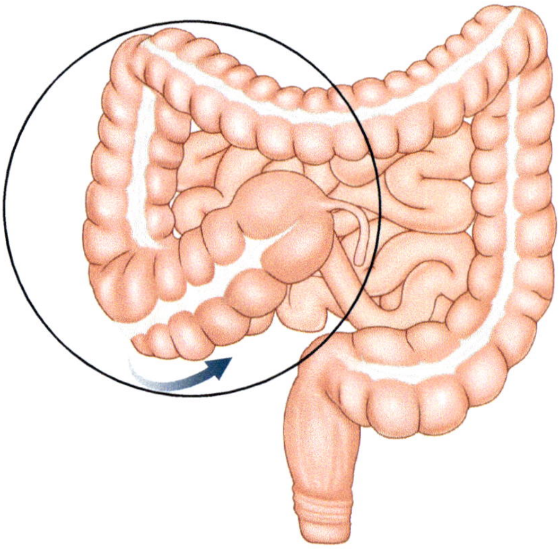

Fig. 40.20 Illustration of cecal bascule demonstrating the anterior-superior folding of the mobile cecum over the proximal ascending colon

Uncommon Types

Ileosigmoid Knotting

- Ileosigmoid knotting is the wrapping of the ileum around the sigmoid colon leading to obstruction (Fig. 40.20).
- Imaging may suggest the diagnosis by a distended sigmoid colon on the right and distended small bowel loops on the left.
- Seventy percent of patients will have gangrenous bowel at surgery.
- Four variants of the ileosigmoid knot have been described.
- The intraoperative options are largely dependent on the overall condition of the patient, the anatomy of the ileosigmoid knot, the state of the bowel segments involved, and the surgeon's experience. It is not uncommon that several segmental resections are required with creation of one or several anastomoses.

Splenic and Transverse Colon Volvulus

- Patients with either a transverse or splenic flexure volvulus will present with symptoms of acute or chronic LBO. Due to the rarity of its presentation, diagnosis is often delayed risking necrosis of the involved segment and increased mortality.
- Treatment typically involves surgical exploration and resection with or without a primary anastomosis. Similar to other types of volvulus, the decision to create a stoma depends on several factors, including the overall condition of the patient and the bowel, the degree of contamination, and the feasibility of the anastomosis.

Acute Colonic Pseudo-Obstruction (ACPO)

- The distinction between functional and mechanical causes of LBO usually requires CE or CT scan. Common findings include proximal colonic dilatation and a transition at or near the splenic flexure.
- The majority of patients with ACPO can be managed conservatively with bowel rest, aggressive fluid and electrolyte replacement, and elimination of offending agents, if possible (Fig. 40.21). In general, supportive measures alone are successful in about 70% of patients with morbidity and mortality rates of 6% and 10%, respectively.
- When supportive measures fail, more advanced treatment options become necessary. Historically, colonoscopic decompression has been the treatment of choice, usually after 3–4 days of failed supportive therapy.

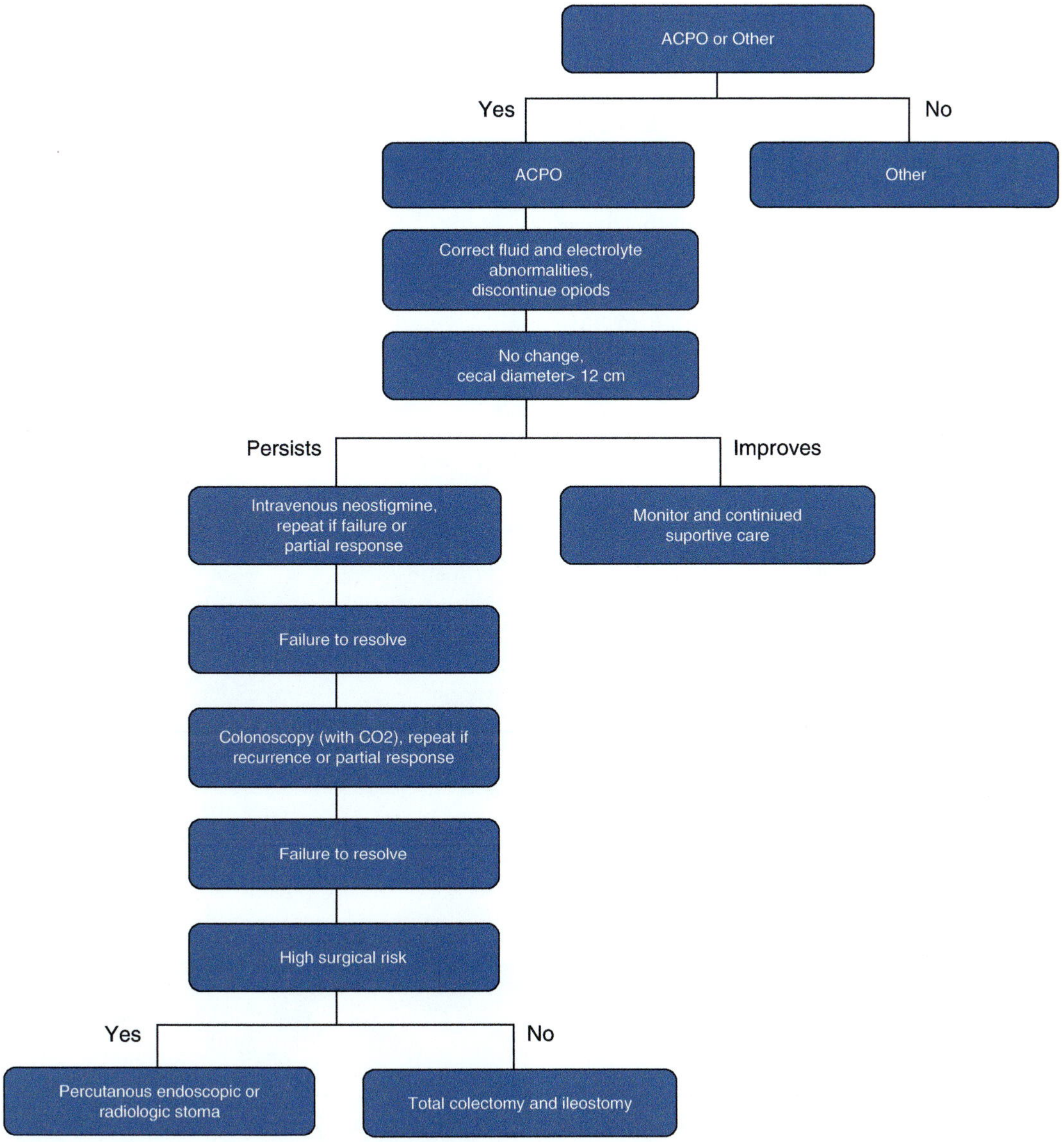

Fig. 40.21 Proposed algorithm for LBO secondary to ACPO

- Multiple prospective studies have validated the use of neostigmine as first-line treatment in ACPO.
- Neostigmine is a reversible acetylcholinesterase inhibitor, thus increasing acetylcholine and promoting intestinal activity. The standard dose is a 2–2.5 mg bolus administered over a 3–5 min period. The onset of action is usually 20–30 min. A repeat dose may be necessary in refractory cases.
- The parasympathetic activity of neostigmine can lead to adverse events, including bradycardia, hypotension, asystole, seizures, restlessness, nausea, emesis, and abdominal cramps. Patients should be closely monitored in a telemetry unit for cardiac arrhythmia. Relative contraindications to its use include recent myocardial infarction, acidosis, asthma, chronic obstructive pulmonary edema, bradycardia, renal insufficiency, and therapy with β-blockers.
- Recurrence rates after neostigmine administration vary from 17% to 38%.
- When supportive and pharmacologic measures fail, endoscopic decompression is recommended.

- Colonoscopy for ACPO should be performed without administration of oral laxatives or bowel preparation and with minimal air insufflation. If available, carbon dioxide (CO2) should be substituted.
- Endoscopic advancement to the level of the hepatic flexure is usually sufficient to achieve decompression.
- Success rates of colonoscopic decompression alone vary ranging from 61% to 95% after an initial procedure and 73–88% after one or more procedures. Recurrences, however, continue to be problematic and have been reported to occur in up to 40% of patients.
- Cecostomy, via a mini-laparotomy or laparoscopy, can provide effective decompression of the colon while minimizing the morbidity of colon resection in refractory ACPO.
- In cases of ischemia or perforation, the extent of colon resection is dictated by the degree of colon involvement. If feasible, enough colon remnant should be left behind as either a mucous fistula or a long Hartmann's pouch, left buried in the subcutaneous tissue or intraperitoneally.

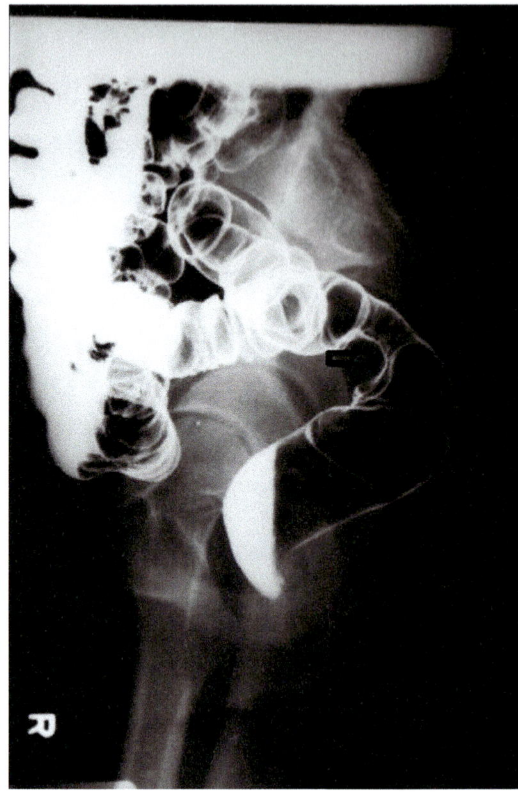

Fig. 40.22 Water-soluble CE demonstrating smooth narrowing at rectosigmoid due to endometrioma. Arrow points to sight of obstruction at rectosigmoid junction

Other

Endometriosis

- The rectum and sigmoid are the most common sites for implantation of ectopic endometrial implants in the gastrointestinal track and may lead to progressive luminal narrowing (Fig. 40.22).
- Typical symptoms include dyschezia, rectal bleeding, and constipation. Bowel obstruction occurs in less than 1% of patients.
- On endoscopy, a submucosal mass may be seen with eccentric wall thickening and narrowed lumen (Fig. 40.23).
- Patients often require a segmental resection and a low or ultra-low colorectal anastomosis performed as a single- or two-stage surgery.

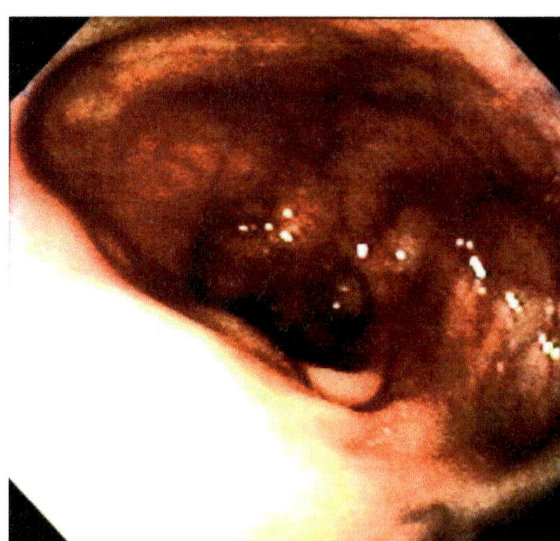

Fig. 40.23 Endoscopic appearance of submucosal causing luminal narrowing

Fecal Impaction

- The diagnosis is often confirmed by performing a digital rectal examination with the hallmark findings of copious hard or clay-like stool in the rectal vault.
- The traditional treatment of fecal impaction involves digital manipulation, enema instillation, or disimpaction under anesthesia. For more proximal impaction, the hydrostatic effects of a water-soluble contrast enema may be diagnostic and therapeutic. Starting a bowel maintenance program, following successful disimpaction, is critical.
- Laparotomy is rarely necessary and required only in the presence of complications such as stercoral ulcer perforation.

Gallstone

- Gallstone ileus, a rare complication of cholelithiasis, is an infrequent cause of mechanical bowel obstruction. The gallstone usually passes through a biliary-enteric fistula and lodges most commonly in the terminal ileum and ileocecal valve. LBO due to a migrating gallstone is even a rarer event, occurring in 4% of all patients presenting with gallstone ileus.
- Typical signs and symptoms of LBO are present in addition to pneumobilia on imaging. CT scan remains the gold standard for diagnosis.
- Surgical exploration and stone extraction via colotomy is often necessary. A simultaneous cholecystectomy is not recommended as patients typically have multiple comorbidities and are at risk of significant perioperative morbidity and mortality.

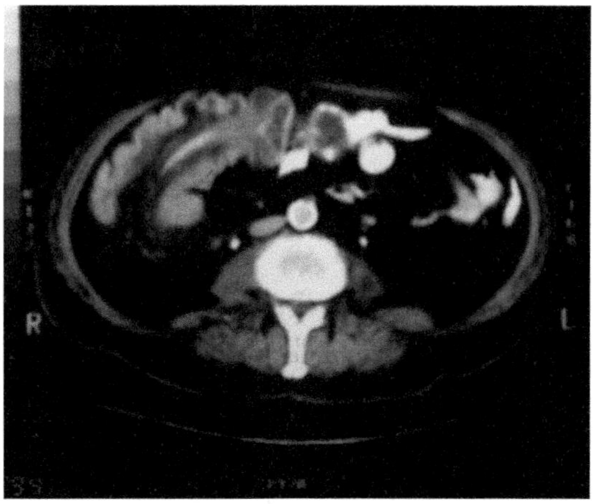

Fig. 40.24 CT scan demonstrating colo-colonic intussusceptions due to a lipoma

Intussusception

- Intussusception is a rare cause of bowel obstruction in adults with the majority occurring in the small bowel or ileocecal valve. Colo-colonic intussusceptions account for 17% of confirmed cases of intussusception.
- The majority of colonic intussusceptions are due to malignant lesions, primarily adenocarcinoma and lymphoma (Fig. 40.24). Benign causes, such as lipoma, adenomas, and Peutz-Jeghers polyps, have also been described.
- Due to the concern over malignancy, hydrostatic reduction is usually not recommended; segmental resection is typically required utilizing oncologic principles.

41 Lower Gastrointestinal Hemorrhage

Brian R. Kann and H. David Vargas

Key Concepts

- Common etiologies of lower gastrointestinal hemorrhage include diverticular disease, angioectasia, ischemic colitis, and neoplasm.
- The primary consideration in managing the patient with acute lower gastrointestinal hemorrhage is ensuring adequate volume resuscitation.
- Patients presenting with massive lower gastrointestinal bleeding should be evaluated for upper gastrointestinal and anorectal sources, via gastric lavage and anoscopy/proctoscopy.
- Screening for active bleeding via CT angiography or ^{99m}Tc-RBC scan increases the likelihood of identifying active bleeding on mesenteric angiography.
- An active bleeding source seen on mesenteric angiography can often be managed with superselective transcatheter embolization.
- The patient with a self-limited major lower gastrointestinal hemorrhage that has stopped should undergo colonoscopy for further evaluation after a mechanical bowel prep.
- In certain circumstances, colonoscopy for the evaluation of active lower gastrointestinal bleeding may be considered; if active bleeding is encountered, therapeutic options include clipping, injection, and argon plasma coagulation.
- The unstable patient with uncontrolled, unlocalized lower gastrointestinal hemorrhage should undergo a total abdominal colectomy, in most cases with an ileostomy.
- The patient with ongoing or recurrent hemorrhage from a localized lower gastrointestinal source may be managed with a targeted, segmental resection.
- Clinical pathways and predictive models may help better guide the management of patients with acute lower gastrointestinal hemorrhage, limiting unnecessary admissions and optimizing the use of resources.

Introduction

- Lower gastrointestinal bleeding (LGIB) refers to the passage of visible blood from the rectum and classically originates from a source distal to the ligament of Treitz.
- LGIB frequently stops spontaneously prior to definitive diagnosis.

B. R. Kann (✉) · H. D. Vargas
Department of Colon and Rectal Surgery, Ochsner Medical Center, New Orleans, LA, USA
e-mail: brian.kann@ochsner.org

S. R. Steele et al. (eds.), *The ASCRS Manual of Colon and Rectal Surgery*,
https://doi.org/10.1007/978-3-030-01165-9_41

Epidemiology

- There are over 1.7 million office visits in the USA for rectal bleeding.
- LGIB is a common cause for hospital admission.
- While LGIB affects both the young and the old, the incidence of LGIB increases dramatically with age as many of the conditions responsible for LGIB, such as diverticulosis coli and angioectasia, increase with time.

Etiologies of Lower Gastrointestinal Bleeding

Benign Anorectal Causes: Hemorrhoidal Bleeding and Fissures

- Hemorrhoidal bleeding accounts for 5–20% of all admissions for LGIB.
- Chronic bleeding from hemorrhoids over time may result in iron-deficiency anemia.
- Hemorrhoids and anal fissures are usually not a likely cause of massive lower GI hemorrhage.

Diverticulosis Coli

- It is estimated that 15% of patients with diverticulosis will develop bleeding as a complication.
- Diverticulosis is generally considered to represent the most common cause of LGIB not of anorectal etiology, accounting for 30–65% of cases.
- Diverticular bleeding is the most likely etiology of major lower GI hemorrhage.
- The presumed pathophysiology for diverticular bleeding involves the erosion of vasa recta through the mucosa at the neck or at the dome of the diverticulum.
- Risk factors that predispose to diverticular bleeding include the use of nonsteroidal anti-inflammatory drugs (NSAIDs), hypertension, and anticoagulant use.
- The diagnosis of a diverticular bleed is often considered presumptive, owing to the presence of diverticulosis on colonoscopy in the absence of another definitive bleeding site.
- Spontaneous cessation occurs in up to 80% of cases.
- The incidence of recurrent bleeding varies and has been noted to be as high as 40%.

Angioectasia

- Angioectasia [also known as angiodysplasia, arteriovenous malformations (AVMs), and vascular ectasias] is dilated, tortuous vascular abnormality of the submucosa (Fig. 41.1).
- The most widely accepted theory proposes that, with aging, low-grade obstruction of the submucosal veins results in incompetency of the precapillary sphincters, producing a small arteriovenous communication.
- Colonic angioectasias more commonly occur in the cecum and right side of the colon, tend to be multiple, and are estimated to be the underlying etiology of bleeding in 3–15% of LGIB episodes.

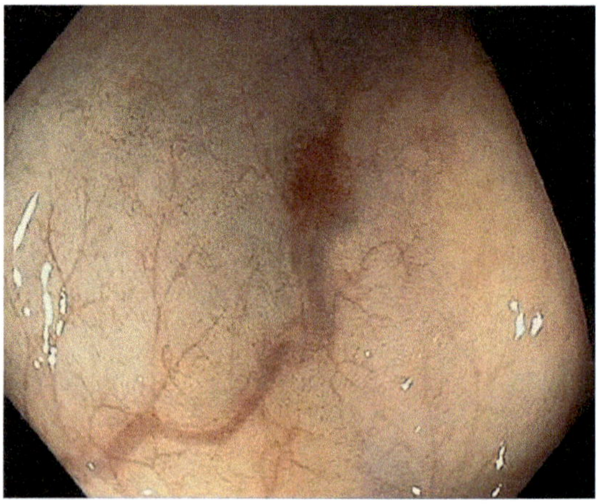

Fig. 41.1 Angioectasia, seen on colonoscopy

- The clinical presentation of LGIB due to angioectasia varies; the color of blood ranges from occult blood to melena to painless hematochezia. Angiodysplasia is characterized by chronic or recurrent LGIB.
- Factors that predispose to bleeding include increased age, comorbid conditions, multiple lesions, and the use of antiplatelet and anticoagulant therapy.
- Recurrent bleeding is associated with multiple lesions, anticoagulation and antiplatelet therapy, the number of prior bleeding episodes, and rate of bleeding (events/year).
- Angioectasias are most commonly found in the jejunum (80%), followed by the duodenum (51%), stomach (22.8%), right colon (11.4%), and ileum (5.4%); nearly two-thirds of patients have lesions in multiple locations.

Ischemic Colitis

- Ischemic injury of the colon is responsible for approximately 10% of cases of LGIB.
- Bleeding typically occurs as a result of reperfusion of an ischemic segment of the bowel, with sloughing of the mucosa and varying degrees of ulceration and necrosis (Fig. 41.2).
- Bleeding generally is less severe when compared to diverticular bleeding or that related to angioectasias.

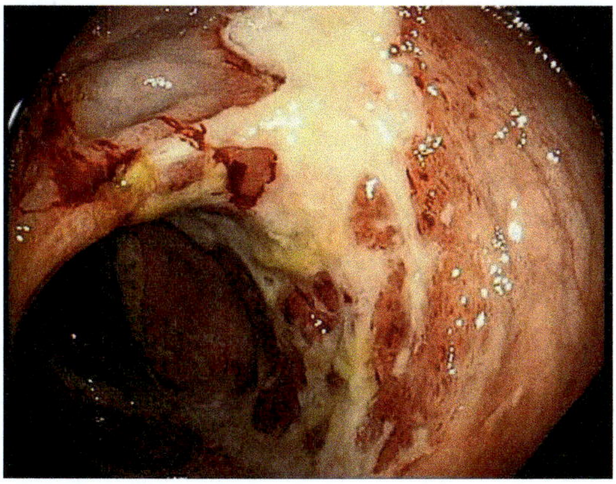

Fig. 41.2 Ischemic colitis, seen on colonoscopy

- "Ischemic colitis" generally refers to a less severe ischemic intestinal injury that tends to be transient and reversible.
- Certain segments of the hindgut appear more vulnerable to this transient interruption of blood flow. These segments classically are referred to as the "watershed" regions:
  - Splenic flexure (Griffiths' point), where vessels originating from midgut (superior mesenteric artery distribution) and hindgut (inferior mesenteric artery distribution) communicate via the marginal artery of Drummond.
  - Rectosigmoid colon (Sudeck's point) where the marginal artery generally is absent and the arterial blood supply is provided by end sigmoidal vessels with less collateral redundancy.
- Patients with ischemic colitis often present with cramping, abdominal pain, and associated tenderness localized to the left side of the abdomen. Typically, patients describe diarrheal stools that become bloody within 24 h of onset and can be either bright red or maroon-colored.
- Generally, bleeding from ischemic colitis is not severe, and blood transfusion is necessary in fewer than 5% of patients. Symptoms generally resolve quickly (within 2–3 days) due to rapid restoration of blood flow, and acute complications requiring surgical intervention occur rarely.
- Conversely, patients experiencing acute mesenteric vascular occlusion due to thromboembolism or mesenteric venous thrombosis, or those suffering from profound hypotension requiring vasopressor therapy (NOMI), are at greater risk for severe and irreversible ischemia, bowel necrosis, and need for urgent surgical intervention.
  - Patterns of ischemia tend to be either pancolonic or isolated right colonic ischemia (IRCI) and are more likely to be associated with small bowel ischemia and infarction.
  - Outcomes following surgical resection are associated with high mortality rates, ranging from 37% to 47%.

Neoplasms of the Large Intestine

- Acute massive hematochezia due to ulceration of the tumor is rare in the setting of colorectal cancer, and colorectal cancer represents less than 10% of all cases of LGIB requiring hospitalization.

Additional Causes of LGIB

- *Post-polypectomy hemorrhage* occurs in less than 1% of colonoscopic polypectomies. However, given the vast numbers of colonoscopies and polypectomies performed annually, this may account for up to 8% of all episodes of LGIB.
- *Inflammatory bowel disease* (IBD) commonly presents with lower gastrointestinal bleeding. However, severe, massive hemorrhage as the primary symptom prompting hospitalization occurs infrequently and accounts for less than 6% of patients.
- *Nonsteroidal anti-inflammatory drugs* (NSAIDs) increase the risk of LGIB, especially in patients with diverticular disease. Remarkably, the prevalence of NSAID use among patients experiencing LGIB remains high, reported to be 86% in one series.
  - The association of NSAID use and LGIB may be the result of a specific effect of the medication on the mucosa or alternatively may exacerbate an underlying condition such as diverticulosis.
- *Infectious hemorrhagic colitides* due to bacterial infection must be considered in the individual experiencing LGIB. Inflammatory diarrhea is characterized by bloody and mucopurulent stool that is often associated with fever, tenesmus, and severe abdominal pain.
  - Common pathogenic bacteria causing inflammatory diarrhea include *Campylobacter*, *Salmonella*, *Shigella*, enteroinvasive and enterohemorrhagic *Escherichia coli*, and *Yersinia* species. In North America, the most common clinically significant strain is *E. coli* O157:H7. The infection causes mucosal injury with resulting bloody diarrhea, which is generally self-limited, requiring only supportive care.
- *HIV-positive patients* may experience LGIB from a variety of potential causes. Viral infections, Kaposi's sarcoma, and sexually transmitted pathogens may cause bloody stools.
- *Radiation injury to the large intestine* can be either acute (< 3 months) or chronic. Chronic injury results in endarteritis obliterans that leads to neovascularization and telangiectasias, most commonly in the rectum.
  - The most common symptom of chronic radiation-induced proctitis remains rectal bleeding, while other associated symptoms include fecal urgency, incontinence, rectal pain, and mucoid discharge.
- *Ulceration of the rectum* has been described as a source of LGIB that can be severe and unrelenting, often requiring urgent colonoscopy and intervention. These ulcerations can result from stercoral injury or de novo in acutely ill patients.
- *Dieulafoy's lesions,* most commonly found in the stomach, may be located elsewhere in the gastrointestinal tract 30% of the time, including the colon, rectum, and small intestine. These lesions represent a rare cause of GI bleeding (1–2%).
  - Characteristic endoscopic findings describe a solitary vessel, histologically normal but large in diameter, without surrounding ulceration. Bleeding can be violent and voluminous and lead to life-threatening hemorrhage.
  - The cause of Dieulafoy's lesions remains uncertain and has occurred in acutely ill hospitalized patients as well as in newborn infants. Approximately 5% of Dieulafoy's lesions occur in the colon and rectum, with the right colon being the most common location.
- *Ectopic varices* represent another rare but sinister cause of LGIB. Ectopic (non-esophageal) varices may occur in up to 70% of patients with portal hypertension and cirrhosis. Rectal varices result from portosystemic shunting and decompression of the inferior mesenteric

vein and superior rectal veins via the middle and inferior rectal veins.

- Rectal varices do not prolapse, tend to be blue-gray in color, and may extend from the rectum superiorly to the squamous epithelium of the anus distally, in distinction to internal hemorrhoids, which may prolapse, tend to be purple in color, and generally do not extend proximally into the rectum.
- When bleeding occurs, hemorrhage can be massive and life threatening, requiring urgent intervention. Medical management includes consideration of decompression procedures such as transjugular intrahepatic portosystemic shunt (TIPS). Endoscopic techniques, such as injection sclerotherapy, as well as interventional radiology techniques, such as embolization, have been reported to be effective. While band ligation has been described as a treatment modality for esophageal varices, rectal varices less commonly are amenable to ligation technique, with variceal size (> 9 mm) being an important predictor of poorer outcome.

- *Obscure bleeding from a small intestinal source* has been estimated to account for 5% of LGIB episodes. Previously an anatomic territory difficult to image endoscopically, the small bowel can now be directly visualized using techniques such as device-assisted enteroscopy (balloon and double-balloon enteroscopy) and video capsule endoscopy. Such technologies prove far more sensitive than contrast studies or computed tomography and can identify many of the varied diagnoses causing bleeding, such as angioectasias, ulcerations, small bowel tumors, and IBD.
  - In younger patients with LGIB, one must always consider Meckel's diverticulum, especially when bleeding is acute and massive. Radionuclide imaging identifying ectopic gastric mucosa assists in confirming this diagnosis.

Table 41.1 summarizes the distribution of causes of LGIB, as reported in a number of large epidemiological studies.

Models Predicting Severity of Lower Gastrointestinal Bleeding

- Patients presenting with LGIB represent a considerable challenge, given the heterogeneous nature of causes, spectrum of severity, and often elusive nature owing to spontaneous cessation of bleeding prior to definitive diagnosis.
- While occasionally dramatic in presentation, the vast majority of patients with LGIB do not require surgical intervention.
- Although predictive models have been developed and validated, it is unclear as to what extent their implementation will impact clinical practice and improve patient outcomes.

Presentation, Evaluation, and Management

- Due to the diversity in underlying etiologies, the presentation of LGIB can range from occult bleeding to life-threatening hemorrhage.
- Of paramount importance is rapid assessment of the patient's hemodynamic stability.
  - Patients presenting with massive gastrointestinal bleeding and signs of hemodynamic instability, chest pain, shortness of breath, or orthostatic hypotension should immediately have two large-bore intravenous lines placed and undergo rapid volume resuscitation with crystalloid while awaiting labs and availability of cross-matched blood; in extreme circumstances, one may consider transfusion with non-cross-matched type O-negative blood.
  - Continuous monitoring of vital signs is essential, and a Foley catheter should typically be placed to monitor urine output.
- Aspiration of frank blood, clot, or coffee grounds from an NG tube should prompt upper endoscopy. A bilious aspirate all but excludes an upper gastrointestinal source, while a clear aspirate is indeterminate, as there could be source of bleeding distal to a contacted pylorus.

Table 41.1 Lower gastrointestinal bleeding: distribution of etiologies

Author Year	Diverticulosis (%)	Hemorrhoids (%)	Neoplasm (%)	Angioectasia (%)	Ischemic colitis (%)	IBD (%)	Colitides (%)	Ulcers (%)	Post-polypectomy (%)	Small bowel (%)	Radiation (%)	Other (%)	Unknown (%)
Longstreth (1997)	41.6	4.6	9.1	2.7	8.7	2.3	5.0					10	11.9
Velayos (2004)	30	12	6	4		4		4	2	6			11
Strate (2003)	30	12	6	3	10	4	8		7		3	7	9
Strate (NIS) (2008)	33.1	20	21.3	6.0	6.6	4.4							11
Gayer (2009)	37.3	21	11.8	2.3		5.4	10.7 (includes ischemic)			8		6.58	3.45
Hreinsson (2012)	23.3	10.4	10.5	3.1	16	11.7				3.1		11	9.2

- A directed history and physical examination should be performed, including an intake of the patient's medications, paying particular attention to NSAIDs, anticoagulants, and antiplatelet agents that may exacerbate bleeding, as well as beta-blockers that may mask the physiologic response to hypovolemia.
- Pertinent points in the history should include onset and duration of bleeding, volume and frequency of bleeding, color of blood (bright red, maroon, or tarry), and presence or absence of clots.
- The presence of significant pain represents a branch point in the evaluation of the patient with LGIB and should prompt earlier cross-sectional imaging if the patient is hemodynamically stable.
- Particular attention should be paid to those who have undergone prior intestinal surgery, due to the possibility of an anastomotic ulcer, and those who have been previously treated with abdominopelvic radiation, implicating radiation proctitis/colitis/enteritis.
- Physical examination should begin with assessment for signs/symptoms of hypovolemic shock.
- Once the patient's volume status has been assessed and appropriate resuscitation initiated, a more directed physical exam should ensue.
- Abdominal examination should focus on the presence of pain, palpable masses, distention, scars from prior surgeries, and hepatosplenomegaly. Stigmata of chronic liver disease, such as jaundice, caput medusa, or palmar erythema, may suggest variceal bleeding.
- Digital rectal examination should be done to assess for the presence of a rectal mass, and anoscopy and/or rigid proctosigmoidoscopy should usually be performed to evaluate for a distal source of bleeding, such as internal hemorrhoids, proctitis, ulcers, or varices.
- Laboratory studies should include a basic chemistry panel, complete blood count, coagulation parameters, and type and cross. Coagulopathies should be corrected via transfusion of blood products and/or factors as appropriate.
- Volume resuscitation of the hypovolemic patient should include bolus infusion of isotonic crystalloid, such as normal saline or lactated Ringer's solution, aiming to restore normotension. Continued hypotension despite aggressive crystalloid infusion should prompt transfusion of packed red blood cells.
- Further transfusion should be guided by the patient's hemodynamic response and change in hemoglobin. A hemoglobin transfusion threshold of 9–10 g/dL has traditionally been employed, especially in patients with significant cardiovascular disease. While data regarding a more restrictive pattern of transfusion specifically in patients with LGIB is lacking, a number of studies in patients with UGIB have demonstrated improved outcomes using a more restrictive threshold, as low as 7 g/dL, in low-risk patients.
- For patients requiring transfusion of multiple units of PRBC, concurrent administration of platelets and fresh frozen plasma may prevent dilutional coagulopathy.

Colonoscopy

- When patients present with a self-limited LGIB, colonoscopy is the diagnostic modality of choice, identifying either a definitive or presumed source of bleeding in 74–100% of cases.
- The major advantage of colonoscopy is the potential for concurrent diagnosis and therapeutic intervention, even in the absence of active bleeding.
- Because most bleeding stops spontaneously, colonoscopy is typically performed semi-electively, usually following a mechanical bowel preparation.
- While the use of a mechanical bowel purge allows for more complete visualization of the colonic mucosa, it also necessitates a delay in performing the procedure. If bleeding has stopped by the time colonoscopy is performed, it is often difficult to know which if any of the potential sources was responsible.

- There is conflicting data regarding the utility of urgent colonoscopy. Early colonoscopy has the potential for therapeutic intervention if a source is identified.
- Colonoscopic interventions for cessation of active bleeding include clipping, band ligation, injection of epinephrine or saline, monopolar or bipolar electrocautery, laser coagulation, or argon plasma coagulation (APC).
- AVMs can be treated either with electrocautery, APC, or laser coagulation. Multiple sessions may be required, and long-term rebleeding rates range from 10% to 39%. One must keep in mind that AVMs in particular are more often located in the thinner-walled right colon, increasing the risk of perforation with any intervention.

Radionucleotide Scintigraphy

- Two techniques can be employed for the detection of active GI bleeding – ^{99m}Tc-sulfur colloid and ^{99m}Tc-labeled RBCs – the latter of which has been shown to be superior for the detection of GI bleeding.
  - ^{99m}Tc-RBC scanning requires labeling a small sample of the patient's blood with technetium, and then injecting it back into the patient's blood stream, followed by scintigraphic scanning. Active hemorrhage is indicated by extravasation and pooling of the radionucleotide tracer (Fig. 41.3).
  - The procedure is noninvasive, carries little risk, and does not require mechanical bowel preparation. Other benefits include its high sensitivity and the slow washout of the tracer, which allows repeat scanning over periods of up to 24 h in instances of intermittent bleeding. This is important to take into consideration, given that rebleeding can be seen in up to 27% of patients after an initial negative ^{99m}Tc-RBC scan.
  - The main drawbacks are that this technique requires some prep time to extract and tag the RBCs (approximately 30 min) and there is no possibility for therapeutic intervention.
  - Detection of bleeding as slow as 0.04–0.05 cc/min has been reported with ^{99m}Tc-RBC scans. Reported accuracy in detection of the anatomic site of bleeding varies widely (41–94%), mainly because of rapid movement of tracer within the lumen of the bowel due to peristalsis and gravity, as well as difficulty discriminating the colon from overlying small bowel.
  - Because of the variability in accurate localization of the anatomic site of bleeding, most algorithms that include ^{99m}Tc-RBC scanning in the evaluation of patients with LGIB use it as a screening study prior to proceeding with mesenteric angiogram rather than as a definitive localizing study.
  - Similarly, owing to the lack of reliability in determining the actual anatomic site of bleeding, segmental resection based on ^{99m}Tc-RBC scan localization alone is often problematic.

Computed Tomography Angiography (CTA)

- With widespread availability of CT scans, CTA has largely supplanted ^{99m}Tc-RBC scanning as the initial means of evaluating most patients presenting with acute LGIB.
- Besides the detection of active bleeding, CTA has the added advantages of being able to localize the site of bleeding and identify any coexisting pathology.
- A positive CTA (Fig. 41.4) should prompt further therapeutic efforts, such as angiographic embolization, or surgical resection for massive hemorrhage.
- The rate of bleeding detected by CTA has been reported to be as low as 0.3 mL/min. The

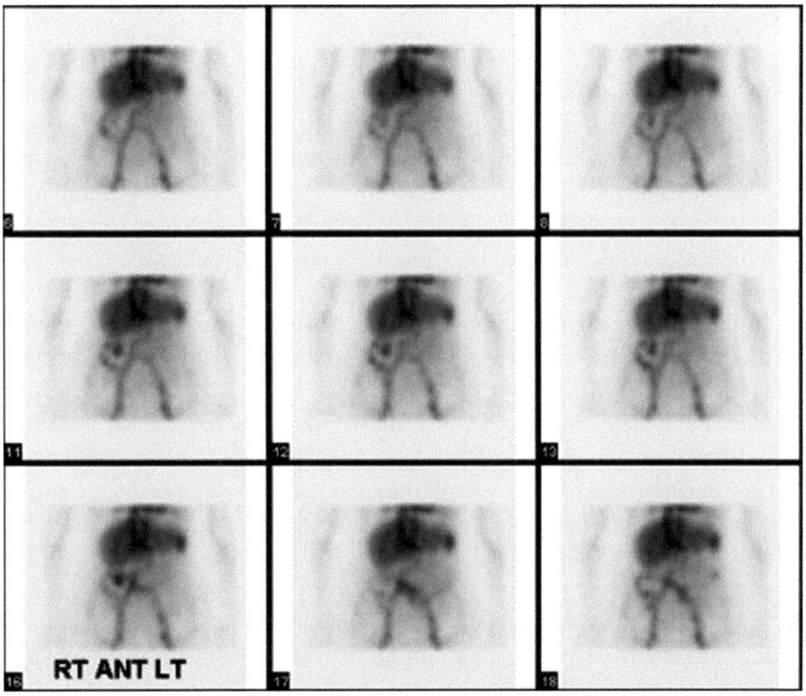

Fig. 41.3 ^{99m}Tc-RBC scan showing active extravasation in the right lower quadrant. RBC, red blood count

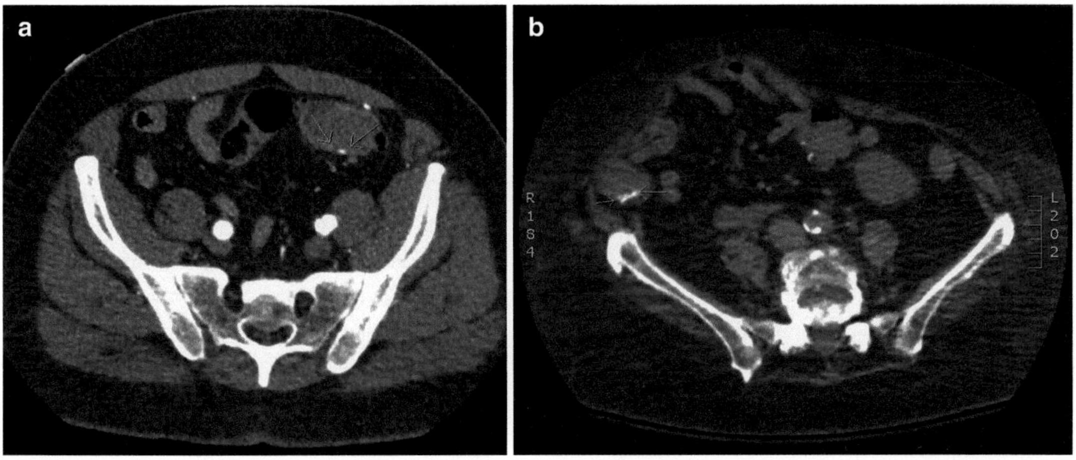

Fig. 41.4 (**a**) CT angiogram showing active extravasation in the sigmoid colon. (**b**) CT angiogram showing active extravasation in the cecum

sensitivity of CTA for localization of a LGIB source is 91–92% when active bleeding is present, though it drops to as low as 45–47% when bleeding is intermittent.

- A major advantage of CTA is its ready availability and ease with which the study can be performed and rapidly interpreted, leading to earlier and more targeted therapeutic intervention.
- The main disadvantage is the small risk of contrast nephropathy, which may limit its use in patients with renal insufficiency.

Angiography

Diagnostic Angiography

- Diagnostic mesenteric angiography is an invasive procedure with a number of potential complications.
- The major advantage is the ability to perform a therapeutic intervention if active bleeding is identified (Fig. 41.5).
- Angiography requires a more rapid rate of bleeding (0.5–1.5 cc/min) than nuclear scintigraphy to detect active extravasation.
- Identification of active bleeding following a positive "screening" ^{99m}Tc-RBC scan or CTA may be hampered by the intermittent nature of most LGIBs and the time delay between the positive scan and the performance of angiography.
- The success of angiographic localization correlates with a hemodynamic instability on arrival, a drop in hemoglobin level $\geq$ 50% from previous admission, and a transfusion requirement of $\geq$5 U of PRBC within 24 h.
- Mesenteric angiography after a positive CTA has been reported to be eight to nine times more likely to be positive when performed within 90 min of the CTA.
- For patients with recurrent intermittent LGIB that continue to defy localization despite multiple diagnostic studies, provocative angiography, which incorporates the use of heparin, thrombolytics, vasodilators, or some combination of these to induce a bleed, has been advocated. Before considering provocative angiography, one must balance the risk of uncontrolled hemorrhage or intracranial hemorrhage against the potential diagnostic and therapeutic benefit.
- The risks associated with diagnostic mesenteric angiography include bleeding, access complications such as vascular injury and pseudoaneurysm, thromboembolic events, and contrast-induced nephropathy. Contraindi cations include contrast dye allergy and renal insufficiency that might limit the ability to administer intravenous contrast.

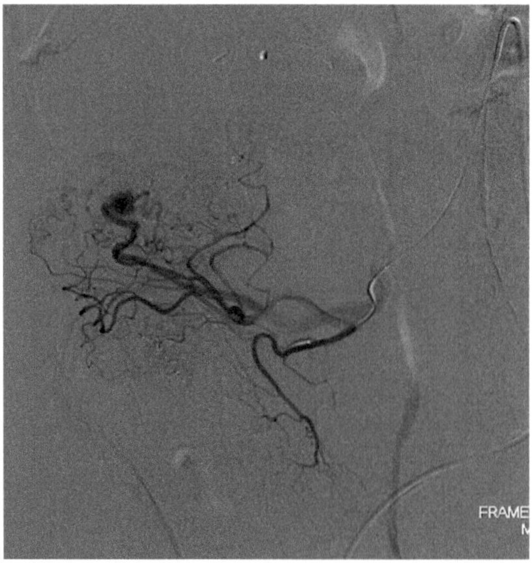

Fig. 41.5 Mesenteric angiogram showing active extravasation from a branch of the ileocolic artery

Therapeutic Angiography

- If a blush or area of obvious extravasation is seen during diagnostic angiography, therapeutic intervention should be attempted.
- Vasopressin infusion via a selectively placed mesenteric arterial catheter to induce vasospasm generally begins at 0.2 U/min and may be increased to 0.4 U/min if bleeding persists. Cessation of active bleeding is seen in up to 90% of patients, though the rate of rebleeding upon discontinuation of the infusion approaches 50%.
- Because of the antidiuretic effect of vasopressin, there is a tendency toward fluid retention and congestive heart failure, so its use in patients with significant cardiac disease becomes somewhat limited, especially considering the significant volume resuscitation many patients with LGIB require.
- With the availability of "microcatheters," transcatheter superselective embolization of target vessels carries a negligible risk of intestinal ischemia. Success rates with cessation of active arterial bleeding range from 50% to 100% with rebleeding rates of 22–24%.

- Complications such as transmural ischemia and stricture formation, which were more common in the past following embolization of larger segmental vessels, now occur rarely with the use of superselective embolization angiography and are usually asymptomatic.
- Due to its efficacy and low risk of complications, superselective embolization is now considered by most to be the first-line angiographic therapy for LGIB. Materials used for embolization include microcoils, polyvinyl alcohol particles, and Gelfoam.

Localization of Small Bowel Bleeding

- When a patient shows signs of ongoing GI bleeding in the face of negative evaluations of both the upper and lower GI tracts, one should consider evaluation for a small bowel source of bleeding. Options include video capsule endoscopy (VCE), double-balloon enteroscopy (DBE), radionucleotide Meckel's scan, and, as a last resort, intraoperative push enteroscopy.
- VCE and DBE have both been shown to have diagnostic yields in range of 55–65% in patients with hematochezia.
- VCE takes significant time to perform and is most commonly utilized to evaluate for an occult source of chronic bleeding, not in the presence of massive LGIB.
- DBE is a technically challenging and time-consuming procedure that should only be attempted by a skilled endoscopist who has training and significant experience with the technique.
- Despite these limitations, DBE compared to VCE has the added benefit of both localization and potential therapeutic intervention if bleeding source is identified. If a site of bleeding is identified but endoscopic intervention is not possible, the endoscopist can mark the site of bleeding with endoclips or tattooing for later identification at the time of possible radiologic or surgical intervention.
- A Meckel's scan relies on uptake of ^{99m}Tc-pertechnetate in ectopic gastric mucosa within the Meckel's diverticulum that has the potential for hemorrhage. The procedure is noninvasive, has minimal morbidity, and has both specificity and PPV approaching 100%, though its sensitivity is much lower at 62%. Concurrent administration of H-2 blockers has been shown to increase the diagnostic yield.

Surgery

- The number of patients who require emergency surgery without a preoperatively localized site of bleeding is less than 5%.
- In hemodynamically unstable patients with refractory, ongoing LGIB, emergent surgical intervention is indicated. Also, patients in whom a source of bleeding has been localized but therapeutic efforts are either unsuccessful or not feasible should be considered surgical candidates, as should those with massive transfusion requirements.
- Six units of PRBC in a 24-h period have traditionally been considered the threshold trigger prompting surgical intervention as massive transfusion increases surgical morbidity and mortality.
- When ongoing massive LGIB hemorrhage is present and a source cannot be localized despite multiple diagnostic studies or if the patient is too unstable for additional diagnostic studies, the patient should undergo exploratory laparotomy.
  - The small bowel should be thoroughly examined to exclude a Meckel's diverticulum or a palpable mass that could be a source of bleeding.
  - Transillumination of the small bowel may reveal small tumors or angiodysplasia.
  - If the patient is stable, an intraoperative colonoscopy can be performed with luminal lavage and irrigation of sequential segments with proximal compression of the colon.
  - Intraoperative push enteroscopy can also be considered if a colonic source is not identified and there is bright red blood and/

or clots in the terminal ileum, though this can be technically challenging and time consuming.
  - If a clear source cannot be identified and there is no obvious source in the stomach or small bowel (and an anorectal source has been excluded), the bleeding source is presumed to be colonic; a total abdominal colectomy should be performed with either an end ileostomy or, in select circumstances, an ileoproctostomy. Rebleeding rates after total abdominal colectomy generally are less than 5%, and modern advances in postoperative ICU care have reduced postoperative mortality to 2–6%.
- When the bleeding site has been localized but endoscopic or angiographic attempts to control it have failed, a targeted segmental resection is indicated, either with primary anastomosis or a stoma, dictated by the patient's clinical condition at the time of surgery. In this scenario, rebleeding rates and mortality are 4–10% and 0–40%, respectively.
  - Compared with subtotal colectomy and ileorectal anastomosis, segmental colectomy provides measurable improvements in postoperative morbidity, frequency of bowel movements, social restrictions, and overall quality of life.
- A "blind" segmental resection without preoperative localization should not be performed. Blind segmental resections have been shown to have mortality rates ranging from 30% to 57% with rebleeding rates of 33–75%.

Summary

- LGIB is a commonly encountered condition, with a number of possible etiologies and several options for evaluation.
- Key points in the management include restoring hemodynamic stability, identifying and localizing ongoing bleeding, and cessation of hemorrhage, either by radiographic or surgical means when necessary.
- There are a number of options in the evaluation of patients with LGIB, which should be individualized to the experience of the evaluating physician and available resources.
- New technologies such as CTA and earlier use of colonoscopy now allow for more rapid and accurate detection of active bleeding; the number of nondiagnostic invasive angiograms has diminished, and pre-angiographic localization of an active bleeding site via CTA helps to facilitate treatment via therapeutic angiography.
- Advances in interventional techniques and the use of microcatheters have improved the efficacy of therapeutic angiography and reduced the risk of post-embolic ischemia.
- Fewer patients are undergoing emergency surgery for non-localized bleeding, and even fewer are requiring subtotal colectomy for non-localized LGIB; those who do require surgery fare much better than in the past, due to improvement in postoperative ICU care.
- An algorithm summarizing the evaluation and management of the patient presenting with LGIB is presented in Fig. 41.6.

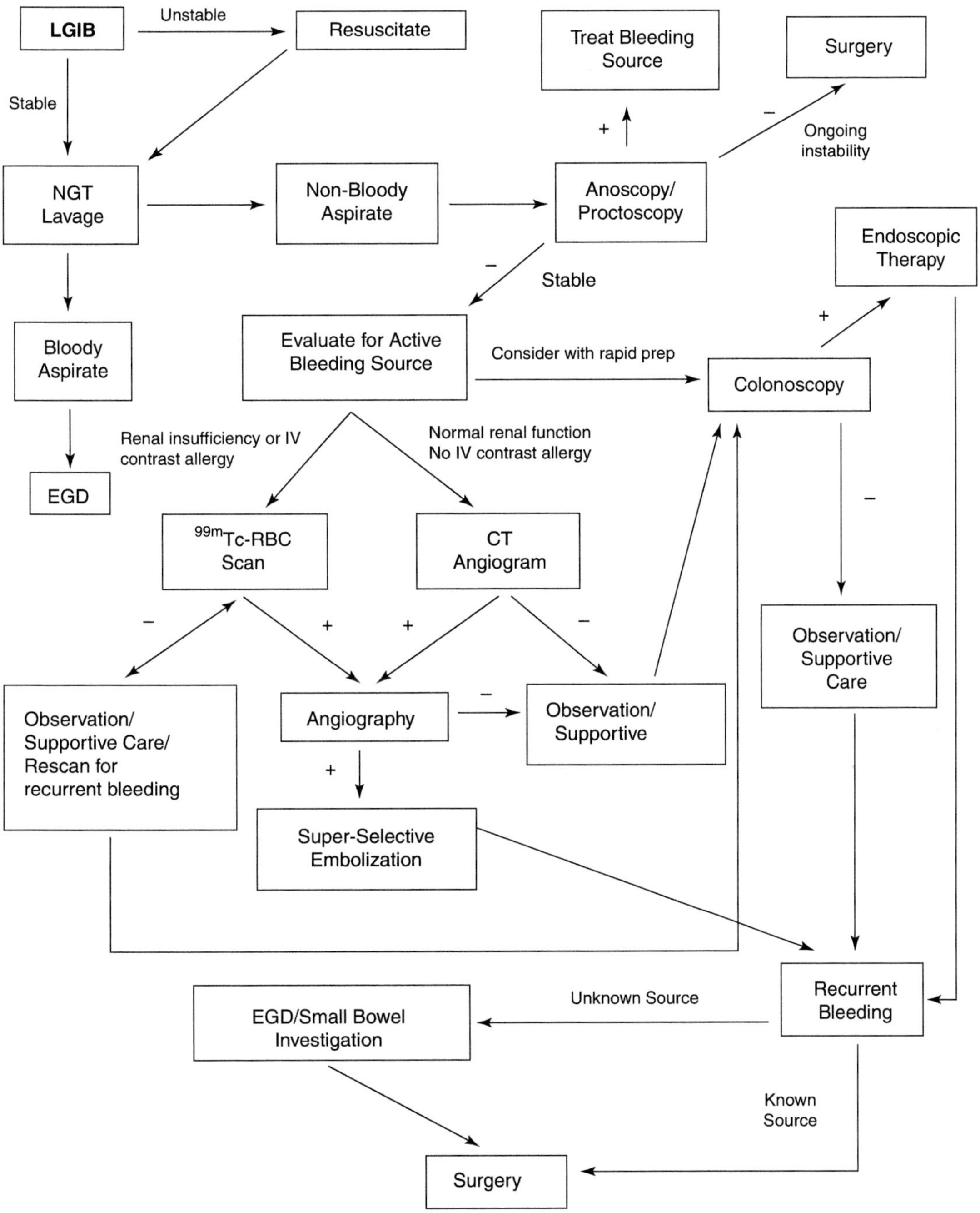

Fig. 41.6 Algorithm for the evaluation and management of the patient with LGIB (lower gastrointestinal bleeding)

42 Endometriosis

Michael J. Snyder

Key Concepts

- Endometriosis is a common cause of young women having major surgery.
- Endometriosis causes infertility, pelvic pain, and dyschezia.
- Laparoscopy has revolutionized the diagnosis of endometriosis.
- Symptomatic endometriosis usually requires surgery.
- Excision of deep pelvic endometriosis is often a combined procedure with gynecologists and urologists.

Introduction

- Endometriosis is a disease characterized by the presence of endometrial glands and stroma outside the uterine cavity.
- It is one of the most common conditions requiring surgery for women during their reproductive years.
- Endometriosis may be associated with disabling pain and intractable infertility.
- Small lesions may cause severe pain and infertility, while larger lesions may be asymptomatic and be found only incidentally during surgery for other diagnoses.
- Diagnosis is typically made or confirmed at laparoscopy or during laparotomy.
- Treatment for endometriosis is usually multimodal and may require surgery in those patients with infertility, pelvic pain, obstruction, or a poor response to hormonal suppression.

Epidemiology

- The true prevalence of endometriosis is unknown.
- There is no noninvasive screening test for endometriosis, and diagnosis depends on the visual or pathologic identification of implants during laparoscopy or laparotomy.
- Various authors have estimated that up to 15% of all women of reproductive age and one-third of infertile women have endometriosis.
- While endometriosis is primarily a disease of the reproductive years, the widespread use of exogenous estrogens and increasing obesity in our society have increased the prevalence in postmenopausal women.
- There is a decreased incidence in women who use oral contraceptives or experience multiple pregnancies.

M. J. Snyder (✉)
Department of Surgery, University of Texas Health Science, Houston, TX, USA
e-mail: michael.j.snyder@uth.tmc.edu

S. R. Steele et al. (eds.), *The ASCRS Manual of Colon and Rectal Surgery*,
https://doi.org/10.1007/978-3-030-01165-9_42

Etiology

- The two most popular theories as to its etiology are coelomic metaplasia or the implantation of viable endometrial cells from retrograde menstruation through the fallopian tubes.
- Retrograde menstruation remains the most plausible explanation for the distribution of endometrial implants; however, while retrograde menstruation occurs in virtually all women, endometriosis affects only a small minority. As such, other factors must be involved to enable the implantation and growth of endometrial tissue.

Clinical Manifestations

- The most common site where endometriosis occurs is the pelvis (Table 42.1).
- Potential sites of implantation in the abdomen include the appendix, small bowel, and diaphragm. Rarely, implantation may occur in the inguinal canal (in patients with hernias), surgical incisions, the vulva, vagina, cervix, or systemically in the lungs, bronchi, or kidneys.
- As the majority of women have disease confined to the pelvis, the most common presenting complaints relate to menstrual irregularities, pelvic pain, and infertility.
- Many women with endometriosis may be completely asymptomatic, and the natural history of the disease in these patients has never been well defined.

Table 42.1 Sites and incidence of endometriosis

Common	Less common
Ovaries 60–75%	Appendix 2%
Uterosacral ligaments 30–65%	Ureter 1–2%
Cul-de-sac 20–30%	Terminal ileum 1%
Uterus 4–20%	Bladder <1%
Rectosigmoid colon 3–10%	Abdominal scars <1%

Rare; diaphragm, inguinal canal, liver, spleen, kidney

Pelvic Pain and Dysmenorrhea

- Pain is the most common symptom of endometriosis, affecting up to 80% of patients subsequently diagnosed with the disease.
- Endometriosis has been discovered in 30–50% of women undergoing laparoscopy for pelvic pain.
- Pelvic pain associated with endometriosis presents as dysmenorrhea, dyspareunia, or chronic noncyclic pelvic pain.
- There are women, however, with extensive endometriosis and little or no pain. Total lesion volume does appear to correlate directly to the degree of pain.
- Symptoms are related to the depth of penetration of the lesion, the type of lesion, and its location.
- Implants involving the uterosacral ligaments and rectovaginal septum are most often implicated.
- The pain is typically most intense just prior to menstruation and lasts for the duration of menstruation. The pain is often associated with back pain, dyschezia, and levator muscle spasm and is more severe with advanced stages of endometriosis.
- Dysmenorrhea occurs in most women with endometriosis.
- Dyspareunia, deep pelvic pain with vaginal penetration, is usually a symptom of advanced endometriosis.
  - Dyspareunia is most pronounced just prior to menstruation and is associated with specific coital positions.
  - The presence of dyspareunia is often indicative of the degree of fixation of the pelvic organs, especially in the cul-de-sac of Douglas and the rectovaginal septum.
- Chronic noncyclic pelvic pain is pain present for longer than 6 months and may be intermittent or continuous. The pain is often associated with both perineural inflammation and uterosacral ligament involvement. Gastrointestinal and urinary complaints may accompany the pain.
- Pain in the shoulder during or just preceding menstruation may be due to endometrial

implants involving the diaphragm. The diaphragms should be inspected during laparoscopy.
- Adhesions, very common in endometriosis, may be associated with pain.
- Adherence of the colon and small bowel along with retroflexion of the uterus from extensive posterior adhesions may occur with consequent back and rectal pain.

Infertility

- Whether endometriosis causes infertility or is the product of uninterrupted menstruation continues to be debated.
- However, moderate to severe disease with mechanical distortion of the fallopian tubes, ovaries, and peritoneum can potentiate infertility.
- Pelvic endometriosis and the resulting inflammatory response can produce dense, fibrotic adhesions that may significantly interfere with both the oocyte release from the ovary and the ability of the fallopian tube to pick up and transmit the oocyte to the uterus.
- Blockage of the tube may produce a hydrosalpinx.
- In moderate or severe endometriosis, the pregnancy rates following surgery are 50% and 40%, respectively, compared to only 7% when expectant management is practiced. Surgical treatment of these patients is clearly beneficial.

Intestinal Symptoms

- Although some women with intestinal endometriosis may be asymptomatic, some degree of intestinal complaints are found in those women with moderate to severe disease.
- Bowel involvement occurs in 12–37% of cases of endometriosis.
- In patients with intestinal endometriosis, the rectosigmoid is involved in over 70%, followed by the small bowel and appendix.
- Rectosigmoid disease often results in alterations in bowel habits such as constipation, diarrhea, a decreased caliber of the stool, tenesmus, or, rarely, rectal bleeding.
  - Such symptoms appear more often around the time of menses and are most likely due to the inflammatory nidus of the endometrial implant.
- Colonic endometriosis can present with obstruction and be maybe difficult to differentiate from other causes of large bowel obstruction, such as Crohn's disease or neoplasm.
- Colonic perforation has been reported during pregnancy from endometriosis.
- Patients with asymptomatic intestinal endometriosis appear to have a benign natural history; consequently, intestinal resection in asymptomatic patients is probably unwarranted.
- Confusion between small bowel endometriosis and Crohn's disease may occur, as both can produce similar laparoscopic, endoscopic, and even histologic findings (Fig. 42.1).
- Small bowel implants involving the terminal ileum are often noted incidentally at the time of laparoscopy and are commonly asymptomatic. Occasionally, acute or chronic small bowel obstruction develops from extensive associated fibrosis.
- Endometrial implants are not infrequently found when the appendix is removed incidentally.
- Endometrial implants may produce acute appendicitis, including perforation.

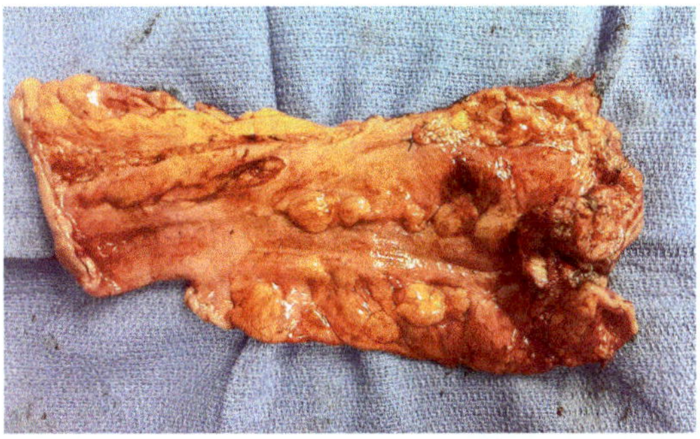

Fig. 42.1 Gross pathologic specimen of endometriosis involving the small intestine. The specimen cut open with the typical appearance of an endometrioma after hormonal therapy inducing diminished vascularity

- Endometriosis of the appendix may also produce a chronic obstruction of the intestinal lumen with formation of a mucocele or periappendiceal inflammatory mass that is difficult to distinguish from a neoplasm.
- Finally, endometrial implants of the appendix and cecum may serve as lead points for an intussusception.

Malignant Transformation

- Malignant transformation of endometriosis may occur; almost 80% of the tumors are ovarian, and two-thirds are endometrial carcinomas.
- In women with known endometriosis, a cyst larger than 10 centimeters, cyst rupture, and a change in the nature of the chronic pelvic pain are potential signs of malignancy.
- The rectosigmoid colon is the most common site for extragonadal tumors arising from endometriosis.
- Treatment of both ovarian and extragonadal tumors is based on the particular stage of the tumor. The prognosis is generally good with tumors confined to the ovary or an extragonadal site having 5-year survivals greater than 60%.

Diagnosis

Physical Examination

- Patients with mild cases of endometriosis may have a normal physical examination; the diagnosis may not even be suspected unless the patient undergoes laparoscopy.
- For patients with pelvic pain, careful bimanual and rectal examination may reveal nodularity or induration especially in the uterosacral ligaments or cul-de-sac.
- Fixed tender retroversion of the uterus in a patient without previous pelvic surgery may raise suspicion for endometriosis.
- Palpation of the ovaries may reveal an ovarian mass.
- The inguinal canal, previous incisions, umbilicus, and lungs can all be potentially involved with endometrial implants.

Laboratory Evaluation

- CA-125 is elevated in women with moderate to severe endometriosis. However, the sensitivity and specificity are poor.

Endoscopy

- As the lesions begin on the outside of the intestine, endoscopic evaluation of the large bowel is often normal except in severe disease or infiltrating nodular endometrial implants.
- Occasionally, serosal involvement with adhesions can lead to obstruction. Endoscopically, the mucosa is generally intact, occasionally associated with significant luminal narrowing.
- Infiltration of the submucosa, while uncommon, may produce nodularity and distortion of the overlying mucosa (Fig. 42.2).
  - These findings may be difficult to visually differentiate from Crohn's disease, ischemia, or malignancy.
- Biopsies of the mucosa, taken in areas of endometriosis, can resemble solitary rectal ulcer or prolapse syndromes.

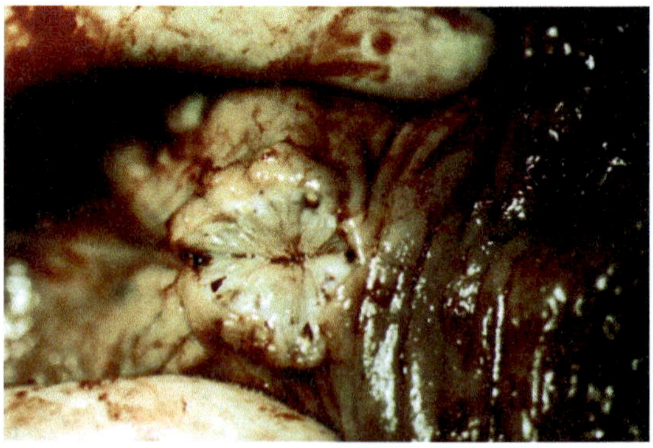

Fig. 42.2 Polypoid endometrial implant of the colon causing mucosal abnormalities

- Rarely is the diagnosis of endometriosis definitively confirmed by endoscopy or from endoscopic biopsies. Colonoscopy is useful in excluding colon cancer from the differential diagnosis.
- Rigid proctoscopy is very helpful in predicting the depth of rectosigmoid involvement in patients with severe endometriosis of the cul-de-sac of Douglas and the associated need for resection in surgical cases.
  - The mucosa is often fixed over an area of submucosal or deep muscular involvement with tethering or puckering and loss of the normal mucosal mobility.

Imaging Techniques

- Imaging techniques are primarily utilized to rule out more common conditions, but there are findings that may suggest the diagnosis of endometriosis.
- The appearance on pelvic ultrasound is highly variable with some lesions being nearly sonolucent and others quite echogenic.
- Endorectal ultrasound is a potentially valuable tool to determine rectal wall invasion by endometrial implants in the cul-de-sac.
- Barium enema with lateral and prone cross-table views of the rectum offers excellent evaluation of the cul-de-sac of Douglas as long as care is taken in ensuring that the balloon is kept in the distal rectum (Fig. 42.3).
- CT evaluation of the pelvic sidewall for endometrial implants is better than ultrasound, but there is still significant overlap between infectious and malignant pathology.
- MRI may be the best noninvasive modality for imaging suspected endometriosis.
  - Colorectal involvement on MRI is strongly suggested when there is disappearance of the fat plane between the rectum and the vagina, loss of the hypointense signal of the anterior bowel wall on T2-weighted images, and a contrast-enhanced mass on T1-weighted images involving the bowel wall.

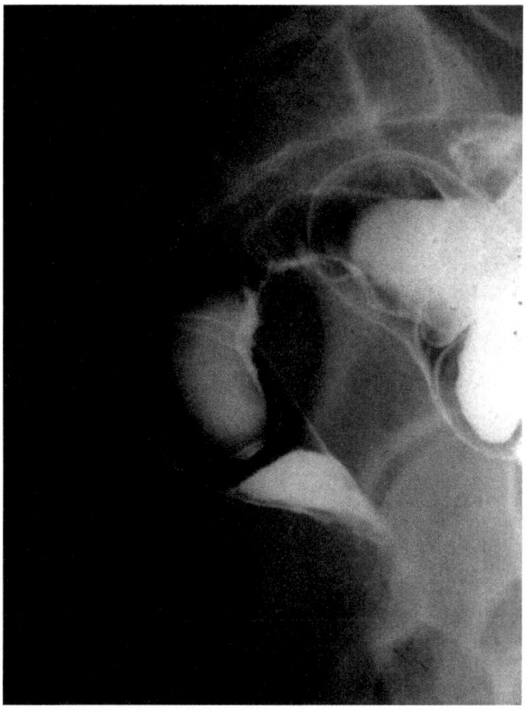

Fig. 42.3 Barium enema demonstrating a rectosigmoid stricture from endometriosis

Laparoscopy

- Laparoscopy is currently the initial approach to many patients suspected of having endometriosis and has revolutionized both its diagnosis and treatment (Fig. 42.4).
- In experienced hands laparoscopic evaluation is 97% sensitive and 77% specific in diagnosing endometriosis.
- Obtaining a biopsy to confirm the visual diagnosis is strongly recommended for at least one lesion and is especially critical for deep disease and endometriomas greater than 3 centimeters in diameter to exclude malignancy.
- A thorough examination of the entire abdomen and especially the pelvis is critical to enable complete assessment of the disease. Both ovaries should be mobilized to evaluate the pelvic peritoneum, and the uterus should be manipulated to allow complete visualization of the cul-de-sac of Douglas, uterosacral ligaments, sigmoid colon, and ureters. It is

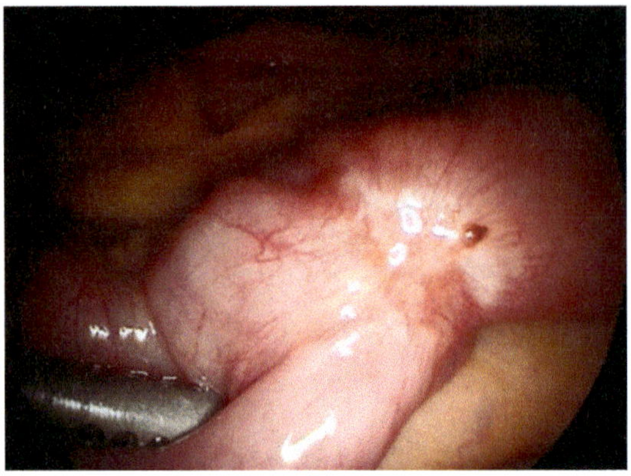

Fig. 42.4 Laparoscopic view of an endometrial implant on the small intestine

important to view the base of the appendix as well as the distal small bowel.

- The findings of endometriosis can be very subtle, and visually normal peritoneum may have microscopic evidence of endometriosis.
- The extent of endometriosis should be carefully documented and staged. The current staging system has been formulated primarily for infertility and was revised by the American Society for Reproductive Medicine in 1998 (Fig. 42.5).
  - Virtually all patients with intestinal lesions requiring resection are Stage IV especially if they have cul-de-sac involvement.
- The classic implant is nodular with a variable degree of fibrosis and pigmentation. The color may be black, white, brown, blue, or even red. The appearance of the lesion may be vesicular, papular, or hemorrhagic (Fig. 42.6).
- Lesions may change color or consistency over time, with red lesions noted early in the course of the disease and blue/black ones typical of older implants. Healed implants appear as fibrotic nodules.
- There are also a wide variety of atypical lesions occasionally associated with positive biopsies. The inability to definitively identify endometriosis through purely visual means necessitates pathologic confirmation of the disease, especially in mild disease.
- Implants in the cul-de-sac of Douglas may be difficult to assess laparoscopically, and the full extent of the implant may not be appreciated until laparotomy. Progressive fibrosis leads to narrowing of the intestinal lumen and occasionally to bowel obstruction.

Treatment

- Treatment options for women with endometriosis are currently based upon the severity and type of symptoms.
- Not all women with endometriosis require treatment.
- Most early endometrial lesions can be ablated or excised at the time of laparoscopic diagnosis. Even complex excisional surgery involving the bowel and ureter can be performed safely via a laparoscopic approach in many patients, especially with mild and moderate disease.

Medical Management

- Medical therapy is designed to treat the symptoms of endometriosis, notably pelvic pain.
- As pelvic pain may have causes other than the endometriosis seen during laparoscopy, a trial of ovarian suppression is often used to help determine the contribution of the pain from the endometrial implants.
- In patients with infertility, with or without pelvic pain, the primary goal is an intrauterine pregnancy; ovarian suppression may allow for laparoscopic removal of smaller endometrial lesions with optimal preservation of ovarian tissue.
- In limited disease, medical therapy is comparable with surgery in terms of relief of symptoms, recurrence of disease, and subsequent pregnancy rates.
- However, hormonal therapies have side effects and often require prolonged treatment.
  - Advanced lesions, especially those with a nodular, proliferative histology will often only partially regress.
  - No current hormonal regimen can completely eradicate these lesions, and upon cessation of therapy, the lesions may again become symptomatic.

Patient's Name ______________ Date ______________

Stage I (Minimal) - 1–5
Stage II (Mild) - 6–15
Stage III (Moderate) - 16–40
Stage IV (Severe) - > 40
Total ______________

Laparoscopy ________ Laparotomy ________ Photography ________
Recommended Treatment ______________
____
Prognosis ______________

	ENDOMETRIOSIS	< 1cm	1–3cm	> 3cm
PERITONEUM	Superficial	1	2	4
	Deep	2	4	6
OVARY	R Superficial	1	2	4
	Deep	6	16	20
	L Superficial	1	2	4
	Deep	4	16	20

POSTERIOR CUL-DE-SAC OBLITERATION	Partial	Complete
	4	40

	ADHESIONS	< 1/3 Enclosure	1/3–2/3 Enclosure	<2/3 Enclosure
OVARY	R Filmy	1	2	4
	Dense	4	8	16
	L Filmy	1	2	4
	Dense	4	8	16
TUBE	R Filmy	1	2	4
	Dense	4•	8•	16
	L Filmy	1	2	4
	Dense	4•	8•	16

•If the fimbriated end of the fallopian tube is completely enclosed, change the point assignment to 16.
Denote appearance of superficial implant types as red [(R), red, red-pink, flamelike, vesicular blobs, clear vesicles], white [(W), opacifications, peritoneal defects, yellow-brown], or black [(B) black, hemosiderin deposits, blue]. Denote percent of total described as R___ %,W__ % and B___%. Total should equal 100%.

Additional Endometriosis: ______________

Associated Pathology: ______________

To Be Used with Normal Tubes and Ovaries

L R

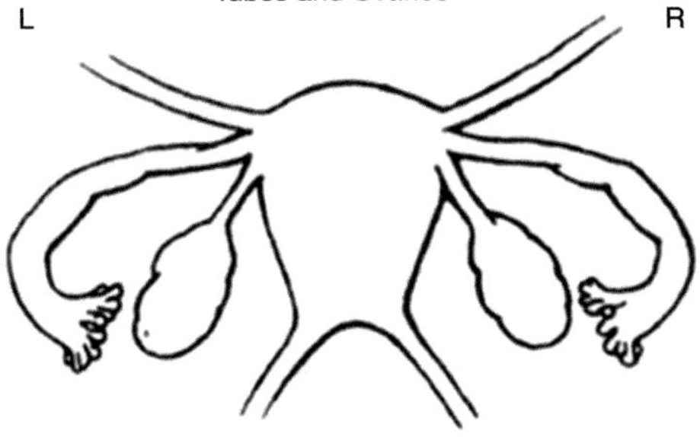

To Be Used with Abnormal Tubes and/or Ovaries

L R

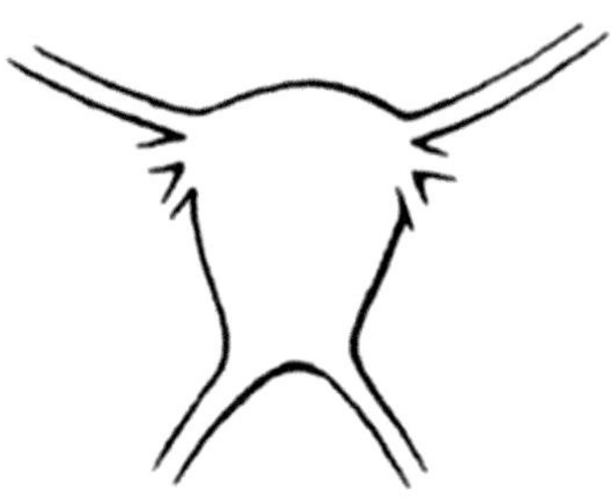

Fig. 42.5 Revised American Society for Reproductive Medicine 1996 classification of endometriosis

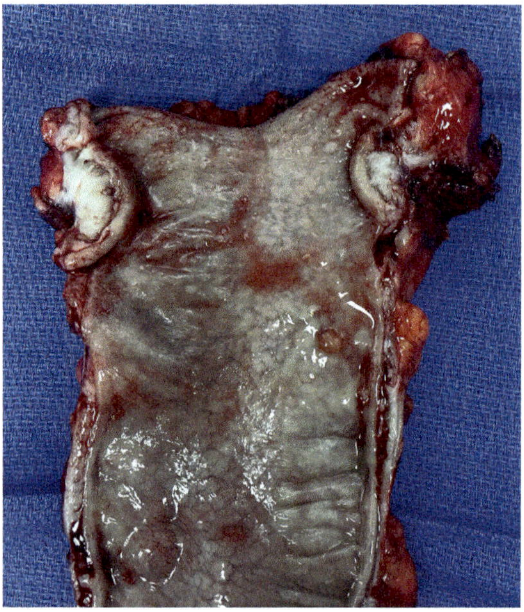

Fig. 42.6 Opened specimen demonstrating the endometrial implant into the bowel wall

Oral Contraceptives

- The usual treatment regimen consists of daily administration for 6–9 months.
  - Another drug regimen involves administration of synthetic progestogens alone.

Danazol

- Danazol lowers peripheral estrogen and progesterone levels by a direct effect on ovarian steroidogenesis and pituitary production of FSH and LH.
- Side effects necessitate discontinuation in less than 5% of patients for short courses, but treatment is poorly tolerated for long-term suppression.

Gonadotropin-Releasing Hormone Agonists

- The introduction of GnRH for endometriosis has improved results primarily by a reduction in side effects.
- Administered either by injection or intranasally beginning in the mid-luteal phase of the menstrual cycle, the current recommended length of therapy is 6 months.
- Pain relief is complete in over 50% of women and significantly decreased in over 90%.
- Laparoscopic evaluation after 6 months of treatment indicates resolution or a significant decrease in size of the lesions in the majority of patients.
- Danazol and GnRH appear to have similar clinical efficacy.
- GnRH is often used as a neoadjuvant or adjuvant therapy combined with surgery. The goal is a reduction in postoperative adhesion formation and recurrence in the pelvis from lesions not visualized or removed at the time of surgery.

Surgical Management

- While the most effective treatment of pelvic pain still consists of surgical castration along with resection of the endometrial implants, many of these young patients strongly desire to maintain their options for pregnancy.
- Currently, surgery is considered conservative only when reproductive potential is preserved. Therefore, the major goal of surgical therapy for endometriosis is to completely excise or ablate the endometrial implants.
- Secondary goals include preservation of ovarian function and minimizing postoperative adhesion formation.

General Principles

- Endometriosis is an invasive disease that can extend deeply into the retroperitoneum and is often surrounded by a rim of fibrosis that may make it difficult to completely assess the true extent of the implant.
- Removal of the lesions requires sharp excision or vaporization with electrocautery and/or the CO2 laser.
- Both techniques have the potential for iatrogenic injury to the intestinal or urinary tracts.
- Utilizing techniques that minimize injury to the surrounding tissue, such as a cutting current to outline lesions to be removed by electrocautery and high power density settings with the CO2 laser, is desirable. Laparoscopic

hydrodissection is also very useful in identifying normal surrounding tissue.
- Meticulous hemostasis and frequent irrigation are critical to maintaining good visualization of the operative field in both open and laparoscopic surgery.
- Tissue planes are often distorted, especially in the cul-de-sac of Douglas, and intraoperative instrumentation of the vagina or proctoscopic evaluation of the rectum may help avoid iatrogenic injury to these structures.
- Minimizing tissue trauma with gentle handling will decrease adhesions and maximize potential fertility.
- Patients undergoing surgery for advanced endometriosis, either by an open or laparoscopic approach, should have a full mechanical and antibiotic bowel preparation.
- Prophylactic antibiotics and other appropriate practices for patients undergoing major abdominal or pelvic surgery are standard.
- Patients are positioned in the low lithotomy position with access to both the vagina and rectum for instrumentation. Ureteral stents are liberally used and are especially useful in women with severe obliterative disease in the cul-de-sac and in reoperative pelvic surgical procedures.

Rectovaginal Endometriosis

- Endometriosis of the cul-de-sac of Douglas that extends into the rectovaginal septum is the most common site of intestinal involvement and may require intestinal resection.
- These lesions are often deep fibrotic nodules that extend from the posterior vagina and anterior rectum to the uterosacral ligaments (Fig. 42.7a–d).
- Small superficial lesions involving the intraperitoneal rectum may be vaporized with the CO_2 laser or electrocautery.
- After the lesion is removed, the bowel wall is carefully assessed. Since most of these super-

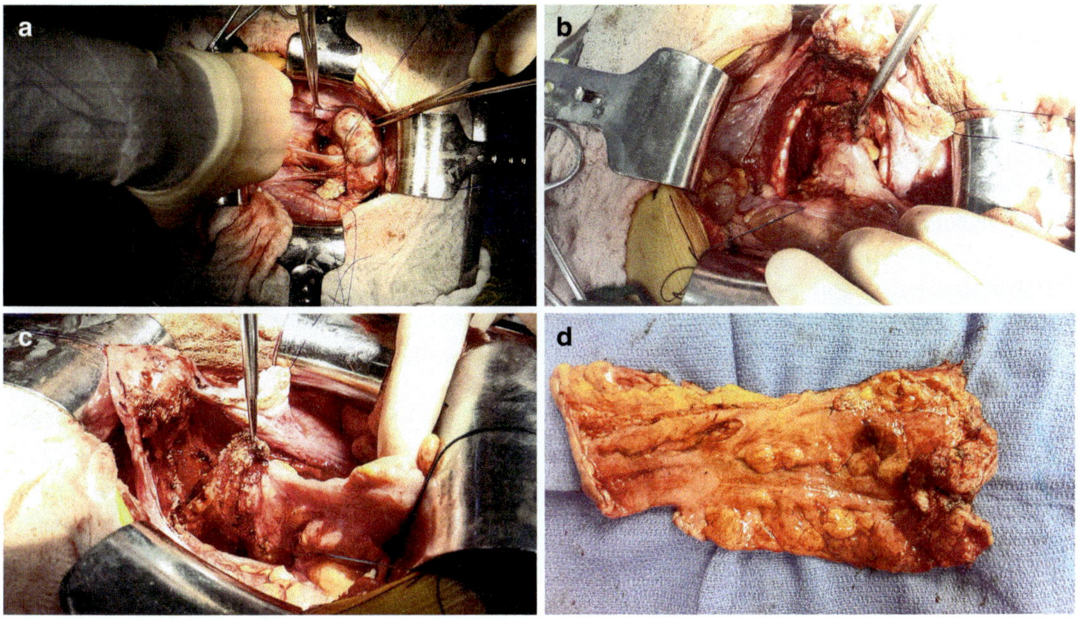

Fig. 42.7 (**a**) Demonstrates the view of the endometrial implants obliterating the pouch of Douglas and an associated large endometrioma on the left ovary at the start of the procedure; (**b**) the large nodule of endometriosis has been dissected from the ureters and posterior vagina (note the lighted ureteral catheters that facilitate the dissection); (**c**) demonstrates visualization of the normal fat within the rectovaginal plane after fully dissecting cul-de-sac of Douglas and mobilizing the lesion rostrally out of the pelvis to allow resection; (**d**) demonstrates sectioning of the specimen to show the typical appearance of an endometrioma after hormonal therapy which induces diminished vascularity of the lesion

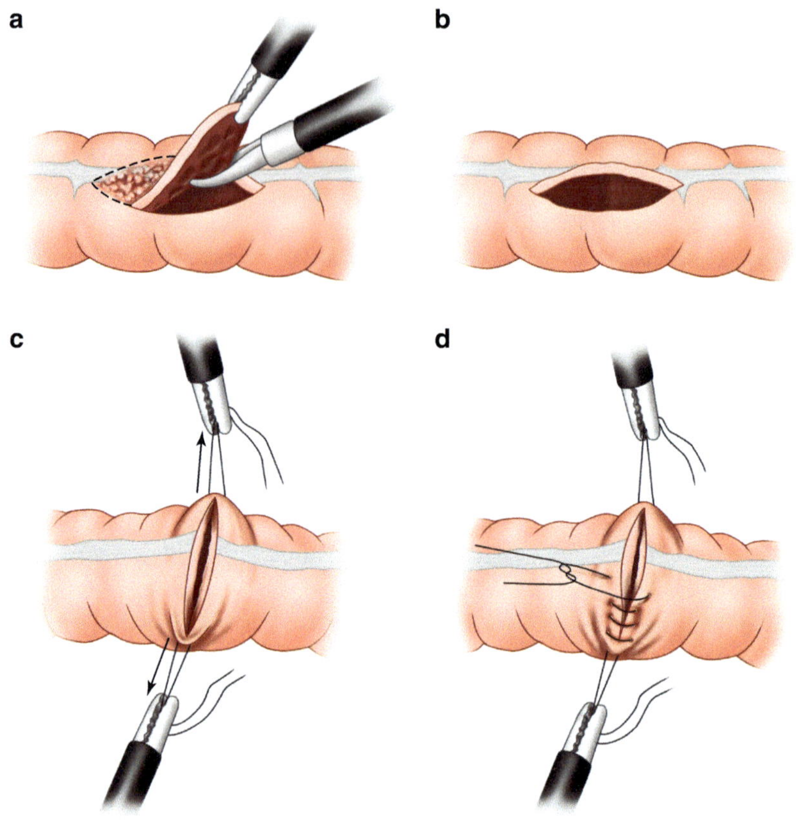

Fig. 42.8 (**a**–**d**) Disc excision of an endometrial implant

ficial lesions can be removed without entering the mucosa, the defects can be closed with Lembert sutures.

- The technique of removing superficial lesions is modified somewhat when it is performed laparoscopically and is termed "shaving." This consists of meticulous removal of the lesion without entering the rectal mucosa.
- Surgical treatment of the deeper lesions is more controversial. Removal of the rectosigmoid with reanastomosis is often technically demanding and should be performed by skilled intestinal surgeons to minimize complications in these young patients.
- Excision of the implant either with a disc of rectal wall (Fig. 42.8) or a formal anterior resection is recommended for women with symptoms related to the endometriosis.
- Both procedures can occasionally be performed laparoscopically if the endometriosis is completely removed.
- The infiltrating nodular endometrial implants involving the rectovaginal portion of the cul-de-sac often invade both the vagina and rectum (Fig. 42.7a–d).
- Since removal of the implant will require resection of a portion of the rectal wall, dissection of the lesion from the vagina allows for en bloc removal of the lesion with the rectal wall.
  - There is often no discernible plane between these lesions and the walls of the rectum or vagina. Care must be taken to avoid penetration of the vaginal wall with possible injury to the cervix, especially in women desiring eventual pregnancy.
  - Often it is advantageous to mobilize the rectum in the posterior and lateral tissue planes to adequately define the lesion before attempting the anterior dissection. After careful dissection of the lesion from the vagina, the normal rectovaginal plane is

reached, and the fixed, hard mass may suddenly become mobile and amenable to resection.

- Disc excision of the anterior rectal wall, by either laparoscopic or open technique, is performed for single lesions usually less than 3 centimeters in diameter.
  - After marking the lesions circumferentially with electrocautery, stay sutures are placed on either side of the endometrial implant.
  - Full-thickness bowel wall excision is then performed with the cutting current electrocautery.
  - Interrupted transverse absorbable sutures are subsequently placed to close the resulting defect.
- Segmental resection of the rectosigmoid is performed for larger lesions or when neoplasia is a concern.
  - Open or laparoscopic excision of these deeply infiltrating rectovaginal lesions is technically demanding. The lack of discernable tissue planes, the intimate association of the rectum and vagina, and the frequent occurrence of distal infiltration of endometriosis down to the mid- to lower rectum make laparoscopic resection challenging.
  - Even in the hands of experienced laparoscopists, rectovaginal fistula requiring ileostomy may occur.

Small Bowel and Appendiceal Endometriosis

- While endometriosis involving the small bowel or appendix is much less common than rectosigmoid disease, careful inspection of these organs is critical in patients with advanced endometriosis to ensure complete removal of all gross disease and to minimize recurrence.
- Superficial small bowel implants may be treated with sharp excision, electrocautery, or the laser.
- Deeper implants may require small bowel resection or ileocecectomy.
- Appendiceal endometriosis is treated with appendectomy.

Results After Surgical Therapy

- Recurrence of endometriosis after surgical excision is difficult to assess because of a wide variability in the operative approach and the need for postoperative laparoscopy to document asymptomatic recurrence.
- While there are no long-term prospective studies to date, the larger studies suggest a histologically confirmed rate of recurrent endometriosis of approximately 19%.
- Gauging the response to surgery by the resolution of preoperative pelvic pain or infertility is easier to measure. Eighty-six percent of patients in a large series had complete or near complete relief of their preoperative pelvic pain.

Combined Medical and Surgical Therapy

- The rationale for preoperative medical therapy conducted over a period of 3–6 months is principally to decrease the inflammation and possibly the size of the endometrial implants.
  - Presumably, this therapy will allow easier excision with diminished adhesion formation.
  - Medical therapy may also reduce the vascularity of endometrial implants.

43 Trauma of the Colon, Rectum, and Anus

W. Brian Perry

Key Concepts

- Primary repair is the treatment of choice for all nondestructive colon injuries.
- Resection and anastomosis is the treatment of choice for most destructive colon injuries.
- Diversion should be considered in patients undergoing damage control laparotomy or who have significant pre-injury comorbidities or significant hemodynamic derangement.
- Primary repair is appropriate for accessible rectal injuries.
- Diversion alone without direct repair is sufficient to treat isolated extraperitoneal rectal injuries.
- Presacral drainage and distal washout are no longer recommended for rectal injuries.
- Anal injuries are often amenable to delayed reconstruction.

Introduction

- The management of the injured colon has evolved considerably over the past century and a half.
- Accumulated wartime experience demonstrates that mortality fell from >90% during the American Civil War to <10% in Iraq and Afghanistan (Fig. 43.1).
- Many factors have led to this improvement, including better transport time (Fig. 43.2), resuscitation, transfusion, antibiotics, and improved surgical techniques.
- Civilian experience has paralleled this and further refined current treatment algorithms.

Colon Trauma

Epidemiology

- Most colon injuries are due to penetrating abdominal trauma.
- Gunshot wounds are most common cause (Fig. 43.3), followed by stabbing and impalement.
- The colon is the second most commonly injured organ in penetrating abdominal trauma, behind only the small bowel.
- Blunt colonic injuries are rare, accounting for <10% of lesions found at laparotomy for blunt trauma, primarily from motor vehicle crashes.
  - Lap belt use, especially without concomitant shoulder harness, increases the risk of visceral injury (Fig. 43.4).

W. Brian Perry (✉)
Audie L. Murphy VA Medical Center,
San Antonio, TX, USA
e-mail: William.perry5@va.gov

S. R. Steele et al. (eds.), *The ASCRS Manual of Colon and Rectal Surgery*,
https://doi.org/10.1007/978-3-030-01165-9_43

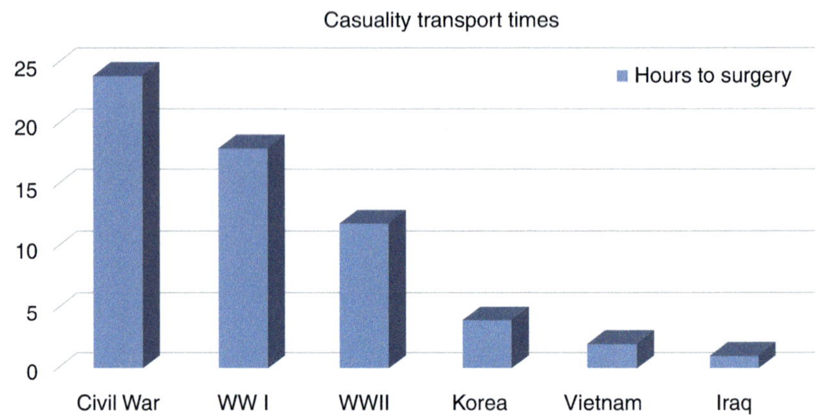

Fig. 43.1 Time from injury to surgical management in American wars

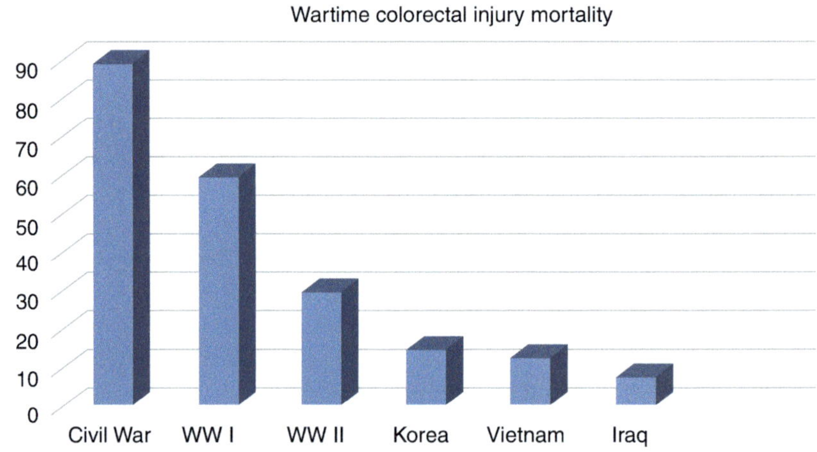

Fig. 43.2 Mortality rate of penetrating colorectal trauma in American wars

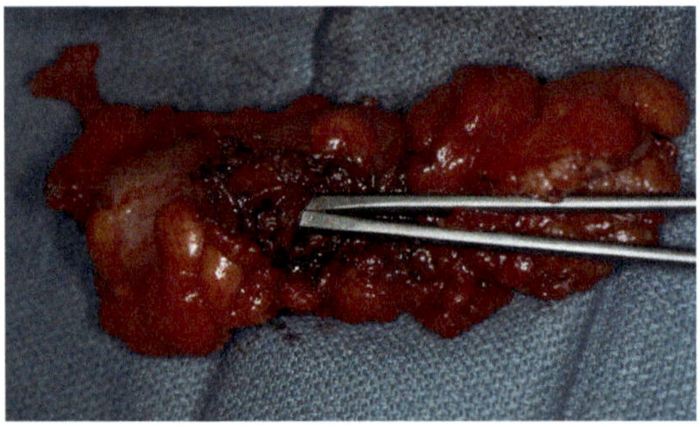

Fig. 43.3 Destructive gunshot wound to the colon

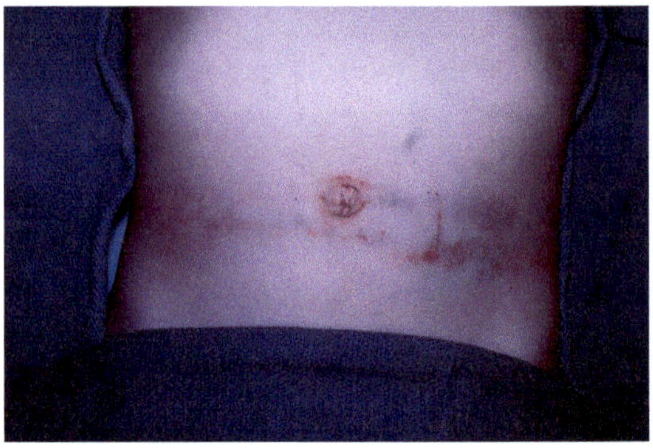

Fig. 43.4 "Seat belt sign" from improperly worn lap belt

- Most blunt injuries are minor, small hematomas or serosal tears; more serious injuries typically involve devascularization due to avulsion from the adjacent mesentery (Fig. 43.5).
- "Blow-out" injuries due to a blast overpressure wave are occasionally seen in victims of explosions, sometimes without external signs of abdominal trauma.

- The American Association for the Surgery of Trauma has published a grading scale for colonic injuries (Table 43.1).

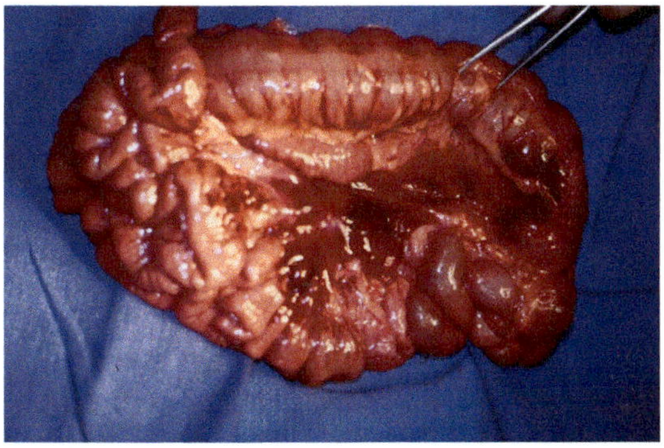

Fig. 43.5 Blunt colonic mesenteric avulsion

Table 43.1 American Association of trauma colon injury scale

Grade	Injury description
I	(a) Contusion or hematoma without devascularization (b) Partial-thickness laceration
II	Laceration ≤50% of circumference
III	Laceration >50% of circumference
IV	Transection of the colon
V	Transection of the colon with segmental tissue loss

Diagnosis

- Prompt abdominal exploration accurately finds the majority of colonic injuries in penetrating anterior abdominal trauma.
- Wounds to the flank or back can cause colonic trauma in the absence of initial peritoneal irritation or hemodynamic instability.
- Computed tomography (CT) with triple contrast is useful for delineating injuries, with 90% sensitivity and 96% specificity.
- Accurate diagnosis of colonic injury is more difficult for a bluntly injured patient, whose examination is often compromised by concomitant brain or spinal cord trauma.
  - Triple contrast CT is the examination of choice in such instances. Free intraperitoneal fluid in the absence of solid organ injury should significantly raise the index of suspicion for bowel injury (Fig. 43.6).
- Laparoscopy has little role in evaluating most penetrating anterior abdominal trauma but may be useful in stable patients with back, flank, or pelvic wounds.

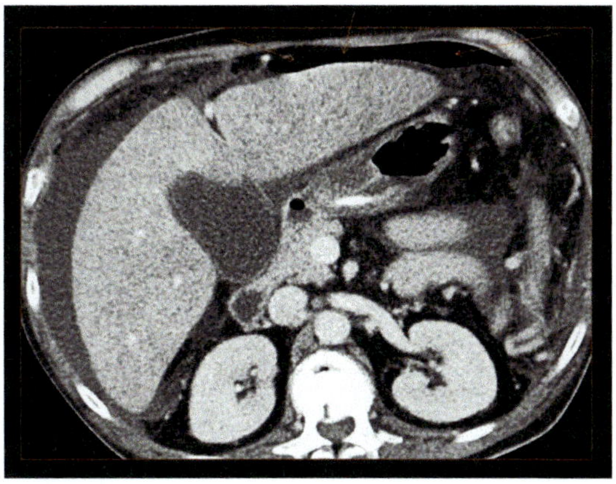

Fig. 43.6 Computed tomography scan of a blunt trauma patient showing free air and free fluid in the absence of solid organ injury. Exploration revealed a cecal injury

History of Military Colon Injury Management

- The accumulated experience of military surgeons has been critical to the evolution of current civilian colon injury management.
- With only a few exceptions, laparotomy was considered futile in the management of penetrating abdominal injury until the early stages of World War I. Laparotomy was accepted by June 1915 and was augmented by more expeditious evacuation of the wounded (Fig. 43.7); mortality decreased from 87% to 40% by Armistice Day.
- In World War II, mortality ranged from 44% for simple suture repair to 100% for resection and anastomosis. As such, the US Army Surgeon General Circular mandated colostomy for penetrating injuries. Regardless of the true impact of this specifically, mortality declined further to around 30%.
- During the Vietnam War, there were multiple series showing the feasibility of resection and anastomosis for right-sided injuries; left colon and rectal injuries were still treated with colostomy. Mortality fell to just over 13%.

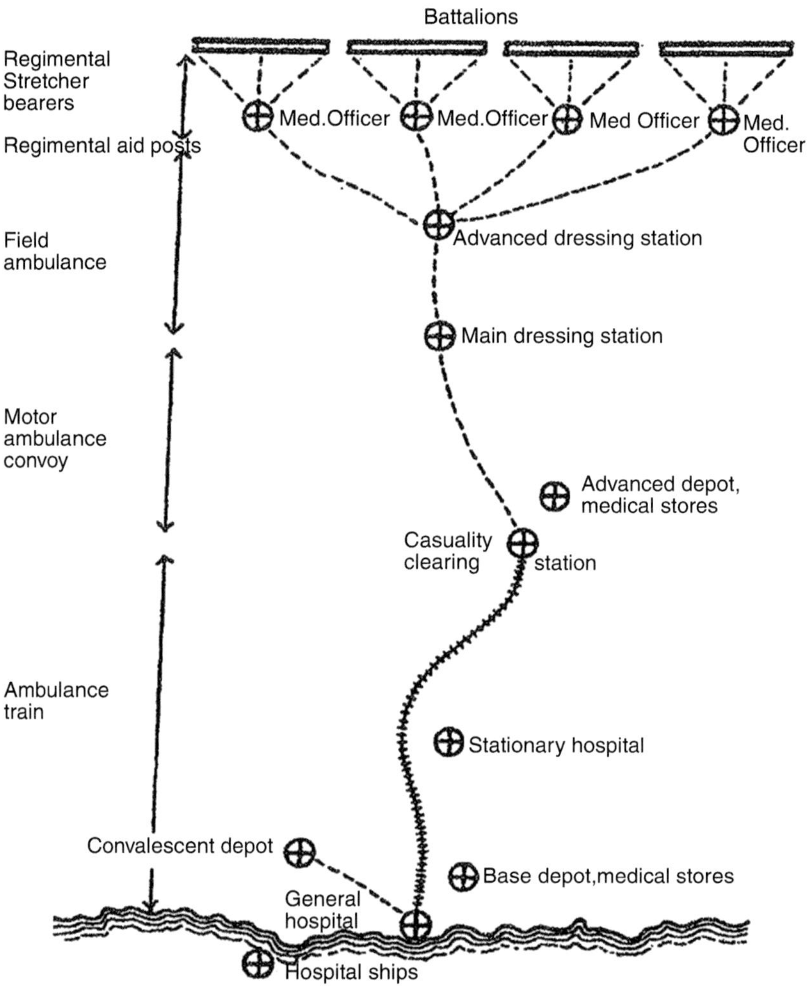

Fig. 43.7 British Army system of casualty evacuation in World War I

- Recent experiences in Iraq and Afghanistan with primary repair or resection and anastomosis demonstrated success in selected cases. However, failure occurred in >15% in one review, reinforcing the concern for primary repair in patients who experience significant hemodynamic derangement pre- or intraoperatively. Despite the challenges of devastating injuries, mortality fell again to 8%.

Current Operative Management

- Civilian experience has paralleled the military experience.
- Accumulated high-quality data have conclusively shown the safety and efficacy of primary repair in patients with Grade II injuries, even in the presence of risk factors such as hypotension, multiple transfusions, and gross spillage (Table 43.2).
- Grade III, IV, and V injuries require resection. The precise criteria for primary anastomosis remain uncertain.
- American Association for the Surgery of Trauma (AAST) conducted a multicenter randomized prospective trial of diversion vs. resection and anastomosis for destructive colon injuries.
  - Colon-related mortality was 1.3%, all in the diversion group.

Table 43.2 Randomized prospective trials of primary repair vs. diversion without exclusion criteria

	Primary repair	Primary repair	Colonic diversion	Colonic diversion
Study	Number of patients	Rate of abdominal septic complications	Number of patients	Rate of abdominal septic complications
Chappuis	28	14.3%	28	17.9%
Sasaki	43	2.3%	28	28.6%
Gonzalez	89	18%	87	21%
Total	160	13.1%	143	21.7%

  - Anastomotic leak rate was 6.6% with no deaths.
  - Severe fecal contamination, transfusion of more than 3 units of blood, and inappropriate antibiotic selection were identified as risk factors for abdominal complications. Shock on admission, delay of surgery, penetrating abdominal trauma index >25, and method of colon management (diversion vs. anastomosis) were not independent predictors of complications.
  - The authors concluded that resection and anastomosis is the treatment of choice in all destructive colon injuries regardless of severity of injury.
- Over the past two decades, the damage control laparotomy (DCL) approach to devastating abdominal trauma has significantly reduced morbidity and mortality. Abbreviated laparotomy and intensive ongoing resuscitation aim to avoid the lethal triad of coagulopathy, acidosis, and hypothermia.
  - An approach utilizing the metabolic status of the patient, the location of the injury, the need for segmental resection, and the condition of the bowel should lead to safe initial restoration of colonic continuity in 70–90% of injured patients (Fig. 43.8).

Technical Considerations

- During the initial exploration for penetrating trauma, control of gross spillage with quick suturing or stapling should occur rapidly, as soon as exsanguinating hemorrhage is stopped. There need not be definitive resection or repair.
- The colon needs to be fully mobilized above and below suspected injuries, with particular attention paid to the flexures and rectosigmoid junction.
- In penetrating trauma, paracolic hematomas must be fully explored; this is less important for blunt injuries unless there are other signs of perforation such as soiling or retroperitoneal emphysema.
- In nearly all cases of penetrating colon injury, the skin is left open, with planned delayed primary closure or secondary closure with a vacuum-assisted closure device.
- Isolated injuries to the more capacious right colon may be amenable to elevation and application of a linear stapler (Fig. 43.9).
- Perforations that are within a few centimeters of each other are best treated by removing the intervening bridge of tissue and performing a single repair (Fig. 43.10).
- There is little difference between stapled and sutured anastomoses (Fig. 43.11).
- Primary anastomosis with proximal fecal diversion with a loop colostomy or ileostomy is an attractive option in protecting high-risk anastomoses; however the data are less clear in the setting of trauma. If chosen, a loop ileostomy is easier to construct and take down.
- Should DCL be necessary, the colon can be left in discontinuity at the initial exploration; creation of a colostomy is not necessary. The abdomen is temporarily closed over nonstick plastic drapes, and a suction method of collecting fluid is fashioned (Fig. 43.12).
- Once restoration of normothermia and correction of acidosis and coagulopathy are accomplished, the patient is returned to the operating

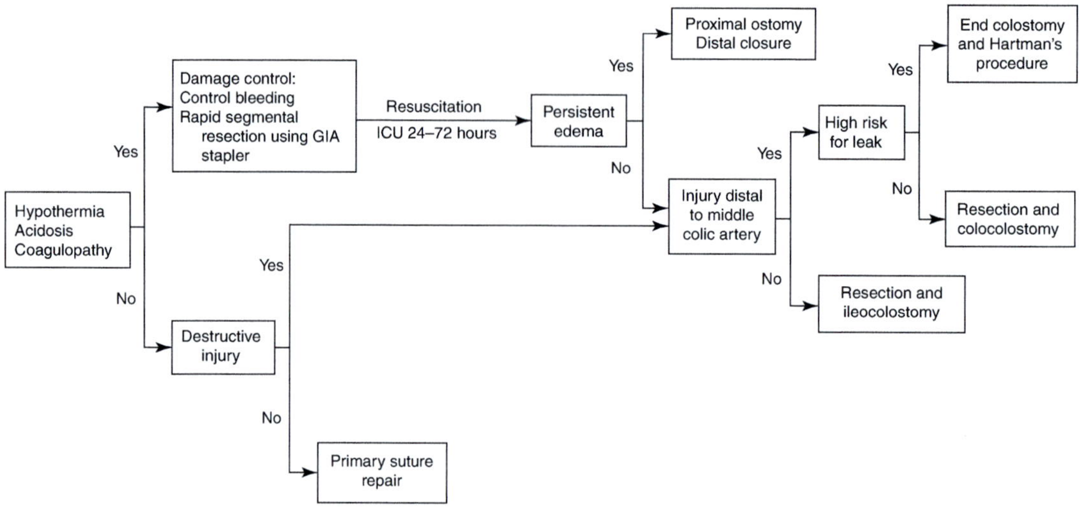

Fig. 43.8 Algorithm for colonic injury management

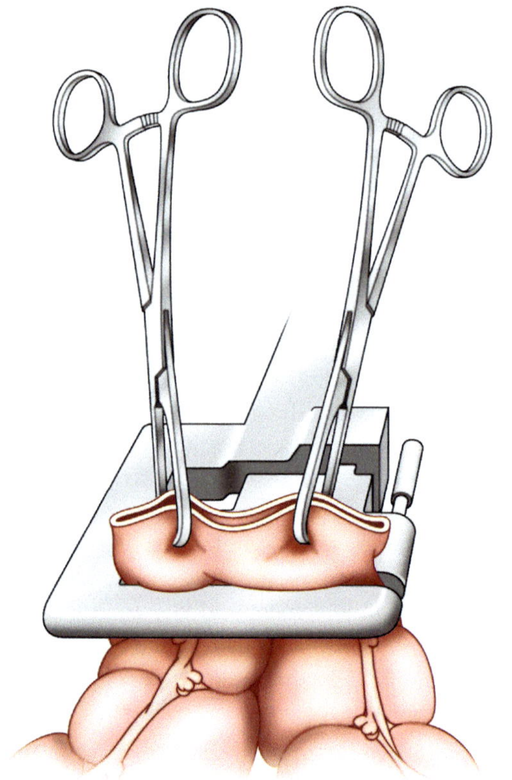

Fig. 43.9 Grade II colon injuries can be elevated and closed with a linear stapler, with care taken not to cause luminal narrowing

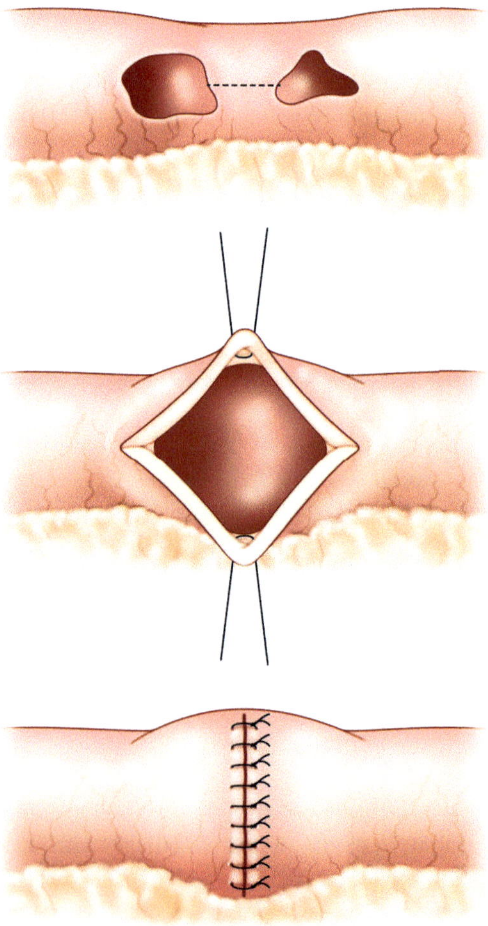

Fig. 43.10 The intervening bridge of tissue between two close perforations can be removed, and the resulting single defect can be closed transversely

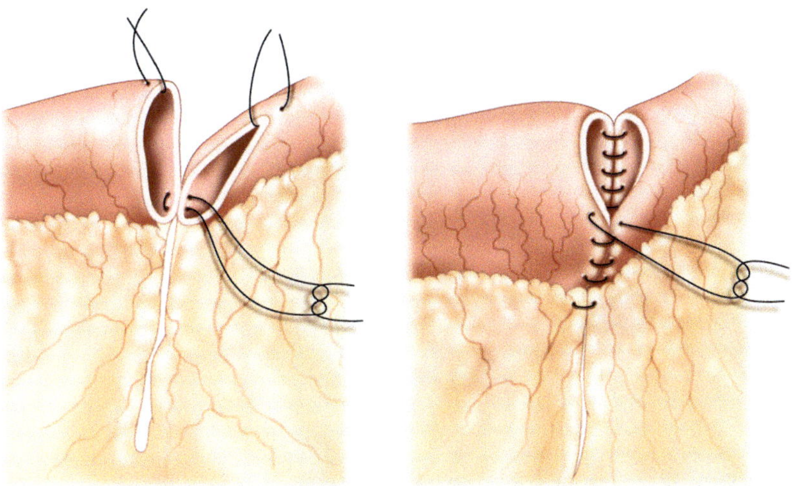

Fig. 43.11 Single-layer hand-sewn colocolostomy

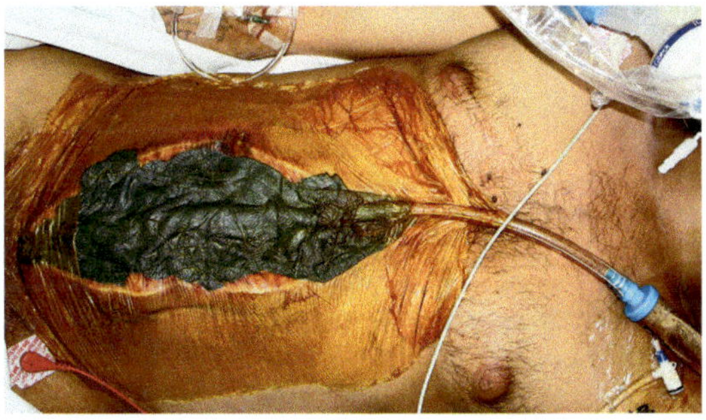

Fig. 43.12 Temporary abdominal closure can be accomplished with towels, a chest tube, and adhesive drapes if wound vacuum-assisted closure materials are not available

room. When possible, the fascial edges should not be allowed to retract causing loss of domain (Fig. 43.13).

- Temporary bridging mesh, either prosthetic or biologic, can be serially tightened at subsequent surgeries, facilitating eventual primary fascial closure (Fig. 43.14).

Rectal and Anal Trauma

Epidemiology

- The majority of rectal injuries are from penetrating pelvic trauma, more than 80% from gunshot wounds in most series. Accidental or intentional impalement, iatrogenic injuries, and rectal foreign bodies account for the rest.
- The rectum may be perforated in blunt force trauma, typically by the intrusion of sharp bony edges from severe pelvic fractures (Fig. 43.15); direct blunt rectal injury in the absence of pelvic fracture is very rare. The anus may be injured in a similar manner.
- The American Association for the Surgery of Trauma has published a grading scale for rectal injuries (Table 43.3).

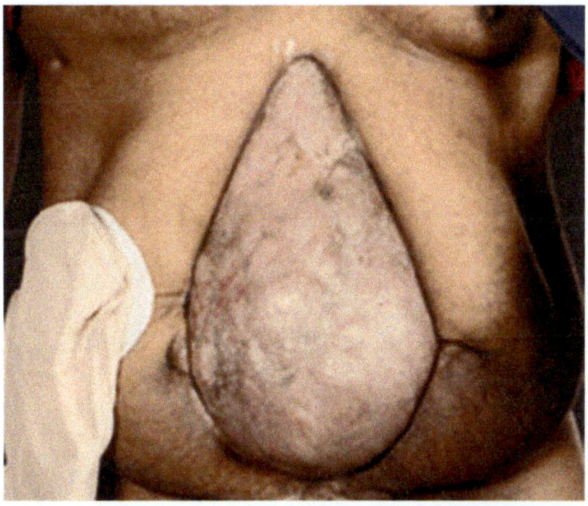

Fig. 43.13 Loss of domain with subsequent skin grafting becomes necessary if the fascial edges are allowed to retract

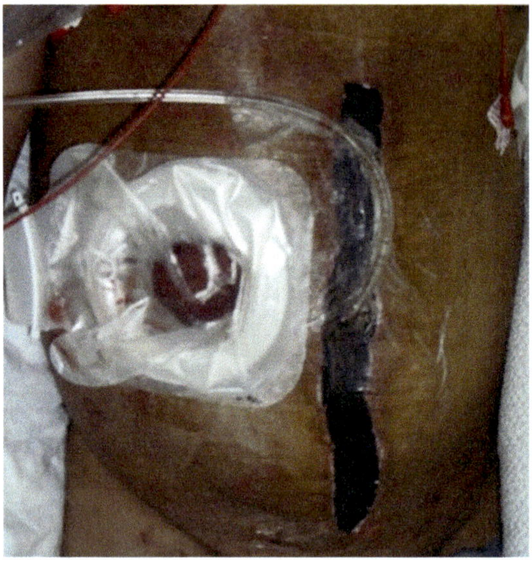

Fig. 43.14 Serial tightening of temporary bridging mesh allows for fascial closure after damage control laparotomy

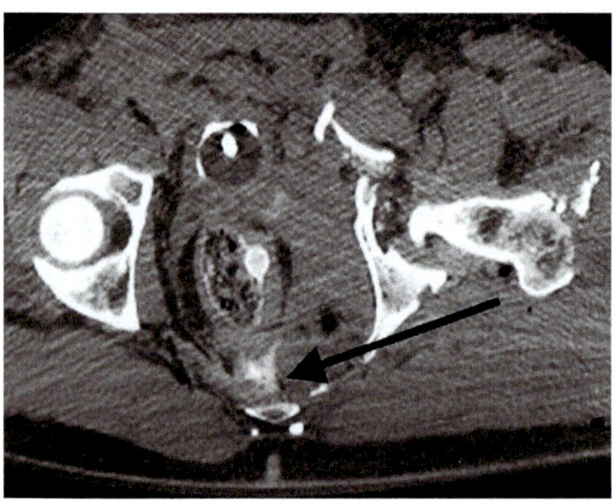

Fig. 43.15 Computed tomography showing rectal injury with contrast extravasation from a severe pelvic fracture

Diagnosis

- The presence of gross blood on digital rectal examination is highly suggestive of rectal injury and mandates further evaluation.
- Sigmoidoscopy, either rigid or flexible, should be performed, with an expected diagnostic accuracy of 80–95%.
- Genitourinary injuries accompany up to a third of rectal injuries; CT scan with bladder and rectal contrast is indicated for preoperative planning in stable patients.
- Certain injury patterns, particularly transpelvic or buttock gunshot wounds, need thorough investigation even in the absence of rectal blood.
- Most anal injuries are obvious on external inspection, although occult sphincter disruption may occasionally occur.

Table 43.3 American Association of trauma rectal injury scale

Grade	Injury description
I	(a) Contusion or hematoma without devascularization (b) Partial-thickness laceration
II	Laceration ≤50% of circumference
III	Laceration >50% of circumference
IV	Full-thickness laceration with extension into the perineum
V	Devascularized segment

Current Management and Technical Considerations

- While not specifically addressed in separate studies, there is consensus that intraperitoneal rectal injuries can be treated as colonic injuries.
- Several studies have shown that small perforations can be safely closed without proximal diversion, either transanally if low enough or from an abdominal approach if minimal rectal mobilization is required.
- Inaccessible injuries are still best managed by proximal diversion; extensive rectal mobilization is not recommended.
- If there is no evidence of intraperitoneal injury, then a loop sigmoid colostomy may be readily constructed.
- Resection with stapling of the rectum distally and end colostomy is required for destructive injuries.
- Abdominoperineal resection is occasionally necessary in devastating open pelvic fracture. These patients typically need damage control surgery with pelvic packing;

ligation or angioembolization of the hypogastric arteries may be necessary (Fig. 43.16a–b).

- Presacral drainage is no longer recommended. Closed suction drains placed in the pelvis after mobilization and repair of mid-rectal injuries at laparotomy may still be useful, as clean tissue planes are not violated.
- Similarly, distal washout of the rectum has not been shown to have any benefit in the routine management of penetrating civilian rectal trauma.
- An algorithm for the management of penetrating civilian rectal injuries, taking into account recent accumulated experience, has been suggested (Fig. 43.17).

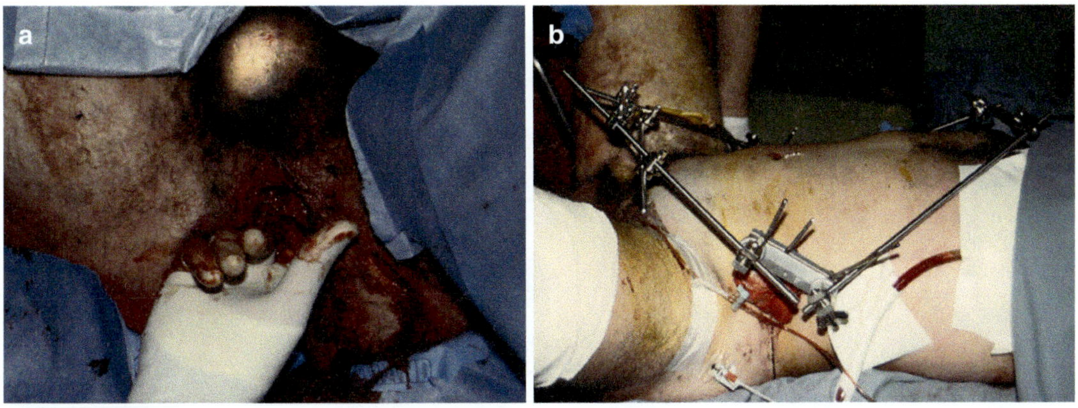

Fig. 43.16 Severe open pelvic fracture with rectal injury. (**a**) Open perineal wound with exsanguinating hemorrhage which required expedient packing and angioembolization. (**b**) Note positioning of external pelvic fixation to allow laparotomy. Attention to colostomy siting is important to decrease the risk of pin tract infections

Fig. 43.17 Algorithm for rectal injury management (43)

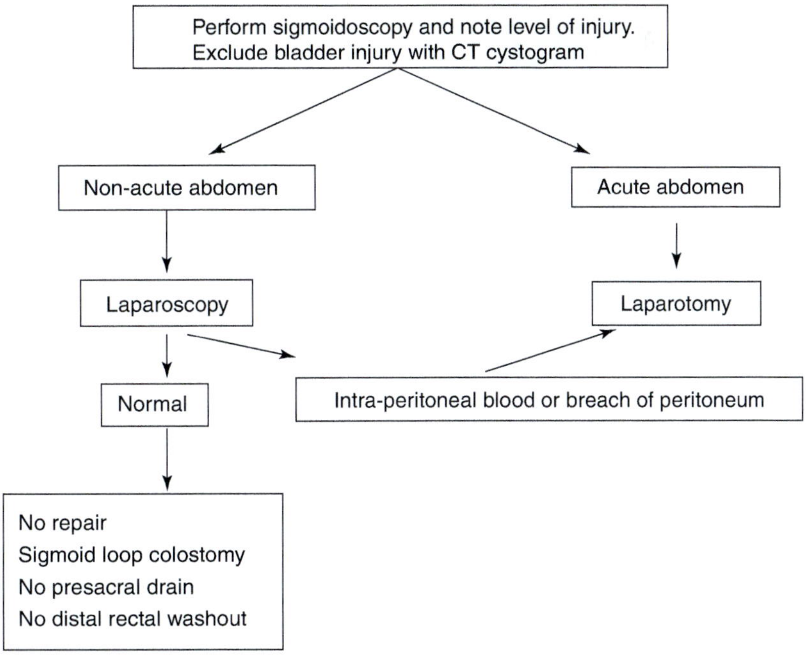

- At laparotomy, small visualized wounds can be primarily repaired while destructive injuries will require resection and end colostomy.
- Anal injuries can be repaired primarily in relatively clean wounds in stable patients; routine proximal fecal diversion is not required.
- For destructive perineal wounds, appropriate debridement and proximal diversion are paramount. A vacuum-assisted wound closure device can be used on the perineum for short periods while serial debridement is ongoing.
  - Marking of the ends of the sphincters with nonabsorbable suture can aid later reconstruction. It is imperative to investigate the genitourinary tract, as many patients will have combined injuries (Fig. 43.18a–e).

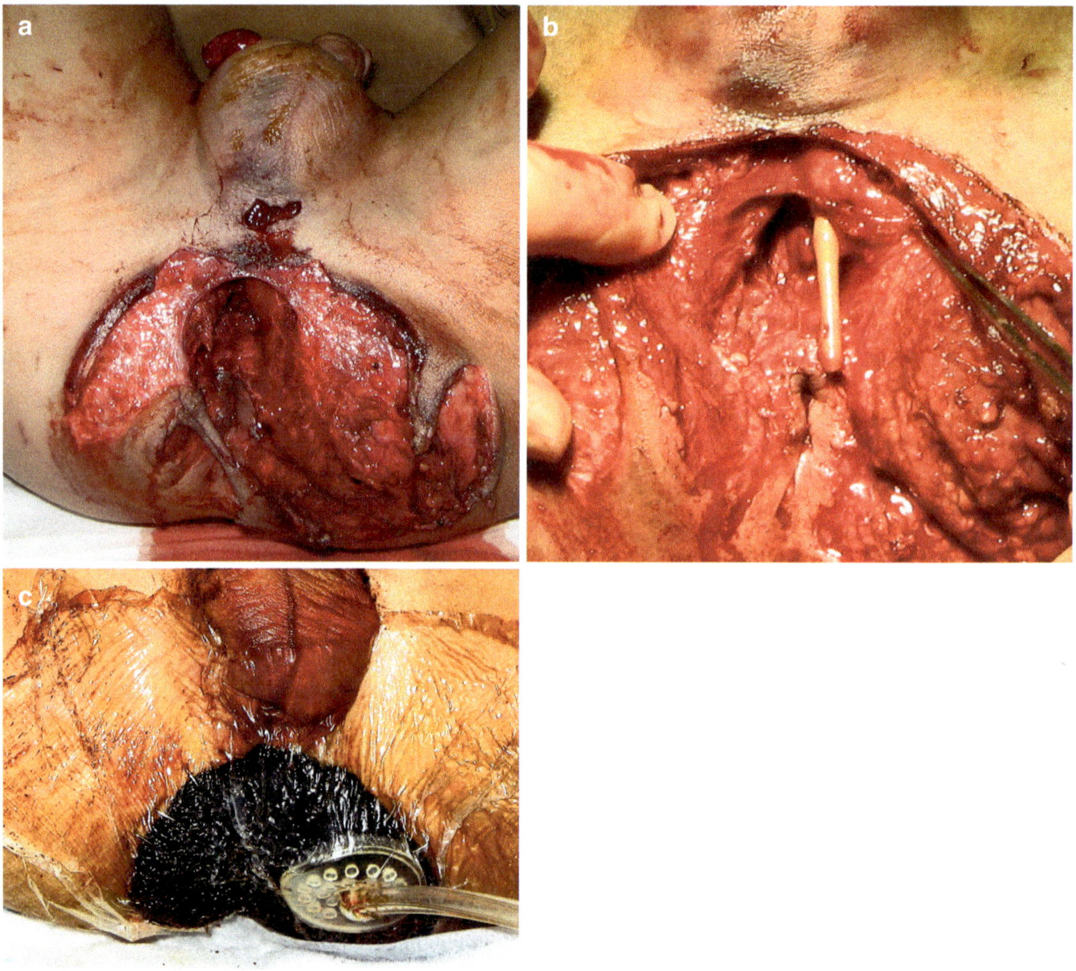

Fig. 43.18 Destructive perineal and anal injury. (**a**) Mortar fragment entered the right hemiscrotum and exited the perineum, causing a massive injury. (**b**) Urethral transection was repaired through the perineum. (**c**) Serial debridements and wound vacuum-assisted closure changes created a healthy wound bed. (**d**) Flaps were constructed to facilitate closure. (**e**) After sphincteroplasty, the final wound closure. Colostomy was closed 6 weeks later and patient had excellent continence

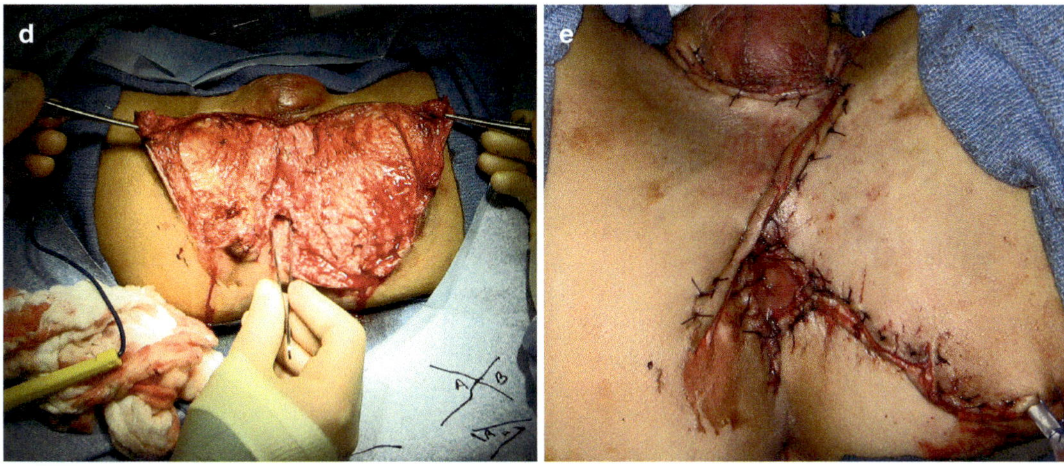

Fig. 43.18 (continued)

Inflammatory Bowel Disease: Pathobiology

44

Tara M. Connelly and Walter A. Koltun

Key Concepts

- The current theory on the etiology of inflammatory bowel disease is an exposure to an environmental factor of host or foreign origin in the individual with a genetic predisposition to dysregulated immunity.
- Over 300 genes and several hundred polymorphisms have been associated with the disease through genome-wide association studies (GWAS). Some are associated with CD, others with UC, and some with both diseases suggesting distinct but overlapping pathobiologies.
- The NOD2 gene, which is involved in bacterial recognition and response, was the first gene to be associated with the disease and is the most commonly associated gene.
- Defects in both innate and adaptive immunity have been demonstrated in murine models and human tissue from patients with the disease.
- Innate immunological processes involved in disease pathobiology include epithelial barrier function including tight junction integrity, autophagy, and pathogen recognition.
- Adaptive immunological processes involved in disease pathobiology include T cell activation, differentiation, and function.
- All main innate and adaptive immunological processes involved in both UC and CD have at least one associated gene known to be correlated with IBD through GWAS.

Introduction

- Ulcerative colitis (UC) and Crohn's disease (CD) are relapsing, inflammatory conditions of the gastrointestinal tract with distinct yet overlapping clinical and pathological features (Table 44.1).
- Although the precise etiology of these two inflammatory bowel diseases is unknown, the current research model suggests that an environmental trigger causes disease in a host predisposed due to intrinsically impaired immunity.
- Significant genetic (allele) associations have been identified in both CD and UC.
- Although the majority of such IBD alleles are associated with both CD and UC, others are exclusive to one or the other disease.
- The combination of these host genetic factors with some environmental stimulus ultimately

T. M. Connelly
Department of Colorectal Surgery, University Hospital Limerick, Limerick, Ireland

W. A. Koltun (✉)
Department of Surgery, Division of Colon and Rectal Surgery, Milton S. Hershey Medical Center, Penn State College of Medicine, Hershey, PA, USA
e-mail: wkoltun@psu.edu

S. R. Steele et al. (eds.), *The ASCRS Manual of Colon and Rectal Surgery*,
https://doi.org/10.1007/978-3-030-01165-9_44

Table 44.1 Biological characteristics of Crohn's disease and ulcerative colitis

	Crohn's disease	Ulcerative colitis
Environmental factors		
Smoking	Risk	Protective
Appendectomy	Risk	Protective
NSAIDs	+++	++
Pathogens	++	+++
Microbiome	++	+++
Genetic predisposition	+++	++
Familial association	+++	++
Number of genes associated with disease	++++	++
Innate immunity		
Mucosal integrity	++	+++
Autophagy	++++	++
Paneth cells	++++	–
Adaptive immunity		
Th1 cells	++++	++
Th2 cells	++	++++
Treg cells	++++	++
Th17 cells	++++	++
Cancer/dysplasia risk	++ (colitis)	++++

leads to an imbalance in the host immune system causing unregulated inflammation and compromise in the gut's mucosal integrity (Fig. 44.1).

The Host Environment in UC and CD

- IBD is more prevalent in more industrialized countries, among higher socioeconomic populations, in urban areas and in geographic regions further from the equator.
- Risk is increased in specific ethnic groups, such as the Ashkenazi Jewish population.
- These epidemiological phenomena suggest a genetic basis for disease, but also a potential role for infectious causes, through exposure to indigenous microbes or pathogens.

Possible Infectious Causes of IBD

- Early observations of families with multiple affected members led to theories of an infectious etiology for IBD.

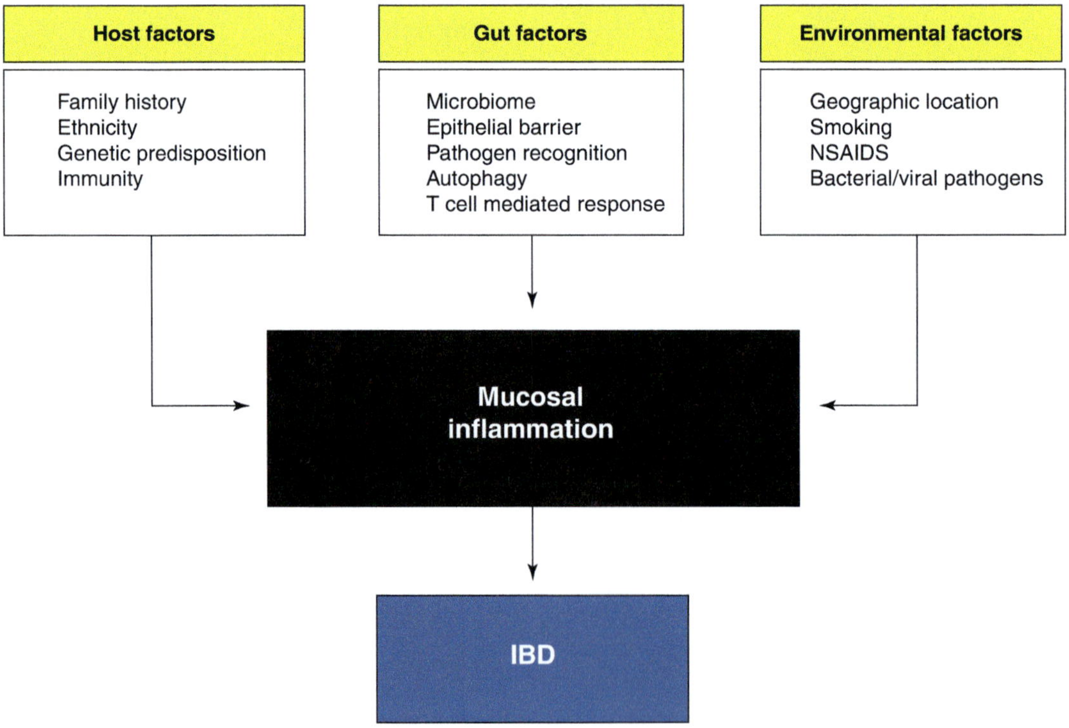

Fig. 44.1 Host, genetic, and environmental factors in the pathogenesis of IBD

- *Mycobacterium avium* subspecies *paratuberculosis* (MAP) causes a CD-like illness in livestock.
- At least 3 viruses (including the common Epstein-Barr and cytomegaloviruses), 6 yeasts, and over 20 bacteria have been associated with IBD.
- The most robust evidence for pathogens in the etiology of IBD is the raised titers of antibacterial and antifungal antibodies including anti-CBir, anti-OmpC, anti-*Saccharomyces cerevisiae* antibodies (ASCA), and perinuclear antineutrophil cytoplasmic antibodies (pANCA) that are well documented in IBD patients.

Smoking

- Of all environmental factors studied, tobacco smoking has the most replicated association with IBD.
  - There is increased risk of disease development and a more aggressive disease course with higher rates of both surgery and clinical recurrence documented in Crohn's patients who are current or former smokers.
  - These associations appear to be "dose dependent" with the strongest association found in current smokers followed by former smokers.
  - In contrast, smoking appears to have a protective effect in UC patients.

Nonsteroidal Anti-inflammatory Drugs (NSAIDs)

- NSAID use has been commonly found to be associated with an increased risk of IBD development.
- Studies on the role of NSAIDs in relapse/flares have produced conflicting results with the exception of aspirin which has not been shown to adversely affect disease activity.
- Avoidance of NSAIDs is currently recommended in most IBD patients.

The Microbiome

- Early exposure to a variety of pathogens is required for the development of a healthy immune system.
- A lack of varied pathogenic exposure, particularly in infancy and early childhood, may lead to an exaggerated immune response when the individual is exposed to these pathogens later in life.
- The inability to induce colitis in murine models with predisposing genetic mutations when raised in germ-free environments is further evidence of a role for the microbiome in disease.
  - Such animals when transferred to a nonsterile environment, populating their intestinal tract with bacteria, rapidly develop colitis.
  - Reduced intestinal microbiota diversity in IBD patients and the improvement of symptoms after fecal diversion have led to studies focused on the role of gut bacterial imbalance or "dysbiosis."
  - Probiotics have a role in the treatment and/or prevention of pouchitis in UC patients with ileal pouch-anal anastomosis (IPAA).
  - Fecal transplantation promotes microbial diversity but has had mixed results in clinical studies of IBD.
  - Microbiome research in IBD will likely be facilitated by the "big data" analytic techniques being used in genome analysis.

Appendectomy

- Meta-analysis has suggested a potential protective role of appendectomy for the development of UC.

The Role for Genetics in IBD

- A genetic predisposition to both UC and CD that has now been well established.
- Up to 40% of IBD patients have at least one affected family member.
- Affected members from "IBD families" are generally concordant for age of onset, location, and disease behavior.
- Genetics appear to play a stronger role in CD than UC. Monozygotic twin concordance rates for CD range from 20% to 50% but only 14–19% for UC.

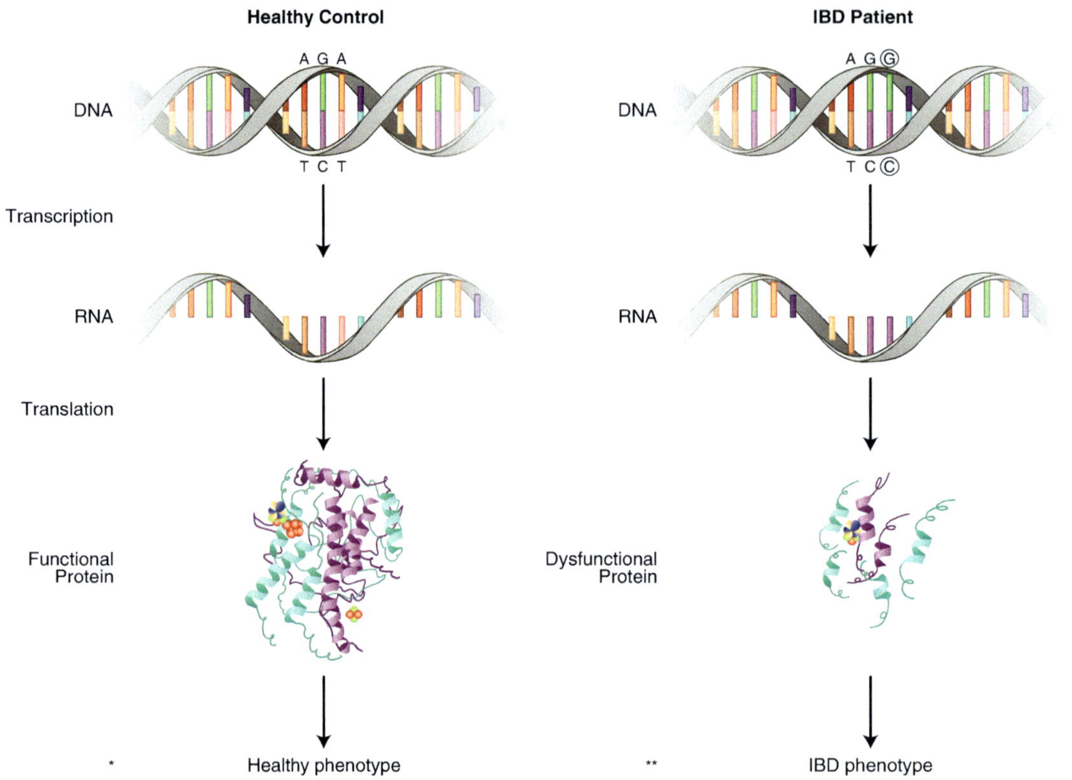

Fig. 44.2 Potential genetic differences between a healthy patient and an IBD patient

- Publically available genetic databases of the most common genetic variants demonstrate significant genetic differences between those with and without IBD (Fig. 44.2).
- To date over 300 SNPs implicating over 150 genetic loci/genes have been associated with IBD (Fig. 44.3).
- No single gene appears to be causative of either CD or UC, and thus inheritance is not the simple Mendelian pattern seen in some diseases.
- Interestingly, several gene associations are shared between IBD and other immune-related diseases such as rheumatoid arthritis, multiple sclerosis, and even leprosy suggesting overlapping pathobiology.

Innate Immunity in Crohn's Disease

- The innate immune system, present from birth, is the first line of host defense against enteric pathogens prior to the activation of adaptive or acquired immunity.
- Three key functions of innate immunity have been demonstrated to play a significant role in CD: (1) epithelial barrier function, (2) pathogen recognition, and (3) autophagy (Fig. 44.4a–c).

Epithelial Barrier Function

- The epithelial barrier forms the interface between the luminal contents of the gut and the organ itself (Fig. 44.4a).
- Mutations in cation transporter genes have been associated with both CD and UC.
- Tight junction abnormalities in IBD patients leading to inflammation and the release of cytokines such as interleukins, TNFα and IFNɣ (Fig. 44.4b).
- Interestingly, abnormal tight junction function has been demonstrated in CD patients before the onset of disease suggesting a pre-existing susceptibility to pathogen invasion due to baseline altered permeability.

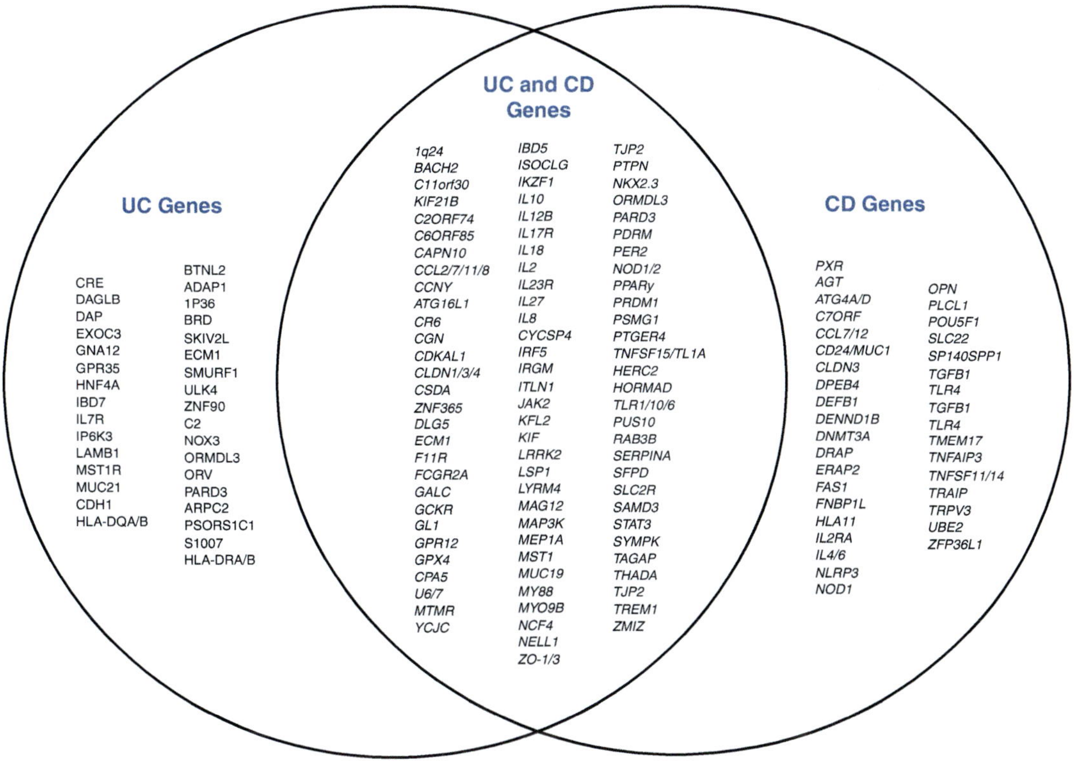

Fig. 44.3 Single nucleotide polymorphisms (SNPs) associated with IBD

Autophagy

- The healthy innate immune system also allows for the congenital ability to recognize certain antigens as foreign with subsequent "autophagy" or autodigestion.
- Toll-like receptors (TLRs) are located within endosomes and on epithelial cell surfaces. Several have been demonstrated to play prominent roles in IBD.
- Through the efficient degradation and recycling of cellular components, the process of autophagy is an energy-conserving mechanism for nutrient supply to the cell (Fig. 44.4c).
- Autophagy is also involved in the adaptive immune system through the differentiation of T and B cells.
- The main site of autophagy is the small intestinal Paneth cell; thus autophagy plays a stronger role in the pathobiology of CD than UC.
- Mutations within several genes involved in this pathway are among the most highly replicated IBD-associated genes (NOD2/CARD15, ATL16L1, IRGM).

Macrophages

- Macrophages are involved in the pathobiology of IBD through two main mechanisms: proinflammatory cytokine secretion and phagocytosis.
- Secretion of cytokines activates natural killer (NK) cells which then secrete interferon gamma (INFy) leading to dendritic cell (DC) activation.
- Once activated, DCs secrete TNFα, resulting in the recruitment of more inflammatory cells to the area.
- When levels of chemokines, cytokines (including IL1 and TNFα), and leukotrienes are elevated, leukocytes traveling within blood vessels cross the endothelial surface to reach the site of inflammation.
- Integrins, which are receptors on the surface of neutrophils, bind to factors such as mucosal addressin cell adhesion molecule-1 (MAdCAM-1) on the endothelium facilitating margination and a homing process. These integrins are the targets of some of the newest pharmacological treatments for IBD.

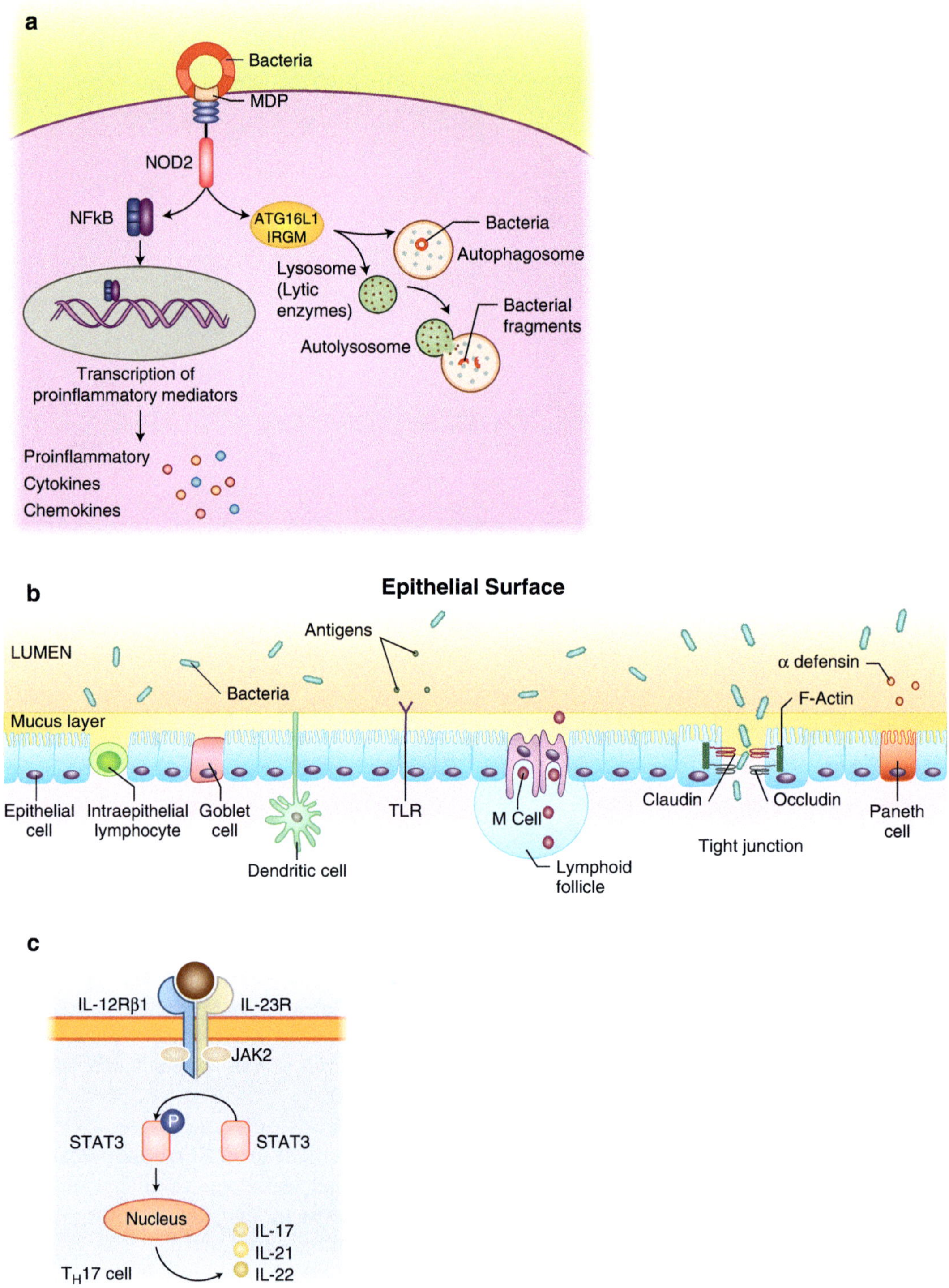
a
Bacteria
MDP
NOD2
NFkB
ATG16L1
IRGM
Bacteria
Autophagosome
Lysosome
(Lytic
enzymes)
Bacterial
fragments
Autolysosome
Transcription of
proinflammatory mediators
Proinflammatory
Cytokines
Chemokines
b
Epithelial Surface
Antigens
LUMEN
α defensin
Bacteria
F-Actin
Mucus layer
Epithelial
cell
Intraepithelial
lymphocyte
Goblet
cell
Dendritic cell
TLR
M Cell
Lymphoid
follicle
Claudin
Occludin
Tight junction
Paneth
cell
c
IL-12Rβ1
IL-23R
JAK2
P
STAT3
STAT3
Nucleus
IL-17
IL-21
IL-22
TH17 cell

APCs: The Bridge Between the Innate and Adaptive Immune Systems

- Antigen-presenting cells (APCs) recognize both host enteric and foreign peptides.
- Dendritic cells (DCs) are the APCs most implicated in the pathobiology of IBD (Fig. 44.4c).

Adaptive Immunity in Crohn's Disease

- Together, the T and B lymphocyte response to the presence of antigen comprises the adaptive immune response.
- T and B lymphocyte activation results in the elimination of pathogens through direct killing, cytokine-mediated pathways, and antibody-meditated killing.
- Differentiation into one of four major subsets is guided by the influence of cytokines in the cellular milieu (Fig. 44.5).

Cytokine Signaling

- Several cytokines play a role in the pathways involved in IBD.
- Some maintain these pathways while others induce or disrupt them.

Innate Immunity in Ulcerative Colitis

- The epithelial barrier plays a greater role in the pathobiology of UC as opposed to CD.
- UC is characterized by a loss of epithelial integrity and damage to the goblet cells, enteroendocrine cells, and enterocytes.
- Impaired tight junction permeability has been associated with an increase in proinflammatory cytokines even in quiescent IBD.
- Autophagy is also involved in the pathobiology of UC but is more studied in CD.
- Integrin mediators on the surface of neutrophils including MAdCAM-1 are also implicated in UC, and targeting of these molecules has been shown to be effective in the treatment of UC.

Adaptive Immunity in Ulcerative Colitis

- During differentiation, a Th2 cell bias leading to increased production of IL4, 5, and 13 has been associated with UC (Fig. 44.5).

Fig. 44.4 (**a**) The Epithelial Barrier. The epithelial barrier comprises the interface between the luminal contents of the gut and the organ itself. In the small bowel, 4 main cells types are found: enteroendocrine cells, mucous producing goblet cells, anti-microbial α defensin secreting Paneth cells and enterocytes. Additional cells of mucosal defense, include M cells shown channeling particles into the underlying lymphoid follicle and a dendritic cell reaching a dendrite between epithelial cells to make contact with lumenal antigens are depicted. The tight junction joining neighboring epithelial cells is comprised of transmembrane proteins that interact with the intracellular actin cytoskeleton is also depicted. In IBD, tight junction abnormalities allow the entry of antigens leading to inflammation and the release of cytokines such as interleukins, TNFa, INFy, which in turn further worsen tight junction permeability. (**b**) Autophagy and NOD2. The recognition and digestion of self and non self particles through autophagy is key to immunity. The figure shows the fusion of a lysosome with a bacteria-containing auto phagosome. This is in part dependent on functioning ATG16L1 and IR6M pathways. The NOD2/CARD15 pathway is also depicted, showing the recognition of MDP on the bacterial wall ultimately leading to NFkB activation that then results in changes in nuclear transcription of relevant inflammatory genes. (**c**) JAK/STAT PATHWAY STATs remain latent in the cell cytoplasm until, in response to signals from growth factors and cytokines through all sorts of receptors, become activated by receptor -associated tyrosoine kinases from the Janus kinase (JAK) family. STATs then dimerize, translocate into the cell nucleus and activate the transcription of inflammatory modulators

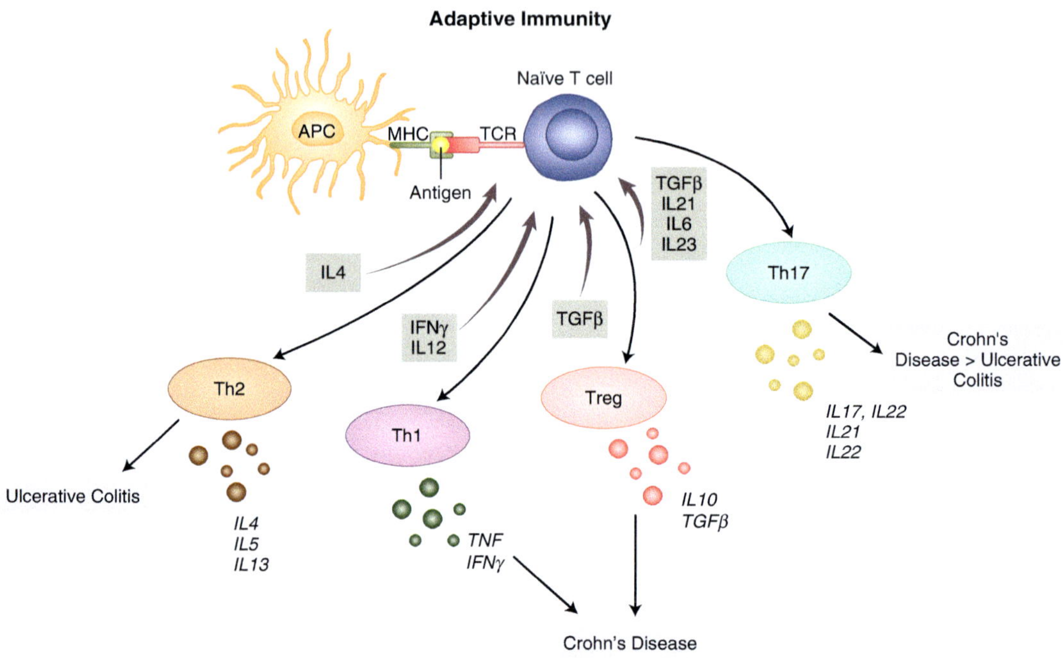

Fig. 44.5 Adaptive immunity in Crohn's disease

Genetic Correlates Suggesting Mechanisms of Disease in IBD

Innate Immunity

Epithelial Barrier

- The MUC family of glycoproteins is the main component of intestinal mucus.
- Murine MUC2 knockout models develop an IBD-like colitis with features of both CD and UC.
- Polymorphisms in several cellular transport genes have been associated with IBD.
- A number of IBD-associated genes including signal transducer and activator of transcription molecules (STATs) can be classified as epithelial integrity genes.
- STATs translocate into the cell nucleus and activate transcription and the expression of various proteins (Fig. 44.4d).

Pathogen Recognition and Autophagy

NOD2/CARD15

- Genes within the autophagy pathway were the first genes to be associated with IBD.
- NOD2/CARD15 is the strongest, most commonly replicated gene association with IBD, especially CD.
- The gene is expressed in several cell types involved in the pathobiology of IBD including intestinal epithelial cells, Paneth cells, dendritic cells, and monocytes.
- Despite having the strongest IBD association, not all IBD patients have a NOD2/CARD15 mutation.

The Adaptive Immune System

- The human leukocyte antigen (HLA), also known as the major histocompatibility complex (MHC), involved in the presentation of antigen to T cells, has been the focus of much study in IBD with a particular focus on HLA-DR subtypes.
- Several cytokines are involved in the pathways involved in IBD. Some maintain these pathways, while others induce or disrupt them.
- The most well-known IBD-associated cytokine is IL10. This cytokine is unique since it has anti-inflammatory properties.

- IL23 is secreted by DCs, monocytes, and activated macrophages and is involved in the Th17 differentiation of naïve T cells and the release of other proinflammatory cytokines.
- The IL23 gene is also associated with other immune-mediated diseases including rheumatoid arthritis and ankylosing spondylitis as well as extraintestinal manifestations in UC.

The Molecular Basis of Malignant Degeneration

- Both UC and CD patients are at an increased risk of developing colorectal cancer (CRC).
- Inflammation is a known risk factor for dysplasia, metaplasia, and progression to carcinoma.
  - IBD-associated dysplasia and CRC is found predominately in tissues with evidence of current or past inflammation; risk is therefore also related to disease extent and duration.
- In IBD, however, this progression is generally unpredictable.
- Like sporadic CRC, IBD-associated CRC involves p53 and adenomatous polyposis coli (APC) mutations and microsatellite instability. However, the sequence of these mutations in progressive malignant degeneration is different between IBD-associated malignancy and conventional CRC (Fig. 44.6).
- Methylation levels have been demonstrated to be higher in human UC-CRC versus sporadic cancer.

Surgical Genetics in IBD

- There are several gene alleles that suggest a predisposition to early surgery in IBD.
- The presence of the IRGM SNP rs4958847 was associated with the more frequent need for repeat ileocolectomy.

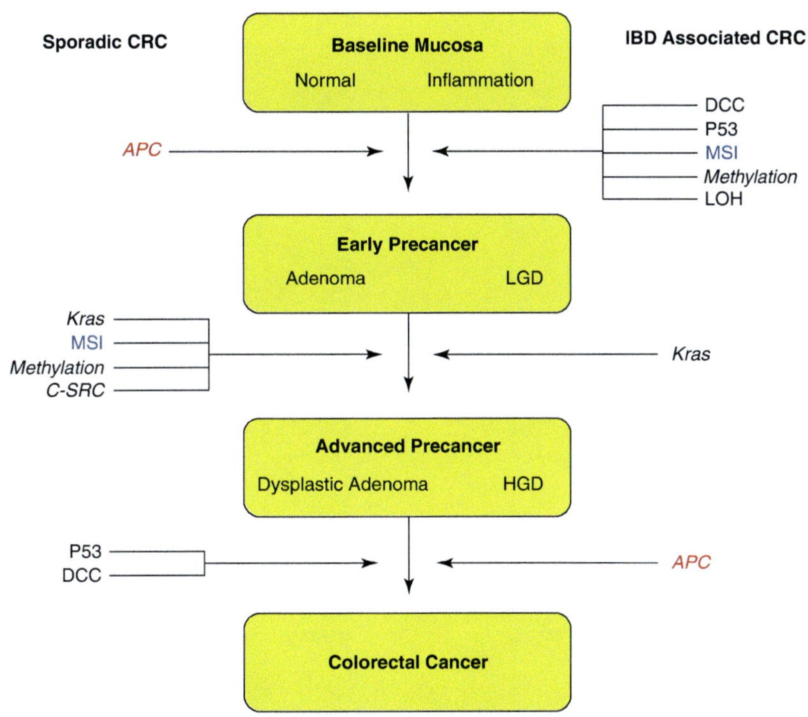

Fig. 44.6 Malignant degeneration in the setting of IBD versus sporadic colorectal cancer

IBD Diagnosis and Evaluation

45

Matthew M. Philp and Howard M. Ross

Key Concepts

- Familiarity with modes of clinical presentation of ulcerative colitis and Crohn's disease allows the clinician to promptly select the most efficient combination of tests.
- Knowledge of histologic findings of ulcerative colitis and Crohn's disease facilitates discussion with other physicians of the care team and tailors specific medical and surgical therapies.
- Serologic tests such as ASCA, pANCA, and fecal markers such as calprotectin are increasingly becoming utilized for diagnosis and treatment effectiveness monitoring.
- High-definition images, chromoendoscopy, confocal laser endomicroscopy, and double balloon enteroscopy add to the ability to diagnose and treat ulcerative colitis and Crohn's disease.
- Capsule endoscopy, computerized tomography, and computerized tomography enterography, magnetic resonance imaging, and magnetic resonance enterography are revolutionizing the care of the IBD patient.

M. M. Philp
Division of Colon and Rectal Surgery, Temple University Hospital, Philadelphia, PA, USA

H. M. Ross (✉)
Department of Surgery, Division of Colon and Rectal Surgery, Temple University Hospital, Philadelphia, PA, USA
e-mail: Howard.Ross@tuhs.temple.edu

Inflammatory Bowel Disease: Diagnosis and Evaluation

Context

- Crohn's disease and ulcerative colitis are collectively referred to as inflammatory bowel disease.
- Though largely different in the distribution of disease and the manner which inflammation affects the gastrointestinal tract, occasionally the diseases overlap both in behavior and in their responses to similar treatments.

Ulcerative Colitis

- The classic presentation of ulcerative colitis is the passage of bloody diarrhea.
- The goal of investigation is to make a specific, prompt diagnosis to facilitate early treatment.
- Patients with prior immunosuppression, foreign travel, or antibiotic use may be more likely to have an infectious colitis.
- Careful abdominal examination and rectal exam should be performed.
- External anal exam may reveal signs of anal Crohn's disease (waxy thickened skin tags, fistulae).
- Infectious colitides that mimic ulcerative colitis and are evaluated via stool culture.
- The colon is evaluated by colonoscopy.

S. R. Steele et al. (eds.), *The ASCRS Manual of Colon and Rectal Surgery*,
https://doi.org/10.1007/978-3-030-01165-9_45

Table 45.1 Extraintestinal manifestations of ulcerative colitis

Site	Manifestation	% of UC patients
Skin	Erythema nodosum	3
	Pyoderma gangrenosum	1.4–5
	Aphthous stomatitis	4
Hepatopancreatobiliary	Primary sclerosing cholangitis	5
	Cholangiocarcinoma	Rare
	Primary biliary cirrhosis	Rare
	Autoimmune hepatitis	Rare
	Portal vein thrombosis	Rare
	Pancreatitis	Rare
Musculoskeletal	Peripheral arthritis	20–40
	Axial	5
	Metabolic bone disorders	2–40
	Myopathy	Rare
Ocular	Episcleritis	Rare
	Uveitis	Rare
	Scleritis	Rare
	Optic neuritis	Rare
Hematologic	Anemia	8–73
Vascular	Venous thromboembolism	Rare
Genitourinary	Urolithiasis	Rare
Pulmonary	Bronchiolitis	Rare
Cardiac	Pericarditis	Rare

  - Classically, ulcerative colitis begins in the distal rectum and extends proximally. The inflammation progresses in a confluent manner and affects only the mucosa, without fissuring, or skip areas.
  - Extraintestinal manifestations can be associated with both ulcerative colitis and Crohn's disease (Table 45.1).

Crohn's Disease

- Crohn's disease can affect anywhere in the digestive tract from the mouth to the anus; the inflammatory process of Crohn's involves the full thickness of the bowel wall.
- These attributes contribute to the clinical behavior of the disease and the varied manners of presentation.
- The most common site of Crohn's disease is an ileocolic distribution, though anal disease and intestinal or colonic disease alone are also regularly seen.
- Stricture, obstruction, fistula, and abscess formation are important sequelae.
- Discontinuous skip areas of involvement are common and are a clear differentiating behavior from ulcerative colitis.

IBD Histology

- The combination of clinical disease activity, endoscopic findings, and histology generates accurate diagnosis.
- Communication with an experienced IBD pathologist enables correct treatment decisions in many situations.

Ulcerative Colitis

- The classic macroscopic finding in ulcerative colitis (UC) is contiguous mucosal inflammation extending from the rectum proximally for a variable distance in the colon (Table 45.2).
- Clinicians should be aware of certain instances where inflammation in UC may not be con-

Table 45.2 Macroscopic features used for the diagnosis of IBD

	Ulcerative colitis	Crohn's disease
Localization GI tract	Especially colon and rectum	Whole GI tract
Ileum	Not except in backwash ileitis	Often involved
Colon	Left > right	Right > left
Rectum	Commonly involved	Typically spared
Distribution GI tract	Diffuse (continuous)	Segmental (discontinuous)
Ulcers	Superficial ulcers	Aphtoid ulcers, confluent deep linear ulcers
Pseudopolyps	Common	Uncommon
Skip lesions	Absent	Present
Cobblestone pattern	Absent	Present
Deep fissures	Absent except in fulminant colitis	Present
Fistulae	Absent except in fulminant colitis	Present
Mucosal atrophy	Marked	Minimal
Thickness of the wall	Normal	Increased
Fat wrapping	Absent	Present
Strictures	Uncommon	Present

tinuous to avoid confusion with Crohn's disease.
  - The cecal cap or patch is an isolated area of inflammation surrounding the appendix.
  - Backwash ileitis is a contiguous ileal inflammation and is correlated with severity of cecal inflammation. Patchy or noncontiguous ileal involvement should raise suspicion for Crohn's disease.
  - Rectal mucosal sparing may result from topical therapy.
- The hallmark of microscopic ulcerative colitis is widespread crypt distortion with a continuous pattern of inflammation (Fig. 45.1).
- The severity of inflammation is worse distally in the colon and limited to the mucosa, with occasional extension into the superficial submucosa.

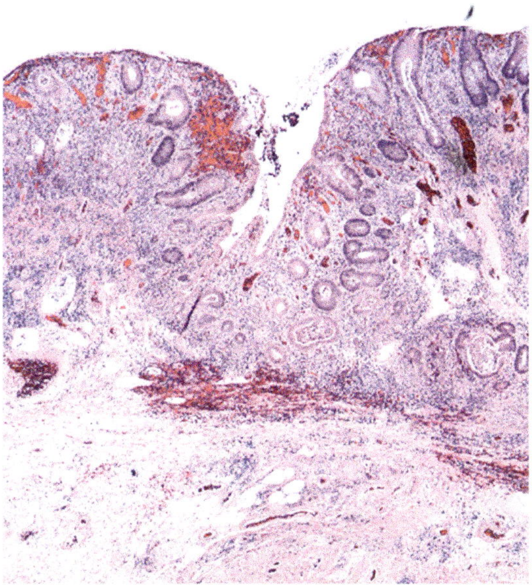

Fig. 45.1 Low-power view of ulcerative colitis showing inflammatory infiltrate confined to the mucosa

- In fulminant UC, ulcer penetration to the muscularis propria with serositis can occur, making it difficult to discriminate from Crohn's disease.
- Crypt abscesses occur more frequently in UC (41%) than in Crohn's disease (19%).
- Basal plasmacytosis is an early feature of UC and can be used to help differentiate it from infectious colitis.

Crohn's Disease

- Crohn's disease (CD) can affect any portion of the gastrointestinal tract. Mostly commonly the ileocolon is involved.
- "Creeping fat" at the mesenteric edge of the bowel is due to transmural inflammation and is strongly correlated with Crohn's.
- Aphthous ulcers are one of the early gross mucosal findings.
- Coalescence and spread of the ulcers leads to the classic cobblestoned mucosal appearance (Fig. 45.2).
- Inflammatory pseudopolyps caused by inflammation and reactive hyperplasia are more common in UC but also occur in Crohn's colitis (Fig. 45.3).

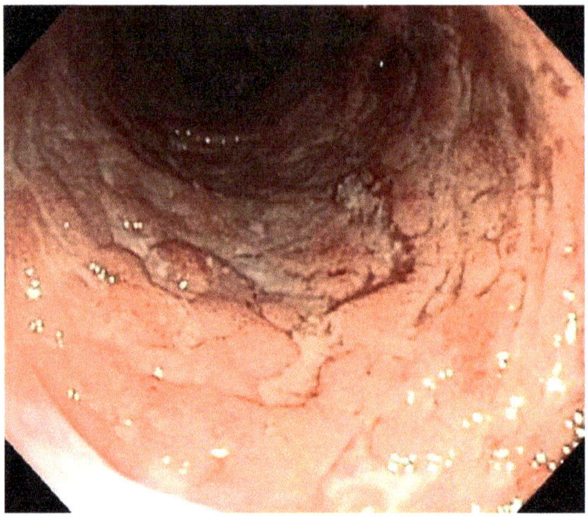

Fig. 45.2 Crohn's disease with cobblestone appearance of the mucosa

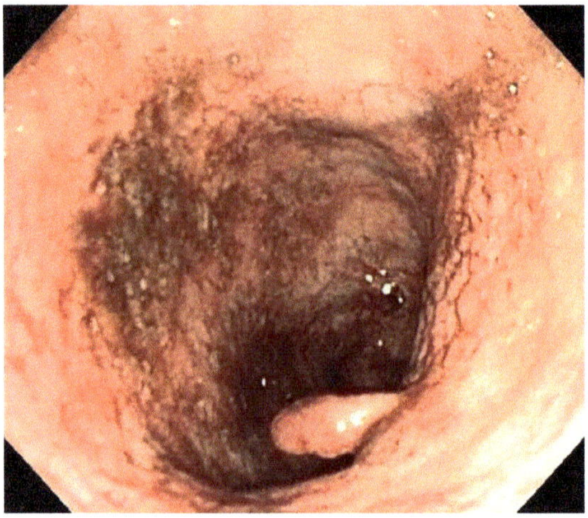

Fig. 45.3 Pseudopolyp in Crohn's disease

- Focal chronic inflammation, granuloma, and localized crypt distortion are some of the commonly accepted microscopic features in Crohn's. Plasma cells and lymphocytes in the lamina propria are hallmarks of colonic inflammation (Figs. 45.4 and 45.5).
- Lymphoid aggregates are common and transmural. Granulomas, although highly suggestive, are not specific for Crohn's, being present in a few as 18% of samples (Fig. 45.5).
- Microscopic differences between UC and CD are listed in Table 45.3.

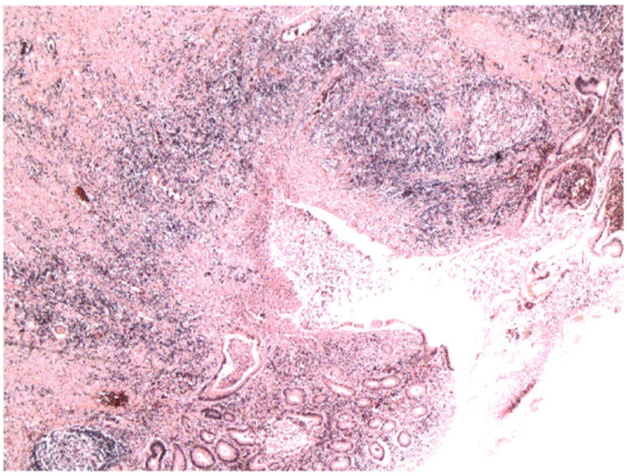

Fig. 45.4 Low-power view of Crohn's disease with lymphocytic infiltration and mucosal ulceration

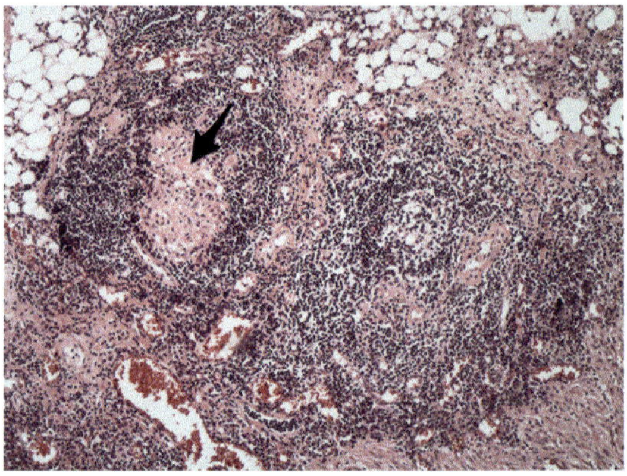

Fig. 45.5 Crohn's disease with full-thickness inflammatory change and lymphocytic infiltration into the serosa and granuloma (arrow)

Indeterminate Colitis

- Often the clinical and histologic features of a patient's disease course may share features of both UC and Crohn's disease.
- The Montreal Working Party recommended that the term indeterminate colitis should be reserved only for those cases where colectomy has been performed and pathologists are unable to make a definitive diagnosis of either CD or UC after full examination.
- The term "inflammatory bowel disease, type unclassified" (IBDU) is suggested for patients in whom there is evidence on clinical and endoscopic grounds for chronic inflammatory bowel disease affecting the colon, without

Table 45.3 Microscopic features used for the diagnosis of IBD

	Ulcerative colitis	Crohn's disease
Crypt architectural irregularity	Diffuse (continuous)	Focal (discontinuous)
Chronic inflammation	Diffuse(continuous) decrease proximally	Focal (discontinuous) Variable
Patchiness	Uncommon	Common
Localization	Superficial transmucosal sometimes in submucosa	Transmural
Serositis	Absent except in fulminant colitis	Present
Lymphoid aggregates	Frequent in mucosa, submucosa	Common, transmural
Granulomas	Absent, except with ruptured crypts	Present
Acute inflammation	Diffuse (continuous)	Focal (discontinuous)
Crypt epithelial polymorphs	Diffuse (continuous)	Focal (discontinuous)
Crypt abscesses	Common	Uncommon
Mucin depletion	Present, pronounced	Uncommon, mild
Neuronal hyperplasia	Rare	Common
Muscular hypertrophy	Absent	Present
Paneth cell metaplasia	Present	Uncommon
Pyloric gland metaplasia	Rare	Present

small bowel involvement, and no definitive histological or other evidence to favor either CD or UC.

- The distinction between UC and Crohn's colitis is highly relevant when considering a patient with an IC or IBDU diagnosis for a restorative proctectomy.
  - Higher rates of pelvis sepsis, pouch fistula, and pouch failure have been reported in patients with IC undergoing ileal pouch-anal anastomosis (IPAA), compared to a UC cohort.
  - However, when the patients ultimately diagnosed with CD are excluded, outcomes for the IC patients are similar to the UC group.

Serology and Markers of Disease

ASCA and pANCA

- Anti-Saccharomyces cerevisiae antibodies (ASCA) and perinuclear anti-neutrophil cytoplasmic antibodies (pANCA) have been extensively studied as biomarkers in IBD.
- pANCA positivity ranges from 2% to 28% in CD patients, while a sensitivity of 56% and specificity of 89% has been reported in UC patients,
- ASCA positivity is found in 39–69% of CD patients and in 5–15% of UC patients.

Fecal Markers

- The presence of calprotectin in stool implies mucosal inflammation.
- Calprotectin has been used in a variety of clinical situations for IBD patients, including diagnosis, prediction of clinical course, monitoring response to therapy, and postoperative surveillance.
- Lactoferrin is similar to calprotectin in that it is neutrophil derived and found in the stool.
- Fecal markers would be a desirable tool for following mucosal healing. There is mounting evidence that mucosal healing is a better target in IBD treatment than control of clinical symptoms.
- In post-resection CD, fecal calprotectin >200 μg/g has been shown to be predictive of endoscopic recurrence at 12 months.
  - Calprotectin was superior to CRP and a clinical disease index (CDAI) for detection of recurrence and monitoring response to treatment.

Inflammatory Markers

- C-reactive protein (CRP), erythrocyte sedimentation rate (ESR), and albumin are three common serum measures of the acute phase of inflammation.
  - Albumin has a long half-life (5 days), limiting its clinical usefulness.
  - CRP has a short half-life (19 h) compared with other acute phase proteins and will therefore rise early after the onset of inflammation and rapidly decrease after resolution of the inflammation.

- Compared with CRP, ESR will peak much less rapidly and may take several days to decrease, even if the inflammation resolves.
- Inflammatory markers are useful in excluding IBD diagnosis in patients with functional bowel disorders.

Endoscopy in IBD

Flexible Endoscopy

- Flexible endoscopy remains the gold standard technique in the initial diagnosis and follow-up management of patients with suspected or established inflammatory bowel disease (Figs. 45.6 and 45.7).
- Endoscopy allows for mucosal inspection and tissue sampling for histology. Therapeutic interventions, such as balloon dilations of strictures, can also be performed.
- Intubation and biopsy of the terminal ileum is especially important in patients with suspected Crohn's disease.
- Endoscopically abnormal areas of the colon should be sampled.
- Biopsy of normal areas is important as well, as presence or absence of microscopic colitis can aid in differential diagnosis.
- Particular attention should be directed to areas of colonic stricture, with historical studies showing 24% of UC and 6% of CD strictures may be malignant.
- IBD patients are known to carry higher risks of procedural complications. This is especially true in patient with advanced age, severe colitis, or during therapeutic interventions.
- Upper endoscopy plays a role in the smaller subset of Crohn's patients that present with esophagogastroduodenal involvement.
- Single and double balloon enteroscopy allow endoscopists to reach far into the small bowel, in both antegrade and retrograde directions.
  - Double balloon enteroscopy has been shown to be similar to CT enterography for the evaluation of Crohn's small bowel disease.
  - Double balloon enteroscopy is invasive, however, and carries a risk of perforation, with major complication rates of around 1% and interventional procedure complication rates of 4–5%.
  - One major advantage is that it can be used for stricture dilation or retained video capsule removal, with relatively good rates of success.
- Beyond initial diagnosis, endoscopy is used for evaluating the response of IBD to medical therapy, monitoring recurrence after surgery, and for dysplasia surveillance in UC.
- Colonoscopy is indicated when there is a major change in symptoms; however, it is well

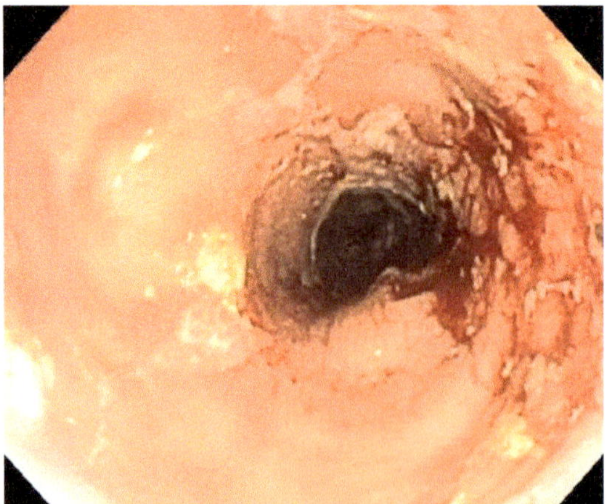

Fig. 45.6 Crohn's colitis of transverse colon

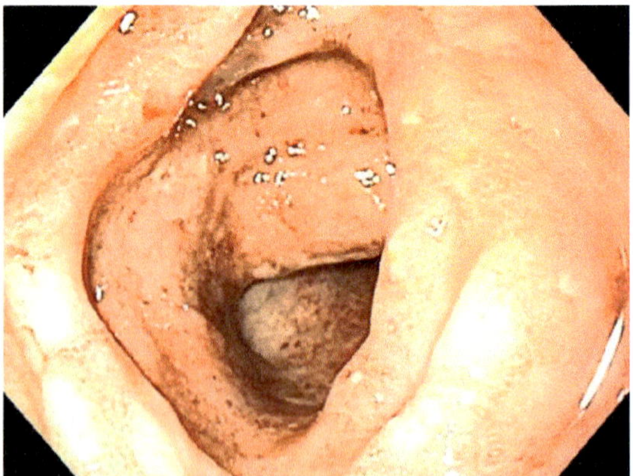

Fig. 45.7 Sigmoid colon in ulcerative colitis

established that clinical symptoms and endoscopic findings may not be congruent.

- Colonoscopy is recommended 6–12 months after surgery for CD, as anastomotic recurrence (Fig. 45.8) is common (60–90% at 1 year).
- Fecal calprotectin may be a useful screening trigger to prompt earlier colonoscopy.
- Early medical intervention in the postoperative CD setting is associated with lower rates of endoscopic recurrence and higher rates of complete mucosal healing.

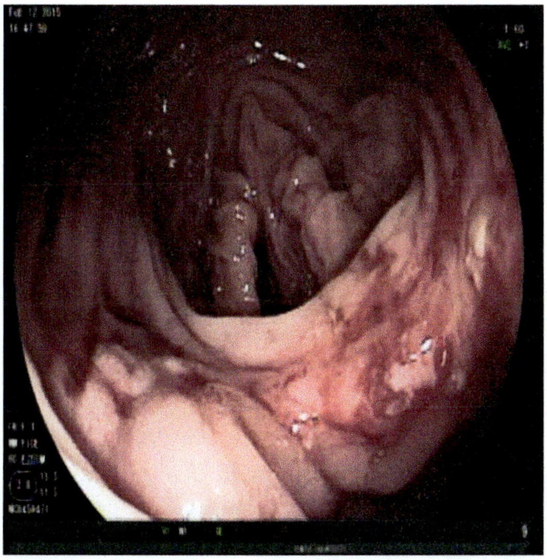

Fig. 45.8 Anastomotic recurrence 2 months after ileocolic resection

- The Rutgeerts endoscopic score (Table 45.4) has been shown to predict the recurrence of symptoms and need for repeat surgery based on the endoscopic appearance of the neoterminal ileum and ileocolonic anastomosis.
- There are many endoscopic scoring systems described for UC. Two of the most commonly used are the Baron and Mayo scores (Table 45.5).
- Colonoscopy is recommended for patients with chronic colitis for dysplasia surveillance.
  - The risk of colorectal cancer surpasses that of the general population after 8–10 years of disease.
  - Although studies linking dysplasia and cancer in UC are more widely available than those on CD, surveillance and treatment paradigms are often similar in the two groups.
  - The Crohn's and Colitis Foundation of America (8–10 years), the American College of Gastroenterology (8–10 years), and the American Society of Colon and Rectal Surgeons (8 years) all have similar recommendations for initiating surveillance colonoscopy in chronic colitis.
  - After a negative study, most recommend 1–2 year interval for repeat examination.
  - After two negative exams, follow-up time can be 1–3 years.

Table 45.4 Rutgeerts score of postoperative endoscopy for CD and corresponding CTE scoring system for postsurgical examination

Rutgeerts	Endoscopic findings	CTE	CTE findings
i0	No lesion in the neoterminal ileum	CTE0	No findings
i1	<5 aphthoid ulcers	CTE1	Minor mucosal irregularities with slight wall thickening and mural contrast enhancement
i2	>5 aphthoid ulcers with normal mucosa in between or skip areas or larger lesions related to anastomosis	CTE2	Mucosal hyperdensity with distinct bowel wall thickening, no stenosis, or stenosis without prestenotic dilatation
i3	Diffuse aphthoid ileitis, with mucosa extensively inflamed	CTE3	Major mucosal abnormalities, distinct bowel wall thickening with target sign and extravisceral signs such as perienteric stranding, comb sign, fibrofatty proliferation, stenosis with prestenotic dilatation, and/or the presence of complications
i4	Diffuse inflammation, large ulcers, nodules, and/or stenoses		

Table 45.5 Baron and Mayo scores for ulcerative colitis

	Baron score	Mayo score
Score 0	Normal mucosa, ramifying vascular pattern clearly visible throughout, no spontaneous bleeding, no bleeding to light touch	Normal or inactive disease
Score 1	Abnormal but not hemorrhagic: appearances between "0" and "2"	Mild disease (erythema, decreased vascular pattern, mild friability)
Score 2	Moderately hemorrhagic: bleeding to light touch, but no spontaneous bleeding seen ahead of instrument on initial inspection	Moderate disease (marked erythema, absent vascular pattern, friability, erosions)
Score 3	Severely hemorrhagic: spontaneous bleeding seen ahead of instrument at initial inspection and bleeds to light touch	Severe disease (spontaneous bleeding, ulceration)

  - After 20 years of disease, recommendations are again every 1–2 years.
  - Patients with primary sclerosing cholangitis (PSC) have higher rates of malignancy and should undergo yearly evaluation.
- The traditional recommendation for endoscopic biopsy for dysplasia surveillance is four-quadrant sampling every 10 cm.
  - Particular attention should be paid to raised lesions or strictures, with sampling of any normal surrounding areas to allow for histologic comparison.
  - Significant pseudopolyposis may make surveillance unreliable by obscuring the mucosa or being too numerable to sample.
  - A typical endoscopic biopsy samples 0.05% of the mucosal surface; a minimum of 33 random biopsies has been shown to result in 80–90% sensitivity for detecting dysplasia, with 64 required for 95%.
- Recent advances in endoscopic technology are changing how dysplasia surveillance is performed.
  - The American Society for Gastrointestinal Endoscopy (ASGE) has recently made strong recommendations that high-definition video equipment be used when using traditional white-light colonoscopy is performed; one retrospective study showed twice as many dysplastic lesions were detected with high-definition equipment rather than standard definition.
  - Chromoendoscopy involves the use of dye applied to colonic mucosa to improve epithelial surface detail and allow for targeted sampling. Two prospective tandem colonoscopy studies have shown chromoendoscopy is 1.8–3.5 times more likely to detect dysplastic lesions than conventional four-quadrant biopsy technique.

Capsule Endoscopy

- For the IBD patient, evaluation of small bowel CD is the most common indication for VCE.
  - Meta-analysis has shown VCE to have higher diagnostic yield than colonoscopy, push enteroscopy, conventional enterography, and CT enterography.
  - Capsule retention is a rare, but feared, complication of VCE, particularly in patients with strictures.
  - Reported rates of capsule retention in CD patients are around 13%; a slowly dissolvable patency capsule exists and is intended to assess patency of the small bowel prior to VCE.
  - The European Society of Gastrointestinal Endoscopy (ESGE) has recommended that VCE be done if deemed necessary to change management in CD and only after cross-sectional imaging and patency capsule evaluation exclude a stricture.

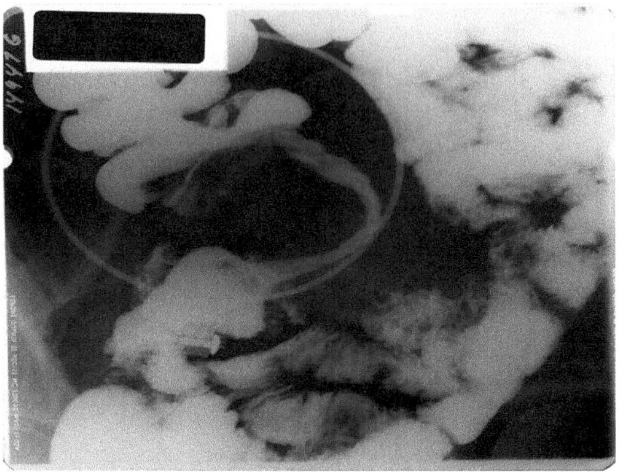

Fig. 45.9 Fluoroscopic enterography study showing terminal ileal stricture in Crohn's disease

Radiology in IBD

Plain Radiography

- Plain radiographs remain a standard for rapid assessment of the IBD patient presenting with acute abdominal symptoms. Free air from hollow viscus perforation, toxic megacolon, or small bowel obstruction from stricture or adhesion can be rapidly and inexpensively confirmed.
- Historically, small bowel follow through (SBFT) studies have been the standard approach to assess active disease (Fig. 45.9).

CT

- CT imaging for UC patients is mostly limited to situations of severe or fulminant colitis.
- CT for CD allows noninvasive assessment of the small and large bowel, as well as possible extraintestinal manifestations of disease.
- CT enterography (CTE) has been shown to be as specific as conventional enteroclysis in diagnosis of Crohn's small bowel lesions, with somewhat less sensitivity.

MRI

- The increased soft tissue resolution delivered by MRI over CT has made it the preferred imaging technique when imaging is required for complex fistulizing perianal CD.

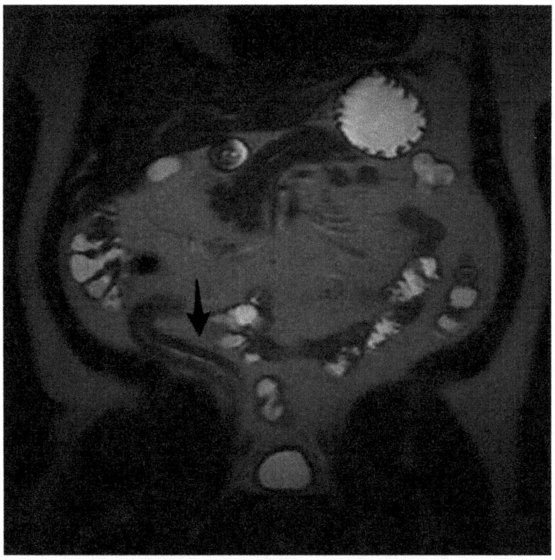

Fig. 45.10 MRE in Crohn's disease. Coronal T2-weighted images demonstrate segmental mural thickening of the terminal ileum (black arrow)

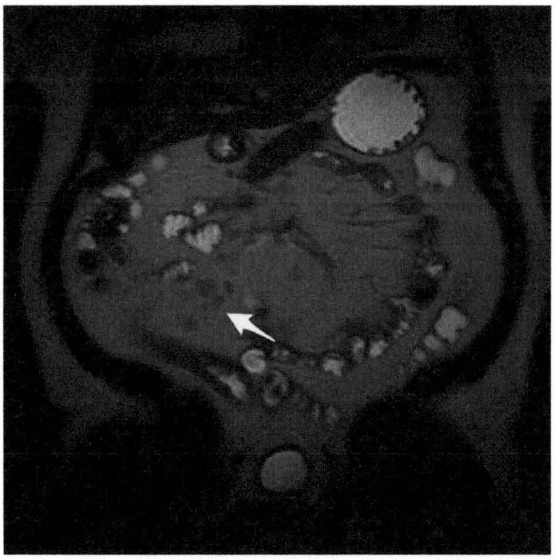

Fig. 45.11 MRE in Crohn's disease. Coronal T2-weighted images with surrounding fibrofatty proliferation and ileocolic lymph nodes (white arrow)

- Multiple image acquisition sequences are taken including T1, T2, and diffusion weighted (Figs. 45.10, 45.11, and 45.12).
- The presence of bowel wall thickening in conjunction with asymmetric mural hyperenhancement is essentially pathognomonic for Crohn's disease (Fig. 45.10).
- The ability of MRE and CTE to detect Crohn's lesions is similar.

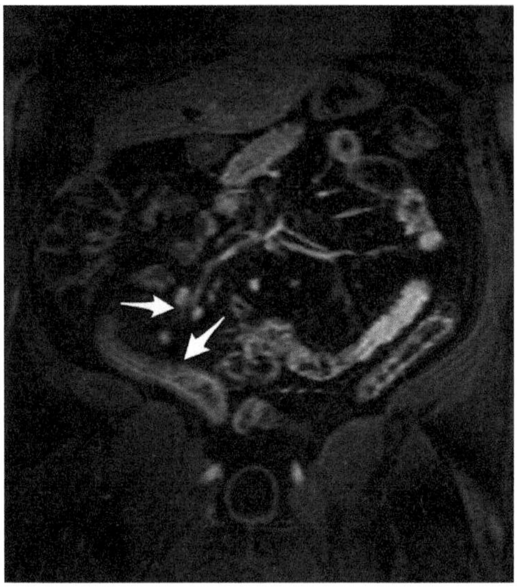

Fig. 45.12 MRE in Crohn's disease. Gadolinium-enhanced coronal T1-weighted image demonstrates mucosal hyperenhancement as well as enhancement of the ileocolic lymph nodes, indicative of active Crohn's disease (arrows)

Ultrasound

- US is a highly operator-dependent imaging method, and correct interpretation requires adequate experience in abdominal and bowel sonography.

Evolving Role of CTE and MRE

- There is concern regarding increasing exposure of patients to ionizing radiation and subsequent risk of malignancy.
  - IBD patients represent a cohort at particular risk for repeated studies employing ionizing radiation.
  - The young IBD patient represents a particular concern.
  - Given the similar clinical usefulness of both CTE and MRE, many advocate for the use of MRE in most situations where imaging is required, especially in the adolescent IBD patient.

Medical Management of Chronic Ulcerative Colitis

46

Stefan D. Holubar and Mattias Soop

Key Concepts
- CUC is highly prevalent in North America and Europe, and its incidence is increasing globally.
- CUC has an unknown etiology, but the pathogenesis is believed to be multifactorial, with an impaired mucosal immune regulation and unknown environmental conditions or trigger(s).
- Surgeons must be familiar with the numerous medical treatments for CUC, including their side effects.
- Mild-to-moderate CUC is typically treated in a bottom-up manner with oral aminosalicylates, and if steroids are required for flares, then the patient is transitioned to AZA/6MP or a biologic agent to wean the steroids.
- Moderate-to-severe disease is typically treated in a top-down manner with combination therapy with a biologic agent and immunomodulator, often under the cover of temporary steroid treatment.
- Patients may require surgery and should be aggressively optimized in terms of anemia, malnutrition, and VTE prophylaxis.
- Pouchitis is common and responds promptly to oral antibiotic use. Patients with "Crohn's-like" picture of the pouch may benefit from additional medical therapy.

Electronic Supplementary Material The online version of this chapter (https://doi.org/10.1007/978-3-030-01165-9_46) contains supplementary material, which is available to authorized users.

S. D. Holubar (✉)
Department of Colorectal Surgery, Cleveland Clinic, Cleveland, OH, USA
e-mail: holubas@ccf.org

M. Soop
Department of Surgery, Salford Royal NHS Foundation Trust, Salford, UK

Manchester Academic Health Science Center, The University of Manchester, Manchester, UK

Part 1: Defining CUC

Introduction

- Chronic ulcerative colitis (CUC) is an idiopathic, recrudescent chronic disease of colonic mucosal ulceration (Fig. 46.1) with a prevalence of well-over 600,000 affected persons in North America.
- CUC is one end of the spectrum of idiopathic inflammatory bowel disease (IBD) (Fig. 46.2).
- The vast majority of patients with CUC will require multiple medications to control disease over the course of their lifetime.

S. R. Steele et al. (eds.), *The ASCRS Manual of Colon and Rectal Surgery*,
https://doi.org/10.1007/978-3-030-01165-9_46

- Symptoms include chronic diarrhea, often bloody, accompanied by tenesmus, defecatory frequency and urgency.
- The urge incontinence that many patients experience is often the most troubling symptom.
- Extraintestinal manifestations are numerous and summarized in Fig. 46.3.

Diagnosis

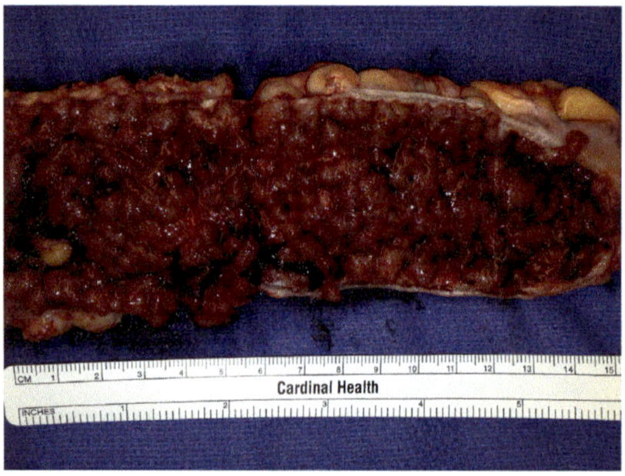

Fig. 46.1 Operative specimen, gross photo. Note ulcerated, hemorrhagic mucosa with severe pseudopolyposis and exposed muscularis, slightly (chronically) thickened bowel wall. (Courtesy of Dr. Stefan D. Holubar MD, MS)

- CUC is diagnosed using a combination of history, physical exam, and colonoscopic and histologic appearance (Fig. 46.4).
- Conditions that may need to be ruled out in the differential diagnosis include irritable bowel syndrome, celiac sprue, and the other colitides.
- Relatives and siblings of patients with IBD may also have either CUC or Crohn's disease.

Colonoscopy

- Mucosal inflammation starts in the rectum (not the anus) and progresses continuously proximally a variable distance.
- Inflammation may be mild, with a granular mucosa with contact bleeding, to more severe with linear ulcerations, to fulminant with severe pseudopolyposis (Fig. 46.1).
- In patients with long-standing disease, the colon may be foreshortened, ahaustral ("lead-pipe colon").
- Biopsies demonstrate acute and/or chronic colitis, with inflamed lamina propria and

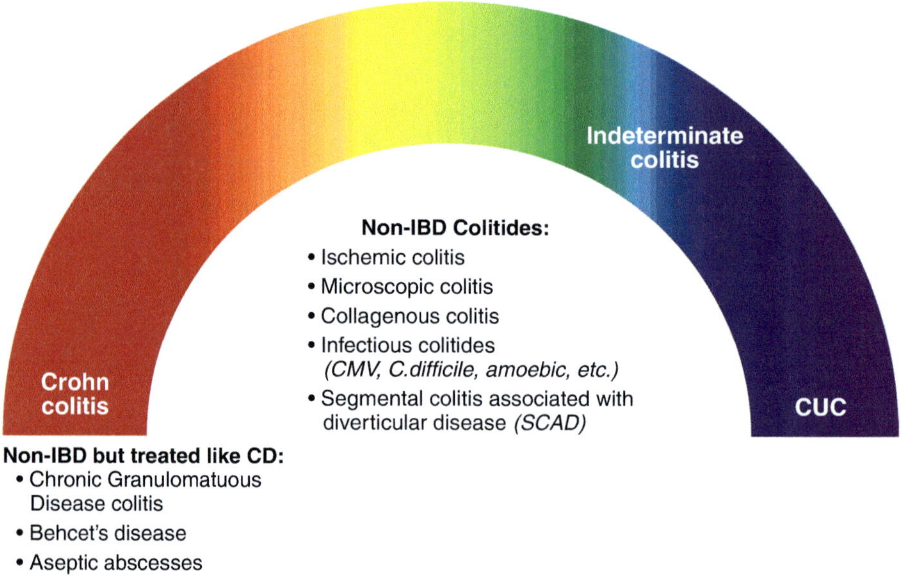

Fig. 46.2 Auto-inflammatory colitis spectrum

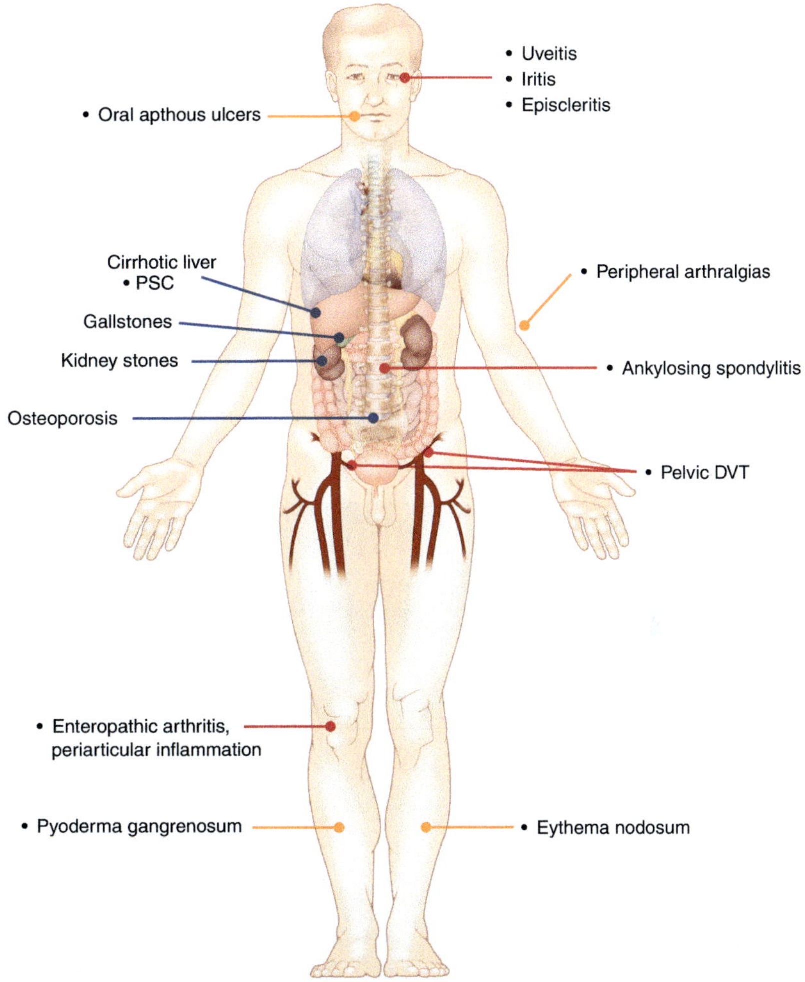

Fig. 46.3 Schematic representation of common extraintestinal manifestations in CUC

distorted crypt architecture. The presence of granulomas generally indicates CD (Fig. 46.4: photomicrograph of CUC vs. CD with granuloma).

Imaging

- Imaging studies such as fluoroscopic small bowel follow-through, magnetic resonance enterography (Fig. 46.5), computed tomographic enterography (CTE, Fig. 46.6), or capsule endoscopy (Video 46.1) may be used to assess for stigmata of Crohn's disease.
- CT and MRI may also demonstrate the extent and severity of colitis. Findings include an edematous, thickened rectal and colonic wall with mucosal hyper-enhancement.

Serology

- Nonspecific serologic inflammatory markers include white blood cell count (WBC), erythrocyte sedimentation rate (ESR), and C-reactive protein (CRP).
  - Both ESR and CRP are sensitive markers of inflammation, inexpensive, and available

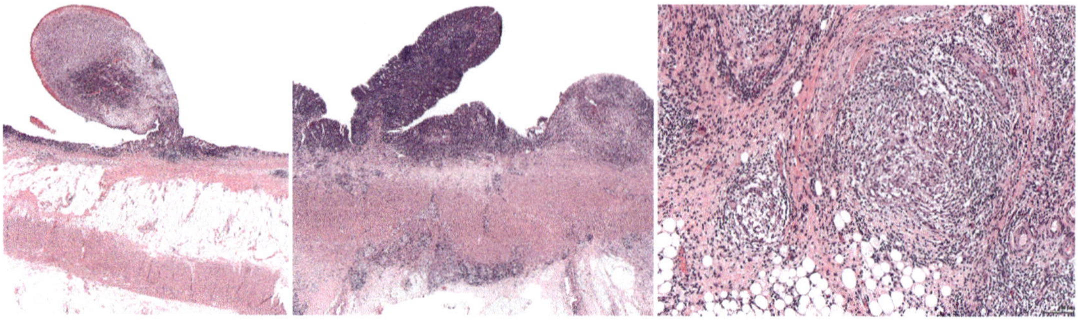

Fig. 46.4 Photomicrograph of CUC vs. CD. H&E stain. Top panel shows severe transmural inflammation and granulomas consistent with Crohn's disease; middle panel shows severe mucosal ulceration consistent with ulcerative colitis; bottom panel shows mucosal inflammation and a pseudopolyp consistent with ulcerative colitis. (Courtesy of Dr. Anthony Senagore)

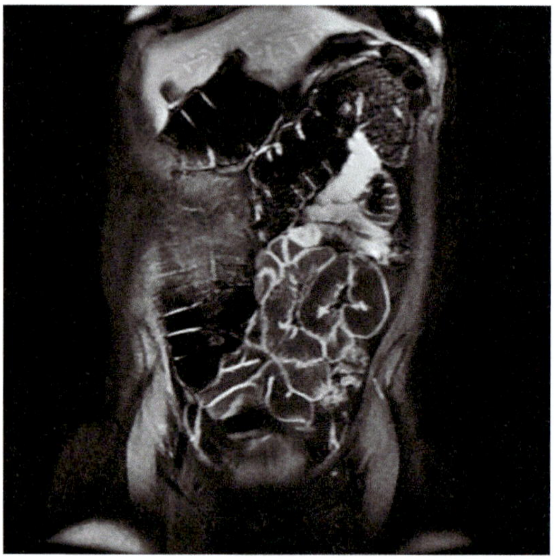

Fig. 46.5 Magnetic resonance enterography, LAVA sequence 70 s post-contrast. Note the normal appearance of the small bowel wall in a CUC patient prior to total colectomy. Specifically the small bowel wall is of normal thickness, and the lack of mucosal or bowel wall hyper-enhancement, with no demonstrable fistula, strictures, or abscesses

in most centers. The main difference is ESR's longer half-life.
- Fecal calprotectin can predict and follow the trajectory of disease flares and predict mucosal healing.

- Prometheus® antigen testing is reserved for cases that are difficult to classify based on traditional criteria.

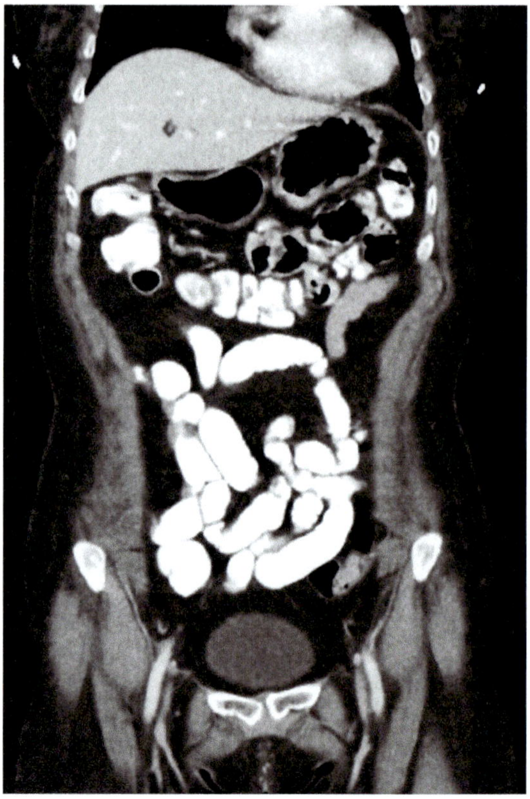

Fig. 46.6 Computed tomographic enterography. Note the normal appearance of the small bowel wall in a CUC patient prior to total colectomy. Specifically the small bowel wall is of normal thickness, and the lack of mucosal or bowel wall hyper-enhancement, with no demonstrable fistula, strictures, or abscesses

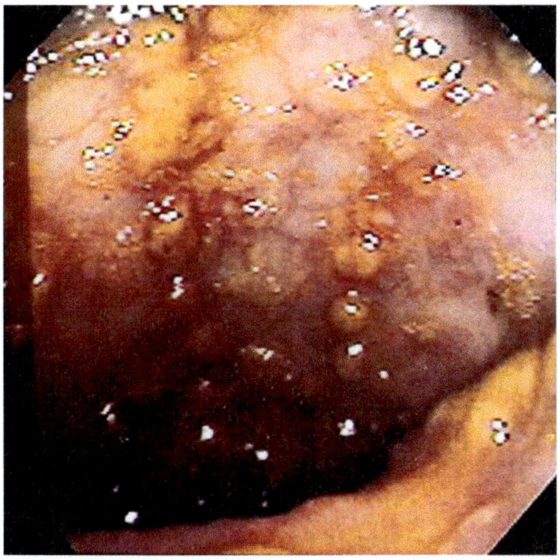

Fig. 46.7 Colonoscopic appearance of pseudomembranous (*Clostridium difficile*) colitis. Note the pale white appearance of the pseudomembranes. (Courtesy of Dr. Anthony Senagore)

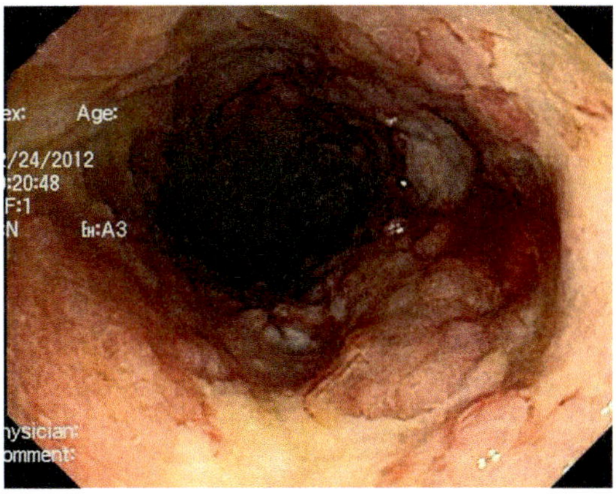

Fig. 46.8 Colonoscopic appearance of CMV colitis in a patient with CUC. Note the classic "punched-out" ulcerations (bottom center of photo) in a background of pseudopolypsis. (Courtesy of Dr. Anthony Senagore)

Infectious Work-Up

- For patients presenting with bloody diarrhea, infectious colitides should be considered.
- Standard stool studies for ova and parasites mainly to assess for *Giardia lamblia* or cryptosporidium in the case of immunosuppressed patients are appropriate.
- *Clostridium difficile* is seen with increased frequency in IBD and can be assessed by endoscopic appearance (Fig. 46.7) or molecular testing.
- Cytomegalovirus (CMV) colitis (Fig. 46.8), with its characteristic "punched-out" ulcerations, is also seen with increased frequency.

Epidemiology

- North America has a relatively high incidence of 8–15 cases per 100,000 persons per year.
- It is estimated that 50,000 new individuals are diagnosed in North America yearly, with an estimated point prevalence of more than 600,000 persons at any given time.
- The incidence of CUC in western societies continues to rise. Risk factors for CUC are summarized in Table 46.1.
- Approximately 70–75% of CUC patients will never require colectomy.
- Unfortunately, the proportion of patients with prolonged remission is only 10%, highlighting the waxing and waning nature of this illness. Approximately 1% of patients live with continuously active disease.

Colorectal Adenocarcinoma

- Patients with CUC are at increased risk of developing colorectal cancer. A rule of thumb is the risk of developing colorectal cancer (CRC) in CUC is 0.5–1% per year after the first 10 years of disease.
- Currently it is recommended that surveillance should commence 8–10 years after onset of colitis (rather than the time of diagnosis).
- Young age at diagnosis, longer disease duration, severity and extent of inflammation, family history of CRC, and the presence of primary sclerosing cholangitis (PSC) are risk factors.

Table 46.1 Epidemiologic risk factors for development of CUC

Category	Risk factor(s)	Comments
Age	Median age of diagnosis = 33 years	Larger studies have disproven bimodal distribution
Gender	Slight male preponderance	–
Genetics	Monozygotic twin concordance = 14–19%, dizygotic concordance 0–7%	If one sibling with CUC, other sibling(s) with 7–17 relative risk of CUC
Geography	Higher prevalence in Northern developed countries but is worldwide	Highest risk areas appear to be North America, UK, Northern Europe, and Scandinavia; rising incidence of CUC in developing countries typically precedes that of CD by 1–2 decades
Race/ethnicity	Caucasians, Ashkenazi Jewish ("Jews of Europe"); incidence rising in Asians and Hispanics	Migration studies suggest that geography is a more important risk factor than race as low-risk groups who migrate to higher prevalence areas then develop a higher prevalence independent of race
Socioeconomic status (SES)	Possible association between increased SES and increased risk of CUC	–
Cigarette smoking	Highly characterized strong, inverse relationship with current smokers at 40% risk reduction for development of CUC	Current smokers with CUC less likely to require hospitalization or colectomy relative to non-smokers
Appendectomy	Highly characterized strong, inverse relationship with patients who have had appendectomy with a 70% risk reduction for development of CUC	Patients who have had appendectomy who do develop CUC may have less severe disease
Antibiotics	Oral antibiotics in prior 2–5 years modestly increase the risk of IBD development	Probable dose-response relationship i.e., the more prescriptions for prior antibiotics, the higher the likelihood of developing IBD
Oral contraceptives	No significant relationship for CUC	Earlier studies suggested a modest increased risk for CUC in prior oral contraceptives
Diet	No significant relationship for CUC	Some studies suggested a link between refined sugar and CD not CUC
Infection	No significant relationship for CUC	Conflicting data for CD but no effect for CUC

Adapted from Loftus EV. Epidemiology of inflammatory bowel disease. In: Talley NJ, editor. GI epidemiology. 2nd ed. Hoboken, NJ: Wiley Blackwell; 2014. p. 273–84

Classification of CUC

- Historically, disease activity was measured by the criteria outlined by Truelove and Witts (Table 46.2).
- More recently the Montreal classification of IBD has become the preferred way to specify disease activity (Fig. 46.9).

Severity

- S0 = clinical remission
- S1 = mild disease: <4 bowel movements per day, no serologic or systemic signs of inflammation
- S2 = moderate: >4 stools per day, some signs of inflammation
- S3 = severe: > = 6 bloody stools daily, pulse >90 beats per minute, temperature > 37.5°C, hemoglobin <10.5 g/100 ml, and ESR > 30 mm/h

Extent

- E1 = ulcerative proctitis
- E2 = left-sided colitis
- E3 = pancolitis
- Endoscopic classification is facilitated by the Mayo Severity Index (Table 46.3).
- The Simple Clinical Colitis Activity Index (SCCAI, Table 46.4) is useful for following patient's symptoms over time.

Table 46.2 Modified Truelove and Witts criteria

Variable	Mild disease	Severe disease	Fulminant disease
No. of stools/day	<4	4–10	> = 10
Blood in stool	Intermittent	Frequent	Continuous
Temperature	Normal	>37.5	>37.5
Pulse	Normal	>90	>90
Hgb	Normal	<75% of normal	Requiring transfusions
ESR (mm/h)	Normal = <30	>30	>30
Abdominal X-ray	Normal	Edema/thumbprinting	Dilation
Abdominal pain	None	Mild diffuse tenderness	Distension and tenderness

Adapted from Mahadevan U. Medical treatment of ulcerative colitis. Clin Colon Rectal Surg. 2004;17(1):7–19
Note moderate disease with features of mild and severe disease

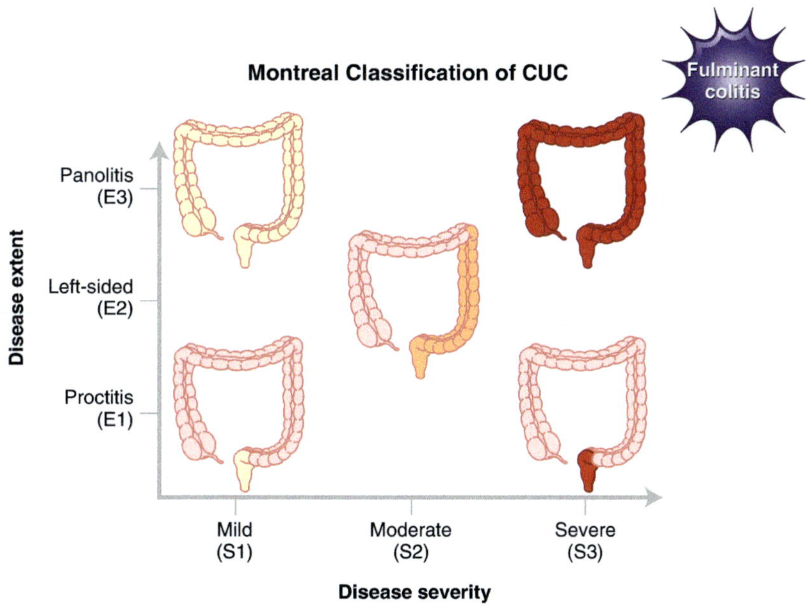

Fig. 46.9 Diagrammatic representation of the Montreal classification of CUC disease severity and extent

Table 46.3 Mayo Severity Index

Variable	Points (range 0–12)			
	0	1	2	3
BM frequency	Normal	1–2 BM > normal	3–4 BM > normal	> = 5 > normal
Bleeding	None	Streaks <50% of BMs	Obvious blood with most BMs	Blood alone
Endoscopy	Normal	*Mild*: erythema, decreased vascularity, mild friability	*Moderate*: marked erythema, lack of vascular pattern, friability	*Severe*: spontaneous bleeding, ulceration
Physicians Global Assessment (PGA)	Normal	Mild	Moderate	Severe

Adapted from Schroeder KW, Tremaine WJ, Ilstrup DM. Coated oral 5-aminosalicylic acid therapy for mildly to moderately active ulcerative colitis. A randomized study. N Engl J Med. 1987;317(26):1625–9

Table 46.4 Simple clinical colitis activity index

	Points (range 0–15)				
Symptom(s)	0	1	2	3	4
Daytime BM frequency	1–3	4–6	7–9	>9	
Nocturnal DM frequency	None	1–3	4–6		
Fecal urgency	None	Hurry	Immediately	Incontinence	
Bloody stools	None	Trace	Occasional frank	Usually frank	
General well-being	Very well	Below average	Poor	Very poor	Terrible
EIMs	1 point per extraintestinal manifestation				

Adapted from Walmsley RS, Ayres RC, Pounder RE, Allan RN. A simple clinical colitis activity index. Gut. 1998;43(1):29–32

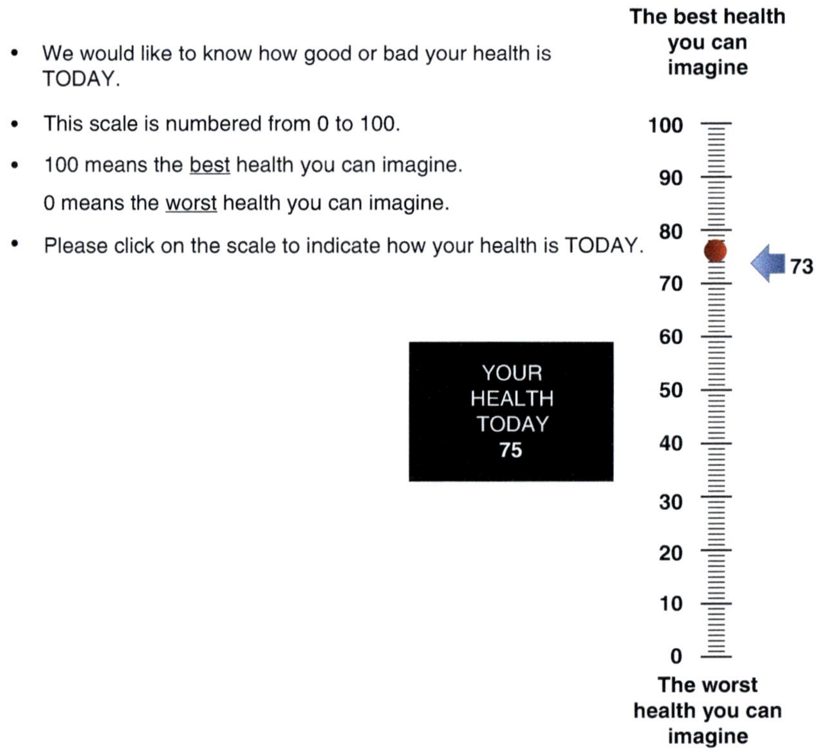

Fig. 46.10 EuroQoL 5D visual analog scale, an example of a rapid, easily administered and interpretable instrument which assesses global health-related quality of life. © Stichting EuroQol Research Foundation

Treatment Endpoints

- The goals of medical therapy include induction of remission, avoiding steroids and improving quality of life (QoL) while avoiding toxicity and preventing neoplasia.
- Maintenance of remission often requires ongoing medical therapy.
- Symptomatic improvement can also be assessed by measuring quality of life (QoL). Instruments to assess QoL may include measures of overall QoL (such as the SF-36 or EuroQoL-5D VAS [Fig. 46.10]), disease (IBD-Q), or symptom-specific (FISI/FIQL).

Cost Considerations

- CUC is known to be a costly disease with medical patients on average consuming $6586 dollars per year, increasing to $15,732–$20,131 in the years prior to surgical intervention.
- The cost-effectiveness of surgery compared with biologic therapy has also been studied,

Table 46.5 Sensitivity analysis of the effect of duration of disease on the cost-effectiveness of infliximab and surgery for severe ulcerative colitis. Quality-adjusted life years based on EuroQoL-5D visual analog scale

Model length	Dominant strategy	Cost of IFX strategy (US dollars)	Cost of surgery strategy (US dollars)	Effectiveness of IFX strategy[a]	Effectiveness of surgery strategy
1 year	IFX	$26,698.45	$63,721.15	0	0
2 years	IFX	$63,648.51	$74,090.32	0.78	0.76
3 years	Surgery	$91,515.26	$82,364.24	1.51	1.50
4 years	Surgery	$112,938.29	$90,277.08	2.19	2.21
5 years	Surgery	$129,786.88	$97,911.94	2.84	2.89
10 years	Surgery	$179,816.82	$132,325.91	5.65	5.98
Lifetime	Surgery	$305,691.59	$270,477.74	16.58	18.34

[a] Quality-adjusted life years based on EuroQoL-5D Visual analog scale

Reproduced with permission from Holubar SD, Piazik B, Xu Kathleen, Dulai P, Tosteson A, Siegel C, Finlayson S. Cost-effectiveness of infliximab versus colectomy for severe ulcerative colitis: a Markov analysis: P-108. Inflamm Bowel Dis. 2012. 7;18:S57–8. © Wolters Kluwer

and early colectomy was found to be a cost-effective treatment compared to maximal medical therapy.

- A sensitivity analysis comparing the cost-effectiveness of infliximab and surgery for severe CUC showed that after 2 years of IFX therapy, surgery increasingly became the dominant strategy (Table 46.5).

Part 2: Specific Treatments

Bottom-Up Versus Top-Down Strategies

- An overview of available medical therapy is shown in Table 46.6.
- "Bottom-up" therapy starts with less expensive, less effective medications which are sequentially added until the desired clinical endpoint is achieved.
- "Top-down" strategy is when patients are initially placed on more aggressive therapies in order to achieve rapid remission, and then agents are sequentially weaned.
  - An example of top-down therapy would be inducing the patient on a biologic and a thiopurine and then attempting to remove the biologic after the patient is clinically improved.

Aminosalicylates (5-ASA Moieties)

- Multiple forms of 5-ASA medications have been developed, mainly in an attempt to reduce side effects.
- 5-ASA medications are administered via enteral or topical formulations.
- There are three release mechanisms: pH (e.g., Asacol®, Lialda®), time release (e.g., Pentasa®), and bacterial cleavage release (e.g., Azulfadine®); these mechanisms dictate the target area of bowel (ileum, colon, or rectum).
- Oral 5-ASA products have been shown to be effective for induction of remission in mild-to-moderate CUC.
- "Bidirectional therapy" with both enteral and per rectal preparations is more effective than either alone.
- Side effects, which are dose-dependent, are mainly dermatologic and gastrointestinal toxicity.

Immunomodulator Therapy (6-MP, Azathioprine)

- Azathioprine (AZA) is the prodrug of 6-mercaptopurine (6-MP), and both act as an immunomodulator and weak immunosuppressant.
- It is important to understand the TMPT metabolic pathway in order to prevent severe toxicity, including life-threatening leukopenia, pancreatitis, and hepatitis (Fig. 46.11).
- In TMPT-deficient patients (prevalence 1 in 300 persons), active metabolites are not efficiently degraded resulting in supra-therapeutic AZA concentrations. Thus, TMPT testing is an integral part of initiating TP therapy.

Table 46.6 Overview of clinical pharmacotherapy for CUC

Class (effect)	Indication	Examples	Dose
5-Aminosalicylates (enteric/topical anti-inflammatory)	Induction *and* maintenance of remission for mild-to-moderate colitis/proctitis	Sulfasalazine	4–6 g PO daily
		Mesalamine Canasa® suppositories	PO: 2.4–4.8 g PO daily PR: 500 mg–1 g per rectum daily
		Olsalazine	1.5–3 g PO daily
		Balsalazide	6.75 g PO daily
Topical corticosteroids (anti-inflammatory)	Maintenance of remission for mild-to-moderate colitis	Budesonide	9 mg PO daily, rectal foam now available
Thiopurine immunomodulators (block purine metabolism)	Induction *and* maintenance of remission for moderate-to-severe colitis	Azathioprine (AZA) 6-MP	AZA: 2.5 mg/kg PO daily (50–150 mg PO q24) 6MP: 1.5 mg/kg daily
Biologic agents (block TNF or leukocyte rolling and adhesion)		Anti-TNF-alpha Antibodies	IFX: 5–10 mg/kg, weeks 0, 2, and 6 and then every 4 weeks Adalimumab: 160 mg week 1, 80 mg week 2, and then 40 every other week
		Anti-integrin Antibodies	Golimumab: 200 mg week 0 and then 100 mg every other week Vedolizumab: 300 mg IV weeks 0, 2, and 6, then every 8 weeks
Systemic corticosteroids (anti-inflammatories)	Rescue therapy for severe colitis[a]	Prednisone	5–40 mg PO daily
		Hydrocortisone	20–300 mg IV daily
Calcinurin inhibitors (immunosuppressives)	Rescue therapy for steroid-refractory severe colitis[a]	Cyclosporine Tacrolimus	2–4 mg/kg daily 0.05 mg/kg twice daily

[a]indicated for induction of remission *not* maintenance of remission. Inability to wean from these agents is an indication for surgery

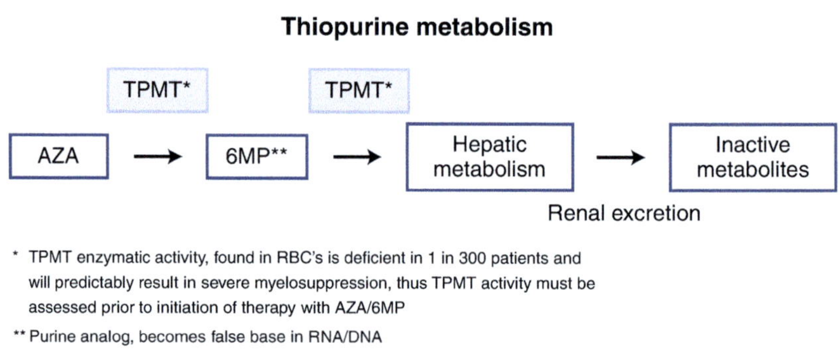

Fig. 46.11 Schematic representation of in vivo thiopurine metabolism

- Immunomodulator therapy may be associated with a marginally increased risk of lymphoma, but the absolute risk is small.
- TPs are effective steroid-sparing medications. They are often started upfront with steroids to induce remission. The steroids are then weaned, and the TP is used as a maintenance drug.
- TPs are often used in combination with biologics in part to prevention of anti-TNF immunogenicity. Thiopurines, in the setting of combination therapy, may also represent an "exit strategy" from chronic biologic therapy.

Biologic Agents

Anti-TNF-Alpha Antibodies

Infliximab (Remicade®)

- IFX is a chimeric mouse/human monoclonal anti-tumor necrosis factor (TNF) alpha antibody. IFX was FDA approved for CUC in 2005 and is now indicated for the treatment of mild-to-severe UC in both adults and children.
- In the ACT-1 and ACT-2 randomized trials assessing the efficacy of IFX for inducing and maintaining remission, 60–69% of patients had successful induction, compared with 29–37% response for placebo.
- The typical loading dose is 5 mg/kg IV at weeks 0, 2, and 6, switching to maintenance dose of 5 mg/kg IV every 8 weeks starting at week 14.
- If a loss of responsiveness occurs and symptoms flare, then the IFX dose can be increased to 10 mg/kg IV every 4–8 weeks.
- Serum drug trough levels are monitored to assure proper dosing; ensuring adequate trough levels may be associated with increased efficacy and decreased risk of colectomy.
- The best outcomes of IFX therapy are seen in combination with other medications such as TPs as demonstrated by the UC-SUCCESS trial with 40% of patients achieving a steroid-free remission, compared with only 2% on monotherapy with either agent; similarly mucosal healing was observed in 63% of combination therapy patients compared with 55% on IFX alone.
- The most widely recognized side effect of IFX is activation of latent infections most notably TB. Thus prior to initiation of IFX therapy, patients are screened with the QuantiFERON® gold assay.
- IFX can make active infections worse and can exacerbate hepatitis B.
- Other adverse reactions include infusion reactions, which can result in flash pulmonary edema or hypersensitivity including anaphylaxis.
- It is highly controversial whether or not biologic agents, and IFX in particular, increase the complication rate of surgery. The half-life of the agents (Fig. 46.12) may provide some guidance for timing of elective surgery.

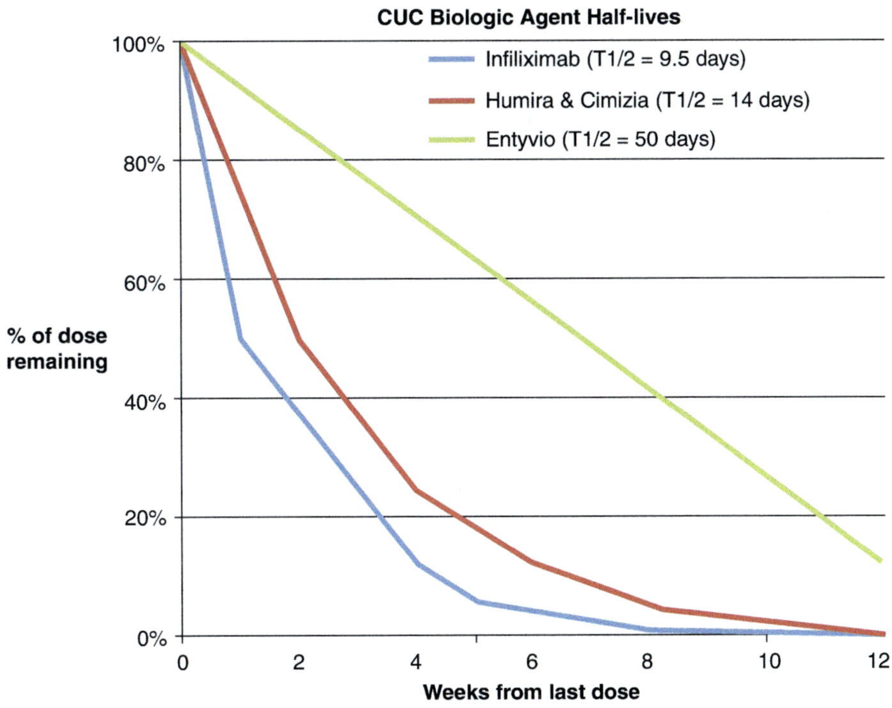

Fig. 46.12 Graphical representation of the theoretical in vivo half-lives of biologic agents used to treat CUC. Note this graph assumes first-order elimination pharmacokinetics

Adalimumab (Humira®)

- This humanized antibody is indicated for induction and maintenance of remission in adults with moderate-to-severe CUC.
- The ULTRA-1, ULTRA-2, and ULTRA-3 trials demonstrated that in patients with moderately to severely active CUC, adalimumab is efficacious in both short- and long-term maintenance of remission for up to 4 years in 60% of patients.
- Loading doses are used (week 0,160 mg; week 2,80 mg; maintenance week 4,40 mg SQ every other week subcutaneously).
- If a sub-optimal response is observed, the dosing interval is often increased to weekly.
- As in IFX, trough levels can be used to monitor and optimize therapy.
- Also as in IFX, the best outcomes are seen with combination therapy with TPs.
- The humanization of the antibody has reduced the side effect profile relative to IFX. Adverse reactions are generally similar to those of IFX and also include local injection site reactions and loss of responsiveness.

Certolizumab Pegol (Cimzia®)

- Cimzia is a partially humanized Fab fragment of an anti-TNF antibody, which is PEGylated.
- Presently it is FDA approved for CD (and RA), *but not approved for CUC.*

Golimumab (Simponi®)

- Simponi is another humanized anti-TNF Ab, which was FDA approved for the induction and maintenance of remission in adults and for patients with loss of responsiveness to IFX and Humira.
- In the PURSUIT-SC study, golimumab was effective for the induction of remission in moderately to severely active CUC, with >51% of patients achieving remission compared with 30% of placebo patients.
- Dosing is usually 200 mg subcutaneously at week 0 and then 100 mg subcutaneously every other week.

Anti-integrin Antibodies

Vedolizumab (Entyvio®)

- Entyvio is an intravenously administered monoclonal antibody to integrin $\alpha 4\beta 7$.
- In 2014, it was FDA approved for the induction and maintenance of remission of both CUC and CD in adults and also for patients with loss of responsiveness to other biologic medications.
- In the GEMINI-I and GEMINI-II studies, vedolizumab resulted in induction of remission in 47% of patients, compared with 25% of placebo, and maintenance of remission in 41% vs. 15% with placebo.
- Dosing, which is intravenous, is 300 mg IV at weeks 0, 2, and 6 and then every 8 weeks.

"Rescue" Therapy

Corticosteroids

- Corticosteroids represent the mainstay of rescue therapy for otherwise medically refractory CUC.
- The mechanism of action is that of nonspecific immunosuppression and immunomodulation.
- Steroids are associated with significant side effects, and they should not be used for maintenance therapy.
- Various formulations are converted to hydrocortisone equivalent doses using readily available online conversion calculators.
- Side effects of steroids include adrenal suppression, water retention, moonlike facies, psychological distress (ranging from agitation and insomnia to frank psychosis), rosacea, buffalo hump, abdominal striations, and osteoporosis.
- One of the most serious and potentially nonreversible adverse effects is osteoporosis, which may not be responsive to calcium or vitamin D supplementation. Patients on repeated courses of corticosteroids need bone density monitoring with dual-energy X-ray absorptiometry (DEXA) scans.

- The CORE-1 study showed that budesonide MMX 9 mg was effective at indication of remission in mild-to-moderate CUC but more limited in maintenance of remission.
- Long-term (2 years) budesonide use was shown to be safe based on bone density and protective if steroid naive.
- Oral steroids are typified by prednisone. Most patients with CUC respond to oral steroids, with only 16% not responding acutely.
- However, systemic steroids have no role for maintenance of remission due to their relatively severe side effect profiles.
- Long-term (> 1 year) corticosteroid treatment is generally contraindicated; inability to wean off chronic steroids represents an indication for surgery.
- IV steroids are indicated for those refractory to outpatient medical therapy. Maximum effective dose is 300 mg hydrocortisone per day. An estimated 60% of patients will respond, usually within 5–7 days.

Cyclosporine/Tacrolimus

- These drugs, used for prevention of graft rejection in solid organ transplantation, are calcinurin inhibitors.
- Calcinurin inhibitors are reserved for use as a rescue agent for severe, otherwise medically refractory, CUC.
- These medications carry a risk of opportunistic infections and are associated with a host of specific adverse reactions; they are potentially nephrotoxic, hepatotoxic, and neurotoxic and may exacerbate hypertension and hyperlipidemia.

Methotrexate (MTX)

- MTX is an antimetabolite, specifically inhibiting folic acid metabolism by competitive inhibition of dihydrofolate reductase (DHFR).
- Aside from being hepatotoxic and myelosuppressive, MTX is also an FDA category X drug, meaning it is teratogenic.

Part 3: Medical Management of Mild-to-Severe CUC

Mild-to-Moderate Distal Colitis/Proctitis (Fig. 46.13)

- Topical mesalamine is the first-line treatment both for inducing and maintaining remission of distal mild or moderate colitis.
  - Foams reach the sigmoid colon, and enemas may even reach the splenic flexure; compliance can be an issue.
  - Although oral aminosalicylates are less effective than topical mesalamine, most patients prefer oral formulations. In moderately severe cases, combining topical and oral therapy is more effective than topical mesalamine alone both in achieving and maintaining remission.
- Topical corticosteroids have similar efficacy in achieving remission in active disease and are an alternative to topical mesalamine. They should not be used for maintenance, however.

Mild-to-Moderate Extensive Colitis (Fig. 46.13)

- For mild or moderate colitis, oral salicylates induce clinical improvement in 60–80% of cases within 4 weeks of therapy.
- In either distal or extensive colitis not responding to 4 weeks of aminosalicylate therapy, a course of oral steroids is indicated.
  - When a clinical response has been achieved, the dose is tapered over several weeks. Although the response rate is around 70%, ~20% develop steroid dependency and cannot be weaned without relapse of symptoms.
- In nonresponders, and in patients who become steroid-dependent, therapy should be started to aid in weaning of prednisone. The two main options at this stage are TPs and biologics.
  - Azathioprine is effective in inducing and maintaining remission, but its effects are

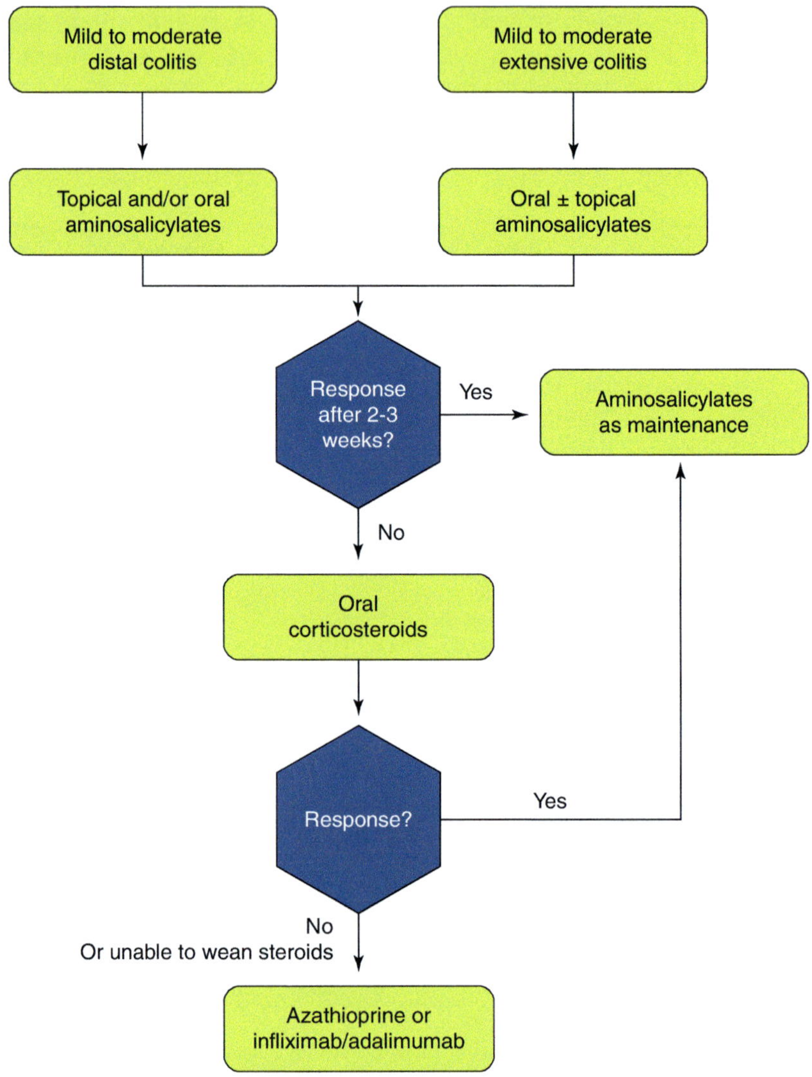

Fig. 46.13 Standard "bottom-up" approach to the management of mild-to-moderate CUC (based on the American College of Gastroenterology 2010 Practice Guidelines)

slow with the time of onset measured in months, requiring overlap with an extended course of oral prednisone.

– Infliximab has been well studied in steroid-refractory mild and moderate colitis; 69% of patients respond to induction treatment. Co-administration of infliximab and azathioprine may be associated with an increased clinical response rate and mucosal healing in moderate and severe steroid-refractory colitis compared to monotherapy with either drug.

- Remission in mild and moderate extensive colitis can be maintained either by oral aminosalicylates, TPs, or infliximab.

Severe Colitis (Fig. 46.14)

- Most patients with severe colitis require hospitalization for stabilization and a course of intravenous corticosteroids, regardless of the extent of disease.

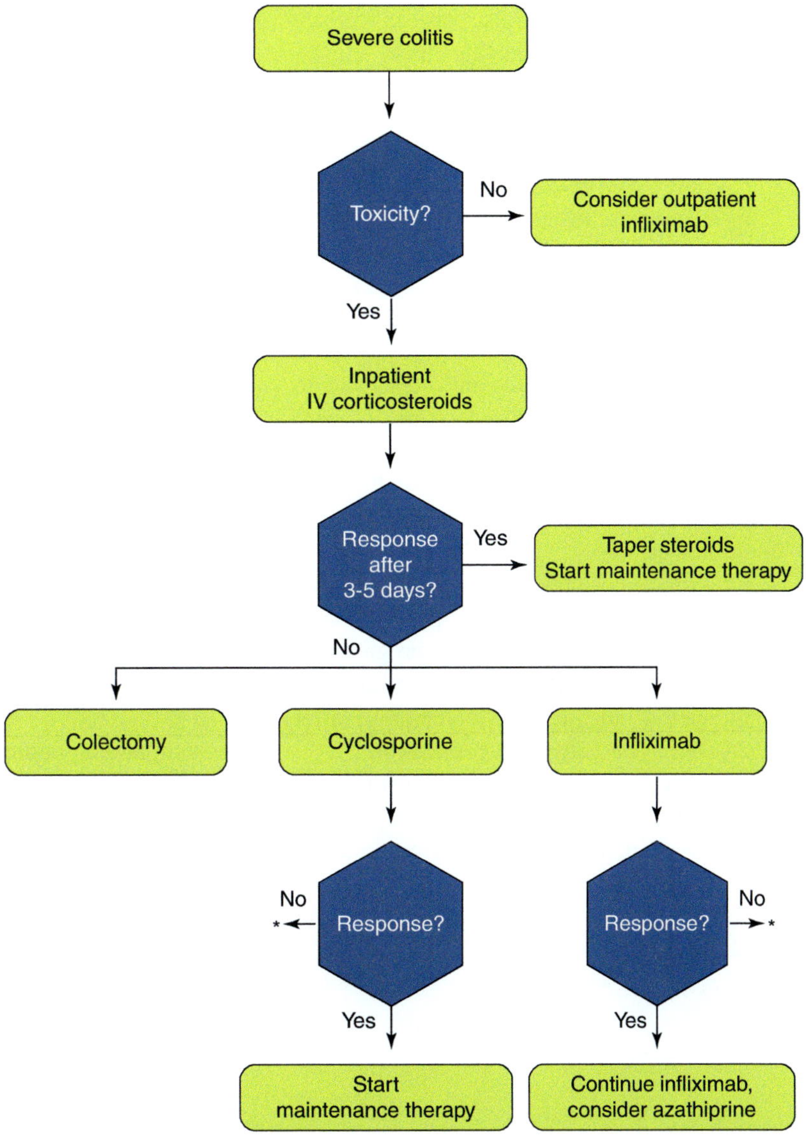

* Colectomy. Selected patients in specialized IBD units may respond to switching from infliximab to cylosporine or vice versa

Fig. 46.14 Standard "bottom-up" approach to the management of severe CUC (based on the American College of Gastroenterology 2010 Practice Guidelines)

- A course of 3–5 days is given with close clinical observation. Consultation with a colorectal surgeon and a stoma therapist is typically advisable during this stage, so that the patient can be in a position to make an informed decision about the next steps by day 3–5 should steroid therapy fail; 20–40% of patients with severe UC will fail to improve on IV corticosteroids.
- Patients will often need supplemental parenteral nutrition support. Continued oral diet is encouraged in most patients, due to the theoretical advantages of short-chain fatty acid provision to the colon. However, bowel rest may be indicated if bowel movements are excessive.
- Thromboembolic prophylaxis is routinely given, and anticholinergic and opioid medications are avoided as possible.

- Importantly, gut infections may exacerbate ulcerative colitis, and treating those aggressively may facilitate induction of remission.
  - Stool samples are obtained for *Salmonella*, *Yersinia*, *Shigella*, and *C. difficile* toxin.
  - Colonic CMV disease is best demonstrated by immunohistochemistry of classic "punched-out" mucosal ulcer biopsies obtained on flexible sigmoidoscopy; leukocyte CMV PCR is sometimes used as a surrogate marker.
- Broad-spectrum antibiotics are often given to patients with toxicity owing to concern about bacterial translocation.
- Patients with megacolon (often defined as colonic dilatation to a diameter > 6 cm) require additional caution.
  - Oral intake is stopped, abdominal signs are closely monitored, and daily plain abdominal films are obtained to assess progression.
  - Failure to respond to corticosteroids is an indication for urgent colectomy after 24–48 h, as is progressive dilatation.
- Fulminant colitis is the advanced form of severe acute colitis and is typically defined as toxic colitis, i.e., colitis with signs of systemic toxicity such as peritonitis, hypotension, impending perforation, and/or end-organ damage such as renal failure.
- Rescue therapy for steroid-refractory severe UC typically includes three options: colectomy, cyclosporine, and infliximab.
  - Intravenous cyclosporine is highly effective in steroid-resistant severe UC, with response rates up to 83%. The issue of recrudescence of colitis following rescue therapy with cyclosporine, in combination with a significant toxicity profile, has led to a reduction in its usage in the biologic era, and presently it is only offered at select centers.
  - Infliximab has emerged as a widely used rescue therapy with response rates in the 50–71% range. One important advantage is that infliximab can be continued long term to maintain remission.
  - A direct comparison confirmed that both cyclosporine and infliximab have high initial response rates when used as rescue therapy in steroid-refractory severe colitis (85 vs. 86%); colectomy rates were also similar at 3 months (18 vs. 21%).
  - The strategy of using surgery as the last resort may actually increase CUC-related mortality, and an undue delay may increase postoperative complications. Patients should be educated about the role and outcomes of surgery.

Medical Management of Crohn's Disease

47

Scott A. Strong

Key Concepts

- Crohn's disease is classified by age at diagnosis, disease location, and disease behavior.
- Disease severity is stratified using a clinical or endoscopic scheme that assesses symptoms and signs or endoscopic appearance, respectively.
- Medical therapy (e.g., 5-aminosalicylate compounds, glucocorticoids, immunomodulators, and biologic agents) should be approached in a "step-up" or "top-down" manner to balance efficacy and toxicity.
- 5-Aminosalicylate compounds are of limited value in the induction and maintenance of remission.
- Glucocorticoids can successfully induce remission, but short- and long-term adverse effects largely limit their usage to management of acute episodes.
- Immunomodulators are of limited use for induction of remission but successfully maintain remission in many patients.
- Biologic agents can induce and maintain remission in patients with moderate-to-severe disease, but the efficacy and safety vary among the different medications.
- Disease prophylaxis after surgery should be individualized according to the patient's risk for recurrence.

Introduction

- The appropriate treatment of Crohn's disease includes a combination of medical and surgical therapy to safely resolve inflammation, lessen symptoms, improve quality of life, and minimize the risk for short- and long-term complications.
- Therapy is usually guided by the age of the patient, anatomic extent of inflammation, disease behavior, symptom severity, treatment response, and risk for adverse effects.
- Operative intervention is generally reserved for patients with disease-related complications or disease that is refractory to medical therapy.

Disease Classification

- The Vienna classification and its modification, the Montreal classification, are based on clinical variables that include age at disease diagnosis, anatomic location of disease, and disease behavior (Table 47.1).

S. A. Strong (✉)
Division of GI and Oncologic Surgery, Northwestern Medicine, Chicago, IL, USA
e-mail: STRONGS@ccf.org

S. R. Steele et al. (eds.), *The ASCRS Manual of Colon and Rectal Surgery*,
https://doi.org/10.1007/978-3-030-01165-9_47

Table 47.1 Vienna and Montreal classification for Crohn's disease

	Vienna	Montreal
Age at diagnosis	A1 below 40 years	A1 below 16 years
	A2 above 40 years	A2 between 17 and 40 years
		A3 above 40 years
Location	L1 ileal	L1 ileal
	L2 colonic	L2 colonic
	L3 ileocolonic	L3 ileocolonic
	L4 upper	L4 isolated upper disease[a]
Behavior	B1 non-stricturing, non-penetrating	B1 non-stricturing, non-penetrating
	B2 stricturing	B2 stricturing
	B3 penetrating	B3 penetrating
		p perianal disease modifier[b]

With permission from: Satsangi J, Silverberg MS, Vermeire S, Colombel J-F. The Montreal classification of inflammatory bowel disease: controversies, consensus, and implications. Gut. 2006;55(6):749–53. Copyright © 2006 BMJ Publishing Group & British Society of Gastroenterology

[a]L4 is a modifier that can be added to L1–L3 when concomitant upper gastrointestinal disease is present

[b]"p" is added to B1–B3 when concomitant perianal disease is present

Disease Severity

- Crohn's disease is caused by immune dysregulation that leads to chronic intestinal inflammation manifesting itself with symptoms including abdominal pain, bleeding, and diarrhea and signs such as anemia.
- The goals of therapy should optimally include induction and maintenance of mucosal healing.
- The Crohn's Disease Activity Index (CDAI) has long been the primary outcome measure to study the impact of medications for the treatment of Crohn's disease. Benchmarks for disease activity were established as follows:

Clinical remission	CDAI <150
Mild disease	CDAI 150–219
Moderate disease	CDAI 220–450
Severe disease	CDAI >450

- Clinical response has been subsequently defined as a reduction from the baseline score of more than 70–100 points.
- The Harvey-Bradshaw Index (HBI) consists of five descriptors including general well-being, abdominal pain, number of liquid stools, abdominal mass, and complications.
  - Remission has been defined as a score of <5.
  - A 3-point change in the HBI correlates with a 100-point change in the CDAI.
- Mucosal healing is an important marker of disease activity since mucosal inflammation often precedes the onset of clinical symptoms.
- The Crohn's Disease Endoscopic Index of Severity (CDEIS) utilizes four descriptors (superficial ulceration, deep ulceration, ulcerated stenosis, and nonulcerated stenosis) to characterize each examined segment (ileum, right colon, transverse colon, left colon, rectum).
  - Complete endoscopic remission has been somewhat arbitrarily defined as a score of <3, endoscopic remission as a score of <6, and endoscopic response as a decrease of >5 points.
- The Simple Endoscopic Score in Crohn's Disease (SES-CD) was developed to overcome the unwieldy nature of the CDEIS.
  - Benchmarks for disease activity have been described as follows:

Remission	0–2
Mild inflammation	3–6
Moderate inflammation	7–16
Severe inflammation	>16

- Unfortunately, both the CDEIS and SES-CD have only a weak correlation with the CDAI.

Medications

- Probiotics, antibiotics, 5-aminosalicylate compounds, glucocorticoids, immunomodulators, and biologic agents are all approved for the treatment of Crohn's disease.

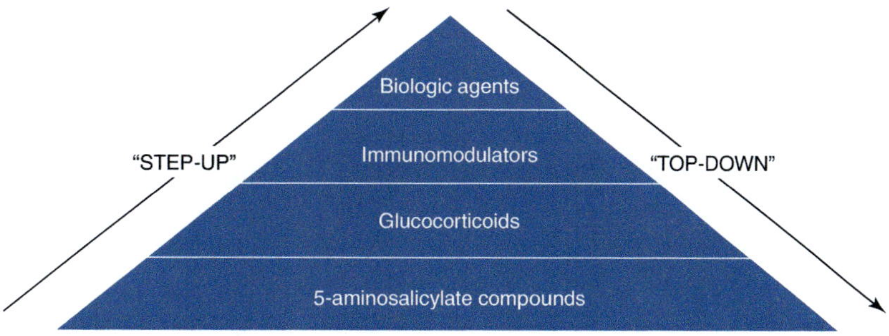

Fig. 47.1 "Step-up" vs. "top-down" models of therapy

- Criteria for disease response should be initially discussed and then measured after a reasonable time interval. The continuation of ineffective drug therapy risks the development of further disease complications.
- "Step-up" therapy is an approach where patients are initially managed with drugs associated with fewer side effects, but might not be as effective as more potent medications linked with greater potential for toxicity.
  - If the initial treatment fails, therapy will be escalated using stronger drugs with the process repeated until the disease is adequately managed or an operation is warranted.
- The "top-down" method is predicated on the hypothesis that using more effective medications from the outset may alter the natural history of Crohn's disease while reducing the likelihood for disease exacerbations, hospitalizations, and operations (Fig. 47.1).

Probiotics

- Probiotics are beneficial microorganisms that can potentially impact the gut's microbiota composition, metabolic activity, and immunomodulation to confer host benefit.
- These bacteria and fungi can alter microbial diversity through competitive inhibition of other microbes, enhance mucosal barrier function via the production of short-chain fatty acids, and interact with intestinal dendritic cells to instigate an anti-inflammatory response.
- Meta-analyses suggest that probiotics are ineffective for both the induction and maintenance of remission in patients with Crohn's disease.

Antibiotics

- Antibiotics may benefit patients with Crohn's disease through the inhibition of pathogenic bacteria and reduction of overall bacterial burden.
- The principal shortcomings associated with antibiotic therapy include lack of specificity associated with therapy, poor insight as to which bacteria should be targeted, and the potential for antibiotic resistance.
- The majority of studies demonstrate improvement with antibiotics only when disease is limited to the colon.
  - Metronidazole, which is active against anaerobic bacteria and some parasites, and ciprofloxacin, especially active against *Enterobacteriaceae* and *Escherichia coli*, are the most frequently used antibiotics.
  - Metronidazole therapy is associated with several side effects that are dose-dependent and occur in up to one-half of patients. These include gastrointestinal intolerance, headaches, metallic taste, and vertigo. Peripheral neuropathy is a rare complication but may be irreversible.

5-Aminosalicylate Compounds

- A number of 5-aminosalicylate (ASA) compounds are available with active 5-ASA released at various locations throughout the intestinal tract depending on the design of each specific drug.
- Sulfasalazine, the original 5-aminosalicylate, is comprised of 5-ASA bound to a sulfapyridine

moiety that detaches when the drug reaches the bacteria of the colon.
  - Sulfasalazine has a number of side effects due to the sulfapyridine moiety, including symptoms such as gastrointestinal upset and headaches. Patients who take sulfasalazine must also take folic acid (1 mg daily) because the medication depletes folic acid stores.
- The role of 5-ASA in treatment or as a maintenance medication is equivocal at best.

Glucocorticoids

- The benefit originates from an ability to modulate the immune response, inhibit expression of adhesion molecules, and decrease trafficking of inflammatory cells to the intestine.
- Glucocorticoids are associated with significant short- and long-term adverse effects that limit their usage to management of acute episodes.
- Budesonide, a glucocorticoid with an extensive first-pass metabolism, was consequently developed because it maximizes the amount of glucocorticoid locally available in the distal ileum and proximal colon but theoretically has minimal systemic accessibility.
- Prednisone is generally prescribed in dosages of 40–60 mg daily for 2–6 weeks to induce remission, although no appropriate dose-ranging studies have been performed.
- Once symptoms are controlled, the drug is tapered.
- The occurrence and severity of most side effects are related to the dose and duration of treatment.
  - Common findings include abdominal striae, acne, cataracts, fluid retention, glaucoma, hyperglycemia, hypertension, insomnia, mood disturbances, moon facies, and weight gain.
  - Musculoskeletal complications, such as myopathy, osteonecrosis, and osteoporosis, are additional side effects.
  - Lastly, adrenal suppression can occur during the course of treatment and contribute to physiologic dependence.

Immunomodulators

- The thiopurines and methotrexate are immunomodulators that can be used to induce remission in patients with active disease, allow glucocorticoid tapering in patients with "steroid-resistant" or "steroid-dependent" disease, and maintain remission in patients with quiescent disease.

Thiopurines

- Azathioprine and 6-mercaptopurine (6-MP) are thiopurines that are known to cause immunosuppression.
- Azathioprine is prescribed at 2.0–2.5 mg/kg, and 6-MP is dosed at 1.0–1.5 mg/kg for daily maintenance therapy.
- Clinical benefit may not be evident until 6–12 weeks after initiation of therapy but tends to be durable.
- Genetic polymorphisms of thiopurine methyltransferase (TPMT), the primary enzyme responsible for 6-MP metabolism, have been identified, and drug metabolite levels can be measured.
- Prior to starting thiopurine therapy, TPMT enzyme activity or genotype should usually be determined because the drugs should be avoided in patients with TPMT deficiency.
- The most common side effect linked to azathioprine and 6-MP is nausea; adverse events include liver function abnormalities, leukopenia, and pancreatitis. Routine monitoring of complete blood counts is recommended.
- Thiopurines have been shown to be effective in maintaining remission.

Methotrexate

- Methotrexate reduces the production of inflammatory mediators.
- Methotrexate (25 mg) is administered weekly by subcutaneous or intramuscular injection. Folic acid (1 mg daily) should be concomitantly prescribed.
- The most frequent side effects reported with methotrexate are gastrointestinal upset and stomatitis.

Table 47.2 Pooled relative risk of inducing and maintaining remission with biologic agents in biologic-naïve patients with moderate-to-severe disease

Biologic agent	Usual maintenance dose	Remission induction		Remission maintenance	
		Relative risk	95% CrI	Relative risk	95% CrI
Infliximab	5 mg/kg IV every 8 weeks	6.11	2.49–18.29	3.31	0.98–14.01
Adalimumab	40 mg SQ every 2 weeks	2.98	1.12–8.18	5.16	1.78–18.00
Certolizumab	400 mg SQ every 4 weeks	1.48	0.76–2.93	2.26	0.38–13.57
Natalizumab	300 mg IV every 4 weeks	1.36	0.69–2.86	4.26	0.71–25.49
Vedolizumab	300 mg IV every 8 weeks	1.40	0.63–3.28	2.20	0.37–13.54

With permission from Singh S, Garg SK, Pardi DS, Wang Z, Murad MH, Loftus EV Jr. Comparative efficacy of biologic therapy in biologic-naïve patients with Crohn disease: a systematic review and network meta-analysis. Mayo Clin Proc. 2014;89:1621–35. © Elsevier 2014

SQ subcutaneous, *CrI* credible interval, *IV* intravenous

  - Leukopenia can also occur, but much less frequently than seen with thiopurine therapy.
  - Rare complications of methotrexate therapy include hepatic fibrosis and hypersensitivity pneumonitis.
- Moderate-quality evidence indicates that methotrexate at a dose of 15 mg weekly is superior to placebo for maintenance of remission in Crohn's disease.

Biologic Agents (See Also Chap. 46)

Antitumor Necrosis Factor (TNF) Agents

- The anti-TNF agents are designed to block the effects of TNFα.
- Three such medications (i.e., infliximab, adalimumab, certolizumab pegol) are currently approved for the treatment of Crohn's disease.
  - Infliximab is permitted for the treatment of moderate-to-severe Crohn's disease.
  - Adalimumab is accepted for the treatment of moderate-to-severe disease and for patients who have lost response to or are intolerant of infliximab.
  - Certolizumab is approved for therapy in patients with moderate-to-severe disease.
- Side effects include an increased risk of infections, such as tuberculosis, as well as autoimmune reactions, heart failure, liver dysfunction, lymphoma, and multiple sclerosis.
- Prior to initiating treatment with an anti-TNF agent, patients should be screened for hepatitis B or tuberculosis infection.

Integrin Receptor Antagonists

- Natalizumab is indicated for inducing and maintaining clinical response and remission in patients with moderate-to-severe Crohn's disease or unable to tolerate conventional therapies and anti-TNF agents.
- Natalizumab should not be used in combination with immunomodulators or anti-TNF medications due to the risk of developing progressive multifocal leukoencephalopathy.
- Vedolizumab is another integrin receptor antagonist indicated for patients with moderate-to-severe disease.
- One systematic review of randomized controlled trials reported that infliximab and adalimumab, but not certolizumab pegol, natalizumab, and vedolizumab, were more likely to induce remission than placebo.
- Similar results were observed for maintenance of remission (Table 47.2).

Induction and Maintenance of Remission

- Infliximab, the combination of infliximab plus azathioprine, adalimumab, and vedolizumab have been found to be superior to placebo for the induction of remission in active disease.
- In comparisons of anti-TNF agents, infliximab plus azathioprine and adalimumab alone were

superior to certolizumab for induction of remission.
- All treatments were superior to placebo for maintaining remission, except for the combination of infliximab plus methotrexate.

Induction of Remission

Mild Disease

- Mildly active Crohn's disease limited to the ileum is often best managed with budesonide.
- Mesalamine and antibiotics in this setting are associated with minimal and no benefit, respectively.
- For mild disease of the colon or ileocolon, sulfasalazine or systemic glucocorticoids can be used.
- Extensive upper gastrointestinal Crohn's disease should be treated with systemic glucocorticoids and immunomodulators.
- Patients with clinical features indicative of a poor prognosis should be offered thiopurines, methotrexate, or anti-TNF therapy used alone or in combination.

Moderate Disease

- Moderately active disease of the ileum should be treated with budesonide or systemic glucocorticoids.
- Antibiotics should be added if features of localized sepsis are noted.
- Systemic glucocorticoids plus an immunomodulator is also a viable alternative.
- Anti-TNF therapy should be considered as an option for patients with active disease that has previously been steroid-resistant or dependent.
- Moderately active colonic disease should be treated with systemic glucocorticoids.
- Anti-TNF therapy with or without thiopurines or methotrexate is an appropriate option for patients who have relapsed with moderately active disease.
- For some patients with only occasional relapsing disease, reintroduction of glucocorticoids with an immunomodulator may be more appropriate.
- Extensive, moderately active upper gastrointestinal disease should be handled with systemic glucocorticoids and immunomodulators.
- For patients who have relapsed, anti-TNF therapy with or without thiopurines or methotrexate is an appropriate option.

Severe Disease

- Severely active ileal Crohn's disease should be initially managed with systemic glucocorticoids.
- For patients who have relapsed, anti-TNF therapy with or without an immunomodulator is an appropriate alternative.
- Severe disease of the colon may be treated with systemic glucocorticoids.
- Patients who have relapsed can be appropriately handled with anti-TNF therapy with or without an immunomodulator.
- Extensive upper gastrointestinal Crohn's disease should be managed with systemic glucocorticoids and immunomodulators.
- For patients who have relapsed, anti-TNF therapy with or without immunomodulators is an appropriate option.
- Patients who demonstrate clinical features predictive of a poor prognosis seem to be the most suitable candidates for early introduction of anti-TNF therapy and thiopurines.
- Surgical alternatives should also be considered at an early stage in patients with moderate-to-severe disease.

Maintenance of Remission

- If remission of an initial presentation has been achieved with steroids, a thiopurine or methotrexate should be considered.
- Oral 5-ASA compounds have not been consistently proven effective in maintenance of remission.
- If remission has been achieved with an anti-TNF agent, maintenance with regular anti-TNF therapy should be offered.
- Patients in a scheduled treatment regimen with regular infliximab infusions appear to do better compared to patients managed using an episodic strategy.
- Combination therapy with infliximab plus a thiopurine is of greater efficacy in achieving and maintaining glucocorticoid-free remission than either infliximab or thiopurines used alone.

- The relapse rate following immunomodulator cessation is nearly 20% at 1 year.
- A de-escalating treatment strategy should be largely limited to patients with a high risk for severe adverse events and patients in deep remission.

Medical Prophylaxis After Surgery

- The cumulative risk for surgery in patients with Crohn's disease is estimated to be 16%, 33%, and 47% at 1, 5, and 10 years, respectively.
- Endoscopic recurrence has been reported in 54% of patients at 5 years; clinical recurrence follows endoscopic recurrence with a prevalence of 28–45% by 5 years.
- Antibiotics, immunomodulator monotherapy, immunomodulator plus antibiotics, and anti-TNF monotherapy reduce the risk of endoscopic recurrence.
- Neither mesalamine nor budesonide is effective in this setting.
- Overall, anti-TNF monotherapy is the most effective pharmacologic intervention for post-operative prophylaxis.

48 Anorectal Crohn's Disease

Stephen R. Gorfine

Key Concepts

- Crohn's disease is an incurable inflammatory condition of unknown cause that can involve any portion of the GI tract. Anorectal involvement is estimated to occur in 25–35% of cases.
- Common manifestations of anorectal Crohn's disease include skin tags, abscesses, fissures, ulcers, fistulas, and strictures. Cancers, both adenocarcinomas and squamous carcinomas, are also possible, occurring with greater frequency than that seen in the general population.
- Evaluation of the Crohn's patient with anorectal disease usually involves examination under anesthesia and imaging studies such as pelvic MRI or ERUS in addition to colonoscopy, enterography, and laboratory studies.
- Any undrained sepsis must be addressed promptly. Incision and drainage of abscesses and placement of drains or setons under general anesthesia are often required.
- Once sepsis has been controlled, medical therapy, which usually includes antibiotics, immunomodulators, and biologics, in combination or as single agents, is generally instituted.
- Fistulizing anorectal Crohn's disease occurs commonly. Fistulas are classified as simple or complex. Simple fistulas can often be treated by lay-open fistulotomy. Complex fistulas are usually treated medically with biologics, often in combination with immunomodulators. Surgical management of complex fistulas can include permanent seton, fibrin glue, fistula plug, endorectal advancement flap, and LIFT procedure. Surgical interventions should be used judiciously as these incur a risk of incontinence and nonhealing wounds.
- Long-standing fistula tracts and strictures should be routinely biopsied to exclude malignant degeneration. Cancers, when found, are generally treated in the same manner as those found in the general population. Total proctocolectomy is a consideration in a patient with extensive Crohn's colitis of long duration found to have a rectal adenocarcinoma.
- Diversion and proctectomy are required in about 10% to 20% of cases.

Introduction

- Crohn's disease (CD) can affect any portion of the GI tract; perianal disease occurs in about 25% of cases.

S. R. Gorfine (✉)
Division of Colorectal Surgery, Department of Surgery, The Mount Sinai Hospital, New York, NY, USA
e-mail: srgny@nyc.rr.com

S. R. Steele et al. (eds.), *The ASCRS Manual of Colon and Rectal Surgery*,
https://doi.org/10.1007/978-3-030-01165-9_48

Incidence and Natural History

- Various perianal lesions are commonly associated with Crohn's disease; these include external tags, fissures, ulcers, abscesses, fistulas, and strictures.
- Anal cancer, either adenocarcinoma or squamous carcinoma, may also complicate perianal CD.
- Symptoms of perianal CD include pain, bleeding, drainage, and incontinence.
- Risk factors for perianal involvement include colonic and especially rectal disease and young age at CD onset.
- In the majority of cases, intestinal manifestations of Crohn's disease will precede anorectal involvement. However in a small number of patients, perianal disease will be the first manifestation of CD.
- The presence of perianal disease suggests a more aggressive CD phenotype.
- Perianal disease is associated with greater disability, more frequent extraintestinal manifestations, and more steroid resistance.

Etiology

- One hypothesis is that inflammation causes a shallow mucosal ulceration which subsequently extends by exposure to stool and the pressure of defecation.
- A second hypothesis implicates infection of anal glands with penetration beyond the intersphincteric space.

Clinical Presentation

- Perianal Crohn's disease manifests as five, often overlapping, conditions.
  - These are anal skin tags, tissue destruction in the form of fissures and ulcers, infective complications consisting of fistulas and abscesses, anorectal strictures, and anorectal cancers.
- Clinical manifestations are exceedingly variable ranging from mildly bothersome anal tags to destructive perianal lesions causing sepsis and incontinence.

Diagnosis

- In addition to a history and physical exam, including a thorough anorectal exam, a colonoscopy and small bowel evaluation will be required.
- The anorectal exam usually includes inspection of the anus and perianal areas, digital anorectal exam, and anoproctoscopy.
- Rectal exam may be limited by patient discomfort, and examination under anesthesia (EUA) may be required.
- In the evaluation of perianal abscess and fistulous disease, a combination of magnetic resonant imaging (MRI) of the pelvis, endorectal ultrasound (EUS), and exam under anesthesia has been shown to yield 100% diagnostic accuracy.

Classification

- The American Gastroenterological Association (AGA) classification may be used:
  - Ulcerations are divided into fissures and ulcers.
  - Only irreversible and fibrous anorectal strictures are included; they may be short, annular, diaphragm-like strictures less than 2 cm in length or longer tubular strictures arising from rectal inflammation.
  - Anal skin tags are either type 1 or type 2.

Skin Tags

- Skin tags are classified into two types.
  - Type 1 are edematous, hard, often cyanotic, tender or not, typically arising from a healed anal fissure, ulcer, or hemorrhoid. These skin tags are caused by lymphedema and often occur in concert with intestinal inflammation.
  - Type 2 lesions are raised, broad or narrow based, single or multiple, soft or firm, and painless (often referred to as "elephant ears"). Elephant ear tags (Fig. 48.1) are common, usually multiple, and are generally asymptomatic except for patient complaints of difficulty cleaning and poor cosmesis.

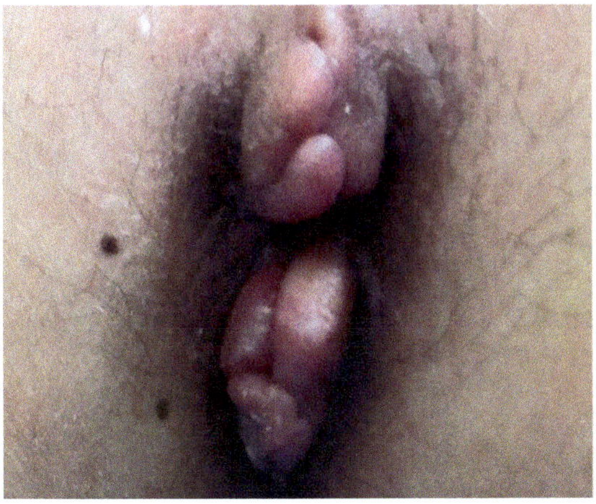

Fig. 48.1 "Elephant ear" tags

Management

- Skin tags associated with CD are generally best managed with benign neglect.
- Excision in some cases can lead to nonhealing, persistent surgical wounds, and a substantially worse problem.

Hemorrhoids

- Symptomatic hemorrhoidal disease is remarkably uncommon in the setting of Crohn's disease.
- The complication rate after hemorrhoidectomy or removal of tags is high. CD patients contemplating hemorrhoid surgery should be free of active anorectal involvement.

Management

- Hemorrhoidal disease in the setting of CD is best managed expectantly.
- Surgical interventions such as rubber band ligation and excisional procedures should only be undertaken when conservative measures have failed and the anorectum is otherwise free of active disease.

Anal Fissure and Ulcer

- In the setting of CD, anal fissures can be idiopathic, similar to those seen in non-CD patients, or "atypical," being Crohn's-related.
- An idiopathic anal fissure is located in the anterior or posterior anal midline at the anal verge (Fig. 48.2).
- Atypical fissures and ulcers are more common among patients with CD. These lesions are often located off the anterior and posterior midline. In many cases there are multiple fissures or ulcers.
- CD fissures have granulating bases and overhanging edges (Figs. 48.3 and 48.4); they can

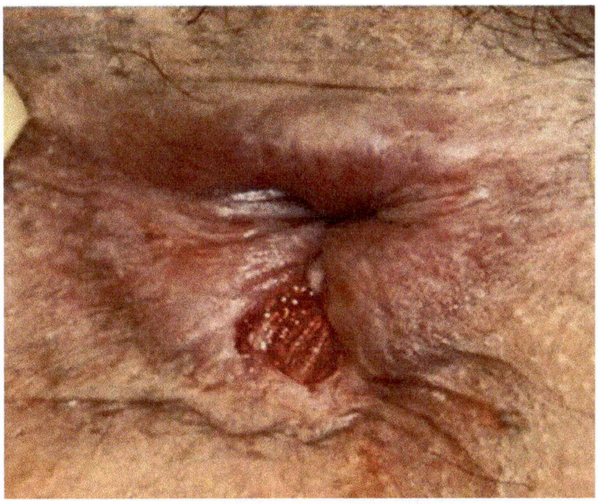

Fig. 48.2 Idiopathic chronic anal fissure. Note "heaped-up" edges and internal sphincter fibers at base

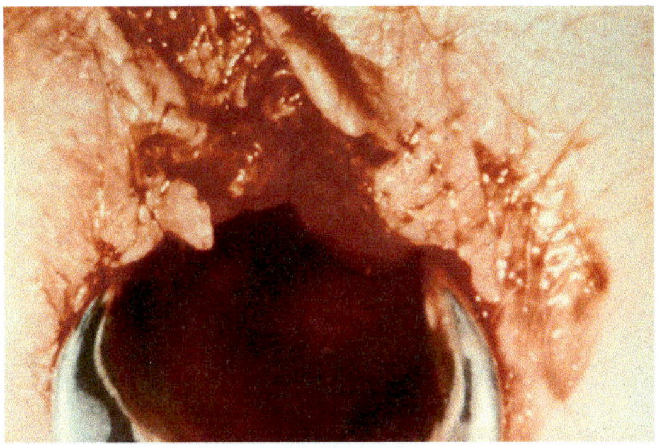

Fig. 48.3 Fissure in Crohn's disease

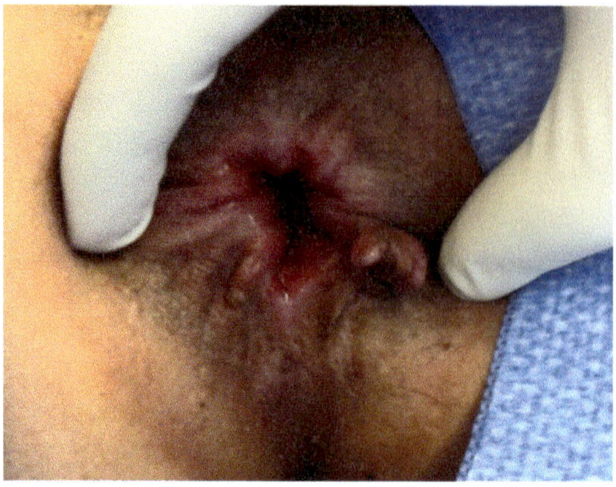

Fig. 48.4 Chronic fissure with associated tag in Crohn's disease

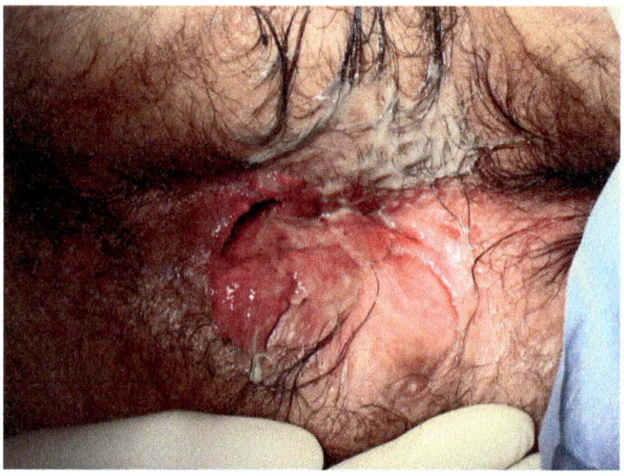

Fig. 48.5 Cavitating Crohn's disease ulcer

extend beyond the anal verge to the perianal skin.

- Large cavitating ulcers with significant tissue destruction are also seen (Figs. 48.5 and 48.6).
  - These lesions are painful in up to 70% of cases.
  - Discharge, pruritus, and bleeding are frequent associated symptoms.
    - Biopsy of these lesions will show non-necrotizing epithelioid cell granulomas, characteristic of CD, in up to 77% of cases.
  - These more extensive fissures and ulcers are thought to result from a direct involvement with Crohn's-related inflammation and are not related to internal anal sphincter hypertonicity.

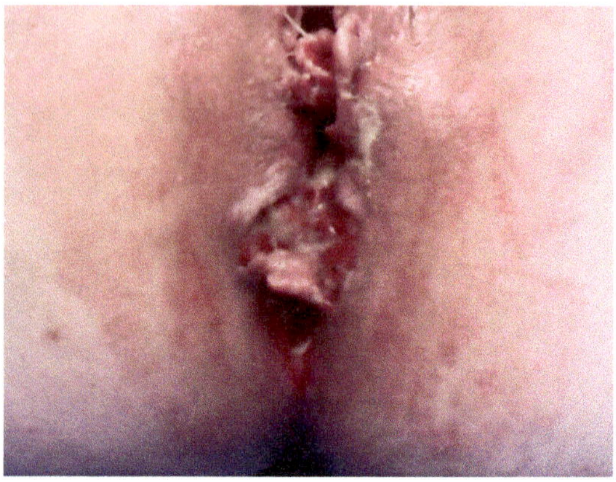

Fig. 48.6 Crohn's disease ulcer

  - Among those patients not known to have intestinal CD, other ulcer-forming anal diseases need to be excluded. These conditions include syphilis, herpes, acquired immunodeficiency syndrome (AIDS), *Neisseria gonorrhoeae*, *Chlamydia trachomatis*, tuberculosis, and leukemic infiltrates.
- Carcinoma and prior radiotherapy may also cause anal ulcerations. Biopsy and microbiologic studies may be necessary to establish the diagnosis.

Management

- Idiopathic fissures in CD patients can be treated in a fashion similar to non-CD patients.
  - Limiting toilet time and use of antidiarrheal medications, when appropriate, is useful.
  - "Chemical sphincterotomy" with topical nitroglycerin, calcium channel blockers, and injected botulinum toxin may be used.
- Surgical treatment should be reserved for CD patients with a single, "characteristic" midline fissure, an elevated resting sphincter tone, and a disease-free rectum.
- Crohn's associated fissures and ulcers present more of a therapeutic challenge. Topical treatments have been used with varying degrees of success including metronidazole 10% and tacrolimus 0.1% cream (Fig. 48.7).

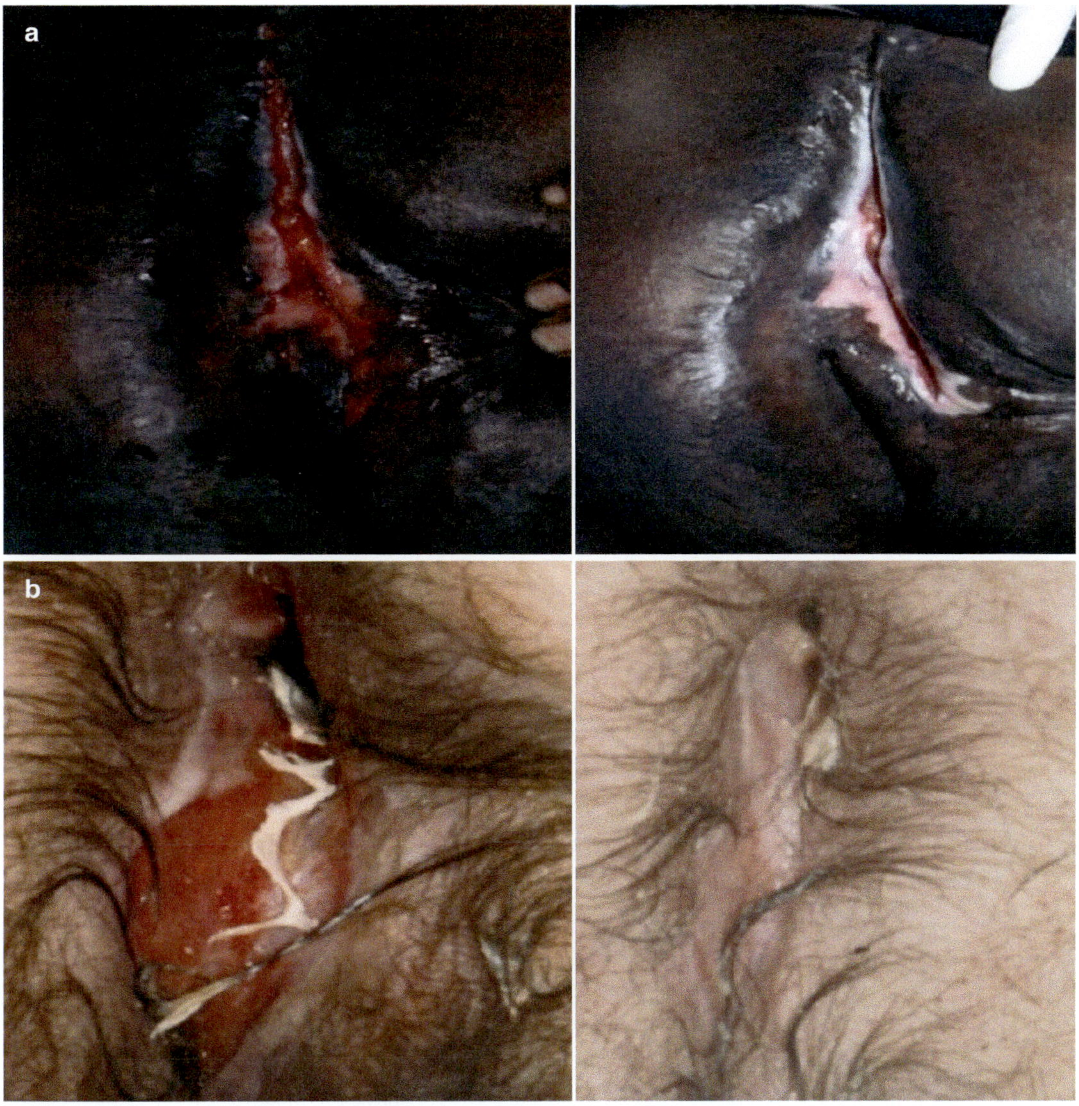

Fig. 48.7 Response to topical tacrolimus for two separate patients (**a** and **b**). Before left, after treatment on right (With permission from Hart AL, Plamondon S, Kamm MA. Topical tacrolimus in the treatment of perianal Crohn's disease: exploratory randomized controlled trial. Inflamm Bowel Dis. 2007; 13(3):245–53 (49) © Wolters Kluwer 2007)

- Corticosteroids, antibiotics, aminosalicylates, and 6-mercaptopurine have been studied for CD perianal ulcerations with inconsistent results.
- Infliximab has become the "gold standard" in the treatment of perianal CD.
- Anti-TNF therapy should be considered as first-line therapy for cavitating ulcers as the long-term outcome is poor, with the risk of anoproctectomy approaching 83% in some studies.

Abscess and Fistula

Abscess

- Perirectal and perianal abscesses can be expected to occur in up to 80% of CD patients.
- Abscesses about the anus and rectum can form in four distinct anatomical locations: the perianal space, the ischiorectal (or perirectal)

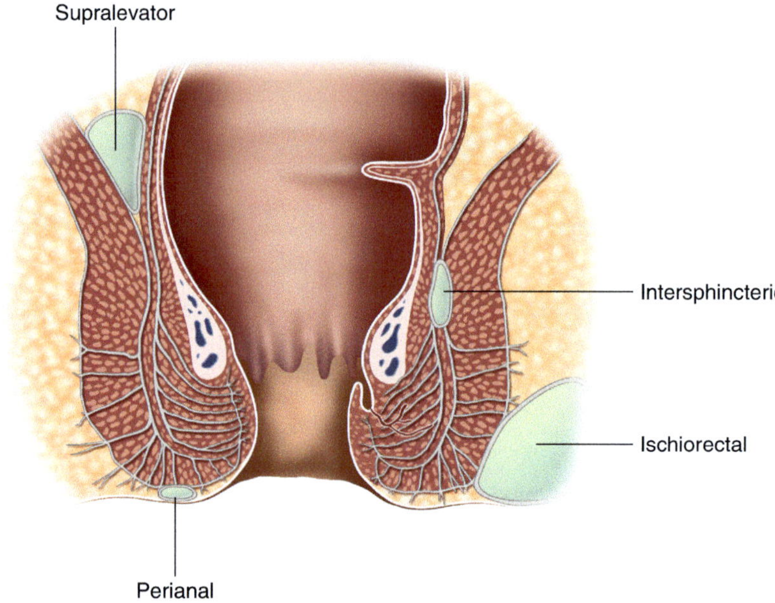

Fig. 48.8 Location of abscesses

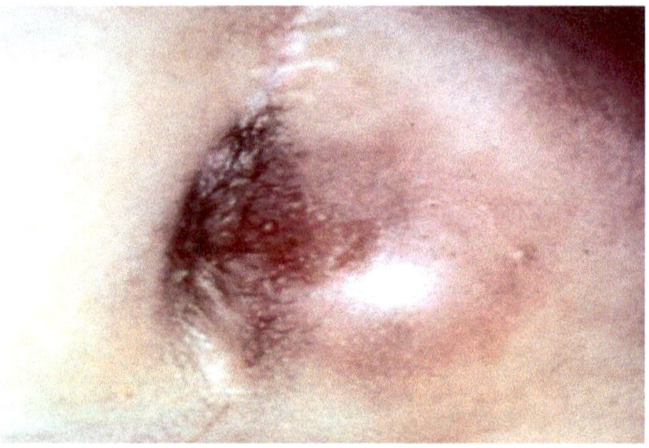

Fig. 48.9 Perianal abscess

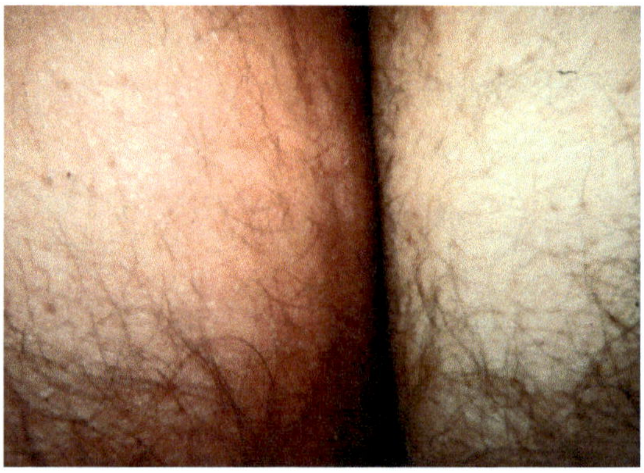

Fig. 48.10 Left perirectal or ischiorectal abscess. Notice left-sided erythema and fullness

space, the intersphincteric (or submucosal) space, and the supralevator space (Fig. 48.8).

- The patient will often present with constant anorectal pain. Fever, chills, and signs of systemic sepsis may also be present.
- Physical exam shows erythema and swelling of the affected side.
- The diagnosis of perianal abscess (Fig. 48.9) and ischiorectal abscesses (Fig. 48.10) is usually fairly easy to establish.
- Submucosal and supralevator abscesses may require imaging studies, such as MRI.
- Induration and tenderness are common findings. Fluctuance is generally a late sign.
- Examination under anesthesia is often required for diagnostic and therapeutic purposes.

Management

- Surgical drainage is indicated; unless the abscess is quite superficial, this is usually best accomplished under general anesthesia in the operating room.
- Superficial perianal abscesses can be drained under local anesthesia in the clinic or emergency department. A cruciate incision will often prevent premature closure of the skin edges.
- Antibiotic therapy is often added, but is not a substitute for adequate surgical drainage.
- The incision for drainage of an ischiorectal abscess should be placed on the buttock, just outside the sphincter complex.

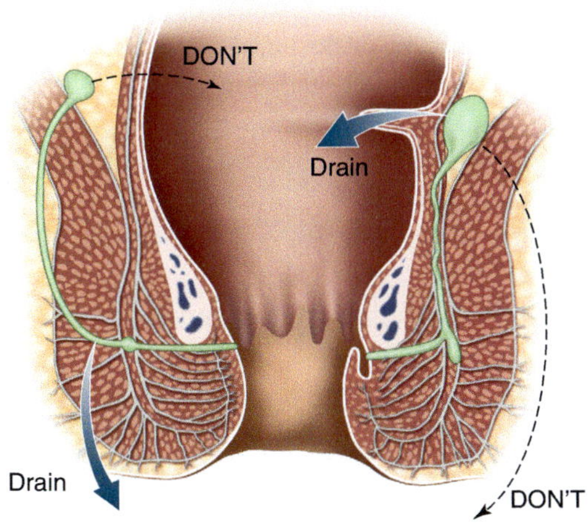

Fig. 48.11 Drainage of supralevator abscess

- Placement of a mushroom or Malecot catheter, or a draining seton if the internal opening of a causative fistula is found, is preferred.
- "Packing" the abscess cavity is contraindicated in virtually all cases, as the packing actually impedes drainage.
- Submucosal abscesses can be successfully drained into the anorectum by incising the overlying mucosa and internal anal sphincter.
- Supralevator extensions of abscesses of cryptoglandular origin should be drained with a mushroom catheter via a perineal incision (Fig. 48.11).
- Abscesses will often lead to anorectal fistulas, whether drained surgically or not.

Fistula

- Fistula formation is probably the most common complication of perianal CD.
- After 10 years of CD, the cumulative incidence of anal fistulas is reported to be up to 33%, and after 20 years it is about 50%.
- CD patients often have complex, branching, and interconnected series of fistulas that are not easily defined, much less objectively classified.
- Fistulas may be divided into two groups: simple and complex.
  - A simple fistula has a low intersphincteric or transsphincteric location and a single, short tract (Fig. 48.12). The internal opening is at or caudad to the dentate line, and the external opening is near the anal verge. Vaginal involvement and abscess are not present.
  - A complex fistula has a single internal opening above the dentate line or multiple internal or external openings. A complex fistula is present when there is vaginal extension, an abscess, multiple openings, and an anorectal stricture or active anorectal CD is present (Figs. 48.13 and 48.14).

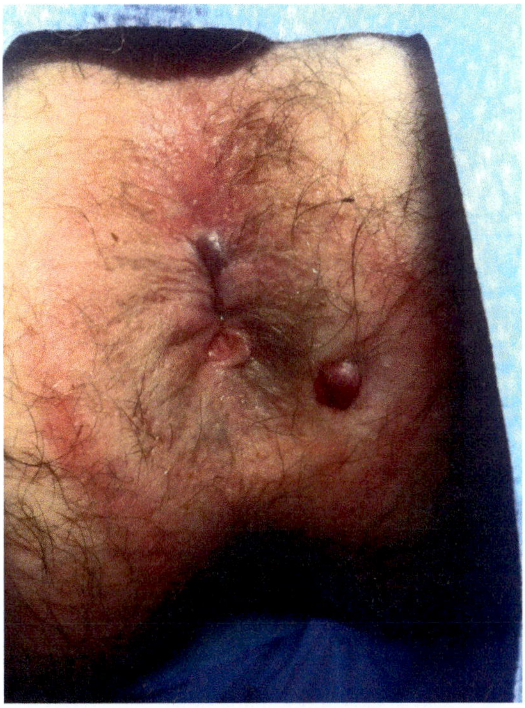

Fig. 48.12 Simple Crohn's disease fistula

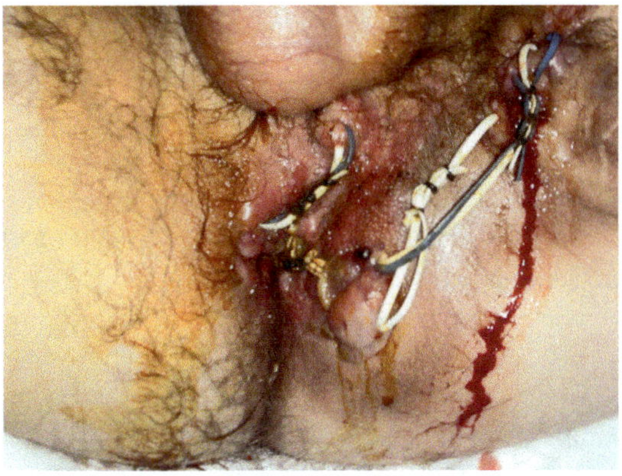

Fig. 48.13 Complex Crohn's disease fistula

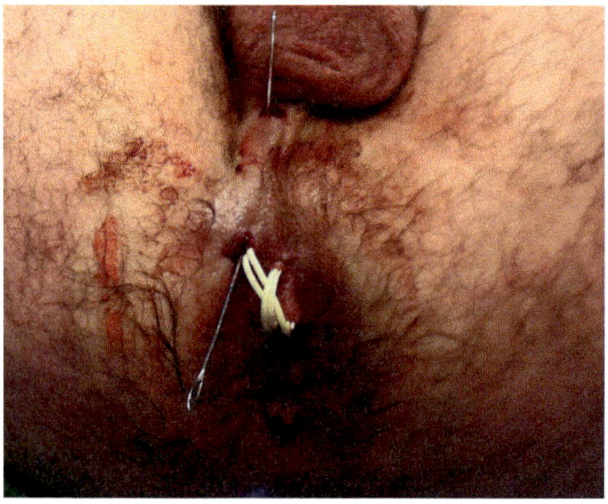

Fig. 48.14 Complex Crohn's disease fistula

Management

- The goals of management include preservation of continence, complete healing, a reduction in the number of septic events, and improvement in the patient's quality of life; these goals are not always met.
- Successful treatment will often require close collaboration among surgeons, gastroenterologists, and radiologists, among others.

Medical Therapy

Aminosalicylates and Corticosteroids

- There is no evidence that aminosalicylates play any role in the treatment of perianal CD.
- Steroids are similarly ineffective and may be contraindicated in the setting of fistulizing perineal disease.

Antibiotics

- Antibiotics are often used as initial treatment in the setting of CD-related fistulous disease.
- Metronidazole is often effective, but is associated with a variety of adverse reactions including nausea, peripheral neuropathy, and paresthesias.
- Ciprofloxacin has demonstrated significant clinical benefits in patients with perianal fistulas.
- Antibiotics are perhaps best used as an effective bridge to biologic therapy.

Immunosuppressives

- Immunosuppressive medications used in the treatment of fistulizing perianal CD include 6-mercaptopurine (6-MP), azathioprine, methotrexate, cyclosporine, and tacrolimus.
  - Several small studies of azathioprine and 6-mercaptopurine found that significantly more patients responded than with placebo.
- Tacrolimus and cyclosporine are calcineurin inhibitors that suppress T-cell activation and interleukin-2 production.
  - Oral tacrolimus was compared to placebo in a randomized, controlled study and found effective for symptomatic improvement, but not fistula remission.
  - Multiple small studies have suggested benefit with cyclosporine and thalidomide.
  - However, use of these agents is limited owing to significant side effects.

Biologics

Infliximab

- Infliximab is a chimeric monoclonal antibody to TNF-α, administered by intravenous infusion, and is the best studied of all the biological agents.
- Efficacy of infliximab in the treatment of fistulizing perineal CD has been demonstrated in multiple randomized, controlled trials.
- Small studies suggest a better response rate, lower recurrence rate, and longer time to recurrence among patients who had a seton placed prior to infliximab treatment. The seton is typically removed after the second infliximab infusion.
- Long-term maintenance therapy (as opposed to episodic therapy) is commonly necessary to prevent fistula relapse.
- Despite clinical improvement, radiographic evidence of complete fistula healing occurs only in a minority of patients.

Adalimumab

- Adalimumab is a completely humanized monoclonal antibody to TNF-α, administered by subcutaneous injection.
- High-quality studies show that adalimumab therapy is associated with a higher rate of fistula closure over time, as compared to placebo.
- Adalimumab may be effective in patients who are infliximab nonresponders or have become infliximab-refractory.

Certolizumab Pegol

- Certolizumab pegol is the PEGylated Fab' portion of a recombinant humanized monoclonal antibody to TNF-α and is administered by subcutaneous injection.
- Certolizumab pegol has also been shown to be effective in the treatment of CD-related fistulas.
- Continuous treatment improves the likelihood of sustained perianal fistula closure.

Natalizumab

- Natalizumab is a humanized monoclonal antibody against the cell adhesion molecule, α4-integrin, and is administered by intravenous infusion.
- Data concerning this agent is limited because of the association with the rare but usually fatal condition, progressive multifocal leukoencephalopathy (PML).

Vedolizumab

- Vedolizumab is a humanized monoclonal antibody specifically designed to inhibit gut $\alpha_4\beta_7$ integrins.
- Owing to gut selectivity, the risk of progressive multifocal leukoencephalopathy is not similar to natalizumab.
- Data for efficacy with CD fistulas is limited.

Surgical Therapy

- Surgical therapy for fistulizing perianal disease needs to be tailored to each individual patient.
- Surgical interventions in CD patients can result in nonhealing perineal wounds, incontinence, and significantly diminished quality of life.
- Surgical management of perianal CD should control perianal sepsis without resort to more extensive procedures when possible.

Seton

- Placement of a loose, draining seton is often the first step in the management of fistulizing perianal CD.
- A silastic vessel loop is passed through the fistula tract and tied to itself outside the anus (Fig. 48.15).

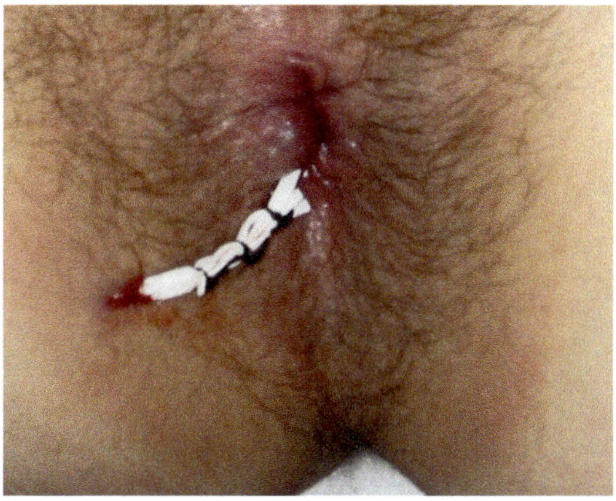

Fig. 48.15 Silastic seton

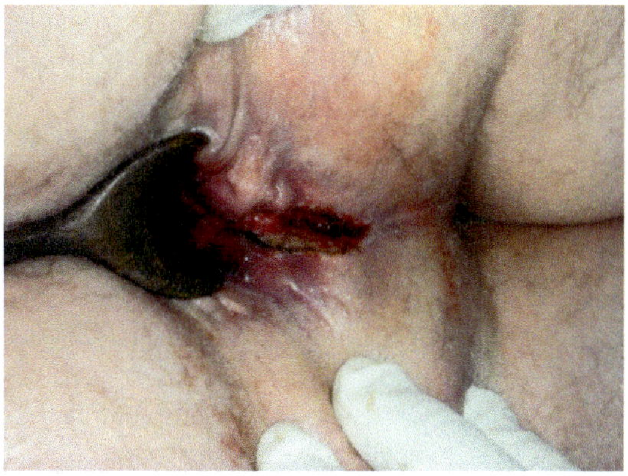

Fig. 48.16 Simple fistulotomy

- The goal of the seton is to promote drainage and prevent recurrence of an abscess.
- Draining setons are generally well tolerated by patients.

Fistulotomy

- Lay-open fistulotomy should be reserved for simple Crohn's fistulas when the anorectum is free of disease (Figs. 48.16 and 48.17).
- Complex fistulas require a more cautious surgical approach. Muscle division in these cases carries a high risk of incontinence and nonhealing perineal wounds.

Fibrin Glue

- Instillation of fibrinogen and thrombin causes a fibrin clot to form within the fistula tract.
- Fibrin glue achieves fistula healing only in a minority of CD cases.

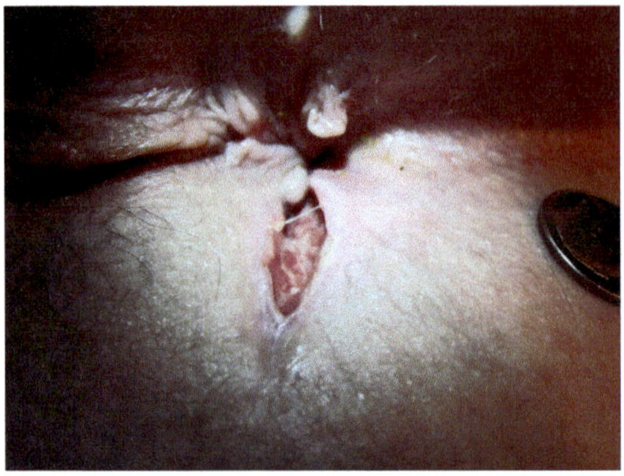

Fig. 48.17 Simple fistulotomy

Anal Fistula Plug

- As with fibrin sealant, the absorbable plug is designed to provide a matrix allowing for the ingrowth of collagen-producing fibroblasts.
- Reported success is wildly variable and data is scant among CD patients.

Adipose Tissue-Derived Stem Cells

- The use of autologous adipose tissue-derived mesenchymal stem cells (ASC) involves injection of the fistula with stem cells recovered from the patient or a healthy donor.
- Early results suggest that ASC could be an effective treatment option for CD fistulas; more evidence is required.

Ligation of Intersphincteric Tract

- Ligation of the intersphincteric fistula tract (LIFT) approaches the fistula tract via an intersphincteric incision; the fistula tract is divided in the intersphincteric space (Fig. 48.18a–f).
- Small studies suggest CD fistulas may be successfully treated by LIFT with minimal wound complications or sphincter injury.

Endorectal Advancement Flap

- A flap of anoderm, submucosa, and a small portion of the internal sphincter is raised proximally so that the flap reaches beyond the internal opening without tension and is sutured to the remaining anoderm (Fig. 48.19a–e).
- Small series have demonstrated reasonable healing rates after advancement flap in CD patients, but less than those seen in cryptoglandular disease.
- While some advocate endorectal advancement flap repair, others point out that surgical outcomes for complex CD fistulas remain disappointing.

Diversion

- In situations where combined medical and local therapy is ineffective in controlling the symptoms of perianal Crohn's disease, fecal diversion, either on a temporary or permanent basis, has an important role.
- Ileostomy and colostomy have both been utilized for this purpose.
- Diversion of the fecal stream from the anorectum may facilitate healing and enables symptomatic control of perianal complications (Figs. 48.20 and 48.21a, b).
- Only a minority of diverted patients ever achieve restoration of intestinal continuity.
- Proctectomy is strongly recommended in instances where the rectum is unlikely to be placed back in continuity owing to the long-term cancer risk.

Proctectomy

- In some instances (10–20%), perineal CD is so severe that proctectomy with permanent diversion is the only viable option.
- Anal stricture and active colonic CD are associated with increased risk of proctectomy and permanent diversion.
- Whenever possible, the perineal approach should utilize an intersphincteric dissection so as to lower the risk of nonhealing of the perineal wound.
- Perineal wound problems can be expected to occur in up to 35% of cases after abdominoperineal resection (Fig. 48.22).
- As perineal disease can be extensive, a staged approach is often warranted. Rectal transection at the level of the levators often allows perineal sepsis to improve for a subsequent, second-stage perineal anoproctectomy.

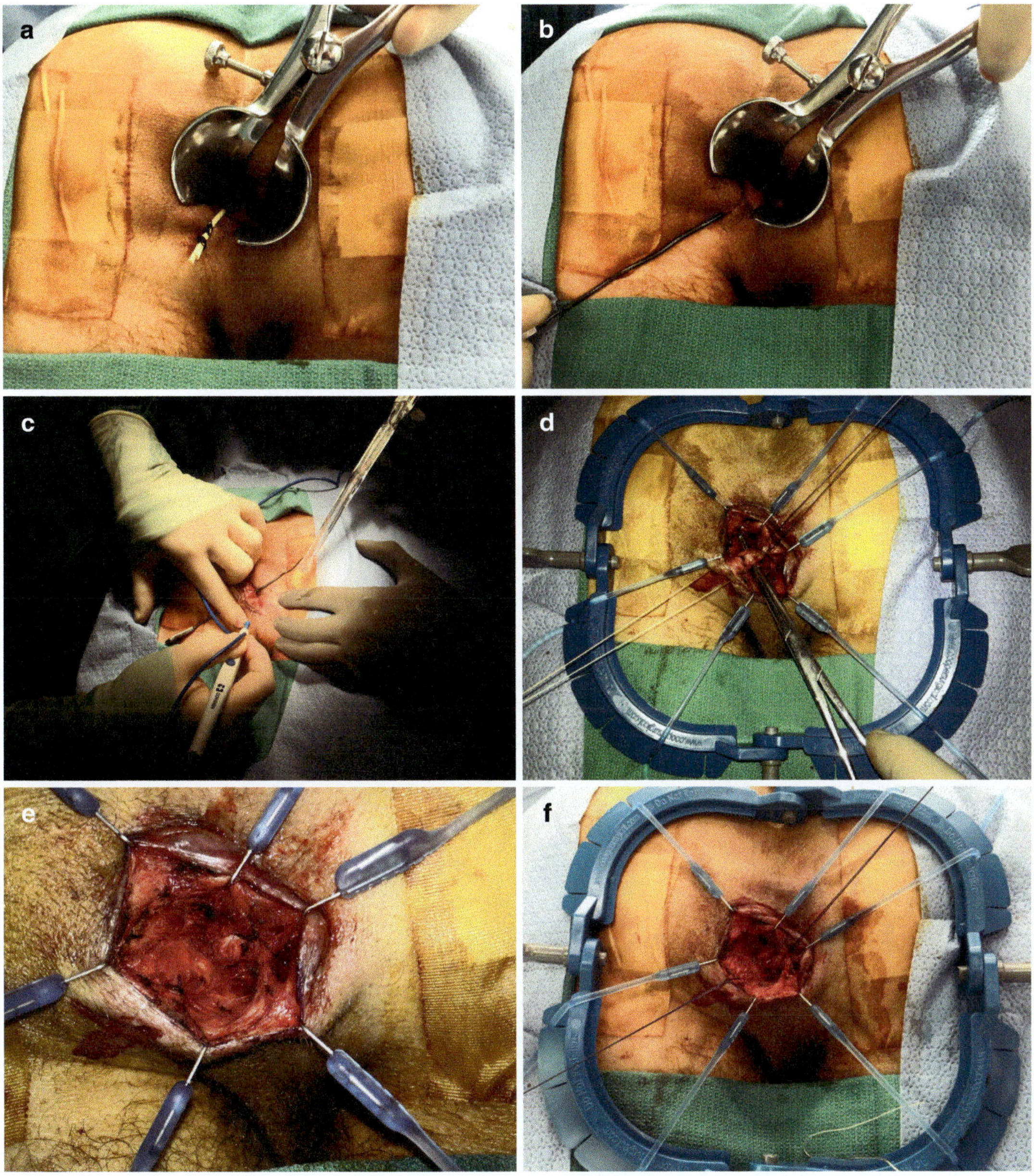

Fig. 48.18 (**a**) LIFT: seton in the fistula tract. (**b**) LIFT: identification of internal opening. (**c**) LIFT: dissection in the intersphincteric groove. (**d**) LIFT: isolation of the tract. (**e**) LIFT: suture ligation of the tract. (**f**) LIFT: ligation of the external sphincter

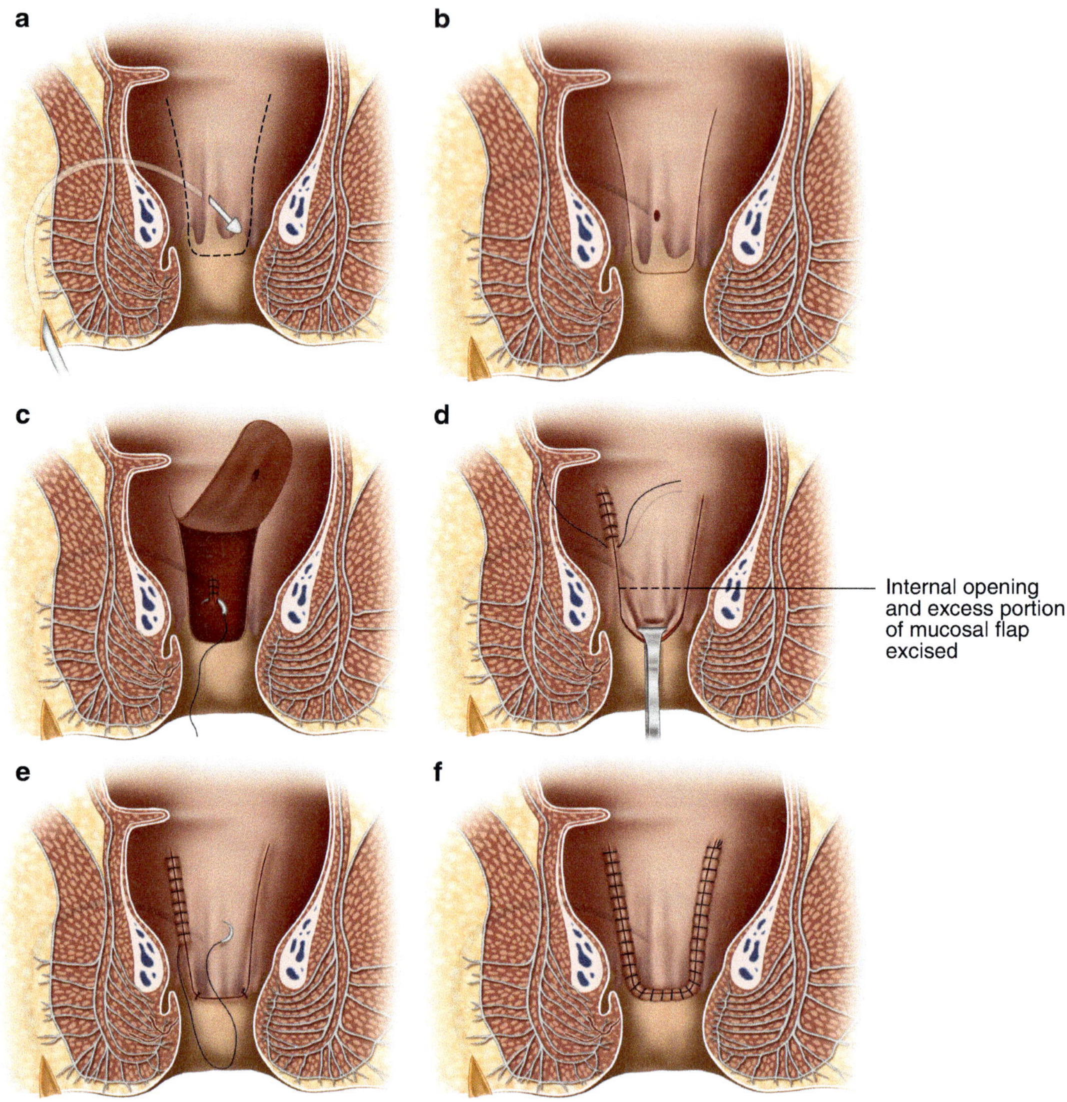

Fig. 48.19 Endorectal advancement flap. (**a**) The probe or seton through the tract and the external opening is widened. (**b**) The internal opening. The flap and area of excess mucosa that will be resected are marked. (**c**) The flap is constructed and the internal opening is closed. (**d**) Excess mucosa resected overlying the fistula. (**e**, **f**) Mucosa is sewn in place in a tension-free manner

- Nonhealed perineal wounds have been managed with a variety of techniques including skin grafting, gracilis, and rectus abdominis myocutaneous flaps.

Anorectal Stricture

- Stricture of the anorectum has been reported in 17% of patients with perineal CD.

Management

- Asymptomatic strictures require no specific therapy.
- Symptoms of obstructed defecation often can be managed with dilatation using a finger, coaxial balloon, or Hegar dilator.
- About half of these patients will eventually come to proctectomy.

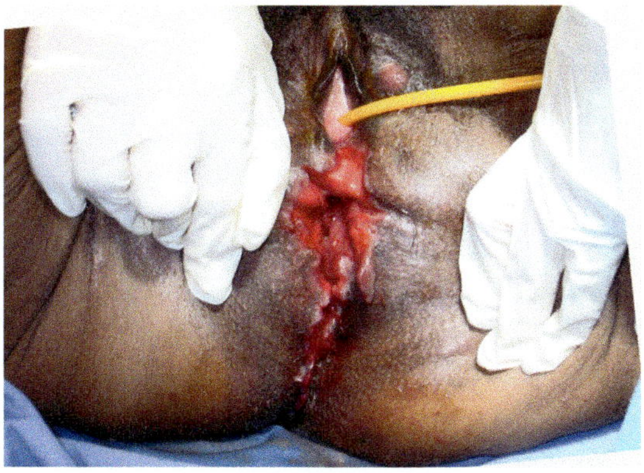

Fig. 48.20 Perineal wounds before diversion

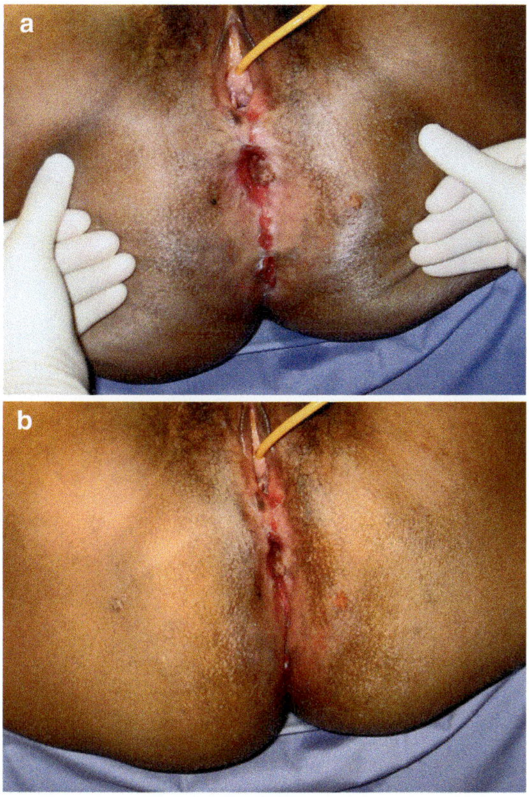

Fig. 48.21 (**a**) Perineal wounds after diversion. (**b**) Near complete healing a few months later

Anal Cancer

- Long-standing perianal disease increases the risk of both anal squamous and adenocarcinomas.

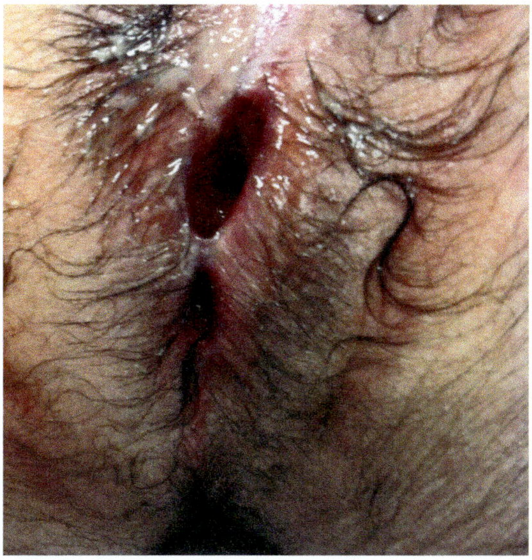

Fig. 48.22 Nonhealed perineal wound 4 years after surgery

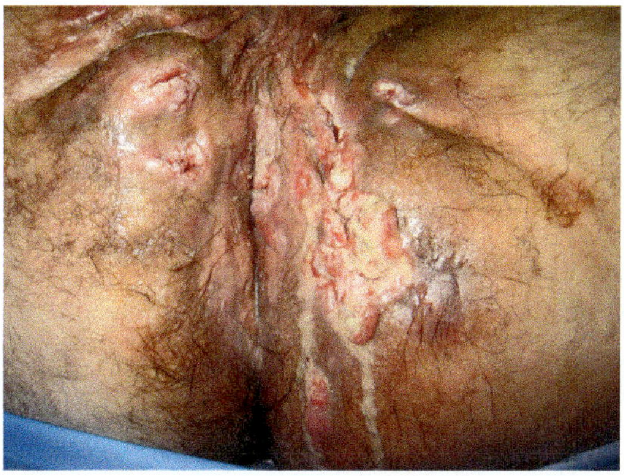

Fig. 48.23 Squamous carcinoma in multiple fistulous tracts

- These lesions can occur within the anal canal or within chronic fistula tracts (Fig. 48.23).
- Cancers are often discovered late; a change in drainage or increased pain in a long-standing fistula tract should raise suspicion and warrants biopsy.
- Physical exam is often misleading in these cases as scarring, induration, and distorted anatomy often coexist.

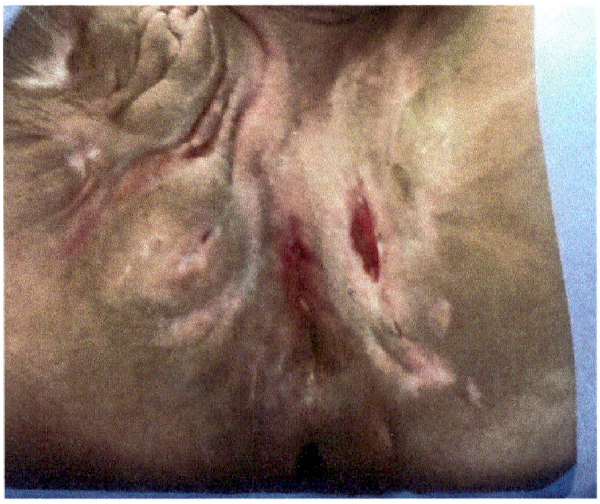

Fig. 48.24 Squamous carcinoma in multiple fistulous tracts after chemoradiation

Management

- Squamous cancers generally are best treated with combined chemoradiation (Fig. 48.24).
- Wide local excision is possible if the lesion is small.
- Adenocarcinomas may require neoadjuvant chemoradiation and then abdominoperineal resection. Consideration should be given to total proctocolectomy in these situations.
- An algorithm of suggested management is presented in Fig. 48.25.

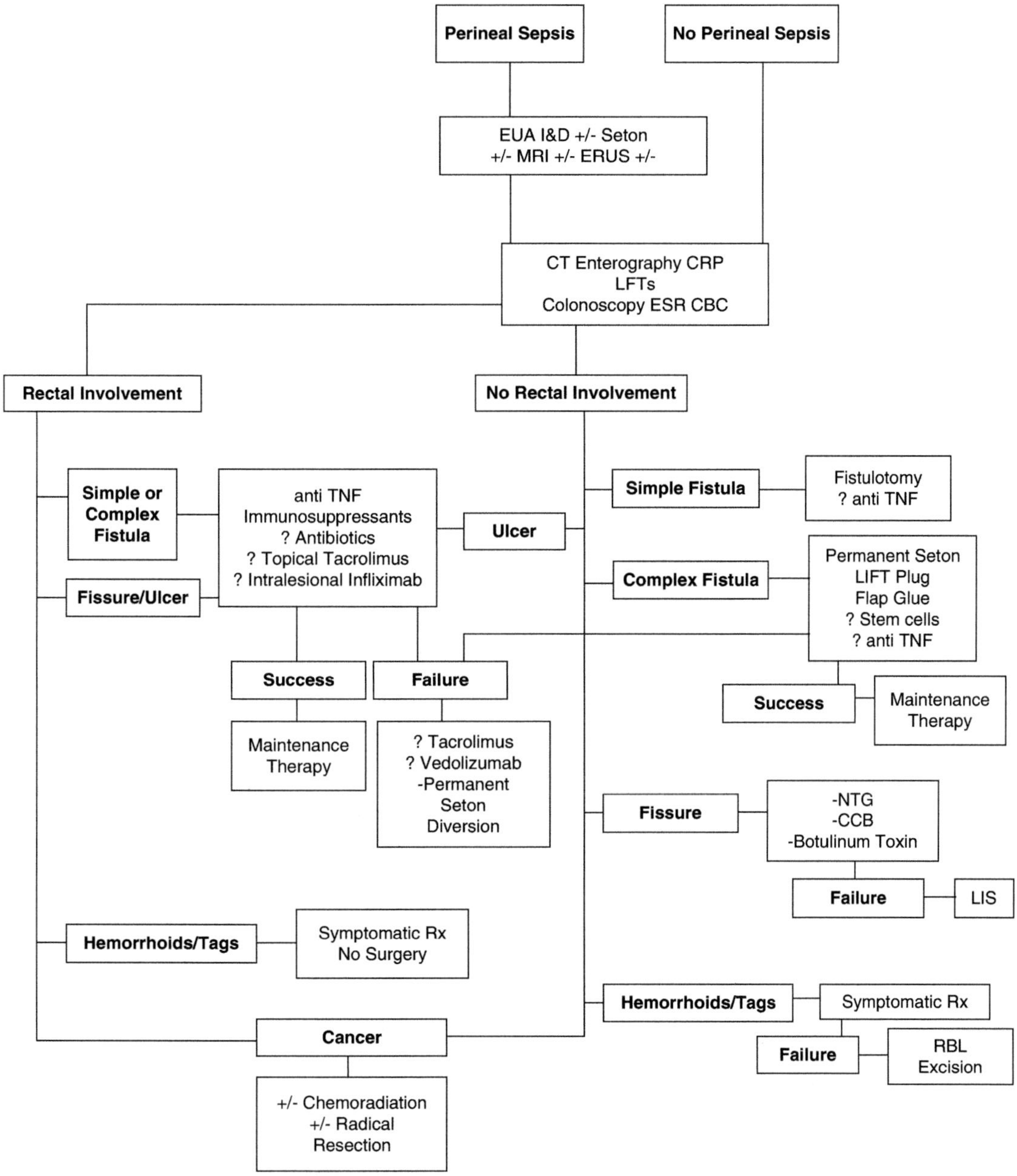

Fig. 48.25 Algorithm for the management of perineal Crohn's disease (*EUA* exam under anesthesia, *I&D* incision and drainage, *MRI* magnetic resonant imaging, *ERUS* endorectal ultrasound, *CT* computed tomography, *CRP* C-reactive protein, *LFTs* liver function tests, *ESR* erythrocyte sedimentation rate, *anti-TNF* antitumor necrosis factor, *LIFT* ligation of intersphincteric tract, *NTG* nitroglycerin, *CCB* calcium channel blocker, *LIS* lateral internal sphincterotomy, *RBL* rubber band ligation)

49 Crohn's Disease: Surgical Management

Roberta Muldoon and Alan J. Herline

Key Concepts

- Crohn's disease is a chronic inflammatory bowel disease which primarily affects the terminal ileum and colon but can involve all portions of the GI tract.
- Surgery is utilized in the treatment of Crohn's disease when medical therapy fails to control the disease or when there are complications from the disease (obstruction, perforation, fistulization, bleeding).
- Preoperative evaluation includes appropriate imaging, nutritional assessment, as well as consideration of current medications and comorbidities.
- Surgical intervention for Crohn's disease should seek to alleviate symptoms while preserving small bowel length whenever possible.
- An ileocolic resection is the most common operative procedure performed on Crohn's patients.
- In cases of toxic colitis, aggressive medical therapy includes corticosteroids and/or rescue infliximab. If the patient fails to respond, total colectomy with end ileostomy is necessary.

Surgery in the Treatment of Crohn's Disease

- Crohn's disease is a chronic transmural inflammatory condition that primarily affects the terminal ileum and colon and however can involve all portions of the gastrointestinal tract.
- Transmural inflammation leads to the complications that are attributed to this disease including strictures, obstructions, fistula, and abscesses.
- Although Crohn's disease is not curable, the goal of treatment is to induce and maintain remission of the disease, to control symptoms, and decrease complications.
- This is accomplished primarily through medications; however, surgery plays an important role in treatment.
- The specific goals of the surgeon are to determine the ideal timing of surgery, maximize patient conditioning to decrease postoperative complications, preserve as much small bowel as possible, and decrease recurrence rates.

Electronic Supplementary Material The online version of this chapter (https://doi.org/10.1007/978-3-030-01165-9_49) contains supplementary material, which is available to authorized users.

R. Muldoon (✉)
Department of Surgery, Vanderbilt University Hospital, Nashville, TN, USA
e-mail: roberta.muldoon@Vanderbilt.Edu

A. J. Herline
Department of Surgery, Georgia Regents University, Augusta, GA, USA

S. R. Steele et al. (eds.), *The ASCRS Manual of Colon and Rectal Surgery*,
https://doi.org/10.1007/978-3-030-01165-9_49

- Thorough planning and preparation, as well as attention to the patient's preoperative state including their overall health status, nutritional status, and current medication are all key factors that affect the outcome of surgery.
- >90% of patients have significant relief or complete resolution of their symptoms after surgery.

Changing Trends in the Era of Immunomodulators and Biologics

- Immunomodulators and biologics may impact the outcomes of surgical intervention.
- The rate of surgical intervention for Crohn's disease has decreased over the years, presumably owing to the advances in medical therapy.
- The longer a patient has the disease, the more likely they are to need surgical intervention.
- Patients that are younger than 40 years of age at the time of diagnosis are more likely to require surgical intervention.
- Patients with terminal ileal or ileocecal disease are more likely to require surgery compared with those that present with colonic disease.
- Those with a penetrating pattern of disease are more likely to require surgery.
- Factors associated with earlier need for surgery included smoking, disease of the small bowel without colonic involvement, nausea, vomiting and abdominal pain at presentation, neutrophil count, and steroid use in the first 6 months of diagnosis.
- Numerous studies have been done looking at the effect medications have had on outcomes.
  - Most studies support the finding that long-term use of anti-TNF therapy decreases the risk of surgery.
  - However, the data needs to be viewed carefully as many factors can confound analysis over time, including length of follow-up and improved diagnostics with earlier detection of the disease in more recent years.

Indications for Surgery

- Crohn's disease is a very complex and heterogeneous disease.
- A multidisciplinary approach including the gastroenterologist, radiologist, and colorectal surgeon is ideal.
- Non-emergent indications for surgery include failure of medical therapy, chronic obstruction, fistulas, abscesses, cancer, and occasionally quality of life issues.
  - The most common of these is failure of medical therapy to adequately control symptoms.
  - Emergent indications include acute obstruction, perforation, hemorrhage, and toxic colitis.

Failure of Medical Management

- Thirty-three to 47% of patients have surgery for Crohn's disease owing to failure of medical management.
- Failure of medical therapy includes failure of the medications to control symptoms and unacceptable side effects from the medications.
- Inability to wean off corticosteroids within 3–6 months is also considered failure of medical management.
- Timing is important to avoid a worsening health status, development of malnutrition or weight loss, or need for escalating steroid dosages; all could have significant deleterious effects on surgical outcomes.

Obstruction

- Approximately 20–25% of surgeries for Crohn's disease are secondary to obstruction.
- Transmural inflammation causes fibrosis and scarring; the resulting stricture can lead to chronic obstruction.
- Since these strictures develop slowly over time, the bowel slowly accommodates to the obstruction.

- Patients may experience intermittent crampy pain, bloating, and intolerance to certain foods.
- Other etiologies of obstruction in Crohn's patients include anastomotic stricture or cancer.
- When a patient presents with obstructive symptoms, it is important to try to differentiate between an inflammatory stricture, a fibrotic stricture, and an anastomotic stricture.
  - An inflammatory stricture usually responds to steroids with symptomatic improvement of the patient without emergent surgical intervention.
  - Fibrotic strictures are more likely to ultimately require surgical intervention.
  - If the obstruction is secondary to an anastomotic stricture, endoscopic dilation may be employed.
- Endoscopic balloon dilation can be considered as part of the therapeutic options for treatment of Crohn's obstructions secondary to strictures.

Perforation

- Free perforation is a rare indication for surgery for Crohn's disease occurring only 1–3% of the time.
- When this does occur, it is usually associated with a complete obstruction or toxic colitis.
- Patients are often septic and require immediate surgical treatment.
- Small bowel perforation is usually best treated with resection and primary anastomosis, with consideration of a proximal diversion.
- Colonic perforation is typically treated by total abdominal colectomy with end ileostomy.

Bleeding

- Massive hemorrhage is a rare event in Crohn's disease accounting for only 2–13% of operations for Crohn's disease.
- The evaluation and treatment are similar to other etiologies of gastrointestinal bleed.
- At presentation, the patient should be resuscitated and stabilized.
- Next, an attempt to localize the source of the bleed is undertaken typically with endoscopic evaluation, bleeding scans, or the use of selective angiography.
- Identification of the source is particularly important in this group of patients so that excessive and unnecessary bowel resection is not performed. Localization with angiography is successful in 40–45% of cases.

Abscesses

- Abscesses are a common indication for surgery in the Crohn's patient and account for 7–25% of surgeries.
- The abscess usually results from microperforation that originates from transmural inflammation of the diseased bowel.
- The most common location in the abdomen is the ileocecal region.
- An inflammatory "mass" may be an abscess or a phlegmon.
  - If there is an abscess, percutaneous drainage should be considered. The majority of patients who develop a spontaneous abscess will ultimately require surgery. If the abscess is small, or not amenable to percutaneous drainage, a trial of antibiotics may be attempted.
  - Percutaneous drainage allows for clinical improvement of the patient and may convert emergent surgery to an elective surgery. If the abscess is successfully controlled with percutaneous drainage, there is a significant decrease in the risk of septic complications following surgery.
- Postoperative abscesses are more likely to be successfully treated with percutaneous drainage alone than spontaneous abscesses.

Fistula

- Fistulas account for 15–24% of surgeries performed for Crohn's disease.
- Fistulas can be internal or external.

- The internal fistulas may be enteroenteric but can also be from the bowel to any surrounding structure or organ such as the bladder, vagina, or retroperitoneum.
- Enterocutaneous fistulas are considered external fistulas. Often, there is a stenotic area in the bowel wall distal to where the fistula originates, which increases the intraluminal pressure.

- Only fistulas that are symptomatic require treatment. For example, a fistula that extends from the terminal ileum to a closely adjacent loop of the small bowel would not necessarily require treatment.
- Enteroenteric fistulas are the most common type of abdominal fistula found in Crohn's disease with the majority originating from the terminal ileum.
- Symptomatic fistulas (e.g., ileosigmoid) are typically treated with excision of the diseased bowel and repair of the non-inflamed bowel wall.
- Enterocutaneous fistulas can occur either spontaneously or as a result of prior surgery.
  - Seventy-five to 85% of enterocutaneous fistulas occur in the post-op period and are secondary to either anastomotic leaks or inadvertent injuries to the bowel.
  - Because this bowel is healthy, the fistula is more likely to close with conservative measures.
  - Fifteen to 25% are spontaneous enterocutaneous fistulas caused by Crohn's disease, radiation, or cancer. These types of fistulas are unlikely to heal without surgical intervention.

Cancer and Dysplasia

- Patients with Crohn's disease have an increased risk of developing cancer in their lifetime.
  - A patient with CD has a two- to threefold increased risk of colorectal cancer compared to the general population.
  - With regard to small bowel cancer, there is an almost 20-fold increase.
  - A number of studies have found a male predominance in the development of cancer in Crohn's disease.
  - The average age at diagnosis is 49–56 years, which is about 10–15 years younger than the average age for sporadic bowel cancers.
  - The mean duration of disease from onset of Crohn's disease to diagnosis of cancer is 20 years.
- Survival seems to be worse for patients with Crohn's disease. Overall, a 5-year survival is approximately 40%.
- There is a higher risk of developing cancer in bypassed segments, which is associated with a poor prognosis.
- There is an increased risk of developing cancer in the area of a stricture. Colonic strictures need to be closely monitored if not surgically resected.
- High-grade dysplasia (HGD) found in patients with Crohn's colitis is an indication for colectomy.

Toxic Colitis

- Severe colitis is a serious and potentially life-threatening condition if not treated appropriately and in a timely manner.
- The addition of dilation of the colon (toxic megacolon) to this compilation of symptoms further increases the risk of complications and can lead to a potentially fatal outcome (Table 49.1).

Table 49.1 Diagnostic criteria for toxic megacolon

Diagnostic criteria
Radiographic evidence of colonic distension
At least three of the following:
Fever >38 °C (101.5 °F)
Heart rate > 120 bpm
Neutrophilic leukocytosis >10.5 × 10^9/L
Anemia
In addition to the above, at least one of the following:
Dehydration
Altered consciousness
Electrolyte disturbances
Hypotension

- A multidisciplinary approach for the treatment of these patients is critical to effectively manage these patients.
- Initial medical management of these patients includes efforts to resuscitate the patient, including intravenous hydration and correction of electrolyte abnormalities, in particular potassium and magnesium. Total parenteral nutrition may be necessary to optimize the nutritional status of the patient.
- It is important to rule out other possible causes of diarrhea including *Clostridium difficile* as well as cytomegalovirus.
- Daily abdominal films should typically be obtained if there is presence of abdominal distension, so colonic dilation can be assessed and monitored.
- Patients with inflammatory bowel disease have a higher risk for thromboembolic disease, so special attention needs to be made for prophylaxis.
- The mainstay of medical therapy is the administration of corticosteroids in a daily equivalent dose of hydrocortisone 300 mg (in divided doses) or methylprednisolone 60 mg (in divided doses).
- Those patients that do not respond or have a decline in their clinical status within 24–72 h of initiation of treatment require emergent surgery. Delays in surgery can lead to increased postoperative complications or worse.
- Mortality rates dramatically increase in those that have suffered a perforation, increasing from 2–8% up to 27–40%.
- The procedure of choice for these patients is a total abdominal colectomy with end ileostomy.
- Emergent proctectomy is rarely indicated for rectal hemorrhage or rectal perforation.

Surgical Considerations

- Surgery for Crohn's disease is not curative, so preserving the small bowel when possible is paramount.
- Recurrence occurs in the majority of patients and so should be considered in operative planning.

Preoperative Evaluation

- Information obtained from the history and physical, past medical, and surgical records, endoscopy, as well as imaging studies will be critical to operative planning and timing.
- Nutritional assessment as well as medication usage deserves special attention as this will effect healing and may increase postoperative complications.
- Preoperative imaging will give information regarding severity, involvement of surrounding structures, concurrent infections, resectability, and possible risk of short bowel syndrome (Fig. 49.1).

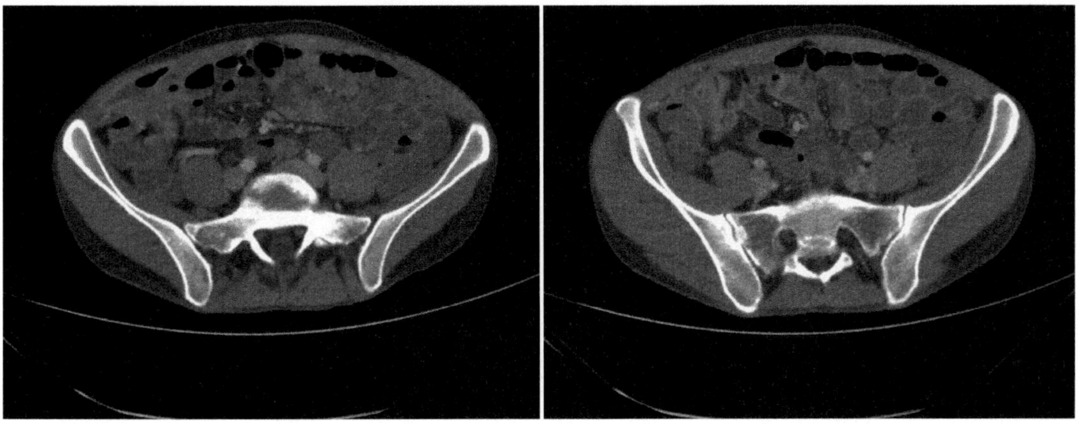

Fig. 49.1 CT scan in a patient with Crohn's disease demonstrating fluid-filled bowel loops, thickened terminal ileum, and a subcutaneous right lower quadrant abscess

History and Physical

- Accurate and detailed information regarding the patient's current symptoms is very important and helpful in deciding if surgery is indicated.
- During the abdominal examination, special attention is paid to areas of tenderness, prior scars, evidence of draining fistula, as well as palpable masses.
- Knowledge of rectal or perianal involvement based on physical examination is often important when planning operative management.

Nutritional Assessment and Role of TPN in Crohn's Treatment

- Poor nutrition has been linked to delayed wound healing, decline in physiologic and psychiatric function, altered immune function, and increased postoperative complications.
- Various markers of nutrition have been evaluated including weight loss, protein depletion, serum albumin, and prealbumin. Each of these has shown a link between malnutrition and poor surgical outcomes.
- Hypoalbuminemia has also been shown to be a good predictor of postoperative morbidity and mortality.
- It is estimated that 80% of Crohn's patients will have some degree of malnutrition; weight loss has been reported in 65–76% of patients with Crohn's disease depending on severity of disease.
- Total parenteral nutrition may be appropriate to improve the patient's nutritional status when enteral feeds are not possible.
- Correction of malnutrition preoperatively lessens the risk of postoperative complications.
- TPN in CD is used also for treatment of intestinal fistulas, for treatment of short bowel syndrome, and for nutritional support when enteric feeds are not possible.
- Complications can be divided into those related to either access, gastrointestinal, metabolic, or infectious.
  - Access-related complications include injuries sustained during insertion of catheters, thrombosis, and embolization.
  - Liver complications are the most important gastrointestinal complication related to treatment with TPN. This includes cholestasis, cholangitis, liver dysfunction, as well as elevation of transaminases.
  - Metabolic imbalances can occur with either excess or inadequate administration of water, glucose, electrolytes, amino acids, fat, and minerals. Close monitoring is necessary to avoid such complications.
  - There can be infectious complications with the most common being catheter-related infection.
- Consideration should be given to either proximal diversion if an anastomosis is formed or the avoidance of an anastomosis with creation of an end stoma in patients who cannot be nutritionally repleted.

Impact of Medications

- A major concern with CD medications is the effect that their immunomodulatory activity may have on surgical outcomes.
- Corticosteroids negatively affect wound healing and increase postoperative complications; 10 mg of prednisone may be a threshold.
- No clear and consistent association between the use of anti-TNF agents and postoperative complications has been established.
- There is no clear association between postoperative complications and the use of thiopurines.

Operative Considerations: Overview

- Complete exploration of the abdomen should typically be performed, assessing the extent of disease as well as involvement of surrounding bowel or other structures.
- Every attempt should be made to preserve uninvolved bowel.

- Care should be taken when handling the bowel and its mesentery because the mesentery can be quite friable and even gentle retraction can lead to troublesome bleeding.
- Typically in the case of fistulas, the diseased bowel loop will need resection, while the "innocent bystander" can be preserved.
- Extent of resection is based on macroscopic disease alone, so a grossly disease-free margin is all that is needed.
- Stapled side-to-side anastomosis may be associated with fewer anastomotic leaks, shorter OR time, as well as lower rate of reoperation for recurrence of disease.

Laparoscopic Surgery and Crohn's Disease

- Laparoscopic surgery has proven benefit over open surgery with respect to return of bowel function, hospital stay, postoperative pain, as well as cosmesis.
- Multiple studies have shown that using the laparoscopic technique in Crohn's patients is both feasible and safe, at least in CD patients with "simple" disease.
- The presence of extensive inflammatory adhesions, multiple areas of diseased bowel, large inflammatory masses, and the presence of fistula and abscesses may necessitate open technique (Video 49.1).
- Contraindications for laparoscopic surgery include hypotension and sepsis, inability to tolerate pneumoperitoneum, an extensive inflammatory mass that would require a large incision for extraction, and those with extensive, complex adhesions.

Operative Considerations for Specific Locations

Upper Small Bowel Disease

- Upper small bowel disease includes any involvement of the small bowel proximal to the terminal ileum.
- Disease in this area, when present, can be quite extensive; this phenotype has a poorer prognosis.
- When the upper small bowel is involved, there may be multiple areas of diseased bowel between areas of normal bowel.
- Surgical options include resection with primary anastomosis, stricturoplasty, or in some instances, when there is significant distal disease present, proximal diversion.
- Resection with anastomosis is commonly the appropriate option if the area to be resected is limited and the patient has not had significant small bowel resections in the past.
- Those loops that have a perforation, associated fistula or abscess, or significant inflammation require resection.
- Resection may also be considered if there are multiple strictures in a short segment of the bowel.
- Resection is carried out to grossly negative margins.
- Stricturoplasty is a method by which obstruction from a stricture in the bowel can be relieved without resection. There are multiple techniques by which this can be accomplished.
  - The Heineke-Mikulicz is the most common stricturoplasty performed and is ideal for short strictures. It is easy to perform with a low complication rate (Fig. 49.2). A variation of this is the Moskel-Walske-Neumayer stricturoplasty (Fig. 49.3).
  - For those strictures that are slightly longer (>10 cm, but <25 cm), a Jaboulay or Finney procedure may be indicated (Fig. 49.4).
  - For those strictures that are even longer (>20 cm), a Michelassi or Poggioli stricturoplasty may be applicable (Fig. 49.5).
- Indications for stricturoplasty include situations where there are multiple strictures; there has been previous significant small bowel resection (>100 cm), in patients that are at risk of short bowel syndrome, duodenal strictures, or recurrent strictures.
- Contraindications to performing a stricturoplasty include severe inflammation, strictures associated with fistulas, abscesses, or a phlegmon or

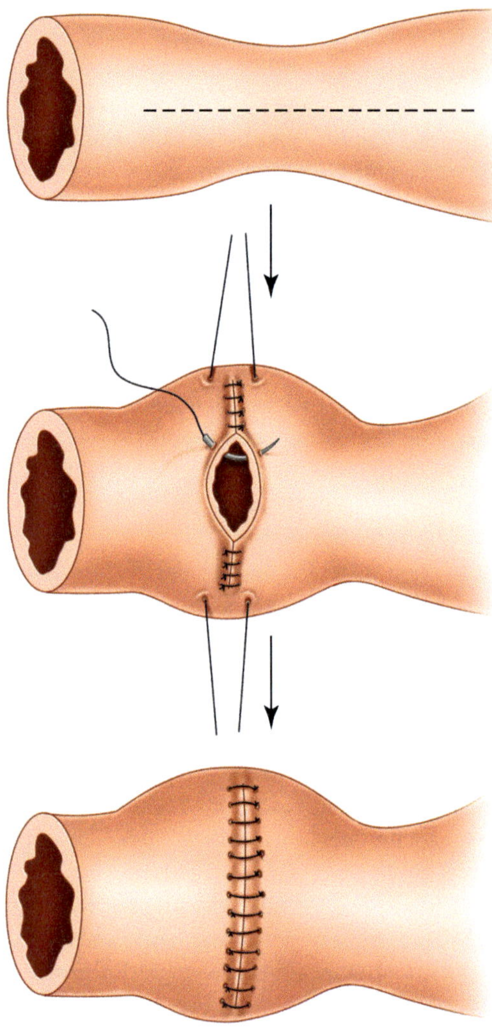

Fig. 49.2 Heineke-Mikulicz stricturoplasty

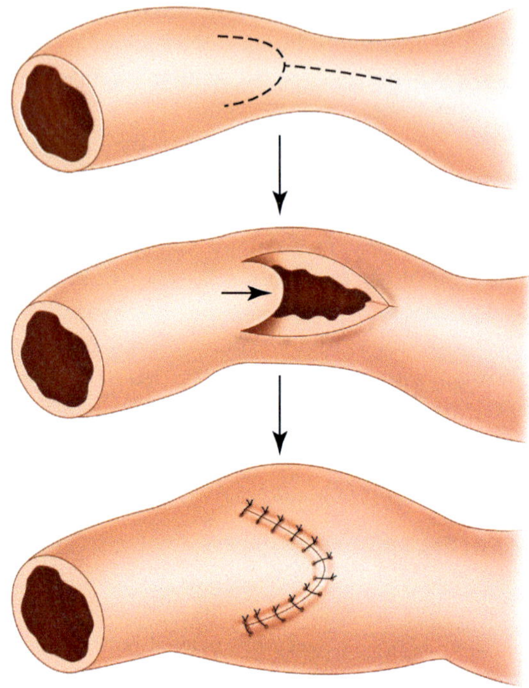

Fig. 49.3 Moskel-Walske-Neumayer stricturoplasty

those with diffuse peritonitis from a perforation. Stricturoplasty should also be avoided if there is concern for cancer and tension or the area of the stricturoplasty is adjacent to an area of resection.

- Multiple studies have suggested comparable recurrence rates to resection.
- In actual practice, the majority of these patients are treated with a combination of resection and stricturoplasty.

Terminal Ileal Disease

- Since terminal ileal disease is the most common location for Crohn's disease to occur, ileocolic resection is the most common operative procedure performed on Crohn's disease patients.
- The point of division is 1–2 cm beyond the palpably thickened bowel. Microscopic negative margins are not necessary (Figs. 49.6 and 49.7).
- Once the bowel has been resected, an anastomosis is typically performed.
- In high-risk situations, the anastomosis may be protected with a diverting loop ileostomy; taking down a loop ileostomy has lower morbidity than laparotomy for takedown of an end ileostomy.

Colonic and Rectal Disease

- Patients requiring an emergent operation for Crohn's colitis typically undergo a total abdominal colectomy with end ileostomy regardless of the presence of rectal involvement.
- Once diverted, symptoms and disease activity will typically subside.

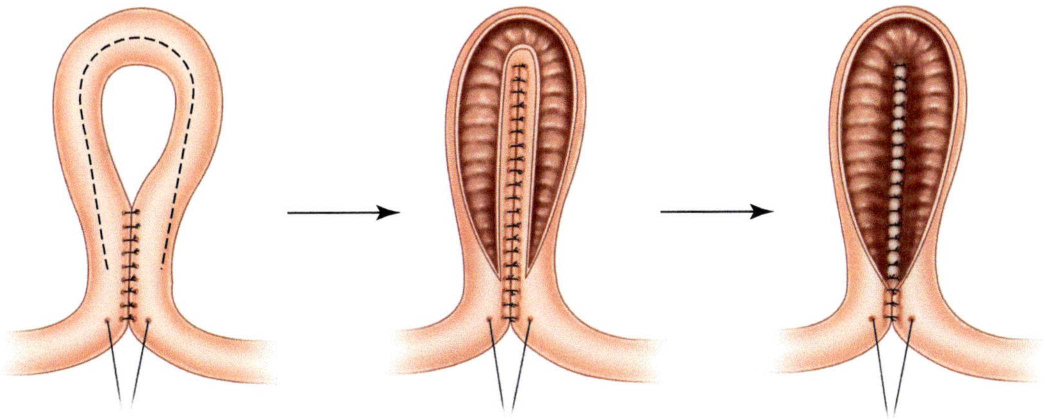

Fig. 49.4 Finney stricturoplasty

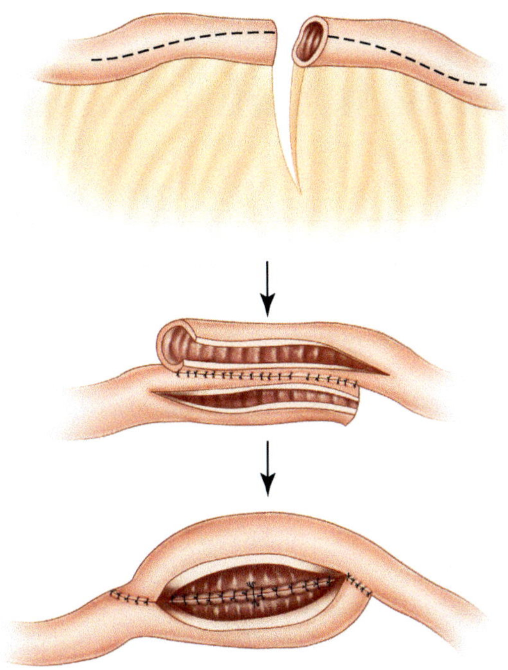

Fig. 49.5 Michelassi stricturoplasty

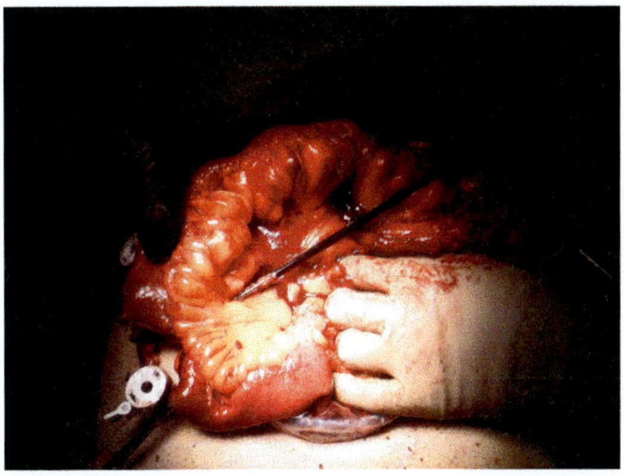

Fig. 49.6 Following laparoscopic mobilization, an energy device is being used to divide the thickened mesentery of a patient with Crohn's disease

- The decision to either leave the rectum in situ, perform an ileorectal anastomosis, or perform a proctectomy can be determined at a later date.
- The decision as to which operation to perform for a patient with Crohn's colitis in the elective setting is more complex as more options are available.
- Patients with refractory colonic and rectal disease typically undergo total proctocolectomy with end ileostomy.
  - The most common complication is perineal wound sepsis (36%).
  - Total abdominal proctocolectomy with a micro-Hartmann's stump and end ileostomy is a viable alternative. At a later date, completion proctectomy can be performed via a perineal approach.
  - Total abdominal colectomy with end ileostomy and delayed proctectomy might be considered in younger patients that are concerned about sexual function and are in their childbearing years. Surveillance of the rectum is necessary until the time of the proctectomy.
- For those patients with Crohn's colitis with rectal sparing, a more limited resection can be entertained. Ileorectal anastomosis may be

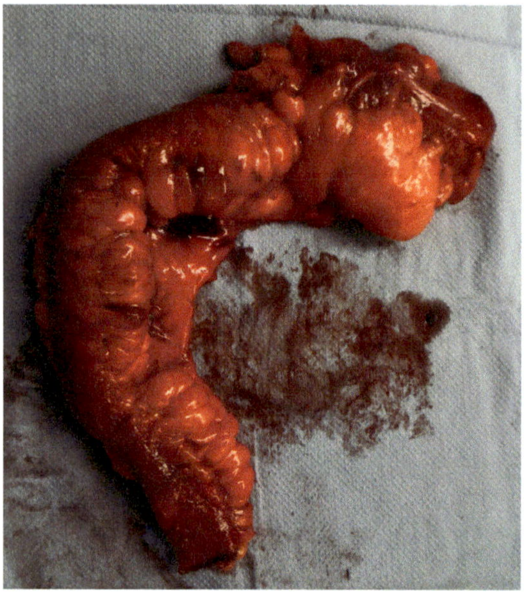

Fig. 49.7 Ileocecectomy specimen in a patient with Crohn's disease

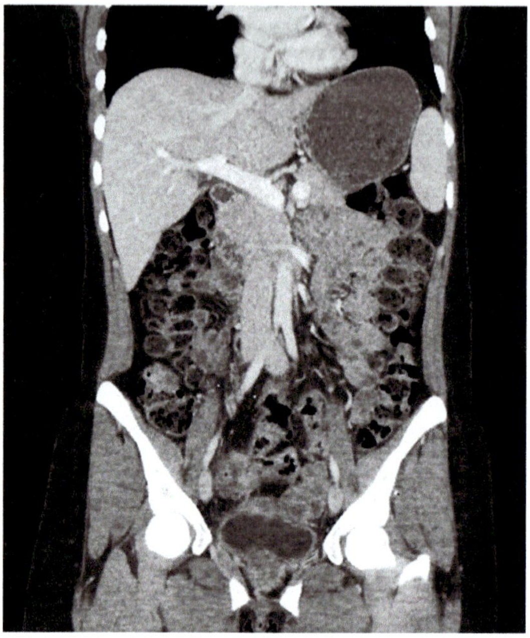

Fig. 49.8 Coronal CT image in a patient with Crohn's disease demonstrating an ileal-sigmoid fistula from the thickened ileum to the sigmoid colon right above the level of the bladder

proposed for selected patients with intact rectal reservoir function.

- Segmental resection for Crohn's colitis is controversial but is appropriate for patients with limited disease.

Special Considerations

Ileosigmoid Fistula

- This is the most common abdominal fistula encountered.
- Most often, the sigmoid colon is not involved with Crohn's disease but happens to be adjacent to the inflamed terminal ileum (Fig. 49.8).
- If there is any question as to active Crohn's disease in the sigmoid colon, a flexible endoscopic exam during surgery should answer the question.
- Wedge resection with primary repair is typically all that is needed.
- Occasionally, the inflammation will be so severe that wedge resection is not safe; in these cases a sleeve resection can be done.

Complex Perineal Wounds After Proctectomy

- Perineal wound complications can be a devastating problem after proctectomy for Crohn's disease leading to postoperative pain, significant wound care issues, and prolonged recovery.
- It has been estimated that the rate of unhealed perineal wounds after proctectomy for Crohn's disease ranges from 23% to 70%.
- Strategies to prevent this complication include smoking cessation prior to surgery, improvement of the nutritional status of the patient, as well as preoperative management of sepsis.
- In cases of severe perianal disease, creation of a low Hartmann's stump instead of complete proctectomy will avoid a perineal wound yet still remove majority of the disease.
- When full resection is necessary, an intersphincteric dissection should be performed

when possible. This decreases the amount of tissue removed as well as leaves well-vascularized muscle to bolster the closure.

- At times, a wide excision is necessary either because of severe perianal disease, significant scarring, or the presence of cancer.
  - In these cases, primary closure may not be possible; wound healing can be achieved with the use of advanced tissue flaps (e.g., gluteus maximus advancement flap, posterior thigh fasciocutaneous flap, chimeric posterior thigh flap, rectus abdominis myocutaneous flap).

Recurrence of Disease

- Recurrence can be described as being endoscopic, clinical, or surgical.
- Postoperative recurrence rates have been shown to be 33% and 44% at 5 and 10 years.
- The rate of surgical recurrence ranges from 9.5% to 20% at 5 years and 18.6% to 44% at 10 years. The rate continues to increase up to 57% at 20 years.
- The strongest predictor of postoperative recurrence is smoking.
- Other risk factors that have been linked to a higher rate of recurrence include prior surgical resection and penetrating/perforating phenotype.
- Risk factors that have had mixed predictive value for postoperative recurrence include gender and location of disease.
- Steroids and probiotics do not appear to have a role in the prevention of postoperative recurrence.
- Mesalamine has been shown to reduce the risk of clinical recurrence when compared to placebo in some studies but not all.
- A randomized control trial demonstrated that those patients who received metronidazole for 3 months after ileocolic resection had a decrease in severity of early recurrence compared to placebo.
- Studies have shown a modest effect impact with thiopurines; one study showed that azathioprine seemed to delay endoscopic postoperative recurrence compared to a historical cohort or placebo groups.
- Biologics have shown the most promise in reducing postoperative recurrence.
  - In one study, endoscopic recurrence rate at 1 year was 9.1% in the infliximab group compared to 84.6% in the placebo group.
  - Clinical recurrence was seen in 0% of the infliximab patients, 38% in the azathioprine patients, and 70% in the mesalamine patients in another study.
  - These studies are relatively small but suggest that infliximab can change the natural history of Crohn's disease.

50 Ulcerative Colitis: Surgical Management

Mukta K. Krane, Erin O. Lange, and Alessandro Fichera

Key Concepts

- Patients with ulcerative colitis should be managed by a multidisciplinary team of gastroenterologists, surgeons, pathologists, enterostomal therapists, and nutritionists.
- Preoperative weight management, improvement of nutrition, and optimization of medical therapy before proceeding with the construction of the ileal pouch-anal anastomosis are critical steps to achieve optimal long-term functional results.
- Laparoscopy should be considered the standard of care for elective surgery for ulcerative colitis.
- While ileal pouch-anal anastomosis should be considered the standard of care in the surgical treatment of ulcerative colitis patients, the surgical plan should be individualized both in terms of staged approach and restoration of intestinal continuity.
- Long-term follow-up of patients with an ileal pouch-anal anastomosis is mandatory, even though the risk of malignant degeneration remains quite low.

M. K. Krane · E. O. Lange
Department of Surgery, University of Washington Medical Center, Seattle, WA, USA

A. Fichera (✉)
Department of Surgery, University of North Carolina, Chapel Hill, NC, USA
e-mail: alessandro_fichera@med.unc.edu

Introduction

- Ulcerative colitis (UC) is an inflammatory intestinal condition characterized by continuous colonic inflammation extending from the rectum proximally.
- While medical therapy is often the first-line treatment, proctocolectomy is curative, and therefore surgery has a pivotal role in the therapeutic armamentarium of UC.

Indications for Surgery

- Approximately 25–30% of patients with UC will undergo surgical intervention in their lifetime, with up to 10% of patients requiring surgery within the first year of diagnosis (Table 50.1).

Table 50.1 Indications for surgery in ulcerative colitis

Elective	Emergent
Failure of medical management	Toxic megacolon
Complications/side effects of medications	Sepsis/fulminant colitis
Dysplasia	Perforation
Invasive cancer	Hemorrhage
Extraintestinal manifestations	
Growth retardation	

S. R. Steele et al. (eds.), *The ASCRS Manual of Colon and Rectal Surgery*,
https://doi.org/10.1007/978-3-030-01165-9_50

Elective Surgery

- Elective indications for surgery include failure of medical management, complications or side effects associated with medications, dysplasia or invasive cancer, extraintestinal manifestations, and growth retardation in children and adolescents.
- High-grade dysplasia (HGD), dysplasia-associated lesion or mass (DALM), or invasive carcinoma in a patient with UC is an absolute indication for surgery.
- Synchronous and metachronous dysplasia and carcinoma are more common in patients with UC than in the sporadic colorectal cancer population.
- The recommended procedure for UC patients with colorectal cancer or HGD is proctocolectomy with end ileostomy or ileal pouch-anal anastomosis (IPAA).
- The need for and timing of surgery in patients with low-grade dysplasia (LGD) remain highly debated.
- Endoscopic mucosal resection and endoscopic submucosal dissection have emerged as possible therapeutic techniques in the treatment of UC-associated dysplasia.
- There are two widely accepted elective surgical options: total proctocolectomy with an end ileostomy or restorative proctocolectomy with ileal pouch-anal anastomosis (IPAA).
- Total abdominal colectomy with an ileorectal anastomosis is a third but rarely used option.
- The choice of elective procedure is individualized based on the patient and the clinical setting.

Emergent Surgery

- Emergent indications for surgery include toxic megacolon, sepsis or fulminant disease not responsive to medical therapy, perforation, and severe bleeding.
  - Perforation and massive hemorrhage occur less frequently than fulminant colitis but are absolute indications for surgery.
  - Toxic megacolon and severe acute flares may respond to intensive medical therapy.
- Toxic megacolon is a life-threatening complication of UC, and there should be a low threshold for surgical intervention.
  - An initial trial of conservative therapy with bowel rest, intravenous fluids, broad-spectrum antibiotics, and close monitoring for 24–48 h may be cautiously attempted.
  - Infliximab and cyclosporine may successfully treat toxic megacolon secondary to UC in 25–40% of patients.
  - Worsening clinical signs or evidence of increasing colon dilation with "thumb printing" or pneumatosis on radiologic imaging are indications for surgery.
- Severity of UC can be characterized as mild, moderate, severe, or fulminant depending on the number of daily bowel movements, systemic symptoms, and inflammatory markers (Table 50.2).
- While advances in medical therapy have resulted in the avoidance or delay of surgical intervention in some patients with severe or fulminant disease, a colorectal surgeon should be consulted.
- Early collaboration between the medical and surgical teams ensures that the patient understands the role of colectomy.
- In patients admitted to the hospital with fulminant UC, steroids and other rescue therapies will often be initiated.
  - Colectomy is generally advocated for clinical deterioration or if there is no significant clinical improvement in 4–7 days.
  - Concomitant infection with cytomegalovirus or *Clostridium difficile* needs to be ruled out and appropriately treated if identified.
- Critical examination of current practice reveals that the threshold for elective surgery is often too high.
  - Three-year mortality in over 28,000 patients hospitalized for UC was 3.7% in the group undergoing elective surgery, while medical management and urgent colectomy groups had similar mortality rates of 13.6% and 13.2%, respectively.

Table 50.2 Ulcerative colitis disease severity scale

	Mild	Severe	Fulminant
Number of bowel movements/day	<4	>6	>10
Rectal bleeding	Rare	Frequent	Profuse and continuous
Hemoglobin	Normal	<75% of normal	Requiring transfusions
ESR (mm/h)	Normal	>30	>30
Body temperature (C)	Normal	> 37.5	> 37.5
Heart rate	Normal	Normal to slightly tachycardic	Tachycardic

Modified from Truelove S.C., Witts LJ. Cortisone in ulcerative colitis; final report on a therapeutic trial. Br Med J. 1955;2(4947):1041–8

  - Urgent surgical intervention for severe colitis is associated with a 40.1% morbidity rate.
- In the emergent setting, the most common procedure performed is a total abdominal colectomy with end ileostomy, leaving the rectum in situ.
- Resection of the diseased colon eliminates the majority of the disease, alleviates symptoms, usually allows the patient to discontinue immunosuppressive medications and return to an improved overall state of health.
- Completion proctectomy with or without an IPAA can then be addressed in an elective setting.
- Resection of the rectum at the time of emergent surgery should be avoided as it hinders future restoration of intestinal continuity and is associated with a higher risk of bleeding, complications, and injury to the autonomic nerves.

Staged Operations

- There are several indications for a staged approach to surgical therapy for UC patients (Table 50.3).
- A two-stage approach (for both open and laparoscopic cases) includes a restorative proctocolectomy with an IPAA and diverting loop ileostomy as the first stage and reversal of the loop ileostomy at the second operation.
- A three-stage approach involves a total abdominal colectomy and an end ileostomy as the first stage, followed by a restorative proctectomy with an IPAA and diverting loop ileostomy as the second stage, and reversal of the ileostomy at the third and final operation.

Table 50.3 Indications for a staged surgical approach

Indications for a staged surgical approach
Obesity
Medical treatment (biologics, steroids)
Fulminant disease/toxic megacolon
Patient comorbidities

- The staged approach to pouch construction among complex UC patients aims to decrease the incidence of pelvic sepsis, often related to a leak at the ileoanal anastomosis, and to minimize long-term sequelae including poor pouch function.
- Pelvic sepsis is a frequent and serious complication of IPAA for UC and is reported to occur in up to 23% of patients.
- Long-term outcomes after IPAA are worsened by the occurrence of pouch-related septic complications.
  - Potential risk factors for postoperative pouch-related septic complications include steroids, infliximab, and immunomodulators.
  - While the role of corticosteroids as a risk factor for postoperative complications is consistently described, the impact of biologics has not been clearly defined to date.
- The theoretical advantage of a three-stage approach is the opportunity to optimize the general medical condition, improve nutritional status, and wean off medical therapy following total abdominal colectomy.
- Patients receiving aggressive medical management generally undergo staged procedures, while primary pouch surgery is offered to healthier patients.

Operative Technique and Surgical Decision-Making

Preoperative Planning

- The patient and family should meet with the surgical team prior to discuss the nature and necessity for the surgery, alternative options, risks and benefits of the procedure, and long-term functional outcomes.
- If a temporary or permanent ileostomy is planned, a certified enterostomal therapist should evaluate the patient for preoperative marking.

Brooke Ileostomy

- When determining the placement of the ileostomy, the patient's abdomen should be assessed in the sitting and standing positions.
- The patient should be seen by an enterostomal therapist for marking.

Operative Details

- A circular incision is made in the skin and carried down through the subcutaneous tissue until the anterior rectus sheath is encountered.
- The anterior rectus sheath is incised vertically, and the rectus muscles are bluntly separated with handheld retractors.
- The posterior rectus sheath and peritoneum are then incised to create an opening that will accommodate two fingerbreadths.
- After ensuring no twisting of the bowel or mesentery, the terminal ileum is delivered through the opening (Fig. 50.1a).
- A full-thickness suture is placed at the open end of the ileum; a seromuscular bite is then taken at the skin level and followed with a subcuticular bite through the dermis (Fig. 50.1b).
- Four to five everting sutures are placed (Fig. 50.1c), with particular care taken at the mesenteric side to avoid injury to the mesenteric vessels.

Operative Considerations

- Stoma-related complications occur in up to 36% of patients, with obesity representing a key risk factor for stoma failure.
- Stoma necrosis, retraction, parastomal herniation, and mucocutaneous separation are among the possible complications of a permanent end Brooke ileostomy.
- The impact of a poorly functioning ileostomy on patient's quality of life must be understood by the surgeon.

Outcomes

- Despite the presence of a permanent ileostomy, HRQOL is very similar to that of the general population.
- A permanent end ileostomy remains a viable option for UC patients requiring surgery and should always be discussed when counseling the patient regarding surgery.

Continent Ileostomy

- Creation of a continent ileostomy, or Kock pouch, involves the building of an ileal pouch with an internal valve to prevent and control the flow of enteric contents.
- This operation should be offered in specialized centers owing to complexity and complication rates.
- Appropriate candidates may include:
  - Patients with locally advanced low rectal cancer that will need adjuvant radiation postoperatively
  - Patients who already have a Brooke ileostomy after proctocolectomy and are dissatisfied with their quality of life
  - Patients that are not candidates for an IPAA because of poor sphincter function
  - Patients who prefer a continent ileostomy to an IPAA as a personal choice
  - Patients who have failed an IPAA but prefer a continence-preserving procedure to a Brooke ileostomy
- Contraindications to this procedure include Crohn's disease, obesity, critically ill patients, and the psychologically unfit patients because of the inability to intubate.

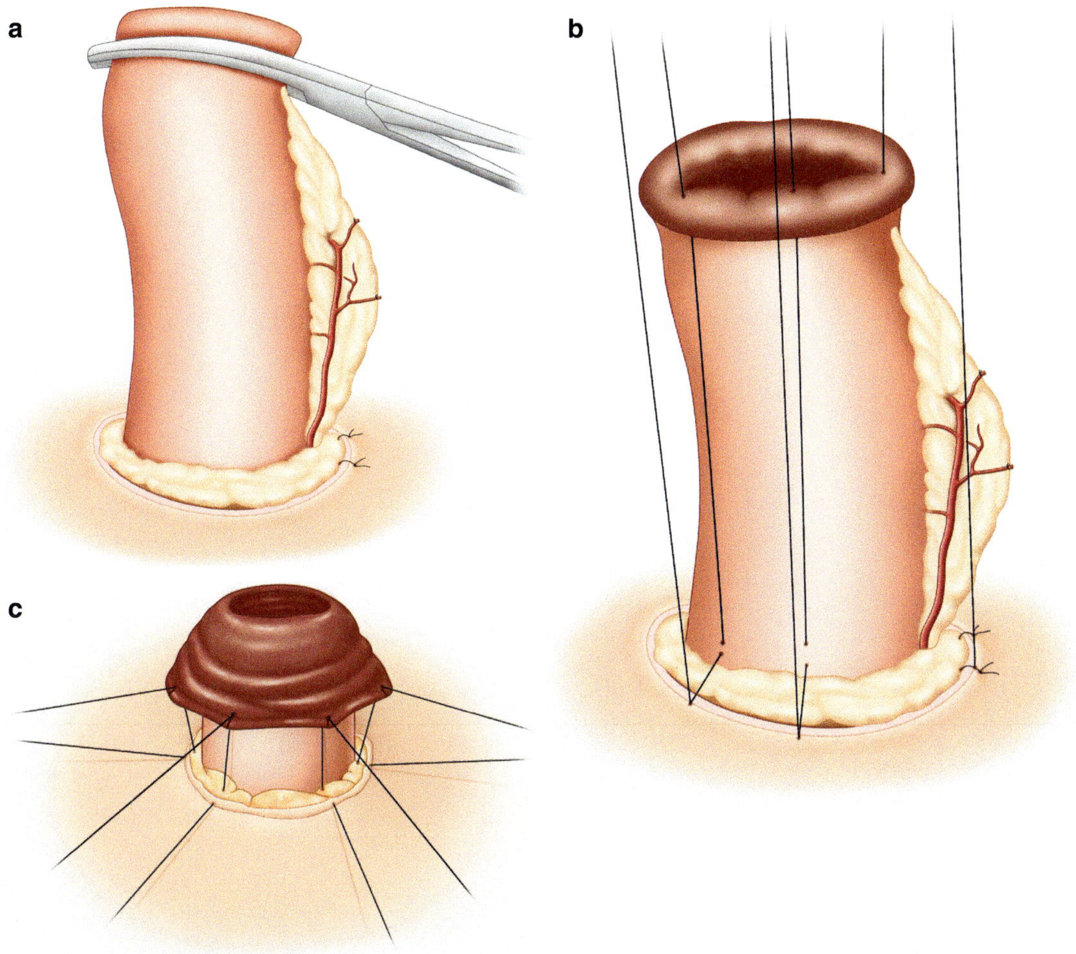

Fig. 50.1 Construction of a Brooke ileostomy. (**a**) The terminal ileum is extracted from the stoma site without tension on the mesentery. (**b**) Sutures are placed along the antimesenteric edge of the ileum and lateral to the mesentery allowing eversion of the bowel. (**c**) Everting sutures are tied, and simple sutures are placed between the ileum and the dermis at the mucocutaneous junction

Operative Details

- About 50 cm of small bowel is used to fashion a Kock pouch (Fig. 50.2).
- The outlet is constructed from the distal 3–5 cm of this segment, the nipple valve is created from the next 18 cm of bowel, and the remaining 30 cm is used for the pouch.
- Excising the peritoneum and mesentery on both sides of the arcade skeletonizes the mesenteric vessels of the small bowel used to build the nipple valve (Fig. 50.3).
- The pouch is generally created in an S-shape by folding the 30 cm length of small bowel into 10 cm limbs with one more cephalad to the other. A posterior row of sutures is placed between each limb and an enterotomy made along the S-shape (Fig. 50.4).
- The incision will be antimesenteric along the middle limb and closer to the mesentery along the two outer limbs. A second posterior layer of sutures is created to re-approximate the cut edges (Fig. 50.5).
- The nipple valve is then created with three passes of a GIA stapler without the knife (two along either side of the mesentery and one along the anterior aspect (Fig. 50.6)).

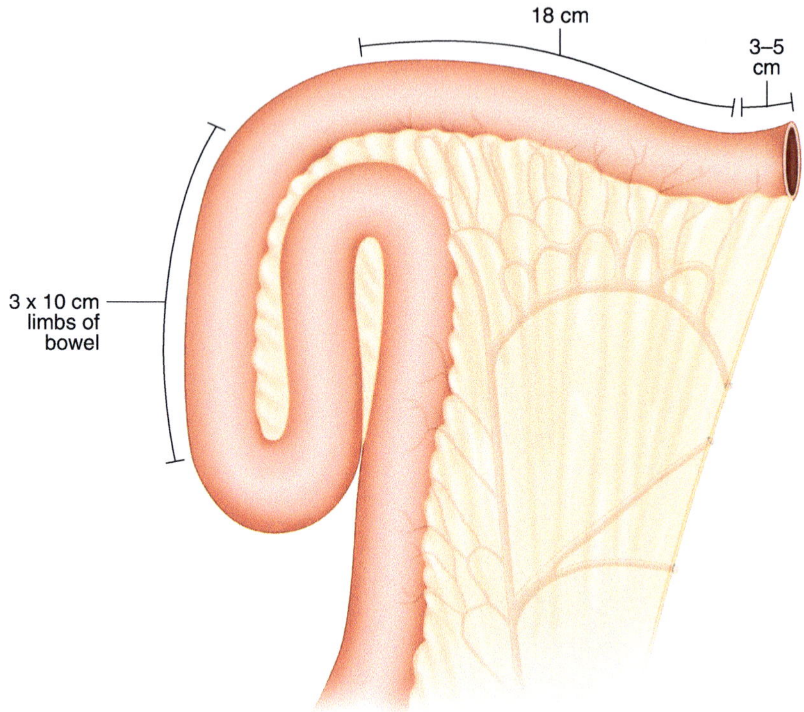

Fig. 50.2 Construction of a Kock pouch – about 50 cm of small bowel is used to create the Kock pouch. The distal 3–5 cm is used for the outlet, the middle 18 cm is used to construct the nipple valve, and the proximal 30 cm is utilized in the creation of the pouch

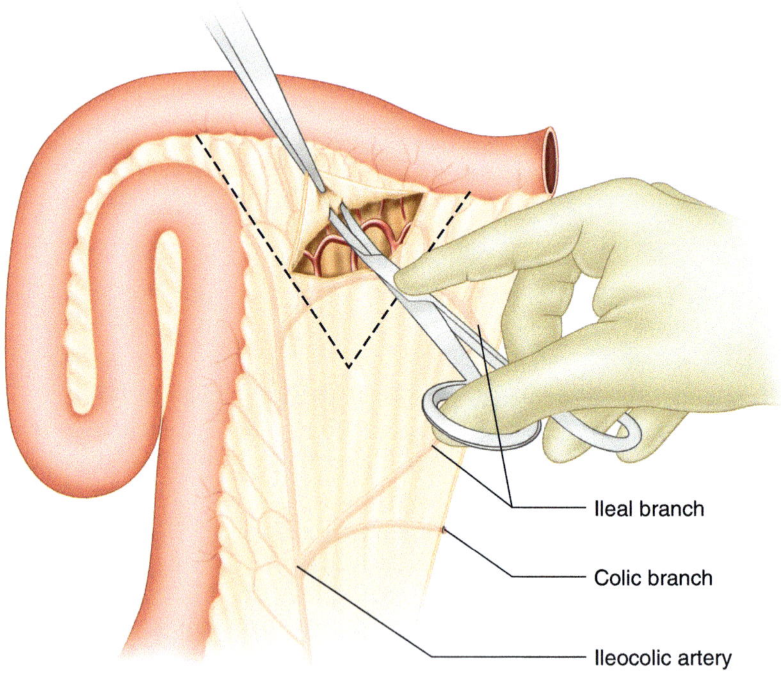

Fig. 50.3 Construction of a Kock pouch – the mesentery of the small bowel to be intussuscepted (marked by dashed lines) is skeletonized assisting the formation of the nipple valve. The blood supply of this segment of bowel is identified with transillumination, and the peritoneum and mesentery on either side of the vasculature are excised

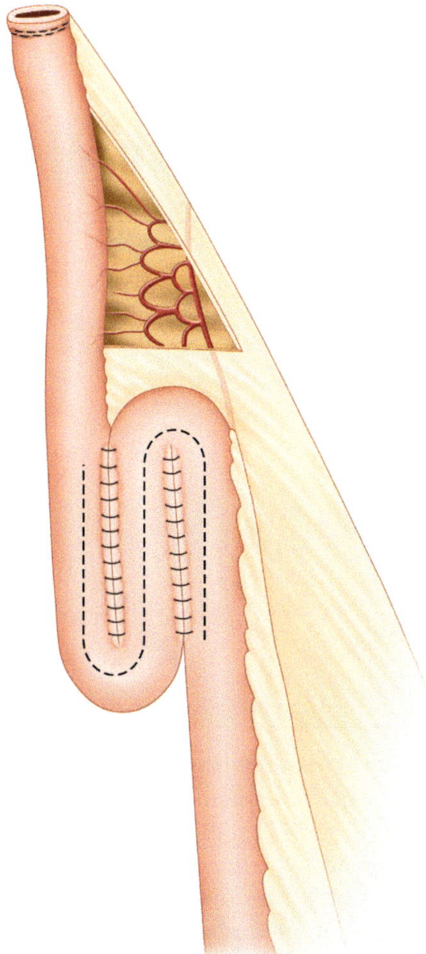

Fig. 50.4 The S-shaped pouch is constructed by folding the proximal 30 cm of bowel into 3–10 cm limbs with sutures placed between the limbs. An enterotomy is made (dotted line) starting at the distal aspect

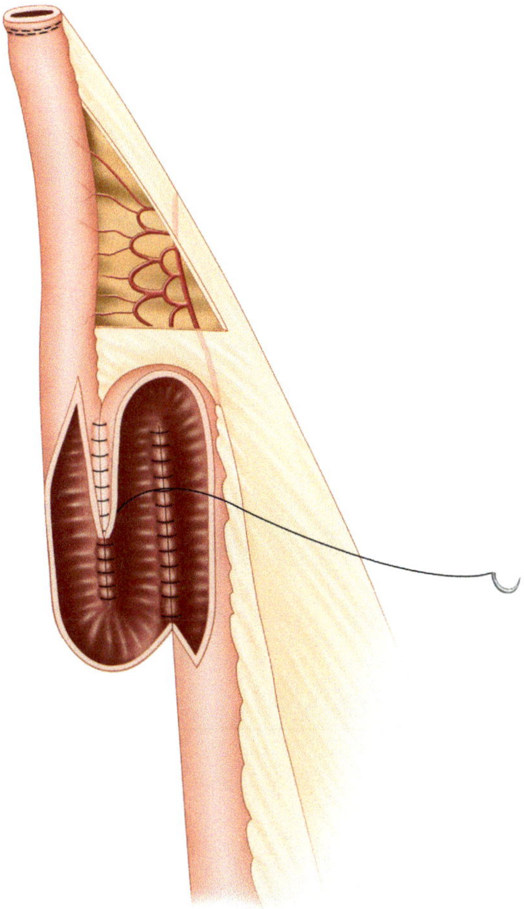

Fig. 50.5 An inner posterior layer is created starting at the proximal end forming the pouch

- A two-layer closure of the anterior portion of the pouch is then performed.
- A circumferential row of interrupted sutures is placed between the outlet and the pouch to help maintain the position of the nipple valve (Fig. 50.7).
- To create the stoma aperture, a small circular incision is made in the skin and carried through the subcutaneous tissue.
- A vertical incision is made in the fascia, the rectus muscle is retracted, and the peritoneum is incised ensuring that the opening can accommodate two fingerbreadths.
- The outlet is brought up to the opening and the pouch secured to the abdominal wall by placing sutures laterally and medially (Fig. 50.8).
- The outlet is transected at a location that will enable the matured stoma to be flushed with the skin.
- A curved Medina catheter is placed into the most dependent portion of the pouch and secured in place by suturing the rubber collar on the catheter to the skin (Fig. 50.9).

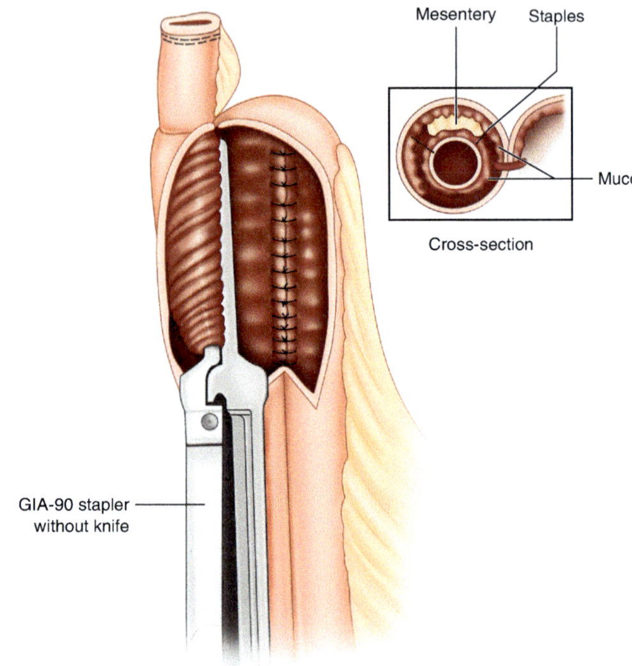

Fig. 50.6 The nipple valve is created with three firings of a GIA 90 mm stapler without the knife

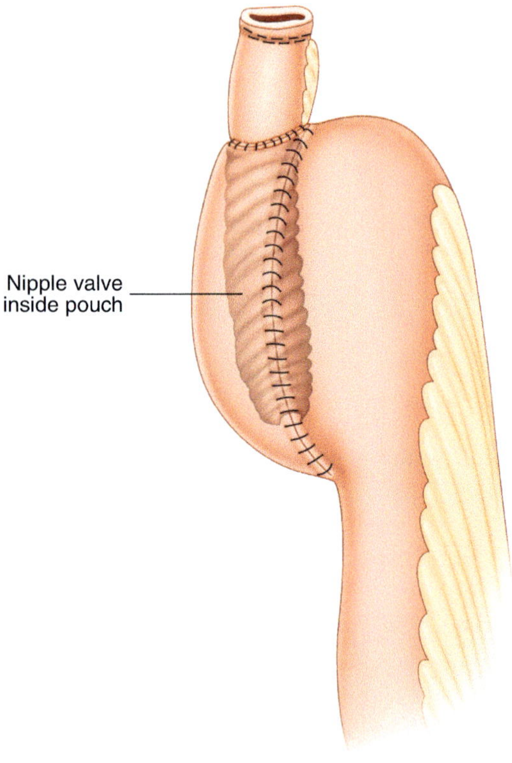

Fig. 50.7 The anterior aspect of the valve is then completed with an inner and outer layer of sutures. To help maintain the nipple valve position, a row of interrupted sutures is placed between the pouch and the outlet

Operative Considerations

- The two main long-term problems with a continent ileostomy are malfunction of the valve and pouchitis.
- Malfunction of the valve causes incontinence and difficult intubation of the pouch and occurs in 11–20% of patients.
- When the continence mechanism fails, the "slipped valve" creates a functional obstruction requiring further surgery.
- The incidence of pouchitis in Kock pouches is nearly identical to that after IPAA, and management is similar.

Outcomes

- Kock pouch procedures have generally fallen out of favor.
- But continent ileostomies in well-selected and properly motivated patients can be durable, with long-term pouch survival rates approaching 80%.
- A well-functioning IPAA appears to be superior to both Brooke ileostomy and Kock pouch in terms of overall quality of life, at least in selected patients.

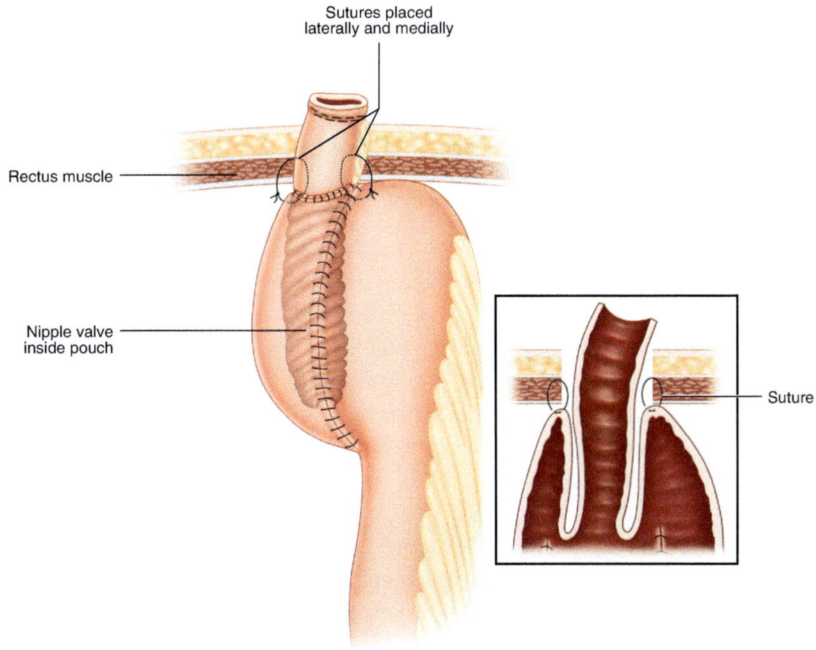

Fig. 50.8 Sutures are then placed between the pouch outlet and the posterior sheath of the abdominal wall on the lateral and medial aspects

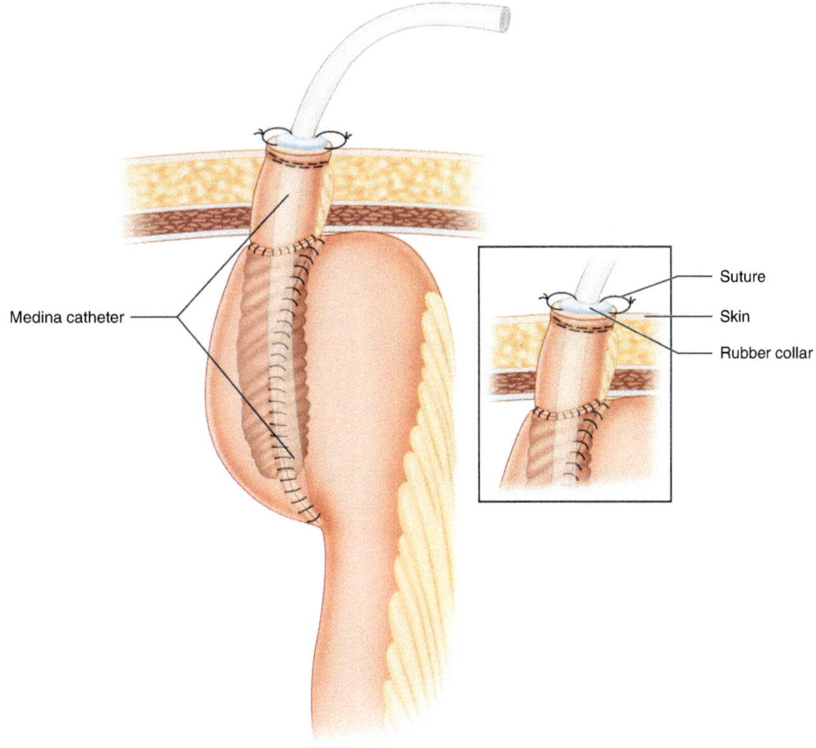

Fig. 50.9 A Medina catheter is placed into the most dependent aspect of the pouch and secured to the skin

Total Abdominal Colectomy with Ileorectal Anastomosis (TAC-IRA)

- IPAA has become the procedure of choice, relegating IRA to a limited role in UC surgery (Table 50.4).
- Advantages of IRA include lack of a permanent stoma, performance of a single stage, less invasive operation, and avoiding pelvic dissection with its associated risk of sexual dysfunction.
- Patient selection is key in assuring long-term favorable outcomes in patients undergoing an IRA. Adequate rectal compliance and normal anal sphincter function are critical for good long-term results.
- TAC-IRA is now generally reserved for patients with limited rectal involvement, good rectal compliance, and no dysplasia or cancer.

Operative Details: Open Approach

- The procedure is performed with the patient in the modified lithotomy position with the legs supported by stirrups, ensuring that all pressure points are appropriately padded.
- The ascending colon and terminal ileum are fully mobilized by incising the lateral peritoneal reflection from the cecum up to the hepatic flexure.
- The transverse colon is separated from its attachments to the stomach with or without preservation of the greater omentum (Fig. 50.10).

Table 50.4 Pros and cons in ulcerative colitis surgery

IRA	IPAA	TPC
+ Function	+ Low cancer risk	+ Cancer risk
+ One surgery	+/– Defecatory function	+ One surgery
+ Low risk of sexual/urinary dysfunction	– Risk of sexual/urinary dysfunction	– Permanent fecal diversion
– Recurrent disease	– Multiple surgeries	– Risk of sexual/urinary dysfunction
– Cancer risk	– Decreased fertility	– Decreased fertility

IRA ileorectal anastomosis; *IPAA* ileoanal pouch-anal anastomosis; *TPC* total proctocolectomy

- Dissection is carried to the splenic flexure exercising care to avoid splenic injury.
- The dissection is then carried along the sigmoid and descending colon, and the splenic flexure mobilization is completed. Care is taken to identify the left ureter and gonadal vessels to ensure their safety.
- The terminal ileum is transected with a GIA stapler, and the mesentery of the colon is ligated and divided.
- The inferior mesenteric artery is generally preserved in order to avoid injury to the hypogastric plexus and preserve adequate blood supply to the rectal stump.
- The rectosigmoid junction is divided at the level of the sacral promontory.
- We generally prefer to create a side-to-end ileorectal anastomosis.
- A flexible sigmoidoscopy is then performed to ensure that the anastomosis is patent, hemostatic, and healthy-appearing, and an anastomotic leak test is conducted.

Operative Details: Laparoscopic Approach

- The procedure is performed with the patient in the modified lithotomy position with the legs supported by stirrups and both arms tucked, ensuring that all pressure points are appropriately padded.
- An infraumbilical (supraumbilical for a hand-assisted procedure) port is placed via an open technique.
- If a laparoscopic approach is feasible, then four additional trocars are placed in the right and left upper and lower quadrants for a straight laparoscopic procedure.
- If the surgeon elects to perform hand-assisted approach, two additional trocars in the bilateral lower quadrants are utilized. The hand-assisted port is placed via a Pfannenstiel incision about two fingerbreadths above the symphysis pubis.
- The cecum is retracted anterolaterally, and the ileocolic artery and vein are identified (Fig. 50.11).
- An incision is made just inferior to the vessels and a mesenteric window created.

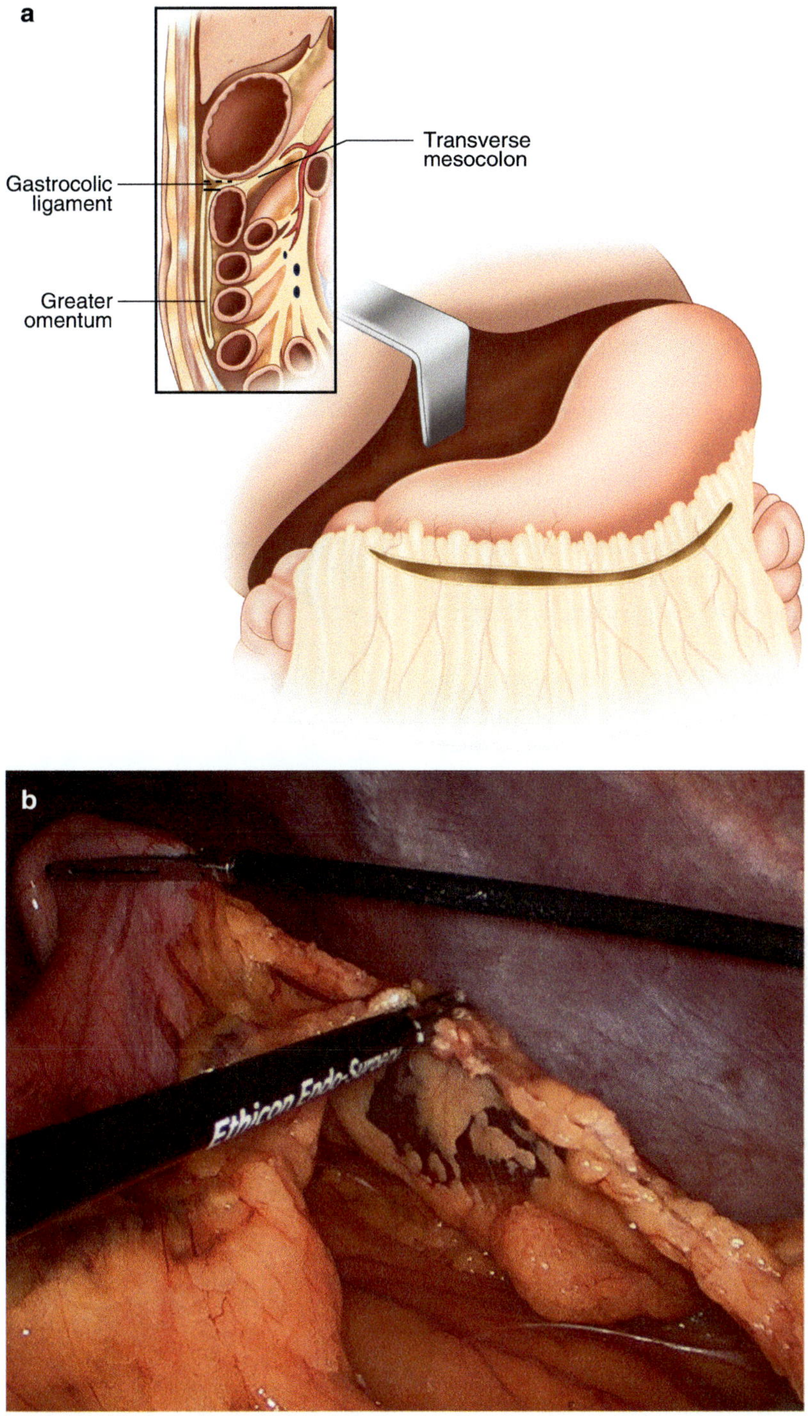

Fig. 50.10 (**a** and **b**) The omentum is divided along the greater curvature of the stomach distal to the gastroepiploic arcade

- The duodenum should be visualized not only to avoid inadvertent injury but because it is an important landmark used to confirm correct identification of the ileocolic artery and vein.
- Mobilization continues superiorly, sweeping down the second portion of the duodenum and separating it from the posterior aspect of the transverse mesocolon (Fig. 50.12).
- The dissection then continues laterally in the plane between the mesocolon and Gerota's fascia. The appendix is then retracted toward the splenic flexure, and the lateral peritoneal reflection is divided from the cecum to the hepatic flexure until the site of medial mobilization is met (Fig. 50.13).
- Dissection continues with serial ligation and division of the transverse mesocolon and omentum caudal to the gastroepiploic arcade (Fig. 50.14a, b).
- Through a combination of blunt and sharp dissection, the splenic flexure is mobilized ensuring no undue traction on the spleen (Fig. 50.15a, b).
- The left mesocolon is serially ligated and divided, and the left-sided peritoneal reflection is incised.
- The sigmoid colon is retracted medially, and the lateral attachments of the sigmoid colon are incised taking care not to injure the left ureter or gonadal vessels.
- The sigmoidal branches are ligated and divided.
- Once the colon has been mobilized up to the rectosigmoid junction, it is extracted through a Pfannenstiel incision, the bowel is transected, and the anastomosis is created.

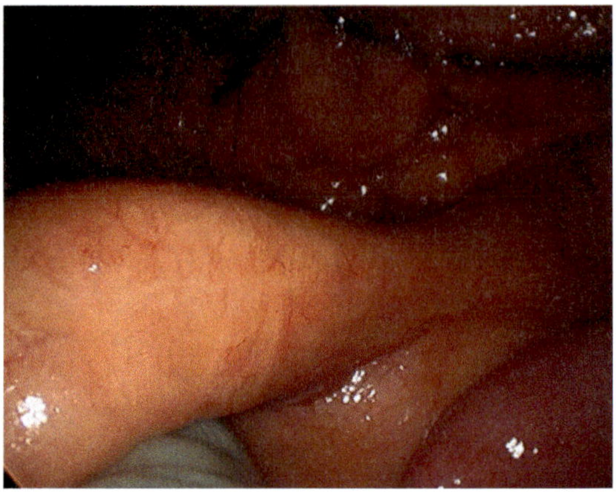

Fig. 50.11 Identification of the ileocolic pedicle

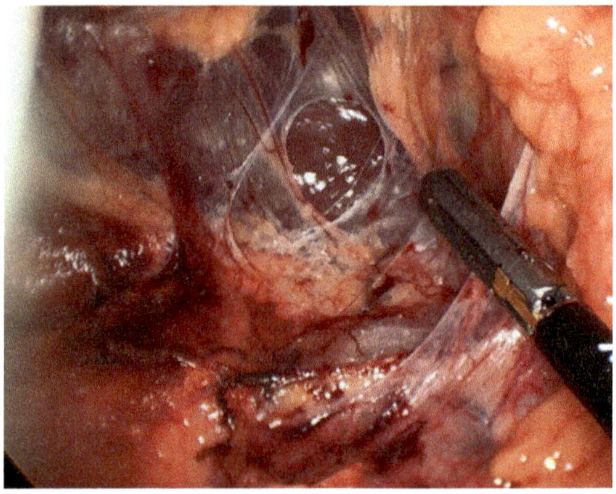

Fig. 50.12 Medial to lateral dissection and creation of the mesenteric window

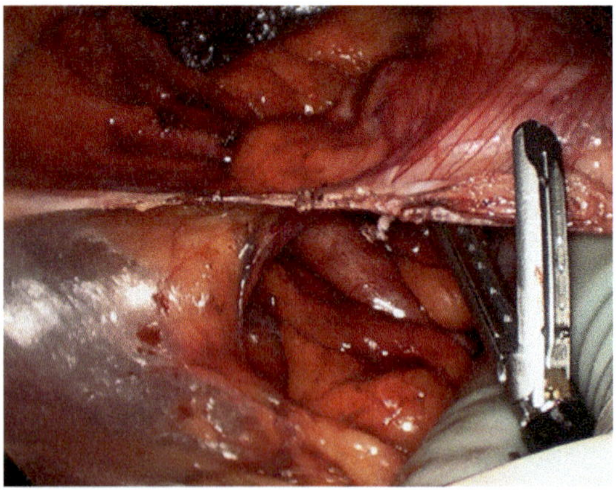

Fig. 50.13 Division of the lateral attachments

Outcomes

- In UC, an IRA is a safe procedure with a reported overall morbidity between 8% and 28%.
- IRA does not involve extensive pelvic dissection, unlike IPAA or total proctocolectomy, minimizing the risk of sexual and urinary dysfunction.
- Disease recurrence in the rectal remnant is significant, and these patients should be monitored and followed up endoscopically.

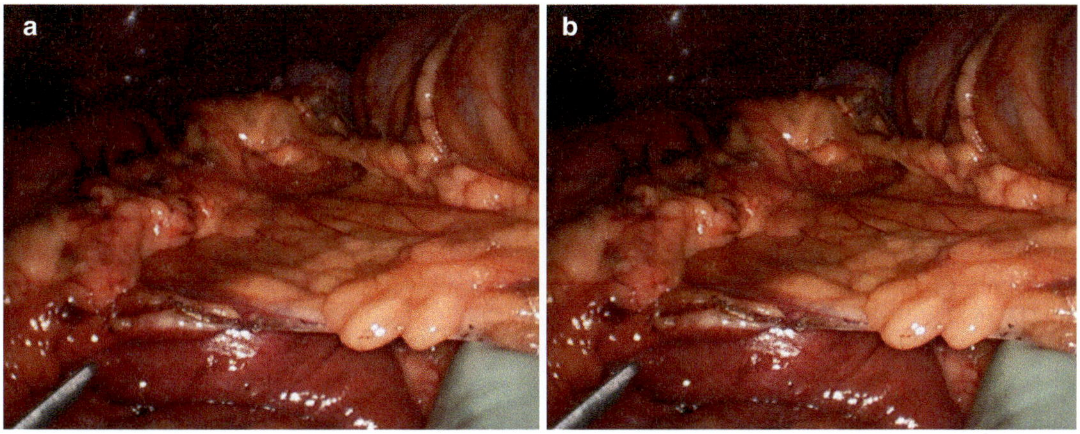

Fig. 50.14 (**a** and **b**) Ligation and division of the transverse mesocolon and omentum caudal to the gastroepiploic arcade

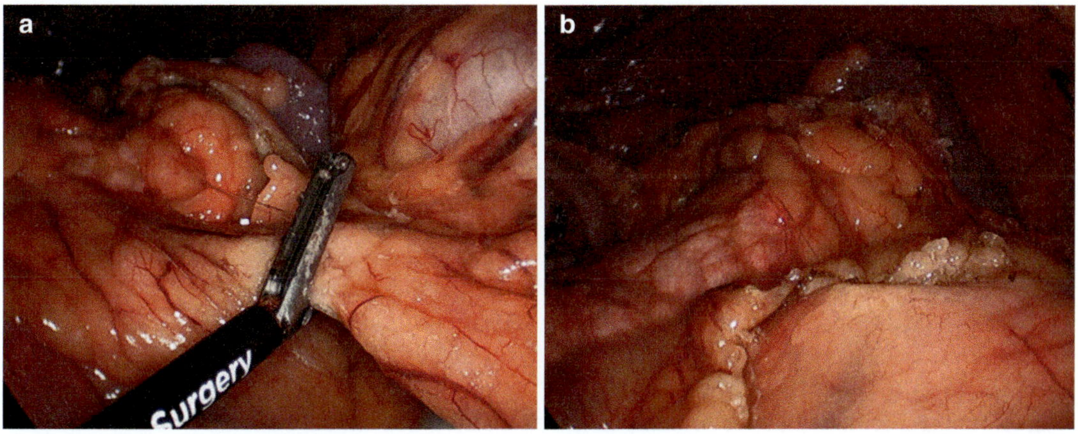

Fig. 50.15 (**a** and **b**) Mobilization of the splenic flexure

- The cumulative probability of having a functioning IRA has been reported as high as 84% at 5 years, 69% at 10 years, and between 46% and 69% at 20 years.
- More than 90% of patients consider that their health status has improved after the operation.
- The main indication for proctectomy is refractory proctitis, followed by dysplasia or cancer, and the development of Crohn's disease. IPAA can often be safely performed in the majority of these patients, thus avoiding permanent fecal diversion.
- Endoscopic monitoring of the rectal remnant is essential given the high rate of disease recurrence and the risk of dysplasia/cancer which increases with time.
- Patients with advanced metastatic disease may benefit from an IRA due to their short life expectancy and the palliative nature of their treatment.

Total Proctocolectomy with End Ileostomy

- By removing all diseased epithelium, proctocolectomy cures patient disease, eradicates the associated risk of malignancy, and eliminates the need for costly medications and time-consuming lifelong follow-up.

- The disadvantages of this operation include the presence of a permanent ileostomy, the potential for nerve injury during pelvic dissection, and the risk of perineal wound healing problems.
- A proctocolectomy with an end ileostomy is indicated in patients who are not candidates for an IPAA (Table 50.5) or perhaps a Kock pouch.
- The operation may also be indicated if other medical problems make a more complex, longer operation too risky.
- Finally a total proctocolectomy is highly appropriate for patients who desire a single operation for cure or whose work and other daily activities make an ostomy appliance easier to manage than frequent bowel movements.
- There are no absolute contraindications to this procedure. However, in the emergent setting, it is advisable to stage the procedure with an initial abdominal colectomy.

Operative Details: Open Proctectomy

- With a staged approach, the initial total abdominal colectomy proceeds as described above with IRA; but rather than creating an ileorectal anastomosis, the rectal stump is left in situ, and the terminal ileum is fashioned into an end ileostomy.
  - The rectosigmoid is transected with a linear stapler at the sacral promontory (Fig. 50.16).
  - A rectal tube may be left in place for 5 days postoperatively to ensure adequate evacuation of rectal contents.
  - The proctectomy with or without ileal pouch can be performed several months later when the patient's overall health improves and they are no longer on medications.
- Rectal dissection begins with division of the terminal branches of the inferior mesenteric artery (the superior rectal arteries) and complete posterior mobilization of the rectum.
- Both the ureters and the sympathetic neural plexus, which lie directly posterior to the inferior mesenteric artery at the pelvic brim, are identified and swept free.
- The terminal branches of the inferior mesenteric artery and vein are ligated and divided at the level of the sacral promontory.
- The parietal peritoneum is incised inferiorly and laterally to gain access to the presacral space between the fascia propria of the rectum and the presacral fascia.
- The rectum is retracted anteriorly and sharp dissection is carried out in the areolar tissue. Care must be taken to ensure that the presacral venous plexus remains covered to avoid bleeding that can often be difficult to stop and may be life-threatening.
- Dissection should be carried down in the posterior plane beyond the coccyx, and Waldeyer's fascia is incised.
- The lateral rectal stalks are then divided as close to the rectal wall as possible to avoid injury to the pelvic plexus.
- Attention is then turned to anterior dissection in the rectovaginal or rectovesicular space posterior to Denonvilliers' fascia.
- At this point, the rectum should be circumferentially mobilized to the levator ani muscles.
- The abdominal wound is closed, the ileostomy is created, and the attention is turned to the perineal dissection.
- A purse-string suture is placed close to the anus at the level of the anal verge.
- A circular incision is made in the intersphincteric groove and carried through the subcutaneous tissue (Fig. 50.17).

Table 50.5 Contraindication to IPAA

Absolute	Relative
Severe fecal incontinence	Severe morbid obesity
Locally advanced low rectal cancer involving the sphincters	Locally advanced low rectal cancer requiring neoadjuvant treatment
Perianal Crohn's disease	Crohn's disease
	Previous extensive small bowel resections
	Personal preference

IPAA ileoanal pouch-anal anastomosis

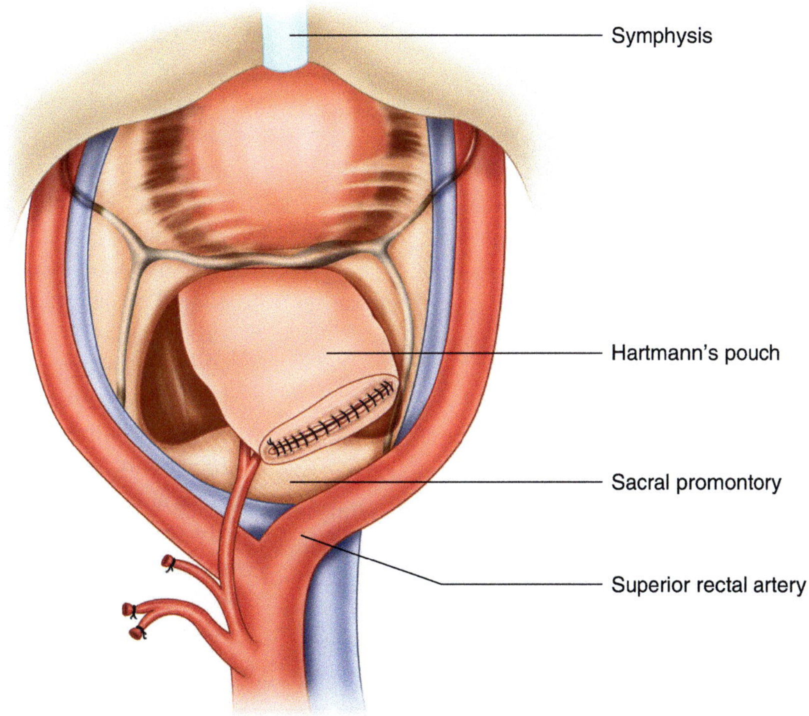

Fig. 50.16 Distal transection at the level of the sacral promontory

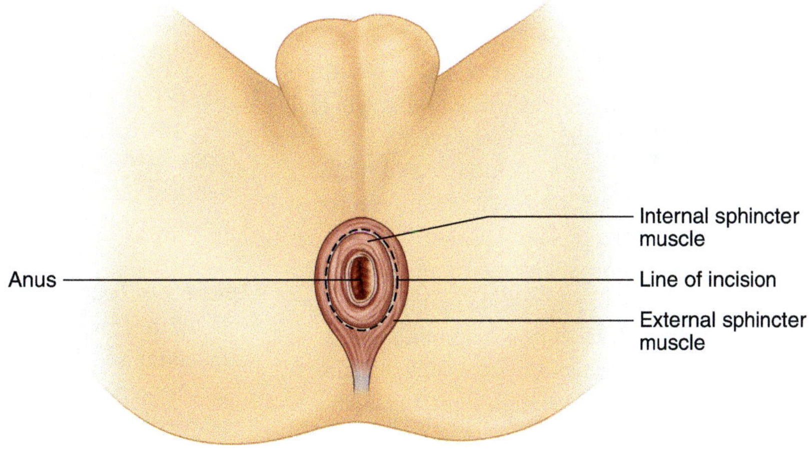

Fig. 50.17 Perineal dissection – circular incision made along the intersphincteric groove

- The anococcygeal ligament is divided and the pelvic cavity is entered posteriorly.
- The incision is extended circumferentially mobilizing the entire distal rectum and anus.
- The specimen is extracted through the perineal opening, and the wound is closed in layers (Fig. 50.18).

Operative Details: Laparoscopic Proctectomy

- As with the open approach, the rectal dissection begins with division of the terminal branch of the inferior mesenteric artery (the superior rectal artery).

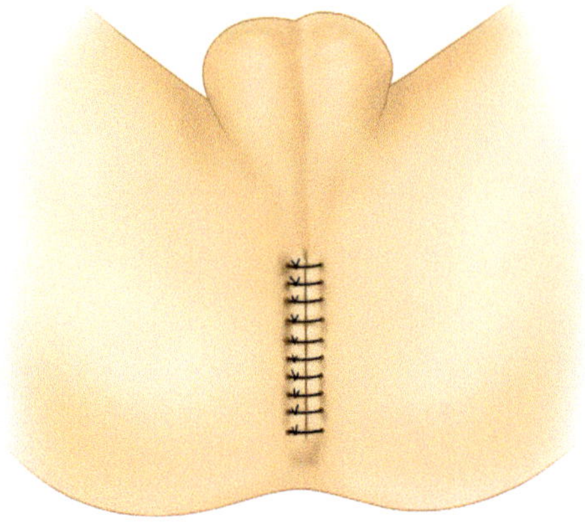

Fig. 50.18 Closure of perineum

- The rectal stump and distal sigmoid colon are retracted superiorly and anteriorly out of the pelvis exposing the inferior mesenteric artery (IMA).
- The peritoneum to the right of the superior rectal artery is incised starting at the sacral promontory and extending cephalad to the origin of the IMA.
- A mesenteric window is created allowing the visualization of the left ureter and gonadal vessels.
- The hypogastric nerves are swept posteriorly, and the superior rectal artery is ligated and divided with a vessel-sealing device.
- The retrorectal space is entered, and the rectum is completely mobilized circumferentially as above down to the pelvic floor.
- After ensuring no twisting of the bowel or mesentery, the cut edge of the ileum is brought out and the end ileostomy matured.
- The perineal dissection proceeds as above with the specimen brought out through the perineal incision.

Restorative Proctocolectomy with Ileal Pouch-Anal Anastomosis (RPC-IPAA)

- Before proceeding with an IPAA, fecal continence should be evaluated particularly in patients presenting preoperatively with impaired function. While it is important to note that continence significantly worsens during a disease flare-up, the report of incontinence should be further discussed and investigated.
- A digital rectal examination performed by the operating surgeon usually provides enough information to decide if more formal evaluation by manometry or endoanal ultrasound should be entertained.
- Problems with defecation prior to surgery (incontinence, diabetic neuropathy, or other neurogenic disorders) should be considered a relative contraindication for IPAA.
- In patients that present with rectal cancer, neoadjuvant chemoradiation therapy does not always represent an absolute contraindication to an IPAA but does clearly worsen long-term outcomes.
  - Postoperative radiation therapy should be avoided at all costs, and it is typically not recommended or utilized.
- In morbidly obese patients with an elective indication for surgery, performing an abdominal colectomy first as part of a staged approach may enable weight reduction surgery before proceeding with the restorative procedure.
- IPAA can be safely offered to selected elderly UC patients who are strongly motivated and possess normal defecatory function. Results seem to be stable over time and comparable to those of younger patients.

Operative Technique

- If the patient is to undergo a RPC-IPAA, the resection of the colon and rectum is performed as above, but the rectum is divided with a TA stapler leaving a short rectal cuff.
- An ileal pouch can be created in the J, S, or W configuration (Figs. 50.19 and 50.20), but J-pouch construction is most common.
- The length of the ileal J-pouch should be about 15–20 cm (Fig. 50.21).
- The stapled end of the terminal ileum is oversewn with 4–0 silk Lembert sutures.
- After ensuring adequate blood supply to the terminal ileum, the apex of the pouch is chosen by bringing the ileum over the pubis and

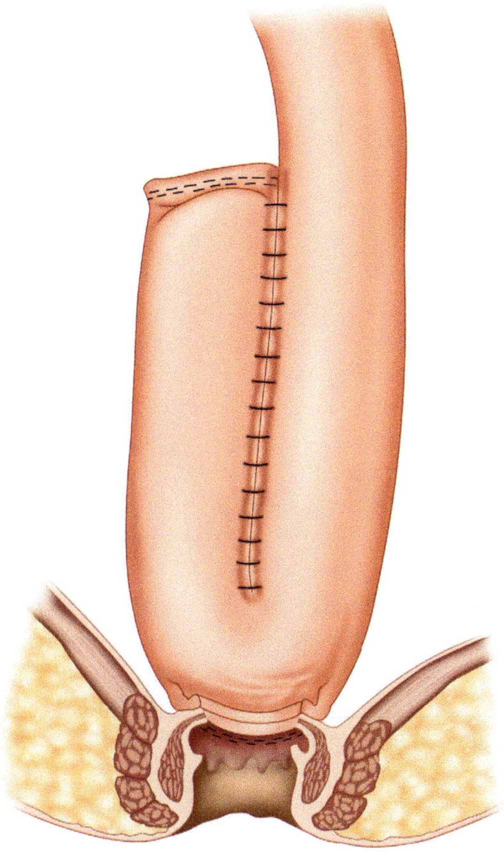

Fig. 50.19 J-pouch configuration

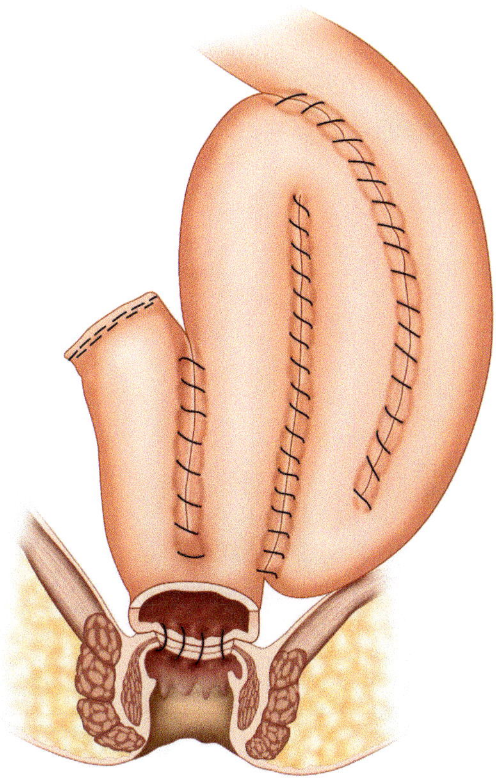

Fig. 50.20 W-pouch configuration

identifying the longest section of the mesentery to enable a tension-free anastomosis.

- The two limbs are approximated, and sutures are placed between the proximal and distal limbs at the ileomesenteric junction (Fig. 50.22a, b).
- Corresponding longitudinal enterotomies are made on the proximal and distal limbs.
- Serial firings with a GIA stapler are used to create the pouch (Fig. 50.23a, b) with care taken to ensure that the mesentery is not included in the staple line (Fig. 50.24).
- The pouch is everted by gently applying Babcock clamps after each staple fire to aid in creating a common channel (Fig. 50.25a, b).
- After the last firing (Fig. 50.26a, b), the staple line is inspected for bleeding (Fig. 50.27a, b) and the pouch reduced with gentle traction on the apical stay suture (Fig. 50.28a–c).
- The anvil of an EEA stapler is brought out through the apex and secured in placed with a purse-string suture (Fig. 50.29).
- The common enterotomy is closed in two layers (Fig. 50.30).
- The EEA stapler is inserted transanally, and after ensuring no twisting of the bowel or mesentery, the ileoanal anastomosis is created.
- A flexible sigmoidoscope is then inserted to inspect the staple lines and perform an anastomotic leak test.
- It is our practice to divert patients with a temporary loop ileostomy for 3 months.

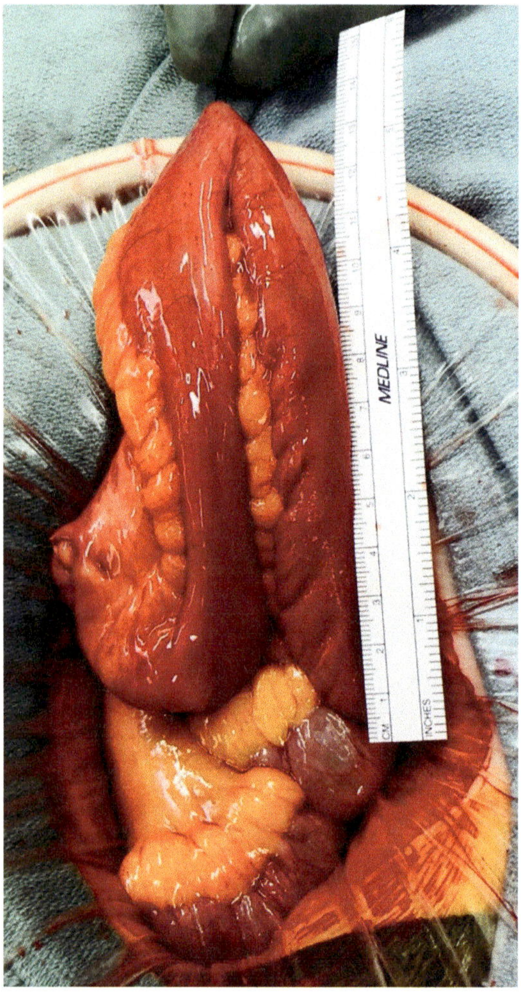

Fig. 50.21 J-pouch should be 15–20 cm in length

Special Considerations

Pouch Configuration

- While the J configuration is most commonly used due to relative technical ease and speed of performance, there is a role for the other two pouches in selected situations.
  - The S-pouch with the long exit limb allows for further reach in tall male patients with short mesentery.
  - The W-pouch has a large capacity and better compliance.

Anastomosis

- A long-standing controversy surrounds the type of the anastomosis and the fate of the anal transition zone (ATZ).
- Stapled IPAA preserves the ATZ including the highly specialized anoderm, decreases trauma to the sphincter mechanism, and may therefore enable better continence.
  - There is less tension on the anastomosis, potentially enabling fewer septic complications, greater ease of construction, and shorter operative times.
  - The disadvantages include the theoretical risk of malignant degeneration of the rectal cuff mucosa and ATZ inflammation.
  - Several comparative long-term studies have reported better functional results for stapled IPAA.
  - No difference in functional results was noted when stapled IPAA was compared to handsewn anastomosis with mucosectomy in a prospective randomized fashion.
- The initial descriptions of IPAA included a mucosectomy to the dentate line with handsewn anastomosis.
  - The dilatation necessary for complete mucosectomy or the eversion of anorectum used to facilitate mucosal removal causes a significant decrease in the maximum resting pressure and increase of the threshold sensation return of the rectoanal reflex and sampling.
  - The entire diseased anorectal mucosa, including the ATZ, is removed, which theoretically should eliminate the risk for future dysplasia and cancer. In actual practice, this is not the case.
- Patients with history of cancer or dysplasia in the colon or rectum are at a higher risk of developing dysplasia in the ATZ.
  - Long-term surveillance to monitor dysplasia is appropriate in this group; if repeat biopsy confirms persistent dysplasia, mucosectomy with pouch advancement is advised.
- Mucosectomy is often advised in the presence of high-grade rectal dysplasia or cancer,

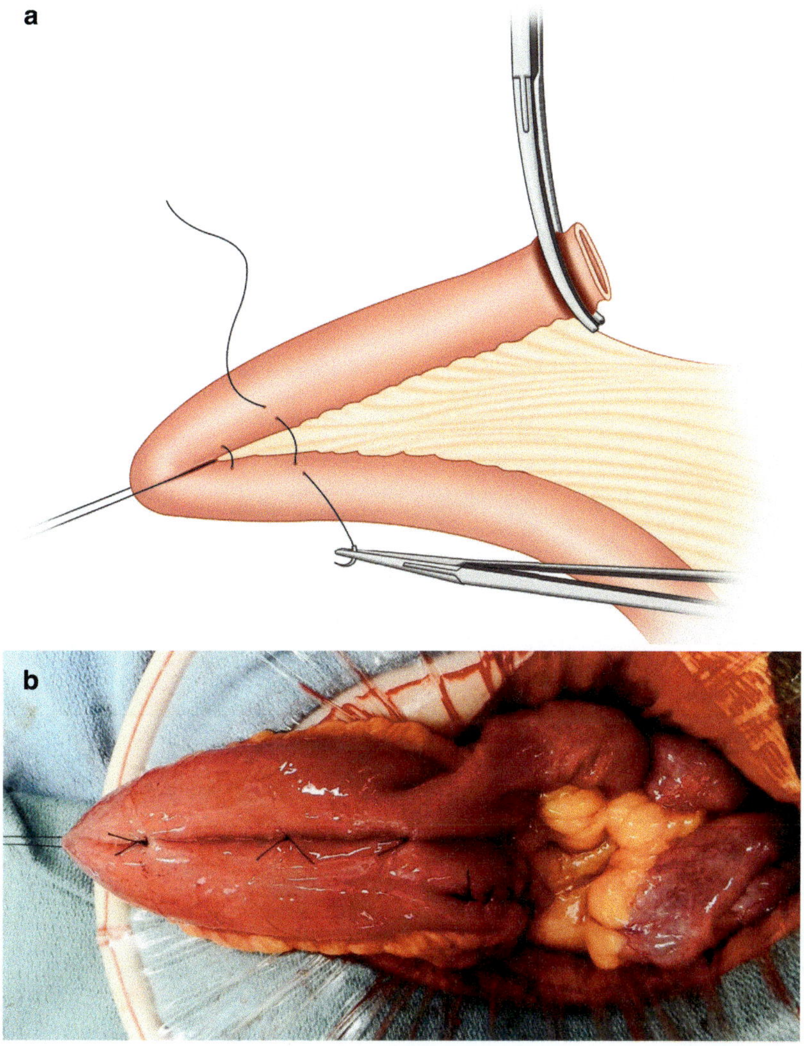

Fig. 50.22 (**a** and **b**) A stay suture is placed along the antimesenteric aspect of the apex of the pouch. Additional sutures are placed between the two limbs of the J-pouch at the ileomesenteric junction

in the pediatric population, and in patients with primary sclerosis cholangitis who are known to have a high risk of dysplasia and cancer.

Optimizing Reach

- An anastomosis between the ileal pouch and anal canal performed under tension is associated with increased risk of dehiscence with severe short-term and long-term sequelae.
- Common techniques include complete small bowel mobilization to the origin of its mesentery, ileocolic vessel ligation close to their origin from the superior mesenteric pedicle, and transverse mesenteric relaxing incisions.
- Leaving the pouch unattached in the pelvis, diverting the patient proximally, and returning at a later date for pouch anastomosis may be considered when standard lengthening measure fails.

Crohn's Disease

- Some patients undergo surgery with a preoperative diagnosis of indeterminate colitis or ulcerative colitis and are found to have Crohn's

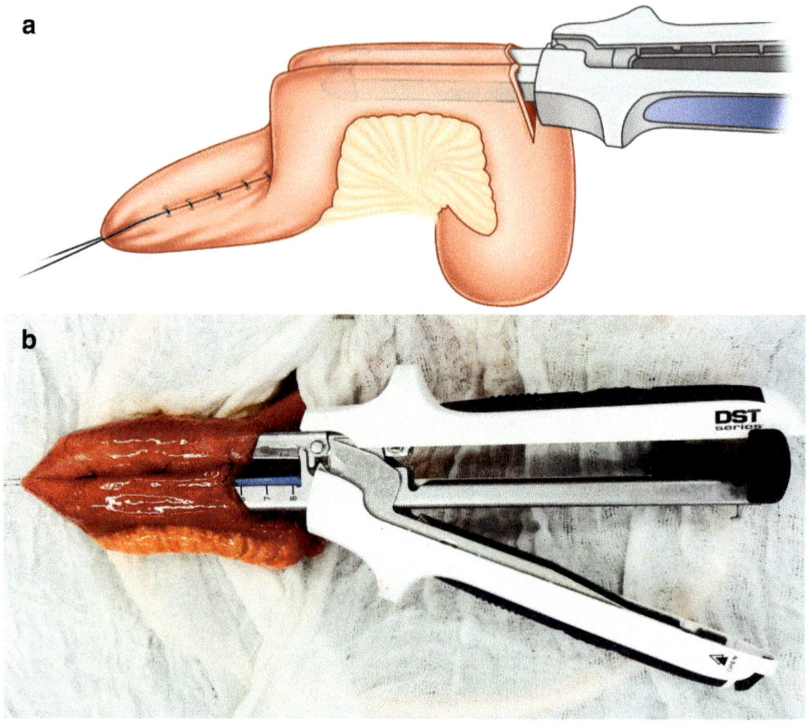

Fig. 50.23 (**a** and **b**) Corresponding longitudinal enterotomies are created on the proximal and distal limbs of the pouch, and the forks of a gastrointestinal stapler are gently inserted into each limb

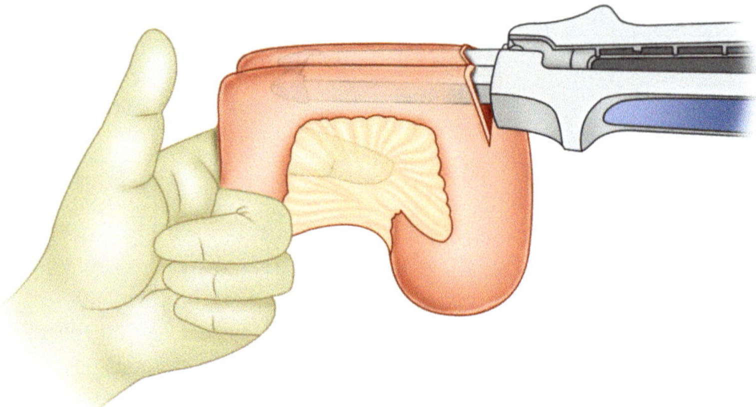

Fig. 50.24 Care is taken to ensure that the mesentery of the ileum is not incorporated into the staple line

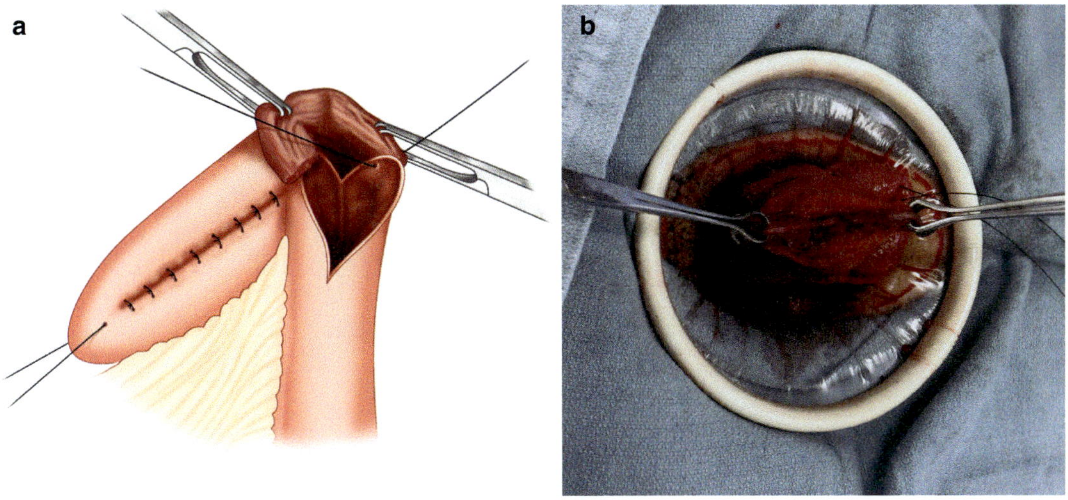

Fig. 50.25 (**a** and **b**) The pouch is everted with the gentle application of Babcock clamps along the staple line until the intact septum is reached

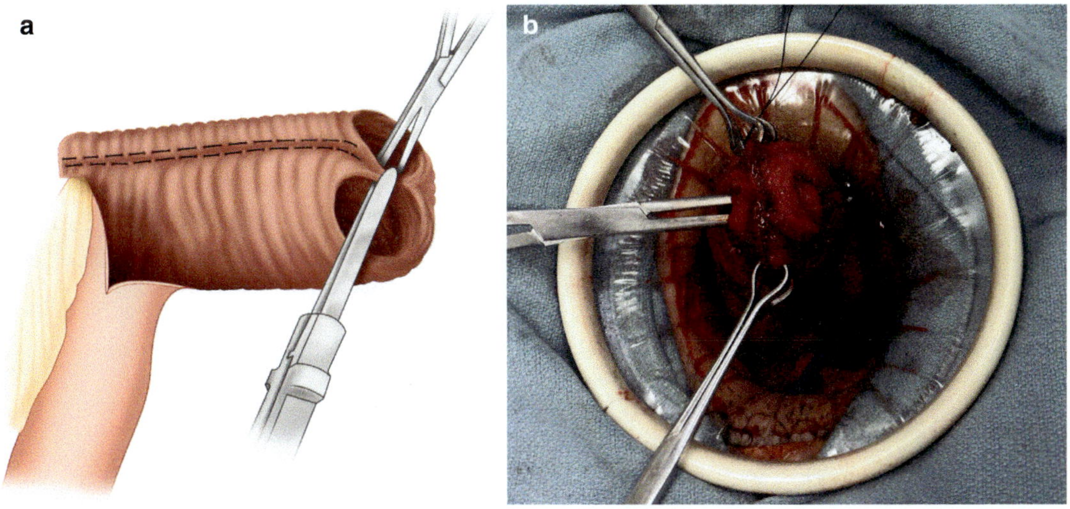

Fig. 50.26 (**a** and **b**) Division of the most distal aspect of the septum is often assisted by gentle passage of a right-angle clamp to guide the stapler

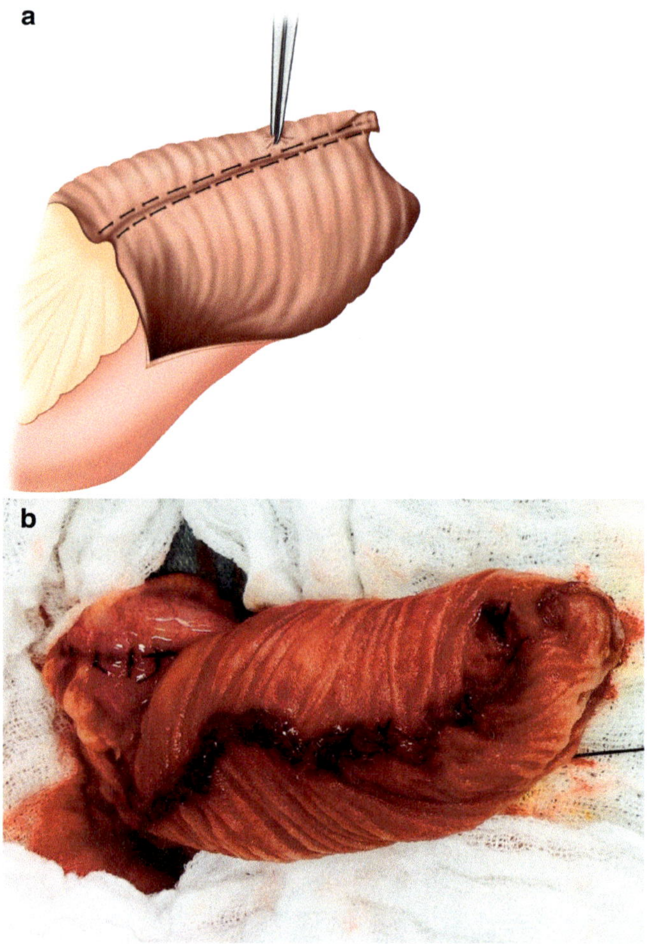

Fig. 50.27 (**a** and **b**) Suture lines inspected to ensure hemostasis

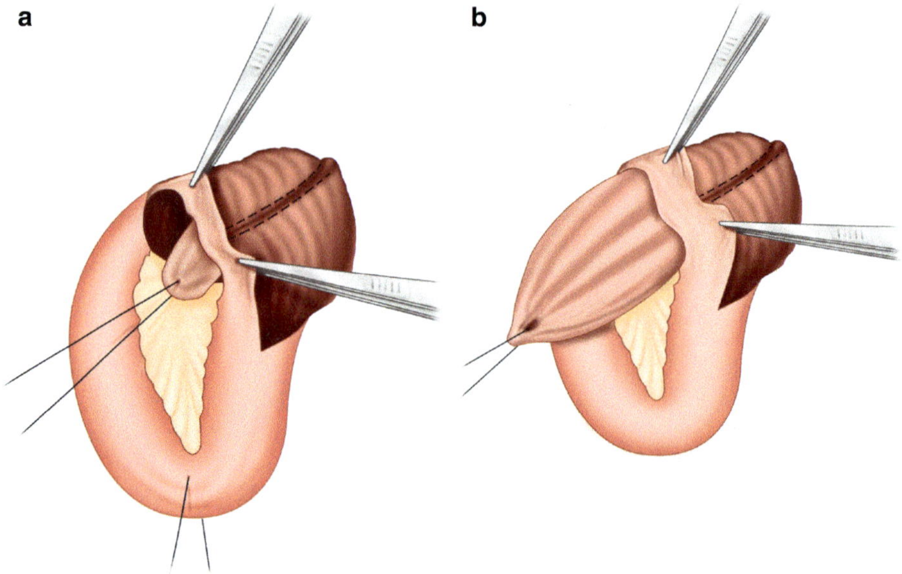

Fig. 50.28 (**a–c**) By placing traction on the apical stay suture and countertraction on the edge of the enterotomy, the pouch is reduced

c

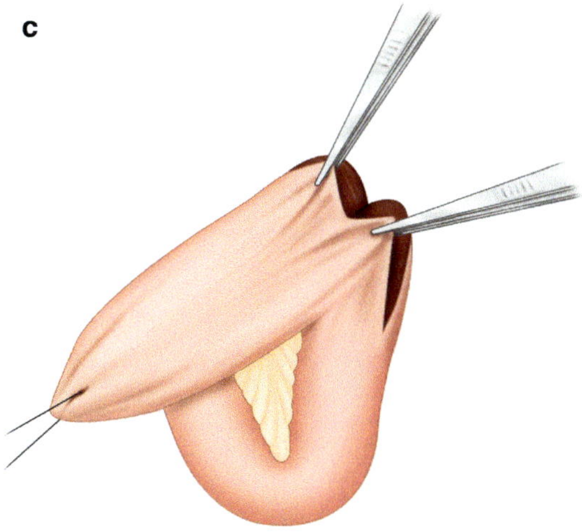

Fig. 50.28 (continued)

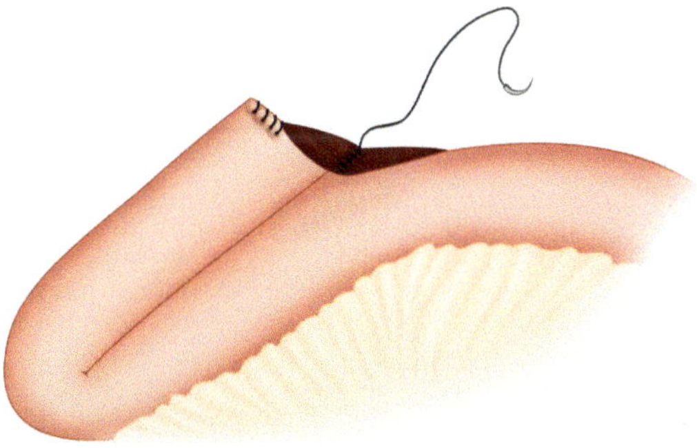

Fig. 50.30 The common enterotomy is closed with a two-layer closure

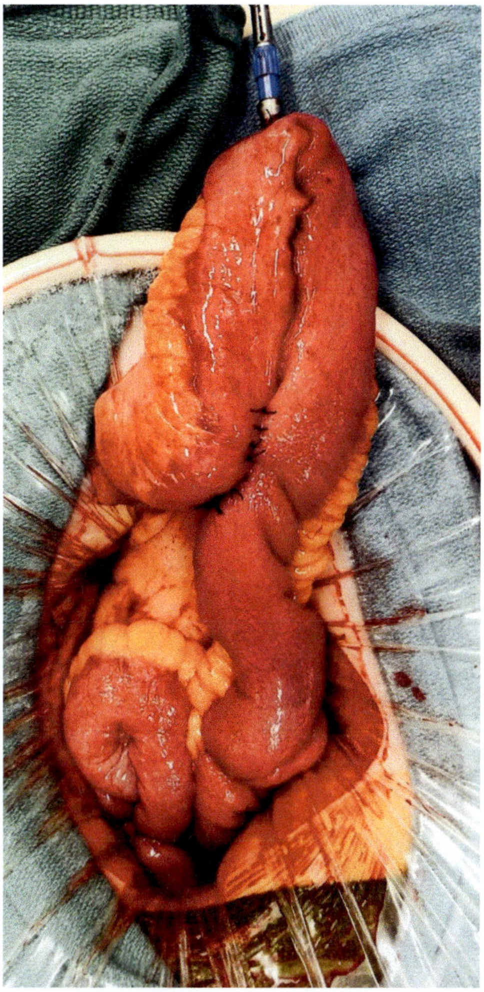

Fig. 50.29 The anvil of an EEA stapler is brought out through the apex

disease on final pathological evaluation of the specimen. Outcomes seem to correlate with clinical features of the disease.

- A highly selected subgroup of patients with Crohn's colitis and no evidence of perineal or small bowel disease may be candidates for an ileal pouch procedure. At present, we do not offer IPAA in our practice to patients with preoperative clinical features of Crohn's disease.

A management algorithm is provided in Fig. 50.31.

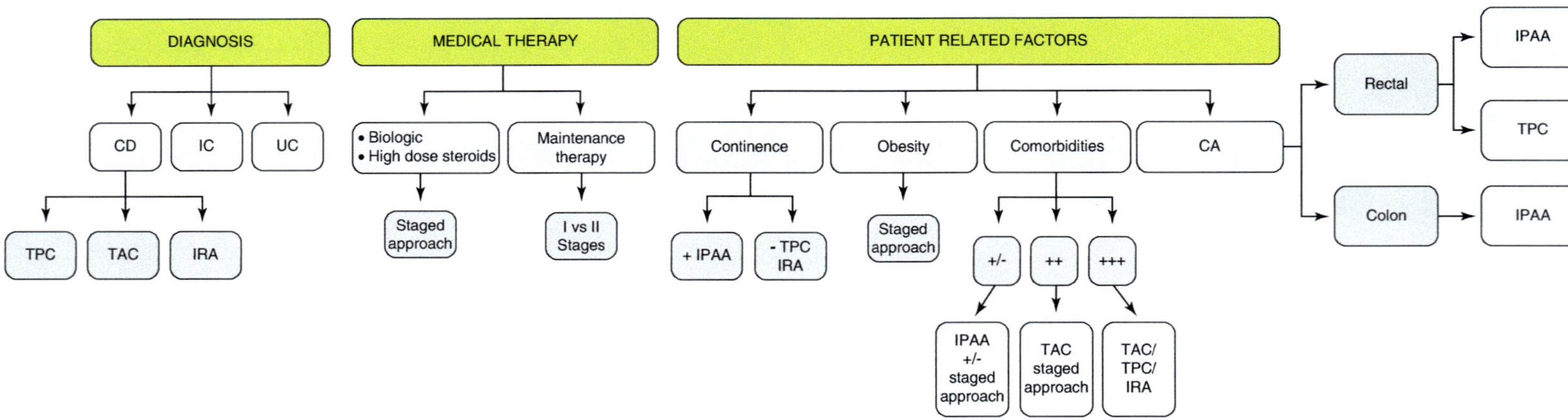

Fig. 50.31 Algorithm showing the approach to colectomy (*CD* Crohn's disease; *IC* indeterminate colitis; *UC* ulcerative colitis; *TPC* total proctocolectomy; *TAC* total abdominal colectomy; *IRA* ileorectal anastomosis; *IPAA* ileal pouch-anal anastomosis; *CA* cancer)

51 Complications of the Ileal Pouch

Daniel L. Feingold and P. Ravi Kiran

Key Concepts

- Pelvic sepsis after pouch surgery is associated with worse function and risks pouch failure. However, prompt management of early postoperative septic complications can preserve pouch function and increase pouch retention rates.
- Technical challenges during pouch surgery include ensuring tension-free reach, preserving adequate blood flow to the pouch, and creating an appropriate diverting ileostomy.
- A three-stage approach is recommended for patients who are malnourished, have severe active colitis, or are under treatment with larger doses of steroids or immunosuppressive medications in order to reduce pouch-related complications.
- The potential diagnosis of Crohn's disease should be considered in any patient presenting with fistulizing disease after pouch surgery as this affects management and prognosis.
- Repeat ileal pouch-anal anastomosis using a revised pouch or a new pouch is a reasonable option for selected patients with pouch failure.
- Mucosectomy at the time of a pouch-anal anastomosis does not prevent future dysplasia or cancer as islands of rectal mucosa may persist.
- Women with ulcerative colitis who undergo total proctocolectomy have a higher rate of infertility than women treated non-operatively, although a laparoscopic approach may reduce this risk.

D. L. Feingold
Department of Surgery, Columbia University, New York, NY, USA

P. R. Kiran (✉)
Division of Colorectal Surgery, Department of Colorectal Surgery, Columbia University Medical Center and Mailman School of Public Health, New York, NJ, USA
e-mail: rpk2118@columbia.edu

Introduction

- Complications after pouch surgery can be grouped into septic versus non-septic-related complications (including mechanical issues).
- Alternatively, IPAA complications can be conceptualized as intraoperative, early postoperative, and late postoperative (Table 51.1).
- Pouch-related complications can significantly affect functional outcomes and patients' quality of life, require multiple corrective procedures, and result in pouch failure.
- Pouch failure may be defined as the need for construction of a permanent stoma with or without excision of the pouch.

S. R. Steele et al. (eds.), *The ASCRS Manual of Colon and Rectal Surgery*,
https://doi.org/10.1007/978-3-030-01165-9_51

Table 51.1 Complications of the ileal pouch

Intraoperative
Problems with reach of the pouch
Pouch ischemia
Problems with stoma creation
Problems with staplers and creating the anastomosis
Early postoperative
Anastomotic leak and pelvic sepsis
Bleeding from the pouch
Late postoperative
Pouch-vaginal fistula
Pouch-perineal fistula
Pouch sinus
Crohn's disease after pouch surgery
Incontinence
Outlet obstruction
Pouchitis and cuffitis
Pouch prolapse
Leak from the tip of the "J"
Dysplasia and cancer after pouch surgery
Small bowel obstruction
Sexual dysfunction
Infertility

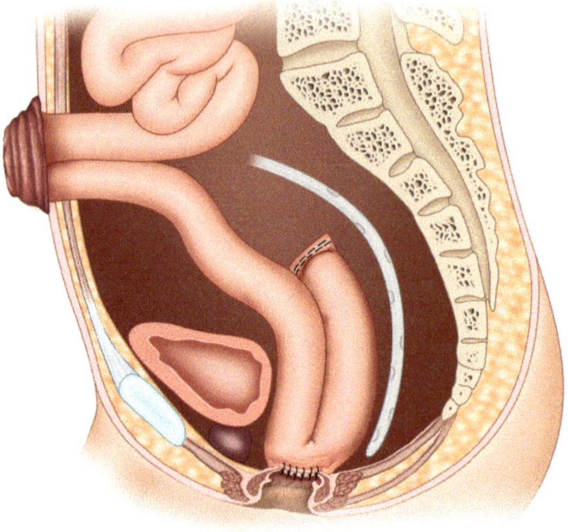

Fig. 51.1 Ileal "J"-pouch-anal anastomosis with defunctioning loop ileostomy

- Preoperative risk factors associated with pouch failure include type of resection (performing a completion proctectomy rather than total proctocolectomy), type of anastomosis (hand-sewn rather than stapled), diagnosis of Crohn's disease, and comorbidities.
- Modifying risk factors to minimize risk of pouch failure should include appropriate medical management leading up to pouch surgery, expeditious surgical management to avoid needing urgent total abdominal colectomy, and medical optimization of comorbidities.
- Body mass index greater than 30 is also associated with septic complications after IPAA, and obese patients should be counseled appropriately in advance of pouch surgery:
  - Performing an initial abdominal colectomy to allow control of disease and achieve weight loss prior to proctectomy and IPAA should be considered.
- Deciding whether or not to operate in stages may impact the risk of complications.
- Healthier patients often undergo a two-stage procedure whereby the pouch is defunctionalized by a loop ileostomy (Fig. 51.1).
- Patients who are malnourished, have severe active colitis, or are under treatment with larger doses of steroids or immunosuppressive agents are recommended to undergo a three-stage procedure.
- Similarly, when the diagnosis is unclear preoperatively, an initial subtotal colectomy may help ascertain the diagnosis of Crohn's disease and determine the suitability of a pouch at the subsequent operation.
- Patients with ulcerative colitis receiving infliximab are at particular risk for developing post-IPAA septic complications; a planned three-stage approach needs to be considered.
- Preoperative pelvic radiation in the setting of colitis-associated cancer is associated with an increased risk of subsequent pouch failure.
- Excessive weight gain (greater than 15% increase) after ileostomy closure in patients with inflammatory bowel disease is also associated with pouch failure, though the underlying mechanism is not clear.

Intraoperative Complications

- The two most common configurations currently used for IPAA are the "J" and "S" pouches which can be anastomosed via stapled or hand-sewn technique (Fig. 51.2).

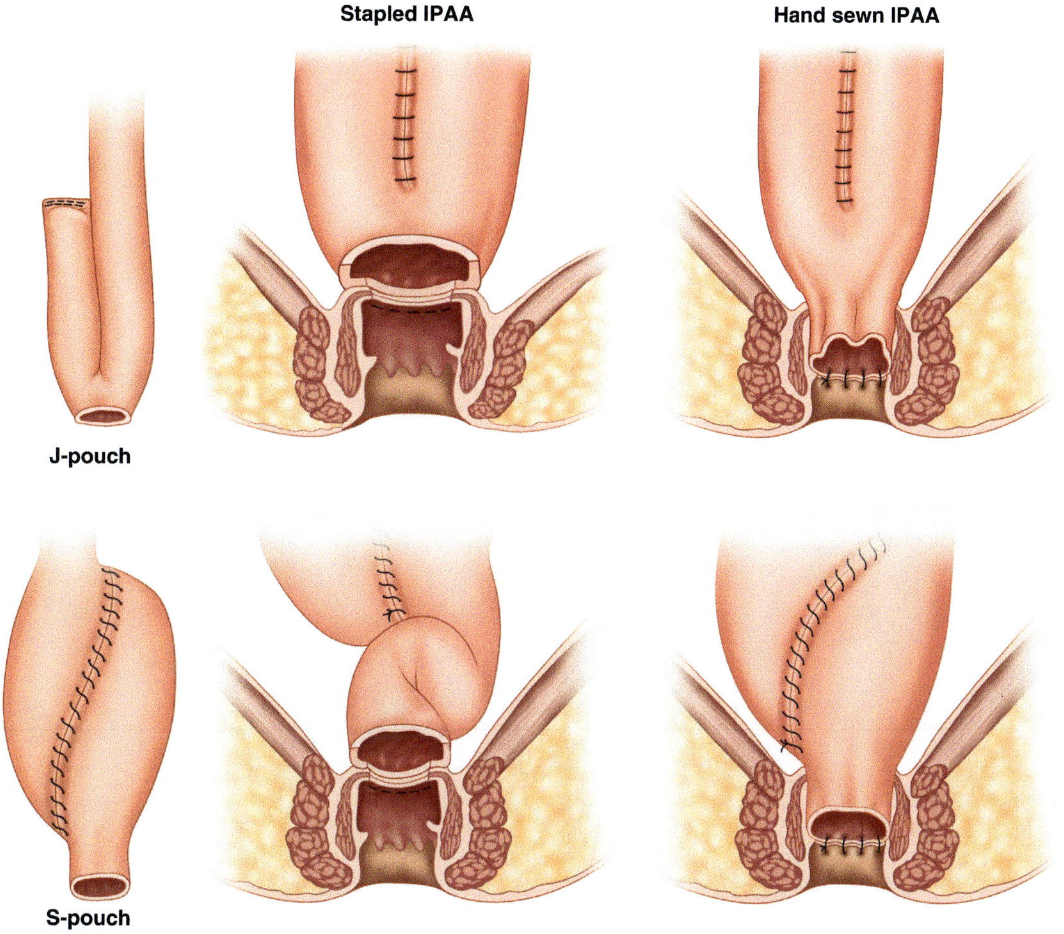

Fig. 51.2 The “J” and “S” pouch configurations used in stapled and hand-sewn anal anastomoses

- A planned mucosectomy with a hand-sewn IPAA is, in general, reserved for patients undergoing redo IPAA, with high-grade dysplasia or cancer involving the distal rectum, or those with familial adenomatous polyposis with polyps carpeting the distal rectum.
- In cases where a mucosectomy and hand-sewn IPAA are planned, an “S” configuration may fit through the pelvic floor anatomy better than a “J” pouch.
- When creating the IPAA, it is critically important to avoid tension across the anastomosis, to maintain correct orientation of the pouch coming down to the low pelvis, to preserve the blood supply to the pouch and the residual anorectum, and to avoid incorporating nearby pelvic structures like the vagina, prostate, and seminal vesicles into the anastomosis.

Problems with Reach of the Pouch

- Ensuring adequate reach of the pouch to the pelvic floor can be difficult and represents one of the more technically challenging aspects of a pouch procedure.
- Tall patients, those with a high BMI, and patients with extensive previous abdominal or pelvic operations are particularly at risk for encountering a problem with reach.
- Weight loss in anticipation of surgery may be helpful.
- Maneuvers to facilitate reach include high ligation of the ileocolic vessels, complete release of the small bowel mesentery from the retroperitoneum, mobilization of the duodenum, and excision of the redundant mesenteric tissue lateral to the superior mesenteric vessels (“jib-sail”).

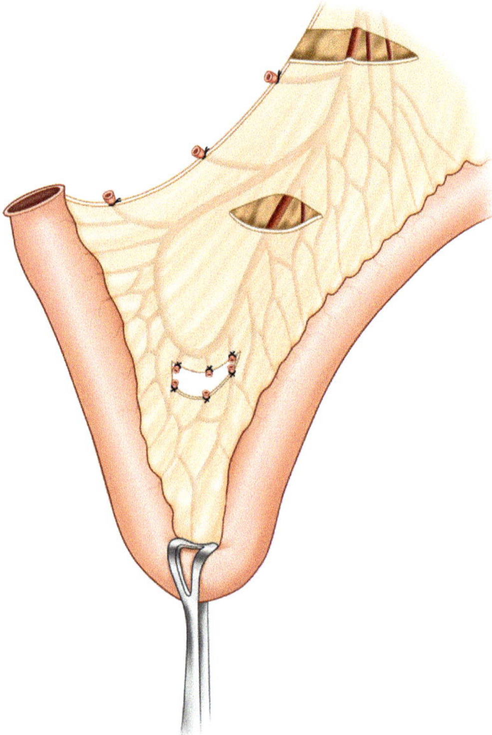

Fig. 51.3 Lengthening of the ileal mesentery in anticipation of "J" pouch construction. The peritoneum is scored to provide additional reach. Selective ligation of the mesenteric arcade can also reduce tension; transillumination of the mesenteric fat can be helpful

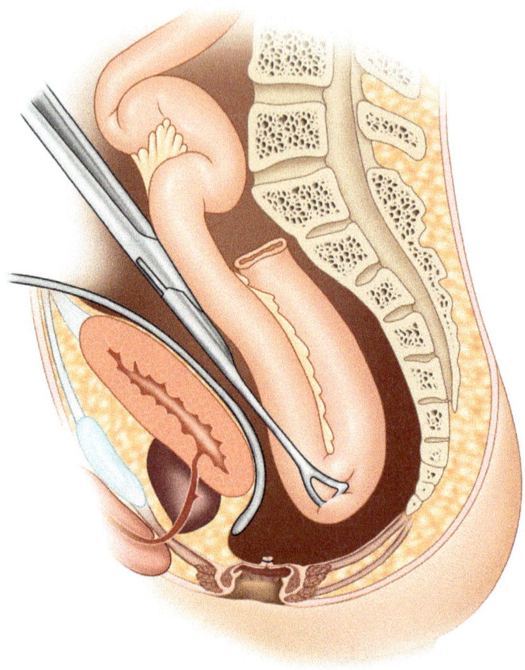

Fig. 51.4 Simulating the reach of the "J" pouch to the level of the anastomosis

- Releasing incisions across the mesentery perpendicular to the small bowel mesenteric vessels supplying the pouch can also provide added reach (Fig. 51.3).
- While sacrificing branches of the SMA or even the main trunk of the SMA may be required to improve reach, these maneuvers can compromise the blood flow to the pouch and are rarely required.
- Difficulty with reach of the pouch can be anticipated before rectal transection by using a long Babcock forceps to simulate the reach of the most dependent part of the bowel into the pelvis (Fig. 51.4).
- Manual palpation through the anal canal helps determine the anticipated reach of the mobilized bowel.
- In certain circumstances, and where the pathology permits, the rectal stump may intentionally be left slightly longer in order to minimize tension at the IPAA.
- If a "J" pouch cannot reach appropriately, changing to an "S" configuration may be advisable as this adds approximately 2 cm of extra reach to the IPAA.
- In rare cases where a pouch is created and insufficient reach cannot be remedied, it is recommended to secure the closed pouch to the pelvis and create a defunctioning ileostomy; this maneuver may allow the pouch to lengthen over time in anticipation of repeat attempt at IPAA.

Pouch Ischemia

- In an effort to provide reach, care should be taken to avoid overzealous skeletonization of vessels within the small bowel mesentery.
- The pouch blood supply can also be injured while scoring the mesentery or by creating a traction injury across the mesentery by creating an IPAA with excessive tension.

- Twisting the pouch around its mesentery as it is brought down to the IPAA can affect arterial inflow and venous outflow causing ischemia or bowel obstruction and should be avoided.
- Confirming correct orientation of the pouch by following the cut edge of the ileal mesentery from the mobilized duodenum to the IPAA can help prevent twisting of the pouch.
- Pouch ischemia requires pouch excision and an attempt at creating another pouch.

Problems with Stoma Creation

- Creating a defunctioning loop ileostomy for an IPAA patient can be challenging especially in patients with difficult reach or a high BMI because the ileal mesentery is fixed.
- One possible option is to defunctionalize using a more proximal segment of the bowel. Patients diverted in this fashion need to be monitored for high ostomy output.
- Anticipating diversion difficulties and discussing potential strategies to address these with the patient allows for setting more realistic expectations and highlights the importance of individualized operative planning requisite for pouch surgery.
- These strategies may include mandating weight loss prior to surgery, trading off the ideal stoma location for one that is functionally better, and instituting a medical regimen early on to preempt high-output stoma issues.

Problems with Staplers and Creating the Anastomosis

- Once the pouch has been created, insufflating the opened, distal end of the pouch with an air-filled bulb syringe as a leak test will alert the surgeon to any structural issues that need to be addressed.
- Prior to firing the circular stapler, it is important to exclude nearby pelvic structures from being incorporated into the stapler mechanism.
- When performing a stapled IPAA, mechanical circular staplers are prone to misfire; an on-table pouchoscopy after creating the IPAA is needed to check the integrity of the anastomosis.
- When a defect in the anastomosis is detected, adequate assistance to facilitate the necessary retraction and exposure, allowing access to the field from the abdomen and the perineum, is needed.
- The specific management in this situation depends on the location, size, and cause of the staple line defect:
  - For a small dehiscence, a defunctioning stoma may be sufficient to allow healing; attempts at suture closure through an abdominal or trans-anal approach should be considered.
  - In the case of a major dehiscence due to stapler misfiring or possibly from a breach in the cuff staple line from inserting the circular stapler too far, the IPAA may have to be taken down and redone.
  - In some situations it may be possible to place a purse string to close the remaining rectal cuff to allow repeat stapling; typically a mucosectomy with hand-sewn IPAA will be required.

Early Postoperative Complications

- Complications related to the anastomosis and pelvic sepsis can affect the long-term function of the pouch.
- Prompt diagnosis and management of these complications is required to preserve pouch function.

Anastomotic Leak and Pelvic Sepsis

- Pelvic sepsis related to pouch surgery is loosely defined as an abdominopelvic or perianal infectious process detected by clinical, radiologic, or operative means within 3 months of IPAA creation or within 3 months of stoma reversal.
- Depending on the manifestations and severity of the infection, pelvic sepsis is associated

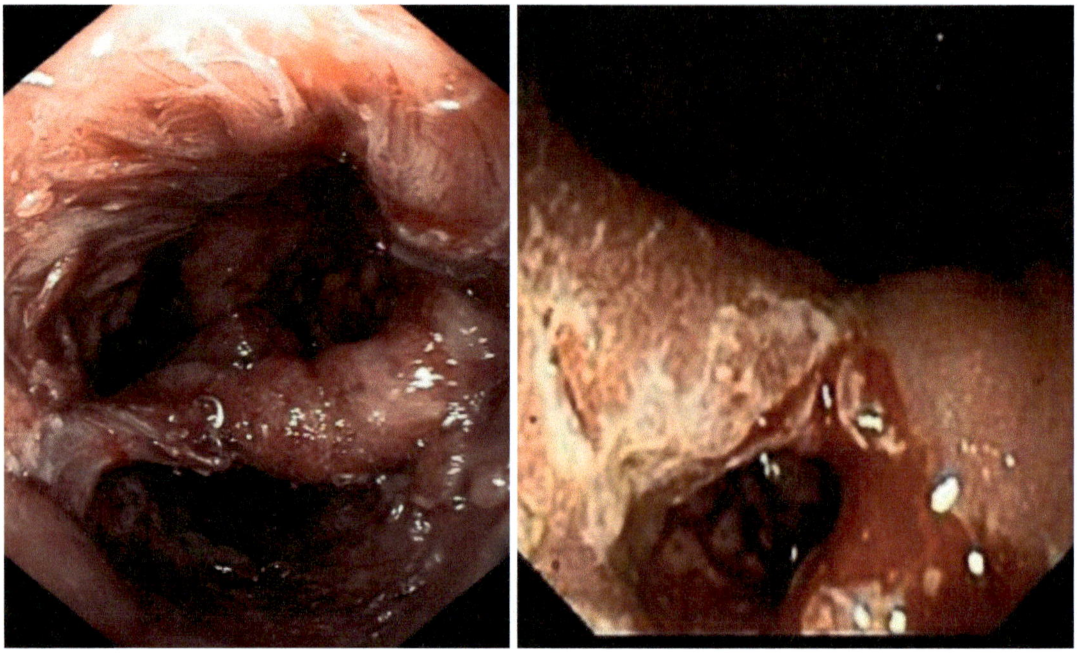

Fig. 51.5 Pouchoscopy demonstrating IPAA dehiscences with posterior defects

with worse functional outcomes, diminished quality of life, and, potentially, pouch failure.

- An anastomotic disruption may be an isolated finding discovered incidentally on pre-stoma reversal evaluation or can present clinically with pelvic sepsis.
- While patients with a pelvic abscess usually exhibit the expected signs and symptoms of infection, some IPAA patients have a more indolent presentation with persistent ileus or fail to meet expected recovery milestones after the surgery.
- Patients with hemodynamic instability and peritonitis require operative exploration to evaluate the anatomy, wash out the field, and effect drainage (Fig. 51.5).
- Patients with less impressive clinical findings can undergo cross-sectional imaging to guide management. CT scan of the abdomen and pelvis with intravenous and water-soluble oral and trans-anal contrast is helpful to diagnose an abscess and an associated leak.
- In patients with an abscess amenable to percutaneous drainage, prompt drainage and broad spectrum IV antibiotic administration may allow for control of the sepsis and may minimize the long-term consequences to the pouch.
- Whether abscess drainage should be performed trans-anally or percutaneously is a matter of debate owing to concerns over the development of an extrasphincteric fistula related to percutaneous drainage.
- When a break in anastomotic integrity is demonstrated coexistent with an abscess, trans-anal drainage through the anastomosis is preferable; however, when the anastomosis is intact, percutaneous CT-guided drainage is preferable.
- This strategy allows prompt drainage of abscesses while minimizing the risk of an extrasphincteric fistula.

Bleeding from the Pouch

- Postoperative pouch bleeding may manifest as bleeding through the anus or up through the loop ileostomy.
- Pouchoscopy with cauterization, clip application, or epinephrine injection usually controls the bleeding.

- In patients with generalized oozing, instilling ice-cold saline with dilute epinephrine into the pouch facilitates hemostasis.

Late Postoperative Complications

- Due to the defunctioning nature of the loop ileostomy, some pouch-related complications do not manifest clinically until after stoma reversal.
- Pre-stoma reversal pouch imaging with water-soluble contrast (done by fluoroscopy or CT scan) and flexible pouchoscopy are routinely performed but do not eliminate the occurrence of late complications.

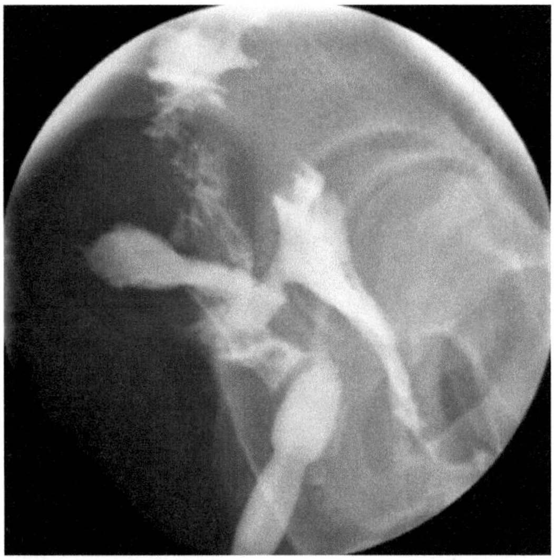

Fig. 51.6 Gastrografin enema demonstrating a pouch-vaginal fistula with contrast filling both structures

Pouch-Vaginal Fistula

- Pouch-vaginal fistula (PVF) is a potentially disabling complication that can cause significantly diminished quality of life.
- The overall risk of PVF ranges from 4% to 16% with pouch failure occurring in as many of 30% of these patients.
- Common symptoms include discomfort, irritation, incontinence, and recurrent vaginal and urinary tract infection.
- In order to tailor the most effective treatment to each patient, the size, nature, and location of the fistula, the state of the perineum and sphincter mechanism, and the configuration, size, and health of the pouch need to be assessed.
- While exam under anesthesia is considered the gold standard study to evaluate PVF, imaging studies are relied on to provide additional information and include water-soluble pouchogram, vaginogram, and pelvic MRI (Fig. 51.6).
- CT or MR enterography can be useful as well to delineate the anatomy above the pouch.
- The potential diagnosis of underlying Crohn's disease should be considered in any patient presenting with fistulizing disease after IPAA, as this affects PVF management and prognosis.
- In practice, differentiating septic complications from Crohn's disease is difficult especially when pathognomonic clinical and histopathological features of Crohn's disease are absent.
- In general, PVF occurring in a colitis patient within 1 year of stoma reversal is likely due to a septic complication of the IPAA, while fistulas presenting beyond the first year should raise the specter of Crohn's disease.
- A thorough review of the history and medical records pertaining to the index IPAA surgery and the postoperative course may provide insight into the potential etiology of the PVF.
- Review of the pathology from the pouch surgery and even from preoperative biopsies may prove helpful.
- Examination under anesthesia allows for assessment of the fistula tract and the associated tissues.
- Active inflammation with induration of the tract and surrounding tissues may respond to drainage and seton placement.
- Medical treatment with antibiotics, anti-inflammatories, and Crohn's disease medications may be required to reduce inflammation in anticipation of a repair procedure.

Treatment Options for PVF

Advancement Flap Repair

- Local repair that may be considered in patients with a low, simple PVF without excessive inflammation:
  - Prone jackknife positioning with general anesthesia provides the best exposure to the field.
  - Placing four-quadrant effacement sutures or using a Lone Star™ retractor (CooperSurgical Inc., Trumbull, CT) further improves exposure.
  - Using appropriately sized Hill-Ferguson retractors in both the vagina and anal canal allows for visualization of the fistula so that a fistula probe can be passed to identify the actual tract.
- In the absence of smoldering infection and if the tissues are supple and healthy, consideration may be given to creating a flap for repair.
- The fistula opening in the pouch is circumscribed, and, after the infiltration of 0.25% bupivacaine with epinephrine, a U-shaped broad-based flap is raised mobilizing mucosa and submucosa with the fistula opening at the apex of the flap.
- The fistula tract is dissected within the pouch-vaginal septum and is excised and the resulting defect is approximated.
- The flap is secured to the pouch-anal mucosa with sutures incorporating the adjoined sphincter mechanism ensuring a tension-free repair.
- If the defect on the vaginal aspect is small, it may be left alone. However, when large, the edges of the defect are freshened and the defect is approximated.
- The success of an advancement flap in the setting of PVF is influenced by the underlying etiology of the fistula, the quality of the tissues involving the fistula, and technical considerations at the time of the repair.
- Flap ischemia, bleeding under the flap, and tension across the flap are to be avoided.
- Patients with a failed advancement flap may be candidates for a redo flap procedure provided any residual local sepsis or ongoing inflammation is addressed and the tissues allow for a redo flap.

Transvaginal Repair

- This can occasionally be attempted when poor access, as with a mild stenosis of the IPAA, impedes repair via the pouch. A vaginal advancement flap repair is performed using similar principles as described above.

Perineal Pouch Advancement

- The anterior half of the IPAA is disconnected from the anal canal and the pouch is mobilized down from the vagina.
- The pouch is re-approximated to the anal canal after freshening and repairing the tissue surrounding the defect in the rectovaginal septum.
- The degree of mobilization obtainable through this technique is often limited given the constraints of operating trans-anally.

Redo IPAA

- Redo IPAA is the definitive treatment option for patients with PVF who have failed prior attempts at repair and desire restoration of the continuity of the intestine.
- Patients with an otherwise healthy perineum, adequate sphincter mechanism, and a low suspicion of having Crohn's disease may be considered for a redo IPAA.
- Redo IPAA is performed via a combined abdominoperineal approach so that the pouch can be disconnected from the prior anastomosis.
- These operations are usually technically challenging, and preoperative planning should consider the placement of ureteral stents to avoid ureteric injury.
- After pouch-anal disconnection, the fistula is excised and debrided to prepare the pouch for

repeat IPAA if the existing pouch is salvageable.

- The pouch may be augmented or refashioned, as required, based on intraoperative evaluation of the health and capacity of the pouch.
- If the status of the pouch is not sufficient, a neoileal pouch may be required.
- Once the pouch is prepared and the vaginal defect is repaired, mucosectomy and repeat IPAA are completed in hand-sewn fashion followed by a protecting loop ileostomy.
- If the greater omentum is available and can be mobilized to reach the low pelvis, an omental pedicle flap is used as an interposition between the pouch and the vagina to potentially reduce recurrent fistulization.
- While salvage procedures are associated with acceptable functional outcomes and quality of life, these outcomes are typically inferior to the results experienced with successful primary IPAA.
- The decision to proceed with redo IPAA requires consideration of anticipated function as well as the individual patient's threshold for long-term stoma avoidance.

Proximal Diversion

- A defunctioning ileostomy is often considered as a temporizing measure to control symptoms and improve the quality of the tissues in anticipation of a local PVF repair or may be performed concomitantly with the repair.
- In certain cases pouch excision with permanent, conventional end ileostomy creation may be recommended.
- Alternatively, conversion of the pouch to a continent ileostomy may be considered in select, highly motivated patients.
- Patients with pouch failure who are not candidates for another restorative procedure are generally recommended to undergo pouch excision as leaving the pouch in situ can cause long-term problems with seepage, anal pain, and overall decreased quality of life.

Pouch-Perineal Fistula

- The evaluation, management, and surgical options for pouch-perineal fistula are similar to those for pouch-vaginal fistula.
- Figure 51.7 illustrates the steps for an advancement flap repair for this kind of fistula.

Pouch Sinus

- Pouch sinus, generally considered an anastomotic leak confined to a blind-ending tract, occurs in 2–8% of patients after IPAA.
- While these tracts may be asymptomatic and incidentally discovered, some patients present with symptoms ranging from minor inflammation to pelvic sepsis, pain, pouch dysfunction, and pouch failure.
- Debridement, unroofing, fibrin glue injection, pouch revision, and redo pouch have all been described with variable rates of healing.
- Symptomatic presentation is associated with a high risk of pouch failure.
- Management is individualized to each patient and depends on the presenting symptoms, size, and location of the sinus as well as other factors such as whether or not the patient is diverted.
- Observation is recommended over intervention, when permitted by clinical circumstances, as these sinuses can resolve spontaneously.
- Patients with a sinus detected incidentally on routine evaluation before stoma reversal are usually recommended to delay reversal for a few months until repeat evaluation demonstrates the sinus has healed (Fig. 51.8).
- Patients with a symptomatic sinus or a nonresolving tract may be managed by trans-anal debridement with drainage, unroofing of the sinus, or glue injection.
- Proceeding with ileostomy reversal may be considered in selected asymptomatic patients

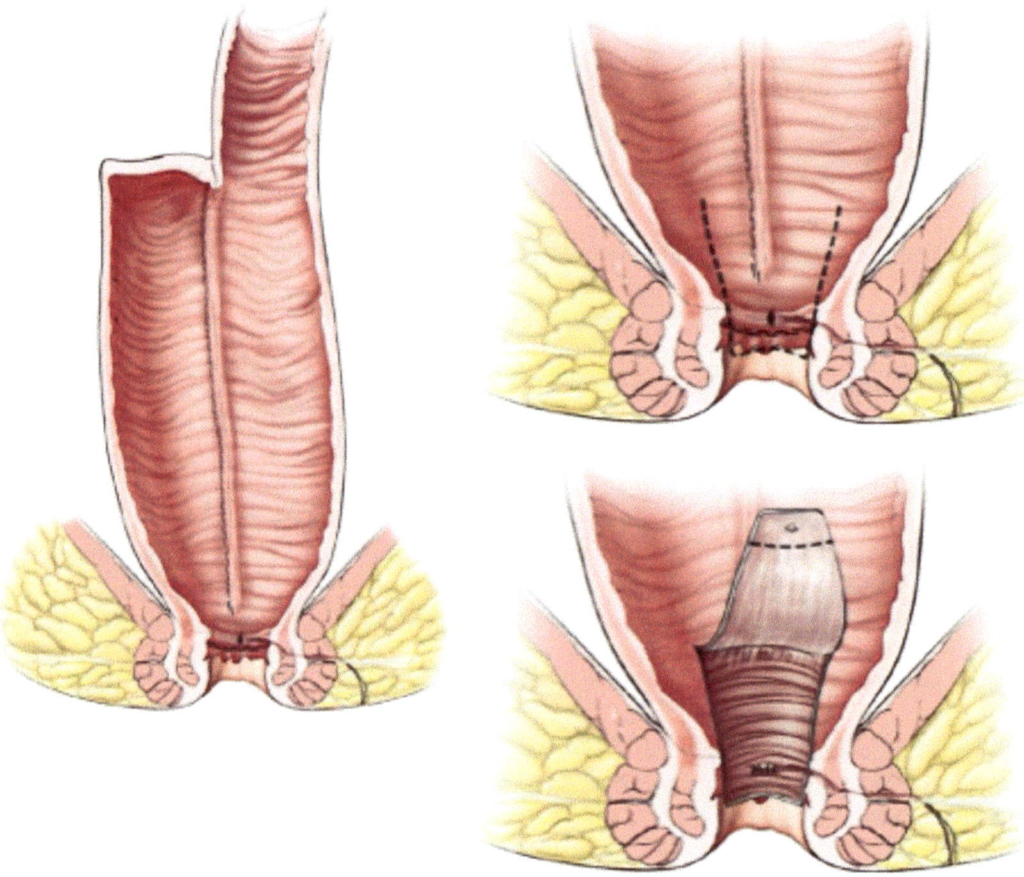

Fig. 51.7 Technique for advancement flap repair of a pouch-perineal fistula

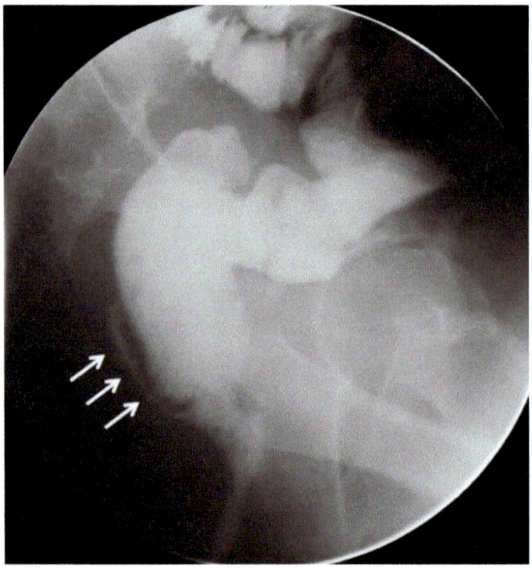

Fig. 51.8 Gastrografin pouchogram demonstrating a posterior sinus (at arrows)

with a persistent small tract who have failed attempts at resolving the sinus.

- Symptomatic patients who fail local attempts to resolve their sinus may go on to require diversion, pouch revision, or redo pouch surgery.

Crohn's Disease After Pouch Surgery

- In general, patients with Crohn's disease are not considered good candidates for IPAA because of the high rates of pouch complications and failure.
- However, a highly select subset of patients with disease entirely confined to the colon and rectum and in whom the small intestine and anoperineum are spared may be candidates for

an IPAA provided patients are thoroughly counseled.
- Pouch patients with presumptive ulcerative colitis or indeterminate colitis may, after developing complications, ultimately be diagnosed with Crohn's disease.
- The diagnosis of Crohn's disease after pouch surgery is usually based on the presence of perianal fistulas unrelated to the surgery, non-necrotizing granulomas on histopathology, or inflammation and ulceration in the afferent limb or in the small intestine on endoscopy in the absence of nonsteroidal anti-inflammatory use.
- Confirming the diagnosis of Crohn's disease after pouch surgery can be challenging.
- In the early postoperative period after restorative proctocolectomy, septic complications related to the pouch may manifest with findings similar to Crohn's disease as reviewed earlier in this chapter.
- Crohn's disease may interfere with pouch function by affecting the body, afferent limb, or anastomosis of the pouch, the perineum, or the proximal small intestine.
- Management depends on the disease manifestations (inflammatory, fibrostenosing, fistulizing) and the resulting symptoms.
- Pouch-related complications in the setting of Crohn's disease are more difficult to resolve compared with complications in patients without Crohn's disease and have a higher rate of pouch failure.
- Treatment relies on a combination of conventional medical therapy for Crohn's disease and surgical intervention tailored to the specific complication at hand.
- Endoscopic balloon dilation may be used for isolated short-segment strictures, reserving surgery for stricturing disease not amenable or responsive to through-the-scope interventions.
- Bowel-preserving stricturoplasty, a cornerstone of Crohn's disease management, if appropriate, is preferred over bowel resection in these cases.
- In the presence of localized disease at these sites, stricturoplasty of the pouch-anal anastomosis, pouch body, and small bowel proximal to the pouch with or without a defunctioning ileostomy may help control symptoms and salvage the pouch.
- Perianal disease may be managed with drainage and medical therapy in anticipation of future surgical intervention.
- Extensive or refractory Crohn's disease may require diversion and possible pouch excision.

Incontinence

- Functional issues after IPAA can significantly impact quality of life.
- Control issues may be due to pouch abnormalities like pouchitis, cuffitis, presacral sinus, or a chronic presacral cavity related to an anastomotic leak.
- Another contributing factor can be weakness of the sphincter mechanism that may have preexisted the IPAA or may be postsurgical in nature from mucosectomy or other operative trauma.
- Evaluation of the pouch, anal canal, and sphincter mechanism can usually elucidate the etiology of these symptoms, and treatment is tailored to the underlying problem.

Outlet Obstruction

- Problems with pouch evacuation may be due to a mechanical or anatomic cause like IPAA stricture, pouch prolapse, or kinking of the outflow of the pouch which can occur in patients with an "S" pouch and a long efferent limb (Fig. 51.9).
- Paradoxical, non-relaxation of the puborectalis muscle can present similarly to mechanical post-IPAA bowel obstruction.
- Treatment of IPAA outlet dysfunction depends on the underlying cause of the symptoms.
- Biofeedback with pelvic floor retraining may be helpful for some patients without a mechanical cause of the symptoms.
- Enemas and intermittent self-intubation to vent or to irrigate the pouch may be useful for patients with obstruction from either anatomic or functional causes.

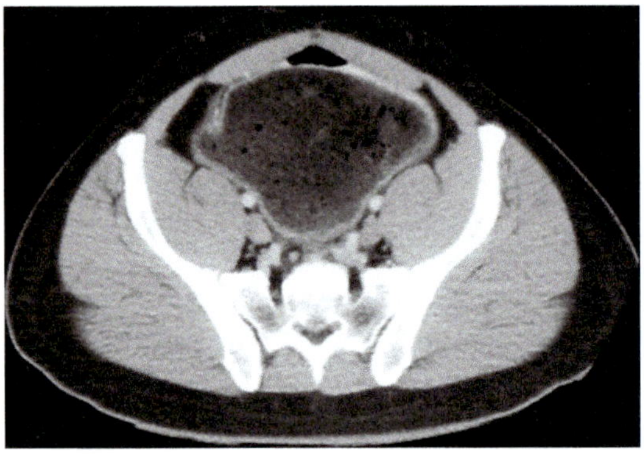

Fig. 51.9 CT scan of a patient with outlet obstruction of an "S" pouch due to kinking of the outflow tract. The pouch is distended with fecalized material

Pouchitis and Cuffitis

- Pouchitis and cuffitis are distinct post-IPAA entities that have similar presentations and treatment options.
- Pouchitis is the most common complication requiring medical treatment after IPAA and occurs much more commonly in pouch patients with ulcerative colitis.
- An estimated 40% of ulcerative colitis patients develop pouchitis after IPAA and some patients develop chronic pouchitis.
- Patients are diagnosed by pouchoscopy and biopsy (Figs. 51.10 and 51.11).
- Treatment for pouchitis and cuffitis is primarily medical and often includes antibiotics, probiotics, anti-inflammatories, and steroids that can be administered orally or trans-anally.
- Patients who exhaust medical therapy and remain symptomatic may benefit from a diverting ileostomy, pouch excision, and possible redo pouch surgery.
- Small focal areas of cuff inflammation may be addressed with ablation.
- Recalcitrant cuffitis may be treated with mucosectomy and pouch advancement or may require redo IPAA if related to a longer segment of retained rectum at the time of the original IPAA.

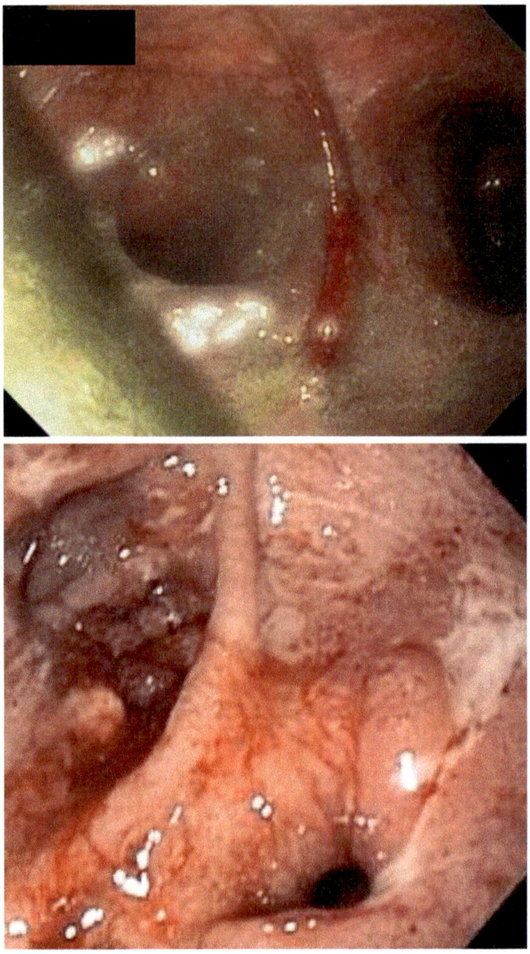

Fig. 51.10 Pouchitis on flexible pouchoscopy. On the left, notice the erythematous mucosa and the watery consistency of the pouch contents. Patients can also have friable, ulcerated, or edematous mucosa as seen on the right. These findings can mimic and may be difficult to differentiate from Crohn's disease of the pouch

Pouch Prolapse

- This is a rare complication occurring in less than 1% of patients after IPAA.
- Diagnosis is usually based on symptoms and physical examination; initial treatment relies on dietary manipulation, bulking agents, and avoidance of straining. Biofeedback may be useful as well.

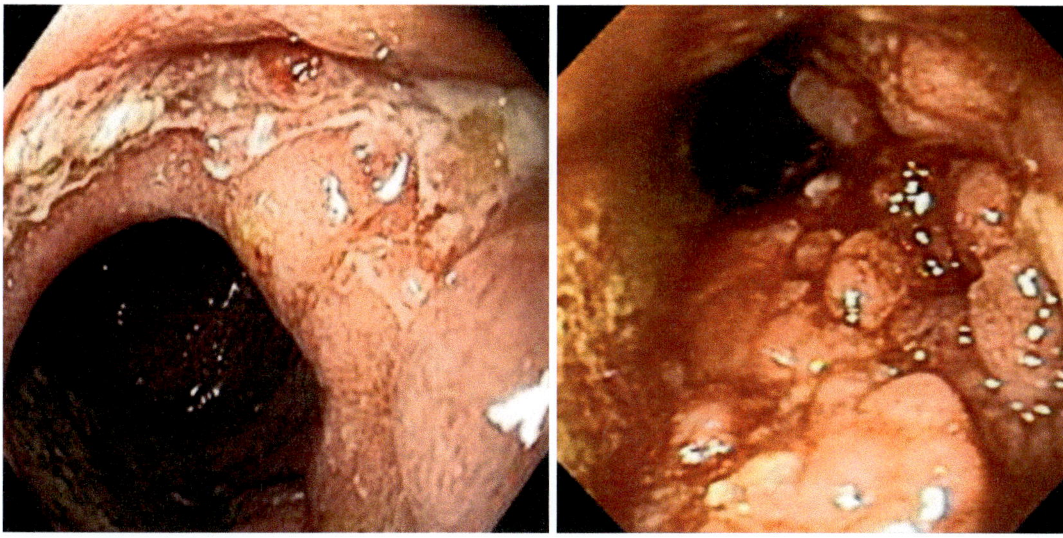

Fig. 51.11 Cuffitis on flexible pouchoscopy. The inflammatory changes are limited to the rectal mucosal remnant and can be severe

- Patients with symptomatic mucosal prolapse may undergo definitive treatment with excision of the redundant mucosa.
- Patients with full-thickness prolapse may require an abdominal approach with fixation of the pouch to the sacrum.

Leak from the Tip of the "J"

- Leak from the tip of the "J" is less common than anastomotic leak after IPAA and occurs in less than 1% of pouch patients (Fig. 51.12).
- Patients present with variable and often nonspecific symptoms of abdominal pain, fever, and changes in pouch output; some patients develop an abscess or fistula.
- These leaks can be difficult to discover on routine pre-stoma reversal evaluation and may not become symptomatic until after the ileostomy is taken down.
- The indolent course associated with this particular pouch complication may explain why some patients are not diagnosed until the time of reoperation.
- Salvage surgery may involve suture repair of the pouch or excision of the tip of the "J" (Fig. 51.13).

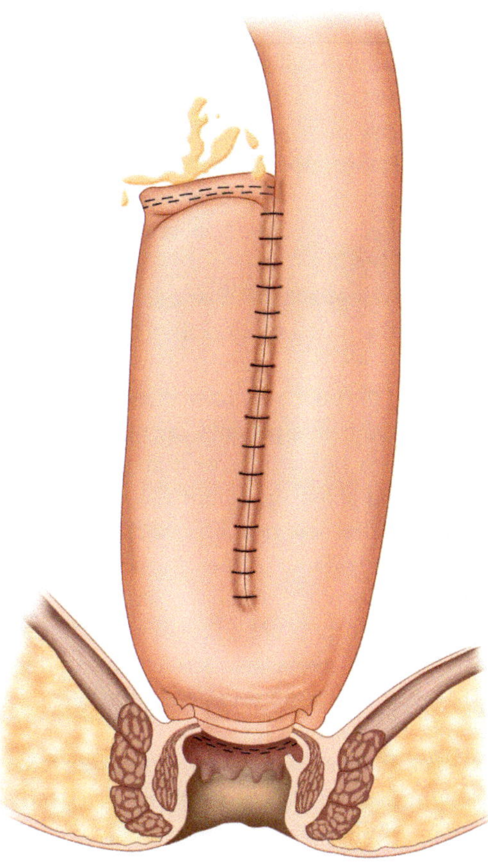

Fig. 51.12 Leak from the tip of the "J"

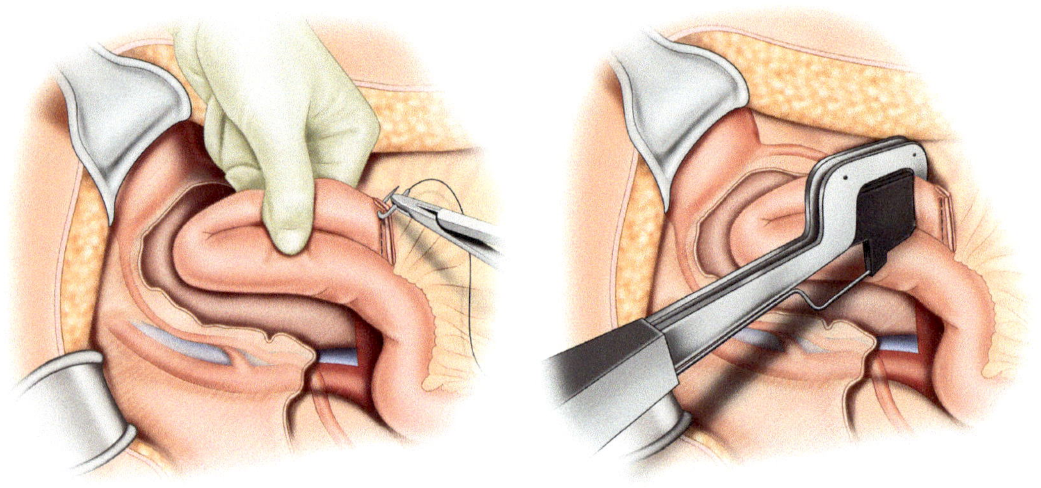

Fig. 51.13 Leak from the tip of the "J" treated with suture repair or excision

Dysplasia and Cancer After Pouch Surgery

- Dysplasia and cancer can develop in the ileal pouch, in the retained rectal mucosa, or in the anal transition zone after IPAA.
- Mucosectomy does not prevent future dysplasia as islands of rectal mucosa may persist even after "complete" mucosectomy at the time of IPAA.
- The development of dysplasia or neoplasia within the pouch of ulcerative colitis patients is extremely rare such that routine surveillance of the pouch is not warranted.
- Ulcerative colitis patients, whether stapled or hand-sewn after mucosectomy, should be counseled about the future risk of malignant degeneration in or near the anal transition zone and can be offered periodic surveillance.
- Prior colorectal dysplasia or cancer and chronic pouchitis are risk factors for developing pouch neoplasia; these patients may benefit from a more targeted pouch surveillance program.
- Pouch patients with focal dysplasia are recommended to undergo ablation or excision and surveillance.
- Patients with cancer will most likely require radical surgery with pouch excision.

Small Bowel Obstruction

- SBO is one of the most common long-term complications after IPAA occurring in as many as 25% of patients.
- Obstruction above the level of the pouch, most commonly due to adhesions, may also be due to volvulus, internal hernia, or stenosis at the site of stoma reversal.
- Laparoscopy, generally thought to reduce the formation of adhesions as compared with open surgery, has not been shown to reduce the long-term incidence of SBO in pouch patients.
- Adhesive SBO in pouch patients is treated with bowel rest, decompression, and exploration with adhesiolysis, if necessary.
- The rate of requiring adhesiolysis appears to be higher in patients with SBO after pouch surgery compared with patients who have had other types of abdominal surgery.

Sexual Dysfunction

- Sexual dysfunction after total proctocolectomy with IPAA may affect up to 20% or more of patients.
- Men may develop erectile dysfunction and retrograde ejaculation.

- Women can experience alterations in sexual desire, arousal, and satisfaction and can suffer from dyspareunia.
- The etiology of sexual dysfunction after IPAA is multifactorial and may involve nerve injury, altered pelvic anatomy, issues related to body image, presence of an ileostomy, and pouch dysfunction.
- In a large retrospective review of sexual function after IPAA, including 762 men and 692 women, 56% of patients reported no change in function, 25% reported having improved function, and 19% had worse function postoperatively.
- Hypogastric nerve injury during pelvic dissection should be avoided in order to reduce the incidence of sexual dysfunction.
- Performing close rectal dissection rather than total mesorectal excision does not appear to improve preservation of sexual function.
- Similarly, laparoscopic pouch surgery, as compared with open surgery, does not influence the risk of sexual dysfunction.

Infertility

- Women with ulcerative colitis have decreased fertility rates after total proctocolectomy compared with women who are managed non-operatively.
- A meta-analysis estimated these patients have a threefold increased risk of infertility. The differences in fecundity are thought due to adhesions and occlusive scarring of the fallopian tubes resulting from the pelvic dissection.
- The higher rate of fertility described after laparoscopic pouch surgery compared with open procedures is thought to be related to decreased pelvic adhesions.
- Women of childbearing age should be counseled appropriately regarding the risk of future infertility and the possible impact of the laparoscopic approach.

Infectious Colitides

52

Frederick R. Lane and Dipen C. Maun

Key Concepts

- Common bacterial colitides are often the result of food-borne pathogens from undercooked meat or contaminated vegetables.
- Parasites are an important pathogen in the differential diagnosis of diarrhea and colitis, especially in patients who have traveled abroad.
- *Cytomegalovirus* can cause a life-threatening colitis usually in the setting of decreased immune status such as HIV or inflammatory bowel disease.
- Travelers to low-income parts of the world frequently have the misfortune of developing acute diarrhea, caused by various forms of *Escherichia coli* in over 50% of cases.
- Diarrhea in the setting of HIV or immunosuppression for transplantation requires an extensive workup for bacteria, viruses, and protozoa.
- Forty-eight million Americans were afflicted with food-borne illness in 2012.
- Bacteria, parasites, viruses, or fungi may cause infectious colitides.
- *Clostridium difficile* colitis has become an increasingly common cause of infectious colitis and should be included in the differential diagnosis for any patient presenting with an acute diarrheal illness.

Introduction

- Infectious colitis is a worldwide cause of morbidity and mortality.
- Estimates suggest that 2–4 billion episodes of infectious diarrhea occur in developing countries annually.

Bacterial Colitides

Campylobacter

- *Campylobacter* typically produces diarrhea and fever.
- The stool may be bloody, and infection may be accompanied by abdominal pain.
- *Campylobacter* results in up to 14% of cases worldwide, with *Campylobacter jejuni* the usual culprit.
- Transmission is commonly through contaminated poultry, but many animals can be infected.
- Infection of the terminal ileum and cecum can mimic acute appendicitis.
- Most illnesses last less than 7 days, but up to 16% of patients may harbor the organism for 2–10 weeks.
- Complications of infection can include hemorrhage, toxic megacolon, pancreatitis, Reiter syndrome, and Guillain-Barre syndrome.

F. R. Lane (✉) · D. C. Maun
Kendrick Colon and Rectal Center, Franciscan St. Francis Health, Indianapolis, IN, USA

S. R. Steele et al. (eds.), *The ASCRS Manual of Colon and Rectal Surgery*,
https://doi.org/10.1007/978-3-030-01165-9_52

- Stool samples with fecal leukocytes and blood support the diagnosis of infectious colitis, but diagnosis of *Campylobacter* is made by culture of the bacteria.
- Colonoscopy may demonstrate segmental edema, loss of vascular pattern, and patchy erythema of the mucosa. These findings are nonspecific and may be difficult to differentiate from that of other colonic mucosal diseases.
- The majority of patients do not require treatment, as the disease is self-limiting.
- Fluoroquinolone antibiotics, which are also active against *Shigella* and other common enteric organisms, can be used empirically. However, resistance to fluoroquinolones is becoming a major problem.
- Azithromycin has been shown to be effective when fluoroquinolone resistance is an issue, while Erythromycin is a third-line choice.

Salmonella

- *Salmonella* can cause both typhoid and non-typhoid illnesses.
- The non-typhoid version causes self-limited diarrhea.
- *Salmonella typhi* and *Salmonella paratyphi* cause typhoid fever, while *Salmonella enteritidis* and *Salmonella typhimurium* are the most common serotypes in the United States.
- The major route of transmission is by the "five Fs": flies, food, fingers, feces, and fomites.
- Contaminated meat and poultry are the main sources of infection.
- Infections with non-typhoidal *Salmonella* present with nausea, vomiting, abdominal cramps, and diarrhea.
  - Symptoms may occur between 8 and 48 h after ingestion of contaminated food.
  - Illness can last up to 3 weeks and bacteremia may occur in up to 10% of patients.
- Typhoid fever can manifest with high fever, delirium, abdominal pain, splenomegaly, and skin rash.
  - Typhoid fever occurs when organisms penetrate the small bowel wall and enter the lymphatics and ultimately the bloodstream.
- Diagnosis is established by identification of the organism with blood culture or cultures from the stool.
- Endoscopic findings in non-typhoidal *Salmonella* infection may include hyperemia, mucosal friability, aphthous erosions, or deep ulcers with segmental involvement.
- Typhoid disease may show punched-out ulcers with slightly raised margins, with the most commonly affected areas being the terminal ileum and right colon.
- Antibiotics are traditionally reserved for patients where bacteremic disease is suspected or would place the patient at marked risk.
  - These are patients who are febrile or toxic, young (3 years old or less), or elderly (65 years or older).
  - Patients with sickle cell disease, inflammatory bowel disease, or acquired immune deficiency syndrome (AIDS) and patients on steroids or hemodialysis should be considered for antibiotic treatment.
  - When indicated, fluoroquinolones are the treatment of choice.

Shigella

- Shigellosis is most commonly a disease of children under 5 years of age but can affect all age groups.
- It is the third most common enteric infection in the United States but is uncommon in Europe.
- *Shigella sonnei* accounts for more than two-thirds of cases in the United States and is typically spread through contaminated food or water or person-to-person contact.
- In developed countries, *Shigella* is seen most frequently in daycare centers, in nursery schools, and in male homosexuals.
- Diarrhea is initially watery without blood, but tenesmus and bloody stools develop 3–5 days after onset.
- Bacteremia is uncommon, but perforation, megacolon, hemolytic uremic syndrome, and severe dehydration may occur.
- Children typically have mild infections, which may last up to 3 days.

- Adults have more prolonged courses, with severe cases lasting 3–4 weeks.
- Symptoms include lower abdominal pain, rectal pain, and diarrhea.
- Stool cultures are needed for diagnosis.
- Colonoscopy shows non-specific erythema, edema, and loss of vascular pattern.
- Antibiotic treatment is always indicated for *Shigella* infections.
- Treatment may be with either ciprofloxacin 750 mg daily for 3 days or azithromycin 500 mg daily for 3 days.

Escherichia coli

- Five groups of *E. coli* cause enteric infections: enteropathogenic *E. coli* (EPEC), enterotoxigenic *E. coli* (ETEC), enteroadherent *E. coli* (EAEC), enteroinvasive *E. coli* (EIEC), and enterohemorrhagic *E. coli* (EHEC).
- EPEC is associated with diarrhea in infants and nursery outbreaks, while EAEC can cause persistent childhood diarrhea.
- ETEC and EAEC (mainly children) are two of the leading causes of traveler's diarrhea.
- EHEC causes hemorrhagic colitis with bloody or mucoid diarrhea and is a common cause of infectious colitis in Western countries, including the United States.
- *E. coli* O157:H7, a subtype of EHEC, is an important cause of acute bacterial colitis, especially from undercooked ground beef.
- Although less common than *Salmonella* or *Campylobacter*, *E. coli* O157:H7 is associated with a higher hospitalization and fatality rate.
- Most cases start with non-bloody diarrhea and resolve spontaneously.
- Some patients will progress to bloody diarrhea, and 5–10% of these can progress to the life-threatening hemolytic uremic syndrome or thrombocytopenic purpura.
- Non-O157 strains have recently emerged as an important cause of infection worldwide.
- Many hospital laboratories are routinely testing for *E. coli* O157:H7 on stool culture; it should be requested in any patient with bloody diarrhea.
- Colonoscopy findings show shallow ulcerations, marked edema, and longitudinal ulcer-like lesions throughout the colon. Inflammation tends to predominate on the right side.
- Clinical data do not support the use of antibiotics for hemorrhagic *E. coli* infection.
  - Rifaximin 200 mg 3 times a day for 3 days may be used for EAEC, as well as fluoroquinolones or azithromycin.

Yersinia

- *Yersinia* can occur from handling of contaminated animals or animal products or ingestion of contaminated food or water (most commonly undercooked pork or contaminated milk).
- Typical symptoms are fever, diarrhea, and abdominal pain, lasting up to 3 weeks.
- The infection may cause mesenteric adenitis or ileitis, mimicking Crohn's disease.
- Extraintestinal symptoms, such as migratory arthritis, Reiter's syndrome, and erythema nodosum, may occur.
- Radiographic and endoscopic findings also may be indistinguishable from Crohn's disease with erosions and ulcerations on the right side of the colon.
- The disease is usually self-limited, but in prolonged cases or patients with extraintestinal manifestations, aminoglycosides, trimethoprim-sulfamethoxazole (TMP-SMX), doxycycline, and fluoroquinolones have all been used successfully.

Vibrio

- *Vibrio* can cause either a cholera or noncholera illness.
- Infections are usually associated with consumption of raw or undercooked shellfish. Most patients with gastroenteritis reported having eaten raw oysters in the week before their illness.
- Patients with *Vibrio parahaemolyticus* infection typically present with diarrhea and abdominal cramps. About half of them have fever and vomiting.

- Stool testing does not typically test for *Vibrio* species but may be specially requested, especially when illness develops within 48 h of ingesting raw or undercooked shellfish.
- Most patients don't require treatment, but tetracycline, fluoroquinolones, aminoglycosides, and third-generation cephalosporins are usually effective.
- *Vibrio cholera* and invasive *Vibrio* infections can cause profuse watery diarrhea, vomiting, and muscle cramps.
- Stool volumes may reach a liter per hour, and this can lead to shock and death within hours without treatment.
- Treatment of cholera includes aggressive fluid replacement. Ciprofloxacin (1 gram orally for one dose) or doxycycline (300 mg orally for one dose) is the antibiotic of choice.

Other Bacterial Colitides

- Tuberculosis is prevalent in the developing world.
  - Patients may present with abdominal pain, weight loss, anorexia, and fever.
  - Because of its predilection for the ileocecal regions, findings frequently mimic Crohn's disease or appendicitis.
  - Cultures are difficult, and a positive skin test is not diagnostic.
  - Endoscopic biopsies of ulcers may be helpful.
  - Classic radiologic signs include a contracted terminal ileum with a wide ileocecal valve (Fleischner sign) and a narrow ileum opening into a contracted cecum (Sterlin's sign).
  - Medical management is complicated and is beyond the scope of this discussion.
  - Surgery is indicated for complications, most commonly obstruction or perforation.
- *Aeromonas* causes diarrhea, most commonly in the tropics. Persistent diarrhea, usually lasting longer than 2 weeks, is common. The disease is usually self-limited. Treatment, in prolonged cases or immunocompromised hosts, is typically with a fluoroquinolone or azithromycin.
- *Bacteroides fragilis* is part of the normal colonic flora, but a subclass that secretes a toxin has been recognized as a cause of acute diarrhea in endemic regions.
- *Arcobacter* is considered an emerging food-borne pathogen.
- *Listeria monocytogenes* is a rare cause of gastroenteritis, most commonly presenting as diarrhea in an immunocompromised patient. Symptoms include diarrhea, nausea, and vomiting, often with fever. Disease is usually self-limited, and antibiotic treatment is not typically indicated but may be used in higher-risk patients.
- *Chlamydia trachomatis* is a common cause of proctitis in homosexual males or women practicing anoreceptive intercourse.
  - It may present with bloody diarrhea, mucopurulent anal discharge, tenesmus, and anal pain.
  - Rectal examination may show extreme tenderness, and sigmoidoscopy may show typical findings of proctitis. The bowel may become fibrotic with progressive disease.
  - Culture for chlamydia can be obtained from stool or rectal swab.
  - Nucleic acid amplification tests (NAAT) are currently considered the gold standard for testing.
  - Azithromycin (1.0 gm orally single dose) and doxycycline (100 mg orally twice daily for 7 days) are highly effective for treatment, with treatment of all sex partners indicated as well.
- *Neisseria gonorrhoeae* is a common sexually transmitted disease that can cause proctitis, especially in homosexual males.
  - Symptoms start about a week after exposure and may include mucoid discharge, rectal bleeding, and diarrhea.
  - Diagnosis is made by rectal swab on chocolate agar (Thayer-Martin).
  - Single-dose ceftriaxone 125 mg IM cures nearly 100% of uncomplicated disease, while fluoroquinolones are an acceptable alternative.
- See Table 52.1 for a summary of treatment for bacterial colitides.

Table 52.1 Treatment of bacterial colitides

Campylobacter	Azithromycin 500 mg daily for 3 days or erythromycin 500 mg 4 times daily for 3–5 days
Salmonella	Mild illness – none. Possible bacteremic disease – levofloxacin 500 mg (or other fluoroquinolones) daily for 7 (immunocompetent) or 14 days (immunocompromised)
Shigella	Ciprofloxacin 750 mg (or other fluoroquinolones) daily for 3 days or azithromycin 500 mg daily for 3 days
EHEC (*E. coli*)	None
EAEC (*E. coli*)	Rifaximin 200 mg 3 times daily for 3 days
Other E. coli	Same as *Shigella*
Yersinia	Same as *Shigella*
Vibrio	Same as *Shigella*
Tuberculosis	Usual TB treatment
Aeromonas	Same as *Shigella*
Traveler's diarrhea	Same as *Shigella*

With permission from DuPont HL. Approach to the patient with infectious colitis. Curr Opin Gastroenterol. 2012;28:39–46. © Wolters Kluwer

- Diagnosis can be made by stool microscopy, antigen detection, PCR, serology, and endoscopy.
- Colonoscopy is preferred over sigmoidoscopy because colitis can be limited to the right side.
  - Bowel preparation should be avoided because it will decrease the detection of the parasites.
  - The mucosa of the colon may have friability, may show classic flask-shaped ulcerations, and may be indistinguishable from inflammatory bowel disease.
  - Microscopic analysis of aspirate from the base of the ulcers or biopsy of the ulcer edges can show the cysts and prove to be diagnostic for amebiasis.
- Treatment of intestinal amebiasis is metronidazole 750 mg PO tid for 10 days (Table 52.2).
- Intravenous antibiotics are reserved for severe cases or those resistant to oral therapy.
- Surgery can be necessary in cases of perforation, peritonitis, and abdominal catastrophe.

Parasitic Colitides

Entamoeba

- Amebiasis is caused by the protozoan parasite *Entamoeba histolytica*.
- Most cases of amebiasis in the United States are from immigrants or travelers returning from an endemic area.
- Infection occurs from ingestion of fecally contaminated food or water or by oral/anal sexual contact.
- Disease presentation can include asymptomatic colonization, diarrhea and dysentery, or liver or brain abscess.
- The majority of patients who ingest cysts from *E. histolytica* remain asymptomatic.
  - A typical incubation period is 2–4 weeks followed by a gradual onset of abdominal pain and bloody diarrhea.
- In rare cases (<0.5%), infection can lead to fulminant colitis, toxic megacolon, or extraintestinal abscess.

Anisakis

- Anisakidosis is primarily caused by *Anisakis simplex* and *Pseudoterranova decipiens*. The majority of the cases in the world (>90%) occur in Japan.
- Infection typically results from the consumption of raw or undercooked fish.
- The majority of patients with anisakidosis present with gastric involvement; only about 4% of cases present in either the small bowel or colon.
- Intestinal anisakidosis presents with vague complaints such as lower abdominal pain, fever, diarrhea, nausea, and vomiting.
- After consumption, the larvae burrow into the intestinal mucosa and cause an intense hypersensitivity reaction with formation of granulomas and infiltration of eosinophils (Fig. 52.1).
- Symptoms can mimic appendicitis, Crohn's ileitis, diverticulitis, gastroenteritis, or other causes of an acute abdomen.

Table 52.2 Summary of parasitic colitis treatment

Diagnosis	Pathogen	Treatment
Amebiasis	*Entamoeba histolytica*	Metronidazole 750 mg PO tid for 10 days
Anisakidosis	*Anisakis simplex Pseudoterranova decipiens*	Albendazole 400–800 mg orally for 6–21 days
Ascariasis	*Ascaris lumbricoides*	Mebendazole 100 mg twice daily for 3 days Albendazole 400 mg X1 dose
Strongyloidiasis	*Strongyloides stercoralis*	Ivermectin at 200 ug/kg per day for 2 days Albendazole 400 mg twice a day for 7 days[a] Thiabendazole at 50 mg/kg daily for 2 days[a]
Trichuriasis	*Trichuris trichiura*	Mebendazole 100 mg twice daily for 3 days Albendazole 400 mg daily for 3 days
Enterobiasis	*Enterobius vermicularis*	Mebendazole 100 mg single dose Albendazole 400 mg single dose
Cryptosporidiosis	*Cryptosporidium*	Nitazoxanide
Balantidiasis	*Balantidium coli*	Tetracycline 500 mg 4 times a day
Giardiasis	*Giardia lamblia*	Metronidazole 250 mg 3 times a day for 7 days Tinidazole 2 g as a single dose
Schistosomiasis	*S. haematobium*, *S. mansoni*, *S. japonicum*	Praziquantel 40 mg/kg single dose
Tapeworm	*Taenia solium* (pork) *Taenia saginata* (beef) *Diphyllobothrium latum* *Hymenolepis nana* *Dipylidium caninum*	Praziquantel 5–10 mg/kg single dose Niclosamide 2 g single dose
Chagas	*Trypanosoma cruzi*	Benznidazole Nifurtimox

[a]Denotes second-line treatment

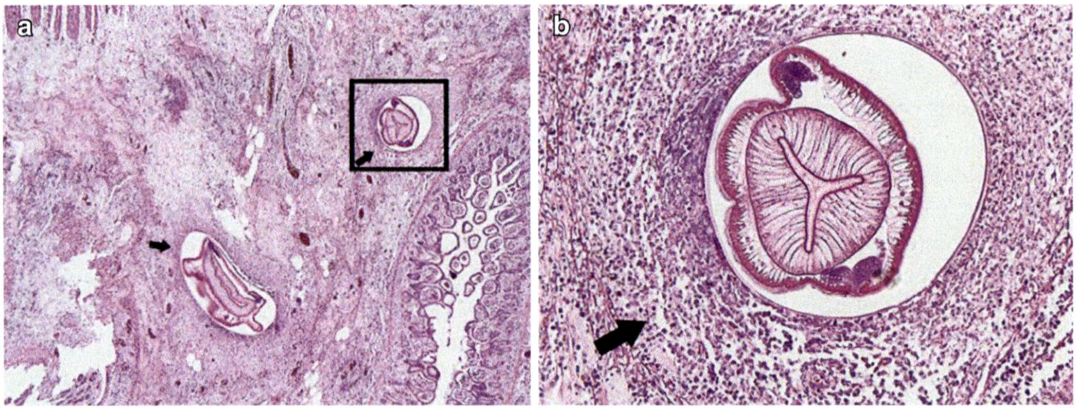

Fig. 52.1 Histopathologic findings show the severe infiltration of inflammation and edema in all layers of the intestinal wall with a submucosal eosinophilic granuloma around larvae (arrows), which were findings of anisakiasis (**a**) (H&E X40), and magnification view of square showed eosinophilic granuloma around anisakiasis larva (**b**) (H&E X200). Kang DB, Oh JT, Park WC, Lee JK. Small bowel obstruction caused by acute invasive enteric anisakiasis. Korean J Gastroenterol. 2010;56:192–5. (Copyright©2008 The Korean Society of Gastroenterology. All Rights Reserved. This is an open-access article distributed under the terms of the Creative Commons Attribution Non-Commercial License (http://creativecommons.org/licenses/by-nc/3.0/) which permits unrestricted noncommercial use, distribution, and reproduction in any medium, provided the original work is properly cited)

- In rare cases, the infection can require surgery due to perforation, intussusception, small bowel obstruction, or pneumoperitoneum.
- If the diagnosis is made prior to surgical intervention, then albendazole 400–800 mg orally for 6–21 days is effective (Table 52.2).

Ascaris

- Ascariasis is caused by the intestinal nematode *Ascaris lumbricoides*. There are more than 1 billion people infected with the parasite worldwide.
- Most patients with ascariasis are asymptomatic.
- As the larvae migrate through the lungs, patients may complain of pneumonia-like symptoms.
- Most patients with intestinal ascariasis are children, because the lumen of the bowel is narrower, allowing for easier obstruction. A common site of obstruction is at the ileocecal valve.
- Large quantities of the worms can lead to the formation of a mass that can intertwine and cause obstruction, volvulus, intussusception, or perforation.
- The diagnosis of ascariasis is made by stool microscopy.
- Treatment is very effective with cure rates as high as 90%. Mebendazole 100 mg twice daily for 3 days and albendazole 400 mg as a single dose are common therapeutic regimens (Table 52.2).
- Obstructed patients with no peritoneal signs can be managed conservatively with hydration and nasogastric tube decompression.
- Surgery is reserved for complicated cases of obstruction and perforation. During laparotomy, the ball of worms can be simply milked into the colon provided there is no perforation or bowel ischemia.

Strongyloides

- Strongyloidiasis is caused by *Strongyloides stercoralis*, another intestinal nematode.
- Hyperinfection can also occur in conditions of immune suppression and results in large numbers of worms traveling through the lungs and intestines.
- Vague pulmonary and abdominal complaints may infrequently be seen as the worms migrate.
- Chronic infection is a result of autoinfection, which can lead to epigastric abdominal pain and diarrhea.
- Strongyloidiasis can sometimes present with a pancolitis and be confused with ulcerative colitis.
- Endoscopic features may include yellowish-white nodules, erythema, and loss of vascular pattern.
- Detecting larvae in the stool makes the diagnosis of strongyloidiasis; however, multiple tests may be necessary. Other options include duodenal biopsy, enzyme-linked immunosorbent assay (ELISA) testing, or bronchial washings.
- All patients with *S. stercoralis* should be treated because of the risk of autoinfection (Table 52.2).

Trichuris

- Trichuriasis is caused by *Trichuris trichiura*, also known as the whipworm.
- There are an estimated 600–800 million infected individuals worldwide, primarily in humid and tropical regions of the world.
- Infection occurs by ingestion of contaminated soil/food.
- Most infected with the whipworm are asymptomatic.
- As the wormload in the cecum and colon increases, symptoms such as diarrhea, tenesmus, and hematochezia can occur. Stools can be watery and will have a characteristic smell.
- Trichuriasis can cause rectal prolapse, and the worms can be visualized on the rectal mucosa (Fig. 52.2).
- Blood loss can lead to anemia and, for unclear reasons, growth retardation.
- Diagnosis is made by identifying the barrel-shaped eggs in the stool or by visualizing the worms on the colonic or rectal wall during endoscopy.

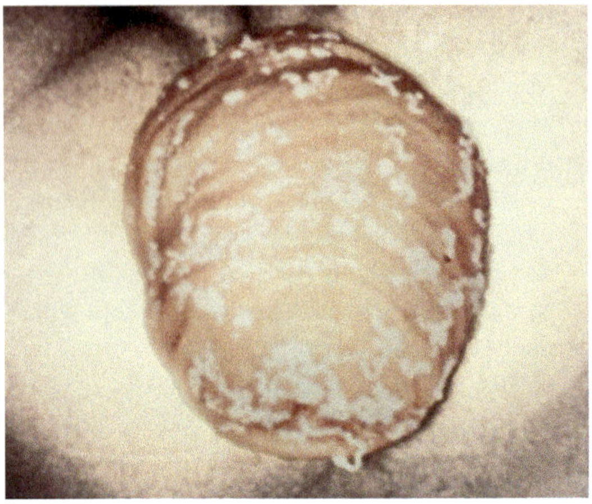

Fig. 52.2 Whipworm and rectal prolapse. Prolapsed rectum from whipworms (Available from http://phil.cdc.gov/Phil/details.asp)

- Treatment is either mebendazole 100 mg twice daily for 3 days or albendazole 400 mg daily for 3 days (Table 52.2).
- Surgery is reserved for cases of rectal prolapse.

Enterobius

- Enterobiasis is caused by the pinworm *Enterobius vermicularis*.
- Unlike other nematodes where infections occur primarily in tropical regions with poor sanitation, enterobiasis is prevalent in all parts of the world including urban areas of the United States and Europe.
- Children are the most commonly affected group.
- Infection occurs by ingestion of eggs. Adult pinworms live in the cecum for as long as 13 weeks.
- About 4 weeks after ingestion, female pinworms migrate to the perianal skin and can lay up to 11,000 eggs.
- The larvae then quickly mature and can cause an intense pruritus ani.
- The intense scratching facilitates fecal-oral transmission to classmates and family members.
- In young girls it is a well-known cause of vulvovaginitis.

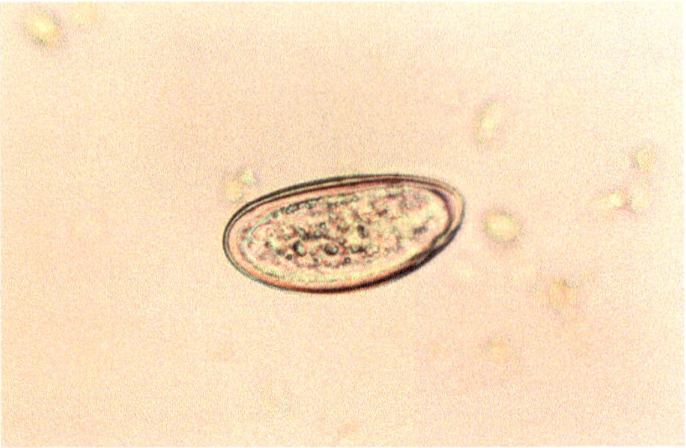

Fig. 52.3 Eggs of *Enterobius vermicularis* on wet mount (Available from http://www.cdc.gov/dpdx/enterobiasis/gallery.html#eggs)

- Diagnosis is typically made by the scotch tape test. This entails taking a strip of clear tape and pressing it against the buttocks. The tape is then transferred to a slide where the eggs can be seen under a microscope (Fig. 52.3).
- Treatment can be with either mebendazole or albendazole (Table 52.2). Usually the entire family is treated empirically.

Cryptosporidium

- Cryptosporidiosis is caused by *Cryptosporidium*, an intracellular protozoan.
- In the 1980s, it became a common cause of debilitating diarrhea in AIDS patients.
- The diarrhea caused by *Cryptosporidium* is usually seen in one of the four settings: childhood diarrhea in developing areas, travelers' diarrhea, debilitating diarrhea in immunocompromised patients, or waterborne outbreaks in developed areas in the immunocompetent host.
- The parasite is ingested in contaminated food or water.
- Disease presentation is hallmarked by explosive watery diarrhea and may be associated with abdominal pain, fever, nausea, and vomiting.
- In immunocompetent hosts, the disease is usually self-limited.
- Immunocompromised patients have a more protracted course which can be debilitating and sometimes life-threatening. In this patient

population, the most common site of extraintestinal infection is the biliary tree, which can cause acalculous cholecystitis or sclerosing cholangitis.

- Diagnosis is made by identifying oocysts in stool or in bodily fluids via microscopy, PCR, ELISA, or loop-mediated isothermal amplification (LAMP).
- Treatment in immunocompetent patients is primarily supportive (hydration, nutrition, and anti-motility agents), as the disease is self-limited. There is no drug or antimicrobial that has been shown to be effective in controlling cryptosporidiosis.
- Nitazoxanide is the only Food and Drug Administration-approved medication and may shorten the clinical course of the disease.
- In AIDS patients, the most effective form of therapy is the institution of highly active anti-retroviral therapy (HAART).
- Cholecystectomy may be useful in cases of acalculous cholecystitis, and endoscopic retrograde cholangiopancreatography (ERCP) may help in cases of sclerosing cholangitis.

Balantidium

- Balantidiasis is caused by *Balantidium coli*, the largest and only ciliated protozoan that infects humans.
- Pigs serve as the main reservoir for human infection, and transmission occurs through ingestion of contaminated food or water.
- Once the parasite is ingested, the cysts embed in the colon causing ulceration and inflammation.
- This can result in asymptomatic infection, non-bloody diarrhea, or severe bloody diarrhea.
- Severe diarrhea can result in large volume loss, peritonitis, and even death.
- Visualizing trophozoites in a stool sample can make the diagnosis. The parasite can also be seen on biopsy specimens of ulcers taken during endoscopy.
- Treatment with tetracycline 500 mg four times a day is usually effective (Table 52.2).
- Surgery is rarely necessary.

Giardia

- Giardiasis is caused by *Giardia lamblia* and is one of the most common parasitic infections in the United States.
- It can occur in almost any country and most climates.
- There are three methods of transmission: waterborne, food-borne, and direct fecal-oral.
- Waterborne transmission occurs when feces contaminate water sources. Infection can occur from drinking from mountain lakes or streams or when fecal matter from children contaminates recreational water, like swimming pools.
- Uncooked foods such as salads and cold meat are the most common food sources.
- Direct fecal-oral is common among children at daycare centers as well as anal-oral encounters in males who have sex with males.
- After ingestion, giardia excysts in the stomach to produce trophozoites (Fig. 52.4). These attach to the small bowel mucosa and can cause villous blunting and crypt hypertrophy.
- Diarrhea usually begins 1–2 weeks after infection.
- Patients tend to have greasy stools with a foul odor and often have other accompanying symptoms such as abdominal cramps, nausea, anorexia, weight loss, vomiting, and fever.

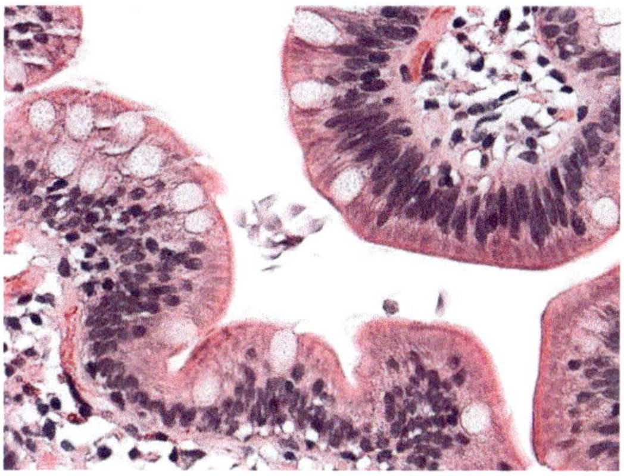

Fig. 52.4 Duodenal giardiasis. Pale pink organisms are identified in the lumen. No architectural distortion or inflammation is seen. (Courtesy of Jeanette R. Burgess, MD)

- Many patients are either asymptomatic or have a benign course.
- Chronic cases, especially in children, can lead to malabsorption and growth retardation.
- Stool ova and parasite examination can easily make the diagnosis.
- Endoscopy to obtain small bowel or duodenal biopsy is sometimes used when stool assays are inconclusive.
- The mainstay of treatment is the nitroimidazole class of drugs. Metronidazole 250 mg three times a day for 7 days is the most common regimen, though not FDA-approved (Table 52.2). Tinidazole 2 g as a single dose is better tolerated.

Schistosomiasis

- Schistosomiasis is primarily caused by three species of trematodes: *Schistosoma haematobium*, *S. mansoni*, and *S. japonicum*.
- It is one of the most prevalent helminthic infections worldwide.
- Depending on the organ that is damaged, schistosomiasis can lead to dermatitis, Katayama fever, obstructive uropathy, bladder cancer, intestinal fistulas and strictures, hepatosplenic disease, pulmonary hypertension, glomerulonephritis, and neural and spinal cord pathology.
- Intestinal schistosomiasis can cause abdominal symptoms such as pain and diarrhea and can lead to more complicated issues such as fistulas, ulcers, and polyposis.
- In rare cases, perforation or obstruction can occur, necessitating the need for surgical intervention.
- Diagnosis is typically made by identification of eggs in the stool by microscopy.
- Serologic assays, radiographs, and endoscopy can also assist in making the diagnosis.
- Colonoscopy may show erosions and petechial and superficial ulcerations, and tissue biopsy can identify the eggs in the colonic mucosa.
- The mainstay of treatment is a praziquantel given as a single dose of 40 mg/kg (Table 52.2). Cure rates in excess of 85% have been described.

Tapeworms

- Tapeworms are cestodes, or parasitic flatworms.
- Patients with *T. saginata* may feel the motile proglottids passing through the anus. Remarkably, they can grow as long as 55 feet (Fig. 52.5).
- Symptomatic patients complain of vague abdominal pain and cramps, nausea, vomiting, anorexia, and weight loss.
- Diagnosis is made by analyzing the parasite using microscopy or by using ELISA or PCR technology.
- Infection with *D. latum* results from eating raw fish.
- Chronic infection can lead to megaloblastic anemia because the broad tapeworm attaches in the ileum.
- The worms can sometimes obstruct small ducts and cause cholangitis, pancreatitis, or appendicitis.
- The treatment for all the tapeworms is a single dose of praziquantel 5–10 mg/kg or niclosamide 2 g (Table 52.2).
- A bowel preparation may be recommended a few hours after treatment to help purge remaining proglottids.

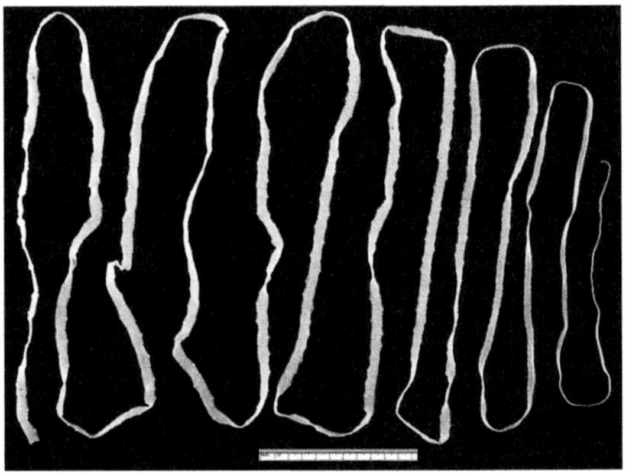

Fig. 52.5 *Taenia saginata* adult worm measures approximately 4 meters in length. These worms may grow to over 50 feet (Available from http://phil.cdc.gov/Phil/details.asp)

Trypanosoma

- Trypanosomiasis (Chagas disease) is caused by *Trypanosoma cruzi*, a flagellate protozoan parasite.
- There are two clinical manifestations of Chagas disease: acute and chronic.
- The acute stage follows parasite entry through the skin. Many patients are asymptomatic, but some may show vague signs like malaise, fever, peripheral edema, periorbital edema, hepatosplenomegaly, and lymphadenopathy.
- After the acute stage, the body enters an indeterminate stage where many stay asymptomatic for life.
- Ten to thirty percent of patients develop symptomatic chronic Chagas disease, which can lead to cardiomyopathy and megadisease, namely, megaesophagus and megacolon.
- For unclear reasons, the parasite causes destruction of neurons in the lining of the gastrointestinal tract, which leads to dilatation and dysfunction. The sigmoid colon is the most affected segment.
- Patients usually complain of constipation and abdominal pain from distention.
- Volvulus and bowel ischemia necessitating surgery can occur in severe cases.
- Treatment for megacolon is primarily conservative with high fiber diet, laxative, and enemas. Fecalomas requiring disimpaction can be common.
- All patients with acute and chronic Chagas should be treated medically. The two drugs available are benznidazole and nifurtimox (Table 52.2). Both have significant side effect profiles with gastrointestinal and central nervous system (CNS) toxicities.

Viral Colitides

Cytomegalovirus

- *Cytomegalovirus* (CMV) is a DNA virus and member of the herpesvirus family.
- The prevalence of the virus is quite high with rates approaching 60–70% in US cities and close to 100% in various parts of Africa.
- Most immunocompetent patients with CMV are asymptomatic, whereas immunodeficient hosts can suffer from life-threatening illness.
- Similar to other viruses in the herpes family, once primary infection occurs, the virus will enter a latent/dormant state.
- It can be challenging to differentiate between reactivation of latent infection versus primary infection.
- In immunocompromised patients, CMV can cause devastating illness to organ systems such as the lungs, liver, brain, gastrointestinal tract, heart, and even skin.
- Colitis related to CMV is most common in patients with AIDS or inflammatory bowel disease.
- Patients can present with ulcers and inflammation in the esophagus and throughout the colon, which can lead to pain, diarrhea, and fever.
- Severe CMV colitis can cause perforation and gangrene requiring urgent surgical intervention.
- Diagnosis of CMV is typically made by biopsy of infected tissue. Cells with CMV have "owl's eye" inclusion bodies, which are pathognomonic (Fig. 52.6).
- Flexible endoscopy is also very useful and can show friability, erythema, and heaped-up tissue resembling a mass (Fig. 52.7).
- PCR assays are available to assist with diagnosis.
- *Cytomegalovirus* reactivation is common in patients with severe colitis, with a reported

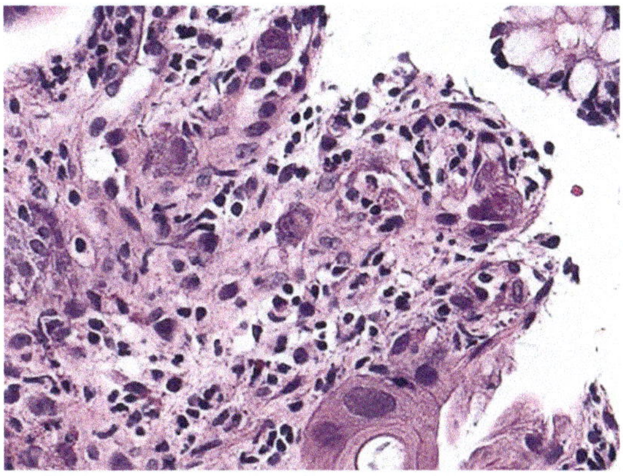

Fig. 52.6 CMV owl's eye inclusion bodies

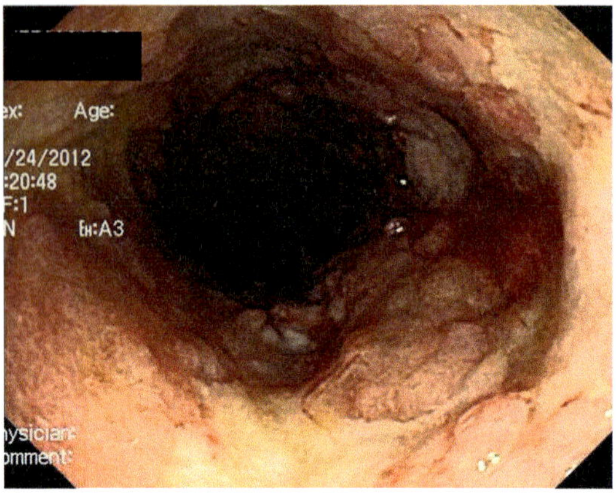

Fig. 52.7 Endoscopic appearance of CMV colitis in the descending colon

prevalence of 4.5–16.6% and as high as 25% in patients requiring colectomy for severe colitis.

- CMV is an important cause of treatment failure in patients with UC.
- There are four main drugs used in the treatment of CMV: ganciclovir, foscarnet, valacyclovir, and cidofovir.

Other Viruses

- Herpes simplex virus (HSV) is also a DNA virus and member of the herpesvirus family.
- There are two main strains, HSV-1 and HSV-2.
- The prevalence of HSV-2 may be as high as 20% in the United States and can approach nearly 50% in countries in South America and Africa.
- HSV-2 is the main cause of recurrent genital infections and proctitis.
  - Patients with proctitis can present with anal pain, bloody discharge, tenesmus, bleeding, sacral paresthesias, and difficulty urinating. The majority of the cases of proctitis are in patients who have rectal intercourse.
  - The disease is usually limited to the distal 10 cm of the rectum. Endoscopic features include ulceration and necrosis.
  - Culturing open sores or rectal aspirate can typically make the diagnosis.
  - PCR tests and serum testing for antibodies can also aid in identifying HSV.
- There is no cure for herpes, but outbreaks can be controlled with acyclovir 400 mg 3 times a day for 7–10 days.
- Other viruses can cause colitis, but they are usually found in immunocompromised or AIDS patients.

Fungal Colitides

Histoplasma

- Histoplasmosis, caused by *Histoplasma capsulatum*, is endemic in the Ohio and Mississippi river valleys.
- Though it is most commonly known for causing a pulmonary infection, *Histoplasma* can lead to progressive disseminated histoplasmosis (PDH) causing life-threatening illness in many organ systems, especially in immunocompromised hosts.
- Gastrointestinal involvement is most common in subacute PDH.
- Ulcerations of the small and large bowel are present in many cases, with the terminal ileum and cecum being the most frequently involved areas.
- Severe cases may have deep ulcerations with pseudopolyps, which may appear similar to adenocarcinoma or inflammatory bowel disease.
- Diagnosis is made by tissue culture or tissue histology showing granulomas and yeast within the mucosa.
- Surgery is reserved for cases of perforation, obstruction, or failure to respond to medical therapy. In many occasions, the diagnosis is not known preoperatively.
- The mainstay of medical treatment is intravenous amphotericin B. Itraconazole may be used in mild cases or when amphotericin is not tolerated.

Candida

- The *Candida* species are not typically pathogenic in patients unless immune systems are compromised.

- Nearly every organ system in the body can be affected by candidiasis.
- Candidal infections of the colon are uncommon as only a handful of case series and case reports have been published in the literature.
- Patients are often very ill with diffuse abdominal pain and diarrhea.
- Flexible endoscopy may show white curd-like plaques on the mucosa.
- Visualizing the budding yeast and hyphae with culture or biopsy makes the diagnosis.
- Treatment depends on the severity of the disease. Fluconazole at varying doses and varying lengths is commonly used.
- Surgery is reserved in cases of perforation or peritonitis.
- Mortality is high in this patient population because of the concomitant immunosuppression.

Other Fungi

- Aspergillosis, caused by the mold *Aspergillus*, is another fungal infection primarily in the immunocompromised patient.
  - Though the most common clinical manifestation is pulmonary, gastrointestinal-invasive aspergillosis is possible in disseminated cases.
  - These patients present with fever, abdominal pain, tenderness, and bleeding.
  - Bowel resection is required in cases of ischemia and bowel perforation.
  - Demonstration of characteristic hyphae from biopsy specimens or from culture makes the diagnosis.
  - Treatment is with voriconazole and a second-line agent is amphotericin B.
- Cryptococcosis, caused by *Cryptococcus neoformans* and *Cryptococcus gattii*, primarily affects the lung and the central nervous system.
  - Risk factors for infection are disease states that cause immunosuppression, such as AIDS, transplantation, steroid use, cancer, and sarcoidosis.
  - Cryptococcus can however affect any organ system in the body.
  - Within the gastrointestinal tract, it can cause colitis and occasional spontaneous perforation.
  - Nodules and ulcers in the stomach and small intestine, which can resemble Crohn's disease, may occur.
  - Diagnosis is made by microscopy of biopsy specimens or culture of bodily fluids.
  - Treatment in severe cases is intravenous amphotericin B.

Special Situations

Traveler's Diarrhea

- Travelers to low-income parts of the world frequently have the misfortune of developing acute diarrhea.
- Disease is characterized by 3 or more unformed stools in 24 h associated with other gastrointestinal issues, such as abdominal cramping, tenesmus, nausea, vomiting, fever, or urgency of bowel movements.
- Cruise ship passengers and staff are at risk for outbreaks of norovirus, which may be difficult to contain once started.
- The average duration of untreated traveler's diarrhea is 4–5 days, with average incapacitation of less than a day. Most travelers are able to continue their activity unaltered.
- More than 10% will present with diarrhea after returning home.
- Traveler's diarrhea is caused by various forms of *Escherichia coli* in more than 50% of cases.
- *Campylobacter*, *Shigella*, and *Salmonella* are the other frequent bacterial etiologies.
- Parasites tend to cause more prolonged diarrhea, with *Giardia lamblia* and *Entamoeba histolytica* the most common.
- Many organisms can cause diarrhea, but bloody diarrhea is typically the result of *Shigella*, *Salmonella*, *E. coli* 0157, *Campylobacter*, and *Entamoeba histolytica*.
- Laboratory investigation is indicated when the diarrhea is severe, bloody, or prolonged.
- This should include stool culture and microscopy looking for parasites. Antigen testing is

indicated if *Giardia*, *Cryptosporidium*, or *Entamoeba* is suspected.

- Prophylactic bismuth subsalicylate has been shown to reduce diarrhea rate by 65% when given 4 times daily but, due to its salicylate component, should be used with caution in patients at risk for bleeding.
- Rifaximin, which is an antibiotic that is poorly absorbed from the intestinal tract, significantly reduced the incidence of traveler's diarrhea in a meta-analysis of over 500 patients.
- The use of probiotics has not been shown to be beneficial.
- Systemic antibiotics reduce the incidence of traveler's diarrhea by more than 90%, with fluoroquinolones most frequently used.
- Concerns about adverse reactions and bacterial resistance make antibiotic prophylaxis controversial, and prophylaxis is not currently recommended for most travelers.
- High-risk patients may benefit from prophylaxis and include patients with a history of stroke, insulin-dependent diabetes mellitus, chronic renal failure, and inflammatory bowel disease as well as patients with ileostomies or colostomies.
- Self-treatment in the event of illness should include oral hydration, treatment with loperamide, and a 1–3-day course of a fluoroquinolone.

Infections in Inflammatory Bowel Disease

- Infectious complications are a major concern in patients with inflammatory bowel disease (IBD).
- Numerous pathogens can play a role in enteric infections, including *Clostridium difficile*, *Salmonella*, *Shigella*, *Campylobacter*, *Escherichia coli*, *Cytomegalovirus*, and *Entamoeba histolytica*.
- These infections increase risk of hospitalization as well as colectomy in patients with inflammatory bowel disease.
- *Clostridium difficile* infection (CDI) in IBD may be atypical and present with bloody stools and in younger patient age.
- CDI should be considered in the absence of diarrhea in patients with constitutional symptoms and leukocytosis.
- Small bowel CDI may occur after colectomy in IBD patients.
  - Medications used to treat inflammatory bowel disease are all associated with infections. Purine antimetabolites predispose to infections by some of the herpes viruses, with *Cytomegalovirus* a major cause of colitis.
  - Immunosuppression with corticosteroids increases the risk of candidal infections.
  - TNF antagonists increase risk of granulomatous infections, such as extrapulmonary tuberculosis.
- CMV infection is very prevalent in patients with inflammatory disease, with an incidence as high as 33%.
  - Many of these patients are "innocent bystanders," and the diagnosis of active CMV disease can be challenging.
  - CMV colitis can clearly complicate IBD colitis and should strongly be considered in steroid-resistant cases.

Diarrhea and HIV

- Nearly all patients infected with HIV develop some sort of gastrointestinal complication.
- Colitis can produce symptoms such as abdominal pain, tenesmus, and urgency. The list of pathogens that can cause colitis is extensive and includes bacteria, viruses, and parasites (Table 52.3).
- Workup of diarrhea in an HIV-infected patient begins with the assessment of the disease itself (i.e., CD4 count and HIV viral load).
- Other tests include stool microscopy for ova, cysts and parasites, bacterial culture, and *Clostridium difficile* toxin and PCR testing for parasites and viruses.

Table 52.3 Pathogens causing enterocolitis in HIV patients

Bacteria
Campylobacter jejuni
Salmonella
Shigella flexneri
Aeromonas hydrophila
Plesiomonas shigelloides
Yersinia enterocolitica
Vibrio
Mycobacterium avium complex
Escherichia coli (enterotoxigenic, enteroadherent)
Bacterial overgrowth
Clostridium difficile
Parasites
Cryptosporidium parvum
Microsporidia
Cystoisospora belli
Entamoeba histolytica
Giardia lamblia
Cyclospora cayetanensis
Viruses
Cytomegalovirus
Adenovirus
Calicivirus
Astrovirus
Picobirnavirus
Human immunodeficiency virus
Fungi
Histoplasma capsulatum

With permission from Bennett J, Dolin R, Blaser MJ. Mandell, Douglas, and Bennett's principles and practice of infectious diseases. 8th ed. Philadelphia: Saunders Elsevier; 2015 © Elsevier

- Colonoscopy allows for visualization and biopsy of the colonic and terminal ileum mucosa for histologic analysis and CMV PCR.
- Not all cases require flexible endoscopy, but in culture-negative patients, endoscopy can help make the diagnosis in 50% of cases.
- An algorithm for evaluating patients with HIV-associated diarrhea is shown in Fig. 52.8.

Diarrhea and Solid Organ Transplantation

- Due to the high levels of immunosuppression needed to prevent graft rejection, solid organ transplantation patients are also at higher risk for infectious gastrointestinal complications.
- Estimates of diarrhea in this population range from 22% to 52%.
- Infectious etiologies are the most common cause of diarrhea in solid organ transplant patients, whereas graft versus host disease (GVHD) is the most common cause of diarrhea in stem cell transplant patients.
- *Cytomegalovirus* (CMV) and *Clostridium difficile* are the two most common culprits.
- Workup typically starts with stool culture, *Clostridium difficile* toxin assay, and blood CMV viral load.
- Colonoscopy can be useful as a second-line test. Other tests include fecal leukocytes, ova and parasites, *Isospora* and *Cyclospora* assays, *Cryptosporidium* antigen screen, and *Norovirus* PCR.
- Treatment of the diarrhea is geared to the identified agent.
- Modifications of immunosuppression dosages and regimen may be required.

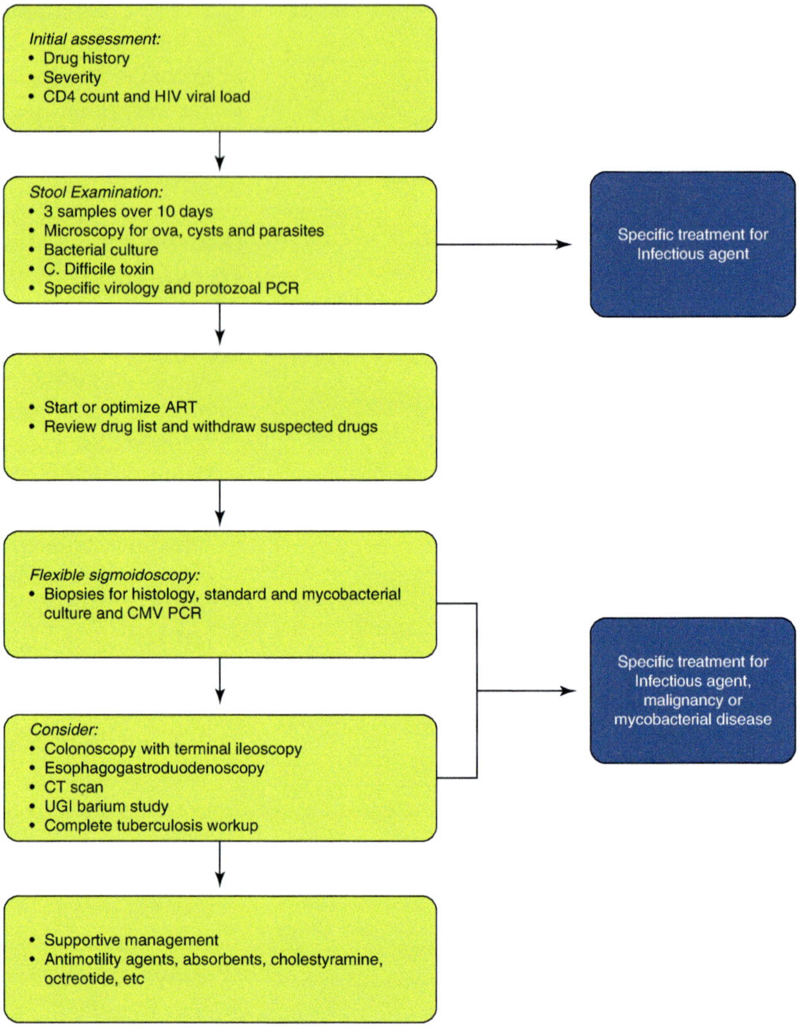

Fig. 52.8 Algorithm showing the management approach to the HIV patient with diarrhea (With permission from Feasey NA, Healey P, Gordon MA. Review article: the aetiology, investigation and management of diarrhoea in the HIV-positive patient. Alimt Pharm There. 2011;34(6): 587–603. © John Wiley and Sons)

Clostridium difficile Infection

53

David B. Stewart

Key Concepts

- The incidence and severity of C. difficile infection is increasing worldwide.
- Testing for C. difficile infection has transitioned to the more sensitive nucleic acid amplification tests (NAATs).
- Exposure to healthcare facilities, prior antibiotic therapy, and proton pump inhibitor usage are common risk factors for infection.
- The preponderance of studies suggests that infection with ribotype 027 is associated with worse disease outcomes.
- The mainstay of therapy is resuscitation and treatment with either metronidazole and/or vancomycin.
- Fecal transfer appears to be a promising potential therapy.
- Surgery can be avoided in most patients but should be considered in cases of continued clinical deterioration despite maximal medical therapy.

D. B. Stewart (✉)
Section Chief, Colorectal Surgery,
University of Arizona - Banner University Medical Center, Tucson, AZ, USA
e-mail: dbstewart@surgery.arizona.edu

Introduction

- Clostridium difficile infection (CDI) has transitioned from being a relatively uncommon diarrheal illness principally limited to those patients rendered immunocompetent from cancer treatment or HIV to a billion dollar per year hospital-acquired infection with a diverse at-risk patient population.
- This epidemiological shift has placed every inpatient at higher relative risk for developing CDI.
- CDI has the potential to reach life-threatening severity, requiring urgent surgical intervention.

Epidemiology

Rising Incidence and Increasing Severity

- During the previous two decades, there has been a population level increase in the incidence of CDI both in the United States and Western Europe.
- C. difficile is the predominant form of antibiotic-associated diarrheal illnesses in acute care facilities.
- In 2009, there were 336,600 hospitalizations which involved CDI either as a primary or a secondary diagnosis, comprising 1% of all hospitalizations in the United States.

S. R. Steele et al. (eds.), *The ASCRS Manual of Colon and Rectal Surgery*,
https://doi.org/10.1007/978-3-030-01165-9_53

- Likewise, the Centers for Disease Control and Prevention (CDC) reported that between 1993 and 2009, hospital stays affected by CDI increased fourfold.
- The impact of this rising incidence on healthcare costs translates into an over 3 billion dollar annual burden to the US healthcare system, when costs from inpatient and outpatient treatments are included.
- Of even greater concern, multiple regions have reported an increase in disease severity.
- The emergence of at least one ribotype of C. difficile (ribotype 027) during outbreaks of severe disease provides further evidence of a change in CDI in healthcare facilities.
  - Certain genetic characteristics of this ribotype suggest that this strain of bacterium may have certain selective advantages toward epidemical forms of the infection.

Clinical Risk Factors for CDI

- The literature is replete with long lists of clinical factors identified as being frequently associated with the development of CDI.
  - In many cases, these risk factors are not causally related to CDI in an independent manner; in most cases the one commonality which they share is a frequent contact with acute or chronic healthcare facilities.
- A distinction must first be made between healthcare facility-acquired CDI and, the rarer form of the disease, community-acquired CDI (CA-CDI).
- A generally accepted definition for CA-CDI centers on the onset of disease at least 12 weeks after any personal contact with a healthcare facility.
- Approximately 35% of patients have not received antibiotics within 40 days of developing symptoms of CDI.
- 14% of CA-CDI patients require an ICU admission, while only 1% require surgery.
- CA-CDI is probably not a disease with a distinct pathophysiology as compared to healthcare-acquired CDI.
- For the remainder of the chapter, unless otherwise specified, CDI will refer to healthcare facility-acquired, healthcare facility-onset CDI.

Advanced Age

- Advanced age is one of the most frequently cited risk factors for CDI; age serves as a risk factor by its association with many other risk factors which are causative.

Contact with a Healthcare Facility

- The primary mode of disease transmission in care settings is person to person through a fecal-oral transmission route.
- The estimated prevalence of asymptomatic colonization of adult patients admitted to an acute care setting ranges from 7% to 26% and may be as high as 5–7% among elderly subjects in subacute or long-term care facilities.

Use of Antibiotics and Their Effect on the Microbiome

- The most important, and the most modifiable, of all risk factors for CDI revolve is the use of antibiotics.
- The manner in which antibiotics effect the development of CDI, however, is much more complex than previously recognized.
- Antibiotics of any class increase the risk of CDI; this risk increases with the number of agents and length of use.
- There are dose-dependent relationships and cumulative dose associations between the use of antibiotics and the development of CDI.
- Second-, third-, and fourth-generation cephalosporins (OR = 2.23–3.2), clindamycin (OR = 2.8), and fluoroquinolones (OR = 1.6) are associated with higher odds of developing CDI.

- The primary difference between healthy and unhealthy gut environments is a matter of microbial population density and diversity.
  - High microbial counts with a high degree of species diversity are associated with relative resistance to CDI.
- While antibiotics reduce floral diversity and density through their indiscriminate killing of bacteria, their effect on the development of CDI may also be mediated by bile salts in the gut.
  - Antibiotics change the proportion of bile salts present in the colon, increasing cholate concentrations, which may result in greater germination of C. difficile spores.

Perioperative Prophylactic Antibiotics and Mechanical Bowel Preparations

- Mechanical bowel preparations do not significantly elevate the risk of CDI.
- The effect that prophylactic parenteral antibiotics have on the incidence of CDI is unclear; however, patients with relatively recent hospitalizations are at risk for developing CDI even after a single dose of prophylactic antibiotics due to their status as an asymptomatic carrier.
- Though infrequent, a single dose of antibiotics can potentially lead to CDI.

Immunocompromised States

- There is a clear association between an immunocompromised state and the development of CDI.

Inflammatory Bowel Disease (IBD)

- CDI is associated with both ulcerative colitis (UC) and Crohn's disease (CD).
- The incidence of CDI in IBD subjects ranges from 6% to 20%.
  - IBD populations may harbor an innate immune dysregulation, which can lead to a chronic dysbiosis.
  - The more frequent need for hospitalizations and antibiotics and the frequent use of immunosuppressive medications produce a merging of host and environmental factors promoting CDI.
- The development of CDI in the setting of a flare of IBD symptoms is associated with a higher rate of surgery.

Proton Pump Inhibitors

- The weight of the current evidence support the concept that PPIs place patients at risk for CDI.
- It is suggested that PPIs promote CDI by alkalinizing the stomach so a greater number of ingested C. difficile survive.
- PPIs (and H2 blockers) may have other mechanisms by which they promote CDI.

Hospital Environmental Factors

- Hand hygiene is effective at preventing the transmission of *C. difficile* (both spores and active bacteria) in acute and subacute care settings.
- Soap and water are better at removing spores from hands than alcohol-based cleansers.
- Isolation techniques for patients with CDI, including dedicated toilets and terminal cleaning programs, can decrease institutional CDI rates.

Microbiological Considerations for Clostridium difficile

Pathogenicity Locus Genes

- *Clostridium difficile* is a variably motile, gram-positive obligate anaerobe.
- That portion of *C. difficile's* genome most responsible for human disease is referred to as

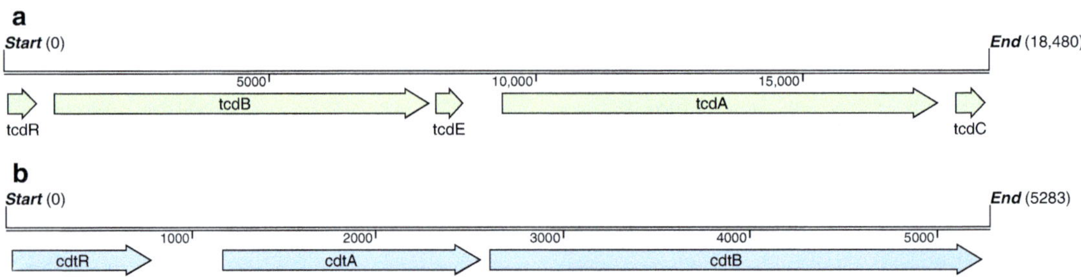

Fig. 53.1 Schematic demonstrating the regulatory and toxin genes of the pathogenicity locus (upper portion) and the binary toxin genes (lower portion)

the pathogenicity locus (PaLoc) (Fig. 53.1), which encodes for toxins A (tcdA) and B (tcdB).

- The presence of binary toxin and a tcdC truncation may be associated with a higher incidence of recurrent CDI.

Diagnosis of C. difficile Infection

Clinical Presentation

- CDI is a toxin-mediated disease whose hallmark feature is diarrhea.
- Asymptomatic carriage occurs among patients and healthcare workers, where exposure to *C. difficile* is endemic.
- Patients who maintain a carriage state without symptoms of CDI have the ability to develop an antibody to toxins A and B.
- For the majority of patients, if there is no diarrhea, there is no CDI.
  - The one notable, albeit rare, exception would be those patients who have such life-threatening colitis from CDI, who have associated ileus.
- Other signs and symptoms (such as tachycardia, abdominal distention, abdominal pain/peritonitis, and hypotension) are variably associated with CDI depending on its severity.
- CT scan findings can include bowel wall thickening, pericolic fat stranding, megacolon, and ascites in severe infections (Figs. 53.2 and 53.3).
- Though segmental colitis with CDI is possible, in most cases, either a left-sided colitis or pancolitis will be observed.

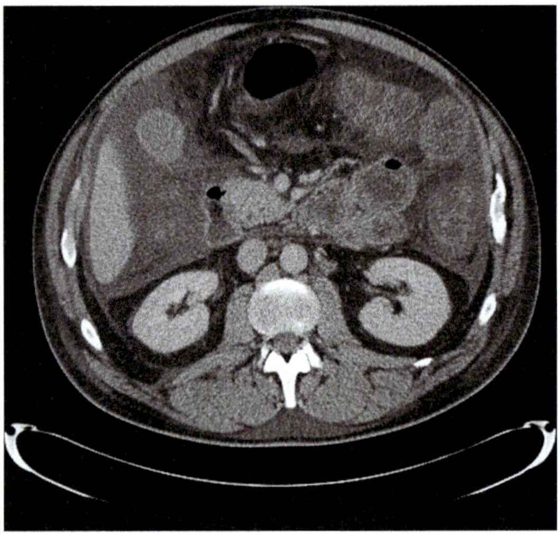

Fig. 53.2 CT findings in a patient with severe, complicated CDI. Note the presence of ascites and the mural thickening of the left colon

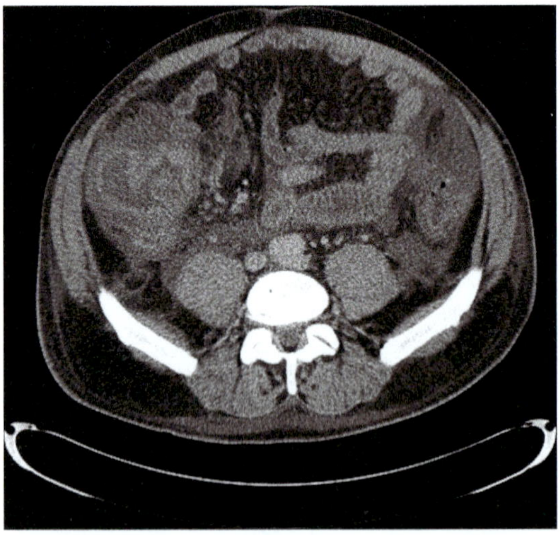

Fig. 53.3 Severe, complicated CDI with characteristic cecal thickening. Colonic wall thickening to this degree is typical of fulminant CDI

- Pneumoperitoneum and portal venous gas are uncommon radiographic features.
- Plain films and ultrasound have little, if any, utility in diagnosing or managing this infection.

Laboratory Diagnosis

- Enzyme immunoassay testing against toxins A and B has > 80% sensitivity and > 90% specificity.
- Many hospitals have transitioned to real-time PCR, which is sufficiently sensitive and specific in diagnosing toxigenic *C. difficile*.
- Routine retesting to confirm eradication of the infection is not recommended as part of routine clinical practice.

Clinical Severity Scores

- There are several clinical severity guidelines, including those published by the Infectious Diseases Society of America/Society for Hospital Epidemiology in America (IDSA/SHEA) and the American College of Gastroenterology.
  - The IDSA guidelines define mild or moderate CDI as being associated with a white blood cell count (WBC) < 15,000 cells/μL and serum creatinine < 1.5 times the patient's premorbid level.
  - Severe CDI is then defined as disease exceeding these two indices, while "severe, complicated" disease is CDI accompanied by hypotension, ileus, or megacolon.
  - The ACG guidelines define mild CDI as diarrhea without other abnormalities, and severe CDI includes those patients with either a WBC ≥ 15,000 cells/μL or a serum albumin of < 3 gm/dL.
  - Moderate CDI then would range between mild and severe disease.
  - Complicated CDI is defined as anyone requiring ICU admission, a temperature ≥ 38.5 °C, ileus, significant abdominal distention, altered mental status, a WBC either > 35,000 or < 2000 cells/μL, a serum lactate > 2.2 mmol/L, or any evidence of organ dysfunction.
- Virtually all of the patients treated by surgeons will fall into the severe, complicated categories of disease, yet most of these patients will not require surgery.
- The more common aberrant WBC finding in CDI is an extreme leukocytosis, with counts of 50,000 cells/μL or higher being common.
- An exaggerated leukocytosis may be driven both by toxigenic and non-toxigenic factors and may not be directly related to the severity of colitis.
- Serum creatinine and lactate levels may better reflect disease severity.

Antibiotic Therapy for CDI

Metronidazole and Vancomycin

- There are primarily two agents used for treating CDI: metronidazole and vancomycin.
- Metronidazole may be provided in a parenteral route and its cost as far lower than oral vancomycin. The dosage should be 500 mg three times daily for 10–14 days.
- For mild CDI, rates of clinical cure are not significantly different between metronidazole and vancomycin.
- Failure to respond to metronidazole therapy within the first 5–7 days of treating mild-to-moderate CDI should prompt a change to vancomycin.
- There is no evidence to support oral vancomycin combined with oral metronidazole, especially for milder forms of CDI.
- For severe CDI, vancomycin has been associated with higher rates of cure (97% vs. 76%, $p = 0.02$).
- Oral vancomycin is dosed at 125 mg four times daily for 10–14 days.
- For severe, complicated CDI, recommendations are for oral vancomycin (if tolerated) 500 mg four times daily.
  - This subset of patients will often require vancomycin enemas due to factors such as an ileus.

  - The addition of parenteral metronidazole at 500 mg every 8 h is also recommended by IDSA/SHEA.
- For recurrent CDI, recommendations are to repeat a course of treatment using the same agent from the preceding course.
- Second recurrences are generally approached with vancomycin given in pulsed or tapered manner.
- More recent data suggests that vancomycin should be used both for first recurrences and all first CDI episodes in patients with inflammatory bowel disease.

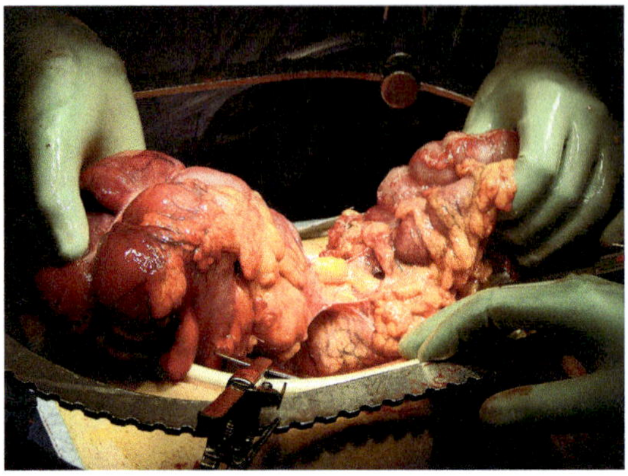

Fig. 53.4 Patient with fulminant CDI with a dilated and thickened colon, with telangiectasias and serositis indicative of severe, transmural inflammation mediated by C. difficile toxins

Fidaxomicin

- Fidaxomicin is a macrocyclic compound which has a more limited spectrum of activity than many other antimicrobials.
- Clinical rates of cure are non-inferior compared to vancomycin (92.1% vs. 89.8%, respectively).
- Lower recurrence rates are observed with fidaxomicin.
- A meta-analysis concluded that while clinical cure rates were quite similar between fidaxomicin and vancomycin (OR = 1.17), relapse rates and sustained cure rates are improved in those treated with fidaxomicin.
- Fidaxomicin is dosed at 200 mg twice daily for 10 days for mild-to-moderate CDI.

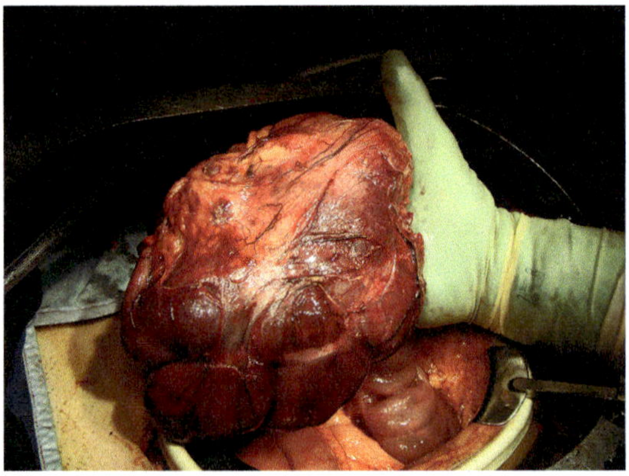

Fig. 53.5 Non-confluent regions of transmural ischemia observed in a patient with fulminant CDI. The combination of bacterial toxins as well as septic shock can produce non-viable large intestine

Surgery for CDI

- The incidence of patients with CDI who require surgery is probably less than 5% (Figs. 53.4, 53.5, and 53.6).
- Although surgery is reserved for patients who have "failed maximal medical therapy," defining when medical therapy has been adequate is often hard to judge.
- A strong association exists between postoperative mortality and preoperative findings of septic shock as well as other manifestations of

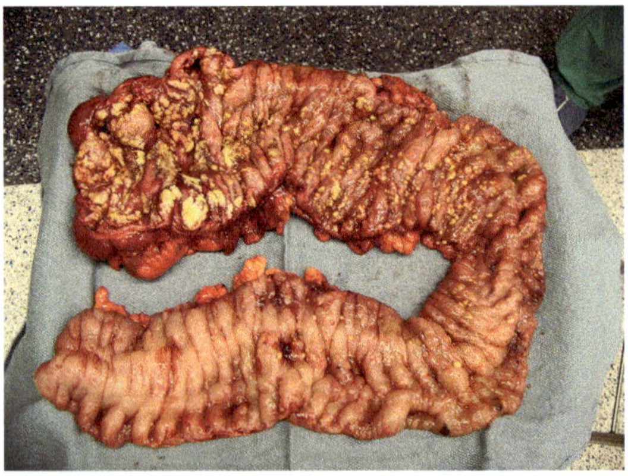

Fig. 53.6 Gross findings of mucosal thickening, inflammation, and pseudopolyps, consistent with severe CDI

organ failure such as acute renal failure and the need for intubation.

- Total colectomy with end ileostomy is the preferred surgery for fulminant CDI failing medical therapy.
- Partial colectomy is associated with an approximately 16% need for reoperation.
- Construction of a loop ileostomy, intraoperative lavage of the colon, and followed by postoperative lavage with intraluminal vancomycin have been successfully applied. The precise indications for this surgical approach are uncertain at the present time.

Fecal Microbiota Transplant (FMT)

- FMT involves the use of donor stool applied to patients with CDI either via a nasogastric/nasoduodenal tube or, more commonly, by lower endoscopy.
- The mechanism of action involves increasing the bacterial population diversity and density, reestablishing healthy microbial communities.
- FMT creates a population shift in 16s rRNA surveys that closely approximate the taxa present in the stool of the FMT donor.
- FMT is effective in breaking the cycle of multiple recurrences of CDI.

Radiation, Microscopic, and Ischemic Colitis

54

Isabelle Raîche and Husein Moloo

Key Concepts

- Microscopic colitis is likely an underappreciated diagnosis. Although there is no "cure," the quality of life for a patient can be improved significantly with treatment.
- Budesonide is the only evidence-based treatment for microscopic colitis.
- Radiation colitis and proctitis range from acute to chronic, which require different management strategies. Patients can present with problems even after 30 years of being asymptomatic.
- Colorectal cancer risk is increased with pelvic radiation, and patients should be screened 5 years after completion of therapy.
- Surgical treatment for radiation proctitis/colitis should be individualized and based on the clinical context of the patient, as morbidity and mortality rates are high.
- Ischemic colitis represents the most common cause of gastrointestinal ischemia. There is a wide clinical spectrum ranging from mild cases with minimal mucosal ischemia to severe cases associated with transmural necrosis.

I. Raîche
Department of Surgery, The Ottawa Hospital, University of Ottawa, Ottawa, ON, Canada

H. Moloo (✉)
Department of Surgery, Ottawa Hospital Research Institute, University of Ottawa, Ottawa, ON, Canada
e-mail: hmoloo@toh.on.ca

Radiation Colitis

Introduction

- It is estimated that approximately 50% of cancer treatment protocols involve the use of radiation.
- With malignancies such as anal cancer increasing and an increasing number of cancer survivors, the colorectal surgeon will continue to encounter postradiation problems.

Pathogenesis of Radiation Injury

- The two main forms of radiation delivery are external beam radiation therapy (EBRT) and brachytherapy.
- External beam is delivered via linear accelerators which produce high-energy x-rays.
  - The planning is typically done in three dimensions with CT (computed tomography) images.
  - Gray (Gy) is the standard unit to indicate the amount of absorbed radiation.
  - Fractionation refers to giving the total dose over multiple sessions; fractionation is done to minimize collateral tissue damage while maximizing tumor destruction.
  - Conformal radiation refers to the use of metal plates (multileaf collimators) to bend the x-rays in order to target the tumor and minimize radiation to normal tissue.

S. R. Steele et al. (eds.), *The ASCRS Manual of Colon and Rectal Surgery*,
https://doi.org/10.1007/978-3-030-01165-9_54

- Brachytherapy refers to placement of the radiation source inside the body – i.e., beads or pellets.
- Radiation damage has been attributed to the "target cell" theory.
  - This theory focuses on the epithelium of the bowel and explains acute effects through damage done to cells that are rapidly proliferating.
  - The delayed effects are explained by damage to other target cells such as endothelial cells or fibroblasts, as their turnover is slower compared to intestinal epithelium.
  - The main addition to this concept is that other tissues/cells are part of the injury process. Therefore alterations to the gut microflora, immune system, microvasculature, and immune system are all thought to play a role in the symptoms induced by radiation.
- Higher BMI is protective against radiation-induced complications.
- Smoking is an adverse risk factor.
- Previous surgery with adhesive tissue fixation, inflammatory bowel disease, diabetes, vascular and collagen vascular disease, and genetic predisposition may also be contributing factors.
- The most important radiation-related factor is dosage.
  - Other factors that play a role are the length of bowel radiated, fractionation, and use of chemotherapy.
- Radiation effects can be considered acute or chronic.
  - Acute symptomatology refers to those that occur during treatment to 6 months after treatment is completed.
  - Chronic radiation symptoms can represent a continuation of the acute phase or occur after an asymptomatic period, commonly 8–12 months after therapy.
  - Radiation-related symptoms can begin 30 years after treatment.

Prevention

- There appears to be a higher rate of chronic problems in patients who experience severe acute proctitis. Severe acute injury leading to chronic changes is termed the "consequential" late effect.
  - However, the absence of acute symptoms does not preclude chronic changes and symptoms from occurring.
- The main goal with radiation delivery is to minimize damage to normal tissues surrounding the tumor.
  - Conformal radiation therapy (described above) is one of the main methods of doing this.
  - Intensity-modulated radiation therapy (IMRT) is a technology whereby different intensities of radiation can be given (high and low) within the planned field.
- Brachytherapy refers to when the source of radiation is implanted into the neoplasm (interstitial brachytherapy) or in a cavity which is close to the neoplasm (intracavitary brachytherapy).
  - It can be used alone or with external beam radiation therapy.
- Proton beam radiation is an area where more research regarding gastrointestinal toxicity is needed; theoretically, photon beam "stops" in the target tissue and collateral damage should be less.
- Patient positioning has been found to be an effective way of reducing radiation to the rectal wall, small bowel, and bladder (i.e., prone, Trendelenburg position).
  - Other strategies employ bladder distension, abdominal wall compression, and determining position based on pretreatment contrast studies.
- Operative maneuvers such as omental slings and tissue expanders can be used to avoid radiation damage post-resection.

Acute Radiation Colitis and Proctitis

- Radiation damages mitotic activity that is occurring in the base of crypts.
  - This can lead to diarrhea because of impaired absorption.
  - The barrier to bacteria is also affected and bacteremia can result.
- Motility is also affected through the creation of giant migrating complexes which reverts to normal after treatment is completed; this contributes to the diarrhea and cramping experienced by patients.
- Diarrhea is the most common acute symptom.
- Other acute symptoms include nausea, tenesmus, fatigue, and abdominal pain.
- Nearly all patients (50–75%) experience symptoms in the acute period, but these symptoms are usually self-limited. Consequently, treatment is usually supportive.
- Diarrhea, for example, can usually be controlled by antidiarrheal medications such as loperamide.
- Dietary modifications such as a lactose-free or low-fat diet may help.
- If first-line antidiarrheals such as loperamide are ineffective, octreotide can be used.

Chronic Radiation Colitis and Proctitis

- Chronic symptoms and complications from radiation can range in severity and quality of life impact.
- The Radiation Therapy Oncology Group (RTOG) and the European Organisation for Research and Treatment of Cancer (EORTC) have devised a grading system (Table 54.1).
- The pathophysiology of these complications is related to ischemic injury which induces fibrosis, atrophy, and vascular damage.
  - Fibrosis is thought to occur because of the reaction of fibroblasts to cytokines, growth factors, and chemokines.

Table 54.1 Late radiation effects on small/large intestine

Grade	Symptoms
0	None
1	Mild diarrhea, mild cramping, bowel movement five times per day, slight rectal discharge or bleeding
2	Moderate diarrhea and colic, bowel movement >5 times per day, excessive rectal mucus, and intermittent rectal bleeding
3	Obstruction or bleeding, requiring surgery
4	Necrosis/perforation, fistula
5	Death

  - Atrophy results from the killing of cells may contribute to malabsorption and strictures.
  - The vascular damage from radiation can lead to dilation of small blood vessels – this is manifested as telangiectasias. There can also be constriction of arterioles which leads to ischemia.
  - Fibrosis can progress over time and worsen the resultant ischemic injury.
  - The small vessel disease is what distinguishes chronic from acute radiation changes.

Diagnosis

- Bleeding can be seen because of telangiectasias or ulcerations from ischemia.
- Malabsorption leading to diarrhea may be caused by mucosal atrophy or strictures, leading to bacterial overgrowth.
- Radiation can also impact the nerves associated with gastrointestinal function and result in accelerated small- and large-bowel motility.
- Ischemic strictures can occur leading to obstruction.
- With full -thickness necrosis of the bowel wall, fistulas or free perforation can result.
- Surgery is complicated by the fact that anastomotic leak rates are higher when irradiated bowel is used.

- Diagnosis is usually made with endoscopy; telangiectasias, atrophy, and friable tissue are often observed.
- Biopsies can rule out processes such as inflammatory bowel disease, ischemic colitis, or drug-induced injury.
- Histologic features of radiation therapy vary with the interval between completion of radiation treatment and onset of symptoms.
  - Acute radiation injury (within 2–3 days after treatment) is characterized by surface epithelial damage, nuclear atypia with bizarre mitoses, attenuation and loss of crypt epithelium, increased apoptosis, and increased eosinophils with eosinophilic crypt abscesses.
  - In the chronic phase of radiation injury, superimposed episodes of ischemia or the presence of mucosal or submucosal fibrosis can mimic primary acute or chronic ischemic colitis.
  - The distinctive features of chronic radiation injury include dilated, thickened, and hyalinized blood vessels, reactive or bizarre-shaped endothelial cells, fibroblasts and myofibroblasts, and foamy cells within the arteries (obliterative arteritis) (Fig. 54.1).

Management

- Treatment of chronic radiation injury to the colon and rectum can be divided into medical, endoscopic, or surgical.

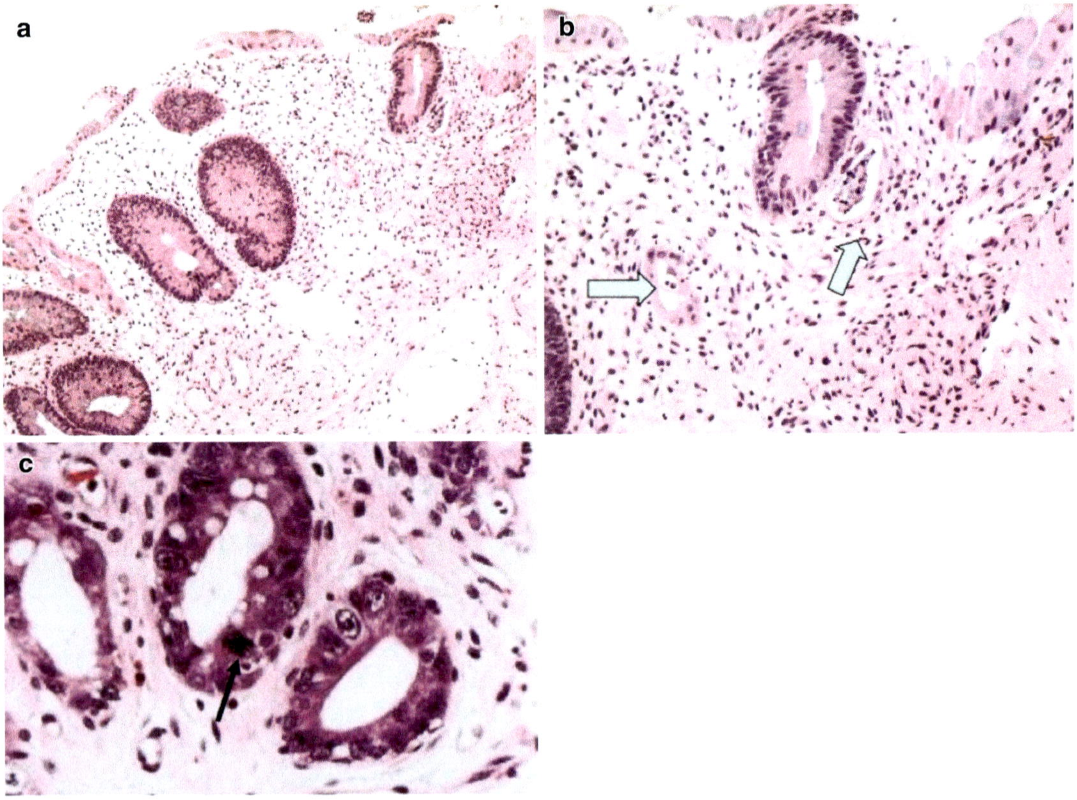

Fig. 54.1 Radiation-induced colitis. Colonic mucosa shows crypt distortion, crypt abscesses (thick arrows), and crypt atrophy, similar with inflammatory bowel disease. The crypt epithelium shows marked mucin depletion, regenerative nuclei, and mitotic figures (thin arrow). Bizarre stromal fibroblasts and endothelial cells may be seen in lamina propria. Vascular injury may be also seen (not shown). Hematoxylin and eosin, 100x, 200x, and 4000x. (Reproduced with permission from Celia Marginean MD)

Medications

- Medical treatment consists of topical versus systemic treatment.
- The main delivery method of topical treatment is via enema per rectum.
  - Sucralfate enemas have been endorsed for the treatment of chronic radiation injury in patients with rectal bleeding.
  - 5-ASA enemas have had mixed results, and there is no clear evidence of benefit.
  - Short-chain fatty acid enemas are of uncertain benefit.
  - Steroid enemas are not consistently been found to be effective in the treatment of radiation proctitis.
- Topical formalin therapy may be used to chemically cauterize the telangiectasias and ulcers that are bleeding and is effective in approximately 80% of cases.
  - The two main methods of delivery are via irrigation of formalin or direct application of a formalin-soaked gauze onto the mucosa usually via a rigid proctoscope.
  - After application, it is recommended that a washout of the formaldehyde is done.
  - Multiple applications may be required to achieve maximal efficacy, especially in those with severe proctitis or taking an antiplatelet agent.
  - Contact with the anoderm should be avoided as formalin can be irritating.
  - Potential complications include anal or pelvic pain, stricture, or rarely rectal wall necrosis and fistula formation.
  - There may be a higher complication rate in patients who have received radiation for anal cancer.
- Various vitamins, loperamide, and hyperbaric oxygen therapy also have some evidence of efficacy.

Endoscopy

- Endoscopic therapy plays a role not only in the diagnosis of radiation injury to the bowel but can be used for treatment.
- APC (argon plasma coagulation) is a safe and effective therapy, with bleeding cessation in 80–90% of cases.
  - APC coagulates to a reliable superficial depth.
  - As with formalin instillation, it can require multiple treatments.
  - Using near the dentate line may cause pain.
  - Complications are rare and typically consist of rectal pain and cramping.
- In one randomized trial comparing APC to formalin, there was no difference in outcomes, and both were found to be very effective in stopping bleeding (94% APC and 100% formalin).

Surgery

- Surgical treatment is required for patients whose symptoms cannot be managed with medical or endoscopic therapy and for complications such as perforation, fistula, or stricture/obstruction.
- Anastomotic leak rates are high when putting two pieces of radiated bowel together and lower if only one of the segments is irradiated.
- Pelvic fistulization can be one of the difficult problems that surgeons can encounter postradiation, most commonly rectovaginal or rectourethral fistulas.
  - Initial fecal diversion will likely be necessary.
  - The approach will then depend on factors such as how high the fistula is and whether it is most amenable to a perineal or abdominal approach.
  - Flap reconstruction for a low rectovaginal fistula (i.e., gracilis or Martius) or a coloanal anastomosis with interposition of well-vascularized tissues such as omentum for a higher fistula may be utilized.
  - In the most severe cases, proctectomy or pelvic exenteration type of procedures may be required.
- Colostomy or ileostomy may also resolve symptoms of pain, tenesmus, sepsis, incontinence, and obstruction and improve quality of

life to the point where further surgical intervention may not be needed.
  - Because dissection can be difficult in an irradiated pelvis, transverse and descending colostomies are safer than a sigmoid colostomy.
  - Diversion does not always help with bleeding, but there has been at least one retrospective study that has shown improvement with a stoma.
- Intestinal resection, diversion, and bypass may all offer symptomatic relief.
- Of the different surgical indications, fistula repair has the lowest success rate (55%) compared to stricture (78%), hemorrhage (64%), and perforation (100%).
- The surgical morbidity rate is a sobering 65% with a mortality rate of 7%.
- Treatment plans should be carefully individualized to the specific patient.

Microscopic Colitis

Introduction

- Microscopic colitis (MC) is a relatively common cause of non-bloody diarrhea.
- Two main types of MC have been described: collagenous colitis and lymphocytic colitis.
- Although milder disorders when compared to other inflammatory bowel disease, MC can have a significant impact on quality of life.

Epidemiology

- The incidence of microscopic colitis is increasing.
- MC has been found in all age groups; however, it is more common in the older population.
- Collagenous colitis is more common in women, while lymphocytic colitis is equally distributed between genders.
- The prevalence of collagenous colitis has been estimated at 39.3 per 100,000 persons vs. 63.7 for lymphocytic colitis.

Etiology and Risk Factors

- The cause of MC has been hypothesized to be multifactorial in origin.

Smoking

- Smoking has been associated with an increased risk of MC (OR 2.12).

Medications

- Evidence regarding the association between MC and medications is equivocal.

Autoimmunity

- In a survey of 116 patients with MC, 30.4% had an autoimmune condition; a particularly strong association was noted with celiac and thyroid disease.

Clinical Manifestations

Clinical Presentation

- Chronic, non-bloody, and watery diarrhea is the hallmark of this disease. It can occasionally lead to fecal incontinence, especially in the elderly.
- Weight loss is also common, being found in 41–46% of patients.
- Abdominal pain is more common in MC patients compared to controls.
- Lymphocytic and collagenous colitis cannot be differentiated based on clinical presentation.

Complications

- MC rarely leads to complications and is not associated with an increased risk of colorectal cancer.

Diagnosis

- Histopathology is the mainstay of diagnosis.
- Because of the nonspecific clinical presentation, the differential diagnosis is wide and includes inflammatory bowel disease, infectious colitis, medication-induced changes, celiac disease, malabsorption, and irritable bowel syndrome.
- Colonoscopy with two or more biopsies in the ascending, transverse, descending, and sigmoid colon, respectively, is the examination of choice.
- There tends to be patchy involvement occurring anywhere in the colon; however the disease is classically more severe in the right colon.
- Up to 30% of rectal biopsies are normal in patients with MC, underscoring the need to obtain biopsies throughout the colon.
- Most patients have a visually normal endoscopic exam, but endoscopic abnormalities have been described in a small number.
- The key histopathologic feature of collagenous colitis is subepithelial collagen layer thickening, although a variety of other microscopic features are associated.
- Findings with lymphocytic colitis include preserved crypt architecture, expanded lamina propria with numerous plasma cells, lymphocytes, and eosinophils. The crypt epithelium shows hyperchromatic, regenerative nuclei (Figs. 54.2 and 54.3).
- Figure 54.4 presents an algorithm to illustrate the pathologic diagnosis of MC.
- Laboratory analysis is usually nonspecific.
- Fecal calprotectin and lactoferrin are not consistently elevated (in contrast to inflammatory bowel disease), which limits their use in the diagnosis of MC.

Management

- There is no curative treatment for MC; the goal of the treatment is to control the symptoms.
- Patients should be advised to stop smoking and avoid any exacerbating dietary factors (dairy product, alcohol, caffeine).
- Long-term remission has been documented in 63–80% of patients.

Budesonide

- In a meta-analysis of nine randomized-controlled trials, budesonide was found superior to placebo to induce clinical and pathological response.
- However, the recurrence rate with treatment cessation is high.

Prednisolone

- Prednisolone is associated with more side effects than budesonide and has not been shown to be superior to placebo.

Cholestyramine and Loperamide

- Antidiarrheals are often recommended as the first line of treatment and seem to have the most benefit in patients with mild symptoms.
- Patients not responding to budesonide or with recurring symptoms should be tested for bile salt malabsorption; affected patients could benefit from cholestyramine.

Aminosalicylates

- Aminosalicylates do not appear to be better than placebo in achieving clinical remission.

Immunosuppressive and Anti-TNF Medications

- These medications are generally reserved for patients refractory to other types of medical management.

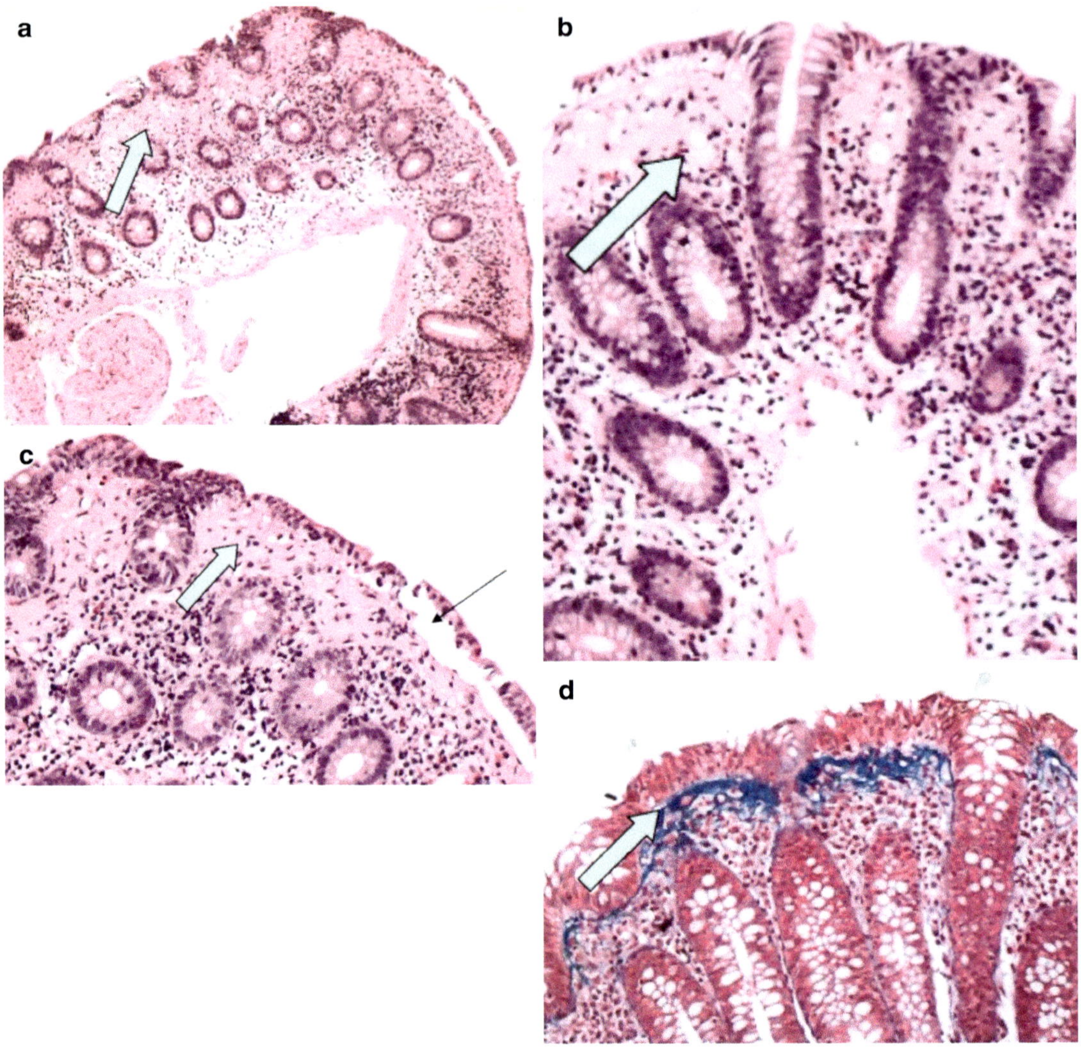

Fig. 54.2 Collagenous colitis. (**a**) Colonic mucosa shows preserved crypt architecture. The lamina propria is expanded by a mixed inflammatory infiltrate, including abundant plasma cells admixed with eosinophils and occasional neutrophils, mostly on the superficial portion underneath the surface epithelium. The crypt epithelium shows regenerative nuclear changes. On several areas, the epithelial collagen layer is moderately thickened. Focally, the collagen band has a lacy appearance and incorporates inflammatory cells and small capillaries. The surface epithelium shows markedly increased intraepithelial lymphocytes and focally is detached (split) from the mucosa. Hematoxylin and eosin, 100x. (**b**) Thick subepithelial collagen layer, incorporating micro-capillaries and inflammatory cells (thick arrows). Hematoxylin and eosin, 200x. (**c**) Thick subepithelial collagen layer, incorporating micro-capillaries and inflammatory cells, with splitting of the surface epithelium (thin arrow). Hematoxylin and eosin, 200x. (**d**) Thick subepithelial collagen layer (blue), incorporating micro-capillaries and inflammatory cells. Masson trichrome stain, 200x. (Reproduced with permission from Celia Marginean MD)

- Thiopurines achieved remission in 41% of patients; side effects included elevated liver enzymes and nausea/vomiting.
- Methotrexate in budesonide refractory MC has yielded conflicting results.
- Any role for anti-TNF therapy is unclear.

Bismuth Subsalicylate

- Bismuth subsalicylate has been widely used, but there is limited evidence confirming efficacy.

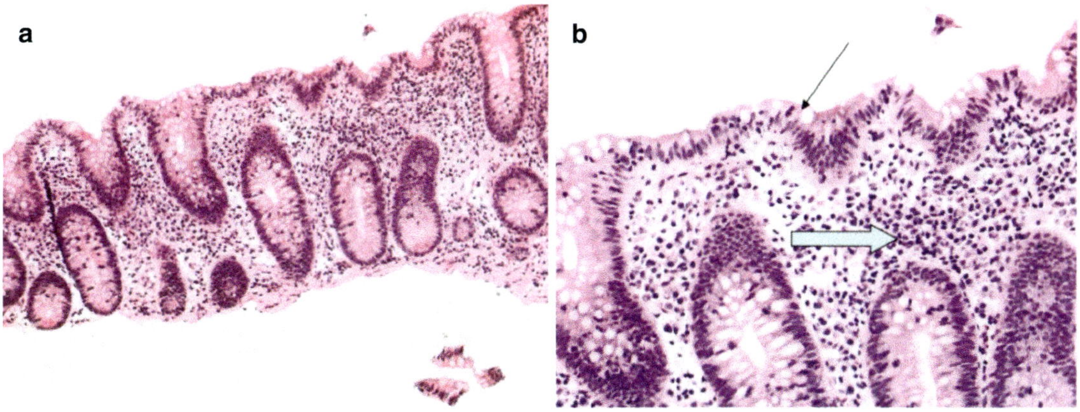

Fig. 54.3 Lymphocytic colitis. (**a**, **b**) The colon shows preserved crypt architecture. The lamina propria is markedly expanded by numerous plasma cells, lymphocytes, and eosinophils (thick arrow). The surface and the crypt epithelium is diffusely infiltrated by numerous lymphocytes (thin arrow). The crypt epithelium shows hyperchromatic, regenerative nuclei. Hematoxylin and eosin, 40x, 100x, and 200x. (Reproduced with permission from Celia Marginean MD)

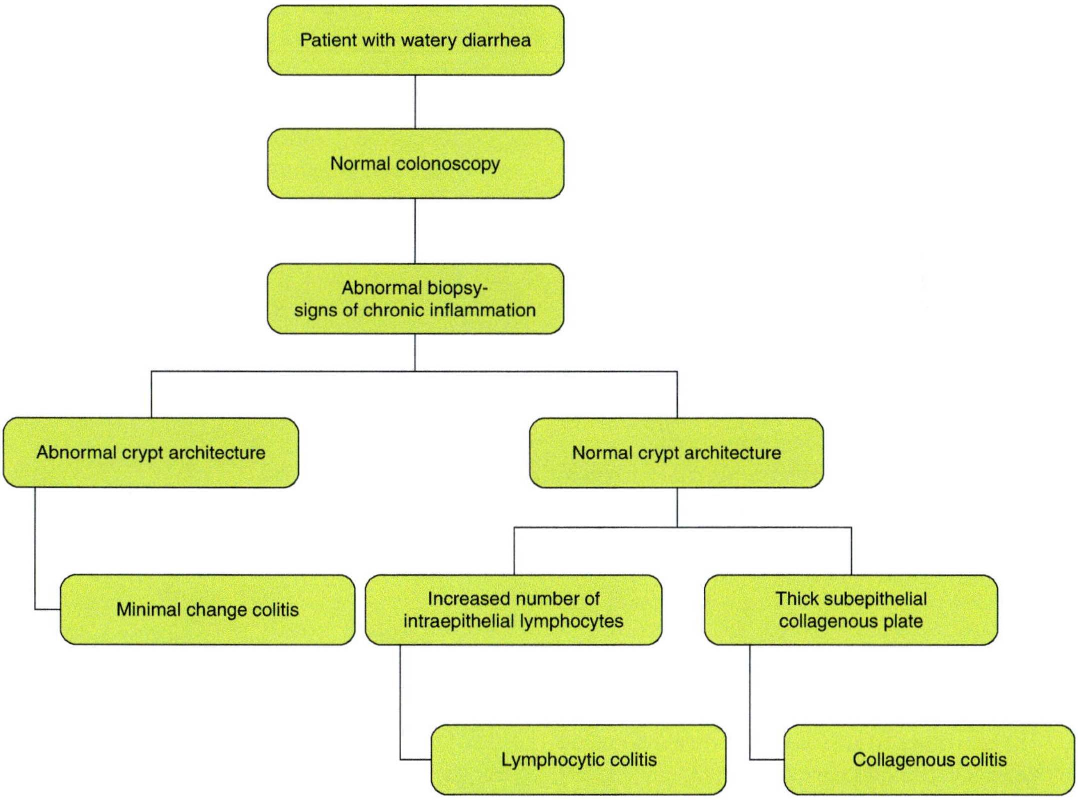

Fig. 54.4 Algorithm for pathological diagnosis. (Adapted from Warren BF, Edwards CM, Travis SPL. 'Microscopic colitis': classification and terminology. Histopathology. 2002;40:374–6)

Surgery

- Surgery has a limited role in the treatment of MC; indications for surgery are ill defined.
- Loop ileostomy, subtotal colectomy, and proctocolectomy with J-pouch have been used to treat severe intractable disease.

Ischemic Colitis

Introduction

- Ischemic colitis (IC) can be defined as "the condition that results when blood flow to the colon is reduced to a level insufficient to maintain cellular metabolic function."
- It is a fairly common disease and usually self-limited.
- Affected patients are often frail which explains the relatively high rate of mortality associated with this disease.

Anatomy and Physiology

- Branches from the superior mesenteric artery and the inferior mesenteric artery supply the colon.
- Splanchnic vessels are among the most reactive in the body, with blood flow varying from 10% to 35% of cardiac output depending on physiologic or pathologic conditions.
- Two watershed regions have been described in the colon where ischemia is most likely: the splenic flexure (area of Griffith) and the rectosigmoid junction (Sudeck's point).

Epidemiology and Risk Factors

- The incidence of IC varies between 4.5 and 44 cases per 100,000 person-years.
- The colon is the most frequent site of gastrointestinal ischemia.
- IC is more common in females and in patients over the age of 65.
- Chronic obstructive pulmonary disease, thrombophilia, history of irritable bowel disease, constipation, diabetes, renal failure, hypertension, extreme exercise, myocardial infarction, and history of vascular disease are all risks factors.
- Multiple drugs increase the risk of developing colonic ischemia (Table 54.2).
- A review of 89,967 patients undergoing AAA repair showed a global incidence of ischemia of 2.2%.
  - Almost 9% of ruptured AAA repair were complicated by IC in contrast to 1.9% of open elective procedures and 0.5% of endovascular repairs.
  - The first manifestation of ischemia in a postoperative patient is often rectal bleeding, generally happening in the first 48 h after surgery.
  - Patients should be investigated with flexible endoscopy.
  - In patients requiring surgery, anastomosis should be avoided to minimize the risk of graft contamination.

Table 54.2 Pharmacologic agents in order of evidence strength (111, 116)

Moderate evidence (further research would likely have an impact on authors' confidence in the estimate effect)	Constipation-inducing medications Immunosuppressive agents Illicit drugs
Low evidence (further research is expected to have an important impact on authors' confidence in the estimate effect)	Antibiotics Appetite suppressants Chemotherapeutic agents Decongestants Diuretics Ergot alkaloids Hormones Laxatives Psychotropic medications
Very low evidence (estimate effect is uncertain)	Digitalis Satins Nonsteroidal anti-inflammatory agents Serotonin agonists/antagonists Vasopressor

Pathophysiology

- Mechanisms of ischemic colitis can be divided into nonocclusive arterial ischemia, embolic or thrombotic arterial occlusion, and mesenteric vein thrombosis.
- The mucosa is the first layer of the bowel to be affected by ischemic change.
- Transient mucosal damage can be seen after 20 min to 1 h of insufficient blood flow with transmural damage occurring after 8–16 h.

Nonocclusive Ischemia

- Nonocclusive ischemia is responsible for 95% of IC cases.
  - Nonocclusive ischemia can be idiopathic without identifiable cause or may be secondary to a medical or surgical condition diminishing colonic blood flow.
  - IC happens on the left side of the colon in >75% of cases but affects the rectum in only 5% of patients.
  - When the ascending colon is involved, the cecum is the most frequently affected colonic segment.
  - Colonic injury and the systemic response to IC are due to both the hypoxic state and reperfusion injury.

Arterial Thrombosis and Emboli-Related Ischemia

- An embolic source of ischemia is a less frequent cause of colonic ischemia.
  - This is often seen with concomitant small bowel ischemia, and the distribution is less likely to follow the zones of the watershed areas.

Venous Thrombosis

- Venous thrombosis is more frequently related with small bowel ischemia; it is the rarest cause of IC.
  - It tends to affect the ascending more frequently than the descending colon.
  - Management is usually non-operative: systemic anticoagulation and occasional catheter-directed thrombolysis.

Clinical Presentation

- Abdominal pain and rectal bleeding are the most frequent symptoms associated with acute IC.
- Nine to twenty-four percent of lower GI bleeds are caused by ischemic colitis.
- Right-sided colitis is less likely to be associated with rectal bleeding.
- IC can evolve from an acute reversible colopathy (70%) to different clinical patterns including gangrene (10%), chronic colitis (18%), and fulminant colitis (2%).
- Strictures develop in 3.3–9.4% of patient – they are asymptomatic in the majority of cases.

Diagnosis

Laboratory Studies

- Results from laboratory studies are often nonspecific, and there is no reliable marker of ischemia.
- Increased white blood count and acidosis are associated with infarction.
- Increased lactate, LDH, CPK, or amylase may indicate tissue damage.
- Stool culture should be sent in patients with uncertain diagnosis as *Salmonella*, *Shigella*, *Campylobacter*, *Yersinia*, and *E. coli* O157:H7, and parasites can cause a similar clinical picture.
- *C. difficile* should be considered even though it is usually not associated with bloody diarrhea.
- *Klebsiella oxytoca* has been found in patients with right-sided hemorrhagic colitis mimicking ischemic colitis.

Imaging

Plain Films and Contrast Enema

- Plain abdominal films can be normal or show nonspecific findings of distention and ileus.
  - Free air can be seen with perforation.

- Classic findings of bowel ischemia (i.e., thumbprinting and pneumatosis) are present in 21–30% of plain films.
- Contrast enemas have a limited use in the acute phase as they may make ischemia worse by increasing intraluminal pressure.

Abdominal CT Scan

- CT scan with intravenous contrast is currently the imaging modality of choice to assess IC.
- The accuracy of CT scan in determining bowel ischemia varies between 74% and 79% depending on the study protocol and the experience of the radiologist.
- The clinical significance of pneumatosis and portal venous gas is controversial.
  - They used to represent a definite sign of bowel wall necrosis and were associated with a dismal prognosis.
  - However, pneumatosis and portal venous gas may be associated with many different conditions.
  - Pneumatosis and portal venous gas indicate transmural necrosis in 62–92% of patients.
  - When portal venous gas and pneumatosis are found in combination with bowel necrosis, the mortality rate is 71%.
- CT angiography has not been found to increase diagnostic accuracy in the acute setting.
  - However, it can be used to rule out superior mesenteric occlusion if clinically suspected.
  - Inferior mesenteric occlusion is of limited clinical significance as it is found in 10% of asymptomatic patients older than 60 years of age.

Endoscopy

- Colonoscopy can be used to confirm the diagnosis of ischemic colitis and to exclude other etiologies.
- Colonoscopy should not be performed in patients with findings of peritonitis or known perforation.
- Findings indicating ischemia at the time of endoscopy include erythema (84% of cases), edema (70%), friability (43%), superficial ulceration (57%), deep ulceration (22%), stenosis (8%), and intraluminal blood (8%).
- In severe and transmural ischemia, the bowel wall may be gray, green, or black.
- However, it is difficult to evaluate the severity of the disease with endoscopy. Endoscopic findings should be integrated into the complete clinical context when making decisions regarding surgical or medical management.
- Histopathologic features of acute ischemic colitis include preserved architecture of the colonic crypts, necrosis of the superficial portion of the crypts sparing the deep portion of the crypts (with or without ghost of crypts), mucin depletion, and reactive changes in the residual crypt epithelium, which may mimic dysplasia.
  - The lamina propria is hypocellular, with very rare or completely absent acute inflammatory cells (neutrophils) and hyalinization.
  - Sloughed necrotic mucosa may produce a microscopic appearance of a pseudomembrane which is composed of fibrin admixed with numerous neutrophils and mucin.
  - Numerous small intravascular hyaline thrombi may be seen in small mucosal capillaries (Fig. 54.5).
  - In more chronic presentations, mucosal atrophy, areas of granulation tissue, and fibrosis may be found.

Arteriography

- Arteriography has a limited use in diagnosis of IC since it is usually an arteriolar disease.

Ultrasound

- Criteria suggestive of colonic ischemia include bowel wall thickening, altered pericolonic fat, and absence of Doppler flow with a thickened bowel wall.
- Repeated exams may be used to follow for healing or progression.
- Ultrasound is user dependent and limited by body habitus and the presence of bowel gas.

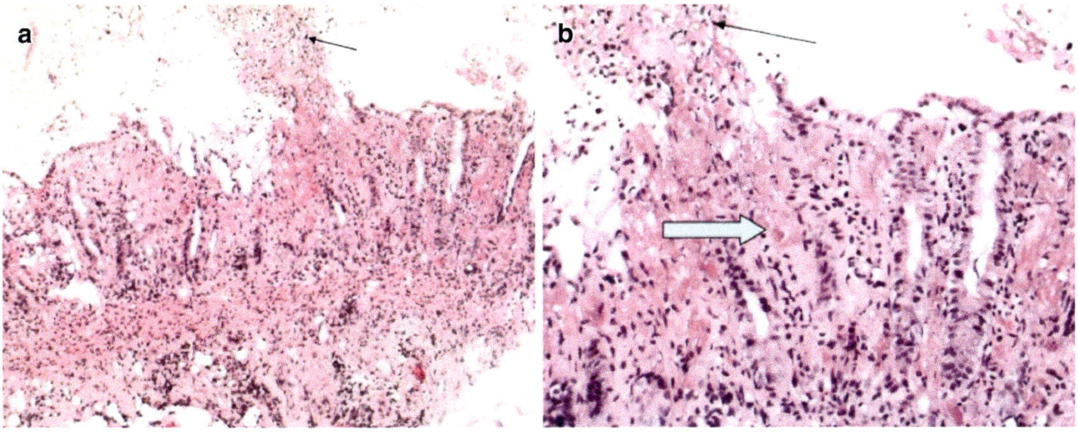

Fig. 54.5 Ischemic colitis. (**a**) Colonic mucosa shows necrosis of the superficial portion of the crypts, sparing the deep portion of the crypts. The lamina propria is hypocellular and shows hyalinization (dense, eosinophilic color). Hematoxylin and eosin, 100x. (**b**) Sloughed necrotic mucosa may produce a microscopic appearance of a pseudomembrane erupting from a crypt, composed of fibrin admixed with numerous neutrophils and mucin (arrows). Numerous hyaline thrombi are seen in small vessels (thick arrow). Hematoxylin and eosin, 200x. (Reproduced with permission from Celia Marginean MD)

Management

General Principles

- Many patients with IC have a self-limited disease and improve without specific intervention.
- Treatment is usually supportive and includes hydration; patients with an ileus may benefit from nasogastric tube decompression.
- Medications should be reviewed, and those promoting splanchnic vasoconstriction should be stopped if possible; cardiac output should be optimized.
- Improvement should be seen in 1–2 days with complete clinical resolution in 1–2 weeks.
- Absence of improvement may suggest development of chronic ischemia or progression toward transmural ischemia.
- After complete resolution of the initial episode, patients should undergo a colonoscopy to ensure compete healing and assess for stricture.
- Asymptomatic strictures can be observed; symptomatic strictures can be managed through surgical resection or endoscopic dilatation.

Antibiotics

- Broad-spectrum antibiotics are recommended as ischemia can lead to bacterial translocation. However, the evidence to support their use is limited.

Antithrombotic

- Anticoagulation is not routinely recommended for patients with ischemic colitis secondary to microvascular pathology or low-flow states.
- If bowel ischemia is due to venous thrombosis or arterial thromboembolic events, anticoagulation is indicated.
  - Patients should be investigated for thrombophilia if no other risk factors are found on history.
- Antiplatelet agents are not generally recommended.

Surgical Management

- Surgical indications include peritonitis, sepsis, radiologic evidence of perforation, suspicion of transmural ischemia on endoscopy, absence of improvement with medical management, and stricture causing obstruction.
- In the acute setting, creation of an anastomosis is controversial especially on the left side.

Prognosis

- Overall mortality rates vary from 4% to 12%.
- In a recent literature review, 19.3% required surgical intervention.
- Mortality has been reported in 39% of patients requiring surgery vs. 6% in those managed medically.
- The recurrence rate is 10% at 5 years and increases with time.
- Clinical factors commonly associated with poor prognosis include right-sided colitis, male gender, peritonitis on presentation, absence of rectal bleeding, and concomitant renal dysfunction.
- Ulceration on endoscopy, tachycardia, and shock in the first 24 h of presentation are strong predictors of poor outcome.

Intestinal Stoma

55

Michael F. McGee and Peter A. Cataldo

Key Concepts

- Preoperative stoma site marking and patient education improve stoma-related clinical outcomes, patient quality of life, and experience, while decreasing healthcare resource utilization.
- The finished stoma should protrude from the skin which improves appliance sealing and decreases complications.
- Optimal care for patients undergoing ostomy surgery includes preoperative and postoperative care by an ostomy nurse specialist, such as a WOCN-certified nurse.
- Early stoma-related complications such as leakage, peristomal dermatitis, and dehydration can often be remedied with stoma care and education.
- Loop ileostomy is preferred over transverse loop colostomy for temporary fecal diversion in most circumstances.
- Stapled and hand-sutured techniques are both acceptable for loop ileostomy closure.
- Asymptomatic parastomal hernias do not mandate repair, while mild symptoms may benefit from appliance modifications or stomal support belt. Suitable-risk patients with significant parastomal hernia symptoms may be candidates for repair.

M. F. McGee (✉)
Section of Colon and Rectal Surgery, Division of Gastrointestinal and Oncologic Surgery, Department of Surgery, Northwestern Memorial Hospital, Chicago, IL, USA
e-mail: MMCGEE1@nm.org

P. A. Cataldo
Department of Surgery, University of Vermont Medical Center, University of Vermont College of Medicine, Burlington, VT, USA

Introduction

- 120,000 stomas are created in North America each year with a prevalence of 450,000–800,000.
- Mastery of preparing, creating, caring for, and reversing stomas is the hallmark of the colorectal surgeon's armamentarium.

Colostomy

Configuration (Fig. 55.1)

- An end colostomy can be permanent or temporary.
- A loop colostomy is typically constructed from redundant sigmoid colon and also can be temporary or permanent. This type of diversion is an excellent choice for palliation due to an obstructing lesion as it creates a distal vent.
- The transverse loop colostomy while easy to construct may have high output or prolapse. It tends to be larger stomas with frequent stoma-related issues.

S. R. Steele et al. (eds.), *The ASCRS Manual of Colon and Rectal Surgery*,
https://doi.org/10.1007/978-3-030-01165-9_55

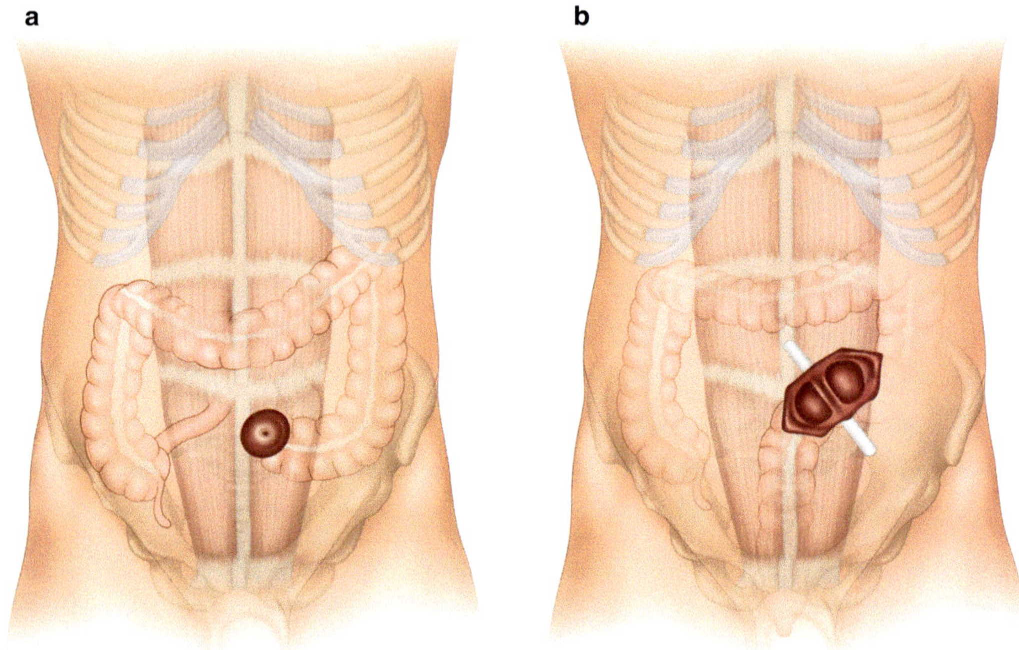

Fig. 55.1 (**a**) End descending colostomy. (**b**) Loop sigmoid colostomy

Physiology

- The majority of the fluid and electrolyte absorption of the 1500–2000 mL that the colon receives from the small intestine is absorbed in the right colon.
- Stool consistency from a stoma depends on where in the colon the stoma is located. Ascending and transverse colostomies tend to have loose stool. Descending and sigmoid colostomies tend to have episodic solid stool.

Small Bowel Stomas

Configuration

- Small bowel stomas may be from the ileum or jejunum.
- These stomas may be temporary or permanent.
- They can be end or loop stomas (Fig. 55.2).

Physiology

- Mean small bowel length is approximately 500 cm (ranging from 275 to 800). The small bowel receives 9–10 L of fluid from the proximal GI tract.
- 2.5 L is reabsorbed from the ileum and the rest in the jejunum.
- Normal end ileostomy output varies from 200 to 1200 mL daily. Stomas located >100 cm proximal to the IC valve can lead to steatorrhea and vitamin B12 deficiency.
- While all small bowel stomas can lead to fluid and electrolyte imbalance, these problems are more common in stomas constructed from the jejunum.

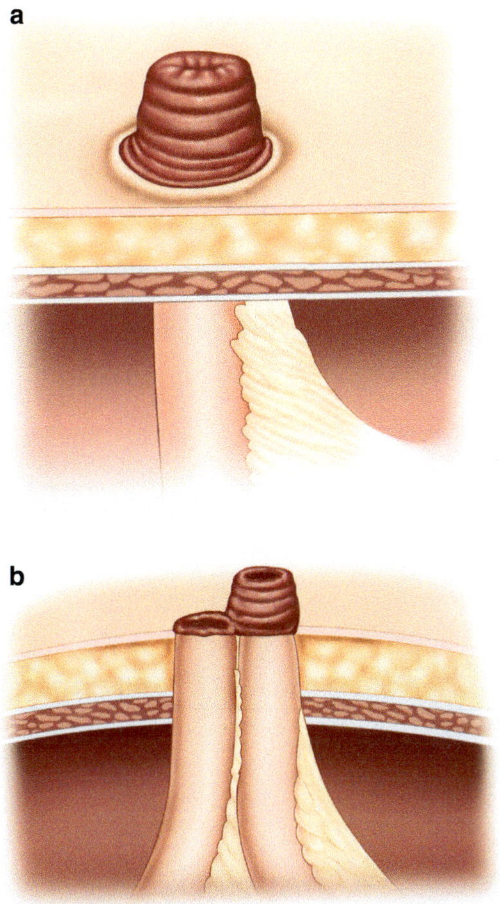

Fig. 55.2 (**a**) End ileostomy. (**b**) Loop ileostomy

Preoperative Considerations for the Ostomate

Stoma Site Marking (Fig. 55.3)

- Creating a stoma in a properly chosen location is the most important predictor of an ostomate's quality of life.
- The ideal site considers body habitus, contours, scars, bony prominences, and the umbilicus standing, sitting, and laying down.
- Patient's lifestyle, occupation, impairments, and preferences should also be considered during the preop marking.
- Efforts are usually made to keep the stoma within the rectus sheath.
- A site should have a 2 inch perimeter of intact skin for an adequate appliance seal.
- The typical site is in the rectus midway between the umbilicus and pubic tubercle, nearly medial to the anterior superior iliac crest.
- After choosing the preliminary site, the patient is asked to sit to ensure they can visualize the site and it is not situated where a skinfold or crease will hinder appliance adherence.
- For patients with a large pannus, a more ideal site may be located in the supraumbilical position.
- When standing consideration includes avoidance of the waistline, pendulous breasts, or hernias.
- If two stomas will be needed (i.e., for fecal and urinary drainage), the patient should be marked on opposite sides at different levels.
- Tattoo or indelible markers (with a protective occlusive dressing to preserve the mark) are then applied to ensure the spot is visible on the day of surgery.

Preoperative Stoma Education

- Traditionally most education regarding stomas occurred in the postoperative period, but evidence suggests preoperative education is equally important.
- Commercially prepared preoperative resources which simulate a stoma can allow patients to practice stoma care.

Technical Considerations of Stoma Creation

Small Bowel: Making the Aperture

- A 2 cm skin disk is excised. The subcutaneous fat is split. The anterior rectus sheath is opened about 3 cm longitudinally. The rectus muscle

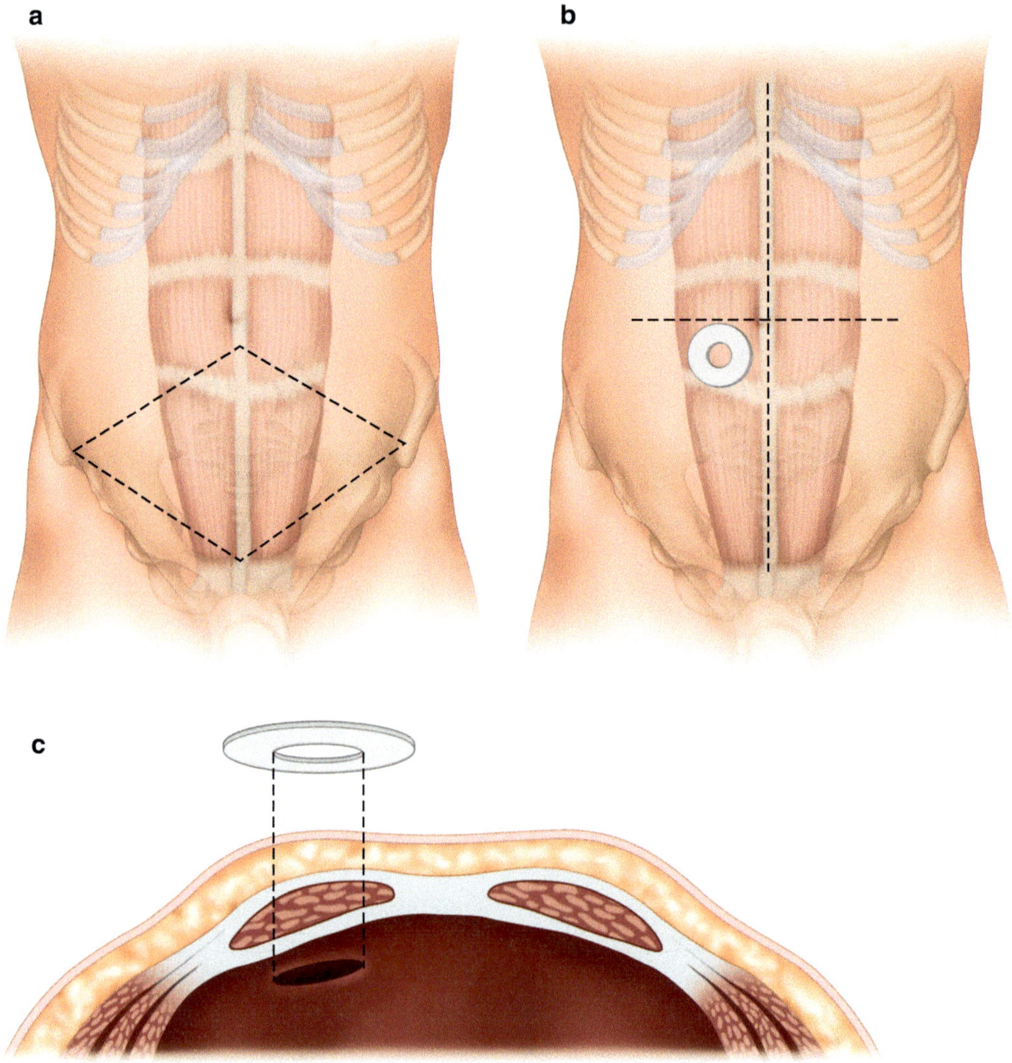

Fig. 55.3 (**a**) The "stoma triangle". (**b**) Intersection of the infraumbilical fat pad and rectus sheath, marked by a stoma siting ring. (**c**) Cross-sectional view of the stoma trephine path and stoma siting ring, fashioned perpendicular to the abdominal wall without veering medially or laterally

is split and the posterior rectus sheath and peritoneum are opened.

- The stoma aperture should easily allow two fingers to pass.
- When constructing a laparoscopic stoma, care must be taken to avoid injury to the underlying abdominal contents when the peritoneum is entered.
- With a laparoscopic stoma, an atraumatic bowel grasper at the apex of the target loop of the bowel and placed directly under the anticipated stoma opening allows easy grasping by a Babcock once the opening is completed.
- An extra small plastic sleeve wound protector may assist delivering the bowel through the abdominal wall.

Small Bowel End Stoma

- After selecting the target bowel, the mesentery is fully mobilized. The bowel with mesentery is carefully delivered 5–6 cm onto the abdominal wall. Care is taken to coax the corresponding mesentery with the bowel.

- A dusky stoma may be related to mesenteric vascular injury, venous outflow occlusion from a narrow trephine, or inadvertent mesenteric interruption. The stoma should be revised before the abdomen is closed if there is concern that there may be a problem.
- After abdominal wounds are closed, the end ileostomy is matured with ideally a 2–3 cm protrusion by everting the bowel back on itself to cover the serosa.
- A fatty mesentery may require careful debulking to allow for eversion.
- Absorbable suture may incorporate a seromuscular purchase and then fix the box at skin level.
- Sutures are placed at skin level through the dermis but not the epidermis to avoid mucosal implants in the skin which will hinder pouching.
- Flush stomas allow effluent to migrate under the stoma appliance and interfere with pouching while simultaneously producing painful, weeping, excoriated skin.

Small Bowel Loop Stoma

- Generally the stoma trephine is slightly larger for a loop stoma than for an end ileostomy (2.5 cm) (Fig. 55.4).
- The mobilized small bowel is marked for orientation and gently advanced through the aperture.
- A plastic stoma rod or temporary support structure is placed just beneath the bowel through the mesentery.

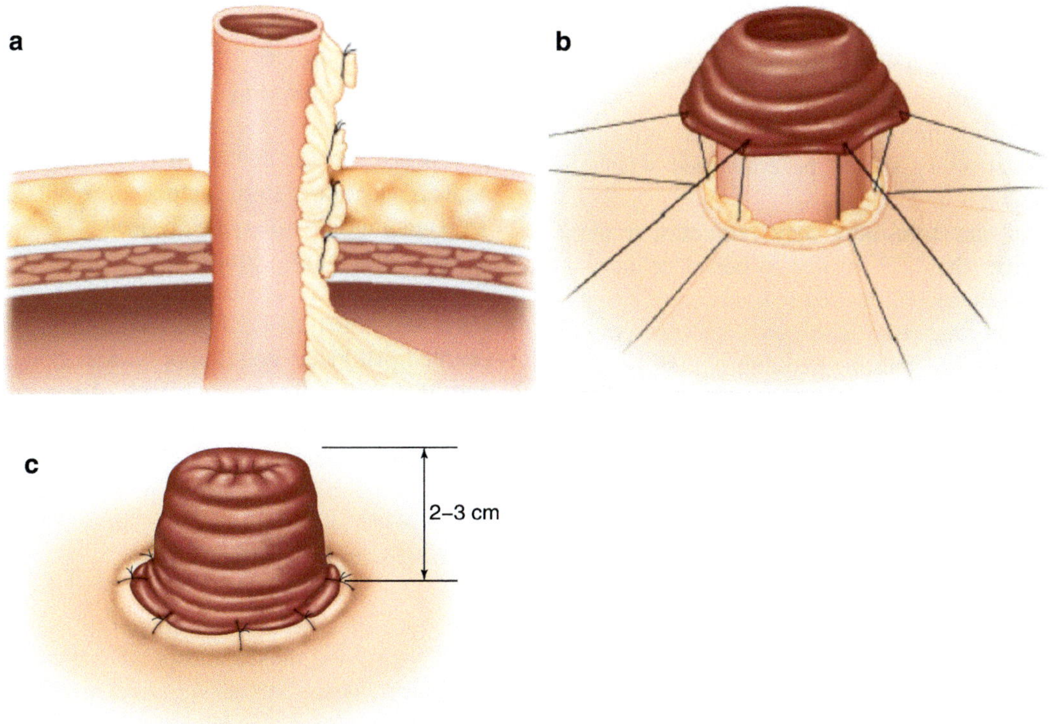

Fig. 55.4 Maturation of an end small bowel stoma. (**a**) An adequately mobilized, tension-free, length of small bowel is eviscerated through the stoma trephine. (**b**) Multiple interrupted absorbable sutures are used to mature the stoma. (**c**) The completed small bowel stoma should ideally protrude 2–3 cm from the skin level

- The distal limb is identified and an incision is made from one point transversely across the antimesenteric surface to the other area where the mesentery meets the bowel with the mesenteric potion of the bowel wall left intact.
- Absorbable sutures are used to secure the defunctionalized portion to the dermis.
- The hood of the other (proximal) side is everted and secured to the other side of the dermis.
- When completed the afferent limb should protrude 2–3 cm above the skin.
- The stoma rod or support is typically removed in 3–5 days.

End Colostomy

- The intended section of the colon for an end colostomy should be completely mobilized. This can be done in an open or laparoscopic fashion.
- When the bowel is brought through the abdominal aperture, several cm of the bowel should reach above the skin in a tension-free manner.
- Confirmation of pulsatile blood from the marginal artery should be confirmed when the colon is divided.
- An end colostomy may require a trephine larger than 2.5 cm due to bowel caliber and mesenteric fat thickness. Excision of epiploic appendages may ease colon passage through the muscle-splitting trephine.
- The everted and matured colostomy should protrude 1–2 cm above the skin.

Loop Colostomy

- A loop colostomy can be done in an open or laparoscopic fashion and requires complete mobilization of the desired segment which is usually sigmoid or transverse colon.
- The trephine is at least 3 cm and the colon should reach several cm above the skin at the desired site.
- The incision to open the colon is along the long axis of the colon (not transverse as with the loop small bowel stoma) and the cut edges matured back to the skin edges.
- The caliber may be large depending on the size of the bowel, postoperative edema, and mesenteric thickness.
- Loop colostomies may be permanent and every detail should be optimized to ensure the best possible ease of care.

Postoperative Care for the Stoma

Early Inpatient Postoperative Care

- The stoma can swell to 2–3 times the end size due to edema. Typically it reaches its baseline size at 4–6 weeks.
- Rods are typically removed from loop stomas at 3–5 days when the tension subsides.
- Thin fluid with a yellow tinge (and without particulate matter) called bowel sweat typically is initially produced from a stoma. A deluge of backed up bowel contents may also initially be produced.
- 30% of new ileostomy patients experience dehydration, and diligence is needed with patient education and early follow-up to address and reduce stoma output and avoid the 15% readmission rate typically seen.
- Patient and family education should begin immediately after surgery. Unpublished data from ACS found that only 53% of newly discharged ostomates could apply a new pouch and 28% could fix a pouch leak. Therefore bridging this gap with home nursing is strongly considered.

Postoperative Outpatient Care

- Periodic stoma assessment (preferably by a WOCN-certified nurse) allows adjustment in equipment as the stoma shrinks and allows treatment of stoma skin irritation.
- A phalange should remain in place 3–5 days. More frequent changes indicate issues with technique, peristomal skin issues, inappropriate appliance, or suboptimal location/construction.

Stoma Appliances

- The stoma appliance consists of an adhesive flange (wafer) that seals to the skin and a one- or two-piece collection bag. In a two-piece system, the bag can be removed with the flange intact—thus allowing inspection of the stoma.
- The flange is composed of a pectin-like wafer ring surrounded by adhesive material. The inner diameter of the ring comes in various sizes and can be trimmed to the exact size of the stoma.
- The collection bag also comes in various sizes and can be clear or opaque. Venting charcoal filters can be placed in the bag to help manage high gas output.
- Specialized products are chosen depending on patient needs. A convex stoma appliance consists of a bowel-shaped wafer that helps "push out" a retracted stoma and augment a seal around the stoma.
- Elastic stoma belts stabilize the appliance to reduce skin leakage.
- Stoma paste and other skin adhesives, protective wipes, topical powders, and other agents assist with difficulties in pouching.

Stoma Complications

- 37% of elective stomas and 55% of emergent operations have complications.
- Early complications include leakage, peristomal dermatitis, and dehydration and are usually remedied with education.
- Late complications such as prolapse, stenosis, and parastomal hernia may require surgery.

Stomal Ischemia: Necrosis, Retraction, and Stenosis

- Poor arterial flow (and sometimes venous obstruction) can lead to ischemia.
- End stomas are more vulnerable to ischemia vs a loop stoma.
- Ischemia of a stoma can run a spectrum from mild to full thickness necrosis.
- It is crucial in a severely ischemic stoma that the bowel is viable at the fascia and more proximal. A well-lubricated clear test tube can be inserted into the stoma at the bedside, while a flashlight is directed down the lumen of the test tube. The extent of the ischemia can be detected through the clean glass.
- Consideration should strongly be given to revise any stoma with subfascial ischemia to avoid intraperitoneal necrosis and perforation.
- An ischemic end colostomy which is viable above the fascia may be observed because pouching the resultant retracted stoma should be possible due to it producing solid stool.
- An end ileostomy with significant ischemia should be revised if feasible in the early postoperative period as a retracted ileostomy is much more difficult to pouch due to the liquid effluent.
- Stoma stenosis may result from long-term ischemia. When stool cannot be expelled or pouching becomes a problem due to retraction, surgical revision may be required (Fig. 55.5).
- Some stomas can be locally revised; however the possibility of requiring an open incision to facilitate mobilization and reduce the chances of a recurrent problem must always be discussed during consent for surgical revision.

Peristomal Skin Disorders

- Peristomal skin disorders are the most common complication for ostomates.
- Most peristomal skin irritation arises from a poorly fitted or improperly sized appliance.
- Effluent (particularly the small bowel) is caustic to the skin leading to weeping, itching, and lack of appliance adherence.
- Patients at particularly high risk for treatable skin problems include those with low health literacy, a poor support system, emergently created stomas, and obese patients.
- Personalized approaches to treating the skin may include change in appliance, convexity, or various means of skin protection.

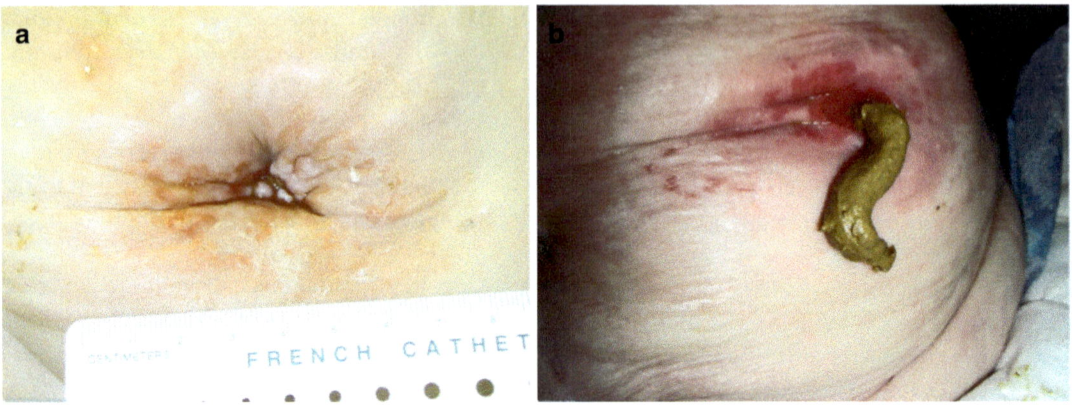

Fig. 55.5 Chronic stoma stenosis (Photo credit: Wound, Ostomy, and Continence Nurses Society (http://www.wocn.org/page/ ImageLibrary))

- Fungal peristomal skin infections appear as reddened shiny patches with satellite papules involving the skin under the appliance flange. Treatment relies on removing the skin moisture and applying antifungal powder with each flange change until the rash resolves (1–2 weeks).

Peristomal Pyoderma Gangrenosum

- Pyoderma gangrenosum is a rare inflammatory skin disease with painful ulcers that have well-defined erythematous and typically undermined borders. It typically begins as a firm pink or purple nodule at the edge of the skin-mucocutaneous border. It rapidly enlarges to a painful ulcer, typically with a raised border, and often with thin bridges of the epidermis spanning the ulcer (Fig. 55.6).
- Pyoderma is associated with inflammatory bowel disease, rheumatoid arthritis, paraproteinemia, and hematologic malignancy or may be idiopathic.
- Pyoderma is more common in women, associated with autoimmune disorders and obesity, or in IBD patients.
- The diagnosis is clinical and requires a high index of suspicion. Biopsy is nonspecific and not helpful.
- There is no standard algorithm for treatment and requires a multidisciplinary approach. Modification of the flange to include an absorbent dressing covered with an occlusive dressing will provide a protective dry barrier and control wound seepage.
- Medical therapy is not standardized and includes debridement with steroid injection, systemic steroids, antibiotics, immunomodulators, and biologics.
- Many patients progress and stoma re-siting is required but re-siting does not guarantee against pyoderma recrudescence.

Peristomal Varices

- Portosystemic venous shunts may also develop between the stoma and the abdominal wall leading to varices in the setting of chronic portal hypertension.
- With peristomal varices the circumferential skin has a subcutaneous blue or purple hue and may have visibly dilated submucosal veins. The skin may easily bleed (Fig. 55.7).
- Peristomal hemorrhage can be temporalized with digital pressure, epinephrine-soaked gauze, or suture ligation.
- Since rebleeding is common, portal decompression with transjugular intrahepatic portosystemic shunting (TIPS) may be indicated. Some patients require hepatic transplant depending on the etiology of the problem.
- If TIPS and liver transplant are not options, injection sclerotherapy, octreotide, and percutaneous embolization have also been employed.

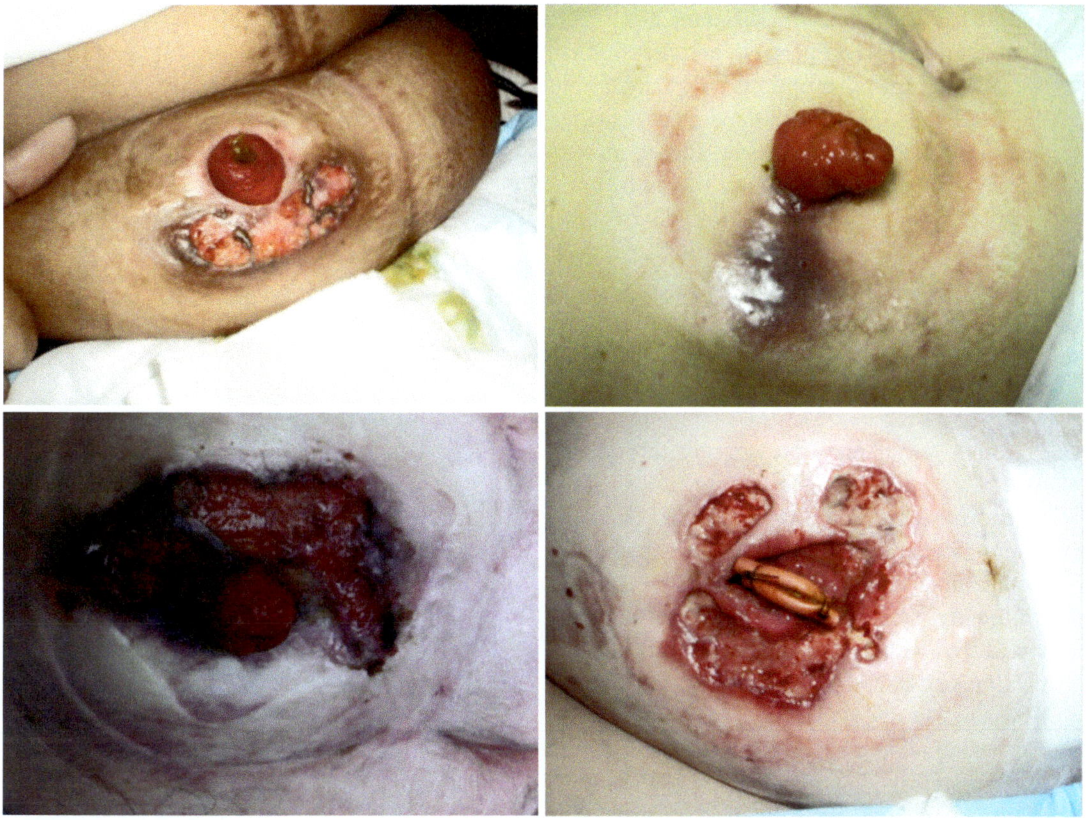

Fig. 55.6 Peristomal pyoderma gangrenosum (Photo credit: Janice Colwell, APRN, CWOCN)

Fig. 55.7 Peristomal varices (Photo credit: Janice Colwell, APRN, CWOCN)

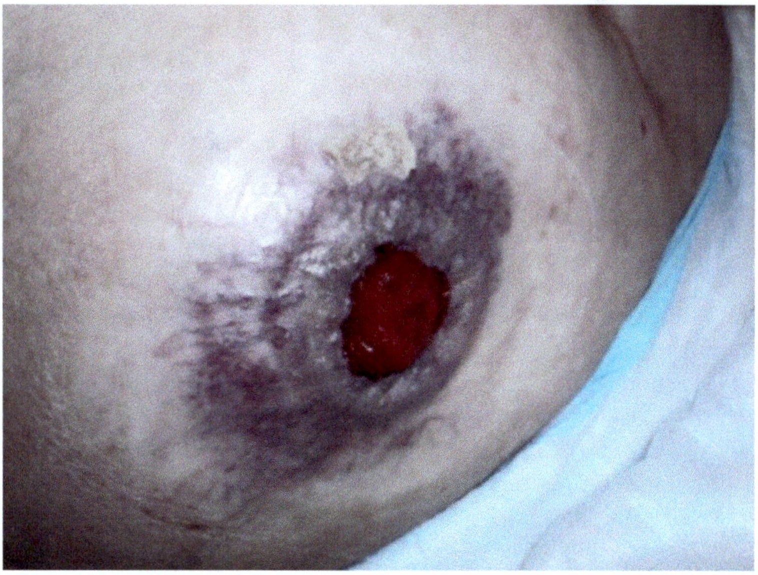

- Surgical mucocutaneous disconnection has been employed when portal decompression is not possible and other options have failed. For this procedure, the bowel is separated from the skin and subcutaneous tissue and then the stoma re-matured. The surgeon should be prepared for significant blood loss associated with this procedure with necessary blood and blood products available.

Stomal Prolapse

- Proximal bowel may intussuscept through a mature stoma and produce prolapse. This can range from a mild cosmetic nuisance to a severe pouching problem. In extreme cases strangulation and incarceration could occur.
- Minimally symptomatic prolapsing stomas are treated with reassurance, appliance modification, and an external fixation device (stoma hernia belt).
- Prolapsing temporary stomas are treated with timely reversal.
- Many techniques have been described for addressing a permanent stoma with symptomatic prolapse. These range from local eversion and then amputation and resuturing of the mucocutaneous junction to various intra-abdominal fixation techniques (Fig. 55.8).
- Typically in a loop stoma the distal end will prolapse; therefore, conversion to an end stoma will alleviate the problem.

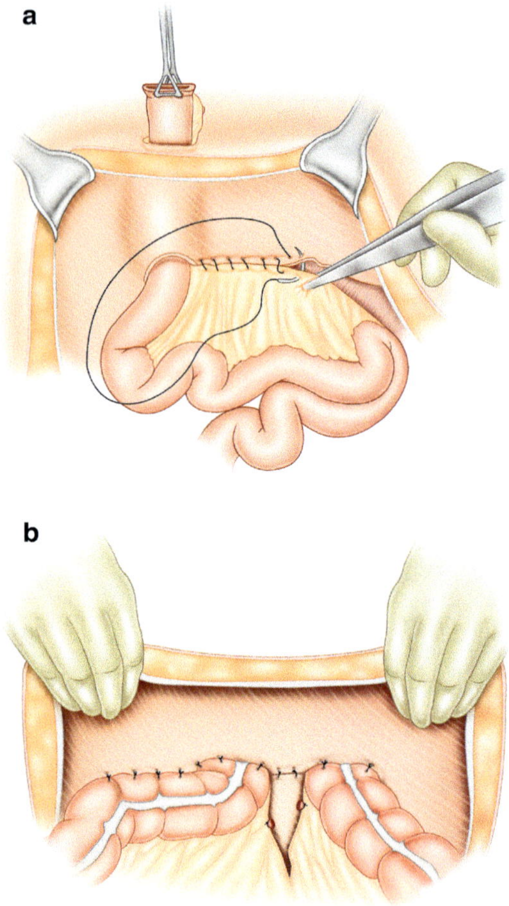

Fig. 55.8 (**a**) Retroperitoneal tunneling of an end ileostomy with suture pexy of the pre-stomal mesentery to limit prolapse. (**b**) Suture pexy of the distal limb of a loop colostomy to mitigate prolapse of the distal limb

Parastomal Hernia

- A parastomal hernia may produce pain, obstruction, disdainful bulge, and pouching difficulties or be asymptomatic.
- Detection may be difficult on physical exam, and "coaching" a patient to strongly Valsalva when asked to hold their breath during a CT exam may aid in detection.
- Repair of a parastomal hernia depends on the degree of symptoms.
- Elective repair is offered to suitable-risk patients with intermittent obstruction, intolerable discomfort, or significant pouching problems.
- Incarcerated hernias with complete obstruction or with signs and symptoms worrisome for strangulation require immediate surgery.
- There are three methods of repair: local, transabdominal, or re-siting.
- While local repair (+/− overlay of mesh) is attractive, it has a high rate of recurrence.
- Re-siting does not prevent hernia formation at the new site.
- Transabdominal mesh underlay repair can be done via an open or laparoscopic approach using biologic or permanent mesh. The contents of the hernia are removed to define the stoma trephine. The mesh is placed intraperitoneal or retro-rectus and secured with tacks or sutures. The bowel

is encompassed within a keyhole slit in the mesh before it is fixed to the surrounding abdominal wall or the mesh placed in the Sugarbaker fashion (secured to the abdominal wall with the bowel brought out at one edge) (Fig. 55.9).

- Some evidence supports the placement of lightweight polypropylene prosthetic mesh at the time of stoma construction is effective in reducing but not eliminating stoma hernias.

Peristomal Abscess

- A peristomal abscess can be seen in the early postoperative period from contamination. Late abscesses may be seen with Crohn's disease.
- Treatment of the abscess is drainage. The drainage catheter should be placed outside the flange or close to the mucosal-skin junction to avoid interfering with the ability to pouch the stoma.
- Evaluation for a fistula is undertaken if drainage persists or recurrent abscesses occur.

High-Output Small Bowel Stomas

- Normal ileostomy output is 800–1200 ml/day, and a high-output stoma is usually seen with small bowel stomas (vs colon).
- Over 50% of high-output stomas resolve within 2 weeks after initial construction.

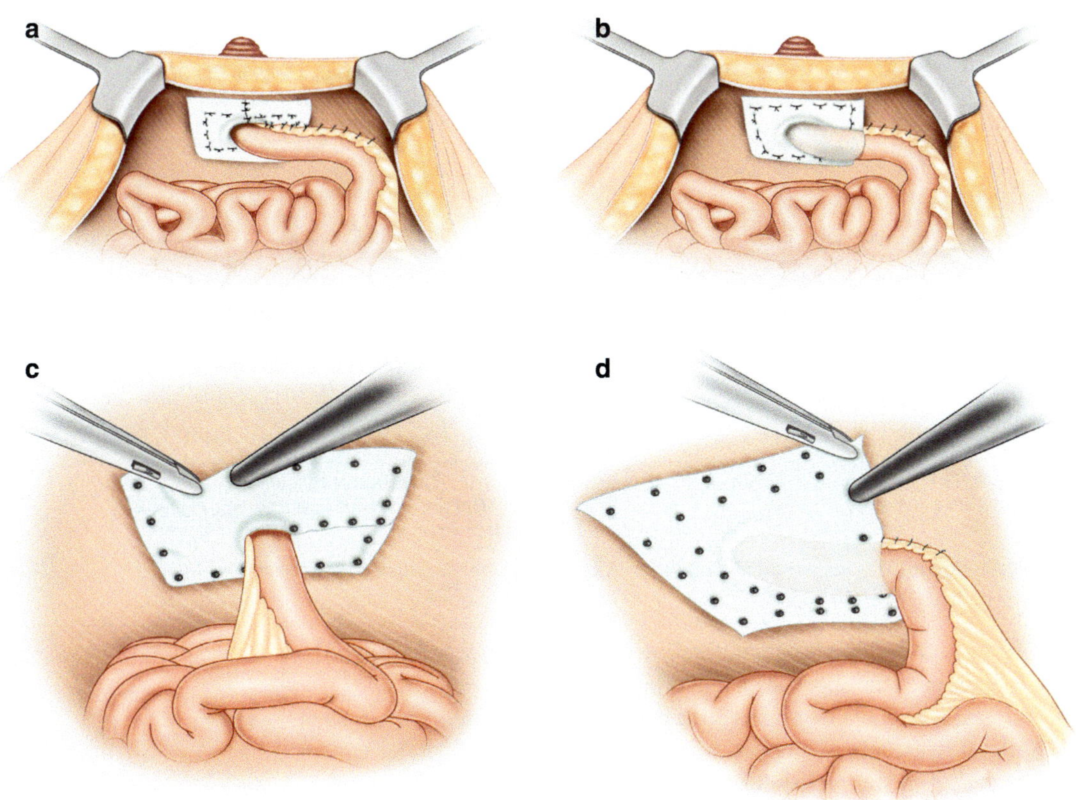

Fig. 55.9 Intra-abdominal parastomal hernia repair with (**a**) open "keyhole", (**b**) open Sugarbaker overlay, (**c**) laparoscopic "keyhole", and (**d**) laparoscopic Sugarbaker techniques with "double crown" tack technique

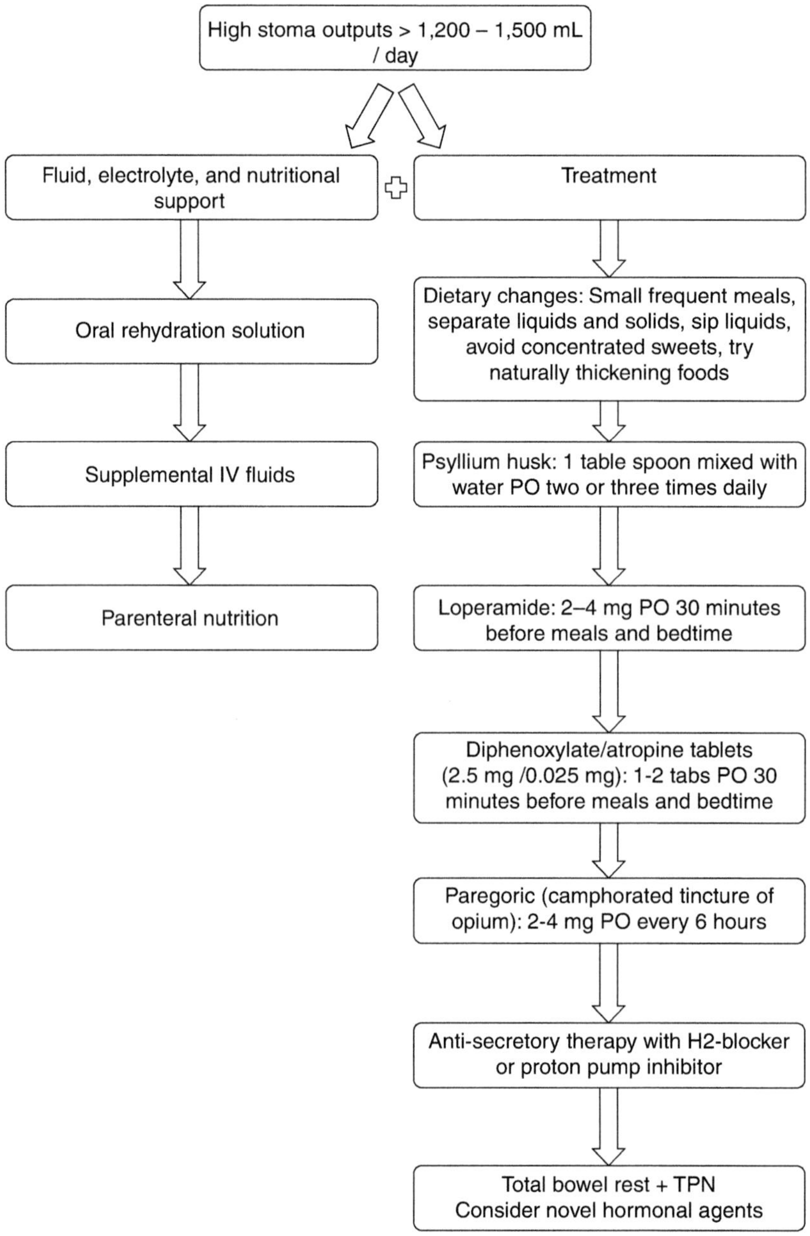

Fig. 55.10 Proposed management algorithm for management of high-output small bowel stomas

- During periods of high output, fluid, electrolyte repletion, and nutritional support may be needed.
- Figure 55.10 is the algorithm for treatment of high-output stomas.
- Table 55.1 is the recipe for oral rehydration solution.
- Table 55.2 lists the common medications and doses to treat high-output stomas.

Stoma Reversal

Preoperative Preparation

- Preoperative evaluation with review of operative and other records, imaging, and endoscopy helps eliminate unexpected intra- and postoperative surprise findings.

Table 55.1 Oral rehydration solution

Ingredients
3/8 tsp salt (sodium chloride)
¼ tsp table salt substitute (potassium chloride)
½ tsp baking soda (sodium bicarbonate)
2 tbsp + 2 tsp sugar (sucrose)
Add tap water to make 1 l
Optional: NutraSweet®- or Splenda®-based flavoring of choice, to taste

Directions: Mix dry ingredients with water and serve. Best sipped slowly over long periods of time

Contains 27 g of sucrose, 70 mEq/L of sodium, 20 mEq/L of potassium, and 30 mEq/L of bicarbonate. The final osmolarity is approximately 245 mOsm/L

tbsp tablespoon, *tsp* teaspoon

Table 55.2 Common medications and doses to treat high-output stomas

Medication	Starting dose	Maximum daily dose
Psyllium	1 tablespoon BID	1 tablespoon TID
Loperamide tab	2–4 mg PO QID	16 mg (4–8 tabs)
Loperamide liquid	2–4 mg PO QID	80 mL (16 mg)
Diphenoxylate-atropine tab	2.5–5 mg PO QID	20 mg (4–8 tabs)
Diphenoxylate-atropine liquid	2.5–5 mg PO QID	40 mL (20 mg)
Codeine tab	15–30 mg PO QID	240 mg (60 mg PO QID)
Codeine elixir	15–30 mg PO QID	240 mg (80 mL)
Paregoric 0.4 mg morphine/1 mL paregoric (45% alcohol)	5 mL PO QID	37.5 mL PO QID (150 mL/day)
Opium tincture 10 mg morphine/1 mL opium (19% alcohol)	0.3–1 mL PO QID	1.5 mL PO QID (6 mL/day)

Adapted from Parekh N, Seidner DL. Medical management of the high output enterostomy and enterocutaneous fistula. In: Fazio VW, Church JM, Wu JS, editors. Atlas of intestinal stomas. New York: Springer; 2012

Timing

- Until more evidence is available (to support closure at <2 weeks), loop ileostomy closure is generally undertaken at 8–12 weeks.
- For patients requiring postoperative chemotherapy, stoma closure may be delayed until the completion, but patients should be carefully monitored for dehydration.
- Timing for closure of end colostomy is contentious and conflicting in the literature. Waiting 3–6 months may facilitate closure particularly in patients who originally underwent an open end colostomy creation.

Technical Consideration of Loop Stoma Reversal

- Most loop stomas can be closed via a circular local incision made just outside the mucocutaneous junction.
- Mobilization is carried into the abdomen and some limited adhesiolysis may be required.
- If the stoma is everted, sharp adhesiolysis is used to flip the everted portion back.
- Serosal tears or enterotomies can be assessed by inserting diluted povidone-iodine solution into each limb and suture repaired.
- Rarely deep bowel injury or tenacious adhesions require a laparotomy.
- A stapled (side to side) or hand-sewn closure can be performed.
- After assuring lack of the bowel adhered to the underlying edges, the fascia is closed.
- Skin closure, purse-string reduction in the circular incisional size, or leaving it open to drainage depends on the surgeon's preference, patient's body habitus, and degree of contamination.

Technical Consideration of End Stoma Reversal

- The surgeon should be prepared for significant adhesions and a hostile abdomen when reversing an end stoma (particularly if constructed via an open approach). The patient should be marked for a temporary loop ileostomy in the event one is needed to protect a difficult colorectal anastomosis. A consideration is given for ureteric stents.

Table 55.3 Stoma reversal complications

Stoma reversal type	Loop ileostomy reversal (%)	Loop colostomy reversal (%)	End colostomy reversal with colorectal anastomosis (%)
Superficial surgical site infection	3–13.5	5–20	14–43.8
Deep space infection/ leak	2–4	2–4	1.5–21
Bowel obstruction/ileus	5–16	4	23
Hernia (clinically diagnosed)	0–50	2–38	3–31

- Intra-abdominally, it is crucial that the distal end of the bowel is the rectum and not the sigmoid. Mobilization in the pelvis may be required to ensure this.
- For a tension-free anastomosis, additional mobilization may be required after the stoma is taken down.
- The anastomosis can be done by suture or stapler. It is important to ensure the stapler reaches the proximal extent of the rectum. If the stapler cannot be advanced fully, further rectal mobilization or resection should be considered. If an end to side (of rectum) anastomosis is done, the staple line must be several centimeters from the proximal rectal resection margin to avoid ischemia.
- Ensuring the vagina and/or bladder is not in the staple line before closing the stapler avoids injury and fistula.
- A leak test also is employed to avoid a postoperative problem.
- An ileostomy is considered when there is significant technical difficulty with the procedure.

Stoma Reversal Complications

- See Table 55.3.

Special Considerations

The Difficult Stoma

- For obese patients, the supraumbilical abdominal wall may be thinner, so placing a stoma in that location may reduce tension on the stoma.
- In some obese patients, a subxiphoid transverse colostomy may be the easiest to construct when all other approaches are not going to be successful.
- Delivery of the bulky tissue associated with a stoma can be done in a stepwise fashion. First the skin, fascia, muscle, and peritoneal opening is created. Next the subcutaneous tissue is elevated and separated off the anterior rectus sheath. The stoma is delivered through the anterior rectus sheath (muscle); then in a second step, the bowel is delivered from the supramuscular position and then through the subcutaneous tissue and onto the skin.
- Use of a plastic sleeve wound protector +/− water-soluble lubricant may decrease the friction and allow the bowel to be passed through.
- A loop end stoma may allow additional reach without ischemia for an ileostomy or colostomy (Fig. 55.11 and 55.12).
- Carefully scoring the mesentery while avoiding injury to the mesenteric vessels can add additional mesentery length (Fig. 55.13).
- Both bowel limbs may be placed through the same skin opening when an anastomosis is not possible in an acute setting. Then at the next surgery both ends can be anastomosed together without a midline incision.
- When forced to compromise, a poor stoma in a good location is the lesser of two evils.
- When the bowel wall is thick and maturation is not possible, securing it to the skin with the serosa left exposed is a possibility. While reactive serositis and stricturing may develop,

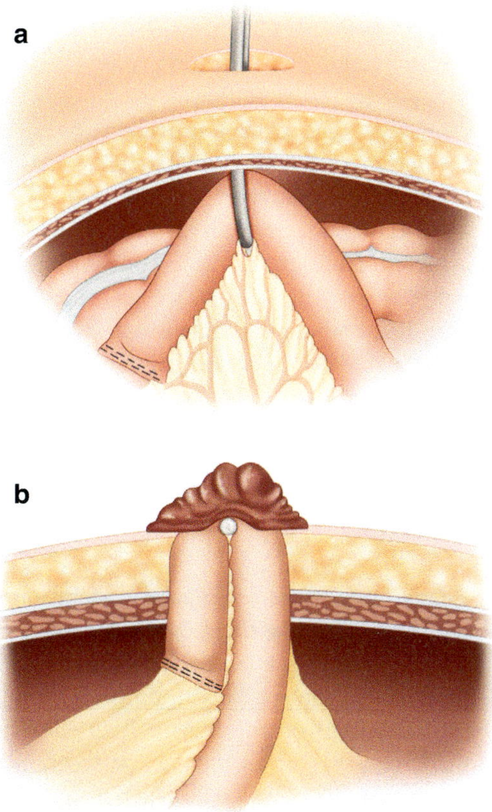

Fig. 55.11 Loop-end ileostomy

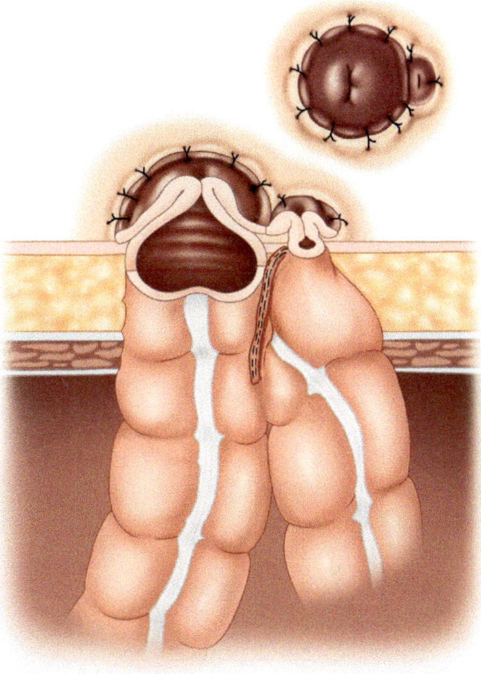

Fig. 55.12 A Prasad-type end-loop colostomy

a revision can be done hopefully with more favorable conditions.

- When a stoma cannot be brought up through the skin, placement in the midline incision should be considered.
- In a loop stoma, when a heavy mesentery or friable bowel leads to the stoma rod tearing through the mesenteric aspect of the bowel, two stoma rods are placed side by side to distribute the tension over a greater surface area. Alternately, the stoma may be braced at the fascia level by passing a long malleable/pliable tube through a skin incision remote from the stoma site and then piercing an avascular portion of the stoma mesentery before piercing the skin on the opposite side of the stoma (Fig. 55.14). The tube is removed after several days.

Temporary Fecal Diversion: Loop Ileostomy Versus Loop Colostomy

- ASCRS clinical guidelines generally recommend loop ileostomy over loop transverse colostomy for temporary fecal diversion.

Genitourinary Stomas

- The ileal conduit is the most common urinary diversion. 10–15 cm of ileum is harvested, 15–20 cm proximal to the ileocecal valve. An ileoileostomy restores continuity, and it is important to remember that the left ureter is tunneled through the sigmoid mesentery. The stoma may be an end or end loop. The tenuous ileal conduit mesentery must be preserved at all costs to prevent conduit infarction. The mesentery will always be inferior to the ileoileostomy (Fig. 55.15).
- Ileal segments may also be used to replace or augment the urinary bladder. A fragile mesen-

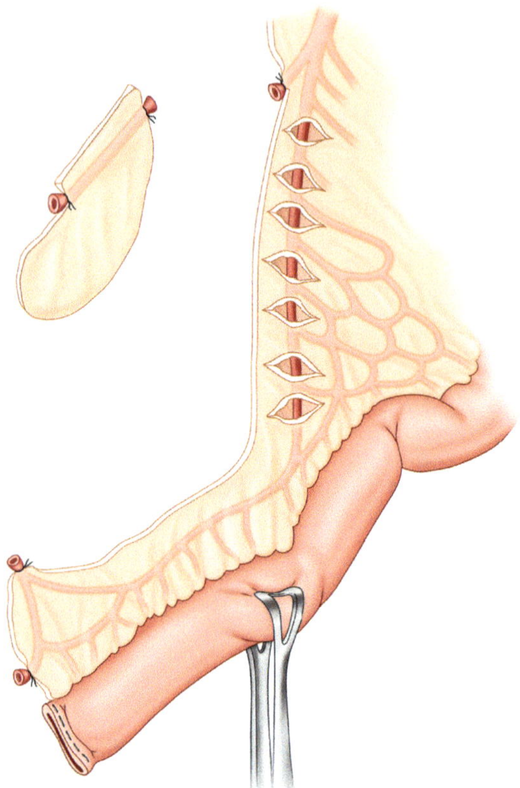

Fig. 55.13 "Pie crusting" of the bowel mesentery to obtain additional length prior to stoma creation. If a difficult end ileostomy is fashioned from the terminal ileum, the surgeon may find it helpful to ligate the ileocolic artery proximally to obtain reach

teric pedicle spans from the closed mesenteric defect toward the pelvis.

- Several catheterizable urinary stomas may be brought to the right lower quadrant or the umbilicus. The cecum is usually harvested and the appendix or terminal ileum used as the channel for catheterization.
- The Indiana pouch is a reservoir constructed from the right colon and ileum. Both ureters are implanted and a narrow skin level stoma is created that serves as a valve to allow for intermittent catheterization (Fig. 55.16).

Ileostomy and Foodstuff Bolus Obstruction

- Edema may cause a temporary occlusion of the bowel at the fascia in the early postoperative period. This is suspected when there is pain around the stoma with thin bilious fluid (bowel sweat) or no effluent. Radiologically there is an abrupt transition in bowel caliber as the bowel transverses the fascia. A 14–18 French Foley may be gently inserted to decompress the bowel. Using a Toomey syringe, small amounts of water are injected and the Foley advanced in that water cushion.

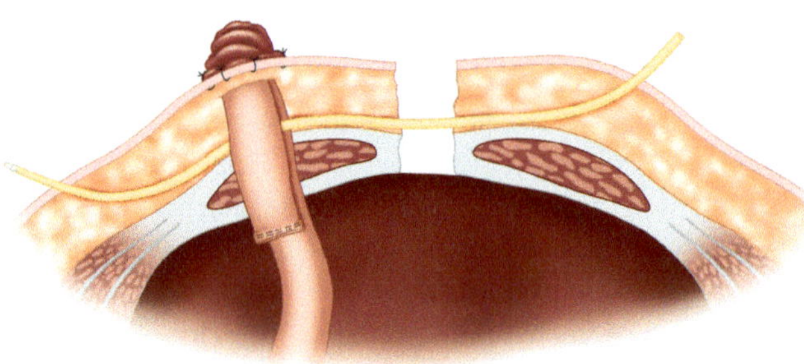

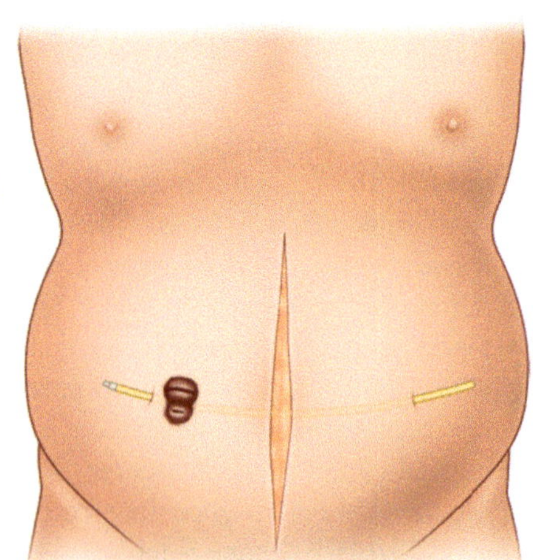

Fig. 55.14 Supporting a difficult loop enterostomy at the fascial level with a filiform catheter

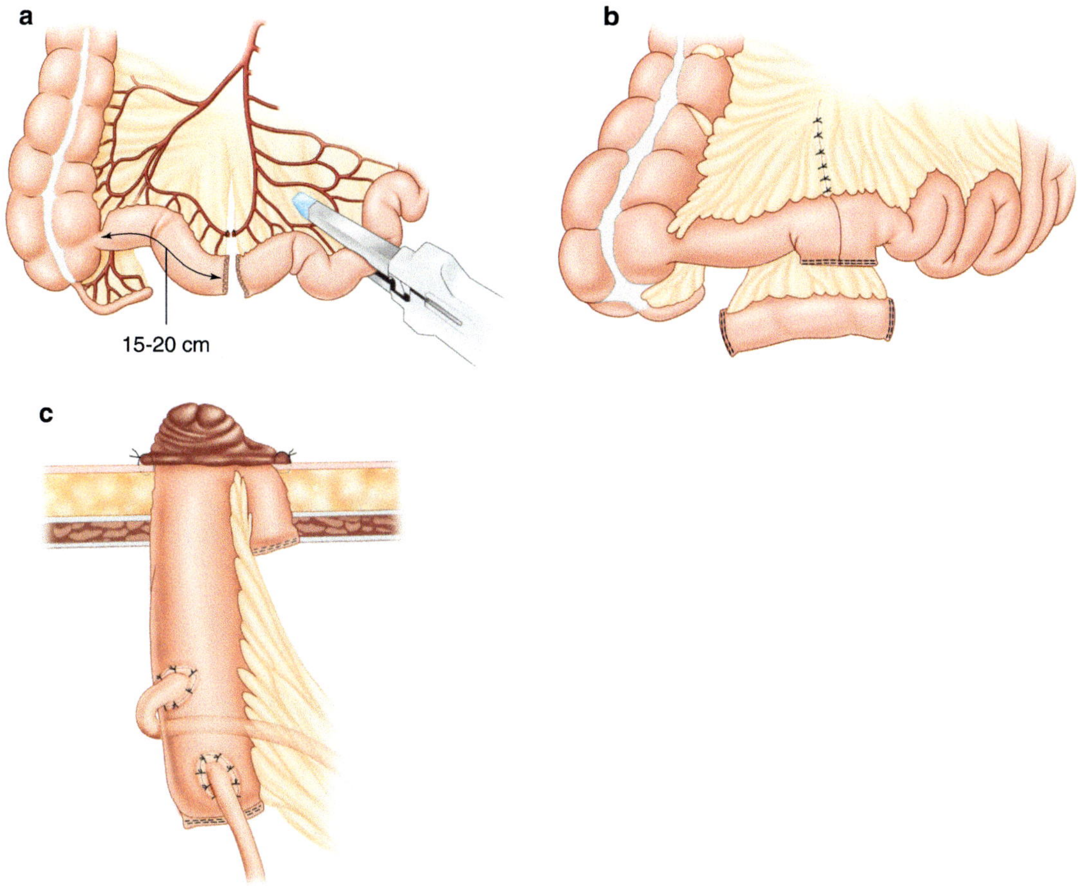

Fig. 55.15 The ileal urinary conduit: (**a**) a segment of mid ileum is resected, (**b**) an ileo-ileostomy is created, and (**c**) the harvested ileal conduit is anastomosed to the ureters and matured as a stoma

The balloon is not inflated. The tube is secured to the appliance.

- A bolus obstruction of nondigestable foodstuff may occur with an ileostomy. Nuts, seeds, sausage casings, or raw produce may become lodged below the fascia. To disimpact this food bolus, a Foley is placed as described above and advanced just beyond the fascia. Slowly 30–50 cc of water is injected until the bolus is dislodged. This process may take 1–2 h.

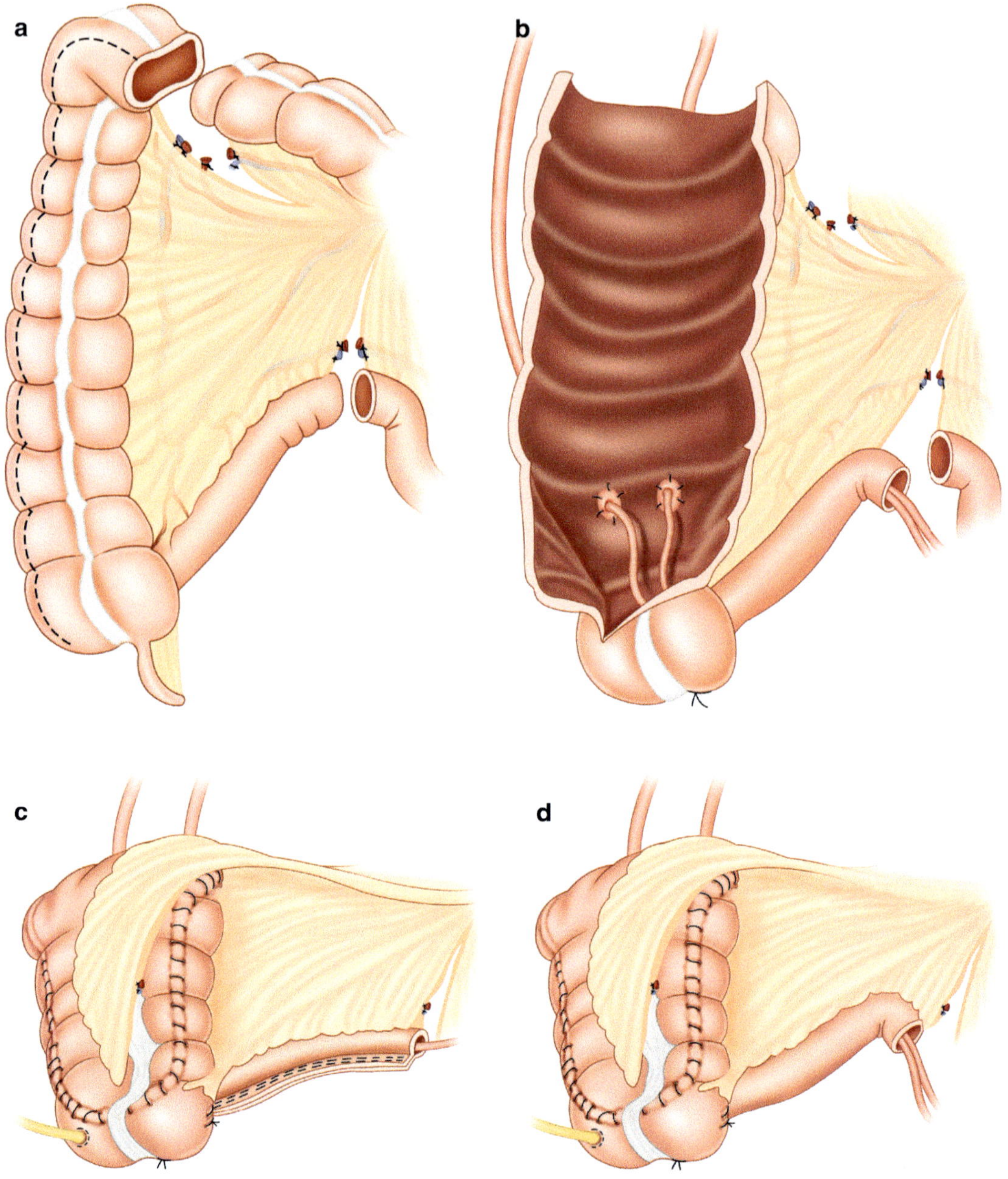

Fig. 55.16 The Indiana pouch

The Turnbull-Blowhole Colostomy
(Fig. 55.17)

- In special circumstances a colectomy with proper fecal diversion is inadvisable. This may occur in a woman with a gravid uterus and fulminant colitis or in a patient with profound comorbidities where a colectomy may be fatal.
- A limited <10 cm upper midline incision can be used to make a loop ileostomy and then a transverse loop colostomy can be brought out via the midline incision. The fascia is closed around the colon before it is opened.
- For those who cannot tolerate a general anesthesia, this procedure can be done via local anesthesia. Using fluoroscopic assistance the colon's position is marked on the skin in order to make the incision directly over the colon.

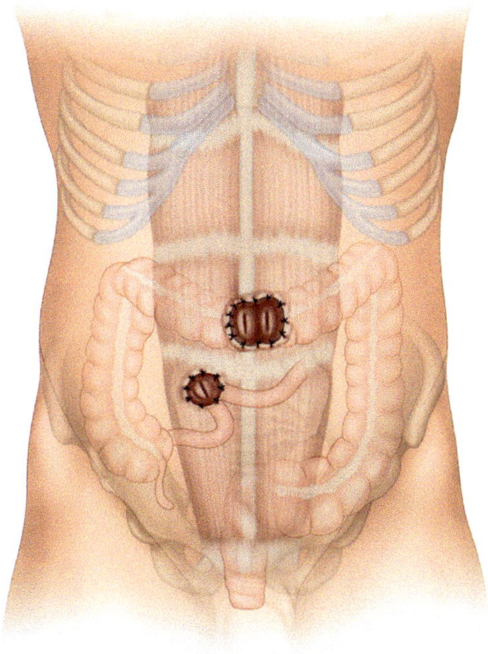

Fig. 55.17 The completed Turnbull blowhole colostomy and loop ileostomy

56 Functional Complications After Colon and Rectal Surgery

Dana M. Hayden and Alex Jenny Ky

Key Concepts

- Low anterior resection syndrome (LARS) is extremely common after proctectomy with a multifactorial etiology including damage to sphincters, variations in RAIR, intestinal motility changes, autonomic and somatic nerve injury, and pelvic floor dysfunction.
- Radiation and pelvic sepsis may contribute to deterioration of bowel function.
- Symptoms may include incontinence to stool or flatus, urgency, fragmentation of stool, difficult evacuation, and a sense of incomplete evacuation.
- Alternative reconstructions utilizing colonic pouch or side-to-end anastomosis may be associated with better bowel function when compared to straight anastomoses.
- Pelvic nerve damage during TME can impair urinary and sexual function as well as bowel function.
- Sexual dysfunction occurs in both males and females and may manifest in women as dyspareunia and failure to lubricate with arousal. In men, erectile dysfunction and retrograde ejaculation may occur.
- Colorectal surgeons may underappreciate the magnitude of bowel dysfunction after rectal cancer resection and its impact on quality of life.
- There is no accepted treatment algorithm for bowel dysfunction after proctectomy; symptom control utilizing medications to slow and bulk stools, protection of the perianal skin, physical therapy, colonic irrigation, and in some cases sacral nerve stimulation are currently recognized therapies.

Introduction

- Bowel dysfunction after colorectal (CRA) or coloanal (CAA) anastomosis is extremely common and underappreciated.
- This dysfunction is termed low anterior resection syndrome (LARS).

Low Anterior Resection Syndrome

Symptoms and Prevalence

- The theory that quality of life is better without a permanent stoma after low rectal resection and CRA or CAA has not been borne out in the literature.

D. M. Hayden (✉)
Department of General Surgery, Loyola University Medical Center, Maywood, IL, USA

A. J. Ky
Mount Sinai School of Medicine, New York, NY, USA

S. R. Steele et al. (eds.), *The ASCRS Manual of Colon and Rectal Surgery*,
https://doi.org/10.1007/978-3-030-01165-9_56

- QOL may be equivalent between those who had an abdominal perineal resection and those with sphincter preservation (low anterior resection [LAR]).
- 50–90% of patients after LAR experience some level of bowel dysfunction postoperatively.
- LARS symptoms include fecal incontinence, urgency, frequent small bowel movements, and clustering of stools. It may also be associated with tenesmus, rectal/anal pain, difficult defecation, impotence, dyspareunia, or debilitating anal skin irritation.
- Diarrhea has the strongest correlation with decreased QOL.
- A definition of LARS is disordered and dysfunctional bowel patterns after rectal resection leading to a detriment in quality of life.
- LARS symptoms may be lifelong with 42% having major LARS symptoms and 22% minor LARS symptoms at 14 years after surgery in one study.

Etiology of LARS

- The exact etiology of LARS is unclear but appears to be multifactorial.
- Reduced rectal reservoir, impaired rectal compliance, abnormal GI motility, partially denervated colon, loss of rectoanal coordination, and impairment of sympathetic and parasympathetic nerve supply have all been implicated in the literature.

Risk Factors for LARS

- Fecal incontinence associated with LARS is multifactorial and has been associated with short anastomotic distance to the anal verge, male gender, younger age, or any form of pelvic sepsis.
- Radiotherapy is a risk factor for LARS.

Evaluation and Bowel Dysfunction After LAR

- The LARS score is calculated from a validated instrument evaluating bowel function after sphincter-preserving rectal cancer surgery (Fig. 56.1).
- A composite score of 0–20 suggests no LARS, while 21–29 is minor LARS, and 30–42 is consistent with major LARS.

Treatment for Bowel Dysfunction After LAR

- There is no specific agreed treatment algorithm for LARS. The current therapy targets distressing symptoms.
- Loperamide, codeine, pelvic floor physiotherapy, biofeedback, and rectal irrigation have been reported to improve symptoms of fecal incontinence and bowel frequency.

Retrograde Colonic Irrigation

- Rectal irrigation of high-volume tepid water is a treatment option for fecal incontinence and fragmentation.
- The side effects are mild and the procedure is inexpensive.

Sacral Nerve Stimulation (SNS)

- SNS improves function by decreasing antegrade colonic motor activity and increasing retrograde activity. The success rate has been reported to be 74%.
- Changes in symptoms include decreased or improved fecal incontinence, nocturnal defecation, fragmentation, urgency, time to defer defecation, and soiling.

The aim of this questionnaire is to assess your bowel function.
Please tick only one box for each question. It may be difficult to select only one answer, as we know that for some patients symptoms vary from day to day.
We would kindly ask you to choose one answer which best describes your daily life. If you have recently had an infection affecting your bowel function, please do not take this into account and focus on answering questions to reflect your usual daily bowel function.

Do you ever have occasions when you cannot control your flatus (wind)?
☐ No, never
☐ Yes, less than once per week
☐ Yes, at least once per week

Do you ever have any accidental leakage of liqiud stool?
☐ No, never
☐ Yes, less than once per week
☐ Yes, at least once per week

How often do you open your bowels?
☐ More than 7 times per day (24 hours)
☐ 4-7 times per day (24 hours)
☐ 1-3 times per day (24 hours)
☐ Less than once per day (24 hours)

Do you ever have to open your bowel again within one hour of the last bowel opening?
☐ No, never
☐ Yes, less than once per week
☐ Yes, at least once per week

Do you ever have such a strong urge to open your bowels that you have to rush to the toilet?
☐ No, never
☐ Yes, less than once per week
☐ Yes, at least once per week

Fig. 56.1 LARS score questionnaire. (Adapted from Emmertsen K, Laurberg S. Low anterior resection syndrome score: development and validation of a symptom-based scoring system for bowel dysfunction after low anterior resection for rectal cancer. Ann Surg 2012;255(5):922–8)

Colorectal Reconstruction and Effects on Function After Colorectal Surgery

- It was speculated that the traditional straight anastomosis led to reduced reservoir volume and contributed to the functional LARS issues. In an effort to improve bowel function, surgeons developed alternative anastomosis with neoreservoirs.

Colonic J Pouch

- The colonic J pouch should be 4–6 cm to reduce problems with incomplete or difficult evacuation (vs the size of the ileal J pouch which is 18–20 cm).
- After having a colonic J pouch, patients in the long term report reduced daily stool frequency, decreased fecal urge incontinence, and less incomplete evacuation, and they used less antidiarrheal medication.

Transverse Coloplasty

- Transverse coloplasty does not confer any functional advantage over a straight anastomosis, and there is minimal indication to reconstruct with this technique.

Side-to-End Anastomosis

- For the side-to-end anastomosis, the anastomosis is created 3–6 cm upstream from the cut edge of the proximal colon (on the antimesenteric side). The open end of the proximal colon is then closed.

- The side-to-end anastomosis seems to have the same functional outcome and benefits as the colonic J pouch.
- Anastomotic leak rates are similar with side-to-end and colonic J pouch reconstructions, but both seem to have a lower rate compared to the straight anastomosis.
- Utilizing a 3–6 cm blind limb seems to reduce evacuation problems.

Sexual and Urologic Dysfunction After Surgery for Rectal Cancer

Nerves of the Pelvis

- The main etiology of sexual and urinary dysfunction after proctectomy is mainly related to direct nerve injury.
- Nerve damage during ligation of the inferior mesenteric artery and dissection in the retrorectal space can damage the superior hypogastric plexus particularly at the sacral promontory and result in retrograde ejaculation.
- Anterolateral pelvic dissection and division of the lateral ligament can damage the pelvic plexus and result in erectile dysfunction.
- Anterior dissection especially on the prostate side of Denonvilliers' fascia can damage the nervi erigentes or cavernous nerves and lead to erectile dysfunction.

Sexual Dysfunction After Surgery for Rectal Cancer

- In men sexual dysfunction after rectal cancer surgery consists usually of erectile dysfunction (ED) and retrograde ejaculation.
- There also can be difficulty with orgasm, libido, and reduced body image.
- Postoperatively in women, sexual dysfunction includes problems with vaginal lubrication, dyspareunia, arousal, and orgasm.
- Other risk factors for postoperative sexual dysfunction include increased operative blood loss, preoperative radiation, anastomotic leak, and presence of a stoma.
- Validated tools to evaluate sexual dysfunction after rectal cancer surgery are the International Index of Erectile Dysfunction (IIEF), the Female Sexual Function Index (FISI), and the EORTC QLQ-30 and EORTC QLQ-CR38 to measure QOL in colorectal cancer patients.
- Treatment of postoperative retrograde ejaculation includes tricyclic antidepressants, antihistamines (chlorpheniramine), and decongestants like ephedrine sulfate and phenylephrine (these help close the bladder neck during ejaculation).
- ED is treated with a trial of sildenafil citrate, tadalafil, or vardenafil. At low dose these medications increase blood flow to the area around the nerves to promote healing.
- For women, medications and creams aimed at improving vaginal lubrication along with pelvic floor physical therapy are the main treatments. Sexual dysfunction in women after rectal cancer surgery has not been extensively studied.

Urologic Dysfunction

- Thirty to seventy percent of patients have bladder dysfunction after pelvic surgery, but this is usually temporary with only 10% requiring medical or surgical treatment.
- Any voiding problem that persists after 3 months may be permanent.

Perianal Skin Irritation After Colorectal Surgery

- Perianal skin irritation is common after rectal cancer surgery due to loose frequent stools and improper wiping techniques.
- Chemoradiation can reduce skin pliability—adding to skin irritation.
- Barrier creams (Desitin™ or Balmex®) applied like frosting to coat the anal area are the first line of therapy to protect the skin. After defe-

cation the goal is to wipe against the cream and avoid wiping it totally off.

- If there is a fungal component adding to the irritation, antifungal powders or creams can be used.
- For severe itching or pain, a short course of steroid cream can provide dramatic relief (but only a short course as it can thin the skin).
- Using wet toilet paper and avoiding the urge to over-wipe are an important advice.
- Management of stool frequency and consistency with fiber to bulk stools and antidiarrheal medication can improve problems with perianal skin irritation.
- Antidiarrheal mediation includes diphenoxylate hydrochloride/atropine and loperamide. Up to eight pills daily of each may be taken, but usually this maximal dose is not required for optimization of stool frequency. This medication should be taken *before* meals.

Common Tests for the Pelvic Floor

57

Dana R. Sands and Amy J. Thorsen

Key Concepts

- Pelvic floor disorders affect a significant portion of the population and account for relevant portion of patients seen in colorectal clinics.
- Proper history and thorough physical examination are the cornerstone of the evaluation of patients suffering from functional disorders.
- Specialized tests to evaluate structure and function augment the evaluation of this complex patient population.

Introduction

- Pelvic floor testing includes anatomic evaluations, functional investigations, and exams that evaluate both function and anatomy.
- Pathology such as neoplastic or inflammatory bowel disease should be ruled out with lower endoscopy when appropriate.

D. R. Sands (✉)
Department of Colorectal Surgery, Cleveland Clinic Florida, Weston, FL, USA
e-mail: sandsd@ccf.org

A. J. Thorsen
University of Minnesota, Minneapolis, MN, USA

History

- A detailed history is the first step in examining the onset, duration, and evolution of symptoms.
- Questions regarding urinary incontinence and vaginal vault prolapse should be discussed.
- Factors that alter stool consistency such as dietary changes, food intolerances, changes in medications, supplements, and surgeries (cholecystectomy, gastric bypass) are investigated.
- Pelvic floor trauma from surgery, childbirth, sexual abuse, or other causes is queried.

Questionnaires

Fecal Incontinence: Four Will Be Reviewed Below

- Cleveland Clinic Florida Fecal Incontinence Score: With this tool there are five frequency categories and each are weighed the same. Besides actual fecal incontinence, this tool includes a determination of pad usage and lifestyle alteration. The range is from 0–20 with zero being totally continent and 20 = total incontinence.
- Vaizey or St. Mark's Incontinence Score: This tool has five frequency categories. The need to wear a pad, constipating medication, and

S. R. Steele et al. (eds.), *The ASCRS Manual of Colon and Rectal Surgery*,
https://doi.org/10.1007/978-3-030-01165-9_57

urgency are given as a single score which does not consider the frequency of use/problem.
- Fecal Incontinence Severity Index (FISI): This is the first score to involve patients in the development. A weighted scale is utilized. Surgeons and patients have different weights assigned to four types of fecal incontinence across five different frequencies.
- Fecal Incontinence Quality of Life Scale (FIQL): This tool measures impact of fecal incontinence on aspects of life. Twenty-nine questions are tabulated into four subscales (lifestyle, coping/behavior, depression/self-perception, embarrassment).

Constipation

- Cleveland Clinic Florida Constipation Score (CCF-CS): Eight variables are assessed with score of 0–30. A score of 15 suggests constipation, and 30 is associated with severe constipation. This is commonly used when assessing obstructed defecation particularly in trials and studies.
- Patient Assessment of Constipation Symptom (PAC-SYM): This assesses symptom frequency and severity based on Rome II Criteria in three symptom subscales (abdominal, rectal, stool) through 12 items on a scale of 0–4 (4 most severe). This does not discriminate constipation subtypes.
- Patient Assessment of Constipation Quality of Life: This consists of 28 items grouped into 4 subscales (physical discomfort, psychosocial discomfort, worries and concerns, satisfaction). Scores range from 0 to 96 (lower scores correspond to better quality of life).

Physical Exam

- Perineal inspection, sensation utilizing pinprick, and the presence of the anocutaneous wink reflex may be the initial parts of the physical exam.
- Digital is performed to detect masses, strictures, fecal impaction, resting tone, squeeze tone, the ability of the puborectalis to relax with strain, rectoceles, and internal intussusception.
- Since other compartments of the pelvic floor can be affected, inspection of the introitus looking for atrophy, lichen sclerosus, cystocele, rectocele, vaginal wall prolapse, or urinary incontinence can be done.
- Bimanual exam of the vagina and rectum may detect an enterocele or sigmoidocele.
- Rectal prolapse may be detected by examining a patient particularly after straining on a commode.

Anatomic Evaluation

Ultrasound 2-D

- Evaluation of anal sphincter integrity can be done with the endoanal ultrasound (US).
- US has replaced needle electromyography in the anatomic assessment for patients with fecal incontinence.
- The internal sphincter is hypoechoic (black), and the external sphincter and puborectalis are hyperechoic (mixed but more white appearance).
- This test may assist when planning surgery or therapy for anal sphincter injury and anal fistula.
- The images are reviewed looking for scarring, thinning, and hypertrophy along with the angle of sphincter disruption.
- Interpretation is operator dependent.

Ultrasound 3-D

- A special probe allows volumetric acquisition of images over 6 cm without movement of the probe. After acquiring, images can be reconstructed and manipulated in coronal, sagittal, and axial planes (Fig. 57.1a and b).

Dynamic US

- Dynamic US uses three separate probes which provide images during four steps (rest, cough, squeeze, push). Video clips are taken. Probes

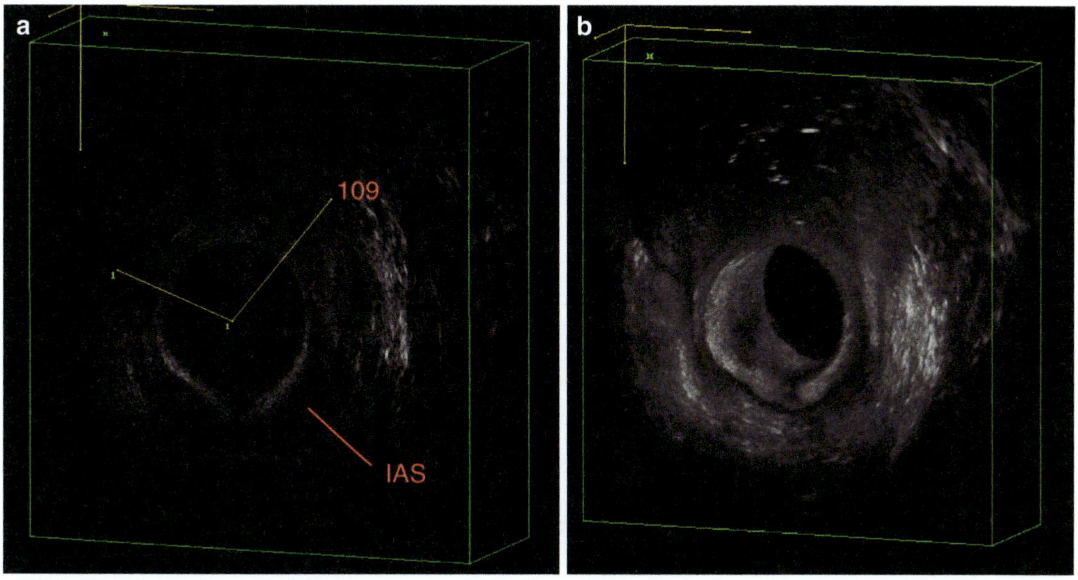

Fig. 57.1 (a) Endoanal ultrasound revealing combined external sphincter defect (measuring 109 degrees) with significant retraction of the internal sphincter (IAS). (b) The external sphincter defect can be more easily appreciated on 3D rendered imaging

are placed transperitoneally, on the perineal skin, transvaginal, and per anus. Some feel the video clips provide data/imaging that is similar to defecography.

MRI

- The appearance of the internal and external sphincter can be assessed with MRI.
- MRI appears to be better at assessing the internal anal sphincter vs US.
- US and MRI seem to have similar detection of external anal sphincter integrity, but MRI may be superior at detecting external sphincter atrophy.
- Due to cost and availability, US is more commonly utilized to evaluate anal sphincters.

Functional Evaluation

Anal Manometry (AM)

- AM is used to evaluate patients with fecal incontinence, constipation, anal pain, fissures, and Hirschsprung's disease.
- No standard protocols exits and age and gender may influence results.
- The probe, placed in the anus, senses pressure. A balloon covers the internal end of the probe and rests in the rectum. There are two types of probes: water perfused (cheaper but potential for making artifact calibration essential) or solid state (expensive and fragile but felt to be more accurate).
- The newest advancement is high-resolution manometry which provides greater detail due to significantly more sensors in a solid-state probe.

Manometry Technique

- The patient is placed in the left lateral position and an enema given if there is a huge stool volume. A digital is done to assess stool burden and any abnormalities or low anastomosis.
- The probe is placed in the anal canal and allowed a period of equilibrium.
- Two systems are in use: water perfused, which has a station pull-through technique where the catheter is inserted to 6 cm and static readings are taken upon withdrawal of every 1 cm, and high resolution, where simultaneous pressure in the entire anal canal at once is recorded.

- Wave patterns that may be observed are slow, ultraslow, and intermediate wave.

Resting Pressure (RP)

- Seventy percent of the RP is from the internal anal sphincter and 30% from external anal sphincter (some also from anal cushions).
- The sphincter length can be calculated by detecting the distance/length where the pressure is at least 5 mm > intrarectal pressure.

Squeeze Pressure

- To measure the squeeze pressure, the external sphincter contraction is measured. The use of accessory muscles should be avoided.
- The duration of squeeze also is noted (the time patient can maintain 50% of maximal squeeze pressure). This may correlate with the ability of the external sphincter to maintain continence.

Cough Reflex

- With a rise in intra-abdominal pressure (cough), there is a reflex contraction of the external sphincter. This is preserved in thoracic spinal injury but lost with cauda equina lesions.

Valsalva

- Relaxation of the external sphincter with strain (Valsalva) facilitates defecation.
- Paradoxical contraction can lead to outlet constipation.
- To determine if there is paradoxical contraction, the intrarectal and intra-anal pressure are compared at rest, squeeze, and strain. In normal defecation, with squeeze the intrarectal pressure < intra-anal and with strain the intrarectal pressure > intra-anal.

Rectoanal Inhibitory Reflex (RAIR)

- To measure the RAIR, the rectal balloon is filled with fluid (typically 50 cc but may be more), and initially the external sphincter will contract followed by internal anal relaxation.
- The RAIR aids in the anal canal sampling mechanism and is an important component of fecal continence.
- The presence of this reflex confirms a functioning myenteric plexus, and its absence is reflective of Hirschsprung's disease and visceral neuropathy.
- Absence to illicit this reflex may be related to a technical factor.

Rectal Sensation

- The rectum does not contain pain fibers but is sensitive to distention via nerves in the pelvic floor mediated via S2–4 nerve roots.
- Incremental increases in filling the rectal balloon are used to assess the sensitivity of the rectum.
- The first sensation, urge to defecate, and maximum tolerated volume (MTV) are recorded.
- Most balloons only hold 300 cc, so if the MTV is 300 cc, it may signal dramatically decreased rectal sensation.

Compliance

- Compliance relates to the dispensability of the rectum.
- It is calculated as the balloon is inflated with change in rectal pressure and change in volume.

Balloon Expulsion

- There is no standard way balloon expulsion is done.
- Generally the balloon is placed in the rectum with the patient in the seated position and about 50 cc of fluid placed in the balloon. The ability and time taken to expel the balloon are measured.
- One minute is the usual cutoff for normal balloon expulsion.

Neurophysiologic Testing

- There are four methods of neurophysiologic testing (concentric needle, monopolar wire, single fiber, and surface anal plug).
- The integrity of the neural motor unit is assessed.
- In areas that have undergone injury, repair, and reinnervation, the action potentials will be prolonged and have polyphasic potentials.

Needle EMG

- Detailed information regarding the electrical activity of the anal sphincter can be obtained by inserting a needle in multiple areas of the anal muscle.
- It is not routinely done as it is painful and generally not well tolerated.

Surface

- Another method to evaluate muscle movement is to place a specialized pad over the muscle and globally assesses movement.
- This technique is useful in the evaluation of constipation and paradoxical contraction. It is used in biofeedback as an aid in treating paradoxical contractions by providing feedback to the patient regarding their muscle movement.

Pudendal Nerve Terminal Motor Latency (PNTML)

- To conduct PNTML, a special probe with an electrode at the tip of the index finger is inserted into the anal canal, and an electrical impulse is delivered to the pudendal nerve at the ischial spine. The time is then noted when the muscle contracts (normal 2.0 +/− 0.2 ms).
- The clinical significance of this test has been debated, and some centers no longer routinely perform this test.

Transit Testing

- Four methods will be discussed to evaluate the transit time of the gastrointestinal tract.

Radiopaque Markers

- There are multiple protocols which use radiopaque markers to assess GI motility, but all require cessation of laxatives 48 h before the start of the test.
- One or two capsules (which contain 24 radiopaque markers) are ingested to start the test.
- The most commonly utilized protocol then requests a KUB on days 1, 3, and 5 after the markers are ingested. 80% of the markers should be expelled by day 5.
- Patients with slow transit constipation will typically have ≥ 20% of markers scattered throughout the colon.
- Patients with pelvic centered constipation will typically have their markers stacked in the rectosigmoid or rectum.

Breath Testing

- This test provides estimation of gastric emptying and orocecal transit.
- Normal orocecal transit is 40–170 min.
- This test can be falsely interpreted in patient with bacterial overgrowth and in the 15–20% of the normal population that does not have the ability to ferment and produce hydrogen (that is measured as part of this test).

Scintigraphy

- Gastric emptying can be measured by calculating the percentage of retained gastric contents of a low-fat meal which contains ^{99}technetium-labeled egg whites. Delayed gastric emptying is defined as >10% of the meal remaining in the stomach at 4 h.
- While the stomach is commonly evaluated with this method of testing, small and large bowel scintigraphy is not routinely used

Wireless Motility Capsules

- This is the newest technology devised to evaluate GI transit. The capsule records temperature, pH, and pressure as it passes through the GI tract and transmits this information to a data receiver worn by the patient. The data can then be downloaded onto a computer.
- All medications that can affect motility are discontinued. The capsule is ingested. After a standardized meal is consumed, the patient is NPO for 6 h to determine gastric emptying time.
- The patient eats normally and records meals, sleep, and defecation.
- Passage from the small bowel into the colon is signaled by a drop in pH or changes in pressure wave frequency of amplitude.
- An abrupt temperature drop occurs when the capsule exits the body.
- This test is standardized and can be performed in an ambulatory setting.

Anatomic and Functional Evaluation

- Dynamic imaging is crucial in evaluating any pelvic floor problems such as obstructive defecation and fecal incontinence.

Defecography

- This test is performed after a patient has rectal contrast (which mimics stool) inserted into the rectum. Then a video is done as the patient defecates the contrast while sitting on a specialized commode.
- By studying the video, dynamic changes in the rectal wall, anal canal, vagina, and other pelvic floor structures can be assessed.
- Some centers add vaginal, bladder, and oral contrast in an effort to better delineate structures.
- The theoretical advantage of this test is that it is done in a position that simulates defecation (sitting). If a patient digitizes to evacuate, this can be replicated during the evacuation phase of the study.

Normal Parameters

- The pubococcygeal line (tip of coccyx to pubis) is a landmark utilized to assess mobility of the pelvic floor. Less than 1/3 of the rectum should be below the line. Pelvic organ prolapse is identified when pelvic viscera descend below this line.
- The angle between the anal canal and the posterior rectum is the anorectal angle. At rest this should be 90°, with squeeze 75°, and with strain 110–180°.
- A lack of relaxation and inability to change the angle with strain may reflect paradoxical contraction (outlet obstruction).
- There can be high intra- and inter-observer variation in the determination of these angles.

Rectocele

- Rectoceles are a common nearly always anterior bulge of the anterior rectal wall into the vagina. A rectocele may be seen in over 93% of asymptomatic women.
- Lateral and posterior rectoceles have also been described in men and women.
- Rectoceles smaller than 2 cm are rarely significant.
- The degree of rectocele emptying during defecography or the need to stabilize/digitate the rectocele for it to empty can be demonstrated during defecography. Retained contrast in the rectocele or being able to empty it with digital manipulation may signal that the rectocele is the etiology of outlet symptoms.

Rectal Intussusception

- Rectal intussusception entails >2 cm invagination of the rectal wall during straining.
- This may be detected in 39% of symptomatic patients and 20% of asymptomatic patients.
- Rectorectal intussusception is usually asymptomatic. Rectoanal intussusception may cause fecal incontinence, obstructed defecation, or rectal pain.

Rectal Prolapse

- Rectal prolapse entails the full thickness of rectum that invaginates and protrudes from the anus.
- This condition may be associated with anterior and middle compartment prolapse.

Enterocele and Sigmoidocele

- An enterocele consists of small bowel loops lying in the pouch of Douglas. Visualization is augmented by giving oral contrast to detect these loops during defecography. If a rectocele is present, opacified loops may be visualized in the rectovaginal septum.
- A sigmoidocele consists of a redundant sigmoid loop filling the pouch of Douglas.
- Both conditions may be associated with the sensation of incomplete evacuation.

Descending Perineum Syndrome

- Perineal hypermobility occurs when the anorectal junction descends more than 3.5 cm during Valsalva.
- This descent can be due to nerve and muscle stretch.
- The position of the pelvis may not correlate with severity of symptoms.

Dynamic MRI

- Some institutions advocate using dynamic MRI to assess pelvic structures instead of defecography.
- The major criticism is that this test is usually done in the supine position which does not simulate normal defecation.
- Open sitting MRI machines have less soft tissue resolution and also loss of detail making them subject to inaccuracies.

58 Evaluation of Constipation and Treatment of Abdominal Constipation

Muneera R. Kapadia and Madhulika K. Varma

Key Concepts

- There are three constipation subtypes which can be differentiated by symptoms and diagnostic testing, although there can be overlap between subtypes.
- Initial treatment of constipation includes behavioral modification and medication.
- Surgical management of constipation is reserved for severe slow transit constipation that is not responsive to medications.

Prevalence

- Two to twenty-seven percent of people have constipation.
- Constipation has a high prevalence in people >65 years.
- Women have constipation 2–3 times more frequently vs males.
- Constipation has a higher incidence in non-Caucasians, those with less education, and lower income.

M. R. Kapadia
Department of Surgery, University of Iowa Hospitals and Clinics, Iowa City, IA, USA

M. K. Varma (✉)
Division of Colon and Rectal Surgery, University of California-San Francisco, San Francisco, CA, USA
e-mail: Madhulika.Varma@ucsfmedctr.org

Etiology of Constipation

- Constipation may have no identifiable cause.
- Constipation can result from dysfunction of any portion of the defecatory process.
- Contributing factors to constipation include diet, medications, neurologic or endocrine disorders, psychosocial issues, colonic disease, or pelvic floor abnormalities.

Constipation Subtypes

- Constipation subtypes may be in isolation or in various combinations.

Slow Transit Constipation

- Slow transit constipation is also called abdominal constipation.
- This is a motility disorder and may involve colon only or also other portions of the GI tract.
- Patients may not move their bowels for days or weeks despite enemas and laxatives.

Normal Transit Constipation

- Normal transit constipation is also called constipation-predominant irritable bowel syndrome (IBS-c).

S. R. Steele et al. (eds.), *The ASCRS Manual of Colon and Rectal Surgery*,
https://doi.org/10.1007/978-3-030-01165-9_58

- Stools progress through the colon normally but are hard, and defecation may be difficult.
- Patients may have abdominal pain and bloating relieved with defecation.

Pelvic Constipation

- Pelvic constipation may be from lack of coordination of the pelvic floor during defecation, rectal hyposensitivity, or impingement leading to inability to fully empty the rectum (such as from rectocele, enterocele, or sigmoidocele)
- Full-thickness rectal prolapse, internal intussusception, or solitary rectal ulcer may be associated with pelvic constipation.

History and Physical Examination

- Table 58.1 lists points that should be elucidated during the history of a patient with constipation.
- Additionally a detailed medical, psychiatric, and surgical history is essential.
- Over the counter medications (including herbal treatments) used to treat constipation are noted.
- The physical exam is usually unremarkable.
- Stool consistency can be described using the Bristol Stool Form Scale (Fig. 58.1).

Diagnostic Testing

- Laboratory testing for patients with constipation include complete blood count, chemistry panel, calcium level, and thyroid function testing.
- Colonoscopy is used to rule out mechanical strictures or malignancy.
- The colonic transit study assesses gastrointestinal motility and can be done with radiopaque mark-

Table 58.1 History for patients with constipation

History for patients with constipation
Bowel habit frequency
Stool consistency
Onset and duration of symptoms
Straining during defecation and need for manual maneuvers
Dietary history
Exercise habits
Laxative use
Medication history
Medical history
Physical and sexual abuse history

Adapted from Lewis SJ, Heaton KW. Stool form scale as a useful guide to intestinal transit time. Scand J Gastroenterol. 1997;32(9):920–4

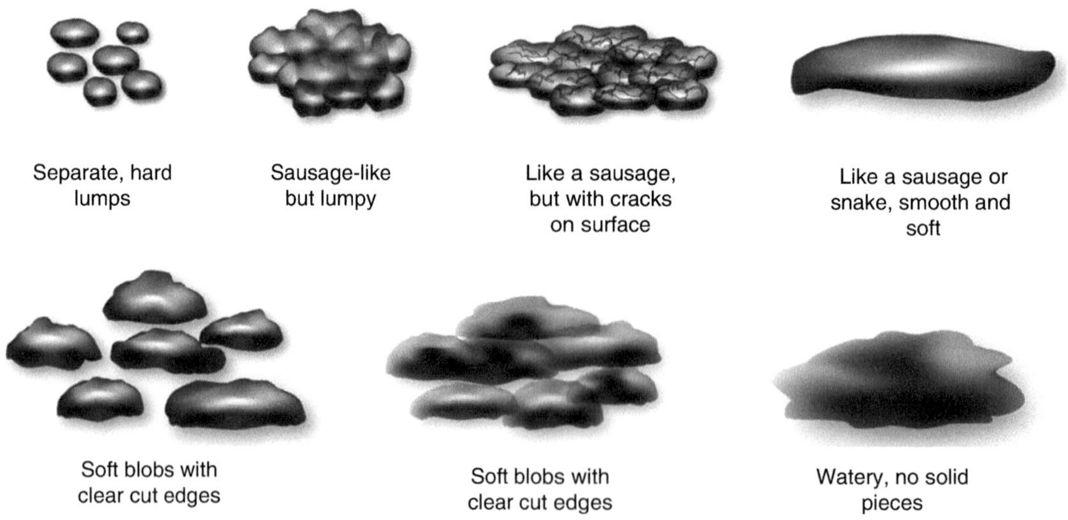

Fig. 58.1 Bristol stool Scale. With permission from Lewis SJ, Heaton KW. Stool form scale as a useful guide to intestinal transit time. Scand J Gastroenterol. 1997;32(9):920–4; Taylor and Francis 1997 (83)

ers, scintigraphy, or capsule studies – but radiopaque markers are the most commonly used.

- During the colonic transit, study patients take no laxatives.
- There are several protocols for the transit study, but typically an abdominal X-ray is obtained on day 5, and if >20% of markers are retained, the study is considered abnormal.
- If the markers are distributed throughout the colon – this is consistent with slow transit constipation.
- Markers distributed mostly in the rectosigmoid suggest obstructive defecation.
- A wireless motility capsule measures pH changes and has been shown to have 87% agreement when compared to radiopaque studies in differentiating slow transit from normal transit.
- Anal manometry is performed particularly looking for a rectal anal inhibitory reflex, nonrelaxation of the pelvic floor, rectal balloon expulsion, and rectal sensitivity (looking at maximum tolerated volume).
- Defecography identifies paradoxical contraction, internal intussusception, rectal prolapse, rectocele, sigmoidocele, and enterocele, all which can contribute to obstructed defecation constipation.

Slow Transit Constipation

- Slow transit constipation is also called colonic inertia.
- Symptoms include markedly reduced stool frequency along with abdominal pain, bloating, nausea, and incomplete defecation.
- The diagnosis of slow transit constipation is confirmed by transit studies.

Medical Management of Slow Transit Constipation

- Treatment begins with appropriate counseling to validate patient complaints and educate patients regarding "normal" bowel habits (normal bowel habits can range from 3 to 20 bowel movements per week).
- Improved hydration, exercise, dietary modification, fiber optimization, and medication modification are the next steps in treatment of constipation.
- Osmotic laxatives promote fluid to be shifted into the colon via osmosis. Lactulose and MiraLAX[R] are commonly used osmotic laxatives.
- Magnesium (Milk of Magnesia[R]) and phosphate (Fleets[R] Phosphosoda) ions can be utilized as an osmotic laxative but are cautiously recommended in patients with renal insufficiency.
- Colonic irritants (senna and cascara) stimulate colonic motility. Long-term use leads to brown mucosal discoloration. Sustained use of anthracene can lead to poor long-term function, and long-term use is discouraged.
- Stool-softening laxatives include mineral oil and docusate.
- Enema and suppository therapy promote defecation through rectal distention and irritation.
- Lubiprostone (Amitiza[R]) activates chloride channels which increases colonic motility.
- Linaclotide (Linzess[R]) increases colonic smooth muscle contraction to promote motility.
- Both lubiprostone and linaclotide are approved to treat slow transit constipation and IBS-constipation in the USA.

Surgical Therapy of Slow Transit Constipation

- Surgery is considered when testing suggests slow transit constipation and nonsurgical therapy has been exhausted.
- Patients may also have generalized intestinal dysmotility which may be associated with recurrent constipation after surgery.
- It is essential that patients have appropriate expectations regarding outcomes and possible postoperative new issues.

Abdominal Colectomy

- Traditionally total abdominal colectomy with an ileorectal (IRA) anastomosis is the surgical treatment for slow transit constipation.

- Possible postoperative issues include ileus, anastomotic leak, persistent constipation, or continued need for enemas or laxatives.
- Studies report approximately 2–3 stools daily after colectomy and IRA.
- Some have reported good results with a variation in the technique with near-total colectomy performed and cecorectal anastomosis or ileosigmoid anastomosis establishing bowel continuity. The aim of preserving this portion of the colon is to reduce concerns of diarrhea and electrolyte abnormalities.
- Some patients may have pelvic floor dysfunction associated with their slow transit constipation. Biofeedback before (or if continued symptoms persist after colectomy) has been used successfully in some patients to address this additional problem.
- Patients with small bowel or gastric dysmotility issues may be offered colectomy and ileorectal anastomosis but must be counseled that postoperatively they could have persistent abdominal symptoms.

Segmental Colectomy

- Some authors have done careful preoperative evaluation noting where markers do not progress through the colon and then performed a segmental colon resection of this area.
- Even though successful outcomes have been reported, radiopaque markers may not be exact, and patients need careful evaluation and counseling.

Proctocolectomy with Ileal Pouch-Anal Anastomosis

- Few patients benefit from proctocolectomy and pouch-anal anastomosis for constipation.
- Careful selection to ensure there is absolutely no issues with pelvic floor relaxation is essential to delineate this limited group of patients.

Ileostomy Creation

- Ileostomy may be offered for patients not sufficiently improved with a colectomy or those with life-altering side effects from surgery (fecal incontinence or diarrhea after colonic resection).
- Patients should be aware that they could have persistent symptoms after ileostomy construction if global intestinal dysmotility is present.

Antegrade Colonic Enema

- Originally described as a treatment for fecal incontinence in children, a washout of the colon via a tube placed in a small stoma leading into the cecum (antegrade colonic enema) has also been used successfully in adults. Satisfaction with this procedure has been reported in about 45%.
- Revisions of the stoma are common secondary to stenosis or leakage.

Sacral Nerve Stimulation

- Sacral nerve stimulation has been shown to increase colonic propagating sequences.
- This treatment is not approved for constipation in the USA.
- While it has been tested outside the USA, results have not been as successful as for fecal incontinence, and further studies are needed to define the patients who will benefit.

Summary

- A treatment algorithm is listed in Fig. 58.2 to outline the evaluation and treatment for constipation.

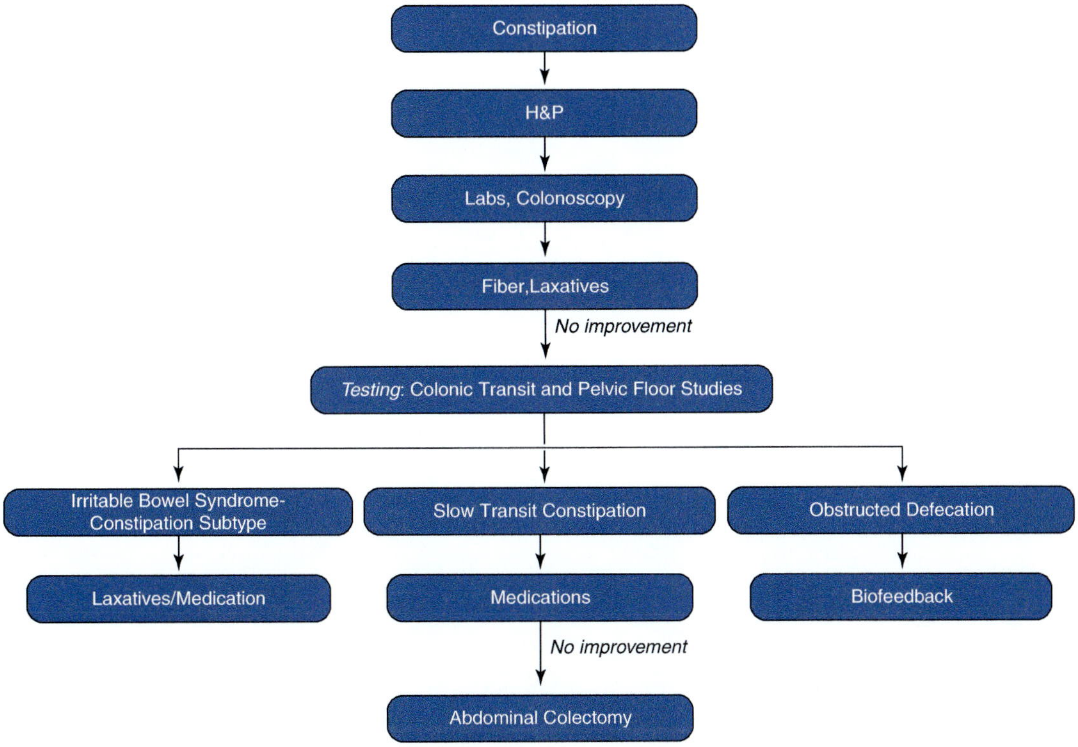

Fig. 58.2 Workup and treatment schematic for constipation

59 Obstructed Defecation

M. Shane McNevin

Key Concepts

- Obstructed defecation syndrome is characterized by excessive straining at stool, incomplete rectal evacuation, and perineal splinting.
- The primary treatment for patients with obstructed defecation is dietary management and pelvic floor physical therapy.
- The primary treatment of patients with overt pelvic prolapse and obstructed defecation is surgical repair of the prolapse.
- Symptoms of obstructed defecation are not as reliably relieved as overt prolapse by surgical repair.
- Ventral mesh rectopexy and stapled transanal rectal resection are alternative surgical procedures which may more reliably relieve obstructed defecation symptoms.
- Sacral nerve stimulation may be an alternative for patients with rectal hyposensitivity and obstructed defecation failing non-operative management.

M. S. McNevin (✉)
Sacred Heart Hospital, Spokane, WA, USA
e-mail: smcnevin@comcast.net

Introduction

- Obstructed defecation is simply constipation in association with pelvic floor disorders.
- Obstructed defecation syndrome is a well-defined symptom complex consisting of excessive straining at stool, the need for perineal splitting, and the sensation of incomplete rectal evacuation.
- Twenty-five percent of women in the USA will have one pelvic floor disorder in their lifetime.

Etiology of Constipation

- A detailed history is important in making the diagnosis of obstructed defecation, and it is important to clarify terminology with the patient as certain terms may have a different meaning to the patient and caregiver.
- The detailed history and physical exam drive further testing and treatment options.
- Endoscopic evaluation is considered when new complaints center on a change of bowel habits.
- Criteria for obstructed defecation syndrome include having >25% of the time any of the following: painful, excessive straining; incomplete or fragmented evacuation; or perineal splinting.

S. R. Steele et al. (eds.), *The ASCRS Manual of Colon and Rectal Surgery*,
https://doi.org/10.1007/978-3-030-01165-9_59

- Patients with obstructed defecation may defecate frequently with symptoms refractory to cathartics.
- Pseudo fecal incontinence may be seen from inability to completely evacuate the rectum.
- Colonic transit study may demonstrate elevated global transit times with delay only in the rectosigmoid area.
- Any disturbance in the complex evacuation process due to pelvic floor anatomic abnormalities, disorders of anorectal sensation, and/or discoordinated pelvic floor musculature will result in symptoms that are associated with obstructed defecation syndrome.

Evaluation of Obstructed Defecation

Endoscopy

- Endoscopy and cross-sectional imaging are used to rule out an intrinsic and extrinsic obstructive lesion, which could also hinder fecal evacuation.

Colon Transit Study

- A colonic transit study may help differentiate types of functional constipation when the history is unclear or disorders coexist.

Balloon Expulsion Study

- Expelling a balloon may be a helpful test and utilized as adjunct when obstructed defecation is suspected.
- Expulsion time >2 min has been shown to correlate with findings from anorectal manometry and electromyography.

Anorectal Manometry

- In the evaluation of obstructed defecation, the most important information from anorectal manometry is the rectal sensory thresholds (first sensation, urge to defecate, and maximal tolerable volume). Rectal hyposensitivity is reflected by an excessively large maximal tolerated volume.
- Presence of the rectoanal inhibitory reflex (RAIR) excludes short-segment Hirschsprung's disease as the etiology of constipation.
- In those patients with obstructed defecation, the mean resting and squeeze pressure may be excessive and associated with non-relaxation of the pelvic floor.

Anorectal Electromyography

- During anorectal electromyography, electrical activity in the pelvic floor muscles is evaluated during rest, squeeze, and strain. Patients with paradoxical puborectalis contraction will contract their anal and pelvic muscles during strain.
- Dynamic defecography may be used to confirm paradoxical contraction.

Defecography

- Defecography can be done via radiologic evaluation with a video taken while defecates on a special commode. Also a magnetic resonance imaging study can be done while the patient squeezes and strains: dynamic MRI. A 3D ultrasonography has also been used to perform defecography.
- Video defecography may show lack of change in the anorectal angle with strain, inability to initiate defecation, and/or inability to fully empty the rectum with strain.
- The goal is to evaluate the precise functional detail of the pelvic floor during defecation.

Interpretation of Test Results

- No one pelvic floor test is diagnostic, and normal individuals can have abnormal testing (with no constipation symptoms).

- Abnormal tests need to be interpreted in conjunction with the history and physical exam.

Etiology and Treatment of Obstructed Defecation

- The most important first step when dealing with patients having obstructed defecation is validation of the symptoms and the significant negative impact they have on the patient's quality of life.
- Reassurance that while their symptoms are obtrusive and debilitating, they are not life-threatening. This may reduce anxiety and fear.
- The treatment goal is to provide as much symptoms relief as possible while exposing them to the least amount of risk.

Hydration/Lifestyle Modification/ Fiber Intake

- In initiation of most treatment for constipation, recommendations include 1–2 liters of non-caffeinated fluid daily and 30–40 grams per day of fiber.
- Modest daily exercise may stimulate colonic motility and increase bowel frequency.
- Cathartic therapy (stimulant or osmotic) is typically ineffective for patients with obstructed defecation.

Pelvic Floor Physical Therapy Retraining

- Pelvic floor retraining is a more appropriate term to describe the comprehensive and complex bowel, bladder, and pelvic floor treatment vs the term biofeedback (biofeedback is simply operant conditioning to reinforce positive behavior).
- No standardized technique or standardized duration of therapy has been reported for pelvic floor retraining.
- The goal is for patients to learn techniques to manage their symptoms.
- Some transition to home programs may be utilized to reinforce points and methods that are taught by the pelvic floor therapist.
- Pelvic floor retraining also includes patient education on dietary management, proper defecation mechanics, and psychological support.

Pelvic Organ Prolapse

Rectal Prolapse: Overt

- Persistence or worsening of obstructed defecation may be seen after abdominal rectopexy where full rectal mobilization is done (with or without the use of mesh).
- Sigmoid resection and preservation of the lateral stalks have been associated with decreased obstructed defecation symptoms.
- Ventral rectopexy has been reported to produce a lower incidence of postoperative obstructed defecation.

Rectal Prolapse: Occult

- Occult or internal intussusception may produce obstructed defecation.
- Diagnosis is typically made during defecography, but internal prolapse may be seen in healthy asymptomatic people.
- Patients initially are treated with the non-operative treatments described above.
- Ventral rectopexy and stapled transanal rectal resection (STARR) are considered for those with life-altering refractory symptoms.

Rectocele

- Eighty percent of adult women have rectoceles and the majority are asymptomatic.
- Symptomatic rectoceles typically require treatment if there is overt vaginal prolapse or functional defecation obstruction.
- While many gynecologists prefer a transvaginal or transperineal approach, colorectal sur-

geons tend to repair rectoceles via a transanal approach.

- When obstructed defecation is the primary symptom driving a rectocele repair, surgical results have varying success in eliminating the defecation problems, and realistic expectations for improvement after surgical reconstruction should be discussed in detail preoperatively with the patient.

Enterocele with or Without Vaginal Vault Prolapse

- An enterocele can lead to obstructed defecation and frequently may coexist with vaginal vault prolapse.
- Pelvic pain and low back pain that is worse as the day progresses while the patient is upright and better laying down, along with dyspareunia, are frequent complaints associated with enteroceles.
- Defecography is usually definitive in seeing the small bowel invade the rectovaginal space.
- For symptomatic patients failing pessary and other conservative measures, an abdominal procedure to obliterate the space is considered. Also associated middle compartment defects can be surgically addressed at the same time.
- Women must be cautioned that successfully closing the space may not improve their defecation issues.

Nonanatomic Causes of Obstructed Defecation

- Dyssynergic defecation is a term used to describe nonanatomic causes of obstructed defecation, but probably obstructed defecation syndrome is a preferable term. These symptoms may be associated with paradoxical puborectalis contraction, rectal hyposensitivity, megarectum, and abnormal perineal descent.

Paradoxical Puborectalis Contraction

- Paradoxical contraction is a term which signifies when the levator ani inappropriately contracts during initiation of defecation. This leads to continued acute angulation of the anorectal angle which effectively blocks defecation.
- Anorectal electromyography and defecography are used for confirmatory testing when the history and exam area suggestive of this problem.
- Dietary modification and biofeedback improve 40–60% of patients.

Rectal Hyposensitivity

- Rectal hyposensitivity may occur with megarectum.
- It may also be associated with patients that have neurological or psychiatric impairment.
- Additionally short-segment Hirschsprung's disease and non-relaxing pelvic floor problems must also be considered when megarectum is detected.
- Patients with rectal hyposensitivity can have obstructed defecation symptoms and may also have stool impaction.
- Diagnosis is confirmed with defecography and anorectal manometry.
- Treatment consists of dietary and behavior therapy. Rectal stimulation with a suppository/enema may also improve symptoms.
- Sacral nerve modulation, while not approved for this indication in the USA, has been successfully used to treat some with this problem.

Fecal Diversion

- Fecal diversion may be offered to those failing all other therapy with life-altering fecal evacuation symptoms.

Conclusion

- A detailed history and symptom-directed physical exam is the single most important test to diagnose and recommend treatment for obstructed defecation.
- Additionally it is important to identify overt pelvic organ prolapse and consider surgical correction (recognizing that the defecation problems may not improve after pelvic organ prolapse is surgically corrected).
- The initial treatment of obstructed defecation itself usually is non-operative and centers around dietary and behavior changes including pelvic floor physical therapy.
- For patients with refractory symptoms, any surgical intervention must be realistic with realistic expectations expressed to the patient.
- Some patients with severely symptomatic obstructed defecation will experience an improvement in quality of life with a stoma.
- Figure 59.1 demonstrates an alorithm for the evaluation and managment of functional constipation.

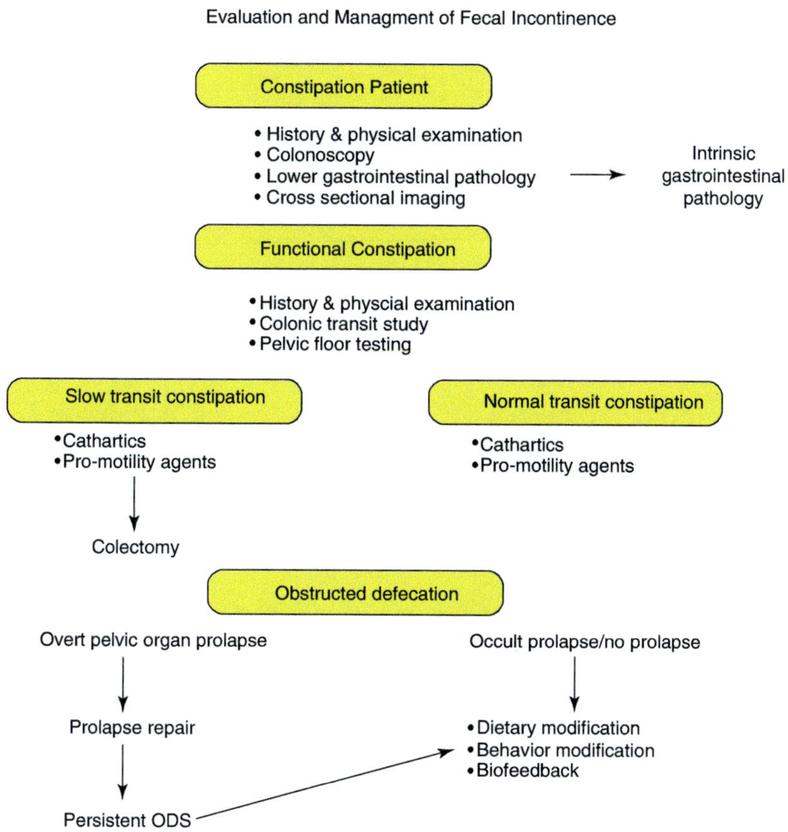

Fig. 59.1 Algorithm for Evaluation and Management of Functional Constipation

Rectal Prolapse

60

Brooke Gurland and Massarat Zutshi

Key Concepts

- Individuals with rectal prolapse may complain of a myriad of symptoms: mucus discharge, rectal bulge, rectal bleeding, fecal incontinence, constipation, tenesmus, pelvic and rectal pain, and pressure. Correction of the prolapse does not guarantee functional improvement.
- Successful outcome measures after rectal prolapse surgery include both prolapse recurrence rates and functional outcomes. The surgeon should be familiar with different abdominal and perineal procedures to choose the best operation for each individual in the setting of initial and recurrent rectal prolapse.
- Laparoscopic ventral rectopexy is associated with functional improvement, low morbidity, and low recurrence rates but has a high learning curve for proficiency and advanced training may be required.
- Robotic rectopexy can be offered safely to patients and has advantages when suturing in the pelvis is required.
- The paradigm for treatment rectal prolapse in the elderly has changed from perineal to abdominal minimally invasive procedures in elderly and high-risk patients.
- Rectal prolapse may coexist with vaginal prolapse and multidisciplinary evaluation, and treatment should be considered in symptomatic patients.

Introduction

- Rectal prolapse is extrusion of the full-thickness circular folds of the rectum through and beyond the anal muscles.
- Occult prolapse or internal intussusception is when the prolapse does not extend beyond the anal muscles.
- In mucosal prolapse, only the anal or rectal mucosa protrudes, and the treatment approach is different.
- Conditions associated with rectal prolapse are laxity of rectal attachments, deep pouch of Douglas cul-de-sac, lack of rectal fixation to the sacrum, and a redundant sigmoid.
- Women are six times more likely than men to have rectal prolapse and the problem peaks in women in their 70s.

Electronic Supplementary Material The online version of this chapter (https://doi.org/10.1007/978-3-030-01165-9_60) contains supplementary material, which is available to authorized users.

B. Gurland
Colorectal Surgery, Stanford University, Stanford, CA, USA

M. Zutshi (✉)
Department of Colorectal Surgery, Lerner College of Medicine, Cleveland Clinic, Cleveland, OH, USA
e-mail: ZUTSHIM@ccf.org

S. R. Steele et al. (eds.), *The ASCRS Manual of Colon and Rectal Surgery*,
https://doi.org/10.1007/978-3-030-01165-9_60

- Men with rectal prolapse tend to have disordered defecation and may have psychiatric issues and developmental delay.
- Women may also have vaginal prolapse and urinary incontinence.
- Of those with rectal prolapse, 50–75% have fecal incontinence, and 25–50% have constipation.

Patient Evaluation

- Evaluation starts with a complete pelvic floor history and physical exam.
- Endoscopy is performed as indicated.
- Constipation should be treated.
- If needed, patients should be examined in the squatting and standing position. If the prolapse still is not visualized, defecating on the commode to view the prolapse and confirm the diagnosis is helpful.
- Patients can be examined for vaginal prolapse and questioned for urinary incontinence. Consideration of a multidisciplinary pelvic floor repair can be discussed/planned with the urologist or urogynecologist.
- Anal physiology testing rarely changes operative strategy. Defecography may reveal associated middle and anterior compartment prolapse that may require treatment.

Non-operative Treatment

- Non-operative treatment is only temporary. Table sugar coated on incarnated prolapse may reduce edema and allow reduction.

Surgical Approaches for Rectal Prolapse

- A wide range of operative procedures are acceptable. The first decision a surgeon must make when individualizing treatment is whether to perform an abdominal versus perineal approach.

Description of Surgical Interventions

Anal Encirclement

- Reducing the prolapse and encircling the anus with a suture or mesh to prevent further prolapse is almost never done due to high recurrence rates and severe outlet constipation it produces.
- For patients with a permanent colostomy and continuous symptomatic prolapse, anal encirclement may be considered.

Perineal Procedures

Delorme

- Stripping the mucosa and then placating the rectal wall (Delorme procedure) is considered for a short segment of full-thickness prolapse in a patient with high surgical risk or "hostile abdomen."
- Recurrence rates are 16–30%.

Perineal Rectosigmoidectomy (Fig. 60.1)

- Also called the Altemeier procedure, a perineal rectosigmoidectomy involves excising

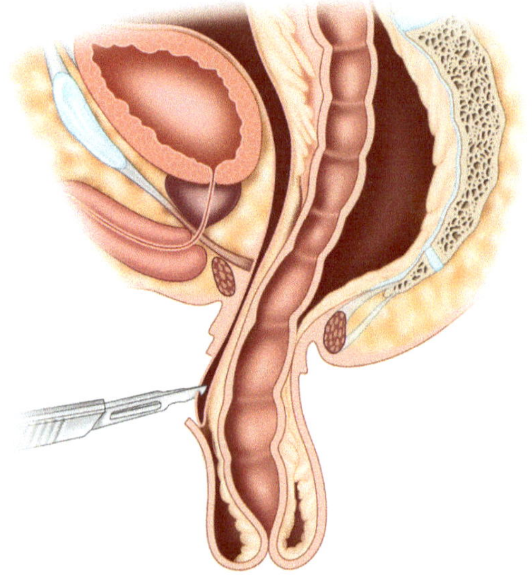

Fig. 60.1 Altmeier procedure. A circular incision is mapped out approximately 2-5 cm cephalad to the dentate line in the rectal mucosa

the extruded prolapse and performing a stapled or hand-sewn anastomosis.
- Fecal incontinence can be exacerbated with this procedure possibly from loss of the rectal reservoir. A levatorplasty may be performed prior to the anastomosis in an effort to improve fecal continence.
- Recurrence rates up to 20% have been reported.

Abdominal Procedures

Transabdominal Rectopexy

- Rectopexy can be done via an open, laparoscopic, or robotic approach and anchors the rectum to the sacrum.
- For the technique, the amount of rectal mobilization varies. Mobilization is on a spectrum and can be as much as fully circumferential or a limited amount posteriorly. The degree of mobilization depends on the procedure and the philosophy of the surgeon.
- Division of the lateral stalks is associated with decreased recurrence but increased constipation (particularly if both stalks are divided).
- Recurrence rates are 0–9%. New-onset constipation is noted in 15%, and 50% describe worsening of preoperative constipation.

Transabdominal Resection Rectopexy

- Sigmoid resection with rectopexy may reduce constipation in those who report preoperative symptoms and counteract the risk of new-onset constipation.
- Sigmoid resection may worsen symptomatic preoperative fecal incontinence.
- For patients with confirmed slow transit constipation and rectal prolapse, total or subtotal colectomy may be considered.

Mesh Rectopexy

- Biologic or synthetic mesh can be attached at various positions on the rectum and then attached to the sacrum to augment fixation.

Ripstein Procedure (Anterior Sling Rectopexy)

- This procedure has been modified from its original description to reduce problems with mesh obstructing the rectum. Currently the midportion of a rectangular strip of mesh is fixed to the sacrum. Each arm is brought around the rectum and sewn (anchored) to the rectum leaving the antimesenteric surface open.
- This procedure, although popular in the past, is rarely performed due to morbidity and the potential for new rectal outlet difficulties.

Posterior Mesh Rectopexy

- Currently, posterior mesh rectopexy is fashioned after the Well's procedure. The rectum is only mobilized posteriorly on the right and with only enough mobilization to allow safe suture or tack placement to the sacrum. The mesh is sutured to the right side of the rectum.
- Recurrence rates are reported to be 3%.

Laparoscopic Ventral Rectopexy

- Laparoscopic ventral rectopexy is currently considered the "gold standard" repair in Europe.
- Mobilization is carried out in the rectovaginal plane to the pelvic floor.
- Mesh (traditionally polypropylene) is sutured to the rectum starting at the pelvic floor and continuing in rows cephalad for about 5 centimeters. Then the mesh is sutured to the sacrum – thus elevating the pelvic floor.
- Besides rectal prolapse, this procedure can be used to address internal rectal prolapse and eliminate rectoceles. It can be combined with vaginal vault suspension (sacrocolpopexy).
- Recurrence rates are reported to be 3.4%. Complication rates vary between 14 and 47%.
- Substantial improvement in fecal incontinence and constipation has been reported.
- Laparoscopically this is a technically demanding procedure due to the need to suture in a

confined space. It has been calculated that 54 cases are needed to gain proficiency as far as reduction in operative time.

- Complications include rectal stricture, rectovaginal fistula, mesh erosion, pain/dyspareunia, and sacral discitis.

Robotic Rectopexy

- Robotic rectopexy improves pelvic visualization and suturing ability.

Rectal Prolapse in the Elderly

- Striking a balance between morbidity and recurrence is important when performing rectal prolapse surgery in the elderly.
- The traditional view for rectal prolapse in the elderly was the perineal approach. However laparoscopic (and robotic) abdominal surgery has challenged that notion.
- Laparoscopic (and robotic) surgery has been proven to be safe in elderly with acceptable morbidity.

Recurrent Rectal Prolapse: What Is the NEXT Operation?

- No algorithm or scheme exits for treating recurrent prolapse.
- Repeat surgery for recurrent rectal prolapse appears to have a higher overall recurrence rate in small limited studies.
- Caution is advised if performing a perineal rectosigmoidectomy if the initial procedure was a resection rectopexy as an ischemic section of distal bowel could be produced. Likewise, if a resection rectopexy is the first procedure, care must be exercised if a perineal rectosigmoidectomy is done for recurrence, and the surgeon must ensure that the colorectal anastomosis is excised to avoid leaving an ischemic segment.
- Mucosal prolapse after an abdominal procedure can be addressed with a Delorme.
- Recurrence after an abdominal procedure may require more extensive rectal dissection than had been performed at the initial operation. When operating for recurrent prolapse, mesh that is securely attached to the rectum can be trimmed but should not be removed as that could lead to perforation.

Combined Vaginal and Rectal Prolapse Procedures

- Combined rectal and vaginal prolapse surgery has been reported to be safe with minimal morbidity.
- While there is theoretical concern regarding bowel resection combined with mesh placement, small studies have shown no increased risk of infection when permanent mesh is used for sacrocolpopexy and the sigmoid is resected.

Solitary Rectal Ulcer Syndrome

- Patient with solitary rectal ulcers presents with defecation difficulty associated with rectal bleeding, tenesmus, mucus discharge, and anal pain.
- Rectal bleeding can be severe enough to require transfusion.
- Typically at endoscopy – ulceration, erythema, or polypoid changes are found anteriorly just above the anal sphincter complex.
- A characteristic pathological finding is fibrous obliteration of the lamina propria. Also there may be thickened muscularis mucosa.
- Colitis cystica profunda is felt to be a related disorder. Pathology reveals mucous cysts lined by columnar epithelium deep in the muscularis mucosa.
- An in-depth history which inquires about straining is crucial for both these entities. Endoscopy with biopsy is essential for an accurate diagnosis.
- Treatment is difficult and centers on dietary optimization and pelvic floor physical therapy to reduce straining.
- Excision and argon plasma coagulation have been described as treatment but recurrence rates are high.

- Some patients benefit from rectopexy, particularly those with internal intussusception demonstrated on defecography. Anterior dissection may be difficult in these patients due to anterior fibrosis and inflammation.
- See Videos 60.1, 60.2, and 60.3.

Evaluation and Treatment of FI

61

Ian M. Paquette and Liliana Bordeianou

Key Concepts

- A thorough history and physical examination, followed by a trial of conservative measures, is the first step to managing FI.
- Preoperative physiology testing may aid in selection of treatment modalities, but does not predict the outcome of treatment.
- Overlapping sphincteroplasty is a successful treatment in patients with complete sphincter disruption.
- Sacral neuromodulation has been demonstrated to be successful in patients with and without a sphincter defect.
- Biomaterial injection and radiofrequency energy delivery appear to provide modest benefit in incontinence scores, but further data is needed to substantiate this.
- The artificial bowel sphincter has demonstrated excellent improvement in incontinence scores, but complications and need for revisions prevent it from being a first-line treatment for FI.

Electronic Supplementary Material The online version of this chapter (https://doi.org/10.1007/978-3-030-01165-9_61) contains supplementary material, which is available to authorized users.

I. M. Paquette
Department of Surgery, Division of Colon and Rectal Surgery, University of Cincinnati Medical Center, Cincinnati, OH, USA

L. Bordeianou (✉)
Department of General Surgery, Massachusetts General Hospital, Boston, MA, USA
e-mail: LBORDEIANOU@mgh.harvard.edu

Introduction

- Fecal incontinence is defined as the uncontrolled passage of feces or gas.
- A recent study indicates that 20% of non-institutionalized people have FI once per year and 9.5% once per month or more. Also the study found that patients prefer the term “accidental bowel leakage” rather than FI.
- Normal continence relies on the interaction of sensory function, sphincter muscle function, pelvic floor muscle coordination, rectal compliance, and consistency of stool.
- Factors associated with FI include obstetrical trauma (occult sphincter damage may be found in 21–35% after vaginal delivery), prior anorectal surgery (fistulotomy, lateral internal sphincterotomy), denervation of the pelvic floor, chronic rectal prolapse, neurologic conditions (spina bifida or myelomeningocele), or a noncompliant rectum (from IBD or radiation therapy).
- A focused physical exam and proctoscopy assesses for obvious sphincter damage, but also to rule out other conditions such as rectal prolapse, inflammation, neoplasm, etc.

S. R. Steele et al. (eds.), *The ASCRS Manual of Colon and Rectal Surgery*,
https://doi.org/10.1007/978-3-030-01165-9_61

Assessment Instruments

- Assessment tools are utilized to track changes related to treatment over time. Grading instruments include the Cleveland Clinic Florida incontinence score, St. Mark's incontinence score, and the Fecal Incontinence Severity Index.
- A 2-week bowel diary also can provide valuable information.
- The most commonly used disease-specific quality of life tool is the Fecal Incontinence Quality of Life Scale.
- While these tools may be cumbersome to use and may underestimate response to surgical treatment, they do provide objective measures to track response to treatment.

Management

- Management of FI always begins with conservative measures.
- Management should be tailored to the patient.

Medications and Lifestyle Modifications

- Conservative measures include:
- Elimination of foods which appear to aggravate stooling symptoms.
- Optimization of stool bulk/consistency with fiber.
- Aggressively treating diarrhea typically with loperamide or diphenoxylate-atropine to slow intestinal motility.
- Select patients may benefit from scheduled enemas.

Biofeedback

- Pelvic floor rehabilitation may be used in conjunction with medical management.
- Unfortunately there is no one regiment making it difficult to compare and assess benefit from this treatment.

Preoperative Testing

- Testing may be done in conjunction with the first visit or after conservative therapy fails, and surgery is being considered.

Anorectal Physiology Testing

- Anorectal physiology testing includes resting and squeeze pressures, sphincter length, rectal compliance, and rectoanal inhibitory reflex. The normal values depend on the equipment and how it is calibrated for each unit.
- Physiologic testing results may not correlate with pre- and postoperative incontinence scores in patients undergoing sphincter repair.
- Physiologic testing may help guide treatment decisions.
- Controversy exits whether pudendal nerve terminal motor latency testing is useful and whether it correlates with response to treatment.

Ultrasound

- Ultrasound is useful to document the presence of an internal and/or external sphincter injury.
- Endoanal ultrasound appears more reliable than transvaginal or transperineal ultrasound in detecting sphincter defects.
- Preoperative use of ultrasound depends on the treatment planned. It may be invaluable before a sphincter repair but add little information before sacral neuromodulation.

Surgical Techniques

General Considerations

- After suboptimal results from conservative therapy, evaluation and testing is strongly considered to guide treatment recommendations.
- Defecography looking for internal intussusception or overt rectal prolapse may be helpful to elucidate an etiology when testing is normal (Fig. 61.1).

Overlapping Sphincteroplasty

- Overlapping sphincter repair remains the mainstay of therapy for women with FI immediately after an obstetrical injury (Fig. 61.2).
- It is also considered for older women with severe FI and a sphincter defect ≤120°.
- 80% of women can expect a reasonable improvement in the short term after sphincteroplasty.
- It is known that efficacy decreases over time after a successful repair, and at 10 years, most will experience significant FI so all must be counseled preoperatively about this.
- Biofeedback after sphincter repair may decrease or slow down deterioration after a successful repair.
- During sphincteroplasty the internal and external sphincter are usually dissected and suture overlapped en bloc. Care is taken to

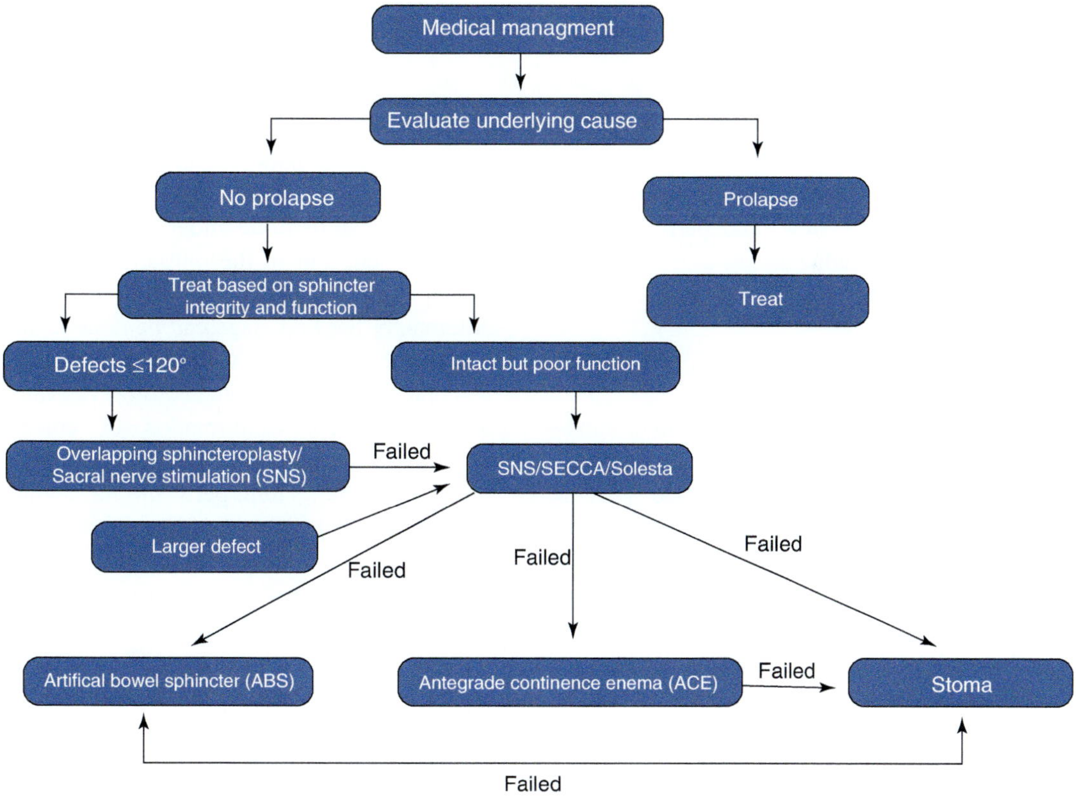

Fig. 61.1 Step-wise algorithm aimed at managing patients presenting with fecal incontinence

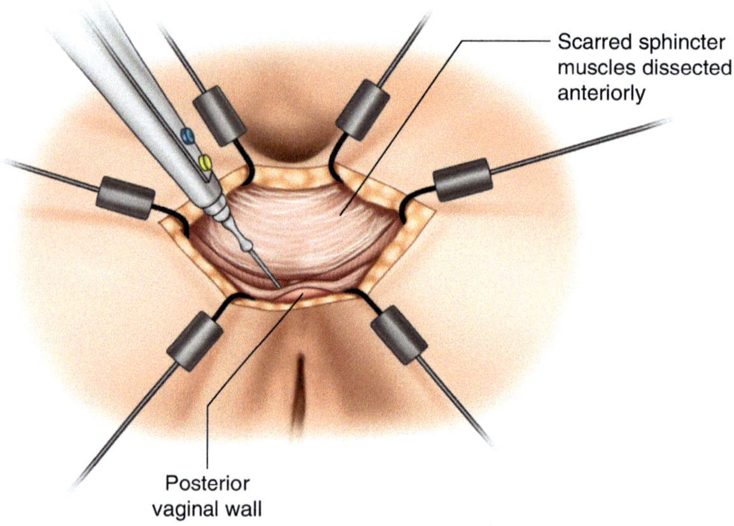

Fig. 61.2 Overlapping sphincteroplasty: scar with attached retracted sphincter muscles are dissected anteriorly

avoid dissection >180° to avoid injury to the pudendal nerves.

- Healing (particularly of the skin) following sphincter repair is slow, and partial wound separation is common.

Sacral Neuromodulation

- The mechanism of action of sacral neuromodulation (SNM) is not fully understood, but it appears to work in an antegrade fashion stimulating affect nerves which in turn send signals to select regions of the brain. Exactly how it modulates the brain is poorly understood. Among other things it may alter colorectal transport and motility (Fig. 61.3).
- SNM reduces the severity and frequency of FI even in patients with sphincter defects up to 120°.
- 35–40% of patients may achieve full continence.
- SNM is performed in two stages. The first stage aims to place a tined electrode utilizing fluoroscopic guidance in the S3 foramen, and this is confirmed with a downward deflection of the toes on the ipsilateral side when stimulation of the lead is applied along with a bellows response (slight tightening of the gluteal and anal muscles). This procedure can be done under local anesthesia with sedation in the outpatient surgery setting.
- Alternately the first stage can be done in the office with a temporary wire and without fluoroscopic guidance (percutaneous nerve evaluation or PNE). Confirmation of correct placement is done by detecting a sensory response in the rectum, perineum, or vagina. In an awake patient in an office setting, it is not feasible to increase the amplitude high enough to elicit a bellows response.
- Following stage I, the patient keeps a diary, and if there is >50% improvement in FI symptoms, the permanent neurostimulator device is implanted. This is also done with local anesthesia and sedation in the outpatient surgical suite.
- The infection rate for SNM implantation is about 11%.
- Drawbacks to this procedure include the need for device revisions. Revisions are usually required for battery replacement or to replace a lead that has migrated.

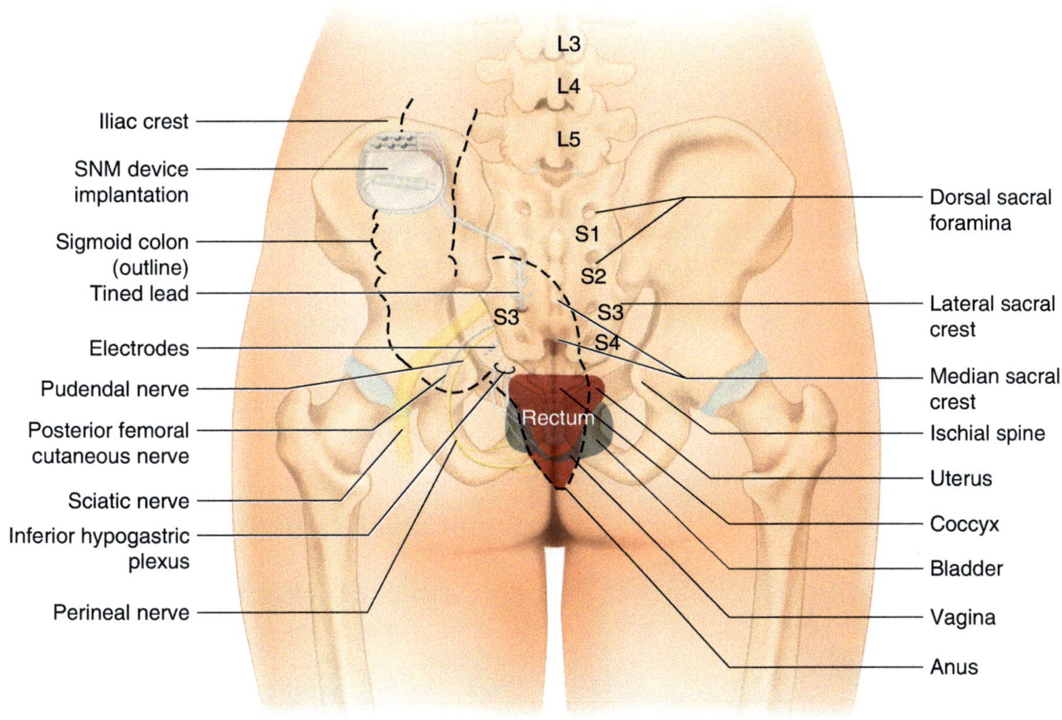

Fig. 61.3 Sacral nerve modulation: the lead is placed through the S3 foramen and the implantable pulse generator is placed below the iliac crest and lateral to the sacrum

- Body MRI is contradicted in patients with a SNM.
- Percutaneous tibial nerve stimulation is another form of neuromodulation that may also be effective in FI, although some recent studies have not produced enthusiastic results.

Sphincter Augmentation Procedures

Radiofrequency Energy Delivery

- Radiofrequency energy can be delivered to the anal canal region with mild sedation either in the OR endoscopy suite.
- The treatment is administered via four curved nickel-titanium needles which form a circle and pierce the anal mucosa and raise the temperature of the internal sphincter to 85 °F. The treatment is administered every 5 mm for four separate levels in the anal canal above and below the dentate. This produces about 16 needle punctures/treatment sites.
- Many studies reveal an improvement in the Cleveland Clinic Florida incontinence score from about 14 pre-procedure to 10 (note 20 is totally incontinent).
- This procedure is contradicted if patients have had previous injection of anal biomaterial.

Biomaterial Injection

- Use of many biomaterial agents to treat FI has been reported in the worldwide literature, but in the USA, NASHA Dx (Solesta[R]) is the only FDA-approved agent.
- This is a stable, non-degrading dextranomer stabilized in hyaluronic acid.
- The exact location and amount of injected material are not standardized, but typically the material is injected in the submucosal space in the upper anal canal.

- It is likely most effective in patients with mild incontinence or seepage.

Sphincter Replacement Strategies

- At the time of this writing, the artificial bowel sphincter (ABS) is currently off the market and may not become available again (Fig. 61.4).

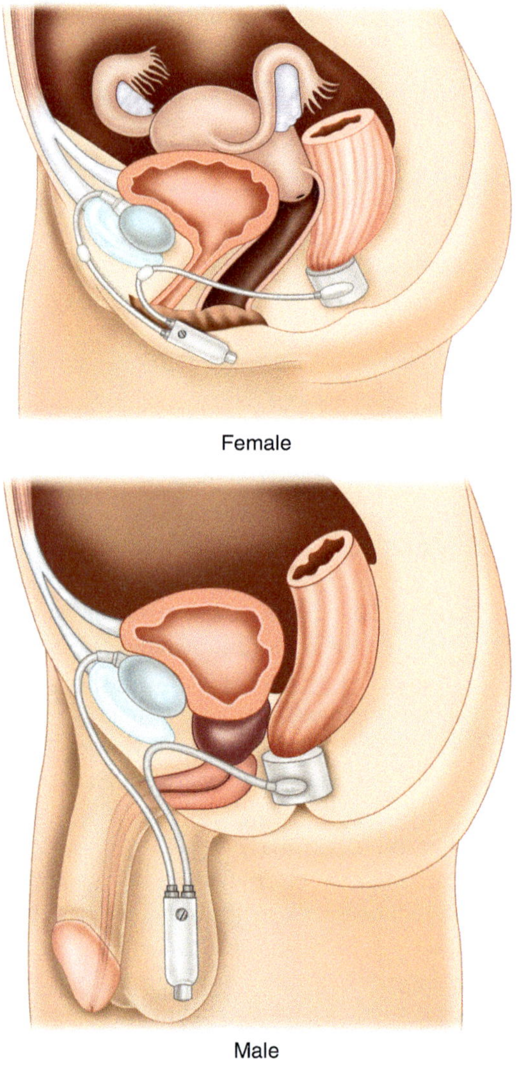

Fig. 61.4 Artificial bowel sphincter placement in males and females. The cuff is placed to encircle the anus, while the balloon is located in the space of Retzius. The button is placed in the labia in females and in the scrotum in males

- The magnetic artificial sphincter (MAS) has been FDA approved, but at the time of this writing, the company is not making it available in the USA to caregivers.
- The MAS contains small magnets on a string that are placed around the upper anal canal. During defecation the pressure from stool forces the magnets apart, and the area expands into the "open" position.
- Preliminary studies demonstrated improvement in fecal incontinence severity scores and improvement in quality of life scores.
- Long-term data on MAS function and retention is not available.

Stoma and Alternatives

- Patients failing other treatments for FI may have improved quality of life with a well-constructed stoma.
- Long term, patients are at risk for stoma-related complications such as stricture, prolapse, skin inflammation, stoma retraction, and hernia. Therefore stoma creation is an option of last resort.
- For select patients a reverse appendicostomy or cecostomy tube placement to administer antegrade colonic enemas (ACE) may be considered.
- For the ACE procedure, patients spend up to 1 h emptying their bowels after irrigation daily or every other day.
- The goal of the ACE procedure is to allow a patient to leave the house without fearing a major FI episode.
- See Videos 61.1, 61.2, and 61.3.

Conclusions

- FI is a common but under-recognized condition.
- Many treatment options are available.
- Future studies comparing cost and efficacy will help shape the future treatment algorithm.
- For now a detailed history and exam enables the doctor to provide personally tailored treatment recommendation.

Functional Bowel Disorders for the Colorectal Surgeons

62

Jennifer M. Ayscue and Anjali S. Kumar

Key Concepts

- Irritable bowel syndrome (IBS) may arise from motility disorders, visceral hypersensitivity, and/or dyssynergy of the brain-gut relationship.
- Treatment for IBS often involves a combination of diet and medications.
- Chronic pelvic pain has multiple names, causes, and anatomic and physiologic features. Similarly treatment options are numerous, but algorithms can be followed.

Introduction

- Disorders discussed in this chapter have roots in physiologic causes but may have a strong psychological component.
- When organic causes are ruled out, these chronic conditions are labeled "functional." Most are poorly understood.

J. M. Ayscue
Section of Colon & Rectal Surgery, Department of Surgery, MedStar Washington Hospital Center, Washington, DC, USA

A. S. Kumar (✉)
Department of Medical Education and Clinical Sciences, Elson S. Floyd College of Medicine, Washington State University, Everett, Spokane, Tri-Cities, Vancouver, WA, USA

Irritable Bowel Syndrome

Epidemiology

- Irritable bowel syndrome (IBS) is the most commonly diagnosed gastrointestinal disorder affecting 3–22% of the population with women affected 1.5–2 times more than men.

Pathophysiology

- Typically a chronic relapsing disease
- Likely caused by a combination of factors that are poorly understood that include immune activation, genetic predisposition, altered intestinal permeability, history of acute gastrointestinal infection, and gut microbiome alterations

Diagnosis and Symptoms

- Diagnosis is based on clinical symptoms after organic causes are ruled out.
- Diagnostic criteria are from a multinational panel of experts and termed the Rome III criteria:
- Recurrent abdominal pain or discomfort at least 3 days per month for the past 3 months

S. R. Steele et al. (eds.), *The ASCRS Manual of Colon and Rectal Surgery*,
https://doi.org/10.1007/978-3-030-01165-9_62

with symptoms >6 months before diagnosis associated with two or more of the following:
1. Improvement with defection
2. Onset associated with change in frequency of stool
3. Onset associated with change in stool form/appearance

- When IBS is felt to be the diagnosis, the only additional testing to consider is serology for celiac sprue as symptoms can be similar.
- Also colonoscopy is recommended for IBS patients >50 years or with specific alarming issues such as bleeding, unintentional weight loss, iron-deficiency anemia, nocturnal symptoms, and family history of selected organic diseases (IBD, colorectal cancer, celiac sprue).
- IBS is further classified into diarrhea and constipation predominant where at least 25% of stools are loose according to Bristol stool scale (diarrhea predominant: IBS-D) or hard and lumpy (constipation predominant: IBS-C). Patients with alternating features at least 25% of the time are IBS-mixed.

Treatment

- Table 62.1 outlines treatment options.
- Diet has been implicated to precipitate symptoms.
- Reduction in the intake of poorly absorbed short-chain carbohydrates (known as fermentable oligosaccharides, disaccharides, monosaccharides and polyols (FODMAPs)) has been shown to reduce symptoms (Table 62.2 further classifies the FODMAP foods and provides simplistic diet recommendations).
- Regular exercise has been shown to improve IBS symptoms. Psychological therapy including hypnotherapy has demonstrated improvement if provided by caregivers experienced in management of this group of patients. Acupuncture showed no demonstrated benefit.

Diarrhea-Predominant IBS (IBD-D)

- Antispasmodics have had some degree of success for postprandial abdominal cramping and loose stools in IBS-D patients but must be balanced against anticholinergic side effects.
- Peppermint oil diminishes visceral hypersensitivity and gut pain sensation with the side effect of reflux.
- Tricyclic antidepressants (TCA) and selective serotonin reuptake inhibitors (SSRI) have been demonstrated to improve global symptoms and pain reduction, but the side effect profile must be carefully balanced; thus these medications require careful selection.

Table 62.1 Treatment options in irritable bowel syndrome

	Mixed IBS	Diarrhea-predominant IBS	Constipation-predominant IBS
Dietary modifications	Lactose free, gluten restriction, low FODMAP	Lactose free, gluten restriction, low FODMAP	Lactose free, gluten restriction
Fiber supplement	Trial (psyllium)	Trial (psyllium)	Trial (psyllium)
Antibiotic, probiotics	Consider trial of antibiotics if it has SIBO, probiotics	Consider trial of antibiotics if it has SIBO, probiotics	Consider trial of probiotics
Peppermint oil	Consider trial	Consider trial	Consider trial
Antidiarrheals/ antispasmodics	Consider loperamide, diphenoxylate atropine	Consider loperamide, diphenoxylate atropine, hyoscyamine	Not recommended
Antidepressants	Consider trial of TCAs, SSRIs	Consider trial of TCAs, SSRIs	Consider SSRIs
Psychological therapies	May consider	May consider	May consider
5-HT3 antagonists	Alosetron (restricted)	Alosetron (restricted)	Not recommended
Prosecretory agents	Not recommended	Not recommended	Trial of linaclotide, lubiprostone
Osmotic laxatives	Not recommended	Not recommended	Trial of PEG, other non-stimulant laxatives

Table 62.2 Examples of foods by varying levels of FODMAP (fermentable oligosaccharides, disaccharides, monosaccharides and polyols)

Food group	Low FODMAPs	Moderate FODMAPs (limit)	High FODMAPs (avoid)
Eggs, meats, poultry, fish	Meats, eggs, fish, shellfish		
Dairy	Low-lactose dairy: cream cheese, half and half, hard cheeses (cheddar, Colby, Parmesan, Swiss, etc.), soft cheeses (Brie, feta, mozzarella, etc.), sherbet, yogurt (Greek), whipped cream		High-lactose dairy: buttermilk, chocolate, creamy/cheesy sauces, custard, ice cream, milk (cow's, goat's, sheep's, condensed, evaporated), soft cheeses (cottage, ricotta, etc.), sour cream
Meat, nondairy alternatives	Nondairy milks, nuts (walnut, macadamia, peanut, pecan, pine), nut butters, tempeh, tofu	<10 almonds <10 hazelnuts	Cashews, beans, black-eyed peas, bulgur, lentils, miso, pistachios, soybeans, soybean milk
Grains	Made with gluten-free/spelt grains		Made with wheat/barley/rye when it's the major ingredient
Fruits	Bananas, blueberries, cantaloupe, cranberries, grapes, honeydew, kiwi, lemon, lime, mandarin, orange, pineapple, raspberries, strawberries	¼ avocado, <3 cherries, ½ grapefruit, ½ pomegranate, <¼ cup shredded coconut, <10 dried banana chips	Apples, applesauce, apricots, blackberries, canned fruit, dates, dried fruits, mango, nectarines, papaya, peaches, pears, plums, prunes, watermelon, avocado
Vegetables	Alfalfa/bean sprouts, bell peppers, carrots, cabbage, cucumbers, eggplant, green beans, kale, lettuce, potatoes, radishes, spinach, squash, tomatoes, zucchini	¼ cup canned artichoke hearts, <3 asparagus spears, 4 beet slices, <½ cup broccoli, <½ cup brussels sprouts, <1 cup savoy cabbage, 1 celery stick, <½ cup green peas, 3 okra pods, <10 pods snow peas, ½ corn cob, <½ cup sweet potato	Artichokes, cauliflower, mushrooms, sugar snap peas
Beverages	Coffee, tea		Made with HFCS, fortified wines (sherry, port)
Seasonings, condiments	Jam/jelly/pickle/relish/salsa/sauce/maple syrup without HFCS, most spices and herbs, homemade broth, butter, chives, cooking oils, mustard, pepper, margarine, mayonnaise, green onion, olives, pesto, salt, seeds, sugar, soy sauce, vinegar		Products with HFCS, agave, garlic, garlic salt/powders, honey, hummus, molasses, onions (not green), onion salt/powders, tomato paste, artificial sweeteners (isomalt, mannitol, sorbitol, xylitol)

- Serotonin subtype 3 (5-HT_3 antagonists) decreases painful gut sensation and decreases motility. Alosetron is restricted (due to the possibility of severe constipation and ischemic colitis) but available for select women with severe IBS-D. Ondansetron is less potent but also has been shown to improve symptoms.
- Loperamide is an effective antidiarrheal to decrease frequency and improve stool consistency, but has not been shown to be effective in treating other troublesome symptoms of IBS-D such as pain.

Constipation-Predominant IBS (IBS-C)

- SSRIs have been shown to improve symptoms of IBS-C with side effects of sexual dysfunction, nausea, drowsiness, agitation, and diarrhea.

- Prosecretory agents such as linaclotide (causes sodium and water secretion and modulation of afferent pain sensors) and lubiprostone (activates chloride channels resulting in chloride and water secretion) have been shown to improve constipation symptoms.
- Laxatives such as PEG formulations can increase the number of bowel movements but do not seem to improve abdominal discomfort and pain.

Chronic Functional Pelvic Pain

- Chronic functional pelvic pain is poorly understood and affects 7% of the population. These symptoms can lead to significant impairment in quality of life, ability to work, and psychological distress.
- Diagnosis depends on a careful history as the physical exam may be unremarkable. Conditions to be ruled out include cryptitis, fissure, abscess, hemorrhoids, solitary rectal ulcer, inflammatory bowel disease, ischemia, prostatitis, and endometriosis, among others.
- There is no consensus regarding usefulness of diagnostic studies for this problem.
- Similarly, there are a wide variety of therapeutic options with difficulty in testing effectiveness due to this problem being multifactorial and difficult to stratify and study.
- Typically pelvic pain disorders are grouped as chronic proctalgia, coccygodynia, and pudendal neuralgia.

Chronic Proctalgia

- The Rome III definition: chronic or recurrent rectal pain or aching lasting at least 20 min in the absence of structural or systemic disease explanations for these symptoms.
- In contrast proctalgia fugax is sudden severe pain in the anorectal region which lasts <20 min and disappears as suddenly as it comes on. Although it can reoccur, the number of episodes typically is few, and thus this is not considered a chronic pain syndrome.
- Chronic proctalgia is further divided by Rome III into levator ani syndrome (when traction on the pelvic floor produces tenderness) and unspecified functional anorectal pain (where painful sensations are absent when the levator ani muscle is palpated during digital exam).
- Psychological factors such as anxiety disorders, depression, and stress along with a history of spinal surgery and childbirth are commonly seen in patients with chronic proctalgia.
- Figure 62.1 outlines the treatment algorithm for this disorder.

Coccygodynia

- Pain arising around the coccyx is termed coccygodynia and is considered chronic if it lasts >2 months.
- Treatment starts with a trigger point injection with steroids and bupivacaine. Pain relief appears to be more effective if these injections are combined with manipulation of the coccyx under anesthesia. This constellation of therapy may be repeated as needed. A select group who fail this less invasive therapy will benefit from coccygectomy.

Pudendal Neuralgia

- Pudendal neuralgia is also termed Alcock's canal syndrome or pudendal canal syndrome.
- In the absence of organic disease, entrapment of the pudendal nerve between the sacrotuberous and sacrospinous ligament or in Alcock's (pudendal) canal is postulated to lead to this painful problem.
- Other risk factors besides entrapment that can give similar chronic pain include herpetic neuropathy, stretch neuropathy, and post radiotherapy neuropathy.
- No imaging abnormalities should explain the pudendal neuralgia.

- Five requirements delineated by a multidisciplinary working group are essential to the diagnosis:
  1. Pain only in the innervation territory of the pudendal nerve.
  2. Pain predominantly experienced or worsened while sitting (in accordance with the nerve compression hypothesis).
  3. The pain rarely awakens the patient at night.
  4. On exam, no objective sensory impairment is noted.
  5. Pain is relieved by anesthetic infiltration of the pudendal nerve.
- Treatment involves nerve injection with steroid and anesthesia, neuromodulation (i.e., sacral nerve modulation, although not FDA approved), nerve ablation, or surgery (neurolysis).
- Regarding surgery, operative approaches for neurolysis include transperineal, transgluteal, transichiorectal, and laparoscopic. Few large studies exist for any of these approaches, but reported success in affected patients has been reported with each approach.
- Augmentation of the canal via transperineal injection of autologous adipose tissue with stem cells to increase the space for the nerve to travel and decrease compression has also been reported in a pilot study with promising results.
- Figure 62.1 also highlights the treatment algorithm for pudendal nerve entrapment.

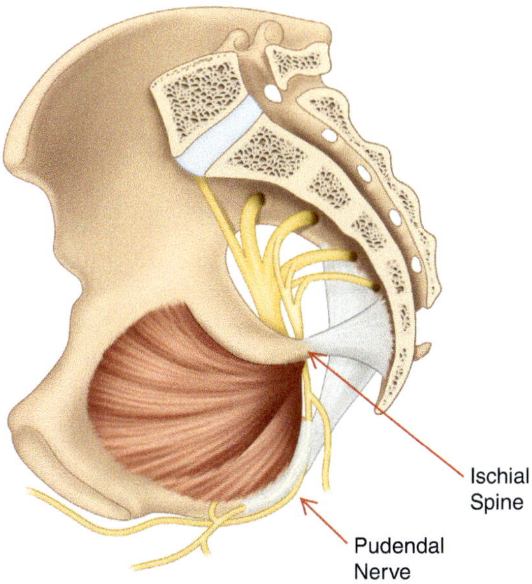

Fig. 62.1 Algorithm for management of chronic proctalgia

Conclusion

- IBS and chronic functional pain represent a spectrum of disease entities that are difficult to diagnose, manage, and treat.
- A systematic approach and multidisciplinary team are essential.
- Surgery is rarely offered.

Middle and Anterior Compartment: Issues for the Colorectal Surgeon

63

Cecile A. Unger and Marie Fidela R. Paraiso

Key Concepts

- Multi-compartment pelvic floor disorders are common and require a multidisciplinary team approach to evaluation and management.
- The levator ani muscles and connective tissue structures of the pelvis provide the main supports to the pelvic floor and pelvic organs.
- Transvaginal repair of pelvic organ prolapse is commonly performed at the time of transperineal repair of rectal intussusception or prolapse.
- The most commonly performed abdominal procedure for pelvic organ prolapse is the sacral colpopexy, which can be performed concomitantly with ventral or other types of rectopexy.
- A transvaginal or transanal approach can be taken to repair a rectocele, but the transvaginal approach is more common and seems to have better outcomes with less morbidity.

Introduction

- Multi-compartment pelvic floor disorders are common in women.
- Evaluation of the anterior, middle, and posterior compartments – thinking about a multidisciplinary approach – should be considered when seeing a patient for a problem involving one compartment.

C. A. Unger (✉) · M. F. R. Paraiso
Department of Obstetrics and Gynecology, Cleveland Clinic, Cleveland, OH, USA
e-mail: UNGERC@ccf.org

Anatomy of the Pelvic Floor

- Levator ani muscles (puborectalis, iliococcygeus, and pubococcygeal) contribute the main support of pelvic organs.
- Connective tissue structures attach the uterus, cervix, vagina, and rectum to the pelvic walls (Fig. 63.1).
- Interactions of the connective tissue and levator ani muscles give structural support to the pelvis.
- Pelvic organ dysfunction is multifactorial, but anatomic understanding is important when thinking about treatment options.

Evaluation of Pelvic Organ Prolapse

- History to elucidate symptoms and physical exam are the cornerstones of diagnosis.
- Physical exam is performed in the lithotomy position, but if needed, standing may provide better representation of the pelvic organ descent.
- The pelvic organ prolapse quantification system (POP-Q) is a validated measure used to

S. R. Steele et al. (eds.), *The ASCRS Manual of Colon and Rectal Surgery*,
https://doi.org/10.1007/978-3-030-01165-9_63

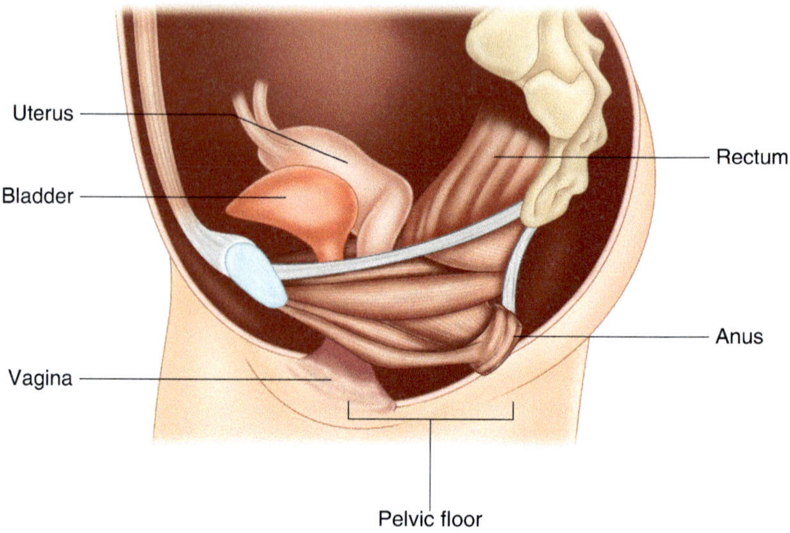

Fig. 63.1 Interaction between the levator ani muscles and the pelvic organs. The levator ani muscles (puborectalis, iliococcygeus and pubococcygeus) contribute to the main support of the pelvic organs and play an important role in the pelvic floor

Table 63.1 Pelvic organ prolapse stages

Stage 0	No prolapse; apex descends within 2 cm of the total vaginal length
Stage 1	Most distal portion of the prolapse descends to a point greater than 1 cm above the hymen
Stage 2	Most distal portion of the prolapse descends within 1 cm of the hymen (above or below)
Stage 3	Prolapse extends more than 1 cm beyond the hymen but no more than within 2 cm of total vaginal length
Stage 4	Complete eversion; extension within 2 cm of the total vaginal length

report prolapse within the vagina **(see** Table 63.1).

- Urinary incontinence is assessed by having a patient cough or Valsalva with a full bladder. Urodynamic testing can also be performed.
- There is a minimal role for routine imagining unless to assist in elucidating possible etiology of posterior compartment defecatory symptoms and their management.

Overview of Urodynamics

- This office-based procedure assesses pressures at which the detrusor muscle of the bladder accommodates during bladder filling, the ability of a patient to suppress micturition at various bladder volumes, and a patient's ability to initiate micturition.
- The procedure is performed in a standard fashion and reported according to published guidelines to facilitate caregiver communication.
- The first stage (*filling cystometry*) examines the relationship of bladder filling and the detrusor muscle. Initially the bladder is filled with saline and pressures recorded when a patient experiences first sensation, first desire to void, strong desire to void, urge, and pain.
- Detrusor contractions are recorded during filling, and rises in P_{det} (defined by subtracting the recorded *abdominal* and *vesical pressure*) may signal *detrusor overactivity* indicative of overactive bladder disorders.
- Bladder compliance is calculated by dividing volume change by change in P_{det} and should remain low during filling. Rises in P_{det} not associated with detrusor contractions signal poor bladder compliance and possible neurogenic bladder disorders.
- The *leak point pressure* measures the urethra's ability to prevent involuntary leakage of urine. *Abdominal leak point pressure* assesses stress urinary incontinence and examines the urethra's ability to avoid leakage as abdominal pressure increases.

- *Uroflowmetry* is the second phase and assesses bladder empting (*voiding phase*). In addition to electronic volume detection and graphical representation of flow patterns, post void residual is measured.

Surgical Management of Middle and Anterior Compartment

- Conservative treatment with a pessary and/or pelvic muscle exercises are usually initiated as the first line of treatment.
- Surgical management of prolapse is recommended if symptoms remain bothersome after conservative therapy. Surgery aims to address all segments of the vagina involved in the prolapse and improve related visceral function to the lower urinary tract, vagina, and anorectum.

Transvaginal Repair

- Anterior compartment prolapse (*cystocele*) refers to the bladders protruding through the anterior vagina. Repair (anterior colporrhaphy) can be performed with native tissue or mesh. Native tissue repair has higher recurrence rates which are weighed against problems with mesh such as erosion.
- Middle compartment prolapse (apical descent of the vagina toward the introitus) can occur before or after hysterectomy and via an extra- or intraperitoneal approach.
- Intraperitoneal approach (can be done at time of vaginal hysterectomy or remote from hysterectomy) suspends vaginal cuff to the uterosacral ligaments.
- Extraperitoneal approach suspends the vaginal apex to the sacrospinous ligament or iliococcygeus fascia below the ischial spines.
- If sexual activity is no longer desired, the vagina can be obliterated in a quick, low morbidity procedure.

Abdominal Repair

- Sacral colpopexy is the most common abdominal procedure and can be done open, laparoscopic, or robotic. The vaginal apex is suspended to the anterior sacral ligament at the pelvic brim with a bridging synthetic or biological graft (Fig. 63.2a and b).
- Pooled data shows sacral colpopexy has superior outcomes to vaginal procedures but has a longer operative time, increased cost, and longer time to return to normal activities.
- This procedure can be done in conjunction with rectal prolapse repairs and the sutures

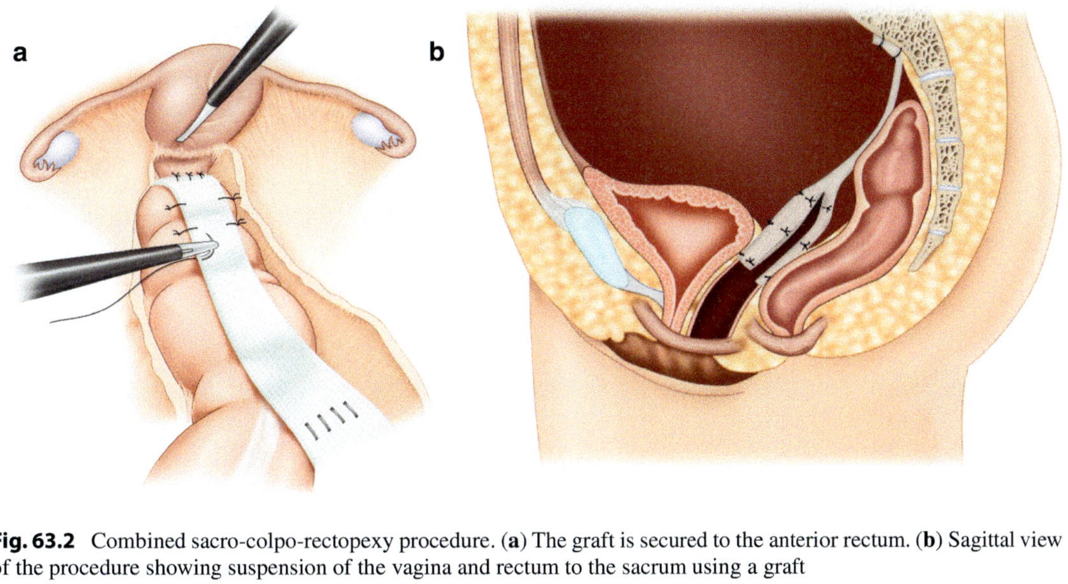

Fig. 63.2 Combined sacro-colpo-rectopexy procedure. (**a**) The graft is secured to the anterior rectum. (**b**) Sagittal view of the procedure showing suspension of the vagina and rectum to the sacrum using a graft

placed at the sacral ligament utilized in both. It is also feasible if sigmoid resection is required. Multidisciplinary approach has been shown in the literature to be safe and effective.
- Spondylodiscitis which is a spectrum of spinal infections is a concern, and a low threshold for obtaining a postoperative CT or MRI for ongoing nondescript low back pain should be considered.
- In a patient with a uterus and still desiring the ability to maintain fertility, suspension of the uterus (hysteropexy) can be done for prolapse.

Surgical Management of the Posterior Compartment: Approach to the Rectocele Repair

- Symptoms associated with rectoceles many times can be managed with diet/medication alteration to avoid constipation and staining, pelvic floor physical therapy, and pessary placement.
- Surgical repair is offered to patients who fail conservative treatment. It is important to ensure the vaginal bulge and defecation emptying problem is not related to physiologic dysfunction such as paradoxical anal contraction during the act of defecation (as that problem should initially be addressed).

Transvaginal

- The most common repair approach is transvaginal.
- The traditional repair has been a midline plication of the vaginal muscularis and rectovaginal tissue +/− levator plication.
- An alternative is the site-specific repair which entails repair of the discrete defect in the rectovaginal septum tissues without levator plication (usually with a finger in the anorectum during surgery to detect the exact area of the defect).
- Transvaginal repairs can be further augmented with a permanent or absorbable graft.
- Dyspareunia and/or persistent or new defecatory problems are possible new problems after transvaginal repair.

Transanal Repair

- The transanal approach is more commonly performed by colorectal surgeons.
- Studies overall show similar alleviation of symptoms with both approaches. Transanal approaches seem to be associated with more clinically diagnosed rectocele recurrences but decreased incidence of dyspareunia (especially if levator plication is performed during the vaginal approach).

Part IV

Miscellaneous

Pediatric Colorectal Disorders

64

Daniel H. Teitelbaum and Peter F. Ehrlich

Key Concepts

- *Cloacal anomalies:* Careful anatomic assessment must be done prior to surgical correction. Long-term follow-up is essential as future gynecological and genitourinary problems may arise that also need corrective action.
- *Anorectal atresias:* Imperforate anal anomalies are commonly associated with both genitourinary and spinal anomalies; both of which may complicate the long-term management and care of such patients. Life-long incontinence may be seen in up to 50% of such patients.
- *Hirschsprung disease:* Surgical correction will often result in a good stooling pattern. Many patients may suffer from recurrent enterocolitis after a pull-through, which requires immediate attention by a surgeon experienced in dealing with this secondary disorder. Children may also occasionally suffer from anorectal incontinence. In general, they need to be followed long-term for similar potential problems.
- *Necrotizing enterocolitis (NEC):* NEC may lead to full-thickness intestinal necrosis, resulting in the loss of a considerable amount of the small and/or large intestine. Even without intestinal loss, an ischemic-associated stricture may occur, which is typically in the splenic flexure region, and may require dilation or resection of this portion of the colon.
- *Inflammatory bowel disease:* Diagnosis and the treatment are quite similar to adults. A key consideration is the need to ensure adequate growth and maturation through adolescence. Often this plays directly into the timing and decision for surgery.
- *Constipation:* Constipation can be challenging and typically can be initially approached with medical management. It is important to rule out Hirschsprung disease and anatomic obstruction. For the most intransigent of cases, some will benefit from an appendicostomy.

Congenital Anomalies

Cloacal Anomalies

- Cloacal anomalies occur in ~1:20,000 live births.
- Embryologically, the cloaca is a transient organ that becomes divided to separate the gastrointestinal tract from the genitourinary tract.
- Clinically, a cloaca involves the urethra, vagina, and rectum empty into a single channel with a single perineal orifice, located on

D. H. Teitelbaum (✉) · P. F. Ehrlich
Section of Pediatric Surgery, University of Michigan
C.S. Mott Children's Hospital, Ann Arbor, MI, USA
e-mail: dttlbm@med.umich.edu

S. R. Steele et al. (eds.), *The ASCRS Manual of Colon and Rectal Surgery*,
https://doi.org/10.1007/978-3-030-01165-9_64

the anterior perineum at the expected site of the urethra (Fig. 64.1).

- Significant abdominal distension may occur due to reflux of urine into the vaginal cavity or excess secretions of the uterus due to maternal hormonal stimulation.
- The exact anatomic delineation will require endoscopy and extensive radiologic workup.

Mechanisms Underlying Cloacal Anomalies

- Normally present in the 4–5-week-old embryo, the cloaca is a derivative of hindgut endoderm.
- A urorectal septum forms at the cranial aspect of the cloaca to divide it into the urogenital sinus ventrally and the anorectum dorsally.

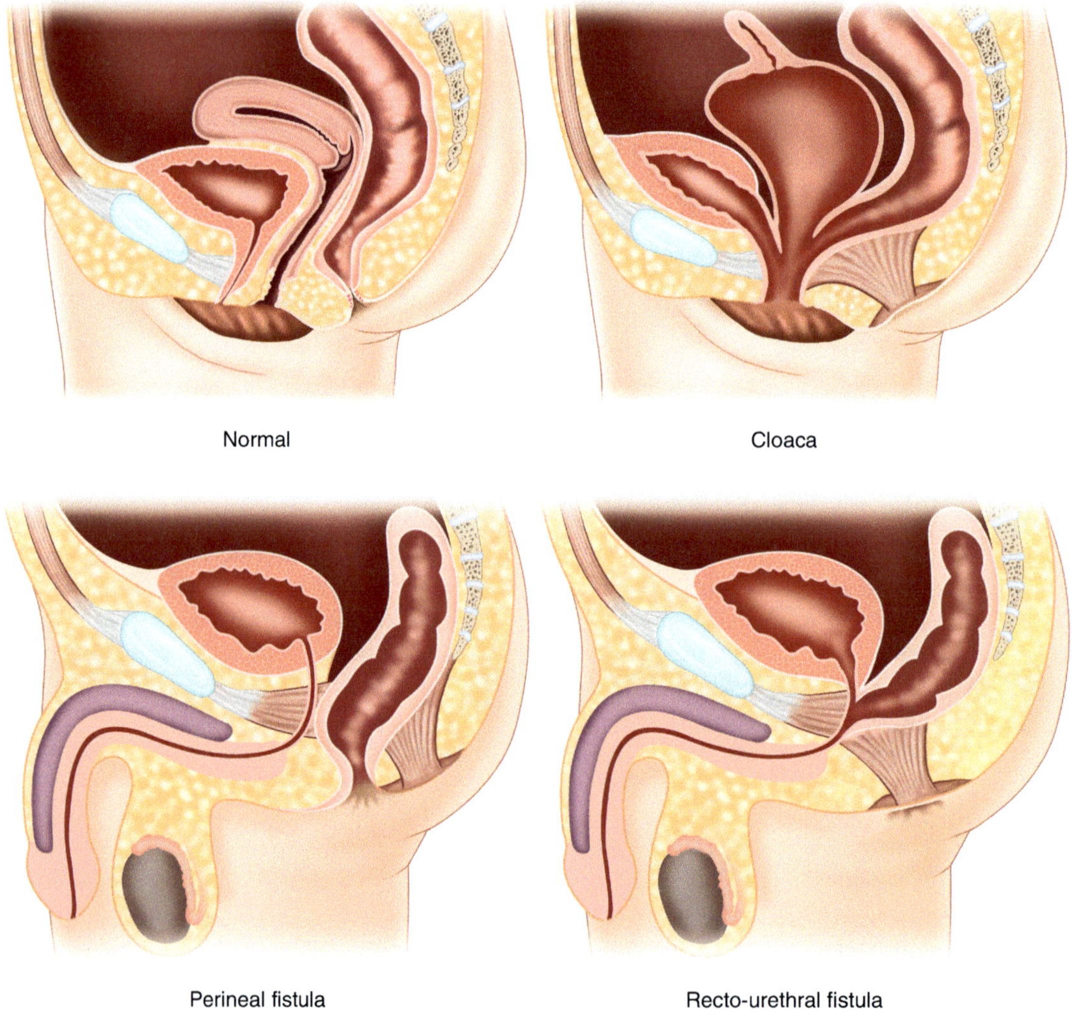

Fig. 64.1 Classification of anorectal atresias. Top left panel Normal cross-sectional appearance of female anatomy. Bottom left panel Male with low imperforate anus (perineal fistula). The rectum is located within most of sphincter mechanism. Top right panel Female with cloaca. Note the rectum, vagina, and urinary tract fuse into a single common channel. Bottom right panel Male with high imperforate anus (rectourethral fistula). There is no plane of dissection between the rectum and urethra

- Once the urorectal septum reaches the perineum, the cloacal membrane dissipates to open the urogenital sinus (becomes the urinary bladder and urethra, with a portion incorporated into the vagina and hymen) and the posterior anorectum.

Current Therapy

- An initial prenatal workup should determine the presence or absence of hydrocolpos (distended vagina filled with fluid).
- Failure to recognize and manage hydrocolpos can lead to serious complications, including vaginal rupture, hydronephrosis (distended and dilated kidney), and sepsis.
- These complications are prevented with early vaginal decompression and drain placement when the colostomy is formed.
- Perforation of either the vagina or uterus may occur in utero, leading to significant abdominal distension, gastrointestinal dysfunction, and respiratory distress.
- Definitive surgery is undertaken once the anatomy has been mapped out using radiologic imaging (fluoroscopy, MRI) and endoscopy.
- Measurement of the channel length is typically assessed with cystoscopy and vaginoscopy just prior to the definitive surgery, and the length of the common channel is a major factor when choosing a definitive surgery.
  - Short common channels (<3 cm) can be repaired with a perineal incision and have less associated morbidities.
  - Long common channels (>3 cm) require a more complicated repair with abdominal and perineal incisions.
- Long-term outcomes depend upon associated anomalies.
- Surgical management will require separation of the rectum from the cloacal channel, with implantation in the center of the remaining sphincter complex, and the introital structures (i.e., vaginal and urethral) are then mobilized as a single unit and brought down to the perineal skin.
- Many children will have lifelong urological and gynecological problems, and patients with imperforate anus have anorectal incontinence in at least 50%.

Anorectal Atresia

- The incidence is estimated to be 1:10,000–1:40,000 live births.
- Anorectal atresia, or imperforate anus, is caused by abnormalities in hindgut development that result in ectopic positioning of the anal opening in the cloaca due to anatomical and/or genetic factors (Figs. 64.1 and 64.2).
- Smaller defects have a more posterior phenotype, such as an anocutaneous fistula, while more extensive defects will lead to more anterior abnormalities.

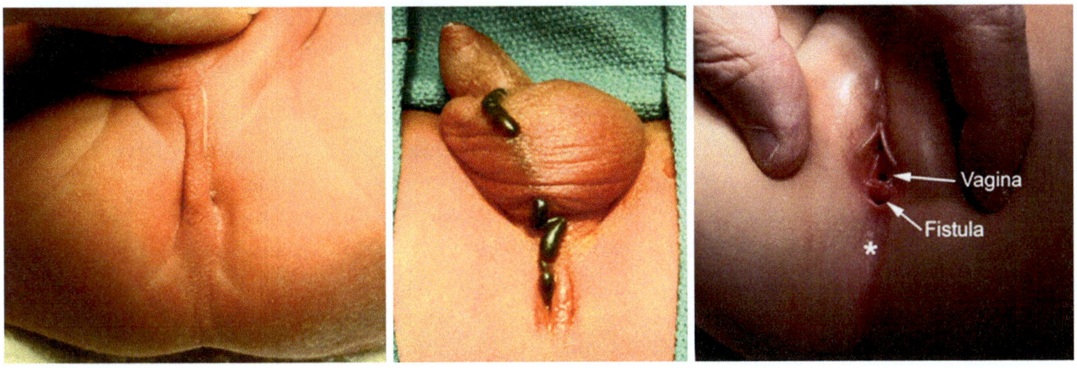

Fig. 64.2 External appearance of perineum in various forms of imperforate anus

- ARMs are associated with the VACTERL complex, which encompasses vertebral defects (e.g., sacral anomalies or hemi-vertebra), anal atresia, cardiac defects (most commonly atrial septal or ventriculoseptal defects), tracheo-esophageal fistula, renal anomalies, and limb dysplasias (e.g., typically a poorly formed radial bone and/or absent thumb).
- Evaluation should include plain films of the vertebral column (cervical to coccyx), ultrasound of spinal cord to rule out a tethered cord, cardiac echo (as the most common defects are atrial septal defects and/or ventricular septal defects, passage of a decompressing tube from the mouth to the gastric lumen may help rule out most types of tracheoesophageal anomalies), and an ultrasonographic exam of the genitourinary system.

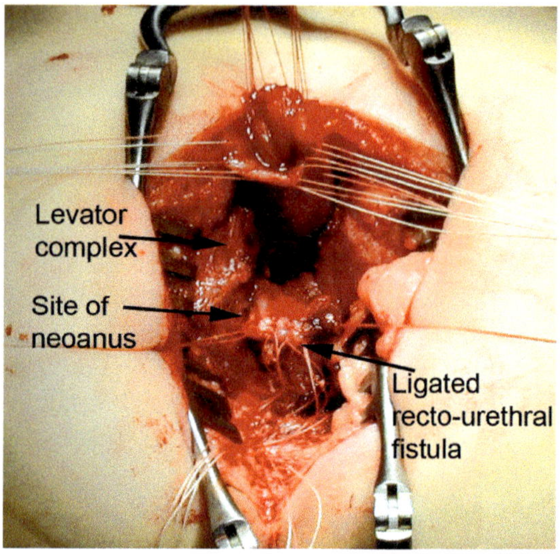

Fig. 64.3 Intraoperative appearance of a posterior sagittal anorectoplasty (PSARP)

Current Therapies

- The initial decision is whether to perform a primary repair or colostomy.
- A post-24-h prone lateral radiograph to visualize the terminal location of the rectum, which may be facilitated with ultrasonography.
- A primary pull-through is feasible if the rectum has descended below the pubococcygeal muscle complex.
- A colostomy should be performed if there is any question of rectal position or when atresias terminate above the pubococcygeal muscle complex.
- Placement of the ostomy should be as proximal as possible in the descending colon to allow sufficient distal rectum to pull-through to the perineum.
- The rectourethral fistula often connects through the child's prostate or sphincter complex of the urinary bladder, and a radiologic contrast study through the colostomy should be performed.
- A posterior sagittal anorectoplasty (PSARP) involves identifying the rectum (typically just above the levator complex), opening it to allow the identification of the rectourethral fistula, dissecting the fistula in the submucosal plane, ligating the fistula, and mobilizing the rectum to allow a pull-through without excess tension.
- A Pena muscle stimulator helps for careful placement of the rectum through the residual sphincter complex (Fig. 64.3).
- Children with anorectal atresia require long-term follow-up, as most will continue to have problems well into adulthood.
- In the few months following surgery, the child will require dilations of the anal canal.
- The most common long-term issues relate to the evacuation of a bowel movement.
  - Lower lesions typically have issues with constipation.
  - Higher fistulas have issues with incontinence.
- Infants having more than three intact sacral vertebral bodies will typically have a reasonable chance for continence.
- Children with imperforate anus with a perineal fistula have issues in the long-term with constipation that will require daily laxative therapy (e.g., polyethylene glycol).
- For infants with poorly formed sacral elements and/or imperforate anal anomalies with a more proximal fistula, incontinence may be at 50% or higher.

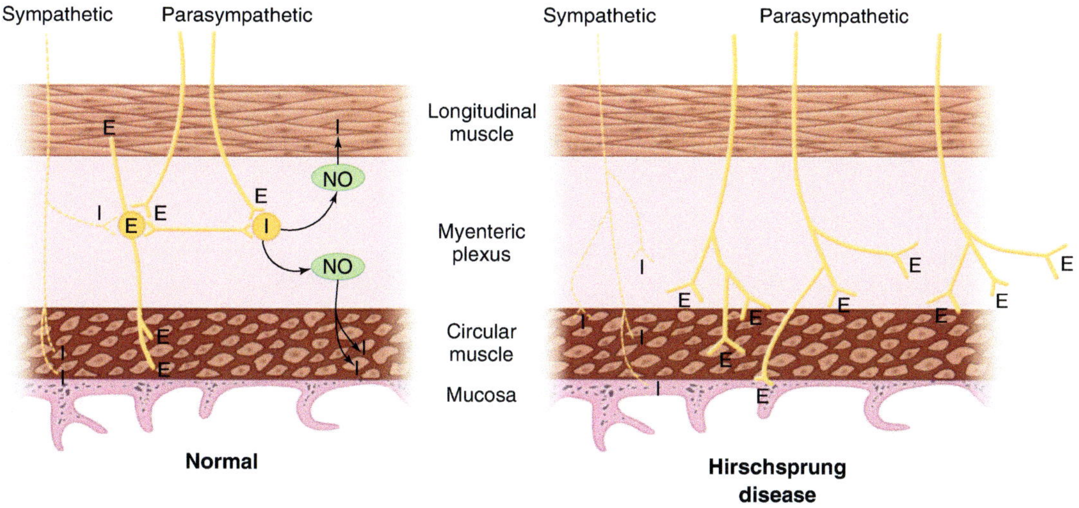

Fig. 64.4 Diagram showing the pathophysiologic processes which drive functional obstruction in Hirschsprung disease. Note in Hirschsprung patients there is predominance of excitatory parasympathetic fibers (causing an increase histologically of hypertrophic nerves) with a loss of intrinsic ganglion cells and a loss of nitric oxide, which is critical for the relaxation of smooth muscle

Hirschsprung Disease

- Hirschsprung disease (HD) is characterized by the absence of colonic ganglion cells, typically in the distal colon (Fig. 64.4).
- HD occurs in ~1:5000 live births, with a male-to-female preponderance of 4:1; total colonic aganglionosis has a stronger association with female patients.
- Infants present with delayed passage of their first bowel movement (meconium), which typically occurs in the first 24 h of life.
- Children present with difficult bowel movements, poor feeding, poor weight gain, and progressive abdominal distension.
- The aganglionic area lacks nitric oxide synthase (NOS) and cannot produce the smooth muscle relaxant nitric oxide, leading to colonic constriction.
- An increased number of stimulatory parasympathetic fibers can also increase the constriction of the distal colon.
- A contrast enema will show a constricted distal rectum with a more dilated proximal colon (the *normal* segment of bowel) (Fig. 64.5).
- Suction rectal biopsy (typically at the bedside), or full-thickness rectal biopsy in the operating room for older children, should be

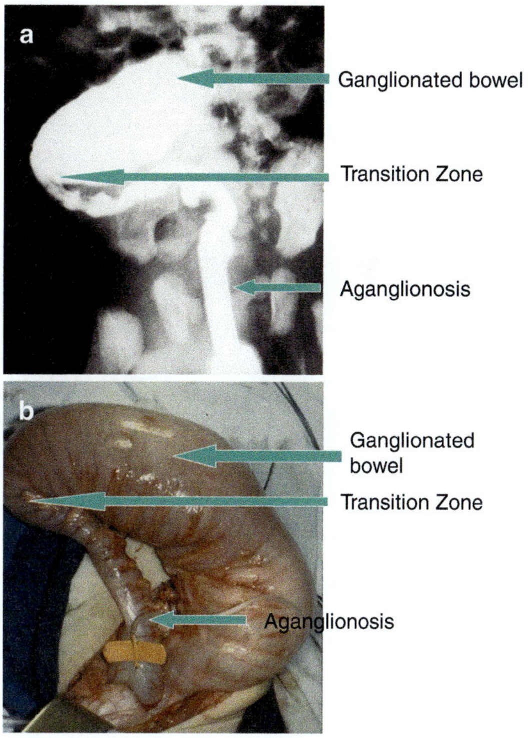

Fig. 64.5 (**a**) Radiographic contrast enema in infant with Hirschsprung disease. Note constricted distal colon representing the aganglionic segment, with a transition zone and proximal, dilated ganglionated colon. (**b**) Operative image of same patient. Note constriction of aganglionic segment and dilation of proximal colon with a hypertrophy of the longitudinal muscle layer

performed to detect hypertrophic nerve trunks and the absence of ganglion cells in the colonic submucosa to confirm the diagnosis.
- Mutations in the *RET* proto-oncogene pathway compromise nearly half of all familial cases and a smaller fraction of sporadic cases, though over 30 genetic mutations have been identified in patients with HD, including mutations in *EDN3* or *EDNRB*.

Current Therapies

- Treatment involves removal or bypass of the aganglionic segment with an anastomosis of proximal, ganglionic bowel.
- The Swenson operation is a full-thickness perineal resection and colo-anal anastomosis.
- The Soave procedure involves a mucosal/submucosal resection distally and a full-thickness resection proximally of the diseased segment, followed by a pull-through procedure within the muscular cuff.
- The Duhamel procedure involves a resection of the proximal diseased bowel with a retrorectal mobilization (leaving the diseased rectum in situ) and performing a retrorectal anastomosis with the rectum and normally innervated bowel.
- Long-term postoperative complications include soiling/incontinence (~5%), constipation, and recurrent enterocolitis.

Acquired Diseases

Necrotizing Enterocolitis

- Necrotizing enterocolitis (NEC) is a leading cause of infant morbidity and mortality in neonatal intensive care units (NICUs) and is the most common premature newborn surgical emergency.
- Infants born with a birth weight of <1000 g and/or < 28 weeks of gestation are at the greatest risk.
- The presence of pneumatosis intestinalis on radiographs or intraoperatively will be seen in most advanced cases; this air may extend into the portal tree (Fig. 64.6).
- NEC is secondary to problems with the GI tract barrier function that initiates an ischemic

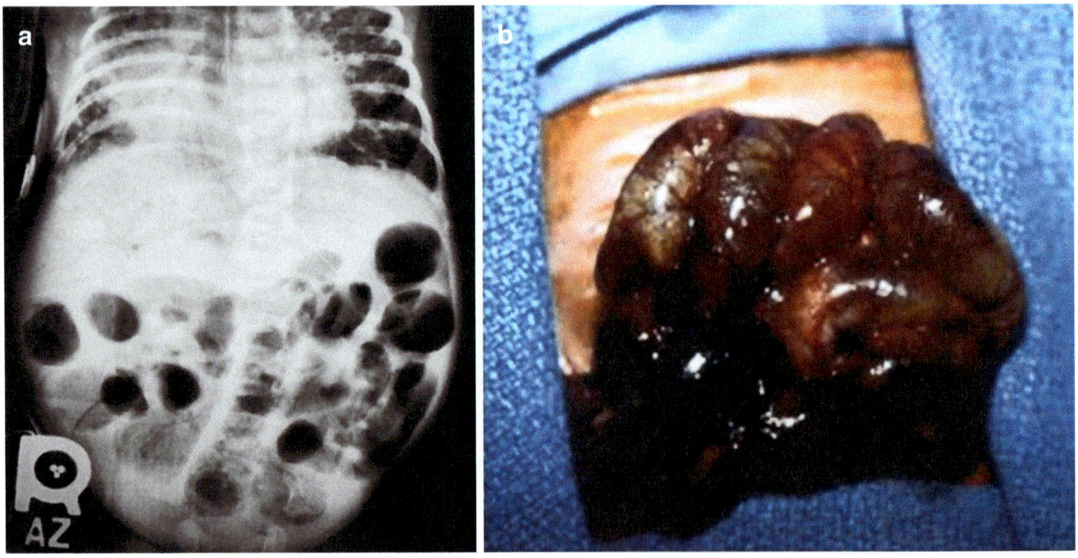

Fig. 64.6 (**a**) Radiograph of a premature neonate with necrotizing enterocolitis. Note diffuse pneumatosis intestinalis and air in the biliary tree. (**b**) Intraoperative appearance of the same neonate showing pneumatosis intestinalis and patchy ischemia/necrosis to the small bowel

cascade with subsequent progressive enteric mucosal and then full-thickness injury.

Current Therapies

- Prevention of NEC should be considered the primary treatment (e.g., breast milk is preventative due to the high concentrations of epidermal growth factor (EGF) and IgA).
- In the absence of a surgical emergency, supportive care involves discontinuing enteral feedings, GI tract decompression, broad-spectrum antibiotics, and administration of intravenous fluids/nutrition.
- Surgery is indicated for clinical signs of perforation (e.g., pneumoperitoneum) or clinical deterioration despite maximum medical treatment.
- The goal of operative treatment is to remove necrotic intestine while preserving bowel length to avoid short bowel syndrome.
- ~50% of neonates undergoing surgery do not survive.
- Performing a percutaneous drainage of the abdomen via a small right lower quadrant incision is an option for very small premature infants an alternative to surgery.

Constipation and Anorectal Incontinence (Fig. 64.7)

- Persistent constipation can lead to fecal retention, impaction, and overflow incontinence.
- Most children pass meconium in the first 48 h of life – a child with "constipation" should be considered to have an organic cause of their constipation or a bowel obstruction until proven otherwise.
- In children outside of the neonatal time period, the vast majority of their constipation is functional.
- Functional constipation is defined as constipation not associated with a congenital anomaly, acquired disease, or medications.
- The Rome III criteria is considered the best method to make an accurate diagnosis of functional constipation.
- Management of functional constipation in childhood includes education especially around toilet training, dietary changes, and oral medications.
- The most commonly used medications are polyethylene glycol or, in more resistant cases, senna glycosides (sennosides).
- Children that are refractory to initial treatment need further workup to rule out an organic cause including a motility assessment, colonic transit, and manometry.
- Nonsurgical treatments that have been reported include abdominal wall transcutaneous electrical stimulation and more recently, the PERISTEEN™ (Coloplast, UK) enema program.

Surgical Treatment for Chronic Functional Constipation

- Most children do not require surgery.
- Common procedures used include the Malone antegrade continence enema (MACE) or other antegrade continence enema procedures such as a cecostomy typically via a Chait® tube (Cook Medical Co.).
- Resection of a megarectum or colon in children has been reported with mixed results, as has a colostomy.
- Sacral nerve stimulation (SNS) has shown promising preliminary results, with ~80% success (currently limited to children over 15 years to date in the USA).

Constipation and Fecal Incontinence in Children with Hirschsprung Disease (HD) or Anorectal Malformations (ARM)

- Constipation and/or fecal incontinence are considerably more challenging to treat in children with HD or ARM.
- In HD, bowel dysfunction has been reported by parents in up to 65% of children; with 42%

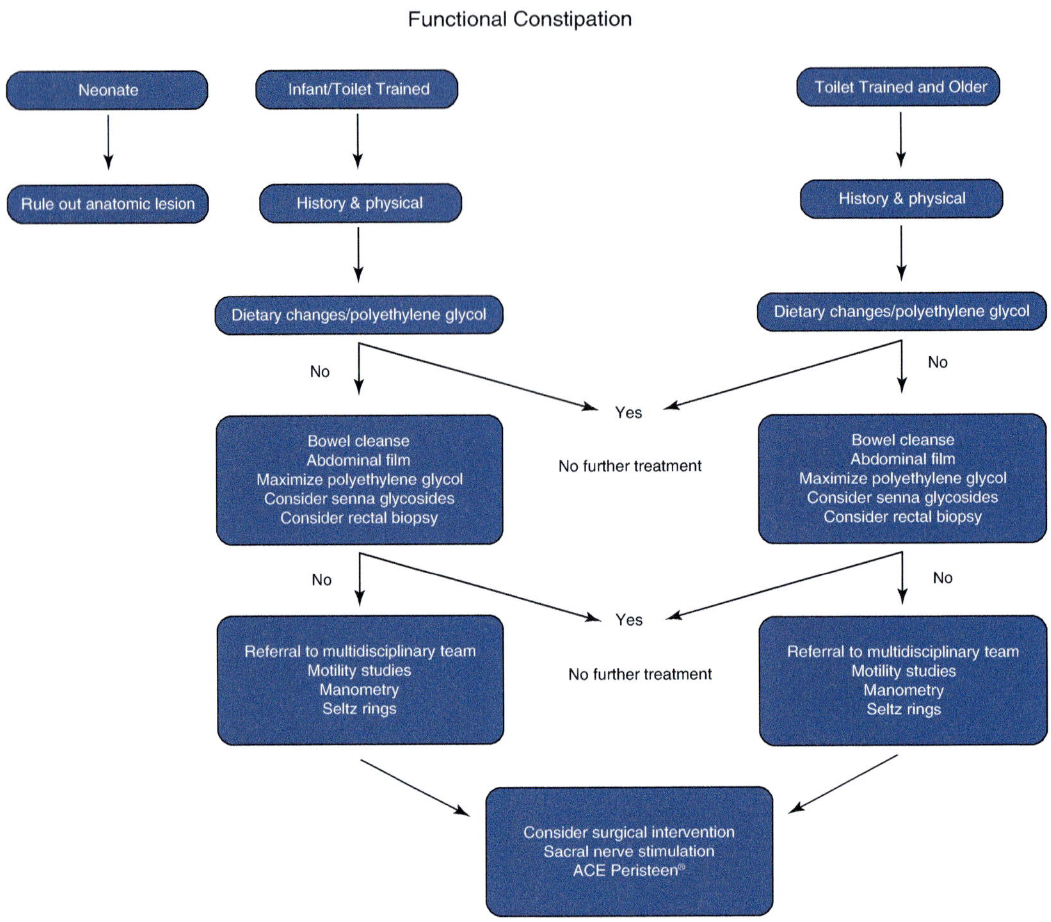

Fig. 64.7 Decision tree in the management of functional constipation. Abbreviations: *ACE* antegrade continent enema

reporting occasional soiling, 12% frequent soiling, 46% no soiling, and constipation occurring in 9%.

- The etiology of constipation or fecal incontinence in children with HD includes enterocolitis, anastomotic issues (including stricture), sphincter dysfunction, and a retained/acquired aganglionic segment.
- Strictures at the anastomotic site (often due to ischemia) may respond to dilatations; however, persistent strictures will require a repeat pull-through.
- Constipation can also be the result of a retained or long aganglionic segment that creates a functional obstruction.
- Constipation and fecal incontinence are even more prevalent in children with ARM, with ~1/3 having voluntary bowel movements and complete evacuation while the remaining requiring some interventions.

Diagnostic Workup and Therapy

- In children with HD and bowel dysfunction, a digital examination, contrast enema, stool studies, anorectal manometry, defecography, motility studies, and endoscopy with biopsies (at 2 cm, 4 cm, and 6 cm) above the anastomosis should be performed to look for a transitional zone or aganglionic tissue.

- For enterocolitis, oral antibiotics (typically metronidazole or intravenous if the child is sick) and a rectal decompression are the first-line treatment options.
- For sphincter dysfunction or aganglionic segments, the initial therapy is a bowel management program, followed by internal anal sphincter botulinum toxin injections.
- Surgical therapy includes posterior myotomy and ACE procedures, and in cases that have failed other treatments, redo pull-through.
- For constipation and fecal incontinence in children with ARM, the initial investigations should include a contrast enema to rule out retention of stool with overflow incontinence, motility studies, defecography, and manometry.
- First line of therapy consists of a bowel management program, though failures requiring surgical may involve an ACE procedure or, for severe cases, a colostomy.

Inflammatory Bowel Disease in Children

- In children, Crohn's and UC can occur at any age, but the peak incidence is in late adolescence to early adulthood, with a slight female predominance.
- The initial symptoms are often systemic in nature without focal gastrointestinal manifestations including fever of unknown origin, arthritis, and chronic microcytic anemia.
- Approximately 35% of children present with delayed growth or development, which can precede the development of any other overt symptoms by months or even years.
- In Crohn's disease, the most frequent distributions are the following: 33% are limited to the small bowel alone, 45% involve both the ileum and colon, 20% have isolated colonic Crohn's, and 1/3 of patients have perianal disease.
- Most Crohn's patients have oral lesions, yet they are rarely severe.
- Children with UC may present with extraintestinal manifestations including polyarthritis involving large joints, but without joint destruction.
- In UC, the severity of inflammation largely parallels the severity of the intestinal component.
  - Colectomy is curative not only of the colitis but also most other extraintestinal manifestations.
  - Colectomy (similar to adults) does not affect bile duct pathology.
- Evaluation in children includes endoscopy with biopsy and magnetic resonance enterography – especially with the concerns of radiation from repeated computed tomography scans CT over time.

Treatment

- The drug choices to treat both Crohn's and UC in children are identical to adults.
- A unique consideration in the medical management of children with IBD is the long-term impact of treatment on growth, bone health, and social development.
- Infliximab use has reduced the need for surgery in children for both Crohn's disease and UC.
- For Crohn's disease, the multicenter REACH trial and the Scottish trial found that overall response rate was 88% and the 8-week remission rate was 59% (REACH trial) and 47% (Scottish trial), respectively.
- For UC, infliximab induced a response in 73.3% of patients, and the overall remission rate at week 54 was 28.6%.
- The surgical indications in the pediatric population for children with Crohn's disease include exsanguinating hemorrhage, perforation, suspected cancer, unresponsive disease, growth retardation, systemic complications, and steroid dependency.

- Surgical indications in children with UC include toxic megacolon, perforation, uncontrolled bleeding, and obstruction.
  - On a more chronic basis, indications include refractive disease, steroid dependency, failure to thrive and impaired psychosocial development, and growth retardation.
- In patients with UC, when a restorative total proctocolectomy is required, most surgeons are performing the ileal pouch-anal anastomosis (i.e., J-pouch).

Considerations for Geriatric Patients Undergoing Colorectal Surgery

65

Kevin R. Kasten and Todd D. Francone

Key Concepts

- The geriatric population is diverse, with varying levels of health status including physiologic reserve and cognitive function.
- Chronological age is a poor marker of functional, physical, and cognitive decline in the elderly.
  a. Fit elderly patients, those without significant comorbidities or cognitive decline, can be managed similar to that of younger patients.
  b. Frail patients are associated with higher morbidity and mortality in both elective and emergent operations.
- Elderly patients undergoing emergent procedures are at high risk (17–31%) for postoperative mortality.
- Minimally invasive surgery is safe and appropriate in the elderly population, allowing them to benefit from the decreased postoperative morbidity, faster return of bowel function, decreased length of stay, and less pain.
- While some assessment models identify age as an independent risk factor for adverse outcomes, a focus on chronologic age substantially limits effective management of the geriatric patient.
- Frailty is used to represent a global limited reserve in the elder population and is a potentially useful tool for predicting poor outcomes.

Introduction

- Over half of all current operations in the United States are performed on patients older than 65 years of age, with estimates of surgical volume increasing from 14% to 47% between 2000 and 2020, due to more elderly patients.
- Elderly patients are less likely to be offered standard-of-care treatment, with advanced chronological age (often inappropriately) considered the main factor for determining surgical intervention, though age does not accurately reflect functional, physical, and cognitive decline.
- Postoperative mortality and morbidity in the older population remain variable, with postoperative morbidity reported as high as 60%.

K. R. Kasten
Department of Surgery, Section of Colorectal Surgery, Atrium Health, Carolinas Medical Center, Charlotte, NC, USA

T. D. Francone (✉)
Department of General Surgery, Section of Colorectal Surgery, Massachusetts General Hospital, Boston, MA, USA
e-mail: tfrancone@partners.org

S. R. Steele et al. (eds.), *The ASCRS Manual of Colon and Rectal Surgery*,
https://doi.org/10.1007/978-3-030-01165-9_65

Current Outcomes in the Geriatric Population

- Elderly have higher rates of comorbidities ranging from cardiovascular disease (e.g., CHF, hypertension) to cognitive decline.
- Elderly colorectal patients undergoing emergent procedures are at high risk for postoperative mortality, ranging between 14 and 31%.
  - The elevated rates are likely related to an increasing number of synchronous comorbidities and lower performance status for this particular subset of the elderly.
  - Mortality is up to ~40% when the patient sustained a postoperative complication, versus 20% without a complication.
- The physiologic reserve of the elderly is clearly less than that of the younger population, with 90-day outcomes for patients over 80 years being worse and mortality of ~13–19%.
- Understanding the relationship between age and comorbidity allows surgeons to stratify appropriate surgical intervention without relying on age alone.
- A NSQIP analysis of surgical patients over 70 years old demonstrated a linear relationship between age and complications, increasing 0.71% per year of age.
- Octogenarians undergoing lower GI procedures demonstrated a 53.5% overall rate of morbidity, with 38.4% requiring postoperative surgical intensive care unit (SICU) admission.
- Common major complications included pneumonia (25%), respiratory failure (15%), and MI (13%), followed by ileus and delayed extubation as common minor complications.
- In addition to specific organ-based complications, elders are prone to delays in functional recovery, in which the return to functional baseline status is often prolonged, and may occur as follows: mental status (3 weeks), timed up and go (6 weeks), activities of daily living (ADL) (6–12 weeks), and grip strength (>24 weeks).
- Age alone should not preclude one's decision to restore intestinal continuity.
- Creation of a stoma is not without risk and may be more detrimental in the elderly population, and quality of life, social impairments, and difficulty in properly managing a stoma bag are all potential issues in the elderly.
- Colostomy closure is a high-risk procedure in most patients regardless of age and comorbidity.

Fecal Incontinence

- The prevalence of fecal incontinence is ~2–5% in patients over 65 years of age, 3–17% in patients over 85 years old, and 50% in institutionalized elders.
- Fecal impaction is a common cause of incontinence in the elderly, as well as constipation from heavy laxative use producing liquid stool and subsequent overflow incontinence around partial or complete impaction.
- Other factors independently associated with fecal incontinence include prior bowel resection, prior hemorrhoidectomy, loose/liquid stool, and constant fecal urgency.
- Treatment depends on etiology, such as appropriate bowel regimen for constipation.
- Other etiologies require appropriate workup with defecography, anal manometry, and endorectal ultrasound to determine management options.
- Biofeedback is a well-described conservative management option for fecal incontinence, with high rates of success in elderly patients.

Diverticulosis/Diverticulitis

- Greater than 65% of patients 80 years or older demonstrate some degree of diverticulosis, and 10–25% of patients develop symptoms consistent with diverticulitis.
- End-stage renal disease (ESRD) in elderly patients (>65 years) undergoing surgical management of diverticulitis is associated

with more emergent surgery, higher rates of complications, and increased ostomy creation.

- Outcomes are worse in elder patients undergoing emergent operations for diverticulitis, with mortality rates of 10.4–12.4% in emergent and 2.4–3.1% in elective cases.
- Early intervention should be considered in certain circumstances given the significant rise in complications associated with urgent/emergent procedures in the elderly population.

Rectal Prolapse

- Surgery should be considered in most cases, with the choice of operation depending upon goals of care, patient comorbidities, and surgeon comfort with treatment options.
- Outcomes for both transabdominal and perineal approaches have been shown similar among young and old groups.
- Laparoscopic and minimally invasive procedures have demonstrated improved outcomes with transabdominal repair in elderly patients with rectal prolapse.

Colonic Volvulus

- Cecal volvulus usually presents in the fifth and sixth decades of life, and sigmoid volvulus at 68 years with a peak incidence in the eighth decade.
- Mortality rates are less than 12% in urgent cases with viable bowel and 30% in urgent cases with nonviable bowel.
- More than 90% of sigmoid volvulus patients are successfully decompressed with endoscopy.
- Treatment is typically resection due to the low risk and high risk of recurrence when non-resectional procedures are performed.
- In patients not fit for operative intervention, percutaneous endoscopic colonic (PEC) tube placement is associated with 75% decompression, along with a 4% mortality and 30% complication rate.

Inflammatory Bowel Disease

- Inflammatory bowel disease (IBD) has a second mode of incidence at 55–70 years.
- IBD in the elderly carries an altered phenotype from younger patients, including involvement of different gastrointestinal sections, poorer response to therapy, higher complications, and higher mortality.
- Despite reported higher morbidity and mortality associated with a restorative proctocolectomy in the elder population, concern also lies with the risk for fecal incontinence and decline in quality of life.
- Data suggests no difference in patient need for surgical resection based upon age at presentation and no difference in rates of surgery for hospitalized IBD patients.

Colon Cancer

- Colon cancer is largely a disease of old age, disproportionately affecting the elderly, with prevalence and incidence increasing significantly into the eighth decade of life (Fig. 65.1).
- When matched for stage and histology, older patients have higher 30-day mortality rates of 8–22%, along with higher complications rates that are almost double that seen in younger populations.
- Select elders will benefit from standard oncologic treatment including surgical resection with or without adjuvant chemotherapy.
- Older persons with stage III disease have been shown to derive the same benefit from adjuvant therapy as their younger counterparts.
  - FOLFOX is well tolerated by the elderly; however, they may not see the same survival benefits of FOLFOX compared to younger patients, so consider infusional 5-FU or capecitabine alone.

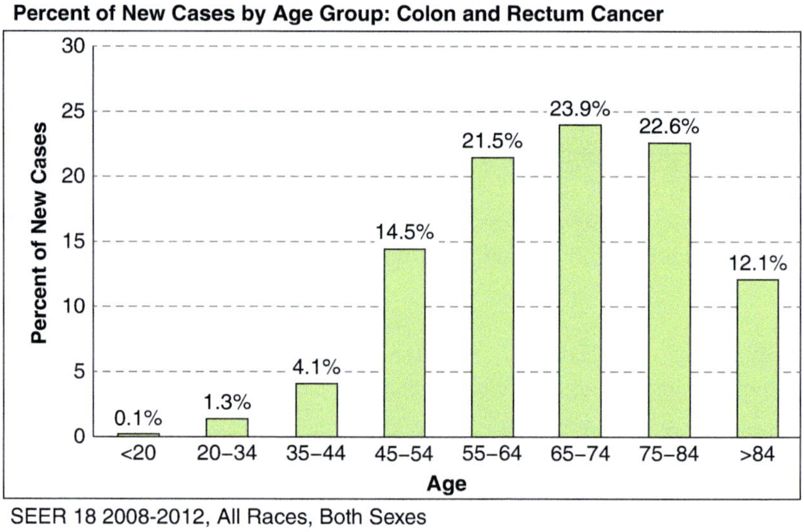

Fig. 65.1 Colon cancer is largely a disease of old age with prevalence and incidence increasing significantly into the eighth decade of life. Colon and rectum cancer represents 8.0% of all new cancer cases in the United States. Available at http://seer.cancer.gov/statfacts/html/colorect.html

- There is little benefit of palliative therapy on overall survival in the elder population.

Rectal Cancer

- For the elderly population, the surgeon should be particularly aware of preoperative fecal incontinence and decreased mobility as restoration of an intestinal continuity with a low anastomosis may worsen the predisposing condition leading to a debilitating and degraded quality of life.
- In the elderly patient population with rectal cancer, fit elders have been shown to tolerate chemoradiotherapy (CRT) similar to that of younger patients.
- Despite the increased morbidity with a pelvic dissection, operative mortality has not been shown to be significantly different among older and younger populations.
- Overall survival for older patients with rectal cancer is worse, though disease-specific survival has not been shown to be worse in elder patients.
- There is increased toxicity with the addition of chemotherapy to radiotherapy, with overall rate of grade 3 toxicity being 34.9%.
- Given the lack of adequate management algorithms in the elderly population, oncologic management of the elderly should be tailored to the individual with an adequate understanding of the patient's underlying functional, physical, or cognitive impairments.

Laparoscopic Surgery in the Elderly

- The benefits of laparoscopy are well established with decreased pain, better cosmesis, early return of bowel function, and shorter hospitalization.
- These benefits extend to the elder population in both benign and oncologic disease with numerous studies validating the benefit of minimally invasive surgery in the elderly.
  - Laparoscopy can reduce postoperative morbidity when compared to open resections (20.2% vs. 37.5%) as well as length of stay (9.5 vs. 13 days).

Re-operative Evaluation in the Geriatric Patient

- Thirty-day mortality significantly increases for each decade through age over 90 years.
- A patient's physiologic age, rather than one's chronological age, has been shown to be a more precise indicator of one's ability to tolerate surgery.

- Because elderly patients are more susceptible to surgical complications, the surgeon must assess optimized modifiable risk factors preoperatively when possible (Table 65.1).

Table 65.1 Preoperative workup for geriatric patients undergoing colorectal surgery

Cardiac assessment
I. Patients with active cardiac conditions require cardiology assessment and workup
II. Patients with over 2 clinical risk factors require heart rate management but do not need cardiac testing unless results will change operative management
III. Patients undergoing low-risk surgery and with more than 3 METs or fewer than 3 clinical risk factors may proceed with surgery
Pulmonary assessment
IV. Encourage smoking patients to quit more than 8 weeks post-op, although 4 weeks may be long enough in some studies
V. Aggressive management of COPD and asthma
VI. Routine CXR and PFTs not indicated
Diabetes and glucose assessment
VII. Obtain baseline glucose level
VIII. Obtain baseline BUN and creatinine
Nutritional assessment
IX. Patients with BMI <18 or unintentional weight loss over 10% in 6 months require evaluation by a registered dietician
X. Preoperative nutritional
Anemia and hematologic assessment
XI. Obtain baseline hemoglobin and hematocrit
Cognitive assessment
– All patients require adequate history from patient and family member
– All patients require cognitive assessment (Mini-Cog)
– All patients require anxiety/depression assessment
– All patients require assessment of alcohol use, identification of possible abuse
– All patients require evaluation of decision-making capacity to ensure informed consent
– Any new findings, or worsening of existing findings, require further evaluation by appropriate geriatrician or mental health-care provider
Laboratory and noninvasive testing
– Unless previously indicated above, routine CBC, BMP, PT/PTT, EKG, and CXR are not required

Adapted from Chow WB, Rosenthal RA, Merkow RP, et al. Optimal preoperative assessment of the geriatric surgical patient: a best practices guideline from the American College of Surgeons National Surgical Quality Improvement Program and the American Geriatrics Society. J Am Coll Surg. 2012;215(4):453–66

- Surgical risk groups are based on the type of surgery and defined as "low," "medium," and "high" risk, with 30-day cardiac event rates (MI and death) of <1%, 1–5%, and > 5%, respectively.
- All abdominal procedures involving the colon and rectum are included within the "medium"-risk group (at a minimum).
- As a reference, one metabolic equivalent of task (MET) is an expended metabolic equivalent at rest, four METs are equivalent to climbing two flights of stairs, and ten METs represent strenuous sports activities (Table 65.2).
- Anything less than four METs is considered poor functional capacity but is not strongly associated with worsened cardiac outcomes in abdominal surgery.
- Patients with greater than four METs do not require further cardiac workup, regardless of risk factors.

Table 65.2 Metabolic equivalents of task

Activity performed	METs
Low-intensity activities	*<3*
– Sleeping	0.9
– Reading/writing	1.6
– Washing, dressing, grooming self, grocery shopping	2.1
– Bowling	3.0
Moderate-intensity activities	*3–6*
– Walking (3.0 mph)	3.3
– Home exercise, light to moderate effort	3.5
– Bicycling, leisure, light effort	4.0
– Dancing	4.5
– Playing volleyball, softball	5.5
High-intensity activities	*>6*
– Hiking, fencing, wrestling	6.0
– Soccer, snowboarding	7.0
– Basketball, jogging	8.0
– Tennis, racket sports	8.5
– Jumping rope	10.0

Table derived using values from Tudor-Locke C et al. website companion, http://appliedresearch.cancer.gov/atus-met/ (Source: 19564664)
Metabolic equivalents are used to measure functional capacity and are often utilized for preoperative risk assessment in surgical candidates of all ages

Cardiac Evaluation

- Overall, the risk of a perioperative cardiac event for patients undergoing a procedure of "medium" risk is less than 1% compared to a 4% risk in patients with known CAD.
- The risk of a cardiac event or death in the elder population is no greater than younger patients.
- Clinical cardiac risk factors include angina, prior MI, heart failure, stroke/TIA, renal dysfunction, and IDDM.
- Exercise tolerance, ambulatory EKG changes, echo changes demonstrating prior MI, valvular disease or left ventricular diastolic dysfunction, and positive stress test have also been associated with increased risk of perioperative cardiac event.
- EKG is required for patients with the presence of cardiac risk factors prior to any surgical intervention.
- Patients undergoing medium-risk surgery (i.e., abdominal) without risk factors should be considered for at minimum an EKG evaluation.
- Echocardiography is not required in patients free of cardiac symptoms but should be considered in patients undergoing high-risk surgery.
- Instead of cardiac catheterization, beta-blockade and statins pre- and perioperatively are strongly recommended prior to non-cardiac surgery.

Goldman Cardiac Risk Index (9 risks)	Points
1. Age > 70 years	5
2. Cardiac History	
Preoperative MI < 6 months	10
3-4. Physical Examination	
3. S_3 Gallop or HJR > 12 cm H_2O	11
4. Significant aortic stenosis	3
5-6. Electrocardiogram	
5. Rhythm other than NSR or atrial ectopy	7
6. VPBs > 5/min	7
7. General Medical Status: one or more of these factors	3
a. pO_2 < 60 or pCO_2 > 50 mmHg	
b. Serum K < 3.0 or HCO_3 < 20 meq/mL	
c. BUN > 50 or creatinine >3.0 mg/dL	
d. Chronic liver disease or delibitation	
8-9. Type of Surgery	
8. Intrathoracic, intraperitoneal, or aorta	3
9. Emergency	4
Possible total points and complications rate	53
Class I: 0.7% cardiac complications & 0.2% mortality	0-5
Class II: 5% cardiac complications & 2% mortality	6-12
Class III: 11% cardiac complications & 2% mortality	13-25
Class IV: 78% cardiac complications & 56% mortality	≥ 26

Fig. 65.2 Goldman Cardiac Risk Index is a tool used to estimate a patient's risk of perioperative cardiac complications. With permission from Goldman L, et al. Multifactorial index of cardiac risk in non-cardiac surgical procedures. N Engl J Med. 1977;297(16):845–50

Pulmonary Evaluation

- Chronic obstructive pulmonary disease (COPD) is the single most important risk factor for the development of postoperative pulmonary failure.
- In patients with history of tobacco abuse, smoking cessation for more than 6–8 weeks is recommended.
- Risk factors requiring further workup include abnormal CXR, high ASA, abnormal respiratory exam, elevated Goldman Cardiac Risk Index (Fig. 65.2), and elevated Charlson Comorbidity Index (Table 65.3).
- Chronic obstructive pulmonary disease (COPD) is the single most important risk factor for the development of postoperative pulmonary failure, with up to 25% of elderly patients with COPD having an operative pulmonary complication and mortality approaching 7%.
- Surgical site is the most significant non-modifiable risk factor for pulmonary complication, with risk increasing as surgical site moves closer to the diaphragm (upper and lower abdominal complication between 13–33% and 0–16%, respectively.)

Table 65.3 Charlson Comorbidity Index – summation of score for given patient provides index

Clinical comorbidity	Item score
Myocardial infarct Congestive heart disease Peripheral vascular disease Dementia Cerebrovascular disease Chronic pulmonary disease Connective tissue disorder Diabetes, without complications Peptic ulcer disease Chronic liver disease (no portal hypertension) Each decade over 40 years	1
Hemiplegia Moderate, severe renal disease Diabetes, with complications Solid organ tumors, cancer Leukemia Lymphoma	2
Moderate/severe liver disease, cirrhosis	3
Malignant tumor with metastases AIDS	6

Charlson Comorbidity Index is the most widely used comorbidity index which was developed to predict the 1-year mortality. Adapted from Charlson ME, Pompei P, Ales KL, MacKenzie CR. A new method of classifying prognostic comorbidity in longitudinal studies: development and validation. J Chronic Dis. 1987;40(5):373–83

Diabetes and Glucose Management

- Over 27% of patients older than 65 carry the diagnosis of diabetes, and another 50% are at risk for development.
- Elderly patients may greatly benefit from strict control of glucose levels below 180 mg/dL.
- Drinking a high-carbohydrate drink 2 h before surgical intervention helps prevent insulin resistance, leading to decreased infectious complications, decreased ileus, less anxiety, and less perioperative discomfort and hunger.
- Hyperglycemia is associated with increased rates of sepsis, surgical site infection, reoperation, and increased LOS.
- There is an increased risk of hypoglycemia in elderly patients attributable to impaired counter-regulatory mechanisms, renal insufficiency, or delay in diagnosis related to delirium and altered mental status which are common in the elder population.

Nutritional Assessment

- Malnourishment affects between 2 and 32% of elderly and has been shown to increase the risk of perioperative complications by sixfold.
- Optimization of nutritional status is highly recommended including the employment of registered dieticians or nutritionists.
- Poor preoperative nutritional status is associated with postoperative delirium and mortality in elderly patients.
- Using BMI or albumin alone to evaluate elderly patients is a poor indicator in clinically ill patients; rather prealbumin, transferrin, and retinol-binding protein provide a more accurate picture of patient nutrition.
- Screening tools which include Subjective Global Assessment (SGA) or Mini Nutritional Assessment (MNA) are also helpful and may provide further insight.

Anemia and Hematologic Disorder Evaluation

- Over 20% of patients >85 years carrying the diagnosis while 16% of men and 10% of women over age 75 are anemic.
- Underlying causes of anemia are split in thirds between malnutrition (iron deficiency accounts for 50%), renal dysfunction, and unexplained anemia.
- A preoperative CBC provides a baseline and allows the surgeon and anesthesiologist to discuss triggers for operative blood transfusion.
- For patients over age 65, preoperative transfusion with hematocrit levels <24% is associated with decreased 30-day mortality.
- For major elective surgeries, consider treatment with iron supplementation, folate supplementation, erythropoietin, or transfusion.

Dementia and Mental Status Evaluation

- Cognitive dysfunction is common in elderly patients, with rates between 5% and 15% in the general population and increasing to >60% in high-risk groups.
- Delirium is defined as a documented change in mental status characterized by reduced environmental awareness and attention disturbance.
  - In patients aged over 70 undergoing abdominal surgery, the overall incidence of delirium was 60% with a 30-day mortality of 20% in those patients.
- Dementia is the single biggest risk factor for postoperative delirium, although multiple additional factors have also been implicated (Table 65.4).
- Treatment should not utilize medications as first-line therapy; rather, avoidance of triggers, reorientation, massage, relaxing music, and one-on-one care with family are recommended.
- If medication is required, Haldol should be initially considered, and the clinician should refrain from restraints except in the most severe cases.

Table 65.4 Risk factors for delirium

Preoperative
Dementia
Age
Malnutrition
Cognitive impairment
Visual impairment
Dehydration
Immobilization
Polypharmacy
Severe illness
Perioperative
Poor fluid status
Poor glycemic control >150 mg/dL
Metabolic derangements
Uncontrolled pain (PCA necessary to improve delirium in elderly patients
Addition of more than 4 new medications
Bladder catheters
Serum urea nitrogen to creatinine ratio >17
Prolonged bed rest
Physical restraints

Current Risk Assessment

- Several risk models have attempted to include markers for physiologic status such as the National Surgical Quality Improvement Program (NSQIP).
- Among other physiologic variables, the model includes age (<65, 65–74, 75–84, 85 or greater) and functional health status (defined as independent, partially dependent, and totally dependent), both of which may help account for elder patients who are frail and reside in nursing homes or assisted living facilities.

Frailty

- Frailty is an age-associated decline in five domains (Table 65.5): shrinking, weakness, exhaustion, low physical activity, and slow walking speed.
- In nonsurgical patients, frailty has been shown to identify those patients at risk for increased falls, disability, hospitalizations, institutionalization, and mortality.
- Frailty has been shown to be independently associated with the development of postoperative complications (OR 2.54; 95% CI 1.12–5.77), length of stay (OR 1.69; 95% CI 1.28–2.23), and discharge to a skilled or assisted living facility after previously living at home (20.48; 95% CI 5.54–75.68).

Table 65.5 Frailty score

Domain	Definition
Shrinking	Unintentional weight loss ≥10 pounds in the last year
Decreased grip strength	Patient squeezed a handheld dynamometer (strength measurement was adjusted for BMI and gender)
Exhaustion	Response to questions about effort and motivation
Low physical activity	Survey about leisure time activities
Slowed walking speed	Speed at which patient could walk 15 feet

Chart adapted from Makary MA, Segev DL, Pronovost PJ, et al. Frailty as a predictor of surgical outcomes in older patients. J Am Coll Surg. Jun 2010;210(6):901–8

Frailty score has been described as an age-associated decline in five domains: shrinking, weakness, exhaustion, low physical activity, and slow walking speed

Table 65.6 Geriatric assessment domains

Domain	Measures
Functional status	(1) Activities of daily living (subscale of MOS physical health) (2) Instrumental activities of daily living (subscale of the OARS) (3) Karnofsky Performance (4) Timed up and go (5) Number of falls in last 6 months
Comorbidity	Physical health section (OARS subscale)
Cognition	Blessed Orientation-Memory-Concentration Test
Psychological	Hospital Anxiety and Depression Scale
Social functioning	MOS Social Activity Limitations Measure
Social support	MOS Social Support Survey: Emotional/Information and Tangible Subscales
Nutrition	(1) Body mass index (2) % Unintentional weight loss in last 6 months

Table 65.7 2012 American College of Surgeons NSQIP and American Geriatric Society proposed checklist

In addition to conducting a complete history and physical examination of the patient, the following assessments are strongly recommended:
Assess the patient's **cognitive ability** and **capacity** to understand the anticipated surgery
Screen the patient for **depression**
Identify the patient's risk factors for developing postoperative **delirium**
Screen for **alcohol** and other **substance abuse/dependence**
Perform a preoperative **cardiac** evaluation according to the American College of Cardiology/American Heart Association algorithm for patients undergoing non-cardiac surgery
Identify the patient's risk factors for postoperative **pulmonary** complications, and implement appropriate strategies for prevention
Document **functional status** and history of **falls**
Determine baseline **frailty** score
Assess patient's **nutritional status**, and consider preoperative interventions if the patient is at severe nutritional risk
Take an accurate and detailed **medication history,** and consider appropriate perioperative adjustments. Monitor for **polypharmacy**
Determine the patient's **treatment goals** and **expectations** in the context of the possible treatment outcomes
Determine patient's **family** and **social support system**
Order appropriate preoperative **diagnostic tests** focused on elderly patients

Adapted from Chow WB, Rosenthal RA, Merkow RP, et al. Optimal preoperative assessment of the geriatric surgical patient: a best practices guideline from the American College of Surgeons National Surgical Quality Improvement Program and the American Geriatrics Society. J Am Coll Surg. 2012;215(4):453–66.
American College of Surgeons' 2012 best practices guidelines for the perioperative care of the geriatric surgical patient

Comprehensive Geriatric Assessment (CGA)

- The CGA generally includes a compilation of validated tools to assess comorbidity, functional status (including the ability to live at home), physical performance, cognitive impairment, psychological status, nutritional status, medication review, and social support (Table 65.6).
- Elements from CGA were found to be associated with an increased risk of poor surgical outcomes and increased length of stay.

Current Recommendations

- In 2012, the American College of Surgeons NSQIP and American Geriatric Society collaborated to create best practice guidelines for the perioperative care of the geriatric surgical patient.
- In addition to conducting a complete history and physical examination, the authors recommended evaluations of preoperative domains which included problems specific to elderly individuals.
- A proposed checklist was drafted for surgeons across all specialties to utilize in the evaluation of a surgical geriatric patient (Table 65.7).

Health-Care Economics

66

Guy R. Orangio

Key Concepts

- In 1965 President Lyndon B. Johnson signed Medicare and Medicaid Amendments (Titles XVIII and XIX) into law.
- In 1987 the Resource-Based Relative Value Scale was instituted as the basis for Medicare Physician-Fee-Schedule.
- All Congressional attempts at controlling the rising cost of health care in America failed.
- The Patient Protection and Affordable Care Act of 2010 mandated Alternative Payment Models
- These Alternative Payment Models require Clinical Integration to be successful in decreasing costs and increasing efficiency and quality in the delivery of Health Care to patients.
- Surgeons will have to understand these new Alternative Payment Models in order to continue to deliver quality cost-effective care to their patients.
- The Relative-Based Relative Value Scale in combination with Quality Metrics will be the foundation of total compensation for surgeons within these new Alternative Payment Models.

G. R. Orangio (✉)
LSU Department of Surgery: Chief Section of Colon and Rectal Surgery, University Medical Center New Orleans, New Orleans, LA, USA

Introduction

- Health- Care Reform has become one of the most important social movements since Franklin Delano Roosevelt signed the Social Security Tax Act (SSTA) of 1935.
- On July 30, 1965, President Lyndon B. Johnson signed Medicare and Medicaid Amendments (Titles XVIII and XIX) of the Social Security Act that instituted a national health program in the United States.
- Health-care expenditures in the United States are at about 18% of the Gross Domestic Product (GDP) and are projected to rise sharply.

Physician Reimbursement

Fee-for-Service (FFS): Resource-Based Relative Value Scale (RBRVS)

- "Fee-For-Service (FFS) *is defined as payment to a provider, usually a physician, who receives a set fee for a particular service-such as performing a physical exam or administering an inoculation-either directly from the patient or from an insurer or other payer. Fee-for-service thus generates payments driven by the volume of services performed.*"
- With the threat of Congress instituting a completely unacceptable method of reimburse-

S. R. Steele et al. (eds.), *The ASCRS Manual of Colon and Rectal Surgery*,
https://doi.org/10.1007/978-3-030-01165-9_66

Table 66.1 Common Current Procedural Terminology (CPT) codes billed by colon and rectal surgeons

CPT Code	Descriptor	wRVU[a]	PE RVU[b]	PLI RVU[c]	Total RVU	Medicare payment $
44140	Colectomy partial with anastomosis	22.59	12.42	4.64	39.65	1370.58
44204	Laparoscopy, surgical; colectomy, partial, with anastomosis	26.42	12.59	5.53	44.54	1592.51
46260	Hemorrhoidectomy, internal, external, two or more columns/groups	6.73	5.65	1.33	13.71	490.20

[a]Work-RVU
[b]Practice expense RVU
[c]Practice liability insurance RVU

ment for physicians, the American Medical Association (AMA) and several specialty societies agreed to supply expert advice to a Harvard research team to design a relative value scale, attempting to reward work and other inputs of resources and correcting biases from historical charges.

- The RUC is an expert panel of physicians that makes recommendations to the government on the resources required to provide medical services and maintain each service's "relativity" to a family of codes and to the entire RBRVS.
- To date there are over 8000 CPT codes listed in the Current Procedural Terminology (CPT) manual.
- Today, the RUC represents the entire medical profession; however, voting members of the RUC are appointed by their national medical specialty societies and usually represent those recognized by the American Board of Medical Specialties or are those that represent a large percentage of physicians in patient care and those that account for high percentages of Medicare expenditures.
- An expert panel of the providers, which in many cases is composed of multiple specialty representatives, discusses the results of the survey, the new or revised "CPT Code" is then presented to the RUC, and finally the Work Relative Value Unit (wRVU) is determined:
  - *The General Formula*
  - *Total RVU = (work-RVU x work GPCI) + (practice expense RVU x practice expense GPCI) + (malpractice RVU x malpractice GPCI)*
  - *Payment total RVU x Conversion Factor (current value 35.8013)*
- The Conversion Factor (CF) calculation is a scaling factor that converts the geographically adjusted number of RVUs for each service in the Medicare physician fee schedule into a dollar payment amount based on the (1) Medical Economic Index, which measures the weighted average annual price changes in the inputs needed to produce physician services, (2) the Sustainable Growth Rate (SGR), and (3) the updated adjustment factor (UAF) (Table 66.1).
- Since 1992, the RBRVS has been the main payment system for Part B and is the basis for the Medicare Physician Fee Schedule.
- The principle of the Physician Fee Schedule (PFS) is that Medicare will pay a standardized "approved amount" for each service regardless of the physician's fee for the service.
- The CMS Physician Fee Schedule remains the basis for commercial insurance company fee schedules throughout America.
- The work-RVU is the current value method of reimbursement for most "employed" physicians today.

Fee-For-Service: Why Did It Fail?

- The Sustainable Growth Rate (SGR) was a failed mechanism intended to constrain Medicare PFS (Part B) spending by adjusting annual physician fee updates.
- Congress passed the Medicare Access and Children's Health Insurance Program Reauthorization Act, which repealed the SGR payment formula and guaranteed the Medicare PFS a 0.5% increase in reimbursements to physicians through 2019.

The Patient Protection and Affordable Care Act of 2010 (P.L. 111–148)

- As a very brief summary of the ACA 2010, it is an approach to expanding access to health-care coverage, and it:
  - *Requires most US citizens and legal residents to have health insurance*
  - *Creates state-based American Health Benefit Exchanges through which individuals can purchase coverage, with premium and cost-sharing credits available to individuals/families with income between 133 and 400% of the Federal Poverty Level (FPL)*
  - *Creates separate Exchanges through which small businesses can purchase coverage*
  - *Requires employers to pay penalties for employees who receive tax credits for health insurance through an Exchange, with exceptions for small employers*
  - *Imposes new regulations on health plans in the Exchanges and in the individual and small group markets. Expand Medicaid to 133% of the FPL*

ACA: Cost Containment Changes

- Administrative changes to health insurance companies, i.e., commercial payers must enact certain provisions in order to simplify delivery and relieve obstructions to the care to their beneficiaries.
- Sweeping changes within Medicare, which mandate the restructuring of payments to all providers (Tables 66.2 and 66.3).
- Decreases funding to disproportionate share hospitals (DSH/Safety Net Hospitals) (Table 66.4).
- The vast majority of these DHS are major academic teaching centers, and this could negatively affect residency programs throughout the United States.
- The final section of Cost Containment is Waste, Fraud and Abuse—where the overriding principle involves decreasing the cost of fraud by expanding over site, increasing the penalties for submitting false claims, and augmenting funding for anti-fraud activities (Table 66.5).

Improving Quality/Health System Performance

- The ACA of 2010 supports comparative effectiveness research by establishing a non-profit Patient-Centered Outcomes Research Institute (PCORI) to conduct research that compares clinical effectiveness of medical treatments.

Table 66.2 Cost containment: Medicare Advantage (MA) Plans restructure payments

MA	Restructure payments based on % of FFS[a]; those with high % of FFS decrease their payments and increase those with a lower % of FFS	Phase in revised payments over 3 years beginning in 2011 for most areas For some areas phase in over 4 to 6 years beginning in 2011
MA	Bonus for those plans receiving four or more stars based on the current five-star quality rating system for MA as much as a double bonus	Beginning 2012
MA	Modify rebate system based on quality rating	Phased in by 2019
MA	Phase in adjustments to plan payments or coding practices related to health status of enrollees (equaling 5.7%)	Phased in by 2019
MA	Require MA plans to submit to secretary of health partial payments if ML ratio is less than 85%	2014
MA	Require secretary to suspend enrollment to MA plan if ML ratio[b] is less than 85% for 2 consecutive years or terminate plan contract if ML ratio is less than 85% for 5 consecutive years	2014
MA	Cap total payments, including bonuses at current payment levels	2014

[a]Medicare fee-for service
[b]Medical loss ratio

Table 66.3 Cost containment: Medicare

Change	Effective date
Reduce annual market basket updates to inpatient hospital, home health, skilled nursing facility, hospice, and other Medicare providers and adjust for productivity	Effective varying dates
Freeze the threshold for income-related Medicare Part B premiums	For 2011 through 2019
Establish a Payment Advisory Board of 15 members (no physicians) to submit legislative proposals containing recommendations to reduce the per capita rate of growth in Medicare spending if spending exceeds a target growth rate	Beginning in April 2013
Reduce Medicare Disproportionate Share Hospital (DSH)[a] payments initially by 75%, and then subsequently increase payments based on percentage (%) of uninsured population and the amount of uncompensated care	Effective January 1, 2015
Eliminate Medicare Improvement Fund[a]	Effective upon enactment
Allow ACOs that voluntarily meet quality thresholds to share in cost savings they achieve for the Medicare program	January 1, 2012
Create an Innovation center (with in CMS) to test, evaluate, and expand Medicare, Medicaid, and CHIP (different payment structures and methodologies to decrease expenditures and/or improve quality)	January 1, 2011
Reduce payments by specified percentages to account for preventable readmissions	Effective October 1, 2012
Reduce payments to certain hospital-acquired conditions by 1%	Effective fiscal year 2015

[a]DSH that treat indigent patients receive at least partial compensation

Table 66.4 Cost containment: Medicaid

Change	Effective date
Increase Medicaid Rebate for Drugs: Brand Name 23.1%, multiple source drugs 13% on average manufacture average price	Effective on enactment
Reduce aggregate Medicaid DSH Allotments	$0.5 Billion 2014 $0.6 Billion 2015 $0.6 Billion 2016 $1.8 Billion 2017 $5.0 Billion 2018 $5.6 Billion 2019 $4.0 Billion 2012 $17.6 Billion total reductions
Reduce aggregate Medicaid to DSH[a] Allotments by developing a methodology to distribute the DSH reductions in a manner that imposes the largest reduction in DSH allotments for states with the lowest percentage of uninsured or those that do not target DSH payments, imposes smaller reductions for low-DSH states, and accounts DSH allotments for 1115 waivers[b]	Effective October 1, 2015
Prohibit federal payments to states for Medicaid services related to health-care-acquired conditions	Effective July 1, 2011

[a]DSH, disproportionate share hospitals/"safety net hospitals"

[b]1115 Waiver Section 1115 of the Social Security Act that gives the Secretary of Health and Human Services authority to approve experimental, pilot, or demonstration projects that promote objective of the Medicaid and CHIP programs. As long as these programs expand eligibility, provide services not typically covered, or use innovative service delivery systems that improve care, increase efficiency, and reduce costs for Medicaid or CHIP programs

Table 66.5 Cost containment: waste fraud and abuse reduction

Change	Effective date
Provider screening	Dates vary
Enhanced oversight periods for new providers and suppliers' initial claims (including enhanced oversight for 90 days)	Dates vary
Moratorium in areas identified as being at elevated risk of fraud in all public programs	Dates vary
Require Medicare and Medicaid providers and suppliers to establish compliance programs	Dates vary
Develop a database to capture and share data across federal and state programs	Dates vary
Increase penalties for submitting false claims	Dates vary
Increase funding for anti-fraud activities	Dates vary

Table 66.6 Improving quality/health system performance: Medicare

Change	Effective date
Establish a national Medicare pilot program to develop and evaluate paying a "bundled payment" for acute inpatient hospital/outpatient services, physician services, and post-acute care services for an episode of care that begins 3 days prior to hospitalization and spans 30 days following discharge	Establish pilot program by January 1, 2013, and expand program, if appropriate, by January 1, 2016
Create Home demonstration program to provide high-need Medicare beneficiaries with primary care services in their home and allow health professionals to share in any savings if they reduce preventable hospitalizations, prevent hospital readmissions, improve health outcomes, improve the efficiency of care, reduce the cost of health-care services, and achieve patient satisfaction	Effective January 1, 2012
Establish a hospital Value-Based Purchasing Program in Medicare to pay hospitals on performance on quality measures. Also, extend physician quality reporting initiative beyond 2010	Effective October 1, 2012
Develop plans to implement Value-Based Purchasing Programs for skilled nursing facilities, home health agencies, and ambulatory surgical centers	Report to Congress due January 1, 2011

Table 66.7 Improving quality/health system performance: Medicaid

Change	Effective date
Demonstration projects in Medicaid to pay "bundled payments" for episodes of care that include hospitalizations	January 1, 2012, through December 31, 2016
Global capitated payments to safety net hospital systems	Effective fiscal years 2010 through 2012
Organize ACOs[a] for pediatric medical providers, and allow them to share in cost savings	Effective January 1, 2012, through December 31, 2016

[a]Accountable Care Organizations

- The law also mandates that Medical malpractice "reform" is an important issue and awards 5-year "grants" to states in order to develop, implement, and evaluate alternatives to current tort litigations, only if the proposals are likely to enhance patient safety by reducing medical errors and adverse events that are likely to improve access to liability insurance (5-year funding began in the fiscal year 2011).
- The improving quality/health system performance reference to Medicare for Alternative Payment Models to providers is shown in Table 66.6.
- The changes to Medicaid payments are just as onerous and are reviewed in Table 66.7.

National Quality Strategy

- The National Quality Strategy was a mandate to "define quality" and also to incorporate quality measures into physician payments as incentives or penalties (Table 66.8).
- This brief overview suggests that the ACA of 2010 is forcing the initiation of Alternative Payment Models and the formation of health-care networks, which in turn forces physicians into clinically integrated networks.

Table 66.8 Improving quality/health system performance: National Quality Strategy

Change	Effective date
Develop a National Quality Improvement Strategy (NQIS) that includes improving the delivery of health-care services, patient health outcomes, and population health	Due to Congress by January 1, 2011
Create processes for development of quality measures involving input from multiple stakeholders for selecting quality measures to be used in reporting to and payment under federal health programs	Due to Congress by January 1, 2011

Alternative Payment Models

The Patient-Centered Medical Home

- Medical home projects focus on providing comprehensive primary care that is patient-centric through better coordination of the care patients receive from all providers.

Accountable Care Organizations

- The ACOs comprise of groups of physicians, other health-care professionals, and facilities that agree to work together to provide high-quality, coordinated care to their patients at measureable levels of savings.
- This model reimburses physicians on a FFS basis, but in order to control the increase in volume, they pay more to physicians who coordinate care and employ information technologies.

Bundled Payment Pilot Projects

- The BCPI is a payment model that allows participating hospitals to enroll in bundled payment agreements with CMS for up to 48 predefined clinical conditions aggregated from Medicare Severity Diagnosis-Related Groups (MS-DRGs).
- The *hospital* is the focal point of the bundle; the bundle is based on an episode of care and includes physician services, post-acute providers, related readmissions, and any ancillary services provided during this episode of care.
- The providers indicate which conditions they want to bundle and propose a discounted price to CMS.
- The principle of the bundled payment model provides a payment for all of the care a patient needs over the course of a defined clinical episode of care.
- Without a definitive way forward, the CMMI/BCPI initiatives for Medicare beneficiaries developed four models of payment (Table 66.9).

Clinical Integration

- Integration of physicians into health-care networks can have ongoing programs to evaluate and modify individual practice patterns because of the high degree of interdependence and cooperation among the physicians within the networks, which in turn will control costs and ensure quality.
- Clinical integration facilitates the coordination of patient care across the "Continuum of Care" in order to achieve quality care; these integrated networks must include six goals of integration. The integrated system must be:
  - Patient-focused
  - Safe
  - Timely
  - Effective
  - Efficient
  - Equitable
- The *National Strategy for Quality Improvement in Health Care (NQS)* was included in the ACA of 2010, and Table 66.10 describes the basis of what is happening right now with quality measures.

Table 66.9 Center for Medicare and Medicaid Innovation: Bundled Payments for Care Improvement (BPCI) payment models

Model	Description	Phase 1	Phase 2	Payment type
1	Involves hospital payments for inpatient stays for most Medicare FFS discharges	Non-risk bearing	Risk bearing	Retrospective
2	Includes all Medicare part A and B payments for the 48 selected clinical conditions	Non-risk bearing	Risk bearing	Retrospective
3	Includes payments only for post-acute claims for participating skilled nursing facility, inpatient rehabilitation facility, long-term care hospital, home health agency, or physician practices	Non-risk bearing	Risk bearing	Retrospective
4	Initial hospitalization, health-care provider fees during the hospitalization, and payments for readmission	Non-risk bearing	Risk bearing	Prospective "lump sum" payment to the participating hospital, which then pays the physicians and other provider groups

Table 66.10 National Quality Strategy priorities and goals

Priority	Goal	Opportunities	Measures
Safer care	Eliminate preventable health-care-acquired conditions	1. Eliminate hospital-acquired infections 2. Reduce the number of serious adverse medication events	Standardized infection ratio for central line-associated blood stream infection as reported by CDC's National Healthcare Safety Network
Effective care coordination	Create a delivery system that is less fragmented and more coordinated, where handoffs are clear, and patients and clinicians have the information they need to optimize the patient-client stewardship	1. Reduce hospital admission and readmissions 2. Prevent and manage chronic illness and disability 3. Ensure secure information exchange to facilitate efficient care delivery	All-cause readmissions within 30 days of discharge Percentage of providers who provide a summary record of care for transitions and referrals
Person- and family-centered care	Build a system that has the capacity to capture and act on patient-reported information including preference-desired outcomes and experiences with health care	1. Integrate patient feedback on preferences, functional outcomes, and experiences of care into all care settings and care delivery 2. Increase use of EHRs that capture the voice of the patient by integrating patient-generated data in EHRs 3. Routinely measure patient engagement and self-management, shared decision-making, and patient-reported outcomes	Percentage of patients asked for feedback
Prevention and treatment of leading causes of mortality	Prevent and reduce the harm caused by cardiovascular disease	1. Increase blood pressure control in adults 2. Reduce high cholesterol levels in adults 3. Increase the use of aspirin to prevent cardiovascular disease 4. Decrease smoking among adults and adolescents	Percentage of patients 18 years or older with ischemic vascular disease whose most recent blood pressure during the measurement year is <140/90 mm Hg Percentage of patients with ischemic vascular disease whose most recent low-density cholesterol is <100 Percentage of patients with ischemic vascular diseases who have documentation of use of aspirin or other antithrombotic during the 12-month measurement period Percentage of patients who receive evidence-based smoking cessation services (e.g., medications)
Supporting better heath in communities	Support every US community as it pursues its local health priorities	1. Increase the provision of clinical preventive services for children and adults 2. Increase the adoption of evidence-based interventions to improve health	Percentage of children and adults screened for depression and receiving a documented follow-up plan Percentage of adults screened for risky alcohol use and, if positive, received brief counseling Percentage of children and adults who use the oral health-care system each year Proportion of US population served by community water systems with optimally fluoridated water

(continued)

Table 66.10 (continued)

Priority	Goal	Opportunities	Measures
Making care more affordable	Identify and apply measures that can serve as effective indicators of progress in reducing cost	1. Build cost and resource-use measurement into payment reforms 2. Establish common measures to assess the cost impacts of new programs and payment systems 3. Reduced the amount of health-care spending that goes to administrative burden 4. Make costs and quality more transparent to consumers	To be determined

Clinical Integration and the Employed Physician: What About Contracting?

- The RBRVS system is and will be a part of the reimbursement to physicians in these Alternative Payment Models.
- Consult an experienced attorney to assist in the legal interpretation and implications of these complex contracts (Table 66.11).
- Compensation models include a fixed salary, base salary plus incentive bonus, treatment for an episode of care or specific services (FFS), capitation per member per month (patients or population), and performance-based pay with increases based on quality of care metrics.
- The method of payment may also be reduced or withheld if "behavior" does not comply with what is required (e.g., financial penalty).
- Most of employed physician salaries are based on a percentile of these national salaries represented by organizations like the MGMA.

Table 66.11 Critical points to consider during contract negotiations

Employment agreements (nonacademic)
Term of agreement
Duties and services
Performance standards
Location of services
Managed care contracts
Total annual cash compensation
Medical malpractice insurance/tail coverage
Salary caps
Compensation per wRVU (the conversion factor for Medicare is $35.082/RVU)
Signing bonus
Guaranteed base + bonus
Pure production
Covenant noncompete clauses
Share of quality/utilization bonuses
Moving expense reimbursement

Fee-for-Service Model: Based on the Work-RVU

- Some contracts will utilize a "production-only" method based on the wRVU and a conversion factor.
- The long-term outlook is not good, primarily because as the health-care dollar reimbursement shifts to value-based purchasing and value-based modifiers, more and more employers will have to "adjust" physician reimbursement according to these modifiers (Appendices 66.1 to 66.3).

Geisinger Health System Physician Compensation Model

- GHS ties employed physician salaries to the care they deliver and to patient outcomes.
- Most of the reimbursement is under a fee-for-service model; however, 20% of the total physician compensation (TPC) is based on performance incentives that are defined annually for each type of clinician.

Base Salary

- GCP defines the base component (80% delivered in monthly paychecks) of each physician's compensation according to factors that describe his/her expected work effort (Table 66.12).

Table 66.12 Geisinger compensation plan: base salary

Work effort: includes teaching, research, and administrative activities measured in wRVUs[a]
Increase or decrease depending on the physicians working above or below the expected ranges
Depends on the physician's experience/specialty market rates
GHS goal is for physician to exceed the 60 percentile for their specialty area in both FFS work unit production and compensation

[a]Work-RVU metric is based on the relative value based upon time, skill, training, and intensity of the service delivered

Performance Incentives for Specialist Physicians

- Each physician in a GHP service line has incentive goals that are developed by the service line members (Table 66.13).
- In this formula this means extremely high levels of productivity do not necessarily translate directly into higher income.
- Innovation, legacy, and growth account for 35% of the incentive compensation and ~7% of total compensation.

Table 66.13 Geisinger compensation plan: performance incentives for specialists

Variable portion of compensation of 20% of incentive payment
Five general areas:
Quality (40%): Defined for each specialty through discussion with specialty leaders and senior management (average 4–5 measures) Innovation (10%): Development (e.g., Wound Care Center) Legacy (10%): Under Geisinger's educational and research mission Growth (15%): Increase in Geisinger's patient population Financial (25%): Directly reflects wRVU recognized under FFS

Massachusetts General Physicians Organization's Incentive Program

- The MGPO is designed as an internal quality incentive program based on several important features that keep physician acceptance and support (Table 66.14).
- These original approaches evolved into the current model, because the targets were initially set at an aggregate level and differed by major commercial payers within the region. In addition, the model was focused only on primary care (Table 66.14).
- Today, the network has over 1700 clinically active physicians who have qualified for the program (Table 66.15).

Table 66.14 Massachusetts General Physicians Organization incentive program

Quality metrics are developed by the institutional management team and by quality leaders of each specialty
Competency in managing performance date and developing measures
Clear communication accompanied by consistent and accessible reporting
A fair process for adjudication appeals to performance decisions
Leaderships' commitment to setting priorities

Table 66.15 MGPO Quality Incentive Program Metrics

Tier	Physicians (%)	Work-RVU	Time-lag measures[a]	Incentive payment $ (annual basis)
One	73	750 or >	Every 6 months	5000.00
Two	19	250–749	Every 6 months	2500.00
Three	8	50–249	Every 6 months	1000.00

[a]Three quality measures are identified: two measures are chosen by program leaders and apply to all physicians. One measure is specialty specific chosen by each clinical department or division

Appendix 66.1

Physician Compensation Model 1: Guaranteed Salary

One-year contract:	$20,000 signing bonus
Base salary	$280.000/26 payments/40-hour workweek
Additional on call per diem	$500–750/day

Appendix 66.2

Physician Compensation Model 2: Work-RVU-Based Compensation

Utilizing a dollar conversion factor is defined as the numeric factor which physicians multiply wRVUs to calculate physician compensation.

Year 1: $40.00/wRVU
Years 2–5: $47/wRVU
Bi-weekly draws approximately: $7000.00 (year 1)
Reconciliations of draw: quarterly and semiannually "true update"

These updates can mean an augmentation for increased production or a "reduction" at the next update for not covering overhead.

Appendix 66.3

Physician Compensation Model 3: Work-RVU Compensation with a Base Salary (Guaranteed)

Five-Year Contract	$20,000 Signing Bonus (returned if terminate Employment before 24 months)
Base Salary Years 1–2	$300,000 which is approximately 6500 wRVUs at $45/wRVU
Base Salary Years 3–5	$300,000 but is subject to adjustment (calculated for a set time period) in advance of the first day of the next employment year and is based on a wRVU, over a period of time the preceding years.
Incentive Bonus Years 1–3	
Work-RVU	**Incentive Compensation/wRVU**
6501–7500	$51
7501–9000	$53
9001–10,500	$55
10,501 or >	$57
Incentive Bonus Years 4–5	is based on wRVUs generated by Physician in excess of Tier One Baseline, which is multiplied by a "conversion factor" per wRVU which will be adjusted/based on an Independent Variable
Salary Cap	approximately $600,000

Ethical Issues in Colorectal Surgery 67

Jason D. Keune

Key Concepts

- Ethics is a formal way of examining what one should do.
- The four principles approach emerged from a common morality of health care.
- A moral dilemma occurs when the moral intuitions of individuals disagree.
- Informed consent is a process that is rooted in respect for patient autonomy.
- Surrogate decision-making is necessary should a patient become incompetent.
- Futility is a concept that is in evolution and should be based on a local definition.
- Disparities in outcomes from colorectal operations vary based on race.
- Financial conflicts of interest are a contemporary problem that has been addressed at the level of the federal government.

Introduction

- Ethics, at its most fundamental, is a way to answer the question, "what should we do?.
- Ethical dilemmas arise against the relatively stable background of an ethical surgical practice due to:
  - As new developments in technology arrive, there is a push to use them, especially in situations where a group of patients were in a position in which no good option was available until the new technology was invented.
  - We live in an increasingly plural society where the cultural, ethnic, and religious differences between a patient and physician can have a shrinking effect on the common moral ground between the two.
  - With an unstable patient, death may be imminent, and there may not be enough time for an ethics consultant to arrive.
  - Communication can also be problematic when time is short.
  - Surgeons cannot easily "undo" their work.

Ethical Reasoning

- The *four principles* approach puts forth what are known as "mid-level" principles: respect for autonomy, justice, beneficence, and nonmaleficence.
- **Respect for autonomy** states that clinicians ought to allow patients to make decisions about their medical care that is both free of coercion and fully informed.
  - Liberty emphasizes that patients should be given the opportunity to decide whether to undergo surgery and just what surgery that should be.

J. D. Keune (✉)
Department of Surgery, St. Louis University School of Medicine, St. Louis, MO, USA
e-mail: jkeune@slu.edu

S. R. Steele et al. (eds.), *The ASCRS Manual of Colon and Rectal Surgery*,
https://doi.org/10.1007/978-3-030-01165-9_67

   - Agency is the quality of granting the patient the knowledge necessary to make the decision and exercising that liberty.
- "First do no harm" is an aphorism that describes the principle of **nonmaleficence**.
- **Beneficence** implores physicians to do positive acts that benefit others.
   - When an act arises from beneficence, but violates respect for autonomy, it is called *paternalistic*.
   - If an act "goes beyond the call of duty," it is known as *supererogatory*.
- **Justice** is concerned with inequality.

Informed Consent

- Informed consent is a process to describe the procedure in detail (as well as the inherent risks, benefits, and alternatives), initiated by the surgeon, which enables the respect for patient's autonomy to be observed when a procedure is being planned or another decision point is reached.

Threshold Elements (Preconditions)

- Competence (to understand and decide)
- Voluntariness (in deciding)

Transformation Elements

- Disclosure (of material information)
- Recommendation (of a plan)
- Understanding (of 3 and 4)

Consent Elements

- Decision (in favor of a plan)
- Authorization (of the chosen plan)
   - The notion of competence rests on an evaluation about whether the patient has the cognitive abilities to both understand information about the procedure and to consider the consequences of the choice to undergo the procedure.
   - Voluntariness is the threshold element that is concerned with freedom from coercion, as patients should be able to make decisions about their care that is free from outside coercive influence.

Surrogate Decision-Making

- When a patient, previously competent about his or her own care, becomes incompetent, someone other than the patient must now be sought to make decisions for the patient.
- Two main questions should be asked:
   1. Who should make decisions for the patient?
   2. How should the surrogate decision-maker best decide?
- Advanced directives are instructions that are provided by patients that give direction to caretakers about how decisions should be made if the patient were to become incompetent.
- A living will is a document prepared by a patient while competent that details the patient's preferences should they become incapacitated.
- The durable power of attorney is a person who is appointed in advance by the patient to act as a surrogate decision-maker.
- With no durable power of attorney, there is typically a hierarchical list: spouse, adult children, siblings, and down the line.

Futility

- The problem of futility arises when the proposed treatment has such a small chance of being efficacious that the surgeon probably ought not perform it.
- The range of what is considered "futile" care tends to focus on lack of efficaciousness, lack of therapeutic "success," or care that is burdensome enough to outweigh any therapeutic benefit of the intervention.

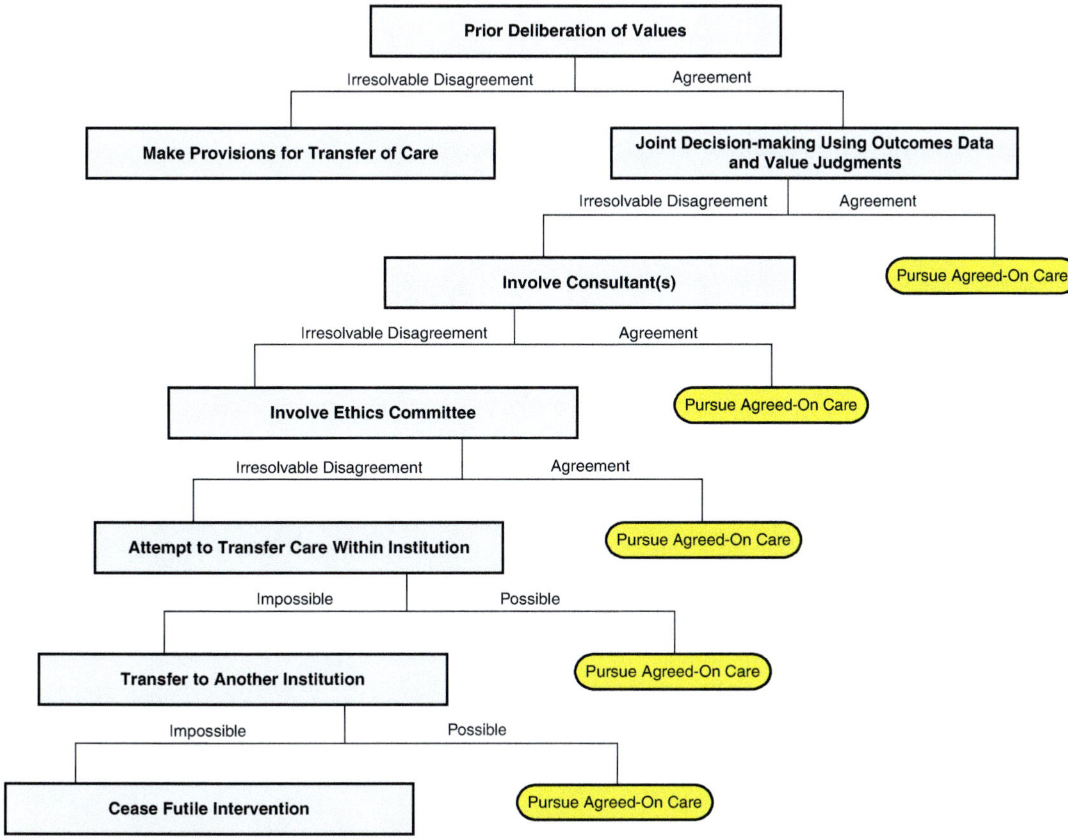

Fig. 67.1 Fair process for considering futility cases. Modified from Plows CW et al. Medical futility in end-of-life care – report of the Council on Ethical and Judicial Affairs. JAMA. 1999; 281:937–941

- Futility was defined in terms of specific *clinical* criteria, either by comparing one group to like patients in whom similar treatments have been useless or with the use of physiological goals.
- The American Medical Association Council on Ethical and Judicial Affairs recommended that a process-based approach to futility determinations should be taken (Fig. 67.1).

Refusal of Care

- With sound mind and proper understanding, refusal of care is a patient's right.
- The strict observation of patient autonomy breaks down, though, when patients consent to a recommended procedure but refuse to have certain elements of the care necessary to perform such procedures.
- Unless the decision is made in an emergency setting, parental consent is needed to perform a procedure on a child.

Outcome Disparities in Colorectal Surgery

- Justice can be thought of at its most fundamental roots as the ability "to be fair."
- In many cases, no matter the question, distinct differences are detected along racial and socioeconomic lines.
- The problem of disparities in surgical outcomes seems to be related to the problem of racial diversity in the surgical workforce.

Physician Financial Conflicts of Interest

- A conflict of interest exists in a state in which there is a dynamic interaction between two differing interests in the same person, such that one interest directly or indirectly impacts his ability to realize and possibly execute a pure motive in the other.
- The conflict of interest problem in the surgical profession comes about especially when one of the two interests is financial and the other is the well-being of the patient.
- The Affordable Care Act, which became law in 2010, includes a section called the "Physician Payment Sunshine Provision," which requires drug, biologics, and medical device companies to report all payments and transfers of value to physicians and teaching hospitals in excess of $10 per instance to the federal government, and is publically disclosed.
- Working with industry also does not equate to an inability to make sound and non-bias judgments regarding patient care.

Conclusion

- For those that have the power to make such significant change in the world, a study of what is right to do seems like a given.
- Ethics should be a part of every surgeon's training, and ethical reasoning should be in every surgeon's toolkit, especially since surgeons are "doers."

Welcome to Litigation

68

Dennis K. Ames

Key Concepts

- In litigation, preparation is the key to a successful outcome.
- Preparation should begin as soon as you become aware of an adverse outcome likely to lead to litigation.
- Don't conduct an independent investigation.
- Never appear at a deposition without consulting an attorney.
- Meet with your attorney early.
- Communicate with your attorney regularly.
- Know what you can expect of your attorney and when.
- Know what is expected of you and when.
- Do your homework; and make yourself available.
- Today's physicians will almost certainly be sued for medical malpractice in his or her career, as general surgeons have a 15.3% annual probability of facing a medical malpractice claim.
- The probability of any such claim leading to an indemnity payment is substantially lower.

Portions of this chapter include material from Judicial Council of California Civil Jury Instructions (CACI), Nos. 200, 208, 219, 221, 501, 505, and 506. Permission to reprint CACI instructions in this publication has been expressly granted by the Judicial Council of California.

D. K. Ames (✉)
La Follette, Johnson, Dehaas, Fesler & Ames,
Santa Ana, CA, USA
e-mail: Dames@ljdfa.com

Preparation: The Key to Success

- If a claim arises from the occurrence of a true surgical misadventure, it may be prudent to posture the matter toward settlement from the outset.
- Preparation should include an early consultation with counsel to discuss the ramifications to you personally and professionally of an early settlement versus proceeding to protracted litigation.
- The reality of litigation is that the "facts" of a case are what the jury says the facts are on its verdict form.
- Effective litigation requires effective accumulation of evidence and effective presentation of that evidence as a result of thorough and focused preparation.

Stages of the Litigation Process

The litigation process can be divided into three stages:

I. Initiation of the litigation process
   A. Notice of an occurrence likely to lead to litigation
   B. Notice of events which suggests that litigation is imminent: Handling requests for medical records
   C. Service of the summons and complaint: Initial meeting with counsel

S. R. Steele et al. (eds.), *The ASCRS Manual of Colon and Rectal Surgery*,
https://doi.org/10.1007/978-3-030-01165-9_68

II. The discovery process
  A. Written discovery
  B. Your deposition
III. Trial

Initiation of the Litigation Process

Notice of an Occurrence Likely to Lead to Litigation

- The litigation process may commence in a number of ways.
  - Unexpected occurrence of something adverse to your patient.
    - The litigation process may be said to be initiated by you, in anticipation of litigation.
    - There are pre-existing protocols and procedures in place (1) to accumulate and preserve the necessary evidence about the event in a timely manner and, (2) as appropriate, to protect the evidence from undue disclosure to the opposition by veiling it within the cloak of one or more legal privileges.
- Typically, with pre-existing procedures for reporting such events for quality assurance purposes, any statement or disclosure made in furtherance of that purpose of quality assurance is privileged from disclosure as a matter of public policy.
- Statements made to a risk management department or to an insurance company representative in anticipation of litigation are typically protected from disclosure by the attorney work-product privilege.

Teaching Points

- The purpose of these pre-litigation procedures is to accumulate reliable evidence that, if litigation does ensue, can then be produced to the assigned counsel to promote the physician's defense.
- This request for a summary of the occurrence will be better served if the summary is prepared soon after the event.
- To avoid question as to why you are preparing a summary of the events outside the medical chart, begin the summary with "The following summary is being prepared in anticipation of litigation, to be provided to my attorney when litigation commences."

Notice of Events Which Suggest that Litigation Is Imminent: Handling Requests for Medical Records

- You may be placed on notice of ensuing litigation for the first time by the patient or her attorney requesting a copy of her medical records from you or by the patient asking that a copy of her records be sent to an attorney.
- The response to the request should include everything that is being requested; to include if requested, this must include the entire record.
- Have a formal, written procedure in place which defines the scope of your medical record for purposes of responding consistently to medical records requests on a day-to-day basis.

Service of the Summons and Complaint: Initial Meeting with Counsel

- The formal civil litigation process starts when the patient files a complaint, has a summons issued, and personally serves the summons and complaint on the physician, giving the physician notice that he has been sued.
- The statement outlining the breach of that duty must, however, provide the defendant with notice of the classification of wrongdoing, which the plaintiff is alleging (i.e., *cause of action.*)
- The allegations of injury generally include general damages or noneconomic damages for physical or emotional injuries (e.g., pain and suffering) and special damages or economic damages for calculable injuries for past and future medical expenses and/or for past and

future loss of earnings, earnings capacity, or financial support.

- A summons is the right of the court to "summon" citizens to answer charges brought against them.
- The complaint will identify each of the defendants who are being sued, but it is the summons which identifies who, among the defendants, is being served and, therefore, who is obliged to respond.
- Before responding to the complaint, the defense attorney must analyze the complaint and the relevant facts and law to determine, among other things.
- Who has been sued?
- Have the defendants been properly identified?
- Was the complaint timely filed, or is it potentially barred by the statute of limitations?
- Has the complaint been timely and properly served, and upon whom?
- Are the causes of action adequately pleaded?
- Does the complaint raise extraordinary causes of action, which require special handling or counseling?

Teaching Points

- You and your office need established procedures to handle legal documents and filings.
  - When a summons and complaint are received, keep the envelope in which it was served.
- Make a notation of when specifically (date and time) it was received and how it was received (by mail or in person).
- Look on the summons to determine who has been served (the doctor, the doctor's corporation, or the practice).
- Notify your insurance company or attorney immediately, and provide a copy of the summons and of the complaint to them.
- Review the complaint to determine whether any extraordinary causes of action (anything besides medical negligence or wrongful death) are listed on the first page of the complaint.
- Look at the last paragraph of the complaint, the prayer, to determine which categories of damages are being requested.
- Confirm with the attorney that an appropriate and timely response has been or will be made on your behalf.
- Confirm that an appointment with the attorney is made, and ask what you need to have available at that first meeting.
- Create a file separate and apart from your medical chart, and keep a copy of the complaint and any other legal correspondence in that separate file.
- Do not speak with anyone (including your partners or office staff) or do any independent research relating to the case, until you have received direction from your attorney.
- Do not alter or supplement your records in any way.
- Judges don't determine what the facts are, juries do.
- Judges decide what the law is and apply the law to the facts as determined by the jury, as such the judge may not adjudicate any factual dispute.

Teaching Points

- Speak with your attorney early, and ask what you need to do "now."
- Learn how long the process is expected to take, and give your attorney your contact information.
- Ask when it will it be necessary for you to be personally involved.
- Be patient! This will take time.

The Discovery of the Process

Written Discovery

- The discovery process is a formalized accumulation and exchange of information which ultimately will be used at trial to educate the jurors about the relevant facts of the case.

- The law allows a party to subpoena or formally request relevant documents, such as medical records or employment records, and to interview opposing parties or witnesses under oath by way of deposition.
- A verification is a signature by the responding party, made under oath or penalty of perjury, which, depending on local rules, may or may not need to be notarized.
- One important purpose of interrogatories is for the propounding party to inquire about additional potential sources of information (e.g., potential witnesses or other sources of documents and records.)
- Expect that you will be asked to answer interrogatories.
- You don't need to wait until you are served with interrogatories, and the time period for responses starts to run, before you begin compiling the necessary information.
- Obtain assurance from your attorney that you will be notified as soon as interrogatories are served and that the notification will include the date by when your preliminary responses will be expected.
- You can expect that at deposition or trial your responses to the interrogatories will be presented to you.

Your Deposition

- Giving an effective deposition requires effective preparation, and you have the right to expect that your attorney will aid you in that preparation.
- A deposition is a recorded question and answer session during which the attorneys for all parties to the litigation, including the opposing party and all co-defendants, have the right to ask you questions.
- A deposition is a "legal," "formal" interview.
- At the conclusion of the deposition, a transcript of the deposition will be prepared by the court reporter, and you will have the opportunity to review the transcript and to make any changes to your answers which you believe are necessary to accurately reflect your testimony.
- The primary liability issue in a medical malpractice trial is whether the physician's care was negligent, i.e., was it below the applicable standard of care?
- The standard of care requires the surgeon to act as other duly competent and careful surgeons would act *under the same or similar circumstances*.
- Ask your attorney to provide you with copies of the relevant records prior to the deposition so that you have the time and opportunity to refresh your recollection.
- The questions asked at deposition must be fair – relatively intelligible and unambiguous; therefore, ask the questioner to rephrase a question if you don't understand it.
- Wait until the questioner has completed his question, think before answering, respond to the question directly, and succinctly; and answer the question which is asked.

Teaching Points

- Always consult with counsel before a deposition, and be represented by an attorney at a deposition, whether you are or you are not a party to the litigation.
- Consult with your attorney sufficiently in advance of your deposition so that if additional record review or preparation is necessary, you have the opportunity to do it.
- Know what your attorney wants you to review prior to the deposition and what she doesn't want you to review or access.
- In every case you should be familiar with the details of your own care, including the substance of all records, consults, or notes which you had available to you at the time of your management of the patient, so that you can reiterate at deposition the basis of your management decisions.
- Understand the difference between giving testimony based upon your memory being refreshed by review of documents and giving testimony based strictly on your acceptance of what the document states. Are you testifying, or is the document testifying?

- Understand in advance whether your attorney intends on your giving expert testimony based on a retrospective analysis or whether you are giving testimony only as a percipient witness, in which case you will testify only regarding thoughts, conclusions, and opinions you actually came to while treating the patient.
- Understand the difference between an estimate and a guess.
- Don't give answers relating to conduct of others which you did not witness or the rationale for the conduct of another, unless that person told you why he did what he did. Knowing *why someone mig*ht do something is not the same *as knowing why this person did* what they did on this occasion.
- Have available at your deposition a list of the documents you reviewed in preparation for the deposition or to refresh your memory, and provide that list to your attorney in advance of the deposition.
- Understand the question before you answer it. If a word used in the question is inherently ambiguous, define the word in your answer to clarify your response.
- Know if your deposition is going to be videotaped, and discuss your attire, accordingly.
- Be prepared to give your best and most complete answers at the deposition so as to avoid the need to make substantive corrections when reviewing the transcript.
- List proposed changes to your deposition on a separate piece of paper, and discuss the proposed changes with your attorney before correcting the original transcript.

The Trial

- It is very important that you be present at trial.
- Answer the question which is asked, and do not insist on attempting to expand or explain your answers, except, as in deposition, by asking, "May I explain?".
- It is the jury's duty to determine the facts of the case, while the judge determines the law of the case.
- The basic standard may be expressed as follows: A surgeon is negligent if he or she fails to use the level of skill, knowledge, and care in diagnosis and treatment that other reasonably careful surgeons would use in similar circumstances.

Teaching Points

- At trial, you are your attorney's best technical asset.
- In preparation for trial, obtain copies of all relevant records and depositions, especially your deposition and all expert depositions.
- Analyze the data with a focus on knowing the circumstances as they existed when you treated the patient; point out where the plaintiff's expert is wrong in his assumption of the facts, and be prepared to support the factual basis of your expert's opinion.
- Know the basic legal standards that will be applied to define "medical negligence," so that you can tailor your testimony to meet that standard.
- Understand the significance of "alternative methods" of treatment.
- Alert your attorney to any schedule conflicts as soon as possible.
- Consult your attorney regarding when exactly the trial is set to begin and when your personal presence is necessary.
- Be present at trial, including jury selection.
- Be cognizant of the opening statements of both sides; it will provide you with valuable insights relating to the proposed testimony.
- Do not react to testimony with gestures or speech. Don't be disruptive of the proceedings or of your attorney's efforts.
- When testifying, direct your responses to the questioner, not to the jury, the judge, or your own counsel.
- Do not expand your answers beyond the question asked, unless you have asked to do so, e.g., "May I explain?".
- Recognize that preparation at each stage requires knowledge of the process and the respective roles of attorney and client; and that preparation is the key to achieving your personal *best result*.

Surgical Education

69

Bradley J. Champagne and Helen M. MacRae

Key Concepts

- The dramatic changes in healthcare and surgical training have forced educators to adopt a new approach with an emphasis on outcomes and competence.
- A major impediment to surgical education is the lack of hospital or administrative support. The fiscal solvency of most academic institutions is more dependent on a high-volume, cost-effective, and efficient department of surgery than ever before.
- Work hour restrictions are another major impediment to training. Residents must now make the most of all learning opportunities, as learners no longer have the "luxury" of unlimited clinical immersion.
- Simulation and surgical skills laboratories will, over time, have an increasing role in training for general technical skills, such as knot tying and procedure-specific skills. The successful application for procedure-specific training with virtual reality systems has recently been demonstrated in several trials.
- Competency-based medical education (CBME) is "an approach to preparing physicians for practice that is fundamentally oriented to graduated outcome abilities and organized around competencies derived from an analysis of societal and patient needs."
- To meet ACGME requirements, multiple assessments will be required to ensure milestone progression along all of the competencies. Assessments that are commonly used include the in-training evaluation report (ITER), 360-degree evaluations (including patient surveys), chart-stimulated recall, oral examinations, multiple-choice examinations, portfolios, and simulations and models.
- Postgraduate medical education now demands an increase in support at a time of waning resource allocation and protected time. In this climate, education often takes a backseat.

Introduction

- One of the developments in medical education over the past decade which will have the largest impact on graduate education has been a shift in the focus from the processes of education to the outcomes of education or development of competencies and attainment of milestones.

B. J. Champagne (✉)
Fairview Medical Center, Cleveland, OH, USA

Department of Colorectal Surgery, Cleveland Clinic, Cleveland, OH, USA
e-mail: Brad.champagne@uhhospitals.org

H. M. MacRae
Department of Surgery, Mount Sinai Hospital, Toronto, ON, Canada

S. R. Steele et al. (eds.), *The ASCRS Manual of Colon and Rectal Surgery*,
https://doi.org/10.1007/978-3-030-01165-9_69

- Simulation-based training has also been used to help accelerate learners' growth in knowledge, skills, and attitudes, prior to entering the clinical arena, and the literature evaluating the use of simulation-based learning will be examined.

Challenges to Surgical Education

- Work hour restrictions require that residents must make the most of all learning opportunities, as learners no longer have the "luxury" of unlimited clinical immersion.
- With fewer duty hours, some learning has moved away from the clinical environment to simulated environments to ensure learning objectives are met and so that residents can make the most of learning opportunities presented to them in the limited hours available.
- Salary-based systems with an incentive-driven compensation plan for increased volumes affect staff time for education and may further impact resident training.
- Remembering that the deficiencies in reimbursement, time commitment, and resource allocation lie more with the system than with the residents can help faculty to deal with some of the frustrations inherent in teaching.

Competency-Based Medical Education (CBME)

- A major focus of new models in postgraduate medical education is a focus on demonstration of attainment of competency, with a shift away from time- and objective-based training to a competency-based framework.
- Programs will have to demonstrate that their trainees have acquired the knowledge, skills, and attitudes of the competencies required for safe and effective practice.
- Competency-based medical education (CBME) is "an approach to preparing physicians for practice that is fundamentally oriented to graduate outcome abilities and organized around competencies derived from an analysis of societal and patient needs. It de-emphasizes time-based training and promises greater accountability, flexibility and learner-centeredness."
  - Ideally, learners will demonstrate progressive attainment of competencies as they move from novice to expert, assembling competencies like building blocks as they develop knowledge, skills, and attitudes.
- A milestone is a defined, observable marker of an individual's ability along a developmental continuum.
- An entrustable professional activity (EPA) is an essential task of a "discipline" that an individual can be trusted to perform independently in a given context.
- EPAs are the tasks or activities that must be accomplished (e.g., manage a patient with rectal cancer), whereas milestones are the abilities of the individual on a continuum (e.g., able to "assess imaging information and justify a TNM-based treatment strategy").

Strategies Outside of the Operating Room

- Nonclinical, or ex vivo, methods of training aim to improve clinical performance by providing practice opportunity in a safe environment.
- Simulation and surgical skills laboratories will, over time, have an increasing role in training for general technical skills, such as knot tying and procedure-specific skills. (Fig. 69.1).
- Dedicated practice with VR simulators has correlated with improved operative times and efficiency of movement for clinical laparoscopic cholecystectomy.
- Using an entire curriculum that addressed multiple aspects of performance, which included procedure-specific simulation, overall laparoscopic colectomy skills have also been shown to enhance.

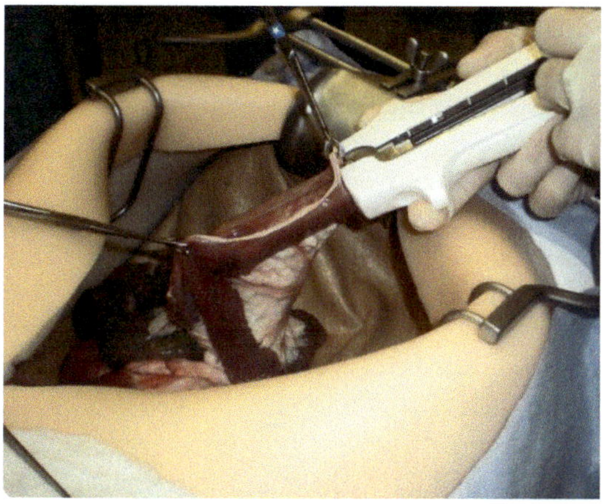

Fig. 69.1 Pelvic Pouch Skills Lab Station at the Institute for Surgery and Innovation at Case Medical Center, Cleveland, OH

Understanding Competency-Based Medical Education (CBME)

- In a pure CBME model, demonstration of defined competence in a time-free model would be used.
- A hybrid model, in which learners move through rotations and other structured learning approaches (such as simulation-based learning), only graduates once milestones are met.
- Summative assessments are used to ensure competencies are attained and residents are progressing satisfactorily with milestone achievement.
- Teachers ensure learners have the necessary learning opportunities and use real-time direct observation to evaluate achievement. (Table 69.1).
- In a time-free model, progression of competence, rather than rotations, is the main organizing structure, with rotations seen as one of many resources to aid learning.
- Milestones are the learning goals, and the role of timed rotations is irrelevant.
- Assessment is focused on documentation of milestone achievement, with summative assessment used to ensure attainment of competencies.

Table 69.1 Comparison of competency-based education and traditional curricular models

Variable	Traditional model	Competency based
Goal of educational encounter	Acquisition of knowledge	Application of knowledge
Responsible for driving process	Teacher	Learner
Assessment	Emphasis on summative	Emphasis on formative with ongoing feedback
Assessment tools	Indirect, proxy assessment	Direct assessment, observation of real tasks of profession
Evaluation standards	Norm referenced (in relation to peers)	Criterion referenced (in relation to objective measures)
Rotations and program completion	Fixed time	Variable time based on demonstration of competence

Adapted from Carraccio C, et al.. Shifting paradigms: from Flexner to competencies. Acad Med. 2002;77;361–7. (24)

- Learners must take ownership of their learning, plotting a course for progression of competence through a variety of learning activities.
- The challenge for programs is to ensure they are documenting enough evaluative feedback to ensure milestone assessment is reliable and valid.

Assessment of Performance

- Assessment of performance during postgraduate training can be either formative (meant to give feedback or direction to learners) or summative (high stakes, end-of-training, such as certification decisions).
- Within a CBME framework, assessment of learning becomes vital to the entire process, and the assessment framework must be robust enough to ensure that developmental milestones are accurately assessed.

Table 69.2 Evaluating outcomes in the core competencies

Core competency	Competency based
Patient care	Direct observation forms, oral examination, chart-stimulated recall, ITERs, 360-degree evaluation, procedure/case logs with reflection, PBAs, OSATS global ratings, portfolios (OSCEs)
Medical knowledge	MCQs, oral examinations, written examinations, chart-stimulated recall, direct observations, portfolios
Practice-based learning and improvement	Portfolios, QI project, 360-degree ratings, MCQs, oral examinations, direct observations
Interpersonal and communication skills	360-degree, patient surveys, direct observations, ITERs
Professionalism	360-degree rating, patient surveys, oral examination, direct observation, ITERs
Systems-based practice	360-degree evaluation, direct observations at care transitions, patient surveys, portfolios

ITER in-training evaluation report, *OSCE* Objective Standardized Certification Examination, *MCQ* multiple-choice question, *PBA* performance-based assessment

- Formative assessment is done frequently, to enhance reliability and validity, and is based around real clinical work.
- Table 69.2 outlines commonly used tools and what competencies are best evaluated through their use.

In-Training Evaluation Report (ITER)

- Assessment during postgraduate training has traditionally relied on the ITER.
- The ITER has the positive attributes of theoretically being comprehensive, being able to assess across all of the competencies, and being relatively easy to use, even in small programs, such as colorectal surgery.
- Qualitative and narrative components on an ITER, if based on specific traits with formative feedback, rather than generalities, can be very useful and have been shown to be a predictor of overall and long-term competence.
- Unfortunately, the educational impact on the learner is poor, especially if ITERs are completed long after the fact, without the opportunity for learners to discuss and reflect on areas needing improvement.
- ITER report quality can be improved with structured feedback to faculty on their ITER completion.

Mini-CEX

- In the mini-CEX, the trainee is responsible for selecting a clinical encounter, where they will ask an assessor to observe them in the real patient setting.
- The assessor collects information on the encounter on a structured evaluation form, with immediate feedback to the resident on their performance.
- Trainees are responsible for selecting from a range of problem groups and assessors, so over time, they have a collection of assessments in their learning portfolio, leading to more stable (reliable) ratings.

360-Degree Evaluation

- The 360-degree evaluation is a measurement tool completed by multiple people, with different perspectives, who each interact with the resident.
- Generally, these are best used for evaluation of competencies such as interpersonal and communication skills, as well as professionalism.
- Usually, 10–20 completed forms are needed for reliable data.

Oral Examinations

- The oral examination has traditionally been used to assess clinical judgment, though medical knowledge, patient care, interpersonal and communication skills, and to an extent, professionalism can also be assessed on an oral examination if it is well structured.

- A structured oral examination is likely best to ensure reasonable reliability for formative or summative assessment.
- A structured oral has reasonable reliability and validity, is educational and acceptable to learners and other stakeholders, and is cost-effective.

Portfolios

- In a learning portfolio, the learner is responsible for developing the portfolio and providing evidence of learning and achievement related to the competencies that have been mastered.
- A learning portfolio might include items such as self-evaluations, articles related to specific outcomes, presentations they have made around a topic, and results of both formative and summative assessments such as the mini-CEX, CARSITE examination, or oral examinations, all helping to support promotion decisions.

Technical Skills Assessment

Logbooks and Case Numbers

- Logbook numbers can be seen as a surrogate for technical skill assessment.
- Case numbers, other than identifying deficiencies, do not give meaningful feedback to residents on where they need to improve.

Procedure-Based Assessment

- Procedure-based assessments (PBAs) are completed via direct observations of entire operations.
- The assessment covers consent, the preoperative planning, preoperative preparation, exposure/closure, intraoperative technique, and postoperative management.
- As the PBA captures performance in a "real-life" environment, it is an ideal form of evaluation to demonstrate milestone achievement; however, the feasibility of its use as a high-stakes assessment is questionable, as residents cannot be left to "fail" the examination.

Simulation/Virtual Reality in Technical Skills Assessment

- Simulation of technical procedures can include non-live animal models, synthetic tissue, computer-based models, cadaveric tissue, live animal, and hybrid platforms.
- VR simulation has been shown to lead to improvements in operative time and "performance," but the impact on patient outcome is unclear.

GAS and L-CAT of the National Training Programme in England

- The National Training Programme (NTP) for Laparoscopic Colorectal Surgery in England used the global assessment scale (GAS) for feedback as part of the training program.
- Once a trainee within the program was deemed proficient, DVD recordings of two independently performed cases were submitted and reviewed by two blinded accredited assessors, using the laparoscopic competency assessment tool (L-CAT).
- The L-CAT is comprised of a 16-item marking sheet (4 task components for each of the 4 domains), incorporating 22 items identified.

Colorectal Objective Structured Assessment of Technical Skills (COSATS)

- The colorectal objective structured assessment of technical skills (COSATS) exam is an assessment tool developed for summative assessment of colorectal technical skills and is a derivation of the objective structured assessment of technical skill (OSATS) examination.

- In the COSATS, the candidate performs tasks specific to colorectal surgery, using a combination of virtual reality and bench models to simulate the selected skills, with performance assessed at each station using a task-specific checklist and a global rating scale, and pass-fail decisions are made based on the performance across eight stations

Global Rating Forms

Several validated global rating forms are available to provide direct feedback to the candidate regarding overall concepts to specific skills within an operation.

How Can CBME Be Applied to Colorectal Residency Training?

- Colorectal milestones have been developed by the American Board of Colorectal Surgery and the ACGME.
- Deficits in technical or other skill sets need to be diagnosed as soon as possible within the training program to ensure adequate progression along the milestones occur.
- Overall, a move to a competency-based curriculum requires assessment to demonstrate that the resident is mastering the component pieces of care (e.g., rectal cancer patient care) and ensuring they move along the milestone progression expected of them.
- As the milestone committee meets, the evidence of competence assessment would be reviewed, and the milestone achievement marked for the resident.
- If there are competencies that are following below expected, targeted learning interventions toward these areas would be implemented.

Conclusions

- Competency-based medical education has arrived and will be an integral part of surgical training.
- We must take responsibility to make trainees understand the importance of both maximizing their learning experience for each case and becoming immersed in the learning environment outside of the operating room.

70 Maintenance of Certification: Current Status and Future Considerations

Jan Rakinic and W. Donald Buie

Key Concepts

- Approximately 6–12% of physicians "fail to meet professional standards of practice" as defined by deficits in knowledge, disruptive behavior, systems problems impeding physicians' care of patients, increasing physician age, problems unrelated to medical care (i.e., licensure issues or allegations of insurance fraud), physical illness, psychiatric illness, and substance abuse.
- The American Board of Colon and Rectal Surgery (ABCRS) ended time-unlimited certificates in 1989 and began issuing certificates that required diplomates in colon and rectal surgery to pass a secure "recertification" examination every 10 years intended to demonstrate continued mastery of content sufficient for specialty practice.
- Parts I (maintenance of unrestricted license and good professional standing), II (lifelong learning and self-assessment), and IV (practice performance assessment and improvement) of the Maintenance of Certification (MOC) were designed to run concurrently in repeating 3-year cycles, with successful performance on the Part III secure specialty examination required at or about every 10 years to maintain specialty certification.
- Part II and Part IV of MOC continue to evolve, with Part II requiring a defined number of CME credits that incorporate a self-assessment activity, which physicians have to pass with a 75% correct grade.
- ABCRS' Part II of MOC self-assessment requirement may be satisfied with, among other activities, completion of the colon and rectal self-assessment program (CARSEP) every 3 years or completion of the surgical education and self-assessment program (SESAP), a product of the American Board of Surgery (ABS).
- Part III of MOC consists of the secure high-stakes examination designed to assess broad knowledge of the specialty (previously the "recertification" exam).
- ABMS and member boards continue to receive criticism regarding the financial and time burden of MOC requirements, redundancy with other professional and regulatory requirements, and most especially lack of relevance to physicians' practices and an absence of proof that MOC produces improved patient outcomes.

Rules are not necessarily sacred; principles are. (Franklin Delano Roosevelt)

J. Rakinic
Section of Colorectal Surgery, Department of Surgery, Southern Illinois University, Springfield, IL, USA

W. D. Buie (✉)
Department of Surgery, Foothills Medical Centre, University of Calgary, Calgary, AB, Canada
e-mail: wdbuie@ucalgary.ca

S. R. Steele et al. (eds.), *The ASCRS Manual of Colon and Rectal Surgery*,
https://doi.org/10.1007/978-3-030-01165-9_70

Table 70.1 ABMS MOC program

The ABMS Program for Maintenance of Certification has four separate parts.
Part 1: Licensure and Professional Standing. Diplomates are required to hold a valid unrestricted medical license in at least one state or jurisdiction in the United States, its territories, or Canada.
Part 2: Lifelong Learning and Self-Assessment. Physicians participate in educational programs that meet specialty-specific standards set by their certifying board and that include a self-assessment component.
Part 3: Cognitive Expertise. Physicians must pass a high-stakes exam to show they possess fundamental practice-related knowledge to provide quality care in their specialty.
Part 4: Practice Performance Assessment and Improvement. Physicians compare their outcomes with peers and national benchmarks.

ABMS American Board of Medical Specialties

Introduction: How We Came to Be Here

- In 2000, ABMS adopted Maintenance of Certification (MOC) as a policy with general standards for its member Boards (Table 70.1).
- Parts I, II, and IV were designed to run concurrently in repeating 3-year cycles, with successful performance on the Part III secure specialty examination required at or about every 10 years to maintain specialty certification.
- It was made clear that ABMS expected Part II of MOC to include a defined number of CME credits that incorporated a self-assessment activity, which the physician had to pass with a 75% correct grade.

The Reasoning and Evidence for Institution of the ABMS MOC Program

- Support of the need for the MOC program estimates that 6–12% of physicians "fail to meet professional standards of practice" including deficits in knowledge, disruptive behavior, system problems, increasing physician age, licensure issues or allegations of insurance fraud, physical illness, psychiatric illness, and substance abuse.
- Five themes including communication, economics, ethics/behavior, knowledge and skills, and competency and assessment had underlying causes such as increasing complexity of healthcare systems, decreasing insurance reimbursement, inadequate staffing, physicians practicing in isolation, problems with documentation and record-keeping skills, failure of teaching team approaches to medical care, and the general punitive approach to physician performance problems.
- Physicians are not very good at assessing their own areas of relative strengths and weaknesses, supporting the concept of activities with scored assessment that can then be used to guide further learning activities.

Is the MOC Program Performing as It Should?

- Part I, maintenance of unrestricted license and good professional standing, involves each physician periodically submitting proof of valid unrestricted licensure and details of medical and specialty training, including board certification in most cases, to secure privileges to practice within most hospitals, healthcare systems, and third-party payer systems.
  - The ABMS MOC program does not contain any provision for how such licensure and professional standing instances might be managed within the program.
  - Part II contains a newly mandated requirement that within each 3-year cycle, a specified number of continuing medical education (CME) credits must include a self-assessment (test) component, with a score 75% or higher required to claim the CME credits.
    - The recognition that many issues with respect to professional standards can be

Table 70.2 The six core competencies defined by ACGME

1. Medical knowledge
2. Patient care
3. Professionalism
4. Interpersonal communication
5. Practice-based learning and improvement
6. System-based practice

ACGME Accreditation Council for Graduate Medical Education

related to one or several of the six competencies (Table 70.2) led ABMS first to encourage, then to require, that Part II activities have a clear definition of the competency or competencies each activity is meant to assess.
    - ABCRS' self-assessment requirement may be satisfied with, among other activities, completion of the colon and rectal self-assessment program (CARSEP) or the American Board of Surgery (ABS) surgical education and self-assessment program (SESAP) every 3 years.
- Part III, the secure high-stakes examination designed to assess broad knowledge of the specialty (previously the "recertification" exam), has remained largely unchanged.
- Part IV, Practice Performance Assessment and Improvement, has been the most difficult part of MOC to address in a way both meaningful to diplomates and also not make overly burdensome.
    - Fulfillment of Part IV was initially attainable without undue burden for most ABCRS diplomates, since participation in NSQIP, SCIP, and a number of other regional and national databases and registries widely available in medical centers was considered acceptable (Table 70.3).
    - ABMS has set up a Multi-Specialty Portfolio Approval Program, dealing with quality projects that may be eligible for Part IV credit.

Table 70.3 Registry participation accepted by ABCRS for Part IV MOC credit

ACS Surgeon Specific Case Log System (with tracking of 30 day complications) https://www.facs.org/quality-programs/ssr
Cancer Quality Improvement Program (CQIP)
Florida Surgical Care Initiative
Hospital Consumer Assessment of Healthcare Providers and Systems (HCAHPS)
Mayo Clinic
Michigan Surgical Quality Collaborative (MSQC)
National Cancer Database (NCDB)
National Surgical Quality Improvement Program ACS (NSCIP)
Ongoing Professional Practice Evaluation (OPPE)
Piedmont Society Program
Press Ganey
Surgical Care and Outcomes Assessment Program (SCOAP) (Washington State)
Surgical Care Improvement Project (SCIP)
University Health System Consortium (UHC)
VHA Surgical Quality Improvement Program (VASQIP)

ABCRS American Board of Colon and Rectal Surgeons; *MOC* Maintenance of Certification

Challenges Presented to Diplomates

- ABMS and member Boards continue to receive criticism regarding the financial and time burden of MOC requirements, redundancy with other professional and regulatory requirements, and most especially lack of relevance to physicians' practices and an absence of proof that MOC produces improved patient outcomes.
- Physicians with fewer resources to devote to the MOC process (lack of practice support for MOC, solo practice, or practice in areas of poverty) appear to be those most at risk for nonparticipation and, therefore, for loss of board-certified status.
- The elements of Part I, Professional Standing, and Part II, Lifelong Learning and Self-Assessment, were perceived as significantly more relevant to practice than Part III, the Cognitive Exam, or Part IV, Practice

Performance Assessment and Improvement activities.
- Frequent critiques of the MOC program as currently designed include a lack of assessment of appropriateness of care and insufficient system-based evaluation.

Challenges for Member Boards

- Compliance with the standards requires significantly more work by each Board's support staff.
- There is a need for website expansion to provide newly mandated diplomate services, as well as to house the growing body of data requiring storage as well.
  - As a direct result of the increased administrative and website workload which are expected to be ongoing requirements, most of the ABMS member boards felt there was no option other than to levy MOC fees to support this unfunded mandate.

Decreasing the Burden of MOC

- Programs such as the American Board of Anesthesiology Part III MOCA minute consist of a continuous dynamic web-based assessment with focused content to assess knowledge and guide the diplomat to appropriate resources.
- Physicians who participated in both MOC and PQRS (Medicare's Physician Quality Reporting System) were eligible to receive a 1.5% bonus in 2011 and a 1% annual bonus between 2012 and 2014, in addition to regular Medicare fees.
- Physicians who choose not to report these quality measures to the PQRS program by 2015 would have their Medicare fees reduced by 1.5% in 2015 and by 2% in 2016.

ABCRS: Current Requirements, Initiatives Under Consideration

- The current requirements for the ABCRS MOC Program are listed in Table 70.4.
- The MOC Committee of the ABCRS is considering changes to the MOC program such as a modular-type Part III examination, or completing a set number of secure multiple-choice questions annually with more timely feedback rather than 200 every 10 years.

Table 70.4 ABCRS MOC required components 2015

Part I. Professional standing (every 3 years)
Documentation of full licensure in the state in which you practice
Documentation of privileges for colon and rectal surgery at your hospital
Letter of recommendation from the chief of staff at your hospital
Part II. Lifelong learning and self-assessment (every 3 years)
90 hours of Category 1 CME credits, 50 with a self-assessment activity (which can include CARSEP or SESAP)
Part III. Cognitive expertise (every 10 years)
MOC cognitive exam.
Part IV. Evaluation of performance in practice (every 3 years); suggested activities include:
Communications and interpersonal skills activities
Clinical practice data – Ongoing participation in a national, regional, or local outcomes database or quality assessment program (**see Table 70.3**)

MOC Maintenance of Certification; *CME* continuing medical education; *CARSEP* Colon and Rectal Self-Assessment Program; *SESAP* Surgical Education and Self-Assessment Program

Quality and Safety in Colon and Rectal Surgery

71

Elizabeth C. Wick and Jonathon Efron

Key Concepts

- Measurement of quality can be separated into structural, process, and outcome-based.
- Quality measures in colorectal surgery are both process and outcome-based.
- Transforming healthcare to a high reliability organization will provide the infrastructure for continuous quality improvement.
- Creating a culture of safety is essential for delivering high-quality care.
- Patient and family engagement has emerged as a new and equally important domain of quality.

Background

- Preventable medical errors represent one of the eight leading causes of death in hospitalized patients.
- In 2001, *Crossing the Quality Chasm: A New Health System for the 21st Century,* provided a framework for how to rework healthcare delivery in the United States (Fig. 71.1).
- To meet these goals, the report outlined ten rules for redesign:
  1. Care is based on continuous healing relationships.
  2. Care is customized according to patient needs and values.
  3. The patient is the source of control.
  4. Knowledge must be shared, and information flows freely.
  5. Decision-making should be evidence-based.
  6. Safety is a system property.
  7. Transparency is necessary.
  8. Needs need to be anticipated.
  9. Waste should be continuously decreased.
  10. Cooperation among clinicians is a priority.
- The 2011 Affordable Care Act's goal was to increase the availability, quality, and affordability of insurance coverage and to be a catalyst for the reinvention of the healthcare system from volume to value-driven.
- A key tool for driving this transition to value instead of volume is the redesign of payment models, with a shift away from fee-for-service reimbursement in favor of global budgets, population health models, and accountable care organizations (ACO).
  - In the years to come, ACOs will likely focus more on surgical care (Table 71.1).

E. C. Wick (✉)
Division of General Surgery, University of California San Francisco, San Francisco, CA, USA
e-mail: Elizabeth.Wick@ucsf.edu

J. Efron
Department of Surgery, Johns Hopkins Hospital, Johns Hopkins University, Baltimore, MD, USA

S. R. Steele et al. (eds.), *The ASCRS Manual of Colon and Rectal Surgery*,
https://doi.org/10.1007/978-3-030-01165-9_71

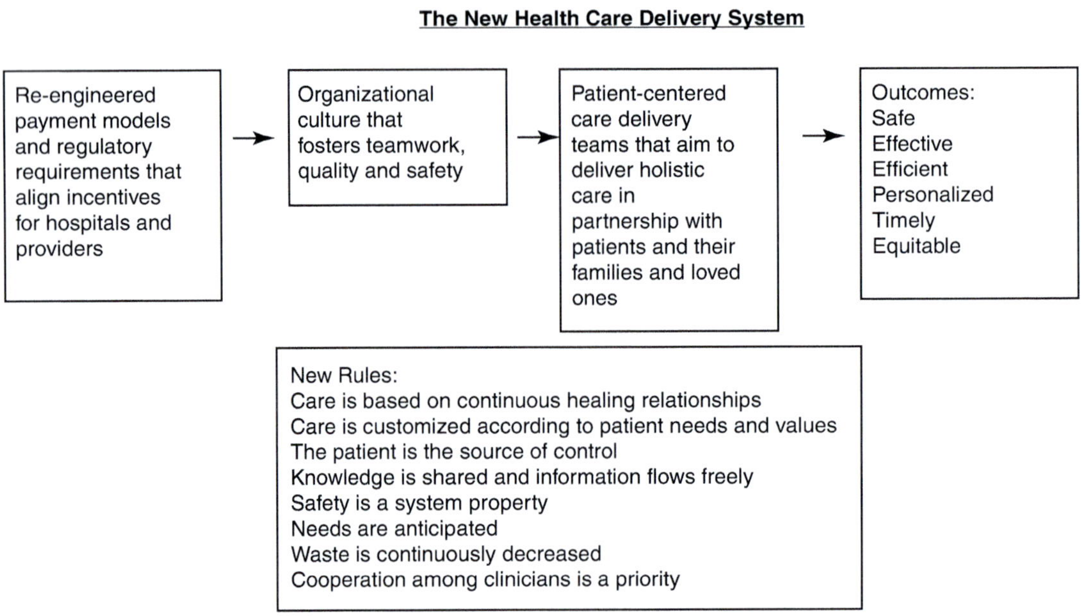

Fig. 71.1 The new healthcare delivery system

Table 71.1 Strategic priorities of 30 medicare ACOs

	Degree of near-term priority											
	Very low		Low		Medium		High		Very high		Don't know or missing	
Strategy	No.	%	No.	%	No	%	No.	%	No.	%	No.	%
Avoid wasted resources due to lack of care coordination	0	0	0	0	3	10	7	23	19	63	1	3
Reduce unnecessary surgery	4	13	12	40	10	33	2	7	1	3	1	3
Manage high-cost or high-risk patients	0	0	0	0	1	3	6	20	21	70	2	7
Reduce overuse of specialists	3	10	8	27	10	33	4	13	4	13	1	3
Reduce unnecessary imaging	0	0	7	23	13	43	3	10	5	17	2	7
Reduce duplicative testing	0	0	5	17	9	30	6	20	9	30	1	3
Reduce avoidable hospital readmissions	0	0	0	0	0	0	5	17	24	80	1	3
Reduce avoidable ED visits	0	0	0	0	1	3	11	37	17	57	1	3

Source: Authors' analysis. Note survey respondents were asked to "Please indicate the priority you are placing on each of the following strategies in the first performance year of your ACO." ED is emergency department

With Permission from Dupree JM, Patel K, Singer SJ, West M, Wang R, Zinner MJ, Weissman JS. Attention to surgeons and surgical care is largely missing from early medicare accountable care organizations. Health Aff (Millwood). 2014 Jun;33(6):972–9. https://doi.org/10.1377/hlthaff.2013.1300. (57) © Project Hope 2014

The Conceptual Model of Quality Measurement: Donabedian Model

- The Donabedian model measures quality by three main types of improvements: changes to structure, process, and outcome (Fig. 71.2).
  - *Structure* refers to the context in which care is delivered—this includes the facility and

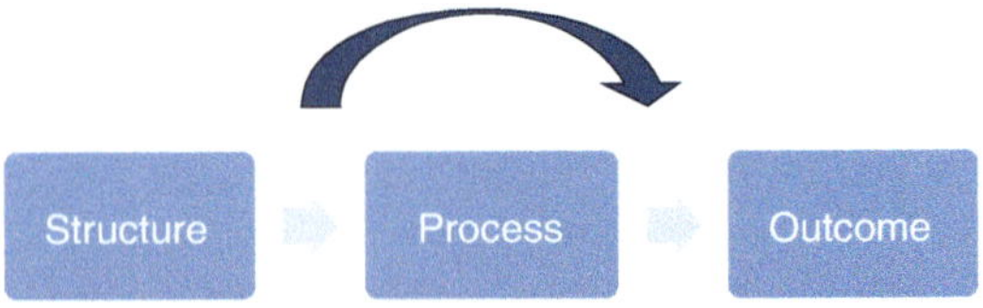

Fig. 71.2 The Donabedian model of quality of care

services, workforce, and payment structure.
  - *Process* is the application of these tools, equipment, and policies/procedures to patients (i.e., good practices and evidence-based medicine).
  - *Outcome* is the result on patients.

Structural Measures

- Structural measures tend to be the most straightforward to assess, such as hospital and surgeon volume, as well as board specialization, association with a reduction in operative morbidity, and 5-year mortality.
- While relatively easy to quantify, the downside of volume as a measure is that it is a proxy measure and not easily "actionable" for quality improvement.
- The ASCRS partnership collaboration with the ACS Commission on Cancer to create the "CoC Rectal Cancer Accreditation Program" is based on five core principles of evidence-based rectal cancer care:
- Total mesorectal excision (TME).
- Measurement of quality of surgery by specific techniques of pathology assessment.
- Specialist imaging techniques identifying those patients at high risk of local recurrence.
- The use of newer more effective neoadjuvant and adjuvant therapies which includes radiotherapy and chemotherapy.
- Multidisciplinary team (MDT) approach that identifies, coordinates, delivers, and monitors the ideal treatment on an individual patient-by-patient basis.

Process Measures

- Advantages of measuring quality through process measures are that most measures are evidence-based, are relatively easy to monitor for compliance, and have imminently actionable results.
- The major downside is that for the most part excellent compliance with surgical process measures has failed to translate into improved outcomes (e.g., SCIP).
- Another example of process measures relevant to the practicing colorectal surgeon is the colorectal cancer measures included in the Commission on Cancer site reports and endorsed by the National Quality Forum (NQF) (Table 71.2).

Outcomes

- The two major types of outcome measures available today are from administrative data and/or clinical registries.
- Administrative data is derived from hospital billing information and relies on the accuracy of the clinical documentation and medical

Table 71.2 Commission on cancer colorectal cancer measures

Colon			
ACT	Accountability	Standard 4.4 90%	(NQF #0223) adjuvant chemotherapy is considered or administered within 4 months (120 days) of diagnosis for patients under the age of 80 with AJCC stage III (lymph node positive) colon cancer.
12RLN	Quality improvement	Standard 4.5 85%	(NQF #0225) at least 12 regional lymph nodes are removed and pathologically examined for resected colon cancer
Rectum			
RECRCT	Quality improvement	Not applicable	Preoperative chemo and radiation are administered for clinical AJCC T3 N0, T4 N0, or stage III; or postoperative chemo and radiation are administered within 180 days of diagnosis for clinical AJCC T1-2 N0 with pathologic AJCC T3 N0, T4 N0, or stage III; or treatment is considered, for patients under the age of 80 receiving resection for rectal cancer

AJCC American Joint Commission for Cancer

coders and is heavily focused on the inpatient stay (e.g., UHC, Premier Advisor, and Medicare.)
- Surgical registry data, usually nurse abstracted, audited, and risk-adjusted, is outstanding for complex clinical variables (e.g., NSQIP) (Appendix 71.1).
- In colorectal surgery, SSIs have emerged as one of the first outcome measures embraced as a national metric.
  - There are three types of SSI defined by NHSN: superficial, deep, and organ space; however, the public reporting metric only includes risk-adjusted *organ* space rates.
- A separate domain of outcome measurement is the patient experience, measured using the Hospital Consumer Assessment of Healthcare Providers and Systems (HCAHPS) survey.
- Composite measures are a more global assessment of quality and include weighted structure, process, and outcome measures (e.g., Leapfrog patient safety score).
- Structure, process, and outcome components of quality measurement all occur within the context of an organization's overall *culture* (i.e., the collective attitudes and beliefs of caregivers), which is increasingly being recognized to be the fourth measurable component to the *structure-process-outcome* model.

Safety

- Patient safety is a discipline that applies safety science methodology toward creating a reliable healthcare delivery system that continuously strives to eliminate adverse events.
- Adverse events occur because of a **breakdown in the system in which we operate** and are **not caused by a single person's actions**.
- A cornerstone of the patient safety movement is limiting blame, and all hospitals are required to have nonpunitive avenues for event reporting as well as forums for discussion and accountability for developing fixes to prevent recurrent events.
- "Systems" thinking in healthcare is the idea that redesigning systems using a combination of clinician input, human factors principles, systems engineering, and health information technology (among others) could result in mistakes being dramatically reduced.

High Reliability Organizations

- Focusing on the principle of high reliability has been proposed as a strategy to transition healthcare from a high-risk, high error rate to a high-risk, low error rate industry.
- High reliability organization theory suggests that proper oversight of people, processes, and technology can handle complex and hazardous activities and keep error rates acceptably low:
  1. HROs are sensitive to operations (continually strive to improve the system).
  2. HROs are reluctant to accept "simple" explanations for problems (do not finger point or accept simple reasons for adverse events).
  3. HROs have a preoccupation with failure (always vigilant and looking for ways to prevent adverse events).
  4. HROs defer to expertise (not committed to hierarchy and training, respect frontline wisdom).
  5. HROs are resilient.

Creating a Culture of Safety

- Culture is to an organization what personality is to an individual—a hidden yet unifying theme that provides meaning, direction, and mobilization.
  1. An acknowledgment of the high-risk, error-prone nature of an organization's activities
  2. A nonpunitive environment where individuals are able to report errors or close calls without fear of punishment or retaliation
  3. An expectation of collaboration across ranks to seek solutions to vulnerabilities
  4. A willingness on the part of the organization to direct resources to address safety concerns

Measuring Safety Culture

- Efforts to foster cultural change within an organization with regard to patient safety have been limited in the past by the inability to measure the impact of any given intervention.
- The Safety Attitudes Questionnaire (SAQ) and the HSOPS (Hospital Survey on Patient Safety Culture) are validated survey instruments that can be used to measure culture in a healthcare setting.
- The surveys consist of a series of questions measuring six domains: teamwork climate, safety climate, job satisfaction, perception of management, stress recognition, and working conditions.
- The ability for all team members, to "speak up" about patient safety concerns, is one of the most important elements of creating a culture of patient safety.

Teamwork and Communication

- According to the Joint Commission, communication breakdown is one of the top 3 root causes of sentinel events such as wrong-site surgery.
- The traditional surgical hierarchy can prevent OR personnel from sharing important patient data and expressing safety concerns.
- The standard workflow of the OR itself presents many opportunities for the loss or degradation of critical information (e.g., handoffs of patient care from the OR to other locations or providers, the surgical count, communication between the surgeon and pathologist).

Measuring Teamwork

- Safety culture surveys can be used to measure teamwork and provide benchmarks for departments or hospitals seeking to measure and improve their teamwork climate.
- Communication and collaboration sections of the surveys reflect OR caregiver views on teamwork and can be used to distinguish meaningful interventions from impractical and ineffective programs.
- Efforts to improve the communication that takes place between physicians and nurses can directly improve the perception of teamwork and collaboration by the OR team.
- Empowering well-respected surgeons to promote principles of teamwork and communication can go a long way toward transforming attitude and behavioral changes in fellow physicians, as well as other members of the surgical team.

Tools for Improving Safety Culture, Teamwork, and Communication

- A hallmark of high reliability organizations is the frequent use of tools such as prompts, checks, standard operating protocols, and communication interventions such as team briefings and debriefings.
- These tools identify and mitigate hazards and allow an organization to complete tasks more efficiently.
- Safety checks and standardized team discussions serve as prompts to help "engineer out" human error, providing quality assurance and improving information flow, and can prevent errors related to omissions.
- Preoperative briefings and checklists are any pre-procedure discussion of requirements, needs, and special issues of the procedure, which can help to facilitate transfer of information between team members.
- The World Health Organization (WHO) has developed a comprehensive perioperative checklist as a primary intervention of the "Safe Surgery Saves Lives" program—an effort to reduce surgical deaths across the globe (Fig. 71.3).
- The comprehensive unit-based safety program (CUSP), an effective tool for improving both safety culture and clinical outcomes, follows five iterative steps: training on the science of safety, identify patient safety hazards, partner with senior executive, learn from defects, and implement tools to improve teamwork and communication.

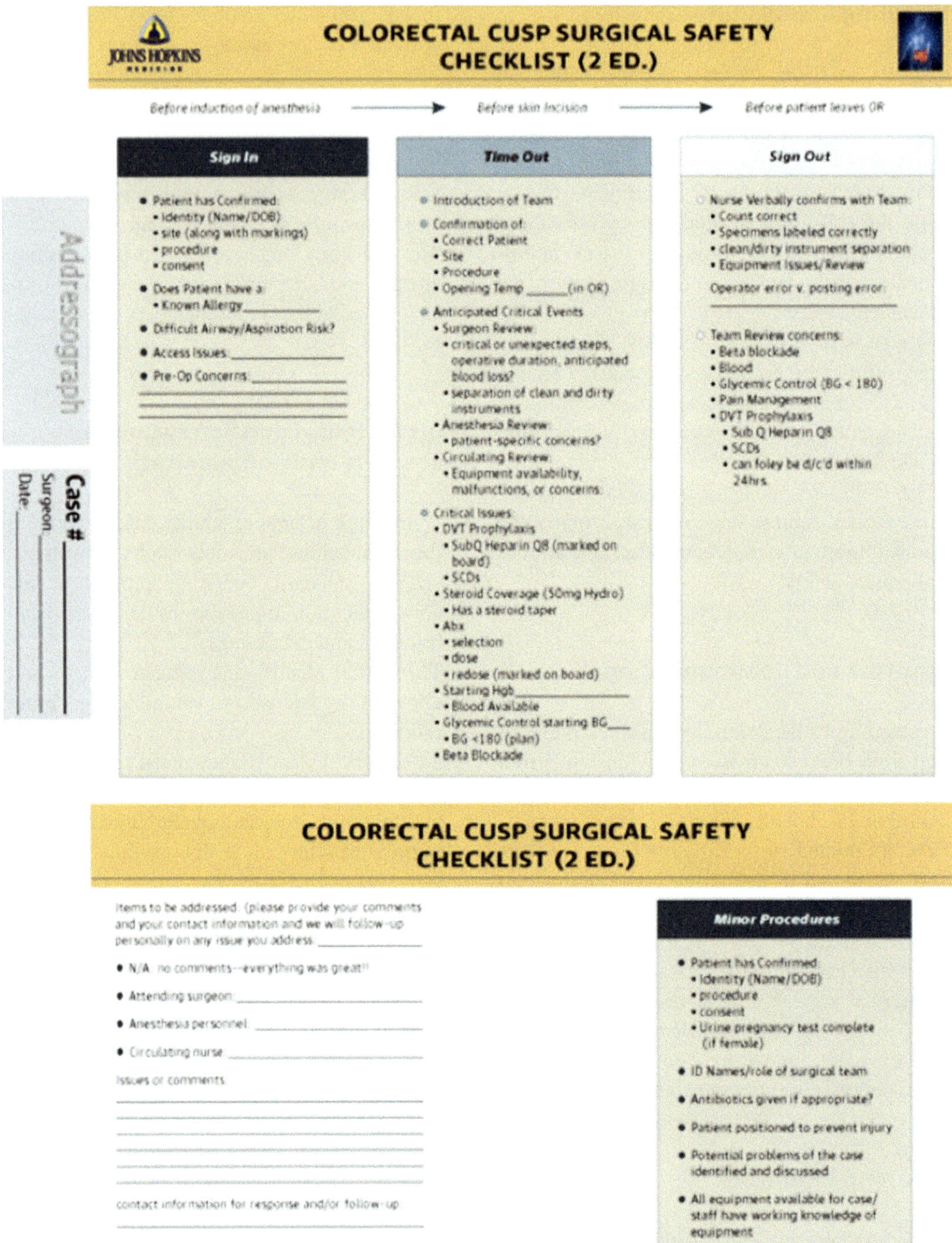

JOHNS HOPKINS MEDICINE

COLORECTAL CUSP SURGICAL SAFETY CHECKLIST (2 ED.)

Before induction of anesthesia → *Before skin Incision* → *Before patient leaves OR*

Addressograph

Case # ______
Surgeon ______
Date ______

Sign In

- Patient has Confirmed:
  - Identity (Name/DOB)
  - site (along with markings)
  - procedure
  - consent
- Does Patient have a:
  - Known Allergy ______
- Difficult Airway/Aspiration Risk?
- Access Issues ______
- Pre-Op Concerns ______

Time Out

- Introduction of Team
- Confirmation of:
  - Correct Patient
  - Site
  - Procedure
  - Opening Temp ______ (in OR)
- Anticipated Critical Events
  - Surgeon Review:
    - critical or unexpected steps, operative duration, anticipated blood loss?
    - separation of clean and dirty instruments
  - Anesthesia Review:
    - patient-specific concerns?
  - Circulating Review:
    - Equipment availability, malfunctions, or concerns:
- Critical Issues:
  - DVT Prophylaxis
    - SubQ Heparin Q8 (marked on board)
    - SCDs
  - Steroid Coverage (50mg Hydro)
    - Has a steroid taper
  - Abx
    - selection
    - dose
    - redose (marked on board)
  - Starting Hgb ______
    - Blood Available
  - Glycemic Control starting BG ___
    - BG <180 (plan)
  - Beta Blockade

Sign Out

- Nurse Verbally confirms with Team:
  - Count correct
  - Specimens labeled correctly
  - clean/dirty instrument separation
  - Equipment Issues/Review

Operator error v. posting error: ______

- Team Review concerns:
  - Beta blockade
  - Blood
  - Glycemic Control (BG < 180)
  - Pain Management
  - DVT Prophylaxis
    - Sub Q Heparin Q8
    - SCDs
    - can foley be d/c'd within 24hrs

COLORECTAL CUSP SURGICAL SAFETY CHECKLIST (2 ED.)

Items to be addressed: (please provide your comments and your contact information and we will follow-up personally on any issue you address ______

- N/A: no comments--everything was great!!
- Attending surgeon: ______
- Anesthesia personnel: ______
- Circulating nurse: ______

Issues or comments:

______

contact information for response and/or follow-up:

______

Minor Procedures

- Patient has Confirmed:
  - Identity (Name/DOB)
  - procedure
  - consent
  - Urine pregnancy test complete (if female)
- ID Names/role of surgical team
- Antibiotics given if appropriate?
- Patient positioned to prevent injury
- Potential problems of the case identified and discussed
- All equipment available for case/staff have working knowledge of equipment

Fig. 71.3 Local adaptation of briefing checklist to colorectal surgery. (With Permission from Hicks CW. Improving safety and quality of care with enhanced teamwork through operating room briefings. JAMA Surg. 2014;149(8):863–8. https://doi.org/10.1001/jamasurg.2014.172. © American Medical Association 2014)

"Never Events" in Surgery

- Never events are errors in medical care that are clearly identifiable, preventable, and serious in their consequences for patients and that indicate a real problem in the safety and credibility of a healthcare facility (Table 71.3).
- Criteria for inclusion as a "never event" include:
  - Unambiguous (i.e., the event must be clearly identifiable and measurable and thus feasible to include in a reporting system)
  - Usually preventable, with the recognition that some events are not always avoidable, given the complexity of healthcare
  - Serious, resulting in death or loss of a body part, disability, or more than transient loss of a body function
  - And any one of the following:
  - Adverse
  - Indicative of a problem in a healthcare facility's safety systems
  - Important for public credibility or public accountability
- Never events are still a significant problem, with a study showing that from 10/1990 to 10/2010, there were 9744 paid malpractice claims for never events in the United States alone; and of these, mortality was reported in 6.6%, permanent injury in 33%, and temporary injury in 59%.
- Retained surgical items in colorectal surgery are usually laparotomy pads, needles, or instruments and occur even when the final count is "correct" or "incorrect"—though this usually occurs when there is poor communication among the operating room team.

Patient and Families as Partners

- One of the hallmarks of the patient safety movement is a new commitment to disclosure of the risks associated with procedures, occurrence of patient safety events, and the recognition of the patient as an essential partner in the delivery of safe, cost-effective care.
- Many believe that shared decision-making is the pinnacle of patient-centered care.
- In surgery, it is generally defined as the patient and physician sharing responsibility in the clinical decision-making process (two-way dialogue) and incorporating the patients' values and beliefs in that process.

Table 71.3 "Never events"

1. Surgical or Invasive Procedure Events
1A. Surgery or other invasive procedure performed on the wrong site (updated) Applicable in: hospitals, outpatient/office-based surgery centers, ambulatory practice settings/office-based practices, long-term care/skilled nursing facilities
1B. Surgery or other invasive procedure performed on the wrong patient (updated) Applicable in: hospitals, outpatient/office-based surgery centers, ambulatory practice settings/office-based practices, long-term care/skilled nursing facilities
1C. Wrong surgical or other invasive procedure performed on a patient (updated) Applicable in: hospitals, outpatient/office-based surgery centers, ambulatory practice settings/office-based practices, long-term care/skilled nursing facilities
1D. Unintended retention of a foreign object in a patient after surgery or other invasive procedure (updated) Applicable in: hospitals, outpatient/office-based surgery centers, ambulatory practice settings/office-based practices, long-term care/skilled nursing facilities
1E. Intraoperative or immediately postoperative/postprocedure death in an ASA Class 1 patient (updated) Applicable in: hospitals, outpatient/office-based surgery centers, ambulatory practice settings/office-based practices

Table 71.3 (continued)

2. Product or Device Events

2A. Patient death or serious injury associated with the use of contaminated drugs, devices, or biologics provided by the healthcare setting (updated)

Applicable in: hospitals, outpatient/office-based surgery centers, ambulatory practice settings/office-based practices, long-term care/skilled nursing facilities

2B. Patient death or serious injury associated with the use or function of a device in patient care, in which the device is used or functions other than as intended (updated)

Applicable in: hospitals, outpatient/office-based surgery centers, ambulatory practice settings/office-based practices, long-term care/skilled nursing facilities

2C. Patient death or serious injury associated with intravascular air embolism that occurs while being cared for in a healthcare setting (updated)

Applicable in: hospitals, outpatient/office-based surgery centers, long-term care/skilled nursing facilities

3. Patient Protection Events

3A. Discharge or release of a patient/resident of any age, who is unable to make decisions, to other than an authorized person (updated)

Applicable in: hospitals, outpatient/office-based surgery centers, ambulatory practice settings/office-based practices, long-term care/skilled nursing facilities

3B. Patient death or serious injury associated with patient elopement (disappearance) (updated)

Applicable in: hospitals, outpatient/office-based surgery centers, ambulatory practice settings/office-based practices, long-term care/skilled nursing facilities

3C. Patient suicide, attempted suicide, or self-harm that results in serious injury, while being cared for in a healthcare setting (updated)

Applicable in: hospitals, outpatient/office-based surgery centers, ambulatory practice settings/office-based practices, long-term care/skilled nursing facilities

4. Care Management Events

4A. Patient death or serious injury associated with a medication error (e.g., errors involving the wrong drug, wrong dose, wrong patient, wrong time, wrong rate, wrong preparation, or wrong route of administration) (updated)

Applicable in: hospitals, outpatient/office-based surgery centers, ambulatory practice settings/office-based practices, long-term care/skilled nursing facilities

4B. Patient death or serious injury associated with unsafe administration of blood products (updated)

Applicable in: hospitals, outpatient/office-based surgery centers, ambulatory practice settings/office-based practices, long-term care/skilled nursing facilities

4C. Maternal death or serious injury associated with labor or delivery in a low-risk pregnancy while being cared for in a healthcare setting (updated)

Applicable in: hospitals, outpatient/office-based surgery centers

4D. Death or serious injury of a neonate associated with labor or delivery in a low-risk pregnancy (new)

Applicable in: hospitals, outpatient/office-based surgery centers

4E. Patient death or serious injury associated with a fall while being cared for in a healthcare setting (updated)

Applicable in: hospitals, outpatient/office-based surgery centers, ambulatory practice settings/office-based practices, long-term care/skilled nursing facilities

4F. Any Stage 3, Stage 4, and unstageable pressure ulcers acquired after admission/presentation to a healthcare setting (updated)

Applicable in: hospitals, outpatient/office-based surgery centers, long-term care/skilled nursing facilities

4G. Artificial insemination with the wrong donor sperm or wrong egg (updated)

Applicable in: hospitals, outpatient/office-based surgery centers, ambulatory practice settings/office-based practices

4H. Patient death or serious injury resulting from the irretrievable loss of an irreplaceable biological specimen (new)

Applicable in: hospitals, outpatient/office-based surgery centers, ambulatory practice settings/office-based practices, long-term care/skilled nursing facilities

4I. Patient death or serious injury resulting from failure to follow up or communicate laboratory, pathology, or radiology test results (new)

Applicable in: hospitals, outpatient/office-based surgery centers, ambulatory practice settings/office-based practices, long-term care/skilled nursing facilities

5. Environmental Events
5A. Patient or staff death or serious injury associated with an electric shock in the course of a patient care process in a healthcare setting (updated) Applicable in: hospitals, outpatient/office-based surgery centers, ambulatory practice settings/office-based practices, long-term care/skilled nursing facilities
5B. Any incident in which systems designated for oxygen or other gas to be delivered to a patient contains no gas, the wrong gas, or are contaminated by toxic substances (updated) Applicable in: hospitals, outpatient/office-based surgery centers, ambulatory practice settings/office-based practices, long-term care/skilled nursing facilities
5C. Patient or staff death or serious injury associated with a burn incurred from any source in the course of a patient care process in a healthcare setting (updated) Applicable in: hospitals, outpatient/office-based surgery centers, ambulatory practice settings/office-based practices, long-term care/skilled nursing facilities
5D. Patient death or serious injury associated with the use of physical restraints or bedrails while being cared for in a healthcare setting (updated) Applicable in: hospitals, outpatient/office-based surgery centers, ambulatory practice settings/office-based practices, long-term care/skilled nursing facilities
6. Radiologic Events
6A. Death or serious injury of a patient or staff associated with the introduction of a metallic object into the MRI area (new) Applicable in: hospitals, outpatient/office-based surgery centers, ambulatory practice settings/office-based practices
7. Potential Criminal Events
7A. Any instance of care ordered by or provided by someone impersonating a physician, nurse, pharmacist, or other licensed healthcare provider (updated) Applicable in: hospitals, outpatient/office-based surgery centers, ambulatory practice settings/office-based practices, long-term care/skilled nursing facilities
7B. Abduction of a patient/resident of any age (updated) Applicable in: hospitals, outpatient/office-based surgery centers, ambulatory practice settings/office-based practices, long-term care/skilled nursing facilities
7C. Sexual abuse/assault on a patient or staff member within or on the grounds of a healthcare setting (updated) Applicable in: hospitals, outpatient/office-based surgery centers, ambulatory practice settings/office-based practices, long-term care/skilled nursing facilities
7D. Death or serious injury of a patient or staff member resulting from a physical assault (i.e., battery) that occurs within or on the grounds of a healthcare setting (updated) Applicable in: hospitals, outpatient/office-based surgery centers, ambulatory practice settings/office-based practices, long-term care/skilled nursing facilities

Appendix 71.1: American College of Surgeons National Quality Improvement Program-Targeted Colectomy and Proctectomy Procedure Measures. With Permission from © American College of Surgeons

AMERICAN COLLEGE OF SURGEONS
NATIONAL SURGICAL QUALITY IMPROVEMENT PROGRAM
PROCTECTOMY
PROCEDURE TARGETED WORKSHEET

***IDN** ____________________ **Cycle Number** ____________________
LMRN____________________ **Case Number** ____________________

DEMOGRAPHICS

Last Name: ______________________ **First:** ______________________ **MI:** _____
Street Address: ____
City/Town: ____________________ **State/Province:** _________ **Zip:** _________ **Country:** _________
Home Phone (____) __________ **Work Phone** (____) __________ **Cell Phone** (____) __________
***DOB:** ______/______/______ *(mm/dd/yyyy)* **Gender:** ☐ *Male* ☐ *Female*
Race: ☐ White ☐ American Indian / Alaska Native ☐ Asian
☐ Black / African American ☐ Native Hawaiian / Other Pacific Islander ☐ Unknown
Ethnicity: Hispanic - ☐ *YES* ☐ *NO* ☐ Unknown **Preferred Language:** ☐ ENGLISH ☐ SPANISH

SURGICAL PROFILE

Principal Procedure ______________________________ **CPT® Code** ____________

Patient Status: ☐ *Inpatient* ☐*Outpatient* **Elective Surgery:** ☐ *YES* ☐ *NO* ☐ *Unknown*

Origin Status:
☐ Not transferred, admitted directly from home
☐ Transfer from other (i.e. Spinal Cord Injury Unit or other facility not listed)
☐ Acute Care Hospital (inpatient status only)
☐ Transfer from outside Emergency Department
☐ Nursing Home/Chronic Care Facility/Intermediate Care Unit
☐ Unknown (if transferred from unknown location or Facility)

Hospital Admission Date: ______/______/______ ***Operation Date:** ______/______/______

Anesthesia Technique:
☐ General ☐Spinal ☐ Epidural ☐ Regional ☐ Local ☐ MAC/IV Sedation ☐None ☐Other ☐Unknown

Additional Anesthesia Technique(s)
☐ General ☐Spinal ☐ Epidural ☐ Regional ☐ Local ☐ MAC/IV Sedation ☐None ☐Other ☐Unknown

***Surgical Specialty:** *(select one)*
1. General Surgery
2. Vascular
3. Thoracic
4. Cardiac
5. Orthopedics
6. Neurosurgery
7. Urology
8. Otolaryngology (ENT)
9. Plastics
10. Gynecology
11. Interventional Radiologist

Surgeon NPI:____________________
Attending Surgeon's Name: ____________________ **Attending Surgeon's IDN:** ____________
LCN: ____________________ **Encounter Number:** ____________

Preoperative Risk Assessment

GENERAL				RENAL		
Height	______	*Inches*	*CM*	Acute Renal Failure w/in 24 hrs	*YES*	*NO*
Weight	______	*Pounds*	*KG*	Currently requiring or on Dialysis w/in 2 wks	*YES*	*NO*
Diabetes Mellitus	*Non-Insulin*	*Insulin*	*NO*	**NUTRITIONAL/IMMUNE/OTHER**		
Current Smoker w/in 1 year		*YES*	*NO*	Disseminated Cancer	*YES*	*NO*
Dyspnea	*Mod. Exertion*	*At Rest*	*NONE*	Open Wound (w/ or w/out infection)	*YES*	*NO*
Functional Health Status	*I*___ *PD* ___	*TD* ___	*Unk* ___	Steroid/Immunosuppressant use for chronic condition	*YES*	*NO*
PULMONARY				>10% loss of body wt. last 6 months	*YES*	*NO*
Vent. Dependent w/in 48 hrs		*YES*	*NO*	Bleeding disorders	*YES*	*NO*
COPD (severe)		*YES*	*NO*	Preop Transfusions (RBC units w/in 72 hrs)	*YES*	*NO*
HEPATOBILIARY				Sepsis w/in 48 hours	*SIRS*	*NO*
Ascites w/in 30 days		*YES*	*NO*		*Sepsis*	
CARDIAC					*Sep Shock*	
CHF w/in 30 days		*YES*	*NO*			
Hypertension req. meds.		*YES*	*NO*			

Tumor Location in the Rectum
☐ N/A ☐ Lower Third ☐ Middle Third ☐ Upper Third ☐ Unknown

Chemotherapy within 90 Days
☐ Yes ☐ No ☐ Unknown

Radiation Therapy within 90 Days
☐ Yes ☐ No ☐ Unknown

Pretreatment Clinical Staging- Primary Tumor "T"
☐ N/A ☐ Tx ☐ T0 ☐ Tis ☐ T1 ☐ T2
☐ T3 ☐ T4 ☐ T4a ☐ T4b ☐ Unknown

Pretreatment Clinical Staging- Regional Lymph Nodes "N"
☐ N/A ☐ Nx ☐ N0 ☐ N1 ☐ N1a ☐ N1b
☐ N1c ☐ N2 ☐ N2a ☐ N2b ☐ Unknown

Pretreatment Clinical Staging- Distant Metastasis "M"
☐ N/A ☐ MO/Mx ☐ M1 ☐ M1a ☐ M1b ☐ Unknown

Complete Evaluation of the Colon Preoperatively
☐ Yes
☐ No-no study identified
☐ No-study was incomplete, obstructing lesion in the colon
☐ No-study was incomplete, entire colon could not be visualized
☐ No-study was incomplete, prep was inadequate
☐ Unknown

Patient Marked for Stoma Preoperatively
☐ Yes
☐ No

Laboratory Data

LABORATORY DATA: ***(report preop lab values closest to the Procedure/Surgery start date & time)***
Preop values should be within 90 days prior to surgery

PREOPERATIVE LAB DATA	Value 90 days	unknown	Date
Serum Sodium (Na)		☐	___/___/___
Blood Urea Nitrogen (BUN)		☐	___/___/___
Creatinine (Cr)		☐	___/___/___
Albumin (ALB)		☐	___/___/___
Total Bilirubin (TB)		☐	___/___/___

Serum Glutamic-Oxaloacetic Transaminase (SGOT)/(AST)		☐	___/___/___
Alkaline Phosphatase (Alk Phos)		☐	___/___/___
White Blood Count (WBC)		☐	___/___/___
Hematocrit (Hct)		☐	___/___/___
Platelets (Plt)		☐	___/___/___
Internat'l Normalized Ratio (INR)		☐	___/___/___
Partial Thromboplastin Time (PTT)		☐	___/___/___

OPERATIVE INFORMATION

Emergency Case: ☐ YES ☐ NO

Wound Classification: ☐ *Clean* ☐ *Clean/Contaminated* ☐ *Contaminated* ☐ *Dirty/Infected*

Surgical wound(s) closure:
☐ All layers of incision (deep and superficial) are fully closed by some means
☐ Only deep layers of incision are closed; superficial layers are left open
☐ No layers of the incision are surgically closed
ASA Class *(circle one)*: *1 2 3 4 5 6 None Assigned (for local anes. only)*

OPERATIVE TIMES: Procedure / Surgery Start: _______:_______ Procedure/Surgery Finish: _______:_______

Pathologic Staging- Primary Tumor "T":
☐ N/A ☐ Tx ☐ T0 ☐ Tis ☐ T1 ☐ T2
☐ T3 ☐ T4 ☐ T4a ☐ T4b ☐ Unknown

Pathologic Staging- Regional Lymph Nodes "N"
☐ N/A ☐ Nx ☐ N0 ☐ N1 ☐ N1a ☐ N1b
☐ N1c ☐ N2 ☐ N2a ☐ N2b ☐ Unknown

Number of Nodes Evaluated
☐ _______________ ☐ Unknown ☐ N/A

Pathologic Staging- Distant Metastasis "M"
☐ N/A ☐ MO/Mx ☐ M1 ☐ M1a ☐ M1b ☐ Unknown

Margins-Radial
☐ N/A ☐ Yes, margin was clear ☐ No clear mass: margin was positive ☐ Unknown

Clear Radial Margin cm
☐ CM_______ ☐Unknown

Margins-Distal
☐ N/A ☐ Yes, margin was clear ☐ No clear mass: margin was positive ☐ Unknown

Clear Distal Margin cm
☐ CM_______ ☐Unknown

Operative Approach:
☐ Open (planned)
☐ Laparoscopic
☐ Laparoscopic with open assist
☐ Laparoscopic with unplanned conversion to open
☐ Robotic
☐ Robotic with open assist
☐ Robotic with unplanned conversion to open
☐ Endoscopic
☐ Endoscopic with open assist
☐ Endoscopic with unplanned conversion to open
☐ NOTES
☐ NOTES with open assist
☐ NOTES with unplanned conversion to open
☐ SILS
☐ SILS with open assist
☐ SILS with unplanned conversion to open
☐ Other MIS Approach
☐ Other MIS Approach with open assist
☐ Other MIS approach with unplanned conversion to open
☐ Combination of approaches not otherwise specified
☐ Combination of Approaches not otherwise specified with open assist

☐ Combination of approaches otherwise specified with unplanned conversion to open
☐ Other
☐ Unknown

ADDITIONAL OPERATIVE PROCEDURES

Other Procedure	CPT
1.	
2.	
3.	
4.	
5.	
6.	
7.	

Concurrent Procedure	CPT
1.	
2.	
3.	
4.	
5.	
6.	
7.	

OCCURRENCES

POSTOPERATIVE OCCURRENCES: ☐ *YES* ☐ *NO*
(Although not required for this program, you may wish to document 'treatment' and 'outcome to date' of the occurrence for internal quality monitoring)

			Date	***Treatments / Outcomes / Comments***
Wound Occurrences				
Superficial Incisional SSI	☐ *YES*	☐ *NO*	___/___/___	__________
Present at Time of Surgery?	☐ *YES*	☐ *NO*		
Deep Incisional SSI	☐ *YES*	☐ *NO*	___/___/___	__________
Present at Time of Surgery?	☐ *YES*	☐ *NO*		
Organ/Space SSI	☐ *YES*	☐ *NO*	___/___/___	__________
Present at Time of Surgery?	☐ *YES*	☐ *NO*		
Wound Disruption	☐ *YES*	☐ *NO*	___/___/___	__________
Respiratory Occurrences				
Pneumonia (PNA)	☐ *YES*	☐ *NO*	___/___/___	__________
Present at Time of Surgery?	☐ *YES*	☐ *NO*		
Intraop **OR** Postop Unplanned Intubation	☐ *YES*	☐ *NO*	___/___/___	__________
Pulmonary Embolism	☐ *YES*	☐ *NO*	___/___/___	__________
On ventilator > 48 hours	☐ *YES*	☐ *NO*	___/___/___	__________
Present at Time of Surgery?	☐ *YES*	☐ *NO*		
Urinary Tract Occurrences				
Urinary Tract Infection (UTI)	☐ *YES*	☐ *NO*	___/___/___	__________
Present at Time of Surgery?	☐ *YES*	☐ *NO*		
Report the most significant level				
Progressive Renal Insufficiency	☐ *YES*	☐ *NO*	___/___/___	__________
Acute Renal Failure	☐ *YES*	☐ *NO*	___/___/___	__________
CNS Occurrences				
Stroke / CVA	☐ *YES*	☐ *NO*	___/___/___	__________
Cardiac Occurrences				
Intraop **OR** Postop Cardiac Arrest req. CPR	☐ *YES*	☐ *NO*	___/___/___	__________
Intraop **OR** Postop Myocardial Infarction	☐ *YES*	☐ *NO*	___/___/___	__________
Other Occurrences				
Transfusion Intraop/Postop (72h of surgery start time) *(transfusion of 1-200 units)*	☐ *YES*	☐ *NO*	___/___/___	# of units transfused: __________
Vein Thrombosis req. Therapy	☐ *YES*	☐ *NO*	___/___/___	__________
Sepsis: Sepsis	☐ *YES*	☐ *NO*	___/___/___	__________
Present at time of surgery?	☐ *YES*	☐ *NO*		
Septic Shock	☐ *YES*	☐ *NO*	___/___/___	__________
Present at time of surgery?	☐ *YES*	☐ *NO*		
Other Postoperative Occurrences (ICD-9 code):			___/___/___	(ICD-9 code) __________

Anastomotic Leak:
☐ No
☐ Yes-Leak, no treatment intervention of any kind documented
☐ Yes-Leak, treated with NPO, antibiotics, TPN or other non-interventional, non-operative means
☐ Yes-Leak, treated with percutaneous/radiological/endoscopic interventional means
☐ Yes-Leak, reoperation
☐ Unknown

Prolonged Postoperative NPO or NGT Use: ☐ Yes ☐ No ☐ Unknown

HOSPITAL DISCHARGE INFORMATION / READMISSIONS / MORTALITY / REOPERATIONS

Acute Hospital Discharge Date: _____/_____/_______ *(mm/dd/yyyy)*

Discharge Destination:
☐ *Skilled Care Facility, not Home* ☐ *Home* ☐ *Expired*
☐ *Unskilled Facility, not Home* ☐ *Separate Acute care (transferred to another acute care facility)* ☐ *Unknown*
☐ *Facility which was Home* ☐ *Rehab*

Post-op ICD.9 Code ______________________ **Diagnosis:** ____

Still in hospital > 30 days: ☐ *YES* ☐ *NO*

Death:
Death during operation OR Postop Death w/in 30 days: ☐ *YES* ☐ *NO*
Date of death: _____/_____/______ ☐ Unknown

Postop Death > 30 days: *(if remained in acute care)* ☐ *YES* ☐ *NO*
Date of death: ______/______/_____ ☐ Unknown

Readmission: (Multiple Readmissions Can Be Entered)

Was there a readmission for any reason within 30 days of the principal operative procedure?
☐ *YES* ☐ *NO* ☐ *Unknown*
If yes, date: _______/______/_______
Information Source *(select one)* ☐ Medical Record ☐ Patient/Family Report ☐ Other

Was this readmission unplanned at the time of the principal operative procedure? ☐ *YES* ☐ *NO*

Was this readmission likely related to the principal operative procedure? ☐ *YES* ☐ *NO*

- If likely related, choose the primary suspected reason (postoperative occurrence)

Superficial SSI	Pulmonary Embolism	Intraop or Postop Cardiac Arrest req CPR	Other: ICD-9 code____________ Free Text:____________________
Deep SSI	On ventilator > 48 hours	Intraop or Postop Myocardial Infarction	
Organ / Space SSI	Progressive Renal Insufficiency	Transfusion Intraop/Postop (72h of surgery start time)	
Wound Disruption	Acute Renal Failure	Vein Thrombosis Requiring Therapy	
Pneumonia	Urinary Tract Infection (UTI)	Sepsis	
Intraop or Postop Unplanned Intubation	Stroke / CVA	Septic Shock	

- If the readmission is unrelated, choose the primary suspected reason (postoperative occurrence)

Superficial SSI	Pulmonary Embolism	Intraop or Postop Cardiac Arrest req CPR	Other: ICD-9 code____________ Free Text:____________________
Deep SSI	On ventilator > 48 hours	Intraop or Postop Myocardial Infarction	
Organ / Space SSI	Progressive Renal Insufficiency	Transfusion Intraop/Postop (72h of surgery start time)	
Wound Disruption	Acute Renal Failure	Vein Thrombosis Requiring Therapy	
Pneumonia	Urinary Tract Infection (UTI)	Sepsis	
Intraop or Postop Unplanned Intubation	Stroke / CVA	Septic Shock	

Unplanned Reoperation:

Did the patient have an unplanned return to the operating room for a surgical procedure w/in the 30 day postoperative period? ☐ *YES* ☐ *NO*

If yes, Surgery Date or Unknown: _____/_____/_______

Source *(select one)* ☐ Medical Record ☐ Patient/Family Report ☐ Other

CPT code _____________

If yes, was the return to the OR for a postop occurrence likely related to the principal operative procedure?
☐ *YES* ☐ *NO*

If yes, record the ICD code _____________ or diagnosis description______________________

Did the patient have a SECOND unplanned return to the operating room for a surgical procedure, w/in the 30 day postoperative period? ☐ *YES* ☐ *NO*

If yes, Surgery Date or Unknown: _____/_____/_______

Source *(select one)* ☐ Medical Record ☐ Patient/Family Report ☐ Other

CPT code _____________

If yes, was the return to the OR for a postop occurrence likely related to the principal operative procedure?
☐ *YES* ☐ *NO*

If yes, record the ICD code _____________ or diagnosis description______________________

Were there more than two unplanned re-operations for a post op occurrence likely related to the principal operative procedure within 30 days? ☐ *YES* ☐ *NO*

FOLLOW-UP

Follow Up Within 30 Days

Were you able to follow the case for the full 30 days? ☐ *YES* ☐ *NO*
(NOTE: Answer yes for death w/in 30 days)

If you were unable to obtain the 30-day follow up information:

A) How many days (0-29) were you able to follow this case? ________

B) Which attempt methods were used for follow-up? Select all that apply.
(A minimum of three attempts should be made to contact the patient)

Method	# of attempts	Method
☐ Phone	________	☐ Documentation
☐ Letter	________	☐ Other

Patient Contact Management:

Contact date: _____/_____/_____ Contact Action: ☐ Phone ☐ Letter ☐ Document ☐ Fax ☐ E-mail ☐ Other

Contact Results:

☐ No Answer	☐ Letter Received	☐ Incorrect Number
☐ Left Message	☐ Talked to Patient	☐ Patient Refused
☐ Letter Sent	☐ Talk to Family	

Contact Notes:

72 Practice Management

Eric M. Haas

Key Concepts

- Lack of awareness about practice management could lead to poor career decisions, financial distress, and surgeon burnout.
- If joining a hospital model, a surgeon may have benefits of a work RVU-based compensation, as well as the support and resources of the institution. However, the surgeon may need to align their personal goals to the goals of the institution and accept lack of autonomy for purchasing and decision-making.
- In the private practice model, the physician is essentially self-employed, their goals and practice mission are basically aligned, and decisions are made real-time to meet the immediate needs of the practice. However, the financial state of the practice figures into decision-making and can limit the physician's ability to realize their goals.
- Revenue in the private practice model is based on professional fee collections and ancillary investments, while the hospital model generates revenue through professional fees, facility fees, downstream revenue, market share, and outcome incentive programs.
- Effective marketing and networking are necessary to develop and maintain relationships with patients and referring physicians.

Introduction

- Practice management is a broad term that covers all daily operations of a surgical practice, including the practice model, office operations, financial planning, patient interaction, personnel, technology, medical records, marketing and business development, coding, billing, reimbursement, practice setup, and compensation.
- A system of consumer (i.e., patient) focus, process control, standards, check and balances, and quality improvement apply to medical practice management.

Practice Models

- An institution-based model encompasses hospital, university, academic institutions, as well as hospital employee and university employee, and integrated healthcare models, such as Kaiser Permanente, which offer not-for-profit health plans and insurance, a tax-exempt shelter for the for-profit medical groups, and physician-owned for-profit partnerships.

E. M. Haas (✉)
Division of Colon and Rectal Surgery,
Houston Methodist Hospital, Houston, TX, USA

The University of Texas Medical School,
Houston, TX, USA

LLP LTD, Houston, TX, USA
e-mail: ehaasmd@houstoncolon.com

S. R. Steele et al. (eds.), *The ASCRS Manual of Colon and Rectal Surgery*,
https://doi.org/10.1007/978-3-030-01165-9_72

- Private practice models include solo and group practices, including single specialty and multispecialty group practices.

Practice Philosophies in Hospital and Private Practice Models

- When choosing a practice model, take into consideration the overall mission and goals of the workplace, the practice environment, compensation and benefits packages, future opportunities and job advancement, performance and production expectations, and levels of autonomy (Table 72.1).

The Hospital Model

- The primary mission of the hospital or institution-based model centers around serving the needs of the community to improve overall patient care and offering value over competitors in the marketplace.
- The hospital administrators' goals are for the hospital system to be profitable, serve the community, achieve local, regional, and national recognition, and advance research and teaching.
- When joining a hospital model, the physician is an employee and as such, loses the ability to make independent decisions regarding staffing, purchasing, recruiting, growth and expansion, and office administration and processes.
- Physician advancement in the hospital model is generally based on a combination of performance evaluations and financial productivity.
  - Financial productivity is assessed on meeting the budgetary calculations of the employed surgeon's proforma, their individual total "cost" with salary, benefits, and overhead.

Table 72.1 Distinctions between the hospital and private practice models

Overall gestalt	Carry out the global goals of the hospital's strategic mission	Concentrate on patient care and the needs of the doctors
Role of the hospital	Employed	Self-employed; voluntary medical staff member to facilitate patient care
Practice philosophy	Physicians exist to help meet the mission of the hospital and assure the hospital is profitable	Hospital exists to help me care for my patients
Management	CEO, CFO, board of directors, vice presidents, and many clinical/administrative department, division, and group heads	Managing partner, practice administrator, office manager
Decision-making process	Formal processes of committees, administration, and the board of directors; decisions take a longer time to make and are met with resistance and often require negotiation for action	Made by individual or group of physicians; decisions often be made to address immediate needs
Time frame of action	Weeks to months for action; layers of bureaucracy to navigate through and consideration of the hospital's strategic plan and budget cycles	Real-time implementation to address current needs
Communication	Bureaucratic, numerous meetings and politics	Autonomist, consensus decision-making
Resources	More resources available, but acquisition more difficult	Limited resources based on financial state of the practice
Culture	Group, formal organization	Individual, informal organization
Staffing	Run by the institution's human resource department. Formal processes for hiring and firing, which may interfere with physician's staffing preferences	Physician has direct control over staffing decisions
Compensation	Salary, relative value unit (RVU) based	Collections based
Outcome metrics	Data acquisition and reporting supported by the hospital system and data widely available; source of revenue for the hospital	Data acquisition not feasible: expensive and labor intensive

- The proforma is composed of the surgeon's calculated cost center, which factors in overhead, salary, and benefits, and is the total costs based on calculated direct and indirect costs attributed or assigned to each individual employed physician.
- Benefits to joining a hospital model include stability and security, having layers of support, experience, and expertise to allow for multidisciplinary care of complex surgical patients, prestige of association with an established, recognized hospital system, having a built-in referral system, and opportunities for mentoring, research, and career development.

The Private Practice Model

- The primary goal of a private practice model is to provide a working environment that fosters best practices in patient care and satisfaction among patients, staff, and physicians – all while proving to be a viable and profitable arrangement.
- The private practice administrator's goals are to provide a sound workflow, a profitable system for the doctors, and high rates of job satisfaction.
- Surgeons in private practice are self-employed and serve as a voluntary medical staff member at the hospital to facilitate patient care.
- Physician advancement is typically based on the individual's productivity measured in patient collections and the time they have been part of the practice.
- Benefits to the private practice model include the freedom of being your own boss, making your own decisions, and implementing changes to meet the immediate needs of the patients and the practice, having no restriction on the ability to invest in ancillary healthcare services, and maintaining any intellectual property and patents on research or devices.

The Basics of Payment, Compensation, Profits, and Billing

- In the private practice model, salary and compensation plans are closely linked to the profitability of the surgeon, which is reflected in the amount of collections they bring into the practice, less the overhead attributed to that surgeon.
- The hospital model generates revenue from professional fees, facility fees, downstream revenue, market share, and outcome incentive programs that are not available in the private practice setting.
- Facility fee reimbursement is the allowable amount of fee that a hospital collects for having the procedure or encounter performed at their institution.
- The downside of employing a surgeon from the hospital perspective is the high associated costs and inefficiencies of management and administration of a doctor's practice.
- The pros and cons of the two main models are seen in Table 72.2.

Table 72.2 Pros and cons of the hospital versus private practice model

Model	Hospital	Private practice
Pros	Stable environment Prestige of institution Mentoring and research opportunities Favorable benefits, RVU compensation Federal incentives for participation in data collection and outcomes metrics	Maintain freedom, autonomy, and personal goals and aspirations Better total compensation Opportunities to supplement income with outside investments Maintain intellectual property over research and devices
Cons	Cannot invest in ancillary care centers Own the individual's intellectual property, research, and patents	No formal benchmarks for outcomes or satisfaction

Compensation

Relative Value Scale System

- Hospital models usually follow a resource-based relative value scale (RVU) to assign numeric value to encounters and procedures based on the difficulty of the service provided, the risk involved, and the overall care requirements of the patient.

- Every procedure and current procedural terminology (CPT) procedure code has an RVU assigned to it for reimbursement rates.
  - Each RVU has three components associated with calculation for payment: physician work (54%), practice expense (41%), and malpractice overhead (5%).

RVU-Based Compensation

- Many institutions use the work component of the RVU system as the basis of their compensation package by calculating a base salary based on an expected amount of production measured as work RVU (wRVU).
- Annual compensation reports and benchmarked trends are available annually from the Medical Group Management Association (MGMA) and the American Group Medical Association (AGMA).
- Hospitals will generally set the wRVU expectations or threshold at 50% MGMA and then use the MGMA salary data to offer a salary commiserate with the 50% level for colorectal surgeons.
- Benefits of the wRVU-based system are that physicians can concentrate more on patient care and less on uninsured rates or insurance type.

Production-Based Compensation

- Production-based compensation is closely linked to surgeon's actual collections rather than wRVU.
- The actual collections will translate into profitability. (Table 72.3).
- Bonus plans are based on excess cash flow once collections attributed to the surgeon are offset by the surgeon's salary and attributed expenses.
- Surgeons need to be very involved in billing and collections because in the production-based compensation model, actual collections received by the practice are the most important factor.

Table 72.3 Example of wRVU payment formula for common colorectal procedures

Common colorectal procedures	wRVU value per unit	Medicare allowable
CPT 99203 – New patient visit, moderate severity	1.42	$110.09
CPT 46221 – Rubber band ligation	2.36	$278.46
CPT 45378 – Screening colonoscopy	3.69	$223.34
CPT 46260 – Surgical hemorrhoidectomy	6.73	$493.84
CPT 44204 – Laparoscopic segmental colectomy	26.42	$1604.27
CPT 44145 – Open low anterior resection	28.58	$1728.83

The conversion factor is 35.7547 for Houston, TX

Non-production-Based Compensation

- Non-production-based compensation is typically a salary-based plan seen in the university academic setting.
- The incentive plan is based on various determinants – patient care production in the form of wRVU, education, research, and academic endeavors.
- Academic centers set the average compensation on MGMA or AGMA benchmarks and then adjust the overall salary based on the percentage of time that is attributed to each of the parameters.

Bonus Structure

- Hospital-based bonuses are usually wRVU-based: Once one reaches the threshold wRVU established in their contract, a bonus is calculated by multiplying each wRVU above the threshold level by a conversion factor.
- The second form of hospital-based bonuses is a collection-based model, where the surgeon recoups a percentage of collections minus expenses once the threshold wRVU number is attained.
- Private practice bonus models usually begin 1 or 2 years after employment and correspond with the surgeon's ability to bring in revenue above expenses.

Budgets, Billing, and Collections

- In a hospital model, a budget is created by the hospital, including expected income and expenses, with quarterly reviews.
  - In the hospital model, the surgeon also surrenders control over billing and collections.
- In private practice, there is no budget per se, rather is a dynamic balance sheet that tracks the current state of the practice's finances without holding any individual accountable for the financial state.
- Billing is the engine of the ship for private practice models.
  - Establishing an in-house billing department should be the final step of independent practice management.
- A financial "checks and balance" system should be in place where numbers and revenue cycles are evaluated to minimize risk of exposure and theft from the practice.

Billing and Coding

- While coding may be auto-generated through electronic practice management systems, the surgeon should be as familiar with the coding points, levels, and compliance.
- If encounters are over- or under-coded, you could expose yourself, your practice, and your institution to scrutiny.
- In the hospital model, compliance officers and coding personnel will review the operative reports and patient encounters to generate the codes to submit to payors.
- In the private practice model, the billing departments may outsource to a third-party billing company or performed in-house.
- Evaluation and management (E/M) codes are the billing codes used to document the patient-doctor encounter such as a history and physical exam.
- For surgical procedures, current procedural terminology (CPT) procedure codes are used where each procedure is assigned a CPT code with descriptors (CPT codes for surgery of the digestive system include 40,490–49,999).

Table 72.4 Common ICD-9 diagnosis codes for colorectal surgery

(078.11) Condyloma acuminatum
(211.3) Benign neoplasms/polyps of the colon
(211.4) Benign polyps of the rectum or anal canal
(153) Malignant neoplasm of colon
(154) Malignant neoplasm of rectum and anus
(455.2) Internal hemorrhoids with other complication
(455.4) External thrombosed hemorrhoids
(455.9) Residual hemorrhoidal skin tags
(555) Regional enteritis
(555.0) Crohn's, small intestine
(555.1) Crohn's, large intestine
(556.9) Ulcerative colitis, unspecified
(562.1) Diverticulosis of colon
(562.11) Diverticulitis of colon, NOS
(564.01) Slow transit constipation
(564.02) Outlet dysfunction constipation
(564.1) Irritable bowel syndrome
(565) Anal fissure and fistula
(565.0) Anal fissure nontraumatic
(566.0) Abscess perianal
(569.1) Rectal prolapse
(569.3) Bleeding rectal
(787.6) Incontinence of feces
(787.99) Change in bowel habits

- For diagnosis, International Statistical Classification of Diseases and Related Health Problems, tenth edition (ICD-10) codes identify the diagnosis on the claim, not the procedure performed. (Table 72.4).
- The approval or denial of services will be relayed to patients in an explanation of benefits (EOB), which is how the insurance company processes a claim.

Setting Up Your Office

Attracting Patients

- The classic 3 A's of medicine continue to be true and pertinent – a physician must be available, affable, and able.
- There are four main methods to attract patients: physician referrals, insurance referrals, word of mouth, and marketing.
- Develop relationships with referring physicians by finding physicians who may not have

Table 72.5 Essential components of an employment contract

	Hospital model	Private practice model	Notes
Reporting structure	X		Responsible party or parties that you directly report to and the chain of command
Partnership tract		X	The criteria to become a practice partner; usually defined by time invested in the practice
Salary and compensation	X	X	Collections based versus RVU based
Bonus structure			Various models exist and can be individualized based on your practice environment
Benefits	X	X	Health and dental insurance, paid time off, retirement, medical malpractice, life, and disability insurance
Continuing medical education (CME)	X	X	Allowance for continuing medical education, including conferences, travel and housing accommodations
Intellectual property	X	X	Rights to research, patents, inventions, and other creations developed during terms of employment
Clinical duties and responsibilities	X	X	Service area of admitting hospitals and practice locations, call coverage
Academic responsibilities	X		Expectations of productivity, presentations, teaching, mentorship, and publications
Secondary income from healthcare-related interests	X		Ownership interests in surgical centers, hospitals, pathology labs, radiology centers, and other healthcare entities
Consulting income	X		Consulting, honoraria, educational courses and lectures, and expert witness legal fees
b. Terms of termination			
Causes for termination	X	X	Defined causes for termination including loss of license, misconduct, fraud, failure to perform duties defined in the contract
Tail coverage	X	X	Malpractice coverage extending after employment to cover any claims made while employed in prior coverage
Cure period	X	X	A specified period of time to adequately and appropriately correct a material breach in duties before termination
Accounts receivable		X	The outstanding payments due to the doctor from patents and insurance companies for charges submitted
Noncompete (restrictive covenant)	X	X	The physician agrees not to practice in competition with their current employer for a defined, time and geographic scope
Non-solicitation of staff	X	X	Agreement not to solicit employees to leave for the benefit of a competitor if employment is terminated
Confidentiality agreement	X	X	Agreement forbidding disclosure of any confidential or proprietary information to a third party in competition with the practice or hospital

an established, "go-to" colorectal surgeon, and set up a face-to-face visit.

- Network to meet referring doctors when starting in practice via office visits or working the doctor's lounge.
  - Make an impression, and try to make a personal connection to have that impression last.
  - Realize that the doctor's staff may just as important as the doctor to obtain future patients.
  - Meeting the other doctors in the hospital can bring a plethora of referrals.
- Provide a presence on the Internet, and have a landing page linking your practice site to the

hospitals website, where potential patients can understand who you are, what you do, and what might set you apart from other surgeons.
- Harness the power of social media on sites like Facebook, Twitter, LinkedIn, Google+, Doximity, Sermo, and doc2doc, which allow direct connections and education to an unlimited number of potential patients and referral sources.
- Encourage satisfied patients to write reviews, on physician and other popular review sites such as Vitals, Healthgrades, RateMDs, and Ucompare.

Playing Nicely with Others

- Alienating other physicians can hurt your reputation and bottom line.
- Consider referring patients who will require medical management to gastroenterology initially, such as Crohn's disease patients, to scope, diagnose, initiate treatment, and medically optimize.
- Align yourself with the general surgeons, show you are not a threat, can work side-by-side with them, and even assist them with undesirable cases.

Staff and Colleagues

- In private practice, hiring and terminating staff and associates are a part of the job.
  - Communicate with a candidate's current or prior employer so you can make an informed decision about hiring them.
- Successful practice management requires effective communication from the staff with patients; take the time to train staff on effective patient communication techniques.

Contracts

- Have a contract attorney review the terms and conditions before entering into any arrangement (Table 72.5).
- While considering a contract, there are two main questions to answer: (1) what am I getting into and (2) what are the options if things do not go as planned.
- The items to deliberate to answer the first question include compensation, bonus structure, benefits, causes for termination, coverage duties and call responsibilities, cure period to address and "cure" issues before termination, tail coverage and insurance, practice restrictions (confidentiality, proprietorship), and the contract term (automatic renewal versus set time frame).
- Understand all option and consequences of early termination.

Considerations When Moving Between Practice Models

- When transitioning from private practice to a hospital system, autonomy changes, the compensation model usually shifts from a collection-based to RVU-based revenue streams, and staffing and administrative support are controlled by the institution.
- The hospital model will almost always have an electronic medical record (EMR) system in place.
- To transition the physical goods from private practice to the hospital system, a bill of sales or purchase agreement is required to negotiate the hard assets of the practice, including furniture, exam tables, computers, manometric equipment, and scopes.

Index

S. Steele et al. (eds.), *The ASCRS Manual of Colon and Rectal Surgery*,
https://doi.org/10.1007/978-3-030-01165-9

F

I

J

K

N

O

Q

R

S